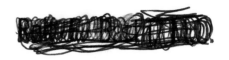

The
Gliomas

The Gliomas

Mitchel S. Berger, M.D.

Professor and Chairman
Department of Neurological Surgery
Director
Brain Tumor Research Center
University of California, San Francisco
San Francisco, California

Charles B. Wilson, M.D., M.S.H.A., D.Sc.

Professor
Department of Neurological Surgery
Principal Investigator
Brain Tumor Research Center
University of California, San Francisco
San Francisco, California

W.B. SAUNDERS COMPANY
A Division of Harcourt Brace & Company
Philadelphia   London   Toronto   Montreal   Sydney   Tokyo

W.B. SAUNDERS COMPANY
A Division of Harcourt Brace & Company

The Curtis Center
Independence Square West
Philadelphia, Pennsylvania 19106

Library of Congress Cataloging-in-Publication Data

The gliomas / [edited by] Mitchel S. Berger, Charles B. Wilson.—1st ed.
p.   cm.

ISBN 0–7216–4825–8

1. Gliomas.   I. Berger, Mitchel S.   II. Wilson, Charles B.
   [DNLM: 1. Glioma.   QZ 380 G561 1999]

RC280.B7G59   1999

616.99′281—dc20

DNLM/DLC   95-42774

THE GLIOMAS   ISBN 0–7216–4825–8

Printed in the United States of America.

Last digit is the print number: 9   8   7   6   5   4   3   2   1

We dedicate this work to those patients and their families who struggle with and fight against this dreaded disease.

M.S.B.
C.B.W.

Contributors

Adriano Aguzzi, M.D.
Senior Lecturer, University of Zürich, Zürich, Switzerland.
Animal Models of Tumors of the Nervous System

Francis Ali-Osman, D.Sc.
Section of Molecular Therapeutics, Department of Experimental Pediatrics, The Brain Tumor Center, University of Texas, M.D. Anderson Cancer Center, Houston, Texas
Human Glioma Cultures and In Vitro Analysis of Therapeutic Response

Michael L.J. Apuzzo, M.D.
Edwin M. Todd/Trent H. Wells, Jr., Professor; Department of Neurological Surgery and Radiation Oncology, Biology, and Physics; University of Southern California School of Medicine; Director of Neurosurgery; Kenneth R. Norris, Jr., Cancer Hospital and Research Institute; Los Angeles, California.
Tumor Removal Devices

Gary E. Archer, Ph.D.
Assistant Research Professor of Pathology, Duke University Medical Center, Durham, North Carolina.
Immunoconjugates

Fred G. Barker II, M.D.
Instructor, Department of Surgery, Harvard Medical School; Assistant in Neurosurgery, Massachusetts General Hospital, Boston, Massachusetts.
Molecular Genetics; Surgical Approaches to Gliomas; Clinical Characteristics of Long-Term Glioma Survivors

M. Josefa Bello, Ph.D.
Instituto de Investigaciones Biomédicas (C.S.I.C.), Madrid, Spain.
Cytogenetics

Mitchel S. Berger, M.D.
Professor and Chairman, Department of Neurological Surgery; Director, Brain Tumor Research Center, University of California, San Francisco, San Francisco, California.
DNA Repair–Mediated Resistance to Alkylating Agents; Positioning During Glioma Surgery; Techniques for Functional Brain Mapping During Glioma Surgery; Extent of Resection and Outcome for Cerebral Hemispheric Gliomas

Mark Bernstein, B.Sc., M.D., F.R.C.S.C.
Associate Professor, Department of Surgery, Division of Neurosurgery, University of Toronto; Head, Division of Neurosurgery, The Toronto Hospital; Toronto, Ontario, Canada.
Closing Procedures and Postoperative Care

Darell D. Bigner, M.D., Ph.D.
Edwin L. Jones, Jr., and Lucille Finch Jones Cancer Research Professor of Pathology (Neuropathology), Duke University Medical Center, Durham, North Carolina.
Immunoconjugates

Keith L. Black, M.D.
Chief of Neurosurgery, Cedars-Sinai Medical Center, Los Angeles, California.
Peritumoral Edema

Peter M. Black, M.D., Ph.D.
Franc D. Ingraham Professor of Neurosurgery, Harvard Medical School; Neurosurgeon-in-Chief, Brigham and Women's Hospital and Children's Hospital, Boston, Massachusetts.
Clinical Presentation, Evaluation, and Preoperative Preparation of the Patient

Lindsey C. Blake, M.D.
Assistant Professor, Senior Fellow, Department of Neuroradiology, University of Washington School of Medicine, Seattle, Washington.
Computed Tomography

A. Blank, Ph.D.
Research Scientist, Department of Pathology, University of Washington, Seattle, Washington.
DNA Repair–Mediated Resistance to Alkylating Agents

Michael S. Bobola, Ph.D.
Assistant Professor, Department of Neurological Surgery, University of Washington; Staff Research Scientist, Department of Surgery, Division of Neurosurgery, Children's Hospital and Medical Center; Seattle, Washington.
DNA Repair–Mediated Resistance to Alkylating Agents

Henry Brem, M.D.
Professor of Neurosurgery, Johns Hopkins University School of Medicine, Baltimore, Maryland.
Treatment of Gliomas Using Polymer-Drug Delivery

Jan C. Buckner, M.D.
Associate Professor of Oncology, Mayo Medical School; Consultant in Medical Oncology, The Mayo Clinic, Rochester, Minnesota.
Systemic Sequelae of Chemotherapy for Gliomas

William M. Chadduck, M.D.
Professor of Neurosurgery, George Washington University, Washington, D.C.
Childhood and Adolescent Gliomas

Thomas C. Chen, M.D.
Assistant Professor, Department of Neurological Surgery, University of Southern California, Los Angeles, California.
Tumor Removal Devices

Timothy F. Cloughesy, M.D.
Department of Neurology, UCLA School of Medicine, Los Angeles, California.
Peritumoral Edema

Stephen W. Coons, M.D.
Staff Neuropathologist, Barrow Neurological Institute, Phoenix, Arizona.
Anatomy and Growth Patterns of Diffuse Gliomas

Walter J. Curran, Jr., M.D.
Professor, Thomas Jefferson University; Chairman, Department of Radiation Oncology, Thomas Jefferson University Hospital; Philadelphia, Pennsylvania.
Issues in the Use of Conventional and Altered Fractionation Radiation Therapy for Pediatric and Adult Gliomas

J. Diaz Day, M.D.
Department of Neurosurgery, Lahey Clinic, Burlington, Massachusetts.
Tumor Removal Devices

Dennis F. Deen, Ph.D.
Professor of Neurological Surgery and Radiation Oncology; Vice Chairman for Research, Department of Neurological Surgery, Associate Director, Brain Tumor Research Center, University of California, San Francisco School of Medicine, San Francisco, California.
Basic Principles of Radiobiology and Radiotherapy

Rolando F. Del Maestro, M.D., Ph.D., F.R.C.S.(C.)
Professor, Department of Clinical Neurological Sciences, Division of Neurosurgery, University of Western Ontario; Chief, Division of Neurosurgery, London Health Sciences Centre; London, Ontario, Canada.
Angiogenesis

Nicolas De Tribolet, M.D.
Professor, Faculty of Medicine, University of Lausanne; Chairman, Department of Neurosurgery, CHUV; Lausanne, Switzerland.
Tumor Immunobiology

Giovanni Di Chiro, M.D.
Chief, Neuroimaging Branch, National Institute of Neurological Diseases and Stroke, National Institutes of Health, Bethesda, Maryland.
Positron Emission Tomography and ^1H Spectroscopic Imaging

William P. Dillon, Jr., M.D.
Professor of Radiology and Neurological Surgery, University of California, San Francisco, San Francisco, California.
Magnetic Resonance Imaging

Edward J. Dropcho, M.D.
Professor, Department of Neurology, Indiana University Medical Center; Chief, Neurology Service, Richard Roudebush Veterans Affairs Medical Center; Indianapolis, Indiana.
Intra-arterial Chemotherapy for Malignant Gliomas

Ira J. Dunkel, M.D.
Instructor, Department of Pediatrics, Cornell University Medical Center; Clinical Assistant, Department of Pediatrics, Memorial Sloan-Kettering Cancer Center; New York, New York.
High-Dose Chemotherapy Followed by Autologous Bone Marrow Rescue for High-Grade Gliomas

Herbert H. Engelhard, M.D., Ph.D.
Associate Professor of Surgery, Division of Neurological Surgery, Northwestern University Institute for Neuroscience, Northwestern University Medical School, Chicago, Illinois.
The Blood-Brain Barrier: Structure, Function, and Response to Neoplasia

Burt G. Feuerstein, M.D., Ph.D.
Associate Professor, Division of Molecular Cytometry, Department of Laboratory Medicine, Brain Tumor Research Center, Department of Neurosurgery, University of California, San Francisco, San Francisco, California.
Tumor Markers in Gliomas

Karen L. Fink, M.D., Ph.D.
Assistant Professor, University of Texas Southwestern Medical Center; Parkland Memorial Hospital; Zale University Hospital; Dallas, Texas.
Tumor Dissemination and Management

Jonathan L. Finlay, M.B., Ch.B.
Department of Pediatrics and Neurosurgery, New York University Medical Center, New York, New York.
High-Dose Chemotherapy Followed by Autologous Bone Marrow Rescue for High-Grade Gliomas

Eric P. Flores, M.D.
Assistant Professor, Department of Neurosurgery, University of Minnesota Hospital and Clinic, Minneapolis, Minnesota.
Antisense Oligonucleotide Targets

William A. Friedman, M.D.
Professor and Associate Chairman, Department of Neurological Surgery, University of Florida, Gainesville, Florida.
Closed Biopsy Techniques

Michael J. Fulham, M.B., B.S., F.R.A.C.P.
Senior Lecturer, University of Sydney Faculty of Medicine, University of Sydney; Attending Neurologist and Director, Positron Emission Tomography Department, Royal Prince Alfred Hospital; Sydney, Australia.
Positron Emission Tomography and ¹H Spectroscopic Imaging

Gregory N. Fuller, M.D., Ph.D.
Assistant Professor of Pathology (Neuropathology), University of Texas, M.D. Anderson Cancer Center, Houston, Texas.
Intraoperative Localization of Tumor and Margins

J. Russell Geyer, M.D.
Professor, Department of Pediatrics, University of Washington School of Medicine, Seattle, Washington.
Gliomas in the Very Young Child

Maria Teresa Giordana, M.D.
Associate Professor of Neurology, University of Turin, Turin, Italy.
Immunologic Cell Markers

Richard L. Gold, M.D.
Department of Radiology, Neuroradiology Section, University of California, San Francisco, San Francisco, California.
Magnetic Resonance Imaging

Michael M. Graham, M.D., Ph.D.
Professor of Radiology (Nuclear Medicine) and Radiation Oncology, University of Washington, Seattle, Washington.
Single-Photon Emission Computed Tomography

Dennis G. Groothuis, M.D.
Department of Neurology, Northwestern University Institute for Neuroscience, Northwestern University Medical School, Chicago, Illinois.
The Blood-Brain Barrier: Structure, Function, and Response to Neoplasia

Stuart A. Grossman, M.D.
Director, Department of Neuro-Oncology, Associate Professor of Oncology, Medicine, and Neurosurgery, The Johns Hopkins Oncology Center, Baltimore, Maryland.
Familial Gliomas

Philip H. Gutin, M.D.
Professor and Chief of Neurological Surgery, Memorial Sloan-Kettering Cancer Center, New York, New York.
Surgical Approaches to Gliomas; Interstitial Radiation and Hyperthermia; Radiosurgery; Central Nervous System Toxic Effects of Radiotherapy

Paula M. Hale, M.D.
Assistant Professor of Pediatrics, Temple University School of Medicine; Attending Physician, Division of Endocrinology, Diabetes, and Metabolism, St. Christopher's Hospital for Children; Philadelphia, Pennsylvania.
Endocrinologic Dysfunction Following Adjunct Tumor Therapy

Walter A. Hall, M.D.
Associate Professor of Neurosurgery and Radiation Oncology, University of Minnesota Hospital and Clinic, Minneapolis, Minnesota.
Antisense Oligonucleotide Targets

Maarouf A. Hammoud, M.D.
Fellow in Neurosurgical Oncology, University of Texas, M.D. Anderson Cancer Center, Houston, Texas.
Intraoperative Localization of Tumor and Margins

Griffith R. Harsh IV, M.D.
Associate Professor, Harvard Medical School; Director, Department of Neurosurgical Oncology, Massachusetts General Hospital, Boston, Massachusetts.
Management of Recurrent Gliomas

David Haynor, M.D., Ph.D.
Associate Professor, Department of Radiology, University of Washington, Seattle, Washington.
The Role of Functional Imaging in the Surgical Management of Brain Neoplasms

John S. Hill, Ph.D., B.Sc.
Chief Scientist, Photodynamic Therapy Laboratory, Department of Neurosurgery, Melbourne Neuroscience Centre, Royal Melbourne Hospital, University of Melbourne, Victoria, Australia.
Photodynamic Therapy

Stephen L. Huhn, M.D.
Assistant Professor of Neurosurgery, Stanford University, Stanford, California.
Clinical Characteristics of Long-Term Glioma Survivors

Mark A. Israel, M.D.
Professor, Departments of Neurological Surgery and Pediatrics; Director, Preuss Laboratory for Molecular

Neuro-oncology; University of California, San Francisco, San Francisco, California.
Molecular Genetics

Kurt A. Jaeckle, M.D.
Associate Professor of Medicine, Department of Neuro-oncology, University of Texas, M.D. Anderson Cancer Center, Houston, Texas.
Intratumoral Administration

Samer E. Kaba, M.D.
Assistant Professor, Department of Neurology, University of Arkansas for Medical Sciences, Little Rock, Arkansas.
Biologic Response Modifiers

Paul Kanev, M.D.
Associate Professor of Neurosurgery and Pediatrics, Pennsylvania State University Medical School, Hershey Medical Center, Hershey, Pennsylvania.
Endocrinologic Dysfunction Following Adjunct Tumor Therapy

Andrew H. Kaye, M.B., B.S., M.D., F.R.A.C.S.
Professor of Neurosurgery, Melbourne University; Professor of Neurosurgery and Director of Neurosciences, Western Health Network; Director, Melbourne Neuroscience Center; The Royal Melbourne Hospital; Victoria, Australia.
Photodynamic Therapy

Patrick J. Kelly, M.D.
Professor and Chairman, Department of Neurosurgery, New York University Medical Center, New York, New York.
Computer-Assisted Stereotactic Laser Resection

Dong H. Kim, M.D.
Assistant Professor, Department of Neurosurgery, Cornell University Medical College, The New York University–Cornell Medical Center, New York, New York.
Tumor Markers in Gliomas

Paul Kleihues, M.D.
Professor, University of Zürich, Zürich, Switzerland; Director, International Agency for Research on Cancer, Lyon, France.
Animal Models of Tumors of the Nervous System

Douglas D. Kolstoe, M.S.
Research Technician, Department of Neurological Surgery, University of Washington, Seattle, Washington.
DNA Repair–Mediated Resistance to Alkylating Agents

Larry E. Kun, M.D.
Professor and Chairman, Department of Radiation Oncology, University of Tennessee College of Medicine; Chairman, Department of Radiation Oncology, St. Jude Children's Research Hospital; Memphis, Tennessee.
Cognitive Deficits

Frederick F. Lang, Jr., M.D.
Department of Neurosurgery, University of Texas, M.D. Anderson Cancer Center, Houston, Texas.
Computer-Assisted Stereotactic Laser Resection

George E. Laramore, M.D., Ph.D.
Professor of Radiation Oncology, University of Washington; Vice-Chairman, Department of Radiation Oncology, Clinical Director, University of Washington Fast Neutron Radiotherapy Project, University of Washington Medical Center, Seattle, Washington.
Particle Beam Therapy

David A. Larson, M.D., Ph.D.
Professor, Departments of Radiation Oncology and Neurological Surgery, University of California, San Francisco, San Francisco, California.
Basic Principles of Radiobiology and Radiotherapy; Radiosurgery; Central Nervous System Toxic Effects of Radiotherapy

Steven A. Leibel, M.D.
Vice-Chairman and Clinical Director, Department of Radiation Oncology, Enid A. Haupt Chair in Experimental Radiation Oncology, Memorial Sloan-Kettering Cancer Center, New York, New York.
Issues in the Use of Conventional and Altered Fractionation Radiation Therapy for Pediatric and Adult Gliomas

B. Lee Ligon, Ph.D.
Senior Editor, Department of Neurosurgery, University of Texas, M.D. Anderson Cancer Center, Houston, Texas.
Intraoperative Localization of Tumor and Margins

Ted Tai-Sen Lin, M.D.
Senior Resident in Neurosurgery, Georgetown University Medical Center, Washington, D.C.
Neurofibromatosis and Other Phakomatoses

Maria Beatriz Sampaio Lopes, M.D.
Assistant Professor of Pathology, University of Virginia Health Sciences Center, Charlottesville, Virginia.
Classification

Walter C. Low, Ph.D.
Professor of Neurosurgery, University of Minnesota School of Medicine, Minneapolis, Minnesota.
Antisense Oligonucleotide Targets

Robert Maciunas, M.D.
Associate Professor of Neurological Surgery and Biomedical Engineering, Vanderbilt University School of Medicine; Associate Professor of Neurological Surgery and Biomedical Engineering, Chief of Neurosurgery Service, Veterans Administration Hospital, Veterans Administration Medical Center; Nashville, Tennessee.
Interactive Image-Guided Surgical Technology for Glial Tumor Resection

Ellen E. Mack, M.D., M.P.H.
Assistant Clinical Professor, Departments of Neurological Surgery and Neurology, University of California, San Francisco, San Francisco, California.
Radiation-Induced Tumors

Lloyd I. Maliner, M.D.
Resident in Neurosurgery, Pennsylvania State University, Hershey Medical Center, Hershey, Pennsylvania.
Deep Venous Thrombosis and Pulmonary Embolism

Kenneth R. Maravilla, M.D.
Professor of Radiology and Neurological Surgery, Director of Neuroradiology, University of Washington School of Medicine, Seattle, Washington.
Computed Tomography; The Role of Functional Imaging in the Surgical Management of Brain Neoplasms

Robert Martuza, M.D.
Professor and Chairman, Department of Neurosurgery, Georgetown University, Washingron, D.C.
Neurofibromatosis and Other Phakomatoses

Masao Matsutani, M.D.
Professor, Department of Neurosurgery, Saitama Medical School, Moroyama, Irumagun, Saitama, Japan.
Cell Kinetics

Leslie D. McAllister, M.D.
Assistant Professor of Neurology, University of Utah, Salt Lake City, Utah.
Intratumoral Administration

Randall E. Merchant, Ph.D.
Associate Professor of Anatomy and Surgery, Virginia Commonwealth University, Medical College of Virginia, Richmond, Virginia.
Intracavitary Immunotherapy

Tom Mikkelsen, M.D.
Senior Staff, Departments of Neurology and Neurosurgery, Henry Ford Hospital; Chief, Neuro-oncology Clinic, Director, Laboratory of Invasion and Molecular Therapeutics, Henry Ford Midwest Neuro-oncology Center; Detroit, Michigan.
Tumor Invasiveness

Gayatry Mohapatra, Ph.D.
Assistant Research Geneticist, Division of Molecular Cytometry, Department of Laboratory Medicine and Brain Tumor Research Center, University of California, San Francisco, San Francisco, California.
Tumor Markers in Gliomas

Richard S. Morrison, Ph.D.
Associate Professor, Department of Neurological Surgery, University of Washington, Seattle, Washington.
Growth Factor–Mediated Signaling Pathways

Raymond K. Mulhern, Ph.D.
Chief, Division of Behavioral Medicine, St. Jude Children's Research Hospital, Memphis, Tennessee.
Cognitive Deficits

H. Stacy Nicholson, M.D.
Assistant Professor of Pediatrics, George Washington University; Staff Oncologist, Children's National Medical Center, Washington, D.C.
Childhood and Adolescent Gliomas

Hiroko Ohgaki, D.V.M., Ph.D.
Chief, Unit of Molecular Pathology, International Agency for Research on Cancer, Lyon, France.
Animal Models of Tumors of the Nervous System

George A. Ojemann, M.D.
Professor of Neurological Surgery, University of Washington School of Medicine, Seattle, Washington.
Techniques for Functional Brain Mapping During Glioma Surgery

Edward H. Oldfield, M.D.
Chief, Surgical Neurology Branch, National Institute of Neurological Disease and Stroke, National Institute of Health, Bethesda, Maryland.
Gene Therapy for Malignant Brain Tumors

Roger J. Packer, M.D.
Professor of Neurology and Pediatrics, George Washington University; Chairman, Department of Neurology, Children's National Medical Center; Professor of Clinical Neurology, Georgetown University; Washington, D.C.; Professor of Neurosurgery, University of Virginia, Charlottesville, Virginia.
Childhood and Adolescent Gliomas

Peter C. Phillips, M.D.
Professor of Pediatrics and Chief of Pediatric Neuro-oncology, Children's Hospital of Philadelphia, University of Pennsylvania, Philadelphia, Pennsylvania.
Pharmacology of Glioma Therapy

Emil A. Popovic, M.B., B.S., F.R.A.C.S.
Neurosurgeon, Melbourne University; Neurosurgeon, The Melbourne Neuroscience Centre; Victoria, Australia.
Photodynamic Therapy

Stephen K. Powers, M.D.
Professor and Chief of Neurosurgery, Pennsylvania State University Medical School, Hershey Medical Center, Hershey, Pennsylvania.
Deep Venous Thrombosis and Pulmonary Embolism

Michael D. Prados, M.D.
Professor of Neurosurgery, Director of Neuro-Oncology Program, University of California, San Francisco, San Francisco, California.
Clinical Characteristics of Long-Term Glioma Survivors

Susan Preston-Martin, Ph.D.
Professor, Department of Preventive Medicine, University of Southern California, Los Angeles, California.
Epidemiology

Zvi Ram, M.D.
The Chaim Sheba Medical Center, Department of Neurosurgery, Tel-Aviv University Sackler School of Medicine, Tel Hashomer, Israel.
Gene Therapy for Malignant Brain Tumors

Juan A. Rey, Ph.D.
Instituto de Investigaciones Biomédicas (C.S.I.C.), Madrid, Spain.
Cytogenetics

Mark L. Rosenblum, M.D.
Professor and Chairman, Department of Neurosurgery, Henry Ford Hospital, Director, Henry Ford Midwest Neuro-oncology Center, Henry Ford Health System, Detroit, Michigan.
Tumor Invasiveness

Raymond Sawaya, M.D.
Professor and Chairman, Department of Neurosurgery, University of Texas, M.D. Anderson Cancer Center, Houston, Texas.
Intraoperative Localization of Tumor and Margins

Davide Schiffer, M.D.
Professor of Neurology and Neuropathology, University of Turin, Turin, Italy.
Immunologic Cell Markers

S. Clifford Schold, Jr., M.D.
Vice-President, Oncology and Neurology, Pharma Research Corporation, Wilmington, North Carolina.
Tumor Dissemination and Management

Charles B. Scott, M.S.
Adjunct Assistant Professor, Jefferson Medical College of Thomas Jefferson University; Senior Biostatistician, American College of Radiology, Philadelphia, Pennsylvania.
Issues in the Use of Conventional and Altered Fractionation Radiation Therapy for Pediatric and Adult Gliomas

Dennis C. Shrieve, M.D., Ph.D.
Assistant Professor of Radiation Oncology, Joint Center for Radiation Therapy, Brigham and Women's Hospital; Harvard Medical School, Boston, Massachusetts.
Basic Principles of Radiobiology and Radiotherapy; Radiosurgery; Central Nervous System Toxic Effects of Radiotherapy

John R. Silber, Ph.D.
Research Associate Professor, Department of Neurological Surgery, University of Washington, Seattle, Washington.
DNA Repair–Mediated Resistance to Alkylating Agents

Richard H. Simon, M.D.
Professor of Surgery (Neurosurgery), University of Connecticut School of Medicine, University of Connecticut Health Center, Farmington, Connecticut.
Pregnancy and Gliomas

Penny K. Sneed, M.D.
Professor, Department of Radiation Oncology, University of California, San Francisco, San Francisco, California.
Interstitial Radiation and Hyperthermia

Alexander M. Spence, M.D.
Professor of Neurology and Pathology (Neuropathology), Adjunct Professor of Neurosurgery, University of Washington School of Medicine, Seattle, Washington.
Glioma Metabolism

Roberto Spiegelmann, M.D.
Lecturer, Departments of Neurology and Neurosurgery, The Sackler School of Medicine, Tel Aviv University, Tel Aviv; Staff Neurosurgeon, The Chiam Sheba Medical Center, Tel Hashomer, Israel.
Closed Biopsy Techniques

Keith J. Stelzer, M.D., Ph.D.
Associate Professor of Radiation Oncology, University of Washington Medical Center; Chief of Radiation Oncology, Seattle Veterans Administration Hospital, Seattle, Washington.
Particle Beam Therapy

David J. Stewart, M.D.
Professor of Medicine and Pharmacology, University of Ottawa; Head of Medical Oncology, Ottawa Regional Cancer Centre-Civic Division, Ottawa, Ontario, Canada.
Hyperosmolar Disruption of the Blood-Brain Barrier as a Chemotherapy Potentiator in the Treatment of Brain Tumors.

Mitsuhiro Tada, M.D., Ph.D.
Neurosurgeon, Department of Neurosurgery, Laboratory of Molecular Brain Research, University of Hokkaido School of Medicine, Sapporo, Japan.
Tumor Immunobiology

Reid C. Thompson, M.D.
Staff Neurosurgeon, Department of Neurosurgery, Cedars-Sinai Medical Center, Los Angeles, California.
Treatment of Gliomas Using Polymer-Drug Delivery

Michael Tymianski, M.D., Ph.D., F.R.C.S.(C.)
Assistant Professor, Department of Surgery, Division of Neurosurgery, University of Toronto, Toronto, Ontario, Canada.
Closing Procedures and Postoperative Care

Raul C. Urtasun, M.D., F.R.C.P.(C.)
Professor of Oncology and Neurosciences, University of
Alberta Medical School; Radiation Oncologist, Department
of Radiation Oncology, Cross Cancer Institute, Edmonton,
Alberta, Canada.
Radiosensitizers

Scott R. VandenBerg, M.D., Ph.D.
Professor of Pathology (Neuropathology) and Neurological
Surgery, University of Virginia Health Sciences Center,
Charlottesville, Virginia.
Classification

Gilbert Vezina, M.D.
Assistant Professor of Radiology, George Washington
University; Director, Neuroradiology, Children's National
Medical Center, Washington, D.C.
Childhood and Adolescent Gliomas

Patrick Y. Wen, M.D.
Assistant Professor of Neurology, Harvard Medical School;
Director of Neuro-oncology, Division of Neurology,
Brigham and Women's Hospital, Boston, Massachusetts.
*Clinical Presentation, Evaluation, and Preoperative
Preparation of the Patient*

Otmar D. Wiestler, M.D.
Professor, Bonn University, Bonn, Germany.
Animal Models of Tumors of the Nervous System

Charles B. Wilson, M.D., M.S.H.A., D.Sc.
Professor, Department of Neurological Surgery; Principal
Investigator, Brain Tumor Research Center, University of
California, San Francisco, San Francisco, California.
*Extent of Resection and Outcome for Cerebral Hemispheric
Gliomas*

Harold F. Young, M.D.
Professor of Surgery, Virginia Commonwealth University,
Medical College of Virginia; Chief of Neurosurgery,
Medical College of Virginia Hospitals, Richmond, Virginia.
Intracavitary Immunotherapy

W.K. Alfred Yung, M.D.
Professor of Neurology, University of Texas Medical
School at Houston; Professor of Neurology, Deputy
Chairman, Department of Neuro-oncology, University of
Texas M.D. Anderson Cancer Center, Houston, Texas.
Biologic Response Modifiers

Michael R. Zalutsky, Ph.D.
Professor of Radiology, Director, Radiopharmaceutical
Chemistry Laboratory, Duke University Medical Center,
Durham, North Carolina.
Immunoconjugates

☐ Preface

The basic science and clinical approaches to neuro-oncology are changing at a steady pace commensurate with progress in other cancer-related disciplines. While progress in the characterization and treatment of certain tumors involving the central nervous system has occurred at an accelerated rate—for example, the germ cell tumors and primitive neuroectodermal tumors—the gliomas as a group have been more challenging in terms of significant gains that affect outcome. This slower momentum notwithstanding, our ability to more readily achieve a diagnosis has improved tremendously as a consequence of new anatomic and metabolic imaging studies, such as magnetic resonance imaging and spectroscopy. The disciplines of neuropathology and molecular biology have grown closer together, and their integration has resulted in a gigantic leap forward in our understanding of the molecular mechanisms responsible for the histologic appearance of the gliomas. We now have a greater understanding of the cellular events responsible for the progression of glial tumors along histologic grades, although we remain largely in the dark about the initial oncogenetic event (or events) that precipitates the critical transformation from normal glial cells to cells having the potential to follow a pathway of progression that results in an aggressive, invasive glioma that may take a patient's life within 12 to 14 months after diagnosis. Technical advances in surgery, radiation oncology, and chemotherapy have permitted physicians to offer patients who have gliomas the most effective of the standard treatments developed to treat this type of brain tumor. In the future, developments now being made in immunotherapy, including tumor vaccines, and in gene therapy will generate a completely different therapeutic strategy and new hope for our patients. The explosion of knowledge in the medical and basic sciences that has taken place over the past two decades has infused the neurosciences with unprecedented interdisciplinary vitality. This book was developed and written with the intention of amalgamating the related disciplines surrounding neuro-oncology in a text that would provide the clinician, the basic scientist, and the allied health care provider with a comprehensive view of the concepts that are emerging and a framework within which to capitalize on them in the hope of making further progress in translational neuro-oncology. This is a very exciting time in the neurosciences and in our evolving understanding of the biology of cancer. With this text, it is our goal to track the advances in neuro-oncology and to provide individuals from all the related neuro-oncology disciplines with the most thorough understanding available of this evolving field.

MITCHEL S. BERGER, M.D., F.A.C.S.
CHARLES B. WILSON, M.D., M.S.H.A., D.Sc.

Contents

SECTION I
Epidemiology/Clinical Genetics/Basic Science

SECTION II
Experimental Therapeutics

SECTION III
Pathology

SECTION **IV**
Diagnostic Imaging

SECTION **V**
Preoperative Assessment and Management

SECTION **VI**
Resection Strategies

SECTION **VII**

Treatment Modalities

SECTION **VIII**

Special Topics

SECTION **IX**
Treatment-Induced Complications

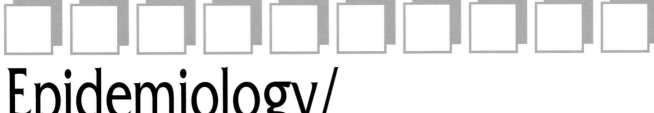

Epidemiology/
Clinical Genetics/
Basic Science

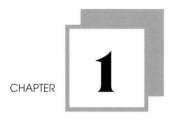

CHAPTER **1**

Epidemiology

Although gliomas are the most common major subgroup of primary nervous system tumors, their etiology is less well understood than is the etiology of the other two major subgroups: meningiomas and neuromas. Both of these are usually benign and are less rapidly fatal than gliomas. Nonetheless, this chapter summarizes what is known about the etiology of gliomas and points out what appear to be promising epidemiologic leads. Reference is made to only a limited number of the hundreds of relevant articles, but for each topic citations include a recent article with a comprehensive bibliography.

About 17,000 U.S. residents are newly diagnosed with primary brain cancer each year, and 11,500 die from this disease.[1] The majority of these brain cancers are gliomas (97% of gliomas arise at intracranial sites). Numerous epidemiologic studies of primary brain tumors have been conducted in recent decades; in most, glioma was the predominant tumor type, but only in recent years have studies commonly analyzed results for glioma separately. Few epidemiologic studies have presented findings for specific subgroups of glial tumors although these subgroups have clearly distinct characteristics, such as median survival following diagnosis and patterns of occurrence in the population.

DESCRIPTIVE EPIDEMIOLOGY

Descriptive data on patterns of brain tumor occurrence are difficult to compare across time periods or across geographic areas because of major inconsistencies both in inclusion criteria and in diagnostic efficiency. Also, few registries have published separate rates for gliomas. Los Angeles County, however, has an unusual resource, the Cancer Surveillance Program (CSP), which enables us to study the distribution of gliomas by demographic characteristics (age, sex, race, address, religion, birthplace, occupation, and industry) and details of the pathologic diagnosis including histologic subtype. The CSP has collected reports on all new gliomas diagnosed in the county population (now about 9 million) since the beginning of 1972. Inclusion criteria have been consistent, and reporting of both benign and malignant tumors has been at least 95% complete since the beginning.[2] In the following sections, data are presented on the 6,950

county residents with gliomas diagnosed from 1972 through 1991. More than 95% of these diagnoses were confirmed histologically—99% in early years and around 90% since 1987, when the CSP joined the state registration system and began enrolling clinically diagnosed cancers at the time of diagnosis. Methods used in the calculation of rates are described in an earlier report.[3]

Spinal Cord Gliomas

In Los Angeles County, only 187 (2.8%) of all 6,950 primary gliomas diagnosed from 1972 to 1991 arose in the spinal cord, and age-adjusted incidence rates are 0.14 new cord gliomas per 100,000 men/year and 0.11 per 100,000 women/year. In both sexes combined, 54% of cord gliomas are ependymomas, 40% are astrocytomas, and only 6% are other types of gliomas.

Brain Gliomas: Age-Incidence Curves and Change in Incidence Rates Over Time

The average annual age-specific incidence rates of all types of intracranial gliomas combined are shown in Figure 1–1. In both males and females, rates decline after a peak before age 10 years, increase after age 25 years, and decline again after age 80 years. This age peak in older age groups formerly occurred at a much younger age both in Los Angeles and in other geographic areas; it has shifted progressively from a peak around age 55 years in registry data before 1955 to a peak at age 80 years in recent Los Angeles data. This shift is likely attributable to substantial underascertainment of brain cancer, particularly in older persons, in earlier decades when imaging tools such as CT scans and MRI were unavailable.[4]

Comparisons of data from different areas of the United States have shown that the shape of the age-incidence curve after age 60 years or so is highly dependent on the autopsy rate.[5] Prior to 1955, rates among those over age 55 years increased steeply with age in data from Rochester, Minn (location of The Mayo Clinic), but decreased in data from other areas (e.g., the Second National Cancer Survey, Connecticut and Iowa). Subsequent analyses showed that the proportion of cases first diagnosed at death was considerably higher in Rochester than in Connecticut, and that when these cases were excluded from the Rochester data, rates declined after age 65 years rather than continuing to rise sharply.[6, 7] These comparisons suggest that brain tumor incidence continues to increase with age throughout life, but that there is often a significant underascertainment of cases in the oldest age groups. Comparisons of brain tumor rates from different registries and across time periods might be more meaningful, therefore, if restricted to age groups under 65 years.

Analyses of international data for ages 35 to 64 years do indicate that the shape of the age-incidence curve is similar across geographic areas, although the level varies.[8] This shape is a straight line on a log-log scale, and the slope (2.6) is the same for males and females, which suggests that incidence increases as a function of age to the 2.6 power. Slopes varied considerably by histologic type as follows: 0.4 for ependymoma; 1.0 for oligodendroglioma; 1.7 for astrocytoma; and 3.9 for glioblastoma.[9] The authors suggest that the significantly higher rate of increase with age seen for glioblastomas compared with other glial tumors is indicative of a different mechanism of carcinogenesis for these highly aggressive tumors.

In the last few years, much debate has focussed on the increase over the past several decades in brain tumor rates, particularly among the elderly. The incidence of primary brain tumors among U.S. residents older than 75 years more than doubled from 1968 to 1985.[10, 11] Similar increases in brain cancer mortality among those older than 65 years occurred in Europe, Japan, and the United States.[12] In Los Angeles County, incidence rates for malignant brain tumors among persons older than 70 years have shown a significantly increasing trend since 1972, due primarily to an increase in glioblastoma multiforme. The annual age-adjusted incidence rates for all ages of Los Angeles males and females combined from 1972 to 1991, are shown in Figure 1–2.

Undoubtedly, much of this apparent increase in brain tumor rates results from more complete diagnosis, but how

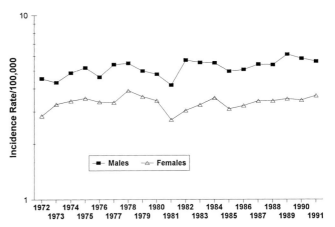

Figure 1–2 Age-adjusted annual incidence per 100,000 persons of histologically confirmed intracranial gliomas in males and females by calendar year, Los Angeles County, 1972–1991, all ethnic groups combined.

much might be attributable to improved diagnosis has been the topic of considerable debate.[13, 14] One particularly thoughtful analysis concluded that the increase in rates is not real but is attributable to the following three factors: (1) the availability of improved imaging; (2) a change in attitude toward care of the elderly; and (3) the introduction of programs such as Medicare, which support diagnostic workup of elderly patients.[15] Advanced imaging techniques such as CT scans and MRI enable doctors to diagnose brain tumors that previously might have been incorrectly diagnosed as strokes, senile dementia, or other neurologic disorders, and recent analyses attribute both the increase in glioma and the decline in stroke rates among the elderly to improved diagnostic accuracy.[16, 17] An analysis of Norwegian data shows that the completeness of brain tumor diagnosis, particularly among the elderly, depends heavily on both the autopsy rate and the use of advanced imaging techniques.[18] An analysis of pediatric brain tumors suggests that the small increase in rates in this age group is also attributable to the wider use of CT.[19] Therefore most, if not all, of the increase in glioma rates seems likely to be an artifact of more complete case ascertainment.

Gender, Ethnicity, and International Variation

Figure 1–3 shows that males, regardless of ethnic group, have higher rates of gliomas. The sex ratio (SR) of male-to-female incidence rates varies considerably by age, glioma subtype, and geographic area.[8] For example, primitive neuroectodermal tumors (PNET; a designation that includes tumors formerly called *medulloblastoma*), which occur predominantly in children, are much more common (SR of up to 2) in boys than girls; in contrast, most other pediatric gliomas have similar rates in both genders (SR of around 1). Table 1–1 includes data on the SR for specific subtypes of glioma common in adults and shows that the SR is higher for ependymoma, oligodendroglioma, and glioblastoma multiforme than for other gliomas. An SR of 1.6 for glioblastoma was also reported from a study of registry data from nine geographic areas in the United States.[8]

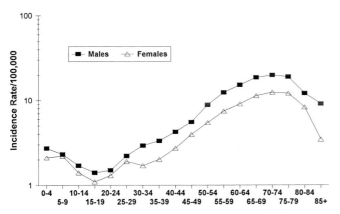

Figure 1–1 Average annual age-specific incidence per 100,000 persons of intracranial gliomas in males and females, Los Angeles County, 1972–1991, all ethnic groups combined. Total cases were 3,855 in males and 2,908 in females.

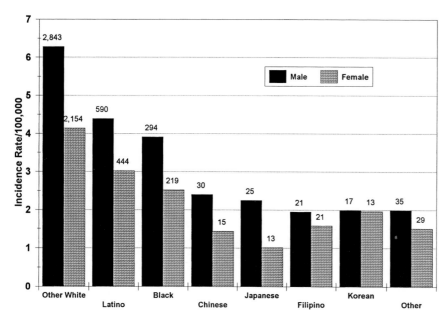

Figure 1-3 Average annual age-adjusted incidence per 100,000 persons of intracranial gliomas by ethnic group and sex, Los Angeles County, 1972–1991. Number of cases is indicated on top of each bar.

In international comparisons, brain cancer rates among whites in Canada, the United States, Europe, the United Kingdom, and Australia are relatively similar, and rates are low in Asian populations. In general, rates of brain and nervous system tumors are highest among whites. Among each other racial group, rates are usually higher in migrant populations than in native populations that remain on the continent of origin. These differences between migrant and native populations, which are most striking for Chinese, black, and Japanese populations, suggest that some change in lifestyle may occur in migrant populations that places them at higher risk for brain tumors, although an increase in diagnostic efficiency may partially explain some of the differences.

Time and Space Clustering

Informal estimates by officials at state health departments indicate that only about 5% of suspected cancer clusters turn out to be statistically significant excesses. Although the identification of such geographic concentrations of brain tumor cases allows the generation of hypotheses regarding potential environmental risk factors, most studies have only a very small number of cases and fail to implicate any suspected factors.[20, 21]

Social Class

Table 1–2 compares brain glioma incidence rates in Los Angeles County by social class. Among males, but not females, there is a clear trend of increasing glioma incidence with increasing social class (as determined by census tract of residence); this trend is seen for white, black, and Chinese males. A similar trend of increasing brain cancer rates with increasing social class (as determined by occupation) was reported for men in England and Wales a few decades ago and for New Zealand males.[4, 22] Because this trend occurs among males but not among females, it seems unlikely that it might relate to factors such as diagnostic efficiency or exposure to diagnostic radiography of the head (e.g., dental x-rays), both of which might be expected to be greater among those in higher social classes.

TABLE 1–1
DISTRIBUTION OF INCIDENT PRIMARY INTRACRANIAL GLIOMAS BY HISTOLOGIC SUBTYPE AND SEX, LOS ANGELES COUNTY, 1972–1991 (ALL ETHNIC GROUPS COMBINED)

Histologic Type (ICDO Codes)	M			F			Sex Ratio
	n	% of Total	Rate	n	% of Total	Rate	
Glioblastoma multiforme (9440–9442)	1,464	38.0	2.14	1,095	37.7	1.32	1.6
Astrocytoma (9400–9421)	1,692	43.9	2.31	1,270	43.7	1.56	1.5
Medulloblastoma (9470–9473)	182	4.7	.25	117	4.0	.17	1.5
Oligodendroglioma (9450–9460)	136	3.5	.17	96	3.3	.11	1.6
Ependymoma (9391–9394)	109	2.8	.15	56	1.9	.07	2.1
Other gliomas (9380–82, 9430, 9443)	272	7.1	.37	274	9.4	.32	1.2
Total gliomas	3,855	100.0	5.39	2,908	100.0	3.55	1.5

ICDO, International Classification of Diseases for Oncology.

TABLE 1–2
PROPORTIONAL INCIDENCE RATIOS AND TOTAL NUMBERS OF CASES* FOR INCIDENT INTRACRANIAL GLIOMAS COMBINED BY SOCIAL CLASS AND ETHNICITY, LOS ANGELES COUNTY, 1972–1989

	Non-Spanish-Surnamed White	Spanish Surnamed	Black	Chinese	Japanese	All races	
M							
1 (High)	127.3	79.5	152.1	207.6	47.6	129.0	(428)
2	107.3	89.2	104.1	118.9	61.6	109.1	(982)
3	98.8	86.1	107.6	175.2	138.7	100.4	(943)
4	91.7	108.9	108.6	62.3	88.0	95.3	(1,344)
5	77.5	104.2	77.4	65.6	174.7	80.0	(343)
6 (Low)	75.8	82.4	99.8	0.0	0.0	79.0	(112)
F							
1	98.4	164.9	34.8	0.0	0.0	102.9	(288)
2	100.7	95.4	91.3	99.8	111.7	102.1	(783)
3	100.8	90.2	91.0	166.4	63.7	100.3	(784)
4	102.4	98.7	107.6	83.2	124.1	100.5	(1,139)
5	95.3	105.7	94.9	128.1	123.3	95.0	(303)
6	72.0	82.2	105.2	0.0	0.0	81.0	(72)

*The numbers in parentheses indicate the number of cases.

Occupation and Industry

Tables 1–3 and 1–4 list all occupations and industries for which a statistically significant excess (and at least two cases) of glioma was observed in Los Angeles County from 1972 to 1991. Occupations with an excess of gliomas among males in both Los Angeles and other regions include engineers; physicians, dentists, and related professionals; and airplane pilots.[4] Industries with a significant glioma excess among males include lumber and wood products, aircraft manufacture, and electrical goods (wholesale). Among females, but not males, in Los Angeles petrochemical workers show an excess.

Although a myriad of epidemiologic studies have investigated the relationship between work in a variety of occupational/industrial settings and brain tumor incidence/mortality,

TABLE 1–3
DISTRIBUTION OF INTRACRANIAL GLIOMAS BY SELECTED OCCUPATIONS, LOS ANGELES COUNTY, 1972–1991, OF NON-SPANISH-SURNAMED WHITE MEN AND WOMEN, AGED 20 TO 99 YEARS

	M		F	
Occupation	n	Proportional Incidence Ratio	n	Proportional Incidence Ratio
Professional, technical, and kindred workers	474	116.0*	195	108.3
Engineers	139	136.6*	4	133.1
Aeronautical and astronautical engineers	42	189.2*	2	301.5
Electrical and electronic engineers	26	150.4†	0	0.0
Agricultural scientists	2	817.6†	0	0.0*
Physicians, dentists, and related professionals	54	142.7†	4	104.9
Physicians, medical and osteopathic	34	142.8†	3	116.1
Teachers of art, drama, and music, university and college	3	479.0†	2	463.2
Teachers, except university and college	21	168.3†	54	106.8
Secondary schoolteachers	3	114.9	6	310.7†
Airplane pilots	7	249.8†	0	0.0†
Office machine operators	2	755.2†	8	106.7
Stenographers	0	0.0	8	372.7†
Apprentice electricians	2	1086.1*	0	0.0*
Telephone linemen, splicers	4	367.4†	0	0.0
Operatives, except transportation	83	79.7†	42	98.2
Clothing ironers, pressers	0	0.0	3	586.1*
Meat cutters, butchers, except manufacturing	10	144.0	2	1380.8*
Solderers	0	0.0	2	1120.8*
Truck drivers	30	63.0†	0	0.0
Construction laborers, except carpenters' helpers	21	159.8†	0	0.0
Service workers, except in private homes	99	79.8†	61	89.7
Food service workers	12	36.4*	27	101.5
Bartenders	3	22.6*	1	95.4

*P < 0.01.
†P < 0.05.

TABLE 1–4
DISTRIBUTION OF INTRACRANIAL GLIOMAS BY SELECTED INDUSTRIES, LOS ANGELES COUNTY, 1972–1991,
OF NON-SPANISH-SURNAMED WHITE MEN AND WOMEN, AGED 20 TO 99 YEARS

	M		F	
Industry	n	Proportional Incidence Ratio	n	Proportional Incidence Ratio
Manufacturing				
Lumber and wood products, except furniture	12	298.2*	2	296.5
Sawmills, planing and milling	7	402.9*	1	338.5
Office and accounting machine manufacture	6	330.9*	1	116.0
Transportation equipment manufacture	181	119.5†	28	92.7
Aircraft and parts manufacture	159	149.8*	26	94.1
Petroleum and coal products	14	81.8	7	291.2*
Petroleum refining	13	80.6	6	268.9†
Transportation, communication, and other public utilities	111	79.1†	26	75.9
Transportation	68	75.3†	8	53.4
Railroads and railway equipment	6	41.1†	0	0.0
Wholesale trade				
Electrical goods	9	272.1*	0	0.0
Machinery, equipment, and supplies	14	176.6†	1	45.6
Retail trade	141	81.0†	106	110.1
Eating and drinking places, retail	20	52.0*	26	104.8
Miscellaneous retail stores	19	169.6†	7	102.0
Retail trade, not specified	6	75.9	9	207.8†
Business management, consulting service	13	193.3†	2	57.3
Auto repair and related services	7	41.8†	1	150.3
Miscellaneous entertainment and recreation	11	84.3	9	213.2†
Offices of physicians	20	163.0†	14	109.9
Legal services	21	112.7	20	169.7†

*$P < 0.01$.
†$P < 0.05$.

repeated studies in various geographic areas have been reported for only a few occupations, including workers in the rubber industry,[23, 24] petrochemical workers,[25, 26] health professionals,[27–29] electrical workers,[3, 30, 31] and agricultural workers.[32, 33] In most of these groups no specific carcinogen has been implicated. Early studies of workers exposed to vinyl chloride, which were inspired by experimental results with this compound, found an increase in brain tumor mortality,[34–36] but recent studies have found no such increase.[37–39] Whether or not the suggested excess of glioma among petrochemical workers is a true excess also remains controversial. Recently, new associations, such as an increased risk of gliomas among women working with cathode-ray tubes,[40] have been suggested by recent studies, but have not been investigated further.

Median Survival

Glioma survival rates vary considerably by histologic subtype and by age. The relative 5-year survival rate in children ages 0 to 14 years is now as high as 60% compared to 35% 20 years ago.[41] In a recent study in the United Kingdom, survival for all brain cancer diagnoses among children under age 15 years was 51% at 5 years and ranged from 13% for unbiopsied brainstem gliomas to 100% for juvenile astrocytomas.[19] Survival rates for all age groups combined also vary considerably by glioma type as shown in a recent analysis for the state of Victoria in Australia.[42] Patients with glioblastoma multiforme have the poorest prognosis (5% survive 5 years), and the proportion who survive 5 years is also low for patients with unspecified tumors (20%) and those whose tumors were not confirmed microscopically (28%). Five-year survival is more likely for patients with ependymoma (65%), oligodendroglioma (61%), medulloblastoma (43%), or astrocytoma (44%). For most histologic subtypes, survival curves for the two sexes are similar.

Clinical Associations

Brain tumors have been associated with various chronic diseases, but few of these suggested concordances have been investigated in more than one or two studies; they are, therefore, neither well-established nor well-understood. Two associations of particular interest that have been found in recent as well as earlier studies are decreases in glioma risk among diabetics[43] and among those with allergic disorders.[40, 43] An excess of brain tumors has been reported in various cohorts of epileptics, and the interpretation of these findings favored by the authors of the reports is that epilepsy is a sign of a slow-growing tumor and that no excess risk is associated with treatment with anti-epileptic drugs.[44–46]

Some studies have found a positive association of serum cholesterol levels and brain cancer,[47–50] but others have found none.[51] However, studies have not evaluated cholesterol intake, and it has been proposed that an existing brain cancer might cause a spurious increase in serum cholesterol concentration.[51]

Summary of the Descriptive Epidemiology

Perhaps the most important finding from our review of the descriptive epidemiology of brain tumors is that the pattern of occurrence varies considerably by histologic type. For all gliomas combined, the SR is greater than 1; incidence peaks before age 10 years and continues to rise again after age 25 years; rates are higher in whites than in non-whites and are lowest in Asians; incidence increases with increasing social class in males but not in females. The male excess of gliomas has often been thought to indicate the etiologic importance of occupational risk exposures. However, the strong positive social class trend casts doubt on this supposition, which assumes that blue collar jobs are most likely to involve carcinogenic exposures.

ESTABLISHED CAUSES

Ionizing Radiation

The occurrence of excess brain tumors after high-dose exposure to ionizing radiation is well established. Children who received CNS radiation during treatment for leukemia have developed an excess of glioma.[52, 53] Two large follow-up studies of children in Israel and New York given x-ray therapy for ringworm of the scalp show them to be at increased risk of both benign and malignant brain tumors.[54, 55] An updated follow-up of the Israeli cohort showed the relative risk (RR) is greatest for nerve sheath tumors (RR = 33.1), intermediate for meningiomas (RR = 9.5), and lowest for gliomas (RR = 2.6).[56] The association with low-dose exposure is more controversial. Prenatal exposure from diagnostic radiography has been related to an excess of pediatric brain tumors in several early studies,[57, 58] and a recent study in Swedish twins found that abdominal x-rays of the mother during pregnancy were associated with an increase in CNS tumors, which appeared not to be confounded by mother's age, obstetric complications, or other factors.[59]

Inheritance

Some gliomas have a relatively clear genetic character, particularly those that occur in association with neurofibromatosis and other phakomatoses (these are the topic of Chapter 3). The familial occurrence of gliomas (discussed in Chapter 2) has also been investigated in several epidemiologic studies. One study found that Connecticut children with central nervous system tumors more often had relatives with nervous system tumors than did control children, but this familial occurrence, although statistically significant, was observed for fewer than 2% of the children with CNS tumors.[60] Medulloblastoma and glioblastoma were overrepresented among children whose relatives had nervous system tumors.[60] What is important to note is that population-based studies that have investigated associations of gliomas with recognized predisposing genetic syndromes and/or with fa-milial aggregations suggest that the proportion of glioma risk attributable to inheritance is no more than 4%.[61, 62]

ETIOLOGIC HYPOTHESIS: *N*-NITROSO COMPOUNDS CAUSE GLIOMAS IN HUMANS

A compelling experimental model developed in the 1970s showed that *N*-nitroso compounds (NOCs) cause nervous system tumors in various species, including monkeys,[63] and that the fetal animal is 50 times more sensitive than the adult animal to this effect.

NOCs and Brain Tumors

EXPERIMENTAL DATA AND RELEVANCE TO HUMANS

NOCs and their precursors are ubiquitous in the environment of our modern industrialized society; they are also among the most potent experimental carcinogens. Ninety percent of the approximately 300 NOCs tested are found to be carcinogenic.[64, 65] This category of compounds contains two major subcategories: nitrosamines, which require metabolic activation, and nitrosamides, which do not. The nitrosamides, in particular various nitrosoureas, are effective nervous system carcinogens,[66] and only two chemicals other than NOCs (propylene imine and propane sultone) induced brain tumors in rats in recent systematic carcinogenicity studies of several hundred compounds.[67] NOCs cause cancer in more than 40 species used experimentally.[65] Because there is no reason to think that man is less susceptible to these compounds it is likely that NOCs cause cancer in humans as well. Although NOC exposures in some occupational settings (e.g., machine shops; tire and rubber factories) can be substantial, most people have low-level, but virtually continuous, exposure to NOCs throughout life. But, because NOCs are the most potent of carcinogens in animals (and likely in humans as well), only small doses are needed to cause cancer.[65]

Neurogenic tumors can be caused by transplacental exposure to ethylnitrosourea (ENU) or by addition of low levels of ENU precursors (ethyl urea and sodium nitrite) to the food and drinking water of a pregnant animal; however, no tumors develop if ascorbate (vitamin C) is also added to the diet.[68, 69] In rodents, these tumors occur in the brain, spinal cord, and peripheral nerves and are of various histologic types, including gliomas. In nonhuman primates, the nervous system tumors that are induced by transplacental exposure arise exclusively in the brain and have a histologic spectrum similar to that of pediatric brain tumors. ENU exposure leads to the formation of O^6-ethylguanine, a mutagenic lesion of DNA that is removed more slowly from brain DNA than from the DNA of other tissues.[70] The inability of the brain to remove this mutagen quickly, coupled with the high rate of DNA replication in the fetal brain, may explain why fetal animals are more sensitive than adults and why the brain is more sensitive than other tissues to the carcinogenic effects of ENU[70]; other investigators argue that this DNA alkylation may not be the key event in tumor development, although it may be a necessary one.[65] It is further thought that these alkylated bases cause base-mispairing and point mutations that lead to uncontrolled expression of oncogenes and growth factor receptors followed by permanently heightened cell proliferation.[71]

Population Exposure to NOCs

Endogenous formation of NOCs in humans, which occurs in the stomach or bladder when both an amino compound and a nitrosating agent are present simultaneously, is likely to be the most important source of population exposure to nitrosamides. Food is a primary source of both highly concentrated nitrite solutions (e.g., from cured meats) and amino compounds (e.g., in fish and other foods, but also in many drugs). When inhibitors such as ascorbate (vitamin C) or α-tocopherol (vitamin E), which are nitrite scavengers, are also present at high concentrations, NOCs are not formed.[71] The level of NOCs in the human body is also influenced by other factors, such as which amino compounds are present, presence of bacteria or other nitrosation catalysts, gastric pH, and other physiologic factors. Uncertainty as to the simultaneous presence of NOC precursors and of inhibitors and/or catalysts of nitrosation make this hypothesis difficult to study epidemiologically. This difficulty is compounded by further uncertainty about what exposure period (during a person's life) is most likely to be etiologically relevant.

Epidemiologic Evidence

Findings from a preliminary study conducted in Los Angeles indicated that the hypothesis that NOCs cause brain tumors in humans deserves further investigation.[72] Other epidemiologic studies of pediatric[73–75] and adult[76–78] glioma patients have provided limited support for this hypothesis. Findings that use of vitamin supplements and/or high intake of fresh fruit or vegetables protect against glioma development might also be interpreted as supportive of the *N*-nitroso hypothesis, although this effect may be due to another mechanism.[72–75, 77, 79] The experimental model and its potential relevance to humans are sufficiently compelling to encourage further investigation of this hypothesis despite the fact that it is a difficult one to test epidemiologically.

OTHER SUGGESTED RISK FACTORS

Parental Occupational Exposures

Excess brain tumors have been observed not only among workers in a number of industries but also among children whose fathers worked in paper and pulp mills, the aircraft industry, the Air Force, printing and graphic arts industries, chemical and petroleum refining, agriculture, and metal-related jobs. Multiple studies have evaluated paternal job exposure to pesticides and hydrocarbons with inconsistent results; however, consistent associations are seen with fathers' exposure to paints. Only some of these studies also looked at mothers' occupations; increased risks have been seen for factory workers, bakers, and persons with job exposure to chemicals. These associations are clearly summarized in a review article,[80] and some subsequent reports have appeared.[81, 82]

Infectious Agents

Although some viruses have been shown to induce brain tumors experimentally, only scattered studies hint at associations of prior viral infections with later glioma development, and recent population-based studies have failed to confirm these associations. Astrocytomas, but not other histologic types of brain tumors, appeared to be associated with positive antibody titers to *Toxoplasma gondii*,[83] but another study failed to confirm this.[84] Reports in the literature of the isolation of viruses or virus-like particles from human cerebral tumors or tumor cell lines are numerous, but whether these findings have etiologic implications is uncertain.[85, 86] People who received polio vaccine contaminated with SV40 did not have more brain tumor development in the 20 years after vaccination, although some histologic types (e.g., spongioblastoma, medulloblastoma) did appear to occur disproportionately.[87]

Neither prospective nor retrospective studies of maternal influenza infection during pregnancy have found a brain tumor excess in offspring.[88, 89] One study reported three medulloblastomas among 9,000 children whose mothers had chickenpox during pregnancy and none among the 9,000 control children.[89] Another study found no association between childhood brain tumors and maternal chickenpox, rubella, or mumps.[90]

ABO Blood Type

There are several studies in the literature of the relationship between blood group and brain tumors, but some have been poorly designed or have reported findings in such a way that they are difficult to interpret. What appears to emerge as a common finding is an excess of blood group A among astrocytoma patients[91, 92] or among men with brain tumors of all types.[93, 94] No explanation has been offered for this association, and studies relying on self-reports of blood group failed to confirm these associations.[43] A smaller proportion of U.S. blacks compared with U.S. whites have blood group A.[95] Whether this relative deficit of type A among blacks may relate to their lower glioma incidence has not been investigated.

Medications

Pediatric gliomas were associated with maternal use of barbiturates during pregnancy in two early studies, but not in more recent ones.[72, 96–98] Associations with other drugs used by mothers of glioma patients include diuretics, antihistamines, and antinausea medications.[72, 98]

Head Trauma

Limited experimental evidence suggests that trauma may act as a co-carcinogen in the induction of gliomas, but epidemiologic studies have found an association of trauma with meningioma but not with glioma.[99] Limited evidence suggests that birth trauma or prior severe head injury increases a child's risk of developing brain tumors.[72, 97, 100] But childhood astrocytoma was not associated with head trauma that resulted in loss of consciousness.[98]

Alcohol

No consistent association with glioma risk is seen across studies for consumption of any type of alcoholic beverage or for all types combined. A case-control study of gliomas in adults observed a significantly elevated risk for consumption of wine and a significant positive dose-response trend (i.e., those drinking more wine had greater brain tumor risk).[101] Studies of childhood brain tumors have also been inconsistent in regard to whether or not an association was seen with mothers' consumption of alcohol during the index pregnancy. Two found no association with alcohol use,[72, 98] but one found an elevated risk among the offspring of mothers who drank beer[100]; NOC levels in beer have been of public health concern in Germany and a few other countries.

Tobacco: Active and Passive Exposure

Case-control studies found no association in Los Angeles between personal tobacco use and glioma occurrence,[99] but in Toronto a significant dose-response was found for use of plain (nonfiltered) cigarettes.[101] Several studies in children have shown slightly elevated risks related to smoking by either or both parents[72, 100, 102] but others found no increase in risk.[98, 103] Non-smoking Japanese women whose husbands smoked were more likely to die of brain cancer, and a significant dose-response relationship was observed.[104]

Electric and Magnetic Fields

Several epidemiologic studies of brain tumor risk in electricity-related occupations have recently been reported, with some suggestion that this association may be stronger for astrocytomas.[26, 105] Three studies have found an association with residential exposure to magnetic fields and pediatric brain tumors,[106–108] but a recent study failed to find such an effect.[109] No excess of brain tumors was seen among Swedish workers on electric trains compared with workers on non-electric trains.[110]

PROSPECTS

Ionizing radiation can cause all three major histologic types of brain tumors: gliomas, meningiomas, and nerve sheath tumors, but the association appears weakest for gliomas.

Nonetheless, minimizing population exposure to x-rays of the head is, at this point, the best prospect for prevention of all three types of tumors. Beyond this, the etiology of gliomas remains largely unknown. New etiologic hypotheses are needed that might explain features of the descriptive epidemiology, such as the male excess and the increasing incidence with increasing social class in males but not in females. To date, no one has offered a hypothesis as to why glioma is most commonly a disease of upper-class white men.

Diet will be an important focus of the next generation of epidemiologic studies of gliomas. Studies to date have included some questions about a limited number of dietary variables, such as the several studies that looked at foods thought likely to be relevant to the *N*-nitroso hypothesis. A number of intriguing associations are emerging from these and other studies, including the suggestion that intake of cured meats, fruit, and vitamin supplements all relate to glioma risk, with fruit and vitamins being protective. Future studies must include more complete dietary surveys to better evaluate associations with various micronutrients, cholesterol, nitrite from cured meats, and other suggested associations.

The prospects for studies of gliomas in children warrant separate discussion. Animal experiments strongly suggest that pediatric gliomas may be caused by exposures during gestation. The hypothesis that NOC may cause brain tumors, which is difficult to test epidemiologically, may more easily be investigated in children, because the relevant exposure period (gestation) is more clearly defined for children than it is for adults and because the effect is likely to be stronger when exposure occurs during the period of rapid development of brain tissue. Hopefully, a large international collaborative study of childhood brain tumors currently under analysis will help to evaluate the *N*-nitroso hypothesis; it may also identify potential risk factors for specific histologic types of pediatric gliomas. As always, these studies will further our understanding of the etiology of these tumors only if the right questions are being asked. For gliomas in particular, it seems possible that some of the crucial etiologic questions have not yet been posed.

REFERENCES

1. Boring CC, Squires TS, Tong T: Cancer statistics, 1992. CA 1992; 41:19.
2. Mack T: Cancer surveillance program in Los Angeles County. Natl Cancer Inst Monogr 1977; 47:99.
3. Preston-Martin S, Henderson BE, Peters JM: Descriptive epidemiology of central nervous system neoplasms in Los Angeles County. *In* Selikoff IJ, Hammond EC (eds): Brain Tumors in the Chemical Industry. New York, The New York Academy of Sciences, 1982.
4. Preston-Martin S, Lewis S, Winkelmann R, et al: Descriptive epidemiology of primary brain tumors in New Zealand, 1948–1988. Cancer Causes Control 1993; 4:529.
5. Percy AK, Elveback LR, Okazaki H, et al: Neoplasms of the central nervous system. Neurology 1972; 22:40.
6. Schoenberg BS, Christine BW, Whisnant JP: The resolution of discrepancies in the reported incidence of primary brain tumors. Neurology 1978; 28:817.
7. Annegers JF, Schoenberg BS, Okazaki H, et al: Epidemiologic study of primary intracranial neoplasms. Arch Neurol 1981; 38:217.
8. Velema JP, Walker AM: The age curve of nervous system tumour

incidence in adults: Common shape but changing levels by sex, race and geographical location. Int J Epidemiol 1987; 16:177.

9. Velema JP, Percy CL: Age curves of central nervous system tumor incidence in adults: Variation of shape by histologic type. JNCI 1987; 79:623.

10. Davis DL, Schwartz J: Trends in cancer mortality: US white males and females, 1968–83. Lancet 1988; 1:633.

11. Greig NH, Ries LG, Yancik R, et al: Increasing annual incidence of primary malignant brain tumors in the elderly. JNCI 1990; 82:1621.

12. Davis DL: International trends in cancer mortality in France, West Germany, Italy, Japan, England and Wales, and the USA. Lancet 1990; 336:474.

13. Ahlbom A, Rodvall Y: Brain tumour trends (letter). Lancet 1989; 2:1272.

14. Desmeules M, Mikkelsen T, Mao Y: Increasing incidence of primary brain tumors: Influence of diagnostic methods. JNCI 1992; 84:442.

15. Modan B, Wagener DK, Feldman JJ, et al: Increased mortality from brain tumors: A combined outcome of diagnostic technology and change of attitude toward the elderly. Am J Epidemiol 1992; 135:1349.

16. Riggs JE: The decline of mortality due to stroke: A competitive and deterministic perspective. Neurology 1991; 41:1135.

17. Riggs JE: Longitudinal Gompertzian analysis of primary malignant brain tumor mortality in the U.S., 1962–1987: Rising mortality in the elderly is the natural consequence of competitive deterministic dynamics. Mech Ageing Dev 1991; 60:225.

18. Helseth A, Langmark F, Mork SJ: Neoplasms of the central nervous system in Norway: II. Descriptive epidemiology of intracranial neoplasms, 1955–1984. APMIS 1988; 96:1066.

19. Stevens MC, Cameron AH, Muir KR, et al: Descriptive epidemiology of primary nervous system tumours in children: A population-based study. Clin Oncol 1991; 3:323.

20. Neuberger JS, Brownson RC, Morantz RA, et al: Association of brain cancer with dental x-rays and occupation in Missouri. Cancer Detect Prev 1991; 15:31.

21. Wilkins JR III, McLaughlin JA, Sinks TH: Parental occupation and intracranial neoplasms of childhood: Anecdotal evidence from a unique occupational cancer cluster. Am J Ind Med 1991; 19:643.

22. Buell P, Dunn JE, Breslow L: The occupational-social class risks of cancer mortality in men. Cancer 1960; 12:600.

23. Mancuso TF: Tumors of the central nervous system: Industrial considerations. Acta Unio International Union Against Cancer 1963; 19:488.

24. Sorahan T, Parkes HG, Veys CA, et al: Mortality in the British rubber industry, 1946–85. Br J Ind Med 1989; 46:1.

25. Thomas TL, Decoufle P, Moure-Eraso R: Mortality among workers employed in petroleum refining and petrochemical plants. J Occup Med 1980; 22:97.

26. Marsh GM, Enterline PE, McCraw D: Mortality patterns among petroleum refinery and chemical plant workers. Am J Indust Med 1991; 19:29.

27. Blair A, Hayes HM Jr: Cancer and other causes of death among US veterinarians, 1966–1977. Int J Cancer 1980; 25:181.

28. Ahlbom A, Norell S, Rodvall Y: Dentists, dental nurses, and brain tumors. Br Med J 1986; 292:662.

29. McLaughlin JK, Malker HSR, Blot W, et al: Occupational risks for intracranial gliomas in Sweden. JNCI 1987; 78:253.

30. Thomas TL, Stolley PD, Stemhagen A, et al: Brain tumor mortality risk among men with electrical and electronics jobs: A case-control study. JNCI 1987; 79:233.

31. Mack W, Preston-Martin S, Peters JM: Astrocytoma risk related to job exposure to electric and magnetic fields. Bioelectromagnetics 1991; 12:57.

32. Musicco M, Filipini G, Bordo BM, et al: Gliomas and occupational exposure to carcinogens: Case-control study. Am J Epidemiol 1982; 116:782.

33. Brownson RC, Reif JS, Chang JC, et al: An analysis of occupational risks for brain cancer. Am J Pub Health 1990; 80:169.

34. Monson RR, Peters JM, Johnson MN: Proportional mortality among vinyl-chloride workers. Lancet 1974; 2:397.

35. Waxweiler RJ, Stringer W, Wagoner JK, et al: Neoplastic risk among workers exposed to vinyl chloride. Ann NY Acad Sci 1976; 27:10.

36. Cooper WC: Epidemiologic study of vinyl chloride workers: Mortality through December 31, 1972. Environ Health Perspect 1981; 41:101.

37. Jones RD, Smith DM, Thomas PG: A mortality study of vinyl chloride monomer workers employed in the United Kingdom in 1940–1974. Scand J Work Environ Health 1988; 14:153.

38. Wu W, Steenland K, Brown D, et al: Cohort and case-control analyses of workers exposed to vinyl chloride: An update. J Occup Med 1989; 31:518.

39. Hagmar L, Akesson B, Nielsen J, et al: Mortality and cancer morbidity in workers exposed to low levels of vinyl chloride monomer at a polyvinyl chloride processing plant. Am J Indust Med 1990; 17:553.

40. Ryan P, Lee MW, North B, et al: Risk factors for tumors of the brain and meninges: Results from the Adelaide Adult Brain Tumor Study. Int J Cancer 1992; 51:20.

41. Crist WM, Kun LE: Common solid tumors of childhood. N Engl J Med 1991; 324:461.

42. Preston-Martin S, Staples M, Farrugia H, et al: Primary tumors of the brain, cranial nerves and cranial meninges in Victoria Australia, 1982–1990; Patterns of incidence and survival. Neuroepidemiology 1993; 12:270.

43. Schlehofer B, Blettner M, Becker N, et al: Medical risk factors and the development of brain tumors. Cancer 1992; 69:2541.

44. Olsen JH, Boice JD Jr, Jensen JPA, et al: Cancer among epileptic patients exposed to anticonvulsant drugs. JNCI 1989; 81:803.

45. Olsen JH, Boice JD Jr, Fraumeni JF Jr: Cancer in children of epileptic mothers and the possible relation to maternal anticonvulsant therapy. Br J Cancer 1990; 62:996.

46. Goldhaber MK, Selby JV, Hiatt RA, et al: Exposure to barbiturates in utero and during childhood and risk of intracranial and spinal cord tumors. Cancer Res 1990; 50:4600.

47. Basu TK, Raven RW, Dickerson JWT, et al: Vitamin A nutrition and its relationship with plasma cholesterol level in patients with cancer. Int J Vitam Nutr Res 1974; 44:14.

48. Abrahamson ZH, Kark JD: Serum cholesterol and primary brain tumours: Case-control study. Br J Cancer 1985; 52:93.

49. Neugut AI, Fink DJ, Radin D: Serum cholesterol and primary brain tumours: Case-control study. Int J Epidemiol 1989; 18:798.

50. Davey-Smith G, Shipley MJ: Plasma cholesterol concentration and primary brain tumours. Br Med J 1989; 299:26.

51. Knect P, Reunanen A, Teppo L: Serum cholesterol concentration and risk of primary brain tumours. Br Med J 1991; 302:90.

52. Meadows AT, Baum E, Fossati-Bellani F, et al: Second malignant neoplasms in children: An update from the late effects study group. J Clin Oncol 1985; 3:532.

53. Neglia JP, Meadows AT, Robison LL, et al: Second neoplasms after acute lymphoblastic leukemia in childhood. N Engl J Med 1991; 325:1330.

54. Modan B, Baidatz D, Mart H, et al: Radiation induced head and neck tumors. Lancet 1974; 1:277.

55. Shore RE, Albert RE, Pasternack BS: Follow-up study of patients treated by x-ray epilation for tinea capitis. Arch Environ Health 1976; 31:17.

56. Ron E, Modan B, Boice J, et al: Tumors of the brain and nervous system following radiotherapy in childhood. N Engl J Med 1988; 319:1033.

57. Stewart A, Webb J, Hewitt D: A survey of childhood malignancies. Br Med J 1958; 1:1495.

58. MacMahon B: Prenatal x-ray exposure and childhood cancer. JNCI 1962; 28:1173.

59. Rodvall Y, Pershagen G, Hrubec Z, et al: Prenatal x-ray exposure and childhood cancer in Swedish twins. Int J Cancer 1990; 46:362.

60. Farwell J, Flannery JT: Cancer in relatives of children with central-nervous-system neoplasms. N Engl J Med 1984; 311:749.

61. Wrensch M, Barger GR: Familial factors associated with malignant gliomas. Genet Epidemiol 1990; 7:291.

62. Bondy ML, Lustbader ED, Buffler PA, et al: Genetic epidemiology of childhood brain tumors. Genet Epidemiol 1991; 8:253.

63. Rice JM, Rehm S, Donovan PS, et al: Comparative transplacental carcinogenesis by direct acting and metabolism-dependent alkylating agents in rodents and nonhuman primates. IARC Sci Publ 1989; 96:17.

64. National Research Council: The Health Effects of Nitrate, Nitrite and N-Nitroso Compounds. Washington, DC, National Academy Press, 1981.

65. Lijinsky W: Chemistry and Biology of N-Nitroso Compounds. New York, Cambridge University Press, 1992.

66. Magee PN, Montesano R, Preussman R: N-nitroso compounds and related carcinogens. In Searle CE (ed): Chemical Carcinogens. Washington, DC, American Chemical Society, 1976, p 491.

67. Maekawa A, Mitsumori K: Spontaneous occurrence and chemical induction of neurogenic tumors in rats—influence of host factors and specificity of chemical structure. Toxicology 1990; 20:287.

68. Mirvish SS: Inhibition of the formation of carcinogenic N-nitroso compounds by ascorbic acid and other compounds. *In* Burchenal JH, Oettgen HF (eds): Cancer: Achievements, Challenges and Prospects for the 1980s, vol 1. New York, Grune & Stratton, 1981, p 557.

69. Tannenbaum SR, Wishnok JS, Leaf CD: Inhibition of nitrosamine formation by ascorbic acid. Am J Clin Nutr 1991; 53:247S.

70. Rajewsky MF, Goth R, Laerum OD, et al: Molecular and cellular mechanisms in nervous system-specific carcinogenesis by N-ethyl-N-nitrosourea. *In* Magee PN, Takayama S, Sugimura T, et al (eds): Fundamentals in Cancer Prevention. Baltimore, University Park Press, 1976, p 313.

71. Bilzer T, Reifenberger G, Wechsler W: Chemical induction of brain tumors in rats by nitrosoureas: Molecular biology and neuropathology. Neurotoxicol Teratol 1989; 11:551.

72. Preston-Martin S, Yu MC, Benton B, et al: N-nitroso compounds and childhood brain tumors: A case-control study. Cancer Res 1982; 42:5240.

73. Howe GR, Burch JD, Chiarelli AM, et al: An exploratory case-control study of brain tumors in children. Cancer Res 1989; 49:4349.

74. Bunin GR, Kuitjen RR, Boesel CP, et al: Maternal diet and risk of astrocytoma in children: A report from the Childrens Cancer Group. *In* Kuitjen RR (ed): Risk Factors for Childhood Brain Tumors. Utrecht, The Netherlands, University of Amsterdam, 1992, p 133, thesis.

75. McCredie M, Maisonneuve P, Boyle P: Antenatal risk factors for malignant brain tumours in New South Wales children. Int J Cancer 1994; 56:6.

76. Burch JD, Craib KJP, Choi BCK, et al: An exploratory case-control study of brain tumors in adults. JNCI 1987; 78:601.

77. Preston-Martin S, Mack W: Gliomas and meningiomas in men in Los Angeles County: Investigation of exposures to N-nitroso compounds. IARC Sci Publ 1991; 105:197.

78. Boeing H, Schlehofer B, Blettner M, et al: Dietary carcinogens and the risk for glioma and meningioma in Germany. Int J Cancer 1993; 53:561.

79. Bunin GR, Kuitjen RR, Rorke LB, et al: Evidence for a role of maternal diet in the etiology of primitive neuroectodermal tumor of brain in young children. N Engl J Med 1993; 329:536.

80. Savitz DA, Chen J: Parental occupation and childhood cancer: Review of epidemiologic studies. Environ Health Perspect 1990; 88:325.

81. Wilkins JR, Sinks TH: Parental occupation and intracranial neoplasms of childhood: Results of a case-control interview study. Am J Epidemiol 1990; 132:275.

82. Kuijten RR, Bunin GR, Nass CC, et al: Parental occupation and childhood astrocytoma: Results of a case-control study. Cancer Res 1992; 52:782.

83. Schuman LM, Choi NW, Gullen WH: Relationship of central nervous system neoplasms to *Toxoplasma gondii* infection. Am J Pub Health 1967; 57:848.

84. Ryan P, Hurley SF, Johnson AM, et al: Tumors of the brain and presence of antibodies to *Toxoplasma gondii*. Int J Epidemiol 1993; 22:412.

85. Bigner DD: Role of viruses in the causation of neural neoplasia. *In* Laerum OD, Bigner DD, Rawjewsky MF, et al (eds): Biology of Brain Tumors. Geneva, Switzerland, International Union Against Cancer, 1978.

86. Corallini A, Pagnani M, Viadana P, et al: Association of BK virus with human brain tumors and tumors of pancreatic islets. Int J Cancer 1987; 39:60.

87. Geissler E, Staneczek W: SV40 and human brain tumors. Arch fur Geschwulstforsch 1988; 58:129.

88. Fredrick J, Alberman ED: Reported influenza in pregnancy and subsequent cancer in the child. Br Med J 1972; 2:485.

89. Bithell JF, Draper GJ, Gorbach PD: Association between malignant disease in children and maternal virus infections. Br Med J 1973; 1:706.

90. Adelstein AM, Donovan JW: Malignant disease in children whose mothers had chickenpox, mumps or rubella in pregnancy. Br Med J 1972; 4:629.

91. Yates PO, Pearce KM: Recent changes in blood-group distribution of astrocytomas. Lancet 1960; 1:194.

92. Selverstone B, Cooper DR: Astrocytoma and ABO blood groups. J Neurosurg 1961; 18:602.

93. Buckwalter JA, Turner JH, Gamber HH: Psychoses, intracranial neoplasms and genetics. Arch Neurol Psychiatry 1959; 81:480.

94. Strang RR, Tovi D, Lopez J: Astrocytomas and the ABO blood groups. J Med Genet 1966; 3:274.

95. Garcia JH, Okazaki H, Aronson SM: Blood group frequencies and astrocytoma. J Neurosurg 1963; 20:397.

96. Gold E, Gordis L, Tonascia J, et al: Increased risk of brain tumors in children exposed to barbiturates. JNCI 1978; 61:1031.

97. Howe GR, Burch JD, Chiarelli AM, et al: An exploratory case-control study of brain tumors in children. Cancer Res 1989; 49:4349.

98. Kuijten RR, Bunin GR, Nass CC, et al: Gestational and familial risk factors for childhood astrocytoma: Results of a case-control study. Cancer Res 1990; 50:2608.

99. Preston-Martin S, Mack W, Henderson BE: Risk factors for gliomas and meningiomas in men in Los Angeles County. Cancer Res 1989; 49:6137.

100. Choi NW, Schuman LM, Gullen WH: Epidemiology of primary central nervous system neoplasms: II. Case-control study. Am J Epidemiol 1970; 91:467.

101. Burch JD, Craib KJP, Choi BCK, et al: An exploratory case-control study of brain tumors in adults. JNCI 1987; 78:601.

102. Gold E, Gordis L, Tonascia L, et al: Risk factors for brain tumors in children. Am J Epidemiol 1979; 109:309.

103. Gold EB, Leviton A, Lopez R, et al: Parental smoking and risk of childhood brain tumors. Am J Epidemiol 1993; 137:620.

104. Hirayama T: Cancer mortality in nonsmoking women with smoking husbands based on a large scale cohort study in Japan. Prev Med 1984; 13:680.

105. Thomas TL, Stewart PA, Stemhagen A, et al: Risk of astrocytic tumors associated with occupational chemical exposures: A case-referent study. Scand J Work Environ Health 1987; 13:417.

106. Wertheimer N, Leeper E: Electrical wiring configurations and childhood cancer. Am J Epidemiol 1979; 109:273.

107. Tomenius L: 50-Hz electromagnetic environment and the incidence of childhood tumors in Stockholm County. Bioelectromagnetics 1986; 7:191.

108. Savitz DA, Wachtel H, Barnes FA, et al: Case-control study of childhood cancer and exposure to 50-Hz magnetic fields. Am J Epidemiol 1988; 128:21.

109. Feychting M, Albolm A: Magnetic Fields and Cancer in People Residing near Swedish High Voltage Power Lines. IMM-rapport 6/92. Stockholm, 1992.

110. Tynes T, Jynge H, Vistnes AI: Leukemia and brain tumors in Norwegian railway workers: A nested case-control study. Am J Epidemiol 1994; 139:645.

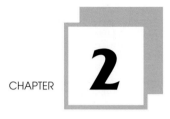

CHAPTER 2

Familial Gliomas

Primary brain tumors are a relatively uncommon malignancy, occurring in approximately 14,000 patients in the United States each year. About half of these are gliomas, which constitute more than 90% of all primary malignant central nervous system tumors.[1] This chapter reviews early data from the National Familial Brain Tumor Registry and published information that suggests that environmental factors may be important in the etiology of these neoplasms. Recognition that primary brain tumors occur in families and that this may provide important clues to the etiology of these disorders should prompt clinicians to investigate the family history of each patient with a primary brain tumor and should encourage researchers to pursue epidemiologic studies to identify factors important in the development of these devastating malignancies.

Despite their relative rarity, the etiology of gliomas has become a focus of scientific activity and public scrutiny. The identification of specific chromosomal abnormalities in primary brain tumors[2] and the association of brain tumors with hereditary diseases, such as tuberous sclerosis,[3] neurofibromatosis,[4] familial polyposis,[5] and Li-Fraumeni syndrome,[6] have prompted researchers to study this malignancy. Recent advances in genetic technology and models of carcinogenesis[7] have also spurred interest in the promotion and progression of these tumors. Research in this area now utilizes chromosomal analysis, fluorescence in situ hybridization (FISH) to detect previously occult genetic changes, polymerase chain reaction-based or Southern blot–based molecular diagnostics, genetic linkage studies, and pedigree construction and analysis.

The debilitating nature of the illness, the high costs associated with the care of patients, the poor results of therapy, and the apparent inability to offer surgical cure even when the tumor is diagnosed early have also stimulated efforts to better understand the underlying cause of this disease. Recent studies noting an increase in the incidence of primary brain tumors has served as another powerful stimulus to consider the etiology of these diseases.[8, 9] Although increases may reflect advances in neuroimaging, a true unexplained age-adjusted increase in the incidence of these tumors in the elderly is likely.

As outlined in the previous chapter, important factors in the etiology of gliomas are poorly understood. Since the 1700s, descriptive observations have been an important source of discoveries in cancer etiology.[10] Examples of descriptive studies that led to formal epidemiologic studies include Ramazzini's observation that breast cancer was more common in nuns (1700), Pott's description of scrotal cancer among chimney sweeps (1775), and Rehn's finding of bladder cancer among aniline dye workers (1895). A few provocative case reports exist in the literature that may provide insight into the etiology of primary brain tumors. These document the familial occurrence of malignant gliomas in the absence of a recognized hereditary syndrome. Von Motz and co-workers[11] described three sisters with grade 3 astrocytomas and Heunch and Blom[12] reported two brothers and a paternal aunt with glioblastoma multiforme. In 1990, three of 32 patients with high-grade astrocytomas on a therapeutic protocol were noted to have first-degree relatives with astrocytic neoplasms.[13] None of these families had known risk factors to predispose them to this illness. In one family, a parent and three children were affected. The odds of these occurring as random events were estimated to be very small.

THE NATIONAL FAMILIAL BRAIN TUMOR REGISTRY

These cases and discussions with experienced clinicians who reported caring for isolated families with similar pedigrees prompted the establishment of the National Familial Brain Tumor Registry at The Johns Hopkins Oncology Center in Baltimore.[14] The initial goals of the registry were (1) to document that primary brain tumors can occur as a familial disorder, (2) to begin to evaluate affected families to gain insight into the etiology of these malignancies, and (3) to serve as a resource to investigators interested in this area of research. Families with two or more first-degree relatives or a husband and wife with primary brain tumors were eligible for inclusion in the registry if they had no evidence of a hereditary syndrome that would predispose them to primary brain tumors. Acoustic neuromas and meningiomas were not considered eligible tumors for purposes of the registry. Informed consent was obtained from the patient or the next-of-kin. Medical records and pathologic slides were obtained for review. In addition, a short questionnaire was completed over the telephone.

The data from this registry are limited by several methodologic factors inherent in the exploratory nature of the registry. Reporting bias and the lack of a well-defined population base for the registry make it impossible to determine the true incidence of familial gliomas. Despite these limitations, 127 cases from 59 families have been collected.[15] These represent 30 parent-child cases, 27 sibling-sibling cases, and 9 husband-wife pairs. The cases were collected from 27 states, the District of Columbia, and Canada. Sixty percent of the patients were male. They had an average age of 49 years and a median of 12.9 years of education. Most lived in urban or suburban settings and the most common occupations of the patients were dairy farmer, teacher, and electrician/telephone line workers. More than 50% of the patients had high-grade astrocytomas.

Common familial malignancies, such as breast cancer and colon cancer, are associated with several important patterns of occurrence. Multiple generations are usually affected, the affected individuals are younger than average for the tumor, and the affected parents and children tend to be diagnosed with the tumor at approximately the same age. The histories of the patients accrued to the National Familial Brain Tumor Registry follow a very different pattern. In general, these tumors were not found in multiple generations. In fact, only one of the 127 affected patients involved a third generation. The remainder were all parent-child, sibling-sibling, or husband-wife cases. In addition, the age distribution of these cases is similar to that expected for all patients with high-grade astrocytomas. Furthermore, in nearly half of the parent-child cases, the child was diagnosed with the malignancy before the affected parent. In many families both family members were diagnosed within the same calendar year. Finally, the occurrence of husband-wife cases argues strongly for a nongenetic factor. In 33% of the husband-wife cases, the diagnosis of the primary brain tumor was made in both patients during the same calendar year following decades of co-habitation.

DATA SUGGESTING POSSIBLE ENVIRONMENTAL CAUSES OF HIGH GRADE ASTROCYTOMAS

Considerable data exist to suggest that astrocytomas can result from environmental exposures. Convincing evidence indicates that therapeutic ionizing radiation can increase the incidence of brain tumors. Ron and Modan[16] reported that Israelis treated with radiation therapy for tinea capitis as children were four times more likely to develop brain tumors than were controls. A study of second neoplasms in 9,720 children after treatment of acute lymphoblastic leukemia demonstrated a 22-fold excess in neoplasms of the central nervous system.[17] These increases were limited to children who had received prophylactic cranial irradiation. Alexander[18] reviewed the risk of brain tumors among workers at 10 nuclear facilities in the United States. This study, which included 1.6 million person-years of observation, estimated a 15% excess risk of primary brain tumors to workers exposed to low doses of radiation. Another study suggests

that airline pilots have a substantially higher mortality than expected from primary brain tumors and speculates that this could result from cosmic radiation.[19]

Primary brain tumors have also been noted in association with other environmental exposures, chemicals, and viruses. Workers exposed to vinyl chloride,[20] pesticides or fungicides,[21, 22] those employed in the rubber industry,[23] and those working with electronics and electrical equipment[24] have a higher than expected incidence of primary brain tumors. In addition, there is increasing scientific and public concern that occupational or residential exposure to extremely low-frequency (ELF) electromagnetic fields[25] and cellular telephones[26] may result in brain tumors.

Chemical carcinogens have long been suspected to cause human brain tumors because certain chemicals are known to induce brain tumors in experimental animals.[27] The prototypical agents for the induction of gliomas following direct injection into brain parenchyma are the polycyclic aromatic hydrocarbons. Nitroso compounds such as *N*-methyl-*N*-nitrosourea and *N*-ethyl-*N*-nitrosourea routinely produce brain tumors in animals following intravenous administration. Other compounds have also been identified to result in the development of primary brain tumors.

In addition, viruses have been implicated in the development of gliomas in rats, dogs, and monkeys. These tumors are most reliably produced by injecting the virus directly into brain parenchyma. Avian sarcoma virus produces glial tumors in rats,[28] Rous sarcoma virus produces gliosarcomas in dogs,[29] and polyomaviruses produce glial neoplasms in monkeys.[30] However, the relevance of these observations in man is still unknown. A recent study of tumor DNA from 80 patients with high-grade astrocytomas was unable to identify DNA sequences from polyomavirus using polymerase chain reaction techniques.[31] However, another virus, Epstein-Barr virus, has been strongly implicated in the development of primary CNS lymphoma in man.[32]

SUMMARY

The data presented in this chapter suggest that brain tumors can occur as a familial disorder. This may happen much more frequently than has been appreciated in this relatively uncommon tumor. In addition, it suggests that family members of patients with brain tumors may be at higher risk of developing these tumors than the general population. Although the data from the National Familial Brain Tumor Registry is purely descriptive, it appears that most patients with familial brain tumors have high-grade astrocytomas. In addition, the clustering in time, the ages of the affected family members, the few generations affected, and the occurrences in spouses suggest that environmental exposures may be important in the etiology of human astrocytomas. Furthermore, ample human and animal data are available to suggest that environmental factors are capable of causing this disease.

Determining the factor or factors responsible for the development of astrocytomas is likely to be difficult. Most patients are exposed to a wide range of potentially important factors during their lifetimes. The period from exposure to the development of a brain tumor is likely to be decades, as evidenced from information available following cranial radiation. The exposures of many of the potential causative agents, such as ELF electromagnetic fields, are difficult to calculate. Furthermore, many patients or families may be genetically predisposed to development of cancers in response to environmental exposures.

Despite these challenges, the rising number of patients being diagnosed with brain tumors and the devastating nature of this disease require an improved understanding of the causes of brain tumors. As progress in epidemiology often depends on recognizing peculiarities in the distribution of illnesses, clinicians caring for patients with brain tumors should be diligent in obtaining family histories and in referring appropriate families to a registry. This will greatly facilitate epidemiologic, genetic, and molecular biologic research on the etiology of brain tumors. The observation that similar genetic abnormalities are often found in heritable and sporadic cases of the same malignancy should also prompt referral of these cases.[33] It is quite possible that these uncommon and unfortunate families may provide new insight on the pathogenesis of this disease. Better understanding of etiologic factors will ultimately result in the development of rational prevention strategies and improved counseling of patients and family members regarding potential risks.

REFERENCES

1. Ries LAG, Hankey BF, Miller BA, et al: Cancer Statistics Review 1973–88. Bethesda, Md, National Cancer Institute, NIH publication No. 91–2789, 1991.
2. Bigner SH, Mark J, Burger PC, et al: Specific chromosomal abnormalities in malignant human gliomas. Cancer Res 1988; 48:405–411.
3. Kapp JP, Paulson G, Odom GL: Brain tumors with tuberous sclerosis. J Neurosurg 1967; 26:191.
4. Rodriguez HA, Berthrong M: Multiple primary intracranial tumor in von Recklinghausen's neurofibromatosis. Arch Neurol 1966; 14:467–475.
5. Turcot J, Despres JP, St Pierre F: Malignant tumors of the central nervous system associated with familial polyposis of the colon: Report of two cases. Dis Colon Rectum 1959; 2:465–468.
6. Li FP, Fraumeni JF: Soft-tissue sarcomas, breast cancer, and other neoplasms: A familial syndrome? Ann Intern Med 1990; 71:747–749.
7. Cho KR, Vogelstein B: Genetic alterations in the adenoma-carcinoma sequence. Cancer 1992; 70(6 suppl):1727–1731.
8. Grieg NH, Ries LG, Yancik R, et al: Increasing annual incidence of primary brain tumors in the elderly. JNCI 1990; 82:1621–1624.
9. Mao Y, Desmeules M, Semencio RM, et al: Increasing brain cancer rates in Canada. Can Med Assoc J 1991; 145:1583–1591.
10. Thorwald J: Science and the Secrets of Early Medicine. New York, Harcourt Brace, 1962.
11. Von Motz IP, Bots G, Endtz LJ: Astrocytoma in three sisters. Neurol 1977; 27:1038–1041.
12. Heuch I, Blom GP: Glioblastoma multiforme in three family members including one case of true multicentricity. J Neurol 1986; 233:142–144.
13. Lossignol D, Grossman SA, Sheidler VR, et al: Familial clustering of malignant astrocytomas. J Neurooncol 1990; 9:139–145.
14. Osman M, Grossman SA, Griffin C, et al: The National Familial Brain Tumor Registry. Proc Am Soc Clin Oncol 1991; 10:124.
15. Grossman SA, Osman M, Hruban RH, et al: Familial gliomas: The potential role of environmental exposures. Proc Am Soc Clin Oncol 1995; 14:149.
16. Ron E, Modan B: Thyroid and other neoplasms following childhood scalp irradiation. In Boice JD, Fraumeni JF Jr (eds): Radiation Carcinogenesis Epidemiology and Biological Significance. New York, Raven Press, 1984.
17. Neglia JP, Meadows AT, Robison LL, et al: Second neoplasms after acute lymphoblastic leukemia in childhood. N Engl J Med 1991; 325:1330–1336.
18. Alexander V: Brain tumor risk among United States nuclear workers. Occup Med 1991; 6:695–714.
19. Irvine D, Davies DM: The mortality of British airway pilots, 1966–1989: A proportional mortality study. Aviat Space Environ Med 1992; 63:276–279.
20. Wasweiler RJ, Stringer W, Wagoner JK, et al: Neoplastic risk among workers exposed to vinyl chloride. Ann NY Acad Sci 1976; 271:40–48.
21. Musicco M, Sant M, Molinari S, et al: A case-control study of brain gliomas and occupational exposure to chemical carcinogens: The risk to farmers. Am J Epidemiol 1988; 128:778–785.
22. Musicco M, Filippini G, Bordo BM, et al: Gliomas and occupational exposure to carcinogens: Case control study. Am J Epidemiol 1982; 116:782–790.
23. Burch D, Craib KJP, Choi BCK, et al: An exploratory case-control study of brain tumors in adults. JNCI 1987; 78:601–609.
24. Thomas TL, Stolley OD, Stemhagen A, et al: Brain tumor mortality risk among men with electrical and electronics jobs: A case-control study. JNCI 1987; 79:223–238.
25. Savitz DA, Wachtel H, Barnes FA, et al: Case control study of childhood cancer and exposure to 60-Hz magnetic fields. Am J Epidemiol 1988; 128:21–38.
26. Burgess J: Cellular phone industry fights cancer allegation. The Washington Post, Jan 30, 1993.
27. Maekawa A, Mitsumori K: Spontaneous occurrence and chemical induction of neurogenic tumors in rats: Influence of host factors and specificity of chemical structure. Crit Rev Toxicol 1990; 20:287–310.
28. Copeland DD, Bigner DD. Glial-mesenchymal tropism of in vivo avian sarcoma virus neuro-oncogenesis in rats. Acta Neuropathol 1978; 41:23.
29. Wodinski I, Kensler CJ, Rall DP: The induction and transplantation of brain tumors in neonate beagles. Proc AACR, 1969, p 99.
30. Houff SA, London WT, McKeever PE, et al: Astrocytomas occurring in another species of new world monkeys following inoculation with JC virus. J Neuropathol Exp Neurol 1982; 41:369.
31. Arthur RR, Grossman SA, Ronnett BM, et al: Lack of association of human polyomaviruses with human brain tumors. J Neurooncol 1994; 20:55–58.
32. Hochberg FH, Miller G, Schooley RT, et al: Central nervous system lymphoma related to Epstein-Barr virus. N Engl J Med 1983; 309:745–748.
33. Levine EG, King RA, Bloomfield CD: The role of heredity in cancer. J Clin Oncol 1989; 7:527–540.

TED TAI-SEN LIN

ROBERT MARTUZA

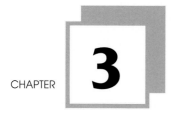

CHAPTER **3**

Neurofibromatosis and Other Phakomatoses

Amongst the phakomatoses, neurofibromatosis is perhaps the one that is most familiar to the general public, thanks in large part to the notoriety of the Elephant Man on stage and screen. The hideous deformities emphasized by these dramas have, in popular perception, become equivalent to the disease itself; yet, ironically, the Elephant Man probably never suffered from neurofibromatosis at all.[1] Indeed, from a medical standpoint, neurofibromatosis represents a far more complex and multifaceted disorder than that which supposedly ravaged poor John Merrick.

Neurofibromatosis is really a heterogeneous family of disorders characterized by neuroectodermal tumors and stereotypical cutaneous pigmentation. Though Riccardi describes seven distinct forms of neurofibromatosis,[1] types 1 and 2 are by far the most numerous and their genetic abnormalities have been identified. Neurofibromatosis type 1 (NF1) is the classic von Recklinghausen's disease, first fully described by its eponym in 1882. Neurofibromatosis type 2 (NF2) represents a separate entity that, traditionally, the literature has failed to distinguish; only recently have formal diagnostic criteria been established for these two disorders.[2]

NF1, clearly the more common of the two neurofibromatoses, has a worldwide incidence of 1 in 3,000 live births,[3] affecting more than 100,000 individuals in the United States alone.[4] It is inherited as an autosomal dominant disorder with a genetic penetrance of 100%[3] but its expressivity is extremely variable. Cutaneous and subcutaneous neurofibromas and abnormal skin pigmentation, known as *cafe-au-lait spots,* are the hallmarks of NF1. The number and location of these characteristic stigmata are varied. Neurofibromas virtually always involve the dermis, but they may occasionally be located in deeper structures, such as larger peripheral nerves and viscera and blood vessels innervated by autonomic nerves.[5] Histologically, the tumors consist of an array of Schwann cells, fibroblasts, neurons, vascular and connective tissue, and mast cells, all interwoven in a complex tangle. Plexiform neurofibromas of larger nerves and the sympathetic chain can cause significant enlargement not only of the nerve itself, but also of the overlying tissues and

affected limbs. These lesions can range from a few to several thousand in number and from millimeters to several centimeters in size; they predominate in the chest, periaureolar, and abdominal regions. It is reported that malignant degeneration of neurofibromas occurs in 13% to 29% of patients with NF1[6]; however, these numbers may be overestimates resulting from the referral base used. Rapid changes in size, shape, and an association with pain can often herald evolution to neurofibrosarcoma, with chances for malignant change estimated at 2% to 5% of NF patients.[4, 7] Conversely, approximately 50% of all neurofibrosarcomas are diagnosed in individuals with NF1.[8] The appearance of neurofibromas differs depending on type, with plexiform lesions occurring congenitally and cutaneous lesions increasing during puberty and adulthood. In most patients, the numbers progress steadily so that by the fifth decade, a plethora of sessile and pedunculated tumors are present.

Cafe-au-lait (CAL) spots are the aptly named integumentary stigmata of NF1 and represent the single most common characteristic of NF1. Fully 94% to 99% of all patients have these markings,[4, 5] usually at birth and certainly by 5 years of age. As with neurofibromas, CAL spots can vary widely in size and location. In a study at the University of Michigan, Crowe and co-workers determined that 78% of NF patients had six or more CAL spots of 15 mm or larger, and this has now become a diagnostic criterion for the disease[4]; it is estimated, however, that 10% of individuals without NF have one CAL spot. Others have noted that despite the congenital nature of these markings, their intensity increases during puberty and pregnancy. Another form of hyperpigmentation common to NF1 patients is freckling of the axilla, buttocks, inframammary areas, and other areas of skin apposition. These stigmata appear later in life, usually not until late childhood or early adolescence. Neither these freckles nor the CAL spots bear any malignant potential, but they serve as an early and rather consistent marker for neurofibromatosis. Lisch nodules represent yet another ubiquitous sign of NF1; these pigmented hamartomas of the iris are asymptomatic and begin appearing during mid-childhood, increasing in number with age to a postpubertal prevalence of 97%. Lisch nodules afflict only individuals with NF1 and are therefore important as a criterion for the diagnosis of the disease.

Aside from cutaneous and pigmentary stigmata, NF1 possesses an extraordinarily broad constellation of signs and associations, including such osseous abnormalities as macrocephaly, sphenoid wing dysplasias, pseudoarthroses of long bones, and kyphoscoliosis. In addition, cognitive and neurologic dysfunctions affect NF1 patients more frequently than usual; 4% have primary seizure disorder,[3] whereas 40% possess some form of learning disability.[5] An equal number suffer from speech difficulties.[5] Within the literature, more obscure associations include megacolon, pruritus, meningocele, and short stature.

Though not traditionally distinguished from von Recklinghausen's neurofibromatosis, NF2 (central neurofibromatosis, bilateral acoustic neurofibromatosis) represents a related, yet clearly distinct, disease entity. It possesses enough similarities with NF1 that its original inclusion is understandable. Patients with NF2 share some of the same cutaneous stigmata as their NF1 counterparts, but to a decidedly lesser extent. Kanter and colleagues found that 42% of their NF2 patients had one or more CAL spots, whereas none had more than six.[4] Martuza and Ojemann[9] encountered six or more CAL spots in only 2 of 15 patients. Moreover, CAL pigmentation tends to be larger and subtler in central neurofibromatosis, so much so that a Wood's lamp may be the only way to detect them. Similarly, the often dramatic profusion of cutaneous neurofibromas in NF1 is largely absent in NF2; they are sparse in most NF2 patients and affect only 30% to 40%.[4, 8] Neither freckling nor Lisch nodules are features of NF2, but almost half of NF2 patients suffer from juvenile subcapsular cataracts. NF2 is a much less common disease than NF1, with a prevalence of only 0.1 per 100,000 persons; within the United States, only about a thousand individuals suffer from it.[4] The pathognomonic lesion for NF2, indeed the feature by which it is often referred to, is bilateral acoustic neuroma. In contrast to acoustic neuromas in nonafflicted patients, these tumors appear two to three decades earlier in individuals with NF2. By the early 20s, patients with NF2 present with unilateral or bilateral hearing loss, facial paresis, imbalance, or tinnitus. In accordance with the diagnostic criteria set by the National Institutes of Health (NIH),[10] detection of bilateral acoustic neuromas necessitates a diagnosis of NF2. A unilateral acoustic neuroma at this age is not diagnostic of NF2, but it requires a thorough investigation for the possibility of central neurofibromatosis.

Genetically, both NF1 and NF2 are inherited as autosomal dominant disorders, the genes responsible for NF1 and NF2 being located to the long arms of chromosomes 17 and 22, respectively. Thirty percent[11] of NF1 cases and approximately 50%[8] of NF2 cases result from spontaneous mutations. The gene for NF1 encompasses 300 kb, and its sequence has been fully deciphered. Similarities with the guanine triphosphate activating protein (GAP) gene suggests that the gene for NF1 plays a role in tumor suppression; its gene product, *neurofibromin,* is a cytoplasmic protein associated with microtubules. It is postulated that the GAP gene encodes for a product that inhibits the p21-*ras* onco-

gene, thereby preventing cellular proliferation. An analogous role for neurofibromin would seem very reasonable; a mutation in the gene would upset this inhibitory equilibrium and result in unregulated cell growth. The molecular basis of NF2 has recently been traced to a deletion within the q12 arm of chromosome 22, a gene encoding a protein belonging to the moesin (membrane-organizing extension spike protein)-ezrin (cytovillin)-radixin family of cytoskeleton-associated proteins. The NF2 gene product, named *merlin* (or, alternatively, called *schwannomin*), links the cytoplasm of a cell with its membrane, playing a crucial role in cellular movement, division, growth, and communication. Inactivation of such a protein results in significant derangement in cell behavior.[12]

The consequences of this dysregulation manifest clinically as the typical stigmata of NF1 and NF2, the neurofibromas and schwannomas described earlier. Yet, in addition to these most common lesions, the neoplasms associated with neurofibromatosis are legion. As mentioned earlier, the older literature on neurofibromatosis did not fully distinguish between the two major forms of the disorder; consequently, concomitant neoplasms were not properly attributed to NF1 vs. NF2. Schwannomas, both intracranial and spinal, predominate in NF2 patients; aside from the hallmark vestibular schwannomas (acoustic neuromas), trigeminal schwannomas occur with secondary frequency. Within the spinal cord, these tumors most commonly affect the dorsal root. Many NF2 patients suffer from multiple lesions throughout the spinal axis. Other extramedullary tumors frequently encountered include meningiomas. Intramedullary lesions are usually ependymomas; rarely, low-grade astrocytomas have been reported. Among non–schwann cell neoplasms, meningiomas and ependymomas are the most prominent intracranial tumors in NF2. In Rubenstein's series of 11 NF2 patients,[3] seven had bilateral acoustic neuromas, six had other cranial nerve tumors, eight had meningiomas (both spinal and intracranial), and nine had multiple spinal nerve root tumors. In addition, two of the patients had low-grade astrocytomas (both in the third ventricle), and five of the patients in the series had ependymomas. The study by Eldridge of 73 persons with central neurofibromatosis[13] yielded 96% with acoustic neuromas and 18% with additional CNS tumors. The diagnosis of NF2 usually occurs by the third decade of life when symptoms of acoustic neuromas become evident, but often, malformative lesions in NF2 remain subclinical,[3] detectable only on microscopic examination. Rubenstein encountered intramedullary schwannosis around the dorsal roots in 9 of 11 subjects in whom Schwann cells and reticulin fibers had infiltrated the spinal cord parenchyma. Schwannosis also occurs within the perivascular sheaths of spinal blood vessels, forming small nodules that expand the surrounding perivascular space. Abnormal proliferation of meningeal cells and microvasculature within the neural parenchyma characterize meningioangiomatosis, resulting in diffuse, microscopic meningiomas throughout the neural axis. Similarly, ectopic ependymal cells were also encountered in the spinal cords of the patients. In all of these cases, the ectopic foci proved structurally identical to symptomatic neoplasms, suggesting the possibility that they are microscopic precursors to future tumors.

The therapeutic mainstay for NF2 remains surgical: the

resection of symptomatic tumors with maximal preservation of function. With acoustic neuromas, the challenge is to identify expanding lesions that threaten hearing and facial sensory and motor function. Fifty percent of NF2 patients present initially with bilateral hearing loss, 21% with unilateral deficits, 10% with imbalance, and 6% with facial paresis.[13] Serial magnetic resonance imaging (MRI) scans are essential in following the variable course of these tumors, with intervention indicated in patients with expanding tumors or increasing dysfunction. Surgical resection of smaller tumors provides the best chance for preservation of hearing and facial motor function. Intraoperatively, monitoring of auditory evoked potentials and facial nerve is necessary. Tumor removal should be weighed against the expense of excessive cranial nerve injury, such as bilateral deafness or serious facial paralysis.[8] Balancing these represents an important challenge in NF2 therapy.

The association between NF1 and rates of malignancy have been studied in numerous series, with results ranging widely between different institutions, from 48% at Memorial Sloan-Kettering Cancer Center, New York,[6] to 3% at the Mayo Clinic.[14] This significant discrepancy can be explained by the sampling bias of various institutions, the figure at Memorial being high because of that hospital's oncologic specialization, the rate at Mayo Clinic representing neurofibrosarcomas exclusively. The commonly accepted rate of malignancy in NF patients is 14%, a composite from nine institutions in Europe and the United States.[7] Another multi-institution study found NF to be the most commonly associated genetic disorder in a population of 5,000 pediatric oncology patients.[15] Aside from hospital-based studies, which tend to select for more seriously affected patients, a study by the National Neurofibromatosis Foundation identified 35 malignancies in 266 NF patients,[16] a rate of about 12%. A 40-year study of NF patients by Sorenson and co-workers[17] in Denmark yielded an overall malignancy rate of 15%. More interesting than the actual figure was the age at presentation in these patients and the type of cancers that developed. The Danish cohort had a mean presentation age of 55 years, fully 13 years younger than the mean age of the general U.S. population. Histologically, the series included 21 CNS tumors (16 gliomas, 2 meningiomas, and 1 malignant neurilemmoma) and 6 PNS tumors (4 neurosarcomas, 1 neuromyxoma, and 1 acoustic neuroma). A quarter of the NF patients were 20 years or younger when the cancer was diagnosed; in the general population only 1% of oncology patients are that age. Nervous system tumors accounted for 47% of all malignancies in the group, whereas the rate in the general population is only 1.7%. Indeed, neurologic malignancies represented the single most common form of cancer in the Danish study; again, the age at diagnosis proved significantly younger, with 76% being discovered by age 40 years compared with 24% in the general Danish population. Of the CNS malignancies, 84% of 19 histologically documented cases were gliomas, 10% were meningiomas, and 6% were malignant neurofibromas.

The Danish incidence for gliomas in NF patients (16/212) reflects that found in many other series throughout the literature. Sorenson and co-workers do not specify whether tumors in patients were classified as NF1 or NF2, as the original cohort was identified between 1924 and 1944. Bras-

field and Das Gupta[6] found brain tumors, all of them gliomas, in eight of 110 patients. Hope and Mulvihill[7] surveyed eight series in the literature and found 55 cases of brain tumors in a total of 1600 NF patients. In the study of Eldridge of NF2 patients,[13] 18% had nonacoustic CNS tumors. The series of Blatt and associates[20] of 121 pediatric NF patients documented 14 with gliomas. A compendium of six series from various pediatric hospitals around the world produced a total of 41 gliomas from 362 patients.[7] In their comprehensive review of the international literature on NF from 1822 to 1965, Rodriguez and Berthrong encountered 48 cases with documented CNS tumors, many of them multiple within the same patient. Of the total, 22 were gliomas, approximately half of which were multiple.[19] Of these tumors, 5.9% were located supratentorially, 3% in the cerebellum, 1.5% in the pons, 11.9% in the medulla, 22.4% in the cervical spinal cord, 23.9% in the thoracic cord, 17.9% in the lumbar cord, 8.9% in the sacrum, 3% in the filum terminale, and 1.5% in the cauda equina. Histologically, Rodriguez and Berthrong noted that 56.3% were ependymomas, 18.7% were astrocytomas, 12.5% were glioblastomas, and 12.5% were nonspecified gliomas. The incidence of ependymomas in the Rodriguez and Berthrong study proves significantly higher than in other studies published since, most of which point to a predominance of astrocytomas in NF patients with CNS tumors. In their study from 1971, Manuelides and Solitaire[20] reviewed the histology of gliomas in 59 NF patients; they concluded that 20 of the gliomas were well-differentiated low-grade astrocytomas, 14 were glioblastomas, 12 were ependymomas, 5 were spongioblastomas, 1 was an astroblastoma, and 1 was an oligodendroglioma. Case reports in the literature indicate that glial tumors associated with NF may occur anywhere that they occur in non-NF patients and that no histologic difference exists between tumors in these populations of patients. A major distinction between gliomas in NF and non-NF individuals is the tendency for multiple tumors in the former. The series of Sorenson and others encountered 6 of 16 glioma patients with more than one CNS tumor; the estimated multiple malignancy rate in the general Danish population is 4%.[21] Ilgren and co-workers[22] reviewed 40 cases of cerebral gliomas in the context of NF and found various combinations of CNS neoplasms; they concluded that both the incidence of multiple tumors and younger age at onset proved significant in individuals with neurofibromatosis.

Ilgren and colleagues reviewed their own series of 89 gliomas in 87 patients with NF. Among these tumors, 11 were cerebral gliomas, 4 were brainstem gliomas, 3 were spinal cord tumors, 11 were third ventricular gliomas, 17 were cerebellar tumors, and 43 were optic nerve gliomas. Histologic examination revealed that among the cerebral gliomas, seven were high-grade astrocytomas, one was a low-grade astrocytoma, and three were of indeterminate grade. The brainstem gliomas proved to be malignant in one case and benign in another. The spinal cord tumors yielded one low-grade astrocytoma, one ependymoma, and one glioma of uncertain grade. Histologic examination of nine of the third ventricular gliomas revealed four malignant astrocytomas and five benign astrocytomas. Cerebellar tumors broke down into 15 astrocytomas (6 of them high-grade astrocytomas) and 2 ependymomas. Clearly, all three series demonstrate that CNS tumors in NF can affect all segments of the neurologic system and can be of a wide histologic variety. Compared with CNS lesions in non-NF patients, Ilgren and colleagues[22] noted that a greater tendency toward malignancy occurred in third ventricular and cerebellar tumors. In the case of cerebellar tumors, only 8% of non-NF patients had malignant histologic characteristics, compared with 50% of NF-associated lesions. Consequently, the 5-year survival rate for persons with NF was 50%, in contrast to a greater than 80% rate in non-NF cases. Similarly, because of the higher grade of third ventricular tumors in NF, the 2-year survival rate in patients in the study of Ilgren and associates[22] proved to be approximately 50%.

In discussing gliomas in the context of neurofibromatosis, special attention must be paid to gliomas of the optic tract. Their incidence in the study of Ilgren and co-workers reflects the fact that they are by far the most common type associated with von Recklinghausen's disease; estimates of their occurrence vary from 10% to 70%.[23] Optic gliomas are pilocytic astrocytomas of the optic pathway that may be located anywhere from the optic globe to the radiations, but they occur most frequently in the optic nerves and chiasm. Traditionally, some clinicians have characterized them as hamartomatous, most notably Hoyt and Baghdassarian in 1969,[24] who advocated conservative treatment because of the tumors' indolent, self-limiting, and non-neoplastic nature.[24] Studies since that time have seriously challenged this viewpoint, but treatment of optic gliomas remains a controversial issue. The histologic study by Stern and colleagues[25] of 34 optic gliomas rejected the idea of their being hamartomatous; invasion of the leptomeninges led the researchers to confirm the neoplastic nature of the tumors. In the study, 55% of patients had NF1, and their tumors bore significant histologic differences from those of individuals without NF. Optic gliomas in NF surrounded the optic nerve in a circumferential-perineural growth pattern without actual invasion, whereas non-NF–associated tumors displayed considerable intraneural astrocytic proliferation and optic nerve distortion. Others have disputed this conclusion, claiming no histopathologic distinction between optic gliomas in either group.[22] That optic gliomas present at an earlier age has been widely observed; the ages of the NF patients of Stern and others[25] averaged 4.9 years at presentation, and the average age of the non-NF patients at presentation averaged 12 years.[25]

The existence of optic gliomas in NF1 patients is unrelated to the presence or severity of other disease stigmata, and visual symptoms may not be commensurate with the actual size of the tumor itself. Most common complaints include decreased acuity, restricted visual fields, strabismus, proptosis, nystagmus, headaches, nausea, and, rarely, diencephalic syndrome. The series of Lewis and colleagues[26] of 217 NF1 patients yielded a 15% rate for optic gliomas, two-thirds of which were clinically silent. Similarly, Listernick and co-workers[27] detected optic gliomas via computed tomographic (CT) scan in 15% of their pediatric patients; in their study, only two patients presented with visual complaints. Because of the symptomatic variability of optic gliomas, current recommendations call for MR or CT imaging of NF1 patients at the time of diagnosis.

The growth of these tumors is variable, and their location and behavior dictate the course of therapy. Many authors have indicated that optic gliomas in NF1 tend to be located in the anterior visual system,[25–27] and indeed, both Lewis and colleagues and Listernick and others found a majority of their patients to be without chiasmal involvement. The multifactorial nature of optic gliomas makes them a therapeutic challenge in terms of timing and modality of treatment. Asymptomatic lesions require careful periodic monitoring, whereas symptoms or size progression requires intervention. Surgically, any unilateral anterior lesion that compromises vision or with which serious proptosis is documented should be resected. Posterior and bilateral lesions should be explored, biopsied, and debulked to relieve any obstructive hydrocephalus that may be present. Surgical intervention should rarely be performed at the expense of increased visual deficit; other modalities such as radiation and chemotherapy are appropriate in the treatment of recurrent unilateral, bilateral, and posterior visual tract disease. Complete surgical resection of unilateral tumors brings a long-term (greater than 10 years) survival rate of more than 85%.[28] Radiation has been the mainstay of traditional nonsurgical treatment; optimal total dosages range from 4,500 to 5,600 cGy. With this radiation dosage, Pierce and co-workers[29] documented a 6-year freedom from disease progression of 88% and a survival rate of 100%. Flickinger and others[30] found the survival rate of their patients at 5, 10, and 15 years to be 96%, 90%, and 90%, respectively; progression-free survival remained 87% at 5, 10, and 15 years.

More recently, chemotherapy has been advocated by some clinicians in the treatment of nonresectable optic gliomas, in view of the toxic effects that radiation incurs on the developing CNS. Permanent radiation-induced cognitive and endocrinologic deficits can be avoided in young children with combination chemotherapy. Two series at Children's Hospital of Philadelphia showed that treatment with vincristine and dactinomycin produced a 100% survival rate at a median of greater than 4 years, with a free-of-progressive-disease rate of 62.5% and normal IQ scores and endocrine function.[31, 32] Petronio and colleagues,[57] using nitrosourea-based agents in addition to vincristine and dactinomycin, reported a favorable response in 15 out of 18 patients at 79 weeks. In all three studies, patients in whom chemotherapy failed went on to receive radiation. Using chemotherapy as a stabilizing modality in the pediatric population is now advocated by many clinicians, thereby deferring radiation effects on the developing CNS.

The neurofibromatoses remain a fascinating and extremely complex constellation of disorders. A thorough familiarity with their stigmata will allow the clinician to treat more expediently their myriad associated disorders. The tendency of neoplastic growth to occur in neurofibromatosis represents a continuing challenge for the neurosurgeon. New techniques have allowed us to decipher the genetic basis for NF1 and NF2, but the current treatments remain largely symptomatic. Until the root cause of neurofibromatosis can be successfully corrected, surgery will remain at the forefront of therapeutic choices. Nevertheless, understanding the molecular mechanisms of the NF1 and NF2 genes may allow for the development of therapy directed at these tumors. Moreover, because similar tumors occur in non-neurofibromatosis patients, these novel therapeutic targets may have much wider application.

Many of the remaining phakomatoses also include characteristic neoplasms of various organ systems, among them the cerebellar hemangioblastoma in von Hippel–Lindau disease (VHL) and the vascular abnormalities of the different neurocutaneous angiomatoses. None of these, however, involves to such a profound degree the glial derangement seen in the neurofibromatoses. As their names suggest, the neurocutaneous angiomatoses are characterized by abnormalities of blood vessels, some of which affect neurologic structures (e.g., the leptomeningeal and trigeminal angiomas in Sturge-Weber syndrome and the midbrain arteriovenous aneurysms of Wyburn-Mason syndrome). Similarly, the hallmark cerebellar hemangioblastomas of VHL arise from primitive vascular tissues within the CNS. The tuberous sclerosis complex (Bourneville's disease) is a notable exception to this. First described by von Recklinghausen in 1862 and later by Bourneville in 1880, tuberous sclerosis complex (TSC) resembles the neurofibromatoses in the prominence of glial neoplasms among its disease manifestations. It is a disorder of unregulated hamartomatous growth in multiple organ systems, including the kidneys, skin, retina, and heart, but it is the cortical tubers that traditionally have been the disease's defining lesion (hence, the name of the disease). Though its history as a pathologic entity is contemporaneous with that of the neurofibromatoses, TSC remains less well understood in many important ways.

TSC is an autosomal dominant disorder whose exact genetic basis remains unknown, despite linkages to the ABO blood group genes on chromosomes 9(9q34) in some familial studies; still others have located the defect to the long arm of chromosome 11.[33] The incidence, too, varies significantly, from 1 in 10,000 live births to 1 in 170,000.[34] The disease's penetrance is estimated at 80% to 100%[8, 34] with a spontaneous mutation rate of 58% to 69%[35, 36] and an expressivity that is impressive in its wide variability. These factors conspire to make TSC a diagnostic challenge despite classic markers such as ash-leaf spots, shagreen patches, or Vogt's triad of seizures, mental retardation, and facial angiofibromas (adenoma sebaceum). Currently, diagnostic criteria for TSC constitutes a rather complex constellation of physical findings, clinical symptoms, and radiologic entities, all of which are categorized as either definitive, presumptive, or suspect diagnostic features. Of Vogt's classic triad, only adenoma sebaceum remains pathognomonic for the disease, along with any of the following lesions: cortical tubers, subependymal glial nodules, retinal hamartoma(s), ungual fibromas, forehead/scalp fibrous plaques, and multiple renal angiomyolipomas. Presumptive and suspect diagnostic characteristics are even more diffuse and varied, the difference between the two being the number of features present in any given individual (Table 3–1). According to Gomez's schema, diagnosis of TSC is suspected with the occurrence of only one of these features, is presumptive with two, and is highly probable with one feature and a first-degree relative afflicted with TSC.[37] This "combination platter" approach to diagnosis is necessary in light of the extreme variability of this disease complex; indeed, a series of 300 TSC patients at the Mayo Clinic revealed that only 29% of them had a full complement of Vogt's triad, whereas 6% had none of the elements at all.[37]

TSC patients may possess a seemingly limitless number of symptomologic permutations, their diagnoses arriving through various mergings of the previously mentioned manifestations. Statistically, 47% to 90% of all TSC patients will have some amount of adenoma sebaceum, with the percentage of individuals increasing after age 4 years.[38] Shagreen patches are found in 21% to 80% of cases, again increasing after the first decade of life. Hypomelanotic macules, the classic ash-leaf spots of TSC, often appear congenitally in up to 2.4% of individuals ultimately diagnosed with the disease. Often these macules are visible only under the Wood's lamp, but an increase in their number and conspicuousness gives this dermatologic manifestation an overall incidence of 89% in all patients with TSC. Various series have established the incidence of ungual fibromas, a mainly postpubertal sign, as varying from 17% to 52%. Aside from dermatologic stigmata, the diagnosis of various TSC lesions has been significantly simplified by advancements in radiology. Clearly, older studies had to rely on autopsy and/or biopsy series to confirm the presence of renal, cardiac, and intracranial lesions of TSC; these neoplasms are now routinely diagnosed by ultrasound, CT, and MRI. Autopsy series have estimated the incidence of renal angiomyolipomas to be about 31 in 46 patients (67%) with TSC, with 13 (28%) of these being multiple[39] and increasing during the second decade of life. Modern imaging studies have approximated the incidence of these tumors at slightly greater than 70%.[40] Autopsies of 36 patients with cardiac rhabdomyomas yielded 11 with pathologic evidence of TSC, giving an association rate of 32%,[41] and, once again, studies with current radiologic modalities have corroborated these figures.[42]

As with all types of intracranial pathologic lesions, CT and MRI have revolutionized the diagnosis of cerebral TSC lesions. In their series of 86 patients with the disease, Houser and co-workers[45] detected 73 with subependymal nodules and/or cortical tubers. Subependymal nodules may be present from birth, calcifying and progressing in size and number with age. Houser and colleagues found most of these lesion to be less than 1 cm in diameter and periventricular in position, corresponding to the classic "candle drippings" descriptions of TSC in the literature. Nodules rarely enhance with contrast and are considered the single most diagnostic CT finding associated with TSC; they are considered to be virtually pathognomonic if they are multiple, calcified, and are encroaching on the lateral ventricles.[46] On MRI, subependymal nodules appear most clearly on T1-weighted images as lesions that are isointense to white matter and slightly hyperintense to deep gray. Separate series estimate the incidence of subependymal nodules on MRI as 74% to 95%.[43, 45]

The same series found cortical tubers in an almost identical percentage of patients undergoing CT imaging and concurred on their position intracranially; 80% to 88% of patients had tubers exclusively in the cerebrum, 12% to 14% had both cerebral and cerebellar tubers, and 0% to 6% had only cerebellar tubers. The actual number of tubers found in individuals with TSC varies tremendously, ranging in the study of Braffman and colleagues from 0 to 60, three-quarters of patients having between 1 and 20 lesions. Like subependymal nodules, tubers may also calcify with age in more than half of patients,[45] consequently appearing hyperdense on CT. Tubers that appear hypodense are thought to be hypomyelinated, and these occur more often in children during the first decade of life; indeed, Houser and col-

TABLE 3–1
DIAGNOSTIC CRITERIA FOR TUBEROUS SCLEROSIS COMPLEX

Pathognomonic features
   Facial angiofibromas*
   Multiple ungual fibromas*
   Cortical tuber (histologically confirmed)
   Subependymal nodules or giant-cell astrocytoma (histologically confirmed)
   Multiple calcified subependymal nodules protruding into the ventricle (radiographic evidence)
   Multiple retinal astrocytomas*

Presumptive features
   Affected first-degree relative
   Cardiac rhabdomyoma (histologic or radiographic confirmation)
   Other retinal hamartoma or achromic patch*
   Cortical tubers (radiographic confirmation)
   Noncalcified subependymal nodules (radiographic confirmation)
   Shagreen patch*
   Forehead plaque*
   Pulmonary lymphangiomatosis (histologic confirmation)
   Renal angiomyolipoma (radiographic or histologic confirmation)
   Renal cysts (histologic confirmation)

Suspicious features
   Hypermelanotic macules*
   ``Confetti'' skin lesions*
   Renal cysts (radiographic evidence)
   Randomly distributed enamel pits in deciduous and/or permanent teeth
   Hamartomatous rectal polyps (histologic confirmation)
   Bone cysts (radiographic confirmation)
   Pulmonary lymphangiomyomatosis (radiographic evidence)
   Cerebral white matter ``migration tracts'' or heterotopias (radiographic evidence)
   Gingival fibromas*
   Hamartoma of other organs (histologic confirmation)
   Infantile spasms

Definite tuberous sclerosis complex
   One primary feature, two secondary features, or one secondary plus two tertiary features

Probable tuberous sclerosis complex
   Either one secondary plus one tertiary feature or three tertiary features

Suspected tuberous sclerosis complex
   Either one secondary feature or two tertiary features

*Histologic confirmation is not required if the lesion is clinically obvious.
From Stern J, Jakobiec FA, Housepian EM: The architecture of optic gliomas with and without neurofibromatosis. Arch Ophthalmol 1980;98:505–511.

leagues[43] found no hypodense tubers in patients older than 30 years and in only 3 of 18 individuals older than 10 years. Tubers usually occupy the white-gray junction, but in more than three-quarters of instances they do not deform the surrounding tissue in any way.[45] Instead, they appear exclusively as signal abnormalities on MRI scans; their peripheries are isointense to gray matter in all sequences, but their inner cores vary according to the age (and the cerebral myelination) of the patient. Tuberous cores in infants and young children are hypointense to premyelinated white matter on long TR/TE images, whereas the opposite is true in older children and adults. Administration of gadolinium contrast enhanced only 3.4% of tubers in the series of Braffman and colleagues.[45]

Characteristic white matter lesions of TSC include radial bands and wedge-shaped abnormalities that extend from the lateral ventricles to the cortical surface in more than 90% of patients studied by MRI.[45] Significantly, many of these lesions lead directly to specific tubers and are proportional to their numbers in some cases. Braffman and others[45] found

between one and ten white matter lesions in 78% of his patients, the radial pattern being almost three times more common than the wedge-shaped one. Neither type exerted mass effect nor did they commonly enhance with contrast. Again, the signal intensities varied according to the age of the patient, much in the same manner as the cortical tubers.

Perhaps the most dramatic intracranial finding associated with TSC is the subependymal giant-cell astrocytoma. As the name suggests, these tumors arise periventricularly, usually along the foramen of Monro, and grow into the lateral ventricles, causing obstruction of the CSF flow in many cases. An estimated 6% to 17%[33, 45] of TSC patients characteristically develop subependymal giant-cell astrocytoma during the second decade of life; Braffman and others noted a mean age of 10.3 years and Shepherd and others[53] a mean age of 13 years. Radiologically, subependymal giant-cell astrocytomas appear as almost midline structures that deform the lateral ventricles, serving as the ostensible source of ventriculomegaly in roughly a third of patients with that finding.[43] Subependymal giant-cell astrocytomas enhance with both CT and MRI contrast, but they are not associated with edema or shift of the surrounding parenchyma, even with very sizable tumors. Calcification is, however, a very common feature. On MRI, T1-weighted scans produce lesions isointense to white matter and hyperintense to gray, whereas T2-weighted scans result in hypointensity.

Through the thicket of multiplicitous lesions associated with TSC, one factor exists to unify them all: the hamartomatous nature of the growths. In skin, heart, kidney, and brain, the hallmarks of this disease lie in the disordered development of organ tissues. Within the brain, the tubers, white matter abnormalities, subependymal nodules, and subependymal giant-cell astrocytomas may be better understood within the context of neuronal and glial migration during fetal development. Various investigators have estimated the developmental insult to occur during the fourth to eighth week of gestation,[46] focusing on a period of cerebral organization.

In normal brain development, neurons of the neocortex originate from the germinal matrix of the periventricular region. There, in the epithelium surrounding the lateral ventricles, progenitor cells undergo terminal mitosis before migrating to the surface of the developing brain. It is important to note that except for the molecular layer (I), all cortical layers arise in an inverse order, with more newly formed neurons populating an increasingly superficial position in the cortex. In accordance to this schema, neurons within layers I and VI are from the same initial migratory phase; those arising subsequently traverse the ever-expanding distance between ventricle and cortical surface to take their prescribed positions within the intervening laminae. This migratory pattern is, under normal circumstances, strictly controlled by complex intercellular interactions, including the crucial one between neurons and radial glia. The latter represents a specialized astroglial population that directs neuronal emigration to the cortical surface, and as such, possesses an extraordinary bipolar morphology, with one process rooted within the mitotically active periventricular zone and the other in the molecular layer. It is along these glial spokes that neurons, fresh from their terminal mitotic divisions, ascend toward the cortical surface.

In TSC, this remarkably ordered progression derails, the monkey wrench within this developmental machinery having yet to be identified. Nonetheless, a histologic examination of the neurologic lesions of TSC provides some understanding of the etiology of the disorder. Richardson has described TSC as a disease in which "the normal, orderly, laminated structure of the cerebral cortex is suddenly interrupted by cytoarchitectural near-chaos."[47] Indeed, specific portions of the TSC brain are an entropic mixture of unusual cells, debatable in lineage and abnormal in distribution, all of which are juxtaposed against areas that are essentially normal in structure. Cortical tubers contain rests of atypical fibrillary astrocytes nestled within a neutropil that is remarkably poor in its density of myelinated fibers. The great numbers of these astrocytes confer on the tubers their characteristic firmness. Within adjacent areas, morphologically primitive neurons predominate; in contrast to the pyramidal cells of normal neocortex, these neurons are multipolar or stellate, with few dendritic spines. The pyramidal cells that are present often contain abnormal orientations and distribu-

tions within the stroma. There exist also the categorically ambiguous giant cells of the TSC tuber, historically the subject of much cytologic debate because of their neuronal and astrocytic features. Under both light and electron microscopy, giant cells possess a confusing complement of features, sometimes containing obvious neurofibrils and Nissl bodies but other times resembling enlarged astrocytes with multiple nuclei.[48] In recent years, immunohistologic studies have helped to clarify the issue; Stefansson and co-workers[51] report that their experience with glial fibrillary acidic protein (GFAP) and neuronal-specific enolase (NSE) produced staining with the latter only, supporting a neuronal lineage for the giant cells.

Structural abnormalities affect the deeper layers of the TSC brain as well; subcortically, atypical neurons, some of them resembling tuberous giant cells, form aggregates of heterotopic gray matter, scattered along the migratory pathway from germinal matrix to cortex. Collections of dysgenic astrocytes extend throughout this same course, these of an astroglial lineage similar to the radially-aligned guide cells of the developing brain. Normally, these bipolar astroglia transform into mature astrocytes; in TSC, they become unusually large cells that maintain a radial orientation, corresponding to the white matter bands and wedges seen on CT and MRI.

In TSC, the deepest layers of the brain harbor the subependymal nodules and giant-cell astrocytomas. These two lesions are closely connected; the latter, according to many, represents continued growth of the former.[47, 49] Histologically, subependymal nodules contain cells reminiscent of those in cortical tubers, although here they are more densely aggregated within a matrix of vasculature, cell processes, and calcific deposits. The astrocytes are of a variety of types: gemistocytic, piloid, even occasionally oligodendrocytic. Present, too, are the extraordinary giant cells of tuberous sclerosis. All of this is enclosed by a layer of ependyma. Both microscopic and immunohistochemical investigation have established the overwhelming predominance of astrocytes within the subependymal nodules,[49] with few cells staining for NSE and many for GFAP.

The reason for continued growth of some subependymal nodules remains unclear, and it is more often convention than pathologic basis that dictates the transformation from a "nodule" to an "astrocytoma." Shepherd and colleagues have stated that "there are no essential differences between subependymal nodules and SEGAs [subependymal giant-cell astrocytomas]." Clinically, a lesion becomes a tumor with the onset of symptoms such as hydrocephalus; radiologically, astrocytomas are those that enhance with CT contrast. Other differences between astrocytomas and nodules are often exceedingly subtle. Microscopic examination reveals astrocytes of gemistocytic and giant-cell variety. Moreover, spindle-shaped, epithelioid, and ganglion-like cells are also present, making for a cytologic admixture more diverse than the term subependymal giant-cell astrocytoma would suggest. Indeed, the exact lineage of some constituent cells, bearing both astrocytic and neuronal features, remains a topic of debate. Immunocytochemical staining by Stefansson and co-workers[49] actually supports a neuronal origin for most of the subependymal giant-cell astrocytoma cells,[51] but the final word remains at issue. No less remarkable is the discordance that often exists between the histology and clinical behavior of these tumors. Mitoses and necrosis, normally the hallmarks of an aggressive neoplasm, may characterize subependymal giant-cell astrocytomas with notably indolent courses.[50] The incidence of these tumors has been reported to be 6%.[51]

The etiology of TSC remains obscure, but the unifying defect responsible for its intracerebral lesions lies in the cells of the germinal epithelium. It is there that multipotential progenitor cells suffer an unknown insult during the earliest days of embryogenesis, between weeks 4 and 8, giving rise to a population of abnormal progeny. Some of these migrate to the cortical surface, doing so in an unregulated and haphazard manner and guided by other cells that are themselves abnormal. Intracellular communication, a factor so crucial in neural development, does not properly occur in TSC; the results are the heterotopic congregations within the white matter of affected cells. The cells that do complete the journey to the cortical surface remain segregated from the normal cytoarchitecture around them, forming instead the tubers of TSC. Some have conjectured that the various lesions of TSC actually constitute a spectrum of cellular differentiation, with the periventricular region being composed of the least differentiated cells.[49] Accordingly, the constituent cells of subependymal giant-cell astrocytomas and subependymal nodules would represent a population too undifferentiated to have been able to migrate.

While the pathogenesis of tuberous sclerosis remains unclear, the consequences of its lesions are better understood. Within the brain, results may range from asymptomatic to extremely severe, with the disease again exerting a great degree of variability. Seizures represent the most common sequelae of the cortical heterotopias, usually occurring during the first year of life. Studies from Europe and the United States have estimated the incidence of seizures amongst TSC patients to be from 80% to 100%.[33, 36, 52] The type, frequency, and chronicity of seizure activity varies, but almost 90% of individuals with infantile spasms continue to experience seizures later in life.[52] Moreover, more than 90% of patients with confirmed seizure activity have cortical tubers on MRI, albeit in locations not necessarily corresponding to abnormal foci on EEG; in 42% of patients a good correspondence does indeed occur.[33] Mental retardation is another well-known consequence of TSC, affecting approximately 50% to 70% of individuals tested.[33, 52] Increasingly, a correlation among radiologic abnormalities, seizures, and mental impairment has been established; Shepherd and colleagues[51] have reported that in their study of 75 patients with TSC, 29 who experienced infantile spasms had a greater number of tubers than those with other forms of seizures. Patients who present with seizures earlier in life and who exhibit greater mental disability also demonstrated more cortical and white matter lesions on scans.[53] Other studies concur; Curatolo and others[52] found a consistent association among seizures, mental retardation, and the number of cortical tubers in TSC patients.

Ultimately, mortality for individuals with TSC results most commonly from renal and CNS disorders. The Mayo Clinic series of 355 patients attributed 12 of 48 deaths to renal disease, including 7 from organ failure, 3 from renal cell carcinoma, and 2 from angiomyolipoma hemorrhage.

Eighteen deaths resulted from CNS pathology: status epilepticus in half of the cases and complications from subependymal giant-cell astrocytomas in the other.[54] Five patients from the latter nine died from increased intracranial pressure; one from tumor hemorrhage and four from various treatment complications. Of the remaining patients, pulmonary disease was responsible for eight deaths and cardiac disease for two (one of which was due to a rhabdomyoma). Eight deaths proved completely unrelated to TSC. Overall, the survival curve for patients with TSC is clearly decreased, with about 65% of the population alive at age 30 years compared with more than 95% of unaffected individuals.

Because of the uncertain nature of tuberous sclerosis, treatment for the disease remains largely symptomatic. Though improved imaging techniques have simplified diagnosis and treatment decisions for intracranial pathologic lesions, the multivariability of TSC has continued to challenge the clinician. Genetic counseling, in particular, is complicated by the variable expression in affected individuals in addition to a significant rate of new mutation. Osborne and co-workers,[36] in a series on TSC patients in Britain, cite cases of nonpenetrance in both siblings and parents and give a recurrence rate of 2% for completely asymptomatic parents with one TSC child.[36] Fleury and colleagues[55] found only 44% of parents with TSC children to possess any signs of the disorder themselves. Management of individuals with tuberous sclerosis should of course reflect the severity of the pathologic signs and symptoms. Anticonvulsant drugs remain the mainstay of seizure therapy, but specific cases may prove amenable to surgical treatment.[56] Surgical intervention is clearly indicated when subependymal giant-cell astrocytomas expand to produce symptoms, largely hydrocephalus in the case of tumors unique to TSC. Because of their indolent nature, recurrence is rare and shunting is usually reserved for cases not amenable to resection.

The tumors that occur with each of the phakomatoses are similar to their solitary counterparts that occur sporadically in the population. Thus, each of these genetic disorders may be seen as a window into the developmental biology and oncogenesis of a particular cell type in the nervous system. It was through the study of NF2 that the gene causing neuromas was discovered. So, too, is it likely to be the case for the other phakomatoses. It is this fact that highlights the importance of these disorders to clinicians and scientists interested in nervous system tumors.

REFERENCES

1. Riccardi VM: Neurofibromatosis: Phenotype, Natural History, Pathology. Baltimore, The Johns Hopkins University Press, 1992.
2. Neurofibromatosis Conference Statement. Arch Neurol 1988; 45:575–578.
3. Rubenstein AE: Neurofibromatosis: A Review of the Clinical Problem. Ann NY Acad Sci 1986; 486:1–13.
4. Kanter WR, Eldridge R, Fabricant R, et al: Central neurofibromatosis with bilateral acoustic neuroma: Genetic, clinical, and biochemical distinctions from peripheral neurofibromatosis. Neurology 1980; 30:851–859.
5. Riccardi VM: Von Recklinghausen neurofibromatosis. N Engl J Med 1981; 305:1617–1626.
6. Brasfield RD, Das Gupta TK: Von Recklinghausen's disease: A clinicopathological study. Ann Surg 1972; 175:86–104.

7. Hope DG, Mulvihill JJ: Malignancy in neurofibromatosis. *In* Riccardi VM, Mulvihill JJ (eds): Advances in Neurology, vol 29: Neurofibromatosis (von Recklinghausen Disease). New York, Raven Press, 1981, pp 33–56.

8. Sampson JH, Martuza RL: Neurofibromatosis and other phakomatoses. *In* Wilkins WH, Rengachary SS (eds): Neurosurgery. New York, McGraw-Hill, 1995, pp 673–685.

9. Martuza RL, Ojemann RG: Bilateral acoustic neuromas: Clinical aspects, pathogenesis, and treatment. Neurosurgery 1982; 10:1–12.

10. NF Conference Statement. Arch Neurol 1988; 45:575–578.

11. Riccardi VM: Neurofibromatosis: Phenotype, Natural History, Pathology. Baltimore, The Johns Hopkins University Press, 1992.

12. Trofatter JA, MacCollin JL, Rutter JR: A novel moesin, -ezrin, radixin-like gene is a candidate for the neurofibromatosis 2 tumor suppressor. Cell 1993; 72:791–800.

13. Eldridge R: Central neurofibromatosis with bilateral acoustic neuroma. *In* Riccardi VM, Mulvihill JJ (eds): Advances in Neurology, vol 29: Neurofibromatosis (von Recklinghausen's Disease). New York, Raven Press, 1981, pp 57–65.

14. D'Agostino AN: Sarcomas of the peripheral nerves and somatic soft tissues associated with neurofibromatosis. Cancer 1963; 8:1015–1027.

15. Bader JL: Neurofibromatosis and cancer. Ann NY Acad Sci 1986; 486:57–65.

16. Bader JL: Increased risk of cancer with neurofibromatosis. Proc Am Soc Clin Oncol 1981; 20:339.

17. Sorenson SA, Mulvihill JJ, Nielsen A: Long-term follow-up of von Recklinghausen neurofibromatosis: Survival and malignant neoplasms. N Engl J Med 1986; 314:1010–1015.

18. Blatt J, Jaffee R, Deutsch M, et al: Neurofibromatosis and childhood tumors. Cancer 1986; 57:1225–1229.

19. Rodriguez HA, Berthrong M: Multiple primary intracranial tumors in von Recklinghausen's neurofibromatosis. Arch Neurol 1966; 14:467–475.

20. Manuelides EE, Solitaire GE: Glioblastoma multiforme. *In* Minckler J (ed): Pathology of the Nervous System. New York, McGraw-Hill, 1971, pp 2026–2071.

21. Storm HH, Jensen OM, Ewertz M, et al: Summary: Multiple primary cancer in Denmark, 1943–1980. Monogr Natl Cancer Inst 1985; 68:411–430.

22. Ilgren EB, Kinnier-Wilson LM, Stiller CA: Gliomas in neurofibromatosis: A series of 89 cases with evidence for enhanced malignancy in associated cerebellar astrocytomas. Pathology Annu 1985; 20:331–358.

23. Riccardi VM: Type I neurofibromatosis and the pediatric patient. Curr Probl Pediatr 1992; 2:66–106.

24. Hoyt WF, Baghdassarian S: Optic glioma in childhood: Natural history and rationale for conservative management. Br J Ophthalmol 1969; 53:793–798.

25. Stern J, Jackobiec FA, Housepian EM: The architecture of optic gliomas with and without neurofibromatosis. Arch Ophthalmol 1980; 98:505–511.

26. Lewis AL, Gerson LP, Axelson KA, et al: Von Recklinghausen neurofibromatosis: Incidence of optic gliomata. Ophthalmology 1984; 91:929–935.

27. Listernick R, Charrow J, Greenwald MJ, et al: Optic gliomas in children with neurofibromatosis type I. J Pediatr 1989; 114:788–792.

28. Tenny RT, Laws ER, Younge BR, et al: The neurosurgical management of optic glioma: Results in 104 patients. J Neurosurg 1992; 57:452–458.

29. Pierce SM, Barnes PD, Loeffler JS, et al: Definitive radiation therapy in the management of symptomatic patients with optic glioma. Cancer 1990; 65:45–52.

30. Flickinger JC, Torres C, Deutsch M: Management of low-grade gliomas of the optic nerve and chiasm. Cancer 1988; 61:635–642.

31. Packer RJ, Sutton LN, Bilaniuk LT: Treatment of chiasmatic/hypothalamic gliomas of childhood with chemotherapy: An update. Ann Neurol 1988; 23:79–85.

32. Rosenstock JG, Packer RJ, Bilaniuk L: Chiasmatic optic glioma treated with chemotherapy: A preliminary report. J Neurosurg 1985; 63:862–866.

33. Gomez MR: Phenotypes of the tuberous sclerosis complex with a revision of diagnostic criteria. Ann NY Acad Sci 1991; 615:1–7.

34. Kuntz N: Population studies. *In* Gomez MR (ed): Tuberous Sclerosis, ed 2. New York, Raven Press, 1988, pp 213–215.

35. Michels V: Genetics. *In* Gomez MR (ed): Tuberous Sclerosis, ed 2. New York, Raven Press, 1988, pp 217–231.

36. Osborne JP, Fryer A, Webb D: Epidemiology of tuberous sclerosis. Ann NY Acad Sci 1991; 615:125–127.

37. Gomez MR: Criteria for diagnosis. *In* Gomez MR (ed): Tuberous Sclerosis, ed 2. New York, Raven Press, 1988, pp 9–19.

38. Rogers RS: Dermatologic manifestations. *In* Gomez MR (ed): Tuberous Sclerosis, ed 2. New York, Raven Press, 1988, pp 111–131.

39. Robbins TO, Bernstein J: Renal involvement. *In* Gomez MR (ed): Tuberous Sclerosis. New York, Raven Press, 1988, pp 133–146.

40. Hoffman AD: Imaging of tuberous sclerosis lesions outside of the central nervous system. Ann NY Acad Sci 1991; 615:94–111.

41. Fenoglio JJ, McAllister HA, Ferrans VS: Cardiac rhabdomyoma: A clinicopathologic and electron microscopic study. Am J Cardiol 1976; 38:241–251.

42. Watson GH: Cardiac rhabdomyomas in tuberous sclerosis. Ann NY Acad Sci 1991; 615:50–57.

43. Houser OW, Shepherd CW, Gomez MR: Imaging of intracranial tuberous sclerosis. Ann NY Acad Sci 1991; 615:81–93.

44. Houser OW, Nixon JR: Central nervous system imaging. *In* Gomez MR (ed): Tuberous Sclerosis, ed 2. New York, Raven Press, 1988, pp 51–62.

45. Braffman BH, Bilaniuk LT, Naidich TP, et al: MR imaging of tuberous sclerosis: Pathogenesis of this phakomatosis, use of gadopentate diglumine, and literature review. Neuroradiology 1992; 183:227–238.

46. Gomez MR, Kuntz N: Pathogenesis. *In* Gomez MR (ed): Tuberous Sclerosis, ed 2. New York, Raven Press, 1988, pp 245–249.

47. Richardson EP: Pathology of tuberous sclerosis: Neuropathologic aspects. Ann NY Acad Sci 1991; 615:128–139.

48. Reagan TJ: Neuropathology. *In* Gomez MR (ed): Tuberous Sclerosis, ed 2. New York, Raven Press, 1988, pp 63–73.

49. Stefansson K, Wollmann RL, Huttenlocher PR: Lineages of cells in the central nervous system. *In* Gomez MR (ed): Tuberous Sclerosis, ed 2. New York, Raven Press, 1988, pp 75–87.

50. Chow CW, Klug GL, Lewis EA: Subependymal giant-cell astrocytoma in children. J Neurosurg 1988; 68:880–883.

51. Shepherd CW, Scheithauer B, Gomez MR, et al: Brain tumors in tuberous sclerosis: A clinicopathologic study of the Mayo Clinic experience. Ann NY Acad Sci 1991; 615:378–379.

52. Curatolo P, Cusmai R, Cortesi F, et al: Neuropsychiatric aspects of tuberous sclerosis. Ann NY Acad Sci 1991; 615:8–16.

53. Shepherd CW, Houser OW, Gomez MR: MR findings in tuberous sclerosis complex and correlation with seizure development and mental impairment. Am J Neuroradiol 1995; 16:149–155.

54. Shepherd CW, Gomez MR, Crowson CS: Causes of death in patients with tuberous sclerosis. Mayo Clin Proc 1991; 66:792–796.

55. Fleury P, de Groot WP, Delleman JW, et al: Tuberous sclerosis: The incidence of sporadic cases vs. familial cases. Brain Dev 1980; 2:107–117.

56. Bebin EM, Kelly PJ, Gomez MR: Surgical treatment for epilepsy in cerebral tuberous sclerosis. Epilepsia 1993; 34:651–656.

57. Petronio J, Edwards MSB, Prados M, et al: Management of chiasmal and hypothalamic gliomas of infancy and childhood with chemotherapy. J Neurosurg 1991; 74:701–708.

JUAN A. REY

M. JOSEFA BELLO

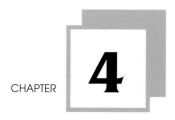

CHAPTER **4**

Cytogenetics

Cytogenetic analysis of human neoplasms has provided data of interest for the understanding of tumor biology and has proven useful in tumor diagnosis, classification, and prognosis. Early cytogenetic studies demonstrated the presence of chromosome alterations in most samples derived from higher-grade malignant tumors, suggesting that somatic genetic changes are important in carcinogenesis. The fact that karyotypic abnormalities are generally more extensive in advanced tumors fits a model of tumor progression in which neoplasms become more aggressive and more malignant with time as a result of the sequential accumulation of genetic changes; this is a multi-step process that implies a clonal evolution.

The demonstration that specific alterations in particular chromosomes are characteristic of certain neoplasms was the main reason for the increased interest in tumor cytogenetics. At present, the diagnosis of chronic myelogenous leukemia (CML) requires, in addition to other studies, a chromosome analysis to determine the presence in bone marrow cells of the chromosomal aberration characteristic of this malignant hematologic disorder: a rearrangement involving chromosomes 9 and 22. Generally, chromosome alterations in tumor cells represent the cytologic expression of a molecular involvement of two main types of genes that participate in tumor development, oncogenes and tumor suppressor genes, and three broad categories of cytogenetic anomalies may be established:

1. Translocations, insertions, and inversions, which commonly contribute to oncogene activation by juxtaposition to other chromosome sequences. A good example is represented by the t(9;22) translocation characteristic of CML.

2. Chromosomal deletions, monosomies, or, in general, the loss of a specific region of a chromosome is correlated with the location of a tumor suppressor gene in the corrresponding region.

3. Trisomies, isochromosomes, and double-minute chromosomes are usually related to gene dose imbalance and gene amplification, which often involve cellular oncogenes.

The objective of the cytogenetic analysis of any histologic

subtype of tumors is the establishment of the recurrent, nonrandom chromosomal abnormalities characterizing the genesis and progression of the tumors under study. In most instances, however, several cytogenetic anomalies involving many chromosomes are found, and the two main types of aberrations should thus be differentiated:

1. Primary aberrations, which are generally nonrandom, regularly present in a tumor cell population and are found recurrently in a series of tumors from the same histologic type. In some instances, these primary aberrations appear as the sole alterations in one tumor type, frequently occur in early stages of carcinogenesis, and may be observed at the time of diagnosis.

2. Secondary aberrations are generally heterogeneous, often occur in addition to the primary changes, and are characteristic of advanced stages of tumor progression. However, when an extensive cytogenetic analysis is possible, it becomes evident that secondary alterations also display a nonrandom pattern of chromosome involvement.

The acquisition of accurate data on the chromosomal characteristics of solid tumors in general, and of malignant gliomas in particular, has been improved by advances in cytogenetic techniques. To obtain the karyotype of the neoplastic cells integrating a tumor, the best method is a direct analysis of the tumor cells in metaphase from the sample under study. This method is called *direct preparation of tumor biopsies*, but the chromosome slides obtained using this technique are of a poor quality, and the quantity of cells in metaphase depends on the mitotic index of the tumor sample, which is generally low in low-grade tumors. To overcome these problems, especially in low-grade tumors, short-term in vitro cultures are used to perform extensive cytogenetic studies. This method increases the possibility of obtaining a sufficient number of high-quality mitoses and allows the performance of consecutive studies. Nevertheless, there are some disadvantages that should be carefully evaluated when performing a cytogenetic analysis after in vitro culture, such as the possible outgrowth of stroma cells rather than tumor cells and the possible addition of in vitro–induced chromosome changes. The possibility of a different in vitro growth rate of tumor cells with a different chromosomal constitution also exists. Whenever possible, cytogenetic analysis of solid tumors should be performed combining both methods on the same biopsy to obtain the pattern of alterations from the direct preparations, which may be improved on with the preparations obtained from in vitro culture. However, in low-grade tumors, only in vitro studies yield a sufficient number of cytogenetically analyzable cells, and normal karyotypes or 45,XO chromosome complements are frequently obtained, as also occurs in many of the low-grade gliomas or even in some high-grade tumors studied. In the next section, a review is presented of the cytogenetic data from about 500 samples derived from almost all histologic subgroups of gliomas. Nevertheless, nearly 40% of these tumors display either normal karyotypes or sex chromosome losses as the sole anomaly, and the chromosomal characteristic should obviously be established on the results from those samples displaying more complex karyotypes. A summary of the cytogenetic findings in each histologic subgroup of gliomas is presented in Table 4–1.

CYTOGENETIC CHARACTERISTICS OF GLIOMAS

Glioblastoma Multiforme (Including Giant Cell Variant)

Banded karyotypes from about 200 glioblastomas have been reported, including 10 pediatric cases.[1–11] Approximately 80% to 85% of tumors arising in adults display near-diploid modal chromosome numbers, and near-triploid or near-tetraploid complements are found in the remaining cases. Normal karyotypes or sex chromosome losses as the sole anomaly have been described in about 15% of samples. The most frequent chromosomal anomalies are numeric deviations: gains of whole copies of chromosome 7 were observed in about 45% of samples, whereas losses of chromosomes 10 and 22 occurred in 35% and 17% of tumors included in this group, respectively. At a lower frequency, losses of chromosomes 13, 14, 17, and 18, and gains of chromosomes 19 and 20 have also been detected. Structural chromosome rearrangements have been identified in about 60% of samples analyzed, and the commonest rearrangement implies deletion or translocation leading to the loss of material from the short arm of chromosome 9, and breakpoints at 9p24–p13 are found in 20% of samples. Less frequently, deletions or unbalanced translocations involve other chromosomes, with the breakpoints clustering to regions 1p36–p32, 7q22–q34, 13q21–q22, 19q13, and 22q13 (Figs. 4–1 and 4–2). Finally, double-minute chromosomes have been observed at variable incidence in glioblastoma multiforme. According to the data from different series, from 12% to 40% of cases display this anomaly.

The findings in ten pediatric glioblastomas[6, 7, 9, 11] may be summarized as follows: normal diploid chromosome complements were found in four cases, and alterations at 9p, 10p, and 22q have been observed in at least one sample. Although these anomalies are similar to those characterizing the gliomas arising in adults, the limited number of pediatric glioblastomas do not allow the establishment of a comparative pattern between both categories of tumors.

GLIOSARCOMA

A few samples derived from gliosarcomas have been studied cytogenetically (six cases).[3, 4, 12] The characteristic anomalies of glioblastomas have also been found in this histologic subtype; that is, gains of chromosome 7 and losses of chromosome 10 were detected in four tumors. Deletions

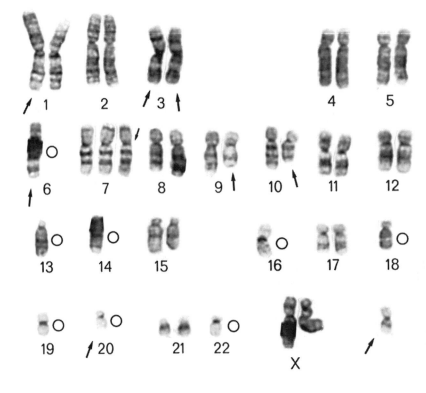

Figure 4–1 G-banded karyotype of a hypodiploid cell from a glioblastoma multiforme displaying several structural rearrangements *(arrows)*, and loss of several chromosomes. Note trisomy 7 and deletion of the short and long arms of chromosome 10.

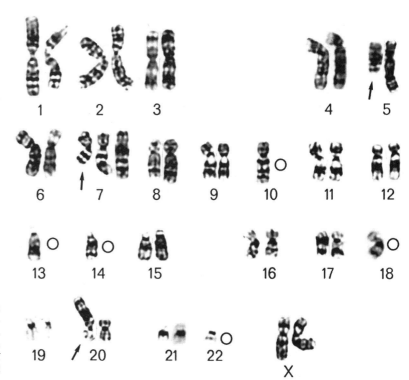

Figure 4–2 G-banded karyotype of a hypodiploid cell from a glioblastoma multiforme showing structural alterations of chromosomes 5, 7, and 20 *(arrows)*, and monosomy for chromosomes 10, 13, 14, 18, and 22. (From Rey JA, Bello MJ, de Campos JM, et al: On trisomy of chromosome 7 in human gliomas. Cancer Genet Cytogenet 1987; 29:323–326.)

or rearrangements of 9p and monosomy or deletion of chromosome 13 presented in two cases, whereas deletion of 1p, double-minute chromosomes, and monosomy 22 were identified in isolated cases. Complex chromosomal abnormalities were found in one tumor from a neonate exposed to heptachlor in utero; the anomalies in this tumor differed from those characteristic of adult gliosarcomas.[12]

Anaplastic Astrocytoma

Banded karyotypes from 43 anaplastic astrocytomas occurring in adults are available.[1–5, 8, 10, 13] About half of these tumors displayed normal diploid or 45,XO chromosome complements. The anomalies detected in the remaining samples are similar to those observed in glioblastoma multiforme, including gains of chromosome 7 (ten cases) and losses of chromosomes 10 (nine cases) and 22 (nine cases). Structural alterations, generally implying loss of material involving 9p, 9q, and 1p, were found recurrently. About 10% of samples displayed double-minute chromosomes.

Cytogenetic data on 22 pediatric anaplastic astrocytomas have been reported.[7, 11] Normal karyotypes were found in 14, and variable abnormalities characterized the remaining eight tumors. According to Karnes and colleagues[7] the main cytogenetic characteristics of these tumors are polyploidy and rearrangement of chromosome 1, whereas Neumann and coworkers[11] could not confirm the presence of trisomy 7 or losses for gonosomes and chromosome 10 (characteristic of adult tumors) in the series of pediatric tumors they studied. Nevertheless, losses of chromosome 22 and deletion of 9p, both also recurrent anomalies in adult tumors, were identified in one sample each.

Pilocytic Astrocytoma

Cytogenetic information on a total of 27 pilocytic astrocytomas is available.[4, 5, 7, 10, 14–16] Either normal karyotypes or sex chromosome losses as the sole anomaly were found in 18 tumors. Three samples displayed single abnormalities as follows: trisomy 7, monosomy 22, and a rearrangement of chromosome 15. In a hyperdiploid tumor (53 chromosomes) only numeric deviations were identified, including gains of chromosomes 5, 7, 10, 11, 12, 20, and 21. The remaining five samples displayed complex karyotypes including multiple alterations. Three of them showed monosomy or deletions of chromosome 22 and two tumors included deletions of 9p. Losses of chromosomes 10 or 17 or alterations of 1p or 19q were found once.

Pleomorphic Xanthoastrocytoma

Three tumors of this histologic subgroup have been analyzed by means of cytogenetic techniques.[4, 14, 17, 18] Two of them displayed polyploid modal chromosome numbers (73–84 chromosomes), both including gains of chromosome 7 and losses of chromosome 10. One of these tumors also displayed deletions of 6q and 9p, whereas monosomy for chromosomes 13, 14, and 22 and a rearrangement of chromosome 15 characterized the other tumor. In the third case, the primary tumor and an untreated recurrent tumor that developed 1 year after the original biopsy were studied.[17, 18] This tumor provides the opportunity to follow the clonal evolution of chromosome aberrations. The primary tumor was characterized by a hyperdiploid chromosome complement, including monosomy 22 and rearrangement of an extra chromo-

TABLE 4–1
SUMMARY OF THE CYTOGENETIC FINDINGS IN GLIOMAS

Histologic Subtype	No. of Cases Analyzed	Chromosome Alteration	No. of Cases
Glioblastoma multiforme	190	NK/45,XO	31
		+7	82
		−10	64
		−22	31
		del(9p)	39
		del(1p)	27
		Alt(7q)	13
		del(13q)	13
		Alt(17p)	10
		Alt(19q)	7
		dmin	34
Gliosarcoma	6	+7	4
		−10	4
		−13/del(13q)	2
		del(9p)	2
		−22	1
		del(1p)	1
		dmin	1
Anaplastic astrocytoma			
Adults	43	NK/45,XO	20
		+7	10
		−10/del(10)	9
		−22/del(22)	9
		del(1p)	5
		Alt(9q)	3
		del(9p)	2
		−17	2
		dmin	4
Children	22	NK/45,XO	14
		−22	1
		del(9p)	1
		polyploidy	4
Pilocytic astrocytoma	27	NK/45,XO	18
		−22/del(22)	4
		del(9p)	2
		−10	1
		−17	1
		del(1p)	1
		Alt(19q)	1
Pleomorphic xanthoastrocytoma	3	+7	3
		−10	2
		−22	2
		del(9p)	1
Subependymal giant cell astrocytoma	1	NK	1
Low-grade astrocytoma (N.O.S.)			
Adults	42	NK/45,XO	31
		+7	5
		−10	1
		−13	1
		−15	1
		−20	1
		−22	1
		dmin	2
Children	31	NK/45,XO	19
		+5	3
		+7	3
		+11	2
		Alt(1p)	3
Oligodendroglioma (low-grade)	38	NK/45,XO	26
		+7	3
		Alt 7q	3
		del(1p)	3
		−10/del(10)	3
		−22/del(22)	3
		Alt 9p	2

TABLE 4–1
SUMMARY OF THE CYTOGENETIC FINDINGS IN GLIOMAS *Continued*

Histologic Subtype	No. of Cases Analyzed	Chromosome Alteration	No. of Cases
Anaplastic oligodendroglioma		NK/45,XO	10
		+7	4
		−22/del(22)	4
		Alt 7q	2
		Alt 1p	2
		Alt 9p	2
		Alt 13q	1
	17	Alt 19q	1
Oligoastrocytoma		NK/45,XO	11
		−22/del(22)	2
		del(1p)	1
		Alt 7p	1
	16	Alt Yp	1
Ependymoma (low-grade) Adults		NK/45,XO	7
		−22/del(22)	6
		−10	3
		del(9p)	2
	17	−11/Alt 11q13	2
Children		NK/45,XO	8
		−22/del(22)	5
		−10/del(10)	3
		−9/del(9)	3
		Alt 1p	3
	24	−11/Alt 11q13	3
Anaplastic ependymoma		NK/45,XO	2
		−22/del(22)	6
		Alt 17	5
		+7	2
		del(10)	2
		del(2)(q34)	2
	13	Alt 13q	2
Myxopapillary ependymoma		Proportional losses 22	2
	4	del(1p)	2

Abbreviations: NK, normal karyotype; Alt, structural alteration; del, deletion; dmin, double-minute chromosomes; N.O.S., not otherwise specified.

some 7 and chromosomes 15 and 20. In the recurrent tumor, aberrations of the telomeres on chromosomes 20 and 22 were observed in all abnormal clones, and the authors concluded that the telomeric associations were the primary event in the cytogenetic evolution of this tumor, leading to the association of chromosomes 15 and 20, or to the loss of a chromosome 22, through the genesis of a ring chromosome 22.

Subependymal Giant Cell Astrocytoma

Only normal metaphases were found in the sole cytogenetically analyzed case included in this histologic subgroup of gliomas.[4] This tumor presented in a 1-year-old girl.

Low-Grade Astrocytoma

Most reports dealing with the cytogenetics of low-grade astrocytomas do not include data on the cytologic characteristics of tumors, and the pathologic diagnosis is not generally

otherwise specified. Thus, we will treat the data from these tumors in aggregate, but we hope that this information will be included in future reports on the subject.

Cytogenetic data from more than 70 of these tumors, including 31 pediatric cases, have been reported.[4, 5, 8, 10, 11, 13–15, 19] Only 26 of the 42 samples from adult patients displayed clonal aberrations, but in 15 cases the loss of a sex chromosome was the sole abnormality detected. Thus, the analysis of the cytogenetic data should be restricted to 11 samples. The only recurrent alteration observed in low-grade astrocytomas from adults is gain of chromosome 7 (five cases) (Fig. 4–3) and double-minute chromosomes (two cases). Losses of chromosomes 10, 13, 15, 20, and 22 and structural rearrangements involving chromosomes 4, 11, 12, 13, 16, 18, and 21 were observed in isolated cases.

Only 12 of the 31 low-grade astrocytomas arising in children displayed aberrations. The most frequent numeric abnormalities were trisomy 5, 7, and 11. One case showed monosomy 22, and trisomy 22 or trisomy 19 were found in single tumors. Structural rearrangements were identified in seven samples, but the only recurrently involved chromosome was chromosome 1, which was involved in translocations in three tumors.

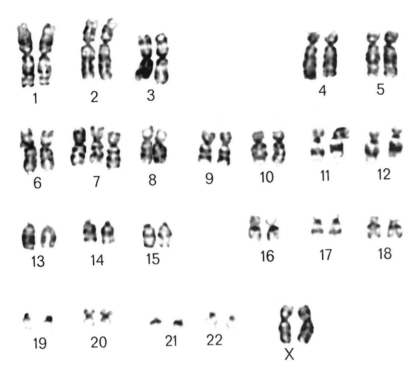

Figure 4–3 · Karyotype (G-banded) from a low-grade astrocytoma characterized by trisomy 7 as the sole chromosomal deviation.

Oligodendroglial Tumors

OLIGODENDROGLIOMA (LOW-GRADE)

Cytogenetic data on 38 low-grade oligodendrogliomas, including eight pediatric tumors, have been reported.[4, 10, 13–16] Normal karyotypes were observed in 16 samples, five of which developed in children, and the loss of the sex chromosomes as the sole abnormality was detected in 10 samples (including one pediatric case). The most consistent anomalies identified in the 12 oligodendrogliomas with complex karyotypes were as follows: gains of chromosome 7 or structural rearrangements of 7q were present in six tumors (Fig. 4–4); variable deletions of the short arm of chromosome 1 were observed in three cases, whereas monosomy 10 or deletions at 10q23 or 10p13 were identified in one sample each. Two cases displayed alterations of 9p, and monosomy of chromosome 22 (one sample) or deletions at 22q13 (two samples) were also observed.

ANAPLASTIC OLIGODENDROGLIOMA

Banded karyotypes have been reported for 17 anaplastic oligodendrogliomas, including one pediatric tumor.[4, 10, 13, 15, 16] In four samples only normal karyotypes were observed, and six additional samples displayed clonal losses of the sex chromosomes as the sole abnormality. Four tumors showed alterations of chromosome 22, which consisted of monosomy or deletions at 22q11 or 22q13. Gains of chromosome 7 were identified in one sample and in isolated cells of three additional tumors. Structural rearrangements of 1p, 7q, 9p, 13q, and 19q have been observed in this tumor type.

OLIGOASTROCYTOMA

Normal karyotypes or random losses were found in six of the 16 mixed oligoastrocytomas with cytogenetic studies

reported in the literature.[4, 8, 14, 15] Five additional tumors displayed losses of the sex chromosomes as the sole clonal anomaly. Structural and/or numeric alterations characterized only five samples: monosomy or structural rearrangement at q13 of chromosome 22 was found in two samples, and deletion of 1p and rearrangements of the short arm of chromosome 7 and Y were identified in one sample each.

SUMMARY OF THE CYTOGENETIC FINDINGS IN TUMORS WITH OLIGODENDROGLIAL COMPONENT

In summary, as shown in Table 4–1, approximately 65% of tumors with a major oligodendroglial component display either normal karyotypes or 45,XO complements. The cases with abnormalities are mainly characterized by alteration of chromosome 7 (gains and/or rearrangements of the long arm), deletions of the short arm of chromosome 1, and monosomy or deletion of chromosome 22 at band q13. A few cases display alterations of 9p, chromosome 10, and 19q.

Ependymal Tumors

EPENDYMOMA (LOW-GRADE)

About 40 cases of banded karyotypes from low-grade ependymomas have been reported and two-thirds of the patients are children.[4, 10, 11, 14–16, 20–25] Normal diploid karyotypes or random losses were observed in 7 of the 17 tumors arising in adults, and the ploidy level of the altered cases was near-diploid in six and polyploid in four. Chromosome 22 was the most frequently involved in losses or structural rearrangements: six tumors displayed either deletions at q13 or monosomy. Other recurrently affected chromosomes were chromosomes 10 (three cases) and 9p (two cases). Chromo-

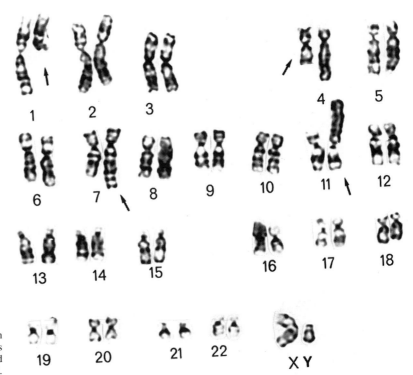

Figure 4–4 Karyotype of a pseudodiploid cell from an oligodendroglioma analyzed with G-banding. Various clonal structurally rearranged chromosomes were identified *(arrows)*. A nonclonal anomaly of 17p was also identified.

some 11 was lost in one tumor and rearranged at q13 band in another sample.

Eight of the 24 samples from tumors occurring in children displayed normal karyotypes. With the exception of two polyploid cases, near-diploid modal chromosome complements characterized the altered pediatric ependymomas. As in the tumors from adults, chromosome 22 was the most frequently altered (five samples). Monosomy 10 (three cases) and abnormalities of 9p (three cases) were also observed. Two samples displayed rearrangements at 11q13, and this was the sole alteration in both instances. Finally, anomalies of 1p were identified in three cases.

ANAPLASTIC EPENDYMOMA

Fewer than 15 banded karyotypes have been reported for this tumor type, including one pediatric tumor.[4, 8, 10, 14, 15, 20, 24, 25] Chromosome anomalies were identified in 11 cases, which primarily displayed a near-diploid modal chromosome number, whereas polyploidy (83 and 75 chromosomes) was found in two cases. Chromosome 22 represents the most frequently altered chromosome in this group of tumors, and monosomy or deletions were identified in six samples. One tumor analyzed by Weremowicz and associates[24] displayed alteration of both copies of this chromosome pair: one chromosome 22 homologue was lost in all cells analyzed and the remaining 22 homologue contained a translocation at band q13.3. Based on these findings, Weremowicz and others[24] proposed that initiation and/or progression of some ependymomas might result from loss or inactivation of a tumor suppressor gene located on the long arm of chromosome 22. Deletions at p13 on chromosome 10, monosomy or deletions of 9p, proportional gains of chromosome 7, deletions at q34 of chromosome 2, and anomalies of chromo-

some 13 have been identified in two samples each, whereas anomalies involving chromosome 17 were observed in five cases. One sample described by Jenkins and others[4] displayed an inversion of chromosome 11 [inv(11)(p11.2;p13)] as the sole abnormality.

MYXOPAPILLARY EPENDYMOMA

Four tumors diagnosed as myxopapillary ependymoma have been described cytogenetically.[14, 15, 26, 27] Two were characterized by polyploid modal chromosome numbers (60 and 76 chromosomes) displaying numeric variations but not structural rearrangements (Fig. 4–5). A proportional decrease in the number of copies of chromosome 22 was evident in both samples. Near-diploid chromosome complements characterized the two remaining samples, which also included structural rearrangements. Deletions of the short arm of chromosome 1 were identified in both tumors, and monosomy 8, trisomy for chromosome 9, and a structural rearrangement at 10q24 were observed in one sample.

SUBEPENDYMOMA

To our knowledge, no sample of this histologic subtype of ependymoma has been studied cytogenetically.

SUMMARY OF THE CYTOGENETIC FINDINGS IN EPENDYMAL TUMORS

A comparative analysis of cytogenetic findings from different ependymoma subgroups shows that the anomalies involving chromosome 22 represent the most frequent alteration; it has been identified in all histologic subgroups of ependymomas. Losses or deletions of chromosome 10 are also present in tumors from all three histologic subgroups,

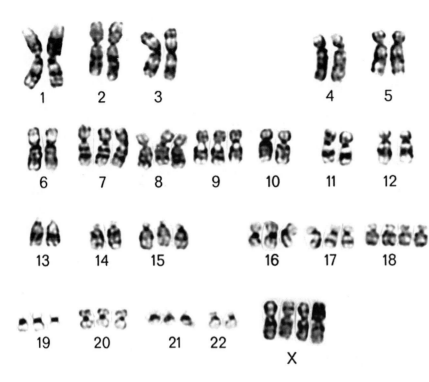

Figure 4–5 Representative G-banded karyotype of a myxopapillary ependymoma. Only numerical deviations are observed. (From Rey JA, Bello MJ, de Campos JM, et al: Chromosomal composition of a series of 22 human low-grade gliomas. Cancer Genet Cytogenet 1987; 29:223–237.)

but two distinct regions seem to be involved (i.e., 10p13 and 10q24). Other recurrent breakpoints are 11q13 and 2q34, which might represent consistent alterations in these neoplasms together with deletions of the short arm of chromosomes 1 and 9 and losses of chromosome 17. Relevant to this issue are the data provided by Rogatto and colleagues,[25] who performed cytogenetic studies on four ependymomas with different degrees of malignancy (grades 1 to 4). Losses of chromosomes 17 and 22 and structural involvement of 2q24–q34 region were found in samples of all grades of malignancy.

INTERPHASE CYTOGENETICS

An alternative approach for the analysis of chromosomal aberrations (primarily numeric deviations) is interphase cytogenetics. The methodology consists of the application of nonradioactive in situ hybridization with chromosome-specific DNA probes to interphase nuclei, thus overcoming the necessity to culture tumor cells when no successful cytogenetic results are obtained by direct-method preparations. Interphase cytogenetics allows detection of the presence of significant populations of nuclei with one (monosomy), two (disomy), or three or more (trisomy, etc.) signals in a sample for a given chromosome. The methodological criteria establish that monosomy is accepted when more than 20% of nuclei display one spot, and trisomy when more than 7.5% of nuclei display three spots. Using this method, Arnoldus and others[28, 29] have reported data on 33 gliomas, including 17 astrocytomas, five oligoastrocytomas, seven oligodendrogliomas, and four ependymomas. The predominant aberrations detected were an overrepresentation of chromosome 7 (13 cases) and an underrepresentation of chromosome 10 (16 cases). These changes occurred in all of the histologic

subtypes of gliomas studied and, in agreement with the data provided by classic cytogenetics, both anomalies were commonly observed in association (in ten cases). Other relatively frequent aberrations were the loss of chromosome 18 (observed in seven cases) and a gain of chromosome 17 (detected in six). Interphase cytogenetics may be a powerful and rapid new tool for the detection of numeric chromosomal deviations and may result in a better understanding of the biologic behavior of gliomas.

TRISOMY 7 IN GLIOMAS

Fact or Artifact?

As mentioned in the previous paragraphs, the gain of one or more complete copies of chromosome 7 is the most frequently observed numeric deviation in gliomas. Two distinct patterns of presentation of this anomaly may be observed: (1) it may present as a solitary abnormality or in association with sex chromosome losses, mainly in certain low-grade tumors; and (2) it may present in addition to other nonrandom anomalies, such as deletions of 1p, 9p, monosomy 10, or double-minute chromosomes. In the latter situation, two possibilities may be observed: (1) the gain of chromosome 7 is noted in the same cells that display the other clonal alterations, and (2) the increased number of chromosome 7 is observed in cellular clones that are different from those that display the characteristic aforementioned alterations.

Gains of chromosome 7 have also been found in a variety of non-glial histologic types of neoplasms[30] as well as in the alleged normal tissue near tumor from patients with tumors of glial origin.[31] These findings have been interpreted to indicate that trisomy 7 might not be a tumor-associated anomaly, particularly when it occurs as the sole abnormality or as an isolated cellular clone in a given tumor. According to Lindström and co-workers,[5] a tendency to gain chromosome 7 seems to be present both in parenchymal and in non-parenchymal cells of brain tumors; this fact, together with the finding of trisomy 7 in short-term cultures of apparent non-neoplastic brain tissue, might be used as an argument against the pathogenetic importance of this anomaly in gliomas. In this respect, as indicated by Lindström and others,[5] the possibility exists that the gain of chromosome 7 might represent a cytogenetic divergence during tumor progression. As mentioned in the previous section, Arnoldus and associates,[28, 29] using interphase cytogenetics, found this aberration in 40% of samples from gliomas studied, whereas it was absent in the nuclei from samples of normal brain tissue analyzed in parallel. Bello and colleagues[32] determined the incidence of gains involving chromosome 7 using cytogenetic and molecular genetic analyses in a series of 57 gliomas; they concluded, in agreement with the data provided by Arnoldus and associates,[28, 29] that the anomaly would be representative of the tumor parenchyma at least in those tumors in which it is observed in association with other chromosomal changes.

Recently, Voravud and others,[33] using interphase cytogenetics, observed increased polysomy of chromosome 7 during head and neck multi-stage tumorigenesis. The data provided interesting information on the possible role played by chromosome 7 gains in malignancy, which might also be applicable to malignant gliomas. The authors found that normal control tissue from individuals free of cancer showed no chromosome 7 polysomy, whereas histologically normal tissue adjacent to the tumors included cells with polysomy for chromosome 7, and the frequency of cells with this anomaly increased as the categories of tissue samples analyzed progressed from histologically normal to premalignant, to hyperplastic/dysplastic, to cancerous. The observation of chromosome number anomalies in the normal and premalignant regions adjacent to the tumors supports the notion of field cancerization, suggesting the existence of multiple independent foci of lesions progressing toward malignant growth. If a similar situation would occur in malignant gliomas, it would explain the cytogenetic results observed in the so-called normal tissue near tumors, and might account for the existence of second or multi-focal glial tumors. However, such studies, which could serve as biomarkers in the determination of the risk of progression to malignancy, have yet to be performed for gliomas.

MOLECULAR GENETIC IMPLICATIONS OF THE CYTOGENETIC FINDINGS

Although a separate chapter of this book deals broadly with the molecular genetic characteristics of gliomas (Chapter 5), the main molecular data are discussed here to give a view of the relationship between both cytogenetic findings and a potential involvement of oncogenes or tumor suppressor genes during glioma development and progression.

Restriction fragment length polymorphism (RFLP) analysis has been used to characterize the chromosomal aberrations in gliomas through the analysis of loss of heterozygosity (LOH) of polymorphic DNA markers at specific chromosomes. Obviously, the main chromosomes subject to this type of analysis have been those frequently lost or deleted, as demonstrated by cytogenetic studies. RFLP analysis for markers located on chromosome 10 has shown that loss of sequences of this chromosome frequently occurs in glioblastoma multiforme and in a lower proportion of low-grade astrocytomas.[8, 16, 34–41] The loss of sequences in this chromosome signifies that the inactivation of a tumor suppressor gene located here seems to be associated with progression toward tumors with the most biologically aggressive behavior, namely glioblastoma multiforme. Similar studies showed loss of heterozygosity involving genomic regions on 9p (in the segment interferon gene–methyl thioadenosine phosphorylase gene) in glioblastomas, anaplastic astrocytomas, and a few oligodendrogliomas.[41–45] The identification of tumors displaying homozygous deletions of this region on 9p speaks in favor of the location here of a tumor suppressor gene, the inactivation of which may represent an important step in the progression of gliomas.

Molecular results compatible with loss of the entire chromosome 22 have been obtained,[34, 35, 46] but in a few instances, loss of heterozygosity was restricted to distal markers located at 22q13[47, 48] confirming that deletions at this level are found in cytogenetic analysis. A tumor suppressor gene located on chromosome 22 should participate in the development of at least some subgroups of gliomas, and a candidate glioma suppressor gene on chromosome 22q arm would be the recently cloned neurofibromatosis 2 gene (NF2).[49, 50] An analysis to determine the mutations involving the coding region of this gene has been performed on 30 astrocytomas and eight ependymomas, and alterations have been seen in only one sample (an ependymoma), which suggests that the NF2 gene is not the 22q tumor suppressor gene involved in astrocytomas.[51] In agreement with previous loss of heterozygosity studies,[47, 48] another gene of this category, distally located to NF2, most likely in the 22q13 region, might be the target of the alterations detected by cytogenetic analysis in gliomas.

Another genomic region where a tumor suppressor gene nonrandomly involved in glioma progression would be located is the short arm of chromosome 1. Loss of heterozygosity studies for markers located on 1p demonstrated a lower than expected incidence of deletions involving this chromosome arm in high-grade gliomas.[16, 34, 35, 37, 52] In contrast, allelic loss at 1p is the most commonly observed anomaly in tumors with a major oligodendroglial component and, as demonstrated by Bello and others,[52] the critical region may be restricted to 1pter–p32. Loss of heterozygosity for 19q is also frequently observed in oligodendrogliomas, but is less specific than the 1p losses, as it is also characteristic of anaplastic astrocytoma and glioblastoma multiforme. According to von Deimling and colleagues,[53] the common region of overlap for the observed deletions includes 19q13.2–q13.3 bands.

In contrast to the scarce cytogenetic evidence for an involvement of chromosome 17 in astrocytic tumors, loss of heterozygosity for loci on this chromosome has been found in both anaplastic astrocytoma and glioblastoma multiforme, involving primarily the region 17pter–p11.2.[54–56] In parallel with these findings, mutational alterations of the *TP53* gene (a tumor suppressor gene located at 17p) have been described in the higher-grade gliomas, suggesting that this could be the target gene for anomalies on 17p.[57–61] Nevertheless, loss of heterozygosity for the distal markers on 17p without alterations of the *TP53* gene has been found in several cases, indicating that a tumor suppressor gene other than *TP53* may be located on 17p and may be involved in progression of gliomas of an astrocytic nature.[52, 62, 63]

The alteration of cellular oncogenes has also been analyzed in human gliomas by molecular genetic technology. Structural alterations and further amplification of the epidermal growth factor receptor gene (EGFR) has frequently been found to characterize glioblastoma multiforme and anaplastic astrocytoma.[64, 65] In some instances a truncated receptor is present, with loss of the extracellular domain. Generally, the amplification of the EGFR gene is associated with the presence of double-minute chromosomes,[65] but this is not the sole cellular oncogene subject to amplification or overexpression as, for example, c-*myc*, -*gli*, and -*ros* have also been altered in a few tumors.[66–68]

The confluence of both cytogenetic and molecular genetic data that are available for malignant gliomas agrees with the hypothesis proposing an accumulation of clonal genomic alterations in a multi-step process during malignant progression in a tumor. According to the data presented in this chapter, the inactivation of five to six tumor suppressor genes located at specific genomic regions is associated with the development of gliomas, and the amplification of the EGFR gene seems to be associated with the late phases of evolution. In some instances, the alteration of those tumor suppressor genes is not expressed as a chromosome anomaly because such submicroscopic anomalies as point-inactivating mutation or microdeletions are not detectable at the level of resolution of the cytogenetic techniques. Doubtless, cytogenetic and molecular data from large series of samples of every histologic subtype of glioma might allow a better understanding of the biologic consequences of these genomic changes and are likely to provide interesting information with potential clinical implications.

CLINICAL IMPLICATIONS OF THE CYTOGENETIC FINDINGS

Cytogenetic analysis has proven useful in diagnosis, classification, and prognosis of patients affected by malignant hematologic disorders.[30] The analysis of cytogenetic results in large series of cases of a given malignancy has allowed the establishment of parameters with clinical significance. In the past, the lack of cytogenetic data for broad series of solid tumors in general, and for gliomas in particular, has represented the main handicap for the undertaking of studies to correlate cytogenetic and clinical characteristics of tumors. Thus, obtaining a large enough body of cytogenetic information, for which statistical studies with significant relevance can be performed, on a series of tumors of each histologic subtype of glioma is the critical point for determining whether any particular cytogenetic anomaly represents a parameter of clinical interest.

Although, as has been mentioned previously in the chapter, cytogenetic data are still limited to a relatively short number of samples from gliomas, several correlation studies have been performed and some interesting preliminary implications have been determined. Al Saadi and Latimer[69] reported longer survival periods in patients with malignant gliomas displaying normal karyotypes or minimal chromosome deviations (i.e., the presence of 45,XO complements as the result of sex chromosome loss). In agreement with these data, the analysis of 41 glioblastomas performed by Kusak and colleagues[70] showed an association between complex karyotypic patterns and biologic aggressiveness of tumors, implying a worse prognosis in terms of recurrence-free survival or overall survival of patients. A similar study by de Campos and others[71] was performed on 13 oligodendrogliomas, and all high-grade tumors and five of seven low-grade tumors were found to display chromosomal abnormalities. Interestingly, all tumors with anomalies were recurrent and the patient subsequently died, whereas in both cases with no alterations, patients remained alive and free of recurrence after treatment at 55 and 87 months of follow-up.

To avoid the establishment of erroneous conclusions, these data should be interpreted with caution due to the small number of cases analyzed in each report. However, the preliminary results seem to suggest a possible prognostic value for the cytogenetic findings, and this information might contribute to obtaining an accurate and perhaps reproducible identification of aggressive glioma subsets. Finally, it must be considered that additional factors, such as tumor location, extent of resection, and treatment programs, may represent critical factors in the prognosis of patients; thus, a multidisciplinary analysis is needed to improve the management of glial tumors.

REFERENCES

1. Rey JA, Bello MJ, de Campos, et al: Chromosomal patterns in human malignant astrocytomas. Cancer Genet Cytogenet 1987; 29:201–221.
2. Rey JA, Bello MJ, de Campos JM, et al: On trisomy of chromosome 7 in human gliomas. Cancer Genet Cytogenet 1987; 29:323–326.
3. Bigner SH, Mark J, Burger PC, et al: Specific chromosomal abnormalities in malignant human gliomas. Cancer Res 1988; 88:405–411.
4. Jenkins RB, Kimmel DW, Moertel CA, et al: A cytogenetic study of 53 human gliomas. Cancer Genet Cytogenet 1989; 39:253–279.
5. Lindström E, Salford LG, Heim S, et al: Trisomy 7 and sex chromosome loss need not be representative of tumor parenchyma cells in malignant glioma. Genes Chromosom Cancer 1991; 3:474–479.
6. Sawyer JR, Swanson CM, Chadduck WM, et al: Evolution of tumor chromosome abnormalities after therapy in a pediatric astrocytoma. Cancer Genet Cytogenet 1991; 53:119–123.
7. Karnes PS, Tran TN, Cui MY, et al: Cytogenetic analysis of 39 pediatric central nervous system tumors. Cancer Genet Cytogenet 1992; 59:12–19.
8. Ransom DT, Ritland SR, Moertel CA, et al: Correlation of cytogenetic analysis and loss of heterozygosity studies in human diffuse astrocytomas and mixed oligo-astrocytomas. Genes Chromosom Cancer 1992; 5:357–374.
9. Sawyer JR, Swanson CM, Roloson GJ, et al: Cytogenetic findings in a case of pediatric glioblastoma. Cancer Genet Cytogenet 1992; 64:75–79.
10. Thiel G, Losanowa T, Kintzel D, et al: Karyotypes in 90 human gliomas. Cancer Genet Cytogenet 1992; 58:109–120.
11. Neumann E, Kalousek DK, Norman MG, et al: Cytogenetic analysis of 109 pediatric central nervous system tumors. Cancer Genet Cytogenet 1993; 71:40–49.
12. Chadduck WM, Gollin SM, Gray BA, et al: Gliosarcoma with chromosome abnormalities in a neonate exposed to heptachlor. Neurosurgery 1987; 21:557–559.
13. Yamada K, Kondo T, Yoshioka M, et al: Cytogenetic studies in 20

human brain tumors: Association of No. 22 chromosome abnormalities with tumors of the brain. Cancer Genet Cytogenet 1980; 2:293–307.

14. Rey JA, Bello MJ, de Campos JM, et al: Chromosomal composition of a series of 22 human low-grade gliomas. Cancer Genet Cytogenet 1987; 29:223–237.

15. Griffin CA, Long PP, Carson BJ, et al: Chromosome abnormalities in low-grade central nervous system tumors. Cancer Genet Cytogenet 1992; 60:67–73.

16. Ransom DT, Ritland SR, Kimmel DW, et al: Cytogenetic and loss of heterozygosity studies in ependymomas, pilocytic astrocytomas, and oligodendrogliomas. Genes Chromosom Cancer 1992; 5:348–356.

17. Sawyer JR, Roloson GJ, Chadduck WM, et al: Cytogenetic findings in a pleomorphic xanthoastrocytoma. Cancer Genet Cytogenet 1991; 55:225–230.

18. Sawyer JR, Thomas EL, Roloson GJ, et al: Telomeric associations evolving to ring chromosome in a recurrent pleomorphic xanthoastrocytoma. Cancer Genet Cytogenet 1992; 60:152–157.

19. Sawyer JR, Roloson GJ, Hobson EA, et al: Trisomy for chromosome 1q in a pontine astrocytoma. Cancer Genet Cytogenet 1990; 47:101–106.

20. Stratton MR, Darling J, Lantos PL, et al: Cytogenetic abnormalities in human ependymomas. Int J Cancer 1989; 44:579–581.

21. Bown NP, Pearson ADJ, Davison EV, et al: Multiple chromosome rearrangements in a childhood ependymoma. Cancer Genet Cytogenet 1988; 36:25–30.

22. Dal Cin P, Sandberg AA: Cytogenetic findings in a supratentorial ependymoma. Cancer Genet Cytogenet 1988; 30:289–293.

23. Sainati L, Montaldi A, Putti MC, et al: Cytogenetic t(11;17)(q13;q21) in a pediatric ependymoma. Is 11q13 a recurring breakpoint in ependymoma? Cancer Genet Cytogenet 1992; 59:213–216.

24. Weremowicz S, Kupsky WJ, Morton CC, et al: Cytogenetic evidence for a chromosome 22 tumor suppressor gene in ependymoma. Cancer Genet Cytogenet 1992; 61:193–196.

25. Rogatto SR, Casartelli C, Rainho CA, et al: Chromosomes in the genesis and progression of ependymomas. Cancer Genet Cytogenet 1993; 69:146–152.

26. Sawyer JR, Crowson ML, Roloson GJ, et al: Involvement of the short arm of chromosome 1 in myxopapillary ependymoma. Cancer Genet Cytogenet 1991; 54:55–60.

27. Kindblom LG, Lodding P, Hagmar B, et al: Metastasizing myxopapillary ependymoma of the sacrococcygeal region: A clinico-pathologic, light and electron microscopic, immunohistochemical, tissue culture, and cytogenetic analysis of a case. Acta Pathol Microbiol Immunol Scand 1986; 94(section A):79–90.

28. Arnoldus EPJ, Noordermeer IA, Peters ACR, et al: Interphase cytogenetics of brain tumors. Genes Chromosom Cancer 1991; 3:101–107.

29. Arnoldus EPJ, Wolters LBT, Voormolen JHC, et al: Interphase cytogenetics: A new tool for the study of genetic changes in brain tumors. J Neurosurg 1992; 76:997–1003.

30. Sandberg AA: The Chromosomes in Human Cancer and Leukemia, ed 2. Norwalk, Conn, Appleton-Lange, 1990.

31. Heim S, Mandahl N, Jin Y, et al: Trisomy 7 and sex chromosome loss in human brain tissue. Cytogenet Cell Genet 1989; 52:136–138.

32. Bello MJ, de Campos JM, Kusak ME, et al: Ascertainment of chromosome 7 gains in malignant gliomas by cytogenetic and RFLP analyses. Cancer Genet Cytogenet 1994; 72:55–58.

33. Voravud N, Shin DM, Ro JY, et al: Increased polysomies of chromosomes 7 and 17 during head and neck multistage tumorigenesis. Cancer Res 1993; 53:2874–2883.

34. James CD, Carlbom E, Dumanski JP, et al: Clonal genomic alterations in glioma malignancy stages. Cancer Res 1988; 48:5546–5551.

35. Fults D, Pedone CA, Thomas GA, et al: Allelotype of human malignant astrocytoma. Cancer Res 1990; 50:5784–5789.

36. Watanabe K, Nagai M, Wakai S, et al: Loss of heterozygosity in chromosome 10 in human glioblastoma. Acta Neuropathol 1990; 80:251–254.

37. Venter DJ, Thomas DGT: Multiple sequential molecular abnormalities in the evolution of human gliomas. Br J Cancer 1991; 63:753–757.

38. Rasheed BK, Fuller GN, Friedman AH, et al: Loss of heterozygosity for 10q in human gliomas. Genes Chromosom Cancer 1992; 5:75–82.

39. van de Kelft E, De Boulle K, Willems P, et al: Loss of constitutional heterozygosity in human astrocytomas. Acta Neurochir 1992; 117:172–177.

40. von Deimling A, Louis DN, Von Ammon K, et al: Association of epidermal growth factor receptor gene amplification with loss of chromosome 10 in human glioblastoma multiforme. J Neurosurg 1992; 77:295–301.

41. Bello MJ, de Campos JM, Kusak ME, et al: Molecular analysis of genomic abnormalities in human gliomas. Cancer Genet Cytogenet 1994; 73:122–129.

42. James CD, He J, Carlbom E, et al: Chromosome 9 deletion mapping reveals interferon alpha and interferon β-1 gene deletions in human glial tumors. Cancer Res 1991; 51:1684–1688.

43. Olopade OI, Jenkins RB, Ransom DT, et al: Molecular analysis of the short arm of chromosome 9 in human gliomas. Cancer Res 1992; 52:2523–2529.

44. James CD, He J, Collins VP, et al: Localization of chromosome 9p homozygous deletions in human glioma cell lines with markers constituting a continuous linkage group. Cancer Res 1993; 53:3674–3676.

45. Bello MJ, de Campos JM, Vaquero J, et al: Molecular and cytogenetic analysis of chromosome 9 deletions in 75 malignant gliomas. Genes Chromosom Cancer 1994; 9:33–41.

46. James CD, He J, Carlbom E, et al: Loss of genetic information in central nervous system tumors common to children and young adults. Genes Chromosom Cancer 1990; 2:94–102.

47. Rey JA, Bello MJ, Jimenez-Lara A, et al: Loss of heterozygosity for distal markers on 22q in human gliomas. Int J Cancer 1992; 51:703–706.

48. Rey JA, Bello MJ, de Campos JM, et al: Abnormalities of chromosome 22 in human brain tumors determined by combined cytogenetic and molecular genetic approaches. Cancer Genet Cytogenet 1993; 66:1–10.

49. Rouleau GA, Merel P, Lutchman M, et al: Alteration in a new gene encoding a putative membrane-organizing protein causes neuro-fibromatosis type 2. Nature 1993; 363:515–521.

50. Trofatter JA, MacCollin MM, Rutter JL, et al: A novel moesin-, ezrin-, radixin-like gene is a candidate for the neurofibromatosis 2 tumor suppressor. Cell 1993; 72:791–800.

51. Rubio MP, Correa KM, Ramesh V, et al: Analysis of the neurofibromatosis 2 gene in human ependymomas and astrocytomas. Cancer Res 1994; 54:45–47.

52. Bello MJ, Vaquero J, de Campos JM, et al: Molecular analysis of chromosome 1 abnormalities in human gliomas reveals frequent loss of 1p in oligodendroglial tumors. Int J Cancer 1994; 57:172–175.

53. von Deimling A, Louis DN, Von Ammon K, et al: Evidence for a tumor suppressor gene on chromosome 19q associated with human astrocytomas, oligodendrogliomas, and mixed gliomas. Cancer Res 1992; 52:4277–4279.

54. El-Azouzi M, Chung RY, Farmer GE, et al: Loss of distinct regions on the short arm of chromosome 17 associated with tumorigenesis of human astrocytomas. Proc Natl Acad Sci USA 1989; 86:7186–7190.

55. Fults D, Tippets RH, Thomas GA, et al: Loss of heterozygosity for loci on chromosome 17 in malignant astrocytomas. Cancer Res 1989; 49:6572–6577.

56. James CD, Carlbom E, Nordenskjöld M, et al: Mitotic recombination of chromosome 17 in astrocytomas. Proc Natl Acad Sci USA 1989; 86:2858–2862.

57. Mashiyama S, Murakami Y, Yoshimoto T, et al: Detection of p53 gene mutations in human brain tumors by single-strand conformation polymorphism analysis of polymerase chain reaction products. Oncogene 1991; 6:1313–1318.

58. Frankel RH, Bayona W, Koslow M, et al: p53 mutations in human malignant gliomas: Comparison of loss of heterozygosity with mutation frequency. Cancer Res 1992; 52:1427–1433.

59. Fults D, Brockmeyer D, Tullous MW, et al: p53 mutation and loss of heterozygosity on chromosome 17 and 10 during human astrocytoma progression. Cancer Res 1992; 52:2987–2990.

60. von Deimling A, Eibl RH, Ohgaki H, et al: p53 mutations are associated with 17p allelic loss in grade II and grade III astrocytomas. Cancer Res 1992; 52:2987–2990.

61. Sidransky D, Mikkelsen T, Schwechheimer K, et al: Clonal expansion of p53 mutant cells is associated with brain tumor progression. Nature 1992; 355:846–847.

62. Saxena A, Clark WC, Robertson JT, et al: Evidence for the involvement of a potential second suppressor gene on chromosome 17 distinct from p53 in malignant astrocytoma. Cancer Res 1992; 52:6716–6721.

63. Biegel JA, Burk CD, Barr FG, et al: Evidence for a 17p tumor related locus distinct from p53 in pediatric primitive neuroectodermal tumors. Cancer Res 1992; 52:3391–3395.

64. Liberman TA, Nusbaum HR, Razon N, et al: Amplification, enhanced expression and possible rearrangement of EGF receptor gene in primary human brain tumors of glial origin. Nature 1985; 313:144–147.

65. Wong AJ, Bigner SH, Bigner DD, et al: Increased expression of the epidermal growth factor receptor gene in malignant gliomas is invariably associated with gene amplification. Proc Natl Acad Sci USA 1987; 84:6899–6903.

66. Trent J, Melzer P, Rosenblum M, et al: Evidence for rearrangement, amplification, and expression of c-myc in a human glioblastoma. Proc Natl Acad Sci USA 1986; 83:470–473.

67. Kintler KW, Bigner SH, Bigner DD, et al: Identification of an amplified, highly expressed gene in human glioma. Science 1987; 236:70–73.

68. Birchmeier C, Sharma S, Wigler M: Expression and rearrangement of the ROS 1 gene in human glioblastoma cells. Proc Natl Acad Sci USA 1987; 84:9270–9274.

69. Al Saadi A, Latimer F: Cytogenetic and Clinical Correlations in Neoplasms of the Human Nervous System. Proceedings of the 74th Annual Meeting of the American Association of Cancer Research, 1983, 24:10.

70. Kusak ME, de Campos JM, Rey JA, et al: Prognostic implications of karyotype pattern in malignant astrocytomas. Am J Hum Genet 1991; 49:243.

71. de Campos JM, Kusak ME, Bello MJ, et al: Karyotype and prognosis in oligodendroglial tumors. Cancer Genet Cytogenet 1991; 52:203.

Mohapatra G, Kim DH, Feuerstein BG: Detection of multiple gains and losses of genetic material in ten glioma cell lines by comparative genomic hybridization. Genes Chromosom Cancer 1995; 13:86–93.

Park JP, Chaffee S, Noll WW, et al: Constitutional de novo t(1;22)(p22;q11.2) and ependymoma. Cancer Genet Cytogenet 1996; 86:150–152.

Park SH, Maeda T, Mohapatra G, et al: Heterogeneity, polyploidy, aneusomy, and 9p deletion in human glioblastoma multiforme. Cancer Genet Cytogenet 1995; 83:127–135.

Pruchon E, Chauvenic L, Sabatier L, et al: A cytogenetic study of 19 recurrent gliomas. Cancer Genet Cytogenet 1994; 76:85–92.

Pylkkänen P, Paetau A, Knuutila S: Chromosome 7 in glioblastoma tissue: Parenchymal vs. endothelial cells. Cancer Genet Cytogenet 1995; 84:73–75.

Sawyer JR, Sammartino G, Husain M, et al: Chromosome aberrations in four ependymomas. Cancer Genet Cytogenet 1994; 74:132–138.

Sawyer JR, Thomas JR, Teo C: Low-grade astrocytoma with a complex four-breakpoint inversion of chromosome 8 as the sole cytogenetic aberration. Cancer Genet Cytogenet 1995; 83:168–171.

Wernicke C, Thiel G, Lozanova T, et al: Involvement of chromosome 22 in ependymomas. Cancer Genet Cytogenet 1995; 79:173–176.

Yamada K, Kasama M, Kondo T, et al: Chromosome studies in 70 brain tumors with special attention to sex chromosome loss and single autosomal trisomy. Cancer Genet Cytogenet 1994; 73:46–52.

ADDITIONAL READINGS

Several reports have provided data of interest on the cytogenetics of human gliomas. The references to these reports are as follows:

Agamanolis DP, Malone JM: Chromosomal abnormalities in 47 pediatric brain tumors. Cancer Genet Cytogenet 1995; 81:125–134.

Bello MJ, Leone PE, Nebreda P, et al: Allelic status of chromosome 1 in neoplasms of the nervous system. Cancer Genet Cytogenet 1994; 83:160–164.

Bello MJ, Leone PE, Nebreda P, et al: Molecular abnormalities of chromosome 19 in malignant gliomas: Preferential involvement of the 19q13.2–q13.4 region. Int J Oncol 1995; 6:655–658.

Bello MJ, Leone PE, Vaquero J, et al: Allelic loss at 1p and 19q frequently occurs in association and may represent early oncogenic events in oligodendroglial tumors. Int J Cancer 1995; 64:207–210.

Coons SW, Johnson PC, Shapiro JR: Cytogenetic and flow cytometry DNA analysis of regional heterogeneity in a low grade human glioma. Cancer Res 1995; 55:1569–1577.

Debiec-Rychter M, Alwasiak J, Liberski PP, et al: Accumulation of chromosomal changes in human glioma progression: A cytogenetic study of 50 cases. Cancer Genet Cytogenet 1995; 85:61–67.

Fujii Y, Hongo T, Hayashi Y: Chromosome analysis of brain tumors in childhood. Genes Chromosom Cancer 1994; 11:205–215.

Harrison KJ, Neumann E, Kalousek DK, et al: Astrocytoma with a unique telomere association. Cancer Genet Cytogenet 1994; 76:33–35.

Hashimoto N, Ichikawa D, Arakawa Y, et al: Frequent deletions of material from chromosome arm 1p in oligodendroglial tumors revealed by double-target fluorescence in situ hybridization and microsatellite analysis. Genes Chromosom Cancer 1995; 14:295–300.

Hecht BK, Turc-Carel C, Chatel M, et al: Chromosomes in gliomatosis cerebri. Genes Chromosom Cancer 1995; 14:149–153.

Hecht BK, Turc-Carel C, Chatel M, et al: Cytogenetics of malignant gliomas: I. The autosomes with reference to rearrangements. Cancer Genet Cytogenet 1995; 84:1–8.

Hecht BK, Turc-Carel C, Chatel M, et al: Cytogenetics of malignant gliomas: II. The sex chromosomes with reference to X isodisomy and the role of numerical X/Y changes. Cancer Genet Cytogenet 1995; 84:9–14.

Li YS, Ramsay DA, Fan Y-S, et al: Cytogenetic evidence that a tumor suppressor gene in the long arm of chromosome 1 contributes to glioma growth. Cancer Genet Cytogenet 1995; 84:46–50.

Magnani I, Guerneri S, Pollo B, et al: Increasing complexity of the karyotype in 50 human gliomas: Progressive evolution and de novo occurrence of cytogenetic alterations. Cancer Genet Cytogenet 1994; 75:77–89.

McKeever PE, Dennis TR, Burgess AC, et al: Chromosome breakpoint at 17q11.2 and insertion of DNA from three different chromosomes in a glioblastoma with exceptional glial fibrillary acidic protein expression. Cancer Genet Cytogenet 1996; 87:41–47.

GLOSSARY*

Autosome: Any chromosome other than a sex chromosome.

Breakpoint: Location of a break in a chromatid or a chromosome, denoted by the exact band involved.

Deletion: Loss of a specific chromosome segment.

Diploidy: The normal composition and number of chromosomes.

Double minute chromosome: Small acentric and paired chromatin fragments of variable size.

Gonosomes: The sex chromosomes, X and Y.

Hyperdiploidy: A number of chromosomes greater than 46.

Hypodiploidy: A number of chromosomes lower than 46.

Insertion: Transfer of a chromosome segment into another chromosome.

Interphase: Portion of the cell cycle during which the cell is not in mitosis.

Inversion: Result of two breaks in the same chromosome, with 180-degree rotation of the segment between the breaks and subsequent fusion of the broken ends.

Isochromosome: Symmetrical chromosome composed of duplicated long or short arms.

Karyotype: Arrangement of chromosomes into various groups according to size, centromere location, and other morphologic features.

Karyotype symbols:
p: short arm
q: long arm
del: deletion
t: translocation
plus (+): gain of a chromosome
minus (−): loss of a chromosome

Marker chromosome: Abnormal chromosome easily identified by its peculiar morphology.

Modal chromosome number: Predominant number of chromosomes in a cell population with a variable number of chromosomes.

---

*Cytogenetic terms are defined according to Sandberg.[30]

Monosomy: Absence of one member of a homologous pair of chromosomes.

Polyploidy: A multiple of the modal number of chromosomes.

Pseudodiploidy: 46 chromosomes with an abnormal karyotype.

Telomere: Terminal region of a chromosome.

Translocation: Breakage followed by transfer of chromosome material between chromosomes.

Trisomy: Presence of an extra (third) copy of a given chromosome in addition to a normal homologous pair.

FRED G. BARKER II

MARK A. ISRAEL

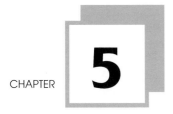

CHAPTER **5**

Molecular Genetics

Cancer manifests itself as uncontrolled cellular proliferation of cells that lack the differentiated features of the tissue in which they arise. Current theories of malignant transformation postulate that this process is a consequence of the sequential accumulation of multiple genetic alterations, each of which contributes to the expression of a tumor's malignant characteristics. The types of genetic alterations found in neoplastic cells may be broadly grouped into two classes: (1) the loss of genetic functions that normally suppress cell division (*tumor suppressor genes*), or (2) the enhanced or inappropriate activity of genes that promote cell division and an anaplastic phenotype (*oncogenes*). Structural alterations or dysregulation of these key genes leads to inappropriate expression of many other genes that encode proteins critical for various aspects of malignancy, including excessive cell division, invasion of neighboring tissues, resistance to antineoplastic therapies, and ability to metastasize.

Both oncogene activation and loss or mutational inactivation of tumor suppressor genes have been reported in human glial tumors. Evidence from cytogenetic studies suggests that the roster of currently recognized genetic alterations in brain tumors forms a subset of the mutations that may eventually be recognized to be important in glial oncogenesis (see Chapter 4 for discussion of cytogenetic studies of gliomas). This chapter reviews molecular genetic alterations known or suspected to be associated with glial neoplasia, beginning with tumors of the astrocyte lineage and progressing to tumors of other histologic types, about which less is currently known.

TUMOR SUPPRESSOR GENES IN ASTROCYTOMAS

Tumor suppressor genes (Table 5–1) are genes whose protein products function to suppress the neoplastic phenotype. Lack of functional tumor suppressor gene products releases the cell from physiologic inhibitory growth controls, thereby contributing to abnormal proliferation. Such genes commonly function in a dominant fashion, such that a single intact copy of the gene is sufficient to maintain the normal phenotype. Whereas a cell with one intact copy and one

defective copy of a tumor suppressor gene may be phenotypically normal, a somatic mutation in the intact copy of the gene results in inactivation of this genetic locus, contributing to tumor development by enhancing the cell's ability to grow in a neoplastic fashion (Fig. 5–1). This model, known as the "two-hit" model of neoplasia, was first proposed by Knudson to explain the familial occurrence of bilateral retinoblastoma.[1]

A variety of inherited predispositions to neoplasia within the central nervous system (CNS) have been proposed as additional examples of this mechanism: neurofibromatosis types 1 and 2, in which astrocytomas and ependymomas, respectively, are observed within the brain and spinal cord; tuberous sclerosis, in which subependymal giant cell astrocytomas are observed; and the Li-Fraumeni syndrome, a rare disorder characterized by the familial clustering of soft tissue sarcomas, breast cancer, and CNS tumors. Von Hippel-Lindau disease, in which cerebellar hemangioblastomas and renal cell carcinoma are seen, and Turcot syndrome, in which colonic polyposis is associated with astrocytomas and medulloblastomas, are additional examples of disorders that have been linked to, or are expected to be associated with, the loss of tumor suppressor gene function. It is likely that some tumors occurring in known kindreds afflicted by familial glioma also arise through the loss of tumor suppressor genes that have not yet been discovered.

The majority of human glial tumors are not associated

TABLE 5–1
TUMOR SUPPRESSOR GENES IMPLICATED IN GLIAL ONCOGENESIS

Gene	Protein Product	Chromosome	References
p53	p53	17p13.1	7, 36–39, 41, 42, 45, 49, 149
NF1	Neurofibromin	17q11.2	106–108
NF2	Merlin	22q12	113, 227
TSC1		9q34	216
TSC2	Tuberin	16p13.3	217
APC	APC	5q21	117
RB1	Rb	13q14	121, 123, 124
CDKN2	p16	9p21	134, 135

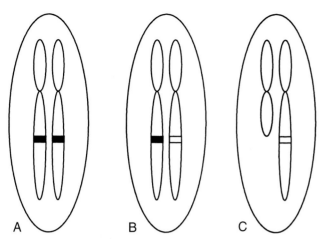

Figure 5–1 The "two-hit" theory of oncogenesis due to loss of tumor suppressor gene function.[1] *A*, Normal cell, with two wild-type alleles for a tumor suppressor gene (black bands). *B*, Typical cell in a person with one wild-type allele (black band) and one germline mutant non-functioning allele (empty band). This cell is phenotypically normal, because the function of tumor suppressor genes is typically dominant. *C*, Tumor cell arising in a patient with an inherited mutant allele. A partial deletion of the chromosome on which the tumor suppressor gene is located has caused the complete loss of tumor suppressor function.

with any known hereditary predisposition to cancer. Although some genetic alterations that have been associated with hereditary cancer syndromes may be important in sporadic tumors as well, the complex process of glial oncogenesis is already known to involve molecular genetic alterations that have not yet been associated with hereditary syndromes. In other tumor types, molecular alterations that are important causes of hereditary cancer syndromes do not seem to play important roles in causing sporadic tumors. An example is the BRCA1 (for *breast cancer 1, early onset*) gene product, which is abnormal in many patients with hereditary breast cancer but appears to be rarely mutated in cases of sporadic breast carcinomas.[2, 3] The present level of understanding of both familial glioma syndromes and sporadic glial tumors is still far from complete.

p53 and the Li-Fraumeni Syndrome

The tumor suppressor gene p53 is the gene most commonly affected in human cancer: it has been found to be mutated in nearly half of all malignant tumors screened to date. Among these tumor types are astrocytomas, anaplastic astrocytomas, and glioblastomas.[4-10] The p53 gene, located on chromosome 17p, encodes a protein of 53 kD known as p53. The p53 protein was first identified as a binding partner of the large T antigen of the DNA virus SV40.[11, 12] Since then, p53 has been found to influence multiple aspects of cellular metabolism including cell cycle control,[13, 14] DNA repair after radiation damage,[5] genomic stability,[15, 16] and the induction of programmed cell death, apoptosis.[17-19]

The p53 protein can induce or repress the transcription of multiple genes whose regulatory regions contain specific DNA sequences to which p53 binds.[20, 21] One such gene, whose expression is induced by p53 and which may mediate several of the apparent effects of p53, is an inhibitor of cyclin-dependent kinases known as p21, WAF1, or CIP1.[13, 14, 17, 22] Cyclin-dependent kinases regulate the passage of cells through the cell cycle. By inhibiting cyclin-dependent kinases, WAF1/CIP1 prevents cells from entering the S phase of the cell cycle, in which DNA is synthesized. WAF1/CIP1 also appears to be part of the pathway through which p53 induces G1 arrest following DNA damage[23, 24] and mediates apoptosis.[17] Although the gene for WAF1/CIP1 is located on chromosome 6p21, a region known to be deleted in some human gliomas,[25] screening of 142 gliomas detected no mutations in the WAF1/CIP1 gene.[26]

The amino-terminal portion of the p53 protein resembles known transcriptional activators in charge and structure, and the primary structure of the carboxyl-terminus suggests a non–sequence-specific DNA-binding function.[10] The intervening portion of the molecule contains domains responsible for binding to various viral oncoproteins (such as the SV40 large T antigen), as well as to sequence-specific DNA binding sites.[8] This portion of the protein is essential for suppression of cell growth.[27] Five regions of the protein have been highly conserved throughout evolution. Inactivating mutations of p53 that occur in human cancers appear to be clustered in these conserved domains. Analysis of the three-dimensional structure of the core portion of the p53 molecule complexed with DNA indicates that many of the mutations found in human cancer affect amino acids that are in direct contact with the bound DNA.[28] Among tumor suppressor genes, p53 is unusual in that many tumor-associated mutations are missense mutations (in which a single peptide residue is replaced by another amino acid) rather than nonsense mutations (in which the protein product is prematurely truncated). The high frequency of dominant-negative missense mutations, resulting in defective p53 proteins that have the capacity to inactivate normal p53 molecules encoded by the nonmutated copy of the p53 gene, may explain this observation. The functional form of wild-type p53 is a dimer or tetramer,[10] and a single defective protein may render the entire oligomeric complex nonfunctional.

Wild-type p53 has a short half-life within the nucleus (less than 30 minutes).[29] Mutant forms have a significantly longer half-life.[30] This difference, as well as the availability of monoclonal antibodies specific for mutant forms of p53,[31] enables the rapid detection of mutant p53 molecules within tumors by immunohistochemical techniques.[32-34] More recent work has shown that wild-type p53 can accumulate within astrocytic tumors that do not harbor mutations of the p53 gene.[35-39] Definitive assessment of p53 function within a specific tumor thus rests on examination of the coding sequences of the gene, and not simply on the presence of immunohistochemically detectable p53 protein in a tumor specimen.

Rapid methods for the detection of p53 point mutations have been developed. The most widely used has been single-strand configuration polymorphism (SSCP) evaluation (Fig. 5–2).[40] More than 400 human astrocytomas and glioblastomas have been examined for p53 mutations by a number of groups using SSCP.[36, 37, 39, 41-56] Several conclusions can be drawn from these series (Table 5–2). The first is that p53 mutations are approximately as common in low-grade diffuse astrocytomas as in glioblastomas: the combined mutation rate in these studies was 40% for grade 2 tumors, 32%

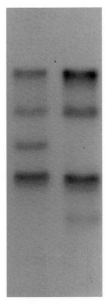

Figure 5–2 Single-strand conformation polymorphism analysis of exon 5 of the p53 gene. Genomic DNA from tumor cell lines is amplified with the polymerase chain reaction using primers specific for exon 5 of the p53 gene. PCR products are then submitted to gel electrophoresis under non-denaturing conditions, allowing single-stranded PCR products to migrate at characteristic individual rates due to secondary structure. *Left lane,* DNA from cell line SF210, which has a point mutation in exon 5. *Right lane,* DNA from cell line T98G, which has a wild-type exon 5 sequence. SF210 DNA displays a band with aberrant migration (third band from top, *left lane*).

for grade 3 tumors, and 27% for grade 4 tumors (see Table 5–2). This may indicate that the mutation of p53 is associated principally with the change from normal tissue to low-grade neoplasia, rather than with progression from low-grade to high-grade tumors—a pattern proposed for other tumor types. In one reported series of low-grade astrocytomas that recurred as more anaplastic gliomas, nearly half of the original tumors displayed p53 mutations, and no new mutations

TABLE 5–2
p53 MUTATIONS IN ASTROCYTIC TUMORS

Patient Characteristic	No. Positive/No. Screened	% Positive
Sex		
Female	27/87	31
Male	40/131	31
Age (yr)		
<40	42/96	44
>40	43/160	27
WHO Grade		
II	31/78	40
III	24/78	32
IV	70/258	27
Loss of heterozygosity (17p)		
No LOH	22/127	17
LOH	42/68	62
Primary vs. recurrent tumor		
Primary	62/189	33
Recurrent	20/52	38

Data pooled from 14 reported series of human astrocytic tumors in patients aged 18 or older.[36, 37, 39, 41, 44, 45, 47, 49–52, 55, 56, 62]

were found in the high-grade recurrences.[57] However, some groups have reported the development of a p53 mutation as a glial tumor progressed to a higher degree of malignancy.[46, 53] This observation would support the clonal evolution model of neoplasia originally proposed by Nowell[58] and elaborated by Fearon and Vogelstein,[59] which proposes that cells accumulate multiple mutations as carcinogenesis progresses. p53 mutations may be an early change in some tumors and a late event in others.[60]

No sex predilection has been noted for p53 mutations in human astrocytic tumors (see Table 5–2). However, the age of the patient is correlated with the frequency of p53 mutation: patients aged 18 to 39 years have a significantly higher rate of p53 mutations than do those aged 40 years or older (see Table 5–2). Pediatric patients are an exception: no p53 mutations were found in two series that examined 24 fibrillary astrocytomas, anaplastic astrocytomas, and glioblastomas occurring in patients aged 1 to 18 years.[61, 62]

Mutational loss of DNA from one of the two alleles encoding the p53 gene can be estimated by examining tumor DNA for loss of heterozygosity (LOH) for structural polymorphisms located in the same chromosomal region as p53 (Fig. 5–3). LOH on chromosome 17p (the location of the p53 gene) was very strongly correlated with mutation in the nondeleted p53 allele in the series cited previously (see Table 5–2). This supports the suggestion that p53 mutations are not simply an epiphenomenon of neoplasia, but that they contribute to the development of the malignant glial phenotype. Two other lines of evidence also support this contention. The first is that restoration of the wild-type p53 gene into a glioblastoma cell line lacking functional p53 transcripts inhibited cell growth.[63, 64] The second is the pre-

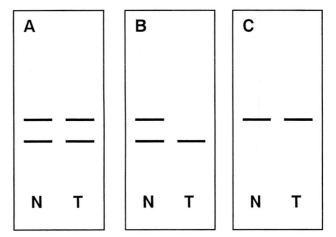

Figure 5–3 Schematic representation of hybridization analysis for restriction enzyme polymorphism loss of heterozygosity. To perform this analysis, DNA isolated from a tumor (T) and from normal somatic cells of the same patient (N) is digested with a restriction enzyme, size fractionated by gel electrophoresis and transferred in situ to a solid matrix and evaluated by hybridization analysis using a locus-specific probe. *A,* This patient's somatic DNA shows heterozygosity for this marker (alleles of two distinct sizes are seen). Because the tumor DNA has both alleles as well, the results are interpreted as showing that there has been no loss of heterozygosity. *B,* This patient's somatic DNA also shows heterozygosity for the marker, but the tumor cells have lost one allele (the upper of the two bands). *C,* This patient's somatic DNA contains two alleles that are the same size, and it is not possible to determine whether the tumor DNA has lost an allele with this assay. The assay is said to be *noninformative.*

disposition for development of a variety of neoplasms, including brain tumors, in patients who inherit one defective copy of the p53 gene.

Germline p53 mutations (mutations borne by every cell in the body) are found in members of families with the Li-Fraumeni syndrome.[65, 66] This syndrome was originally defined as an excess of sarcomas, breast cancer, brain tumors, leukemia, and adrenocortical carcinoma within a kindred.[67–70] Most of the brain tumors that occur in these families are astrocytomas or glioblastomas, although medulloblastomas and choroid plexus tumors also occur.[68, 70] Germline p53 mutations have also been described in patients belonging to families that do not conform to the syndrome originally described by Li and Fraumeni. These include patients with childhood leukemia,[71] breast cancer,[72–74] sarcomas,[75–78] and second malignancies.[79, 80] Despite the heterogeneous clinical manifestations of germline p53 mutations within a family, brain tumors (principally of the astrocytic lineage) remain one of the three most frequent malignancies in these kindreds.[67] Glial tumors in patients with germline p53 mutations tend to occur before age 44 years (27 of 28 tumors in 43 kindreds),[65] and they may have a tendency to begin as low-grade neoplasms.[62, 81–83] It has recently been suggested that glioma patients with multifocal tumors, a second primary malignancy, or a family history of cancer are at increased risk for carrying a germline p53 mutation.[48] This intriguing suggestion, with its implications for screening in asymptomatic family members of the proband with glioma,[84, 85] awaits confirmation by other groups.

Given the apparent importance of p53 mutations in the pathogenesis of glial tumors, several groups have investigated p53 mutation as a potential prognostic factor in patients with gliomas. Some studies relying on immunohistochemical detection of the p53 protein (a putative marker of a mutated p53 gene) in gliomas of various grades have found that immunohistochemically detectable p53 expression predicted poor survival in low-grade astrocytomas,[34, 86] but this finding was not confirmed by other groups of researchers in patients with low-grade astrocytomas[87] or grade 3 and 4 astrocytomas.[41] Reports that analyzed survival of glioma patients by the presence or absence of actual p53 gene mutations have found no statistically significant difference in survival between the two groups.[52, 56, 57]

p53 and the MDM-2 Protein

As noted in the preceding text, p53 was discovered as a cellular protein that bound the SV40 large T oncoprotein.[11, 12] Other proteins, such as the human papilloma virus E6 oncoprotein[88, 89] and the cellular protein MDM2, also have the ability to bind and inactivate the p53 protein. MDM2 was discovered by cloning a highly amplified gene from a spontaneously transformed derivative of mouse 3T3 cells that displayed *m*ultiple *d*ouble *m*inute chromosomes,[90] hence its name. The MDM2 protein binds to the acidic activation domain of p53 and inhibits the ability of p53 to promote transcription.[91, 92] Overexpression of MDM2 protein makes 3T3 cells tumorigenic[93] and immortalizes primary rat embryo fibroblasts, contributing to their oncogenic transformation.[94] MDM2 is thus capable of acting as an oncogene, a gene whose protein product promotes the neoplastic phenotype when overexpressed.

MDM2 gene amplification has been detected in a significant proportion of human sarcomas.[95–97] MDM2 appears to be amplified only in sarcomas that lack p53 mutations.[95, 96] Tumors in which p53 is already inactivated through mutation seem to gain no further growth advantage through MDM2 overexpression. Several groups have examined human gliomas and glioma cell lines for MDM2 amplification.[52, 98–100] Reifenberger and co-workers[98, 101] reported that 10% to 15% of glioblastomas and anaplastic astrocytomas and 7% of glioblastoma cell lines displayed amplification of MDM2, whereas two other groups did not find amplification in any of 57 gliomas examined.[37, 99] In a fourth study, MDM2 amplification was detected in only one tumor (a glioblastoma) out of 120 adult and childhood gliomas examined.[52] Complicating the interpretation of these infrequent positive findings is the observation that genes close to MDM2 on chromosome 12q13–14 are frequently co-amplified in the same amplicon. These genes can include the *gli* oncogene, the CDK4 cyclin-dependent kinase gene (see following section), and other genes of potential importance for oncogenesis.[100, 101] The *gli* oncogene was expressed in a rearranged form in the one glioblastoma that displayed MDM2 amplification in the series of Rasheed and colleagues.[52] Whether one of these genes or another within this same amplicon is important in the oncogenesis of glial tumors is presently unclear.

NF1

NF1 is a large gene (approximately 300 kb, including about 50 exons) located on chromosome 17q11.2.[102] Individuals who inherit a defective copy of this gene have a distinctive syndrome known as von Recklinghausen's neurofibromatosis or neurofibromatosis type 1. This disorder is discussed in detail elsewhere in this book (see Chapter 3). Patients with neurofibromatosis are predisposed to development of pilocytic astrocytomas of the optic pathways (see following text) as well as diffuse astrocytomas of the cerebral hemispheres.[103, 104]

The NF1 gene encodes a protein of 280 kD known as *neurofibromin*.[102] The normal function of this protein may be to inhibit or antagonize the activity of p21-ras, a known oncoprotein.[105] Two forms of the NF1 transcript have been described, and the pattern of expression in sporadic glioblastomas may differ from that seen in normal brain.[106] Only one somatic mutation of the NF1 gene was observed (in a malignant astrocytoma) out of 28 sporadic glial tumors in which the NF1 domain with homology to guanosine triphosphatase (GTPase)-activating proteins was evaluated.[107, 108] Mutations were sought in this region because of the presumed importance of the interaction between neurofibromin and the GTPase-activating protein in regulating p21-ras.[109, 110] However, no large series of glial tumors screened for somatic mutations in the remainder of the NF1 gene has yet been reported, and a role for this gene in the oncogenesis of sporadic glial tumors thus remains speculative.

NF2

The NF2 gene, located on chromosome 22q12, is mutated in patients with neurofibromatosis type 2, a disorder characterized by the occurrence of bilateral acoustic neuromas and multiple meningiomas.[111, 112] Although astrocytic tumors are infrequent findings in patients with neurofibromatosis type 2, the loss of this chromosomal region in some malignant gliomas has prompted the suggestion that this tumor suppressor gene may be involved in the production of sporadic glial tumors.[113] SSCP screening of 30 astrocytic tumors, however, failed to disclose any mutations in the NF2 gene.[113] Based on these preliminary data, it seems unlikely that alterations in the NF2 gene contribute frequently to the genesis of sporadic astrocytomas.

Turcot Syndrome and the APC Gene

Turcot and co-workers[114] first described the occurrence of CNS tumors (a glioblastoma and a medulloblastoma) in two members of a kindred with familial polyposis. Multiple reports have since been made of an association between CNS tumors and familial colonic polyposis, but the mode of inheritance remains uncertain. The discovery of a gene on chromosome 5p, which is mutated in patients with adenomatous polyposis coli (the APC gene),[115] has led to speculation that this gene may be responsible for the manifestations of Turcot syndrome, and may have some importance in astrocytic neoplasia. Hamilton and others[116] studied four kindreds with glioblastomas and colonic tumors. They found no APC mutations, but two families had germline mutations in the DNA mismatch repair genes hMLH1 and hPMS2. Mori and others[117] examined germline DNA from three patients with adenomatous polyposis coli and brain tumors (two medulloblastomas and an astrocytoma) for mutations in the APC gene. None of the patients had a family history of brain tumor. All three patients had germline APC mutations. Examination of DNA from the two medulloblastomas revealed no mutation in the other APC allele. Tumor DNA from the astrocytoma was not examined. No somatic mutations of the APC gene were detected in a large number of sporadically occurring glial tumors that were screened in this report, suggesting that structural alterations of the APC gene may not play an important role in glial oncogenesis.[117]

RB1

The retinoblastoma gene, RB1, is a well-characterized tumor suppressor gene located on chromosome 13q14. Patients with hereditary retinoblastoma have a germline mutation in one RB1 allele: both copies of the RB1 gene are mutated or deleted in tumor tissue from these patients as well as in sporadic retinoblastomas.[118, 119] The cytogenetic observation that some glioblastomas are associated with loss of 13q[120, 121] and the observation that some hereditary retinoblastoma patients also develop brain tumors[122] have prompted speculation that this gene may be important in the pathogenesis of sporadic glial tumors.

Several groups have addressed this question using differ-ent methods. Hamel and colleagues[123] evaluated expression of the Rb protein in glioblastoma cell lines and primary tumors. They found that 1 of 4 anaplastic astrocytomas and 2 of 3 glioblastomas evaluated lacked detectable Rb expression, whereas all lower-grade tumors had detectable Rb expression.[123] Henson and co-workers[124] detected LOH at the RB1 locus in 30% of high-grade astrocytomas, compared with 0% in low-grade gliomas. Four high-grade gliomas with LOH for RB1 had point mutations within the remaining RB1 allele, as assessed by SSCP. Venter and others[121] found that 4 of 9 glioblastomas studied had LOH for the RB1 locus. In one of these four tumors, evidence was present of deletion of a portion of the remaining RB1 allele. In this study, no benign tumors showed allelic loss at the RB1 locus. Tsuzuki and colleagues[125] reported mutations in the RB1 gene in 15 of 52 astrocytomas of grades 2 through 4.

These findings suggest a role for RB1 inactivation in the formation of glial tumors and raise the possibility that RB1 loss or mutation may be a late event in glial carcinogenesis.

p16 and the 9p Tumor Suppressor Gene(s)

Cytogenetic studies of human gliomas and glial tumor cell lines have identified frequent deletions or rearrangements of the short arm of chromosome 9p.[126–131] This suggests that a tumor suppressor gene is located within this region. These deletions have frequently included the interferon-α and interferon-β gene clusters at 9p21–9p22, leading to the suggestion that these may be the genes whose deletion confers the observed growth advantage. This argument has received support from the observation that introduction of the interferon-β gene into a glioblastoma cell line lacking its expression causes growth inhibition.[132]

Other genes important for cellular proliferation may also be affected by a deletion on 9p. One such gene, known as p16 or CDKN2, encodes a 16 kD protein initially isolated as an inhibitor of CDK4, a cyclin-dependent kinase whose normal action is to promote cell division.[22] The CDK4 gene appears to be amplified in several different human tumors, including some glioblastomas,[101, 133] suggesting that overexpression of this gene may contribute to the oncogenic transformation of some cell types. Disruption of the physiologic inhibition of cyclin-dependent kinases is a mechanism of oncogenic action similar to that proposed for p53, which (in its functional form) can induce the expression of WAF1/CIP1, a known inhibitor of cyclin-dependent kinases.[13, 14, 17] The similar mechanism proposed for CDKN2 action has led to the suggestion that CDKN2 may be a tumor suppressor gene located on chromosome 9p that is important in glial oncogenesis.

The CDKN2 gene has been reported to be inactivated through mutation or homozygous deletion in a high proportion of human glial cell lines[134] and primary glial tumors.[135] Deletion of both CDKN2 alleles is a much more common mechanism of inactivation of this gene in glial tumors than is the combination of deletion of one allele and point mutation of the other allele, as is seen in tumors with p53 inactivation. High-grade glial tumors in which RB1 has been inactivated are less likely to contain CDKN2 deletions.[136] CDKN2 participates in the same cell-cycle regulatory pathway that includes RB1, so that CDKN2, and RB1 inactivations are probably functionally redundant. The occurrence of mutations in the CDKN2 gene in some kindreds with familial melanoma[137] makes this gene an interesting candidate for the recently reported syndrome of familial melanoma and astrocytoma.[138]

PROTO-ONCOGENES AND ONCOGENES IN ASTROCYTOMAS

In addition to tumor suppressor genes, whose normal function is to suppress cellular proliferation, several known oncogenes have been implicated in the development of astrocytic tumors (Table 5–3). Proto-oncogenes are genes that function normally to mediate growth and development. When mutated or inappropriately expressed, these genes may have a dramatically altered function or their normal function may be exaggerated or dysregulated, contributing to tumorigenesis (Fig. 5–4). This process is known as activation of the proto-oncogene. Activated proto-oncogenes are known as oncogenes.

Many proto-oncogenes function normally as receptors for growth factors. These genes may be amplified or overexpressed in either their native form or in a mutated form. For example, a mutated transmembrane growth factor gene that lacks the extracellular portion of the protein and is thereby constitutively activated may be expressed. This structural alteration removes the normal activation requirement for the presence of the receptor's physiologic ligand and results in a continuous signal for cell growth. Growth factors and their receptors are discussed in detail elsewhere in this volume (Chapter 6). This chapter highlights their role and the role of other growth-controlling genes as oncogenes important in the pathogenesis of glial tumors.

The EGF Receptor

Gene amplification, leading to either increased numbers of the native or mutated forms of a proto-oncogene, is an

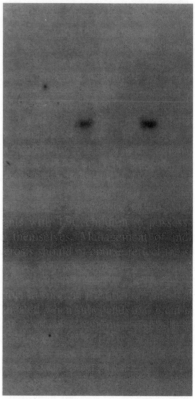

Figure 5–4 Northern blot analyses of messenger RNA (mRNA) for PDGFB expression. mRNA can be detected from total RNA that is prepared from tumor cell lines, size fractionated by gel electrophoresis, and transferred in situ to a solid matrix and hybridized with a specific probe. Two cell lines (U251–O and U343–2:6) express high levels of the c-*sis* proto-oncogene, which encodes the PDGFB chain. (From LaRocca RV, Rosenblum M, Westermark B, et al: Patterns of proto-oncogene expression in human glioma cell lines. J Neurosci Res 1989; 24:97–104.)

TABLE 5–3
PROTO-ONCOGENES IMPLICATED IN GLIAL ONCOGENESIS

Gene	References
Growth factors and receptors	
EGFR	139, 141, 142, 144
PDGF/PDGFR	161, 163, 229
FGF2/FGFR	166–169
IGF1/IGF1R	175–179
c-erbB-2	160
Hepatocyte growth factor receptor (met)	207
Other proto-oncogenes	
TGFB	187–190
myc	196, 197
ras	196
ros	199, 200, 204
gli	205

important mechanism of proto-oncogene activation. The oncogene most frequently amplified in glioblastomas, the EGFR gene, encodes the epidermal growth factor receptor.[139, 140] This transmembrane protein, of molecular weight 170 kD, contains an extracellular domain that binds EGF or TGFA (transforming growth factor-α), a transmembrane domain, and an intracellular domain with tyrosine kinase activity. About 36% of glioblastomas display EGFR amplification, compared with only 7% of anaplastic astrocytomas and 3% of astrocytomas.[140]

EGFR genes amplified in glioblastomas are frequently mutated, encoding shortened forms of the native EGFR molecule.[139, 141 – 144] These deletions can affect either the intracellular or the extracellular portion of the protein.[141] The actual portion of the gene deleted seems to be nonrandom, as several tumors examined have shown very similar deletions.[141, 142] The open reading frame for the native protein is infrequently disrupted by these deletions.[145] Some such mutated proteins have been shown to lack the ability to bind EGF, and these receptors may have constitutive tyrosine kinase activity.[144, 146] Because EGFR mutations often form a new splice junction within a portion of the gene encoding the extracellular domain, a novel peptide sequence may be presented extracellularly in cells that express these modified receptors. It has been possible to generate monoclonal antibodies specific for one such modified protein. These antibodies may prove to be useful for future approaches to diagnostic imaging or targeted antineoplastic therapy.[147]

It has been suggested that EGFR amplification in glioblastoma is exclusively associated with chromosome 10 deletions and that tumors with this combination of characteristics are unlikely to have lost portions of chromosome 17p; in this series, patients with EGFR amplification and loss of chromosome 10 were older than patients with a loss of 17p.[148] Rasheed and others[52] also found that p53 mutations were almost never present in tumors overexpressing EGFR, although another group noted the combination of both findings in 22% of glioblastomas.[45] Lang and colleagues[149] noted EGFR amplification in 7 of 34 glioblastoma samples; 2 of these 7 tumors had p53 mutations by SSCP analysis.

The prognostic importance of EGFR amplification within a glioblastoma remains unclear. Although some groups have found that EGFR amplification was associated with a poor outcome,[150–154] others have disagreed.[155–158] All series have been relatively small. If EGFR amplification is associated with older age in glioblastoma patients,[148] a worse prognosis would be expected, as older age is a strong predictor of shorter survival in this disease (see Chapter 61 for prognostic factors in gliomas).

A gene closely related to EGFR is the Neu or c-erbB-2 gene, which encodes a 185 kD transmembrane receptor.[159] Although overexpression of this gene has been detected in astrocytic tumors of various grades, the gene has not been found to be amplified in glial tumors, and overexpression is not clearly related to prognosis.[160]

PDGF and Its Receptors

Another growth factor receptor encoded by a putative proto-oncogene known to be expressed in some gliomas is the platelet-derived growth factor receptor (PDGFR).[161] Platelet-derived growth factor (PDGF) exists in three isoforms, and there are two known forms of PDGF receptor: PDGFRA and PDGFRB. PDGF is expressed by many glioblastomas, and some glioblastomas also express PDGFRA, forming a potentially important autocrine stimulus for proliferation in these tumors.[162] Amplification of PDGFR genes is much less common than EGFR amplification. One group found PDGFRA amplification in 4 of 50 glioblastomas,[163] and only 1 glioblastoma with PDGFR amplification was found in another series of 120 glial tumors.[52] In one glioma, amplification of PDGFRA was found in conjunction with deletion of the portion of the gene encoding the extracellular domain, analogous to the EGFR findings discussed previously.[164] Although PDGFRB may be overexpressed in endothelial

cells within glial tumors, glial cells themselves do not appear to overexpress this gene.[162]

FGF and Its Receptors

Basic fibroblast growth factor (FGF2) is a mitogen and an angiogenic factor that is expressed by nontransformed astrocytes.[165] Transformed astrocytes appear to express increased amounts of FGF2.[166–168] Both transformed and nontransformed astrocytes also express two forms of a high-affinity receptor for FGF2: FGFR1 and FGFR2.[169–172] It has been proposed that FGF2 serves as an autocrine growth factor in astrocytic tumors.[169] Introduction of an antisense mRNA to FGF2 has been shown to decrease growth in two astrocytoma cell lines,[173, 174] which supports this suggestion.

IGF1 and Its Receptor

Another growth factor and receptor combination implicated in the genesis and progression of glial tumors is insulin-like growth factor 1 (IGF1) and its high-affinity receptor, IGF1R.[175–177] Trojan and colleagues[178, 179] have shown that transfection of rat C6 glioma cells with an antisense mRNA for IGF1 abolishes their tumorigenicity. Interestingly, when transplanted into an animal already bearing a C6 tumor, these transfected cells appear to confer on the host animal an immune response to the nontransfected tumor that causes its rejection.[179] The IGF1 receptor has also been shown to be necessary for growth of the human glioblastoma cell line T98G.[180] Transfection of C6 glioma cells with antisense mRNA for the IGF1 receptor has a similar effect to that noted with IGF1 antisense treatment: transfected cells lose tumorigenicity and become immunogenic.[181]

TGFB

The transforming growth factor-β (TGFB) family of proteins has complex roles in cellular proliferation and differentiation,[182] and may play important roles in the pathogenesis of glial tumors. TGFB1 was identified as a factor capable of inducing anchorage-independent growth in nontransformed rat kidney cells.[183] TGFB2 was initially isolated from media that had been conditioned by a glioblastoma cell line as a factor that suppressed T cells.[184–186] Both TGFB1 and TGFB2 are expressed by glial tumor cells.[187, 188] Paradoxically, TGFB1 suppresses growth of human astrocytes and glioma cell lines, but it also enhances glial tumor cell migration and invasiveness in vitro.[189]

Both TGFB1 and TGFB2 have powerful immunosuppressant properties. These include the ability to inhibit T-cell–mediated tumor cytotoxicity, lymphokine-activated killer- and natural killer-cell activation, and B-cell function.[190, 191] T cells from glioblastoma patients (both from peripheral blood and those that have infiltrated the tumor itself) have an impaired response to mitogens,[192] and a variety of cell-mediated immune functions are abnormal in these patients.[193] It has been suggested that these deficits are due to TGFB2 secretion by the tumor.[194] Transfection of early-passage glioblastoma cell lines with antisense oligonucleotides to TGFB2 inhibits TGFB2 production, which results in increased cytotoxicity and proliferation of autologous peripheral lymphocytes in mixed cultures.[195]

Other Proto-oncogenes

Several other oncogenes have been reported to be amplified or overexpressed in human gliomas or glial tumor cell lines. The c-*myc* proto-oncogene, which encodes a transcription factor, was overexpressed in 86% of glioblastomas compared with 5% of low-grade glial tumors in one study.[196] A number of glial cell lines also express high levels of c-myc mRNA.[197] However, amplification of the c-myc gene itself is a rare event in human gliomas: only 2 of 185 glial tumors in two series displayed c-myc gene amplification.[52, 149] The closely related N-myc oncogene has been reported to be amplified in 2 of 47 glioblastomas.[198]

Overexpression of the Ha-*ras* and N-*ras* protein products, cell-membrane-associated GTP-binding proteins, have also been reported in gliomas (71% of high-grade tumors, compared with 0% of low-grade tumors).[196] As with c-*myc*, amplification of the N-*ras* gene at the DNA level is only rarely detected in human glioma specimens.[149] The c-*ros* oncogene, which encodes a transmembrane receptor with tyrosine kinase activity, has been found to be overexpressed in a number of glioblastoma cell lines[199]; however, overexpression has been found only rarely in primary glial tumors.[200–203] A cytosolic tyrosine kinase, with homology to ros, that is not found in normal glial tissue, has recently been described in glioblastomas.[204]

Other oncogenes rarely found to be amplified or overexpressed in glial tumors include the *gli* gene, which encodes a DNA-binding protein with a zinc finger motif,[52, 205, 206] and the *met* gene, which represents a receptor for hepatocyte growth factor.[207] The significance of these rarely amplified genes is presently uncertain.

OTHER TUMOR TYPES

Pilocytic Astrocytomas

These tumors frequently occur in the optic pathways of patients with neurofibromatosis type 1, leading to the hypothesis that the NF1 gene might be important in the genesis of sporadic pilocytic astrocytomas. One study identified deletion of chromosome 17q (the location of the NF1 gene) in 20% of pilocytic astrocytomas,[208] the majority of which were sporadically occurring tumors. One pilocytic astrocytoma in this series that showed loss of heterozygosity for 17q loci arose in a patient with neurofibromatosis type 1.[208] Structural analysis of the NF1 gene in these tumors has not yet been reported. Deletion or mutation of the p53 locus is very rare in pilocytic astrocytomas.[36, 39, 47, 51, 52, 61]

Pleomorphic Xanthoastrocytomas

Little is known about the genetic basis of these rare tumors. One pleomorphic xanthoastrocytoma (PXA) has been re-

ported in a patient with neurofibromatosis type 1,[209] but the NF1 gene has not yet been examined in a PXA. The cytogenetic observation of chromosome 22 loss in a single PXA suggests that the NF2 gene may be important in the development of these tumors.[210]

Subependymal Giant Cell Astrocytomas

These uncommon tumors seem to occur only in patients afflicted by tuberous sclerosis (TS), an autosomal dominant condition characterized by a number of hamartomatous lesions that are rarely seen sporadically.[211, 212] This disorder has been mapped to two distinct chromosomal regions, one on 9q34 (known as the TSC1 locus) and the second on 16p13.3 (TSC2).[213–216] A candidate gene on 16p13.3, with homology to a known GTPase-activating protein, has been cloned, and deletions within the gene have been confirmed in patients with TS.[217] LOH for markers located near TSC2 was found in one subependymal giant cell astrocytoma (SGCA) from a TS patient, suggesting that the normal TSC2 allele was lost in this tumor.[218] In an SGCA from another patient, whose TS appeared to result from a maternally inherited TSC1 allele, the paternal (normal) copy of the TSC1 region was found to be deleted.[219] Both TS loci have thus been implicated in the tumorigenesis of SGCAs.

Desmoplastic Astrocytoma of Infancy

Desmoplastic astrocytoma of infancy (DCAI) is a rare tumor, and little is known of its molecular genetic basis. One group reported no p53 mutations in four cases studied.[220]

Oligodendrogliomas

A number of oligodendrogliomas, anaplastic oligodendrogliomas, and mixed oligoastrocytomas have been examined for mutations at the p53 locus. Only 5 of 53 oligodendrogliomas or anaplastic oligodendrogliomas in four studies were found to have p53 mutations.[52, 55, 221, 222] The observation that 75% of oligodendrogliomas are positive for the p53 protein by immunohistochemistry is thus of uncertain significance.[223]

EGFR amplification has also been sought in tumors of the oligodendrocyte lineage. None of 21 oligodendrocytomas and only 1 of 11 anaplastic oligodendrogliomas demonstrated EGFR amplification in five series.[52, 139, 141, 143, 153]

Although cytogenetic studies of oligodendrogliomas have shown frequent deletions of chromosome 19q, which suggests a tumor suppressor gene at this location, a putative tumor suppressor gene has not yet been isolated.[224–226] The occasional deletion of chromosome 9p in oligodendrogliomas[127] suggests that the CDKN2/p16 locus may be lost in some oligodendroglial tumors, but this question has not yet been examined systematically.

Ependymomas

Loss of chromosome 22q has frequently been noted in cytogenetic studies of ependymomas.[224] The NF2 gene has been mapped to chromosome 22q, and patients with neurofibromatosis type 2 are predisposed to development of ependymomas. Rubio and co-workers[113] examined eight sporadic ependymomas for NF2 mutations. One mutation was found in a tumor that also had lost the remaining wild-type allele.[113] Another group found no NF2 mutations in 20 sporadic pediatric ependymomas.[227]

Only one p53 mutation that caused an alteration in protein sequence was found in 59 ependymomas evaluated by five groups.[50, 52, 221, 222, 227] One patient with a germline p53 mutation in whom an anaplastic ependymoma developed has also been reported.[228]

Of 10 ependymomas and 15 ''ependymal tumors'' screened for amplification of EGFR or other oncogenes in two series,[52, 101] none had detectable amplification or alterations.

ACKNOWLEDGMENTS

The authors thank the Preuss Foundation, the Betz Foundation, and the Nissen family for their support of the research included in this chapter. F.G.B. was supported by NCI training grant CA 09291.

REFERENCES

1. Knudson AG: Mutation and cancer: Statistical study of retinoblastoma. Proc Natl Acad Sci USA 1971; 68:820.
2. Miki Y, Swensen J, Shattuck-Eidens D, et al: A strong candidate for the breast and ovarian cancer susceptibility gene BRCA1. Science 1994; 266:66.
3. Futreal PA, Liu Q, Shattuck-Eidens D, et al: BRCA1 mutations in primary breast and ovarian carcinomas. Science 1994; 266:120.
4. Harris CC, Hollstein M: Clinical implications of the p53 tumor-suppressor gene. N Engl J Med 1993; 329:1318.
5. Karp JE, Broder S: New directions in molecular medicine. Cancer Res 1994; 54:653.
6. Levine AJ, Perry ME, Chang A, et al: The 1993 Walter Hubert Lecture: The role of the p53 tumour-suppressor gene in tumorigenesis. Br J Cancer 1994; 69:409.
7. Louis DN: The p53 gene and protein in human brain tumors. J Neuropathol Exp Neurol 1994; 53:11.
8. Prives C, Manfredi JJ: The p53 tumor suppressor protein: Meeting review. Genes Dev 1993; 7:529.
9. Soussi T, Legros Y, Lubin R, et al: Multifactorial analysis of p53 alteration in human cancer: A review. Int J Cancer 1994; 57:1.
10. Zambetti GP, Levine AJ: A comparison of the biological activities of wild-type and mutant p53. FASEB J 1993; 7:855.
11. Lane DP, Crawford LV: T antigen is bound to a host protein in SV40-transformed cells. Nature 1979; 278:261.
12. Linzer DI, Levine AJ: Characterization of a 54K dalton cellular SV40 tumor antigen present in SV40-transformed cells and uninfected embryonal carcinoma cells. Cell 1979; 17:43.
13. el-Deiry WS, Tokino T, Velculescu VE, et al: WAF1, a potential mediator of p53 tumor suppression. Cell 1993; 75:817.
14. Harper JW, Adami GR, Wei N, et al: The p21 Cdk-interacting protein Cip1 is a potent inhibitor of G1 cyclin-dependent kinases. Cell 1993; 75:805.
15. Livingstone LR, White A, Sprouse J, et al: Altered cell cycle arrest and gene amplification potential accompany loss of wild-type p53. Cell 1992; 70:923.
16. Yin Y, Tainsky MA, Bischoff FZ, et al: Wild-type p53 restores cell cycle control and inhibits gene amplification in cells with mutant p53 alleles. Cell 1992; 70:937.
17. el-Deiry WS, Harper JW, O'Connor PM, et al: WAF1/CIP1 is induced in p53-mediated G1 arrest and apoptosis. Cancer Res 1994; 54:1169.
18. Lowe SW, Schmitt EM, Smith SW, et al: p53 is required for radiation-induced apoptosis in mouse thymocytes. Nature 1993; 362:847.
19. Yonisch-Rouach E, Resnitzky D, Lotem J, et al: Wild-type p53 induces apoptosis of myeloid leukaemic cells that is inhibited by interleukin-6. Nature 1991; 352:345.
20. Mack DH, Vartikar J, Pipas JM, et al: Specific repression of TATA-mediated but not initiator-mediated transcription by wild-type p53. Nature 1993; 363:281.
21. Vogelstein B, Kinzler KW: p53 function and dysfunction. Cell 1992; 70:523.
22. Serrano M, Hannon GJ, Beach D: A new regulatory motif in cell-cycle control causing specific inhibition of cyclin D/CDK4. Nature 1993; 366:704.
23. Slebos RJ, Lee MH, Plunkett BS, et al: p53-dependent G1 arrest involves pRB-related proteins and is disrupted by the human papillomavirus 16 E7 oncoprotein. Proc Natl Acad Sci USA 1994; 91:5320.
24. Dulic V, Kaufmann WK, Wilson SJ, et al: p53-dependent inhibition of cyclin-dependent kinase activities in human fibroblasts during radiation-induced G1 arrest. Cell 1994; 76:1013.
25. Liang BC, Ross DA, Greenberg HS, et al: Evidence of allelic imbalance of chromosome 6 in human astrocytomas. Neurology 1994; 44:533.
26. Koopman J, Maintz D, Schild S, et al: Multiple polymorphisms, but no mutations, in the WAF1/CIP1 gene in human brain tumours. Br J Cancer 1995; 72:1230.
27. Pietenpol JA, Tokino T, Thiagalingam S, et al: Sequence-specific transcriptional activation is essential for growth suppression by p53. Proc Natl Acad Sci USA 1994; 91:1998.
28. Cho Y, Gorina S, Jeffrey PD, et al: Crystal structure of a p53 tumor suppressor-DNA complex: Understanding tumorigenic mutations. Science 1994; 265:346.
29. Gronostajski RM, Goldberg AJ, Pardee AB: Energy requirement for degradation of tumor-associated protein p53. Mol Cell Biol 1984; 4:442.
30. Finlay CA, Hinds PW, Tan T-H, et al: Activating mutations for transformation by p53 produce a gene product that forms an hsc-70-p53 complex with an altered half-life. Mol Cell Biol 1988; 8:531.
31. Gannon JV, Greaves R, Iggo R, et al: Activating mutations in p53 produce a common conformational effect: A monoclonal antibody specific for the mutant form. EMBO J 1990; 9:1595.
32. Ellison DW, Gatter KC, Steart PV, et al: Expression of the p53 protein in a spectrum of astrocytic tumours. J Pathol 1992; 168:383.
33. Haapasalo H, Isola J, Sallinen P, et al: Aberrant p53 expression in astrocytic neoplasms of the brain: Association with proliferation. Am J Pathol 1993; 142:1347.
34. Jaros E, Perry RH, Adam L, et al: Prognostic implications of p53 protein, epidermal growth factor receptor, and Ki-67 labelling in brain tumours. Br J Cancer 1992; 66:373.
35. Koga H, Zhang S, Kumanishi T, et al: Analysis of p53 gene mutations in low- and high-grade astrocytomas by polymerase chain reaction-assisted single-strand conformation polymorphism and immunohistochemistry. Acta Neuropathol 1994; 87:225.
36. Lang FF, Miller DC, Pisharody S, et al: High frequency of p53 protein accumulation without p53 gene mutation in human juvenile pilocytic, low grade and anaplastic astrocytomas. Oncogene 1994; 9:949.
37. Newcomb EW, Madonia WJ, Pisharody S, et al: A correlative study of p53 protein alteration and p53 gene mutation in glioblastoma multiforme. Brain Pathol 1993; 3:229.
38. Rubio M-P, von Deimling A, Yandell DW, et al: Accumulation of wild type p53 protein in human astrocytomas. Cancer Res 1993; 53:3465.
39. Wu JK, Ye Z, Darras BT: Frequency of p53 tumor suppressor gene mutations in human primary brain tumors. Neurosurgery 1993; 33:824.
40. Orita M, Suzuki Y, Sekiya T, et al: Rapid and sensitive detection of point mutations and DNA polymorphisms using the polymerase chain reaction. Genomics 1989; 5:874.
41. Chozick BS, Weicker ME, Pezzullo JC, et al: Pattern of mutant p53 expression in human astrocytomas suggests the existence of alternate pathways of tumorigenesis. Cancer 1994; 73:406.
42. Chung R, Whaley J, Kley N, et al: TP53 gene mutations and 17p deletions in human astrocytomas. Genes Chromosom Cancer 1991; 3:323.
43. del Arco A, Garcia J, Arribas C, et al: Timing of p53 mutations during astrocytoma tumorigenesis. Hum Mol Genet 1993; 2:1687.

44. Frankel RH, Bayona W, Koslow M, et al: p53 mutations in human malignant gliomas: Comparison of loss of heterozygosity with mutation frequency. Cancer Res 1992; 52:1427.

45. Fults D, Brockmeyer D, Tullous MW, et al: p53 mutation and loss of heterozygosity on chromosomes 17 and 10 during human astrocytoma progression. Cancer Res 1992; 52:674.

46. Hayashi Y, Yamashita J, Yamaguchi K: Timing and role of p53 gene mutation in the recurrence of glioma. Biochem Biophys Res Commun 1991; 180:1145.

47. Hunter SB, Bandea C, Swan D, et al: Mutations in the p53 gene in human astrocytomas: Detection by single-strand conformation polymorphism analysis and direct DNA sequencing. Mod Pathology 1993; 6:442.

48. Kyritsis AP, Bondy ML, Xiao M, et al: Germline p53 gene mutations in subsets of glioma patients. JNCI 1994; 86:344.

49. Louis DN, von Deimling A, Chung RY, et al: Comparative study of p53 gene and protein alterations in human astrocytic tumors. J Neuropathol Exp Neurol 1993; 52:31.

50. Mashiyama S, Murakami Y, Yoshimoto T, et al: Detection of p53 gene mutations in human brain tumors by single-strand conformation polymorphism analysis of polymerase chain reaction products. Oncogene 1991; 6:1313.

51. Ohgaki H, Eibl RH, Schwab M, et al: Mutations of the p53 tumor suppressor gene in neoplasms of the human nervous system. Mol Carcinog 1993; 8:74.

52. Rasheed BK, McLendon RE, Herndon JE, et al: Alterations of the TP53 gene in human gliomas. Cancer Res 1994; 54:1324.

53. Sidransky D, Mikkelsen T, Schwechheimer K, et al: Clonal expansion of p53 mutant cells is associated with brain tumour progression. Nature 1992; 355:846.

54. von Deimling A, Eibl RH, Ohgaki H, et al: p53 mutations are associated with 17p allelic loss in grade II and grade III astrocytoma. Cancer Res 1992; 52:2987.

55. Tenan M, Colombo BM, Pollo B, et al: p53 mutations and microsatellite analysis of heterozygosity in malignant gliomas. Cancer Genet Cytogenet 1994; 74:139.

56. Kraus JA, Bolln C, Wolf HK, et al: TP53 alterations and clinical outcome in low grade astrocytomas. Genes Chromosom Cancer 1994; 10:143.

57. van Meyel DJ, Ramsay DA, Casson AG, et al: p53 mutation, expression, and DNA ploidy in evolving gliomas: Evidence for two pathways of progression. JNCI 1994; 86:1011.

58. Nowell PC: The clonal evolution of tumor cell populations. Science 1976; 194:23.

59. Fearon ER, Vogelstein B: A genetic model for colorectal tumorigenesis. Cell 1990; 61:759.

60. Aguilar F, Harris CC, Sun T, et al: Geographic variation of p53 mutational profile in nonmalignant human liver. Science 1994; 264:1317.

61. Litofsky NS, Hinton D, Raffel C: The lack of a role for p53 in astrocytomas in pediatric patients. Neurosurgery 1994; 34:967.

62. Chen P, Iavarone A, Fick J, et al: Constitutional p53 mutations associated with brain tumors in young adults. Cancer Genet Cytogenet 1995; 82:106.

63. Mercer WE, Shields MT, Amin M, et al: Negative growth regulation in a glioblastoma tumor cell line that conditionally expresses human wild-type p53. Proc Natl Acad Sci USA 1990; 87:6166.

64. Mercer WE, Shields MT, Lin D, et al: Growth suppression induced by wild-type p53 protein is accompanied by selective down-regulation of proliferating-cell nuclear antigen expression. Proc Natl Acad Sci USA 1991; 88:1958.

65. Malkin D, Li FP, Strong LC, et al: Germ line p53 mutations in a familial syndrome of breast cancer, sarcomas, and other neoplasms. Science 1990; 250:1233.

66. Srivastava S, Zou ZQ, Pirollo K, et al: Germ-line transmission of a mutated p53 gene in a cancer-prone family with Li-Fraumeni syndrome. Nature 1990; 348:747.

67. Birch JM, Hartley AL, Tricker KJ, et al: Prevalence and diversity of constitutional mutations in the p53 gene among 21 Li-Fraumeni families. Cancer Res 1994; 54:1298.

68. Garber JE, Goldstein AM, Kantor AF, et al: Follow-up study of 24 families with Li-Fraumeni syndrome. Cancer Res 1991; 51:6094.

69. Li FP, Fraumeni JF Jr: Soft tissue sarcomas, breast cancer, and other neoplasms. A familial syndrome? Ann Intern Med 1969; 71:747.

70. Li FP, Fraumeni JF Jr, Mulvihill JJ, et al: A cancer family syndrome in 24 kindreds. Cancer Res 1988; 48:5358.

71. Felix CA, Kappel CC, Mitsudomi T, et al: Frequency and diversity of p53 mutations in childhood rhabdomyosarcoma. Cancer Res 1992; 52:2243.

72. Borresen AL, Andersen TI, Garber J, et al: Screening for germ line TP53 mutations in breast cancer patients. Cancer Res 1992; 52:3234.

73. Coles C, Condie A, Chetty U, et al: p53 mutations in breast cancer. Cancer Res 1992; 52:5291.

74. Sidransky D, Tokino T, Helzlsouer K, et al: Inherited p53 gene mutations in breast cancer. Cancer Res 1992; 52:2984.

75. Brugieres L, Gardes M, Moutou C, et al: Screening for germ line p53 mutations in children with malignant tumors and a family history of cancer. Cancer Res 1993; 53:452.

76. Iavarone A, Matthay KK, Steinkirchner TM, et al: Germ-line and somatic p53 gene mutations in multifocal osteogenic sarcoma. Proc Natl Acad Sci USA 1992; 89:4207.

77. Toguchida J, Yamaguchi T, Ritchie B, et al: Mutation spectrum of the p53 gene in bone and soft tissue sarcomas. Cancer Res 1992; 52:6194.

78. McIntyre JF, Smith-Sorensen B, Friend SH, et al: Germline mutations of the p53 tumor suppressor gene in children with osteosarcoma. J Clin Oncol 1994; 12:925.

79. Felix CA, Strauss EA, D'Amico D, et al: A novel germline p53 splicing mutation in a pediatric patient with a second malignant neoplasm. Oncogene 1993; 8:1203.

80. Malkin D, Jolly KW, Barbier N, et al: Germline mutations of the p53 tumor-suppressor gene in children and young adults with second malignant neoplasms. N Engl J Med 1992; 326:1309.

81. Srivastava S, Tong YA, Devadas K, et al: Detection of both mutant and wild-type p53 protein in normal skin fibroblasts and demonstration of a shared ''second hit'' on p53 in diverse tumors from a cancer-prone family with Li-Fraumeni syndrome. Oncogene 1992; 7:987.

82. Sameshima Y, Tsunematsu Y, Watanabe S, et al: Detection of novel germ-line p53 mutations in diverse-cancer-prone families identified by selecting patients with childhood adrenocortical carcinoma. JNCI 1992; 84:703.

83. Scott RJ, Krummenacher F, Mary JL, et al: Vererbbare p53-Mutation bei einem Patienten mit Mehrfachtumoren: Bedeutung für die genetische Beratung. Schweiz Med Wochenschr 1993; 123:1287.

84. Li FP, Garber JE, Friend SH, et al: Recommendations on predictive testing for germ line p53 mutations among cancer-prone individuals. JNCI 1992; 84:1156.

85. National Advisory Council for Human Genome Research: Statement on use of DNA testing for presymptomatic identification of cancer risk. JAMA 1994; 271:785.

86. Pardo FS, Hsu DW, Hedley-Whyte ET, et al: High p53 expression is prognostic of overall survival in adult supratentorial astrocytoma patients. J Neurooncol 1993; 15:S19.

87. Iuzzolino P, Ghimenton C, Nicolato A, et al: p53 protein in low-grade astrocytomas: A study with long-term follow-up. Br J Cancer 1994; 69:586.

88. Scheffner M, Werness BA, Huibregtse JM, et al: The E6 oncoprotein encoded by human papillomavirus types 16 and 18 promotes the degradation of p53. Cell 1990; 63:1129.

89. Lechner MS, Mack DH, Finicle AB, et al: Human papillomavirus E6 proteins bind p53 in vivo and abrogate p53-mediated repression of transcription. EMBO J 1992; 11:3045.

90. Cahilly-Snyder L, Yang-Feng T, Francke U, et al: Molecular analysis and chromosomal mapping of amplified genes isolated from a transformed mouse 3T3 cell line. Somat Cell Mol Genet 1987; 13:235.

91. Momand J, Zambetti GP, Olson DC, et al: The mdm-2 oncogene product forms a complex with the p53 protein and inhibits p53-mediated transactivation. Cell 1992; 69:1237.

92. Oliner JD, Pietenpol JA, Thiagalingam S, et al: Oncoprotein MDM2 conceals the activation domain of tumour suppressor p53. Nature 1993; 362:857.

93. Fakharzadeh SS, Trusko SP, George DL: Tumorigenic potential associated with enhanced expression of a gene that is amplified in a mouse tumor cell line. EMBO J 1991; 10:1565.

94. Finlay CA: The mdm-2 oncogene can overcome wild-type p53 suppression of transformed cell growth. Mol Cell Biol 1993; 13:301.

95. Cordon-Cardo C, Latres E, Drobnjak M, et al: Molecular abnormalities of mdm2 and p53 genes in adult soft tissue sarcomas. Cancer Res 1994; 54:794.

96. Leach FS, Tokino T, Meltzer P, et al: p53 mutation and MDM2 amplification in human soft tissue sarcomas. Cancer Res 1993; 53:2231.
97. Oliner JD, Kinzler KW, Meltzer PS, et al: Amplification of a gene encoding a p53-associated protein in human sarcomas. Nature 1992; 358:80.
98. Reifenberger G, Liu L, Ichimura K, et al: Amplification and overexpression of the MDM2 gene in a subset of human malignant gliomas without p53 mutations. Cancer Res 1993; 53:2736.
99. Saxena A, Clark WC, Robertson JT, et al: Evidence for the involvement of a potential second tumor suppressor gene on chromosome 17 distinct from p53 in malignant astrocytomas. Cancer Res 1992; 52:6716.
100. He J, Reifenberger G, Liu L, et al: Analysis of glioma cell lines for amplification and overexpression of MDM2. Genes Chromosom Cancer 1994; 11:91.
101. Reifenberger G, Reifenberger J, Ichimura K, et al: Amplification of multiple genes from chromosomal region 12q12-14 in human malignant gliomas: Preliminary mapping of the amplicons shows preferential involvement of CDK4, SAS, and MDM2. Cancer Res 1994; 54:4299.
102. Marchuk DA, Collins FS: Molecular genetics of neurofibromatosis 1. *In* Huson SM, Hughes RAC (eds): The Neurofibromatoses: A Pathogenetic and Clinical Overview. London, Chapman & Hall, 1994, p 23.
103. Hughes RAC: Neurological complications of neurofibromatosis 1. *In* Huson SM, Hughes RAC (eds): The Neurofibromatoses: A Pathogenetic and Clinical Overview. London, Chapman & Hall, 1994, p 204.
104. Riccardi VM: Neurofibromatosis. *In* Gomez MR (ed): Neurocutaneous Diseases: A Practical Approach. Boston, Butterworths, 1987, p 11.
105. Andersen LB, Fountain JW, Gutmann DH, et al: Mutations in the neurofibromatosis 1 gene in sporadic malignant melanoma cell lines. Nat Genet 1993; 3:118.
106. Mochizuki H, Nishi T, Bruner JM, et al: Alternative splicing of neurofibromatosis type 1 gene transcript in malignant brain tumors: PCR analysis of frozen-section mRNA. Mol Carcinog 1992; 6:83.
107. Tenan M, Colombo BM, Cajola L, et al: Low frequency of NF1 gene mutations in malignant gliomas (letter). Eur J Cancer 1993; 29A:1217.
108. Li Y, Bollag G, Clark R, et al: Somatic mutations in the neurofibromatosis 1 gene in human tumors. Cell 1992; 69:275.
109. Martin GA, Viskochil D, Bollog G, et al: The GAP related domain of the neurofibromatosis type 1 gene product interacts with ras p21. Cell 1990; 63:843.
110. Xu G, Lin B, Tanaka K, et al: The catalytic domain of the neurofibromatosis type 1 gene product stimulates ras GTPase and complements ira mutants of *S. cerevisiae*. Cell 1990; 63:835.
111. Rouleau GA, Merel P, Lutchman M, et al: Alteration in a new gene encoding a putative membrane-organizing protein causes neurofibromatosis type 2. Nature 1993; 363:515.
112. Trofatter JA, MacCollin MM, Rutter JL, et al: A novel moesin-, ezrin-, radixin-like gene is a candidate for the neurofibromatosis 2 tumor suppressor. Cell 1993; 72:791.
113. Rubio M-P, Correa KM, Ramesh V, et al: Analysis of the neurofibromatosis 2 gene in human ependymomas and astrocytomas. Cancer Res 1994; 54:45.
114. Turcot J, Després J-P, St Pierre F: Malignant tumors of the central nervous system associated with familial polyposis of the colon: Report of two cases. Dis Colon Rectum 1959; 2:465.
115. Groden J, Thliveris A, Samowitz W, et al: Identification and characterization of the familial adenomatous polyposis coli gene. Cell 1991; 66:589.
116. Hamilton SR, Lin B, Parsons RE, et al: The molecular basis of Turcot's syndrome. N Engl J Med 1995; 332:839.
117. Mori T, Nagase H, Horii A, et al: Germ-line and somatic mutations of the APC gene in patients with Turcot syndrome and analysis of APC mutations in brain tumors. Genes Chromosom Cancer 1994; 9:168.
118. Horowitz JM, Park SH, Bogenmann E, et al: Frequent inactivation of the retinoblastoma anti-oncogene is restricted to a subset of human tumor cells. Proc Natl Acad Sci USA 1990; 87:2775.
119. Friend SH, Horowitz JM, Gerber MR, et al: Deletions of a DNA sequence in retinoblastomas and mesenchymal tumors: Organization of the sequence and its encoded protein. Proc Natl Acad Sci USA 1987; 84:9059.
120. Jenkins RB, Kimmel DW, Moertel CA, et al: A cytogenetic study of 53 human gliomas. Cancer Genet Cytogenet 1989; 39:253.
121. Venter DJ, Bevan KL, Ludwig RL, et al: Retinoblastoma gene deletions in human glioblastomas. Oncogene 1991; 6:445.
122. Draper GJ, Sanders BM, Kingston JE: Second primary neoplasms in patients with retinoblastoma. Br J Cancer 1986; 53:661.
123. Hamel W, Westphal M, Shepard HM: Loss in expression of the retinoblastoma gene product in human gliomas is associated with advanced disease. J Neurooncol 1993; 16:159.
124. Henson JW, Schnitker BL, Correa KM, et al: The retinoblastoma gene is involved in malignant progression of astrocytomas. Ann Neurol 1994; 36:714.
125. Tsuzuki T, Tsunoda T, Sakaki T, et al: RB gene mutations in human astrocytomas. Brain Pathol 1994; 4:423.
126. Ichimura K, Schmidt EE, Yamaguchi N, et al: A common region of homozygous deletion in malignant human gliomas lies between the IFN alpha/omega gene cluster and the D9S171 locus. Cancer Res 1994; 54:3127.
127. Bello MJ, de Campos JM, Vaquero J, et al: Molecular and cytogenetic analysis of chromosome 9 deletions in 75 malignant gliomas. Genes Chromosom Cancer 1994; 9:33.
128. James CD, He J, Carlbom E, et al: Chromosome 9 deletion mapping reveals interferon alpha and interferon beta-1 gene deletions in human glial tumors. Cancer Res 1991; 51:1684.
129. James CD, He J, Collins VP, et al: Localization of chromosome 9p homozygous deletions in glioma cell lines with markers constituting a continuous linkage group. Cancer Res 1993; 53:3674.
130. Ransom DT, Ritland SR, Moertel CA, et al: Correlation of cytogenetic analysis and loss of heterozygosity studies in human diffuse astrocytomas and mixed oligo-astrocytomas. Genes Chromosom Cancer 1992; 5:357.
131. Sugawa N, Ekstrand AJ, Ueda S, et al: Frequency of IFN beta 1 gene loss in 47 primary human gliomas. Noshuyo Byori 1993; 10:161.
132. Mizuno M, Yoshida J, Sugita K, et al: Growth inhibition of glioma cells transfected with the human beta-interferon gene by liposomes coupled with a monoclonal antibody. Cancer Res 1990; 50:7826.
133. Khatib ZA, Matsushime H, Valentine M, et al: Coamplification of the CDK4 gene with MDM2 and GLI in human sarcomas. Cancer Res 1993; 53:5535.
134. Kamb A, Gruis NA, Weaver-Feldhaus J, et al: A cell cycle regulator potentially involved in genesis of many tumor types. Science 1994; 264:436.
135. Barker FG, Chen P, Furman F, et al: p16 Deletion and mutation analysis in human brain tumors. J Neurooncol 1996 (in press).
136. Ueki K, Ono Y, Henson JW, et al: CDKN2/p16 or RB alterations occur in the majority of glioblastomas and are inversely correlated. Cancer Res 1996; 56:150.
137. Hussussian CJ, Struewing JP, Goldstein AM, et al: Germline p16 mutations in familial melanoma. Nat Genet 1994; 8:21.
138. Kaufman DK, Kimmel DW, Parisi JE, et al: A familial syndrome with cutaneous malignant melanoma and cerebral astrocytoma. Neurology 1993; 43:1728.
139. Libermann TA, Nusbaum HR, Razon N, et al: Amplification, enhanced expression and possible rearrangement of EGF receptor gene in primary human brain tumours of glial origin. Nature 1985; 313:144.
140. Fuller GN, Bigner SH: Amplified cellular oncogenes in neoplasms of the human central nervous system. Mutat Res 1992; 276:299.
141. Ekstrand AJ, Sugawa N, James CD, et al: Amplified and rearranged epidermal growth factor receptor genes in human glioblastomas reveal deletions of sequences encoding portions of the N- and/or C-terminal tails. Proc Natl Acad Sci USA 1992; 89:4309.
142. Wong AJ, Ruppert JM, Bigner SH, et al: Structural alterations of the epidermal growth factor receptor gene in human gliomas. Proc Natl Acad Sci USA 1992; 89:2965.
143. Chaffanet M, Chauvin C, Laine M, et al: EGF receptor amplification and expression in human brain tumours. Eur J Cancer 1992; 28:11.
144. Ekstrand AJ, Longo N, Hamid ML, et al: Functional characterization of an EGF receptor with a truncated extracellular domain expressed in glioblastomas with EGFR gene amplification. Oncogene 1994; 9:2313.
145. Wong AJ, Zoltick PW, Moscatello DK: The molecular biology and molecular genetics of astrocytic neoplasms. Semin Oncol 1994; 21:139.
146. Humphrey PA, Wong AJ, Vogelstein B, et al: Amplification and expression of the epidermal growth factor receptor gene in human glioma xenografts. Cancer Res 1988; 48:2231.

147. Humphrey PA, Wong AJ, Vogelstein B, et al: Anti-synthetic peptide antibody reacting at the fusion junction of deletion-mutant epidermal growth factor receptors in human glioblastoma. Proc Natl Acad Sci USA 1990; 87:4207.

148. von Deimling A, von Ammon K, Schoenfeld D, et al: Subsets of glioblastoma multiforme defined by molecular genetic analysis. Brain Pathol 1993; 3:19.

149. Lang FF, Miller DC, Koslow M, et al: Pathways leading to glioblastoma multiforme: A molecular analysis of genetic alterations in 65 astrocytic tumors. J Neurosurg 1994; 81:427.

150. Hiesiger EM, Hayes RL, Pierz DM, et al: Prognostic relevance of epidermal growth factor receptor (EGF-R) and c-neu/erbB2 expression in glioblastomas (GBMs). J Neurooncol 1993; 16:93.

151. Torp SH, Helseth E, Dalen A, et al: Relationships between Ki-67 labelling index, amplification of the epidermal growth factor receptor gene, and prognosis in human glioblastomas. Acta Neurochir (Wien) 1992; 117:182.

152. Hurtt MR, Moossy J, Donovan-Peluso M, et al: Amplification of epidermal growth factor receptor gene in gliomas: Histopathology and prognosis. J Neuropathol Exp Neurol 1992; 51:84.

153. Schlegel J, Merdes A, Stumm G, et al: Amplification of the epidermal-growth-factor-receptor gene correlates with different growth behaviour in human glioblastoma. Int J Cancer 1994; 56:72.

154. Leenstra S, Bijlsma EK, Troost D, et al: Allele loss on chromosomes 10 and 17p and epidermal growth factor receptor gene amplification in human malignant astrocytoma related to prognosis. Br J Cancer 1994; 70:684.

155. Pigott TJ, Robson DK, Palmer J, et al: Expression of epidermal growth factor receptor in human glioblastoma multiforme. Br J Neurosurg 1993; 7:261.

156. Dorward NL, Hawkins RA, Whittle IR: Epidermal growth factor receptor activity and clinical outcome in glioblastoma and meningioma. Br J Neurosurg 1993; 7:197.

157. Bigner SH, Burger PC, Wong AJ, et al: Gene amplification in malignant human gliomas: Clinical and histopathologic aspects. J Neuropathol Exp Neurol 1988; 47:191.

158. Diedrich U, Soja S, Behnke J, et al: Amplification of the c-erbB oncogene is associated with malignancy in primary tumours of neuroepithelial tissue. J Neurol 1991; 238:221.

159. Dougall WC, Qian X, Peterson NC, et al: The neu-oncogene: Signal transduction pathways, transformation mechanisms and evolving therapies. Oncogene 1994; 9:2109.

160. Schwechheimer K, Laufle RM, Schmahl W, et al: Expression of neu/c-erbB-2 in human brain tumors. Hum Pathol 1994; 25:772.

161. Maxwell M, Naber SP, Wolfe HJ, et al: Coexpression of platelet-derived growth factor (PDGF) and PDGF-receptor genes by primary human astrocytomas may contribute to their development and maintenance. J Clin Invest 1990; 86:131.

162. Hermanson M, Funa K, Hartman M, et al: Platelet-derived growth factor and its receptors in human glioma tissue: Expression of messenger RNA and protein suggests the presence of autocrine and paracrine loops. Cancer Res 1992; 52:3213.

163. Fleming TP, Saxena A, Clark WC, et al: Amplification and/or overexpression of platelet-derived growth factor receptors and epidermal growth factor receptor in human glial tumors. Cancer Res 1992; 52:4550.

164. Kumabe T, Sohma Y, Kayama T, et al: Amplification of alpha-platelet-derived growth factor receptor gene lacking an exon coding for a portion of the extracellular region in a primary brain tumor of glial origin. Oncogene 1992; 7:627.

165. Constam DB, Fontana A: Not only glioblastoma cells but also untransformed glia cells express transforming growth factor beta. Schweiz Arch Neurol Psychiatr 1993; 144:225.

166. Takahashi JA, Mori H, Fukumoto M, et al: Gene expression of fibroblast growth factors in human gliomas and meningiomas: Demonstration of cellular source of basic fibroblast growth factor mRNA and peptide in tumor tissues. Proc Natl Acad Sci USA 1990; 87:5710.

167. Zagzag D, Miller DC, Sato Y, et al: Immunohistochemical localization of basic fibroblast growth factor in astrocytomas. Cancer Res 1990; 50:7393.

168. Stefanik DF, Rizkalla LR, Soi A, et al: Acidic and basic fibroblast growth factors are present in glioblastoma multiforme. Cancer Res 1991; 51:5760.

169. Morrison RS, Yamaguchi F, Saya H, et al: Basic fibroblast growth factor and fibroblast growth factor receptor I are implicated in the growth of human astrocytomas. J Neurooncol 1994; 18:207.

170. Lai C, Lemke G: An extended family of protein-tyrosine kinase genes differentially expressed in the vertebrate nervous system. Neuron 1991; 6:691.

171. Peters KG, Werner S, Chen G, et al: Two FGF receptor genes are differentially expressed in epithelial and mesenchymal tissues during limb formation and organogenesis in the mouse. Development 1992; 114:233.

172. Ueba T, Takahashi JA, Fukumoto M, et al: Expression of fibroblast growth factor receptor-1 in human glioma and meningioma tissues. Neurosurgery 1994; 34:221.

173. Morrison RS: Suppression of basic fibroblast growth factor expression by antisense oligodeoxynucleotides inhibits the growth of transformed human astrocytes. J Biol Chem 1991; 266:728.

174. Murphy PR, Sato Y, Knee RS: Phosphorothioate antisense oligonucleotides against basic fibroblast growth factor inhibit anchorage-depen dent and anchorage-independent growth of a malignant glioblastom cell line. Mol Endocrinol 1992; 6:877.

175. Glick RP, Gettleman R, Patel K, et al: Insulin and insulin-like growth factor I in brain tumors: Binding and in vitro effects. Neurosurgery 1989; 24:791.

176. Antoniades HN, Galanopoulos T, Neville-Golden J, et al: Expression of insulin-like growth factors I and II and their receptor mRNAs in primary human astrocytomas and meningiomas: In vivo studies using in situ hybridization and immunocytochemistry. Int J Cancer 1992; 50:215.

177. Lowe WL Jr, Meyer T, Karpen CW, et al: Regulation of insulin-like growth factor I production in rat C6 glioma cells: Possible role as an autocrine/paracrine growth factor. Endocrinology 1992; 130:2683.

178. Trojan J, Blossey BK, Johnson TR, et al: Loss of tumorigenicity of rat glioblastoma directed by episome-based antisense cDNA transcription of insulin-like growth factor I. Proc Natl Acad Sci USA 1992; 89:4874.

179. Trojan J, Johnson TR, Rudin SD, et al: Treatment and prevention of rat glioblastoma by immunogenic C6 cells expressing antisense insulin-like growth factor I RNA. Science 1993; 259:94.

180. Ambrose D, Resnicoff M, Coppola D, et al: Growth regulation of human glioblastoma T98G cells by insulin-like growth factor-1 and its receptor. J Cell Physiol 1994; 159:92.

181. Resnicoff M, Sell C, Rubini M, et al: Rat glioblastoma cells expressing an antisense RNA to the insulin-like growth factor-1 (IGF-1) receptor are nontumorigenic and induce regression of wild-type tumors. Cancer Res 1994; 54:2218.

182. Massagué J: The transforming growth factor-beta family. Ann Rev Cell Biol 1990; 6:597.

183. Roberts AB, Anzano MA, Lamb LC, et al: New class of transforming growth factors potentiated by epidermal growth factor: Isolation from non-neoplastic tissues. Proc Natl Acad Sci USA 1981; 78:5339.

184. de Martin R, Haendler B, Hofer-Warbinek R, et al: Complementary DNA for human glioblastoma-derived T cell suppressor factor, a novel member of the transforming growth factor-beta gene family. EMBO J 1987; 6:3672.

185. Fontana A, Hengartner H, de Tribolet N, et al: Glioblastoma cells release interleukin 1 and factors inhibiting interleukin 2-mediated effects. J Immunol 1984; 132:1837.

186. Schwyzer M, Fontana A: Partial purification and biological characterization of a T cell suppressor factor produced by human glioblastoma cells. J Immunol 1985; 134:1003.

187. Naganuma H, Sasaki A, Satoh E, et al: Improved bioassay for the detection of transforming growth factor-beta 1 and beta 2 in malignant gliomas. Neurol Med Chir 1994; 34:143.

188. Olofsson A, Miyazono K, Kanzaki T, et al: Transforming growth factor-beta 1, -beta 2, and -beta 3 secreted by a human glioblastoma cell line. Identification of small and different forms of large latent complexes. J Biol Chem 1992; 267:19482.

189. Merzak A, McCrea S, Koocheckpour S, et al: Control of human glioma cell growth, migration and invasion in vitro by transforming growth factor beta-1. Br J Cancer 1994; 70:199.

190. Kuppner MC, Hamou M-F, Sawamura Y, et al: Inhibition of lymphocyte function by glioblastoma-derived transforming growth factor-beta 2. J Neurosurg 1989; 71:211.

191. Palladino MA, Morris RE, Starnes HF, et al: The transforming growth factor-betas. A new family of immunoregulatory molecules. Ann N Y Acad Sci 1990; 593:181.

192. Miescher S, Whiteside TL, Carrel S, et al: Functional properties of tumor-infiltrating and blood lymphocytes in patients with solid tumors: Effects of tumor cells and their supernatants on proliferative responses of lymphocytes. J Immunol 1986; 136:1899.

193. Roszman T, Elliott L, Brooks W: Modulation of T-cell function by gliomas. Immunol Today 1991; 12:370.

194. Maxwell M, Galanopoulos T, Neville-Golden J, et al: Effect of the expression of transforming growth factor-beta 2 in primary human glioblastomas on immunosuppression and loss of immune surveillance. J Neurosurg 1992; 76:799.

195. Jachimczak P, Bogdahn U, Schneider J, et al: The effect of transforming growth factor-beta 2-specific phosphorothioate-anti-sense oligodeoxynucleotides in reversing cellular immunosuppression in malignant glioma. J Neurosurg 1993; 78:944.

196. Orian JM, Vasilopoulos K, Yoshida S, et al: Overexpression of multiple oncogenes related to histological grade of astrocytic glioma. Br J Cancer 1992; 66:106.

197. LaRocca RV, Rosenblum M, Westermark B, et al: Patterns of proto-oncogene expression in human glioma cell lines. J Neurosci Res 1989; 24:97.

198. Wong AJ, Bigner SH, Bigner DD, et al: Increased expression of the epidermal growth factor receptor gene is invariably associated with gene amplification. Proc Natl Acad Sci USA 1987; 84:6899.

199. Birchmeier C, Sharma S, Wigler M: Expression and rearrangement of the ROS1 gene in human glioblastoma cells. Proc Natl Acad Sci USA 1987; 84:9270.

200. Wu JK, Chikaraishi DM: Differential expression of ros oncogene in primary human astrocytomas and astrocytoma cell lines. Cancer Res 1990; 50:3032.

201. Mapstone T, McMichael M, Goldthwait D: Expression of platelet-derived growth factors, transforming growth factors, and the ros gene in a variety of primary human brain tumors. Neurosurgery 1991; 28:216.

202. Watkins D, Rouleau GA: Oncogenes and glial tumors. Rev Neurol 1992; 148:402.

203. Watkins D, Dion F, Poisson M, et al: Analysis of oncogene expression in primary human gliomas: Evidence for increased expression of the ros oncogene. Cancer Genet Cytogenet 1994; 72:130.

204. Wu JK, Wang JK: Increased expression in human astrocytomas of a 100 kDa protein with sequence homology to the ros tyrosine kinase domain. Neurol Res 1993; 15:316.

205. Kinzler K, Bigner SH, Bigner DD, et al: Identification of an amplified, highly expressed gene in a human glioma. Science 1987; 236:70.

206. Xiao H, Goldthwait DA, Mapstone T: A search for gli expression in tumors of the central nervous system. Pediatr Neurosurg 1994; 20:178.

207. Wullich B, Muller HW, Fischer U, et al: Amplified met gene linked to double minutes in human glioblastoma. Eur J Cancer 1993; 14:1991.

208. von Deimling A, Louis DN, Menon AG, et al: Deletions on the long arm of chromosome 17 in pilocytic astrocytoma. Acta Neuropathol 1993; 86:81.

209. Ozek MM, Sav A, Pamir MN, et al: Pleomorphic xanthoastrocytoma associated with von Recklinghausen neurofibromatosis. Childs Nerv Syst 1993; 9:39.

210. Sawyer JR, Roloson GJ, Chadduck WM, et al: Cytogenetic findings in a pleomorphic xanthoastrocytoma. Cancer Genet Cytogenet 1991; 55:225.

211. Shepherd CW, Scheithauer BW, Gomez MR, et al: Subependymal giant cell astrocytoma: A clinical, pathological, and flow cytometric study. Neurosurgery 1991; 28:864.

212. Kwiatkowski DJ, Short MP: Tuberous sclerosis. Arch Dermatol 1994; 130:348.

213. Henske EP, Ozelius L, Gusella JF, et al: A high-resolution linkage map of human 9q34.1. Genomics 1993; 17:587.

214. Sampson JR, Janssen LA, Sandkuijl LA: Linkage investigation of three putative tuberous sclerosis determining loci on chromosomes 9q, 11q, and 12q. The Tuberous Sclerosis Collaborative Group. J Med Genet 1992; 29:861.

215. Povey S, Burley MW, Attwood J, et al: Two loci for tuberous sclerosis: One on 9q34 and one on 16p13. Ann Hum Genet 1994; 58:107.

216. Sampson JR, Harris PC: The molecular genetics of tuberous sclerosis. Hum Mol Genet 1994; 3:1477.

217. European Chromosome 16 Tuberous Sclerosis Consortium: Identification and characterization of the tuberous sclerosis gene on chromosome 16. Cell 1993; 75:1305.

218. Green AJ, Johnson PH, Yates JRW: The tuberous sclerosis gene on chromosome 9q34 acts as a growth suppressor. Hum Mol Genet 1994; 3:1833.

219. Carbonara C, Longa L, Grosso E, et al: 9q34 loss of heterozygosity in a tuberous sclerosis astrocytoma suggests a growth-suppressor-like activity also for the TSC1 gene. Hum Mol Genet 1994; 3:1829.

220. Taratuto AL, Sevlever G, Schultz M, et al: Desmoplastic cerebral astrocytoma of infancy (DCAI) (abstract). Brain Pathol 1994; 4:423.

221. Ohgaki H, Eibl RH, Wiestler OD, et al: p53 mutations in nonastrocytic human brain tumors. Cancer Res 1991; 51:6202.

222. Hsieh LL, Hsia CF, Wang LY, et al: p53 gene mutations in brain tumors in Taiwan. Cancer Lett 1994; 78:25.

223. Kros JM, Godschalk JJ, Krishnadath KK, et al: Expression of p53 in oligodendrogliomas. J Pathol 1993; 171:285.

224. Ransom DT, Ritland SR, Kimmel DW, et al: Cytogenetic and loss of heterozygosity studies in ependymomas, pilocytic astrocytomas, and oligodendrogliomas. Genes Chromosom Cancer 1992; 5:348.

225. von Deimling A, Louis DN, von Ammon K, et al: Evidence for a tumor suppressor gene on chromosome 19q associated with human astrocytomas, oligodendrogliomas, and mixed gliomas. Cancer Res 1992; 52:4277.

226. von Deimling A, Nagel J, Bender B, et al: Deletion mapping of chromosome 19 in human gliomas. Int J Cancer 1994; 57:676.

227. von Haken M, White E, Kalra R, et al: Molecular genetic analysis of chromosome 17p and 22q deoxyribonucleic acid markers in pediatric ependymoma (abstract). Neurosurgery 1994; 35:565.

228. Metzger AK, Sheffield VC, Duyk G, et al: Identification of a germ-line mutation in the p53 gene in a patient with an intracranial ependymoma. Proc Natl Acad Sci USA 1991; 88:7825.

229. Vassbotn FS, Ostman A, Langeland N, et al: Activated platelet-derived growth factor autocrine pathway drives the transformed phenotype of a human glioblastoma cell line. J Cell Physiol 1994; 158:381.

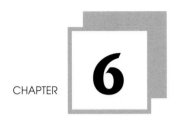

CHAPTER **6**

Growth Factor–Mediated Signaling Pathways

NEOPLASTIC TRANSFORMATION AND PROGRESSION ARE A MULTI-STEP PROCESS

The development of many human cancers is now attributed to the progressive accumulation of multiple genetic changes. These alterations include the inactivation of tumor suppressor genes and the activation of oncogenes (Fig. 6–1). Recent results have demonstrated an important interplay between tumor suppressor genes and genes that regulate transition through the cell cycle.[26, 48] Mutations that result in a loss of cell cycle control contribute to genetic instability, resulting in chromosomal rearrangements and gene amplification. Conversely, restoration of cell cycle control has been shown to diminish the frequency of gene amplification.[81, 175] Genetic instability is presumed to result in the generation of phenotypic variants that possess a selective growth and survival advantage over normal cells.[112] The growth advantage attributed to malignant cells may result in part from the activation of growth factor–signaling pathways.

Ample evidence suggests that a similar mechanism of tumorigenesis, involving multiple genetic changes, occurs in tumors derived from the central nervous system (CNS).[60, 91, 124, 140] These tumors have been shown to exhibit mutations or loss of important cell cycle control genes such as

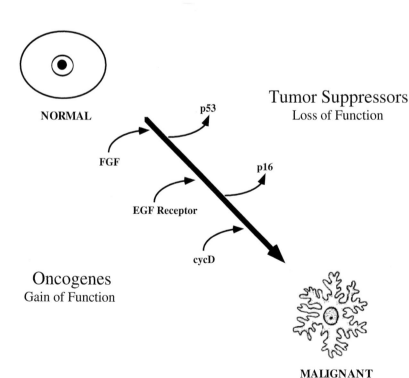

Figure 6–1 Neoplastic transformation in many human cancers is now attributed to the progressive accumulation of multiple genetic changes. Some of the more significant genetic alterations include the inactivation of tumor suppressor genes and the activation of oncogenes. Certain tumor suppressor genes are now known to be capable of arresting cell-cycle progression by directly or indirectly influencing the activity of kinases required for cell division. The induction of growth factors, growth factor receptors, and other signal transduction intermediates results in the generation of positive growth signals. The induction of positive growth regulators in the absence of factors that promote cell cycle arrest leads to uncontrolled cellular proliferation.

p53.[109, 140] They also exhibit significant changes in the expression of mitogenic and angiogenic proteins, which presumably endow astrocytoma cells with a selective growth advantage in the absence of proteins that promote cell cycle arrest. A number of well-defined growth factors, along with their cognate receptors, have been identified in malignant astrocytes. Although growth factor expression in astrocytes is anticipated as part of their normal physiologic function,[46, 100, 158, 167] good evidence exists that indicates that altered growth factor expression is related to abnormal patterns of cellular proliferation, invasiveness, and vascularity. Studies that define the contribution made by growth factor–signaling pathways to the phenotype of malignant astrocytes are essential to understanding the biology of transformation in the CNS. Alterations in growth factor–growth factor receptor expression may provide important diagnostic and prognostic information, but they may also yield new therapeutic targets for inhibiting the growth of malignant astrocytes.

MULTIPLE GROWTH FACTORS AND GROWTH FACTOR RECEPTORS HAVE BEEN IDENTIFIED IN HUMAN ASTROCYTOMAS

A diversity of growth factors and growth factor receptors have been identified in human astrocytoma tissue biopsies and in astrocytoma cells in culture (Table 6–1). The presence of growth factors in these cells may be related to the direct activation of tumor cell proliferation or to the recruitment of new blood vessels. It must not be overlooked, however, that certain growth factors are expressed as part of a repertoire of normal astrocyte activities and are maintained following neoplastic transformation. Much of the work in this field is directed at defining the growth factor pathways that are causally related to the transformed phenotype. In this regard, clear evidence is present for the simultaneous expression of both a ligand and the cognate receptor for the ligand in astrocytoma cells, which suggests the presence of potential autocrine loops. In this instance, a malignant astrocyte would produce a growth factor that stimulates its own proliferation after binding and activating the appropriate receptor on the same cell (Fig. 6–2). Autocrine loops represent a method for directly stimulating tumor cell growth. This would also include the production of growth factor receptors that are constitutively activated in the absence of a ligand. A second functional subset of growth factors has also been identified in astrocytomas. These are growth factors that are produced by malignant astrocytes without the simultaneous expression of the cognate receptor. These growth factors are presumed to have important paracrine functions mediating the recruitment of new blood vessels or influencing immune responses. Receptors for this class of ligand have now been identified on endothelial cells contained within the tumor parenchyma. A third mechanism also exists by which growth factors may influence tumor development in the CNS. This involves malignant astrocytes expressing receptors for ligands they do not synthesize. As a result of tumor cell–endothelial cell interactions, *activated* endothelial cells within the tumor could provide additional growth factors to stimulate the proliferation of malignant astrocytes.

It is obvious that growth factor–signaling pathways are going to play an important role in the development of astrocytomas at several different levels. A more precise understanding of their role in this process requires careful analysis of levels of expression, cellular distribution, temporal expression, and molecular structure in the tumor and in the normal brain. The following review attempts to summarize current knowledge in these areas and in progress being made

TABLE 6–1
ASTROCYTOMAS EXPRESS MULTIPLE GROWTH FACTORS AND GROWTH FACTOR RECEPTORS

Growth Factor/ Receptor	Cellular Distribution	Alteration
TGFA	Tumor cell	ND
EGFR	Tumor cell	Amplification, overexpression, rearrangement
FGF1	Tumor cell	Overexpression
FGF2	Tumor cell/endothelial cell	Overexpression
FGF9	Tumor cell lines only	ND
FGFR1	Tumor cell	Overexpression and shift in alternative RNA splicing ($\alpha \rightarrow \beta$ isoform)
FGFR2	Present in LGA + AA biopsies	Possible gene deletion or transcriptional suppression in GBM
PDGF A-chain	Tumor cell	Overexpression
PDGF B-chain	Endothelial cell	Overexpression
PDGFRA	Tumor cell	Overexpression
PDGFRB	Endothelial cell	Overexpression
IGF1	Tumor cell/cyst fluid	Biopsies express 2 alternatively spliced mRNAs
IGFR	Tumor cell lines	ND
TGFB1	Tumor cell lines	ND
TGFB2	Tumor cell (biopsies and cell lines)	Overexpression
TGFBR	Tumor cell lines	ND
VEGF	Tumor cell	Overexpression
flk-1	Endothelial cell	Overexpression
flt-1	Endothelial cell	Overexpression

Abbreviations: TGFA, transforming growth factor-α; EGFR, epidermal growth factor receptor; FGF, fibroblast growth factor; FGFR, fibroblast growth factor receptor; PDGF, platelet-derived growth factor; PDGFR, platelet-derived growth factor receptor; IGF, insulin-like growth factor; IGFR, insulin-like growth factor receptor; TGFB, transforming growth factor-β; TGFBR, transforming growth factor-β receptor; VEGF, vascular endothelial growth factor; LGA, low-grade astrocytoma; AA, anaplastic astrocytoma; GBM, glioblastoma multiforme; ND, not determined or demonstrated.

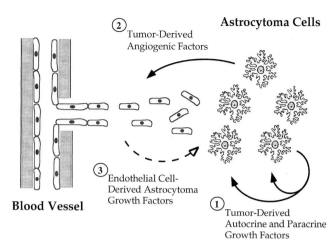

Figure 6–2 Astrocytoma cells express a large assortment of growth factors and growth factor receptors. Some tumor cells are capable of enhancing their own growth by producing growth factors that activate receptors on their own cell surface (*1*). This is referred to as an *autocrine growth pathway*. Growth factors released from one tumor cell can also activate the growth of neighboring tumor cells via a *paracrine growth pathway*. Both of these pathways directly activate tumor cell growth. Tumor development is augmented by enhancing the blood supply to the tumor. Tumor cells can promote new blood vessel development by elaborating growth factors (angiogenic factors) that stimulate endothelial cell proliferation and migration (*2*). Endothelial cells contained in the astrocytoma express proteins not expressed by endothelial cells in non-transformed brain tissue. Some of these proteins include growth factors and their cognate receptors, such as PDGF B-chain and the PDGF-B receptor. Astrocytoma cells express a PDGF receptor that is responsive to PDGF B-chain homodimers. Therefore, *activated* endothelial cells within the tumor can produce growth factors that stimulate the growth of astrocytoma cells (*3*).

in controlling astrocytoma growth by targeting select growth factor–signaling pathways.

ASTROCYTOMA GROWTH FACTORS

Basic Fibroblast Growth Factor

Basic fibroblast growth factor (FGF2) belongs to a family of structurally related polypeptide mitogens.[9, 127] Nine members of this family have now been identified on the basis of amino acid sequence homologies. FGF2 is a multifunctional protein recognized primarily for its mitogenic and angiogenic properties. On the basis of cell culture studies, FGF2 has been shown to be mitogenic for a wide range of cell types derived from mesoderm and neuroectoderm. In addition to the many in vitro studies, FGF2 has also been demonstrated to be active in numerous in vivo models of angiogenesis and wound healing.[9, 127] FGF2 also exhibits potent neurotrophic actions, promoting the survival and differentiation of neurons from the peripheral and central nervous system.[21, 100, 155, 158] In general, the FGF family of proteins expresses an extremely diverse range of actions. They have the capacity to induce, inhibit, and maintain the differentiation of many cell types in culture. Furthermore, substantial evidence indicates that FGF family members display distinct temporal patterns of expression, with some members playing an important role during early development.[74]

A role for FGF in tumor development is supported by observations that transfection of cells with the FGF2 gene increases autocrine growth in monolayer culture and in soft agar.[5, 107, 128] In addition, several recently described oncogenes discovered in human tumors encode proteins structurally related to the FGF family.[15, 31, 84, 141, 146, 179] Elevations in FGF2 and FGF1 (acidic FGF) have been detected in several human tumors, including glioblastomas,[8, 79, 88, 117, 143, 148, 177] gastric carcinoma,[113, 150] renal cell carcinoma,[22] and pancreatic cancer.[169] The overexpression of one or more of these FGF family members is associated with increased malignancy in glioblastomas[88, 147] and pancreatic cancer.[169] Elevated levels of FGF2 have also been demonstrated in the urine of patients with bladder cancer and, purportedly, in the urine of patients with cancer outside of the urinary tract.[108] These results strongly suggest that overexpression of FGF family members by tumor cells may contribute to their accelerated growth.

At least two FGF family members, FGF1 and FGF2, have been identified in astrocytoma cells.[8, 79, 88, 99, 117, 143, 148, 177] FGF9, the last FGF family member to be identified, was purified from a glioblastoma cell line.[94, 106] Further analysis of FGF9 in situ should provide more information about its role in normal glia and astrocytomas. FGF2 appears to be the only FGF family member expressed by normal astrocytes. Although the first reports suggested that FGF2 was synthesized by neurons,[62, 119] recent immunocytochemical analyses employing several well-defined FGF2-specific antibodies have demonstrated that FGF2 is principally expressed by astrocytes.[46, 167] In marked contrast, FGF1 appears to have a neuronal localization,[25, 28, 134, 144, 165] which suggests that these two related factors may have unique actions within the CNS.

FGF1 and FGF2 expression are elevated in malignant astrocytomas in comparison to normal brain.[8, 79, 88, 117, 143, 147, 177] FGF expression within astrocytic tumors has been localized to malignant astrocytes and endothelial cells by in situ hybridization histochemical and immunocytochemical techniques. The mechanism accounting for elevated FGF levels in astrocytomas is not clear. Increased rates of transcription could account for the increase, but there is no direct evidence to support this mechanism. There is evidence that FGF2 messenger RNA (mRNA) is stabilized in glioblastoma cells in culture, which accounts for elevated levels of mRNA.[104] This mechanism could conceivably account for elevated FGF2 mRNA levels in astrocytomas in situ. A more intriguing hypothesis to account for increased FGF2 expression has recently been proposed. Murphy and Knee[103] have provided evidence for the existence, in astrocytoma cells, of a naturally occurring antisense RNA transcript derived from the FGF2 gene. An antisense transcript could potentially regulate the availability of a specific sense (coding) mRNA transcript. High levels of the antisense transcript would be expected to lower the availability of sense mRNA; conversely, low levels of the antisense transcript would result in elevated levels of sense mRNA. Low levels of the FGF2 antisense transcript were observed in glioblastoma cell lines expressing high levels of FGF2 mRNA. Conversely, a human breast cancer cell line that contained very low levels of FGF2 mRNA expressed abundant levels of the antisense transcript. These results suggest that alterations in the ratio of sense to antisense transcripts could lead to elevated FGF2 levels in some transformed cells.

Good evidence exists to indicate FGF2 expression in astrocytoma cells is linked to increased proliferation and invasiveness. This has been evaluated in part by suppressing endogenous FGF2 expression in astrocytoma cells using FGF2-specific antisense oligonucleotides.[97, 105] The application of antisense oligonucleotides resulted in significant growth suppression in two different glioblastoma cell lines. Antisense oligonucleotides directed to two different sites of FGF2 mRNA were effective in suppressing cell growth. Sense-strand control oligonucleotides were ineffective. Treatment with FGF2-specific antisense oligonucleotides reduced FGF2 protein content by almost 70%, whereas sense oligonucleotides had no effect on FGF2 protein levels.[97] Thus, the growth inhibitory actions of FGF2 antisense oligonucleotides appeared to be specific and to result from the formation of specific hybrids between the oligonucleotides and their respective mRNA.

FGF2 activity has also been suppressed using neutralizing monoclonal antibodies.[98, 149] The application of neutralizing antibodies suppressed astrocytoma cell growth in soft agar culture and in nude mice. The results of studies using neutralizing antibodies imply that FGF2 release or secretion may be related to an autocrine pathway promoting astrocytoma growth.

Any contribution made by FGF proteins to disease progression could involve either a direct stimulation of tumor cell proliferation and invasiveness or, concomitantly, increased vascularization resulting from enhanced endothelial cell proliferation and migration. The evidence just presented suggests that FGF2 expression in astrocytoma cells can directly influence astrocytoma cell growth independent of any effects on vascularity. These studies imply that FGF2 expression potentiates phenotypic malignancy in transformed human astrocytes.

FGF Receptors

The biologic responses of FGFs are mediated through specific high-affinity transmembrane receptors. Four structurally related genes encoding high-affinity FGF receptors (FGFRs) have been identified.[56, 66, 72, 116, 131] In addition to high-affinity binding sites, cells exhibit low-affinity FGF binding sites,[69] which have been characterized as extracellular heparan sulfate proteoglycans.[102, 156] Binding to the low-affinity glycosaminoglycan sites appears to be obligatory for binding of FGF to high-affinity receptors and for biologic activity.[70] Cells deficient in heparan sulfate biosynthesis are not able to bind or respond to FGF2.[123, 172] However, the addition of either free heparin or heparan sulfate restores high-affinity binding of FGF2.[172] These results demonstrate that heparin-like low-affinity sites play an important role in the regulation of FGF2 activity and in the response of cells to FGF2.

Structural features common to members of the FGFR family include a signal peptide, two or three immunoglobulin (Ig)-like loops in the extracellular domain, a hydrophobic transmembrane domain, and a highly conserved tyrosine kinase domain split by a short kinase insert sequence. Overall, the proteins encoded by the four FGFR genes are strikingly similar. The most closely related proteins are FGFR1 and FGFR2 (72% amino acid identity), whereas FGFR1 and

FGFR4 are the least closely related (55% identity). Given the structural similarities, it is not surprising that each of the FGFRs can bind several different types of FGFs. However, several reports have been published of cell- and tissue-specific expression of FGF receptors and responsiveness to different FGF family members.[67] One mechanism for generating this selective responsiveness to different FGF family members involves altering the ligand binding specificity or affinity through alternative splicing of RNA, thereby producing several receptor isoforms from a single gene.

Structural variants of FGFR1 and FGFR2 are, in fact, generated by alternative splicing of their RNA transcripts.[19, 53, 66, 68] The divergent receptors generated by this process manifest different ligand-binding specificities and affinities.[14, 90, 137, 164, 173] One common structural variation that involves the second half of the third Ig-like disulfide loop of FGFR1, FGFR2, and FGFR3 dramatically alters the ligand-binding properties of these receptors.[11, 164] Another splicing variant results in FGFRs containing either two or three Ig-like domains in the extracellular region.[23, 54, 68, 126] Alternative RNA splicing involving both the first and third Ig-like domains is subject to cell- and tissue-specific processing that reflects the changing FGF requirement that occurs during tissue growth and differentiation.[68, 126, 130, 164] Changes in ligand-binding affinity and specificity resulting from alternative splicing are also likely to be important in some types of human cancers that rely on FGF family members to sustain growth and invasiveness.[168, 171]

The presence of FGF receptors in human astrocytomas has been well documented. FGF binding sites have been identified on astrocytoma cells in culture using radiolabeled FGF2,[99] and FGFR mRNA transcripts have been identified in human astrocytomas using Northern blot and PCR analysis.[149, 168] At present, only evidence for expression of FGFR1 and FGFR2 in astrocytic tumors has been found.

The transformation and malignant progression of astrocytes has been associated with significant changes in FGFR expression. Analysis of normal white matter specimens and normal brain adjacent to malignant tumor and to low-grade astrocytomas suggests that FGFR2 is the principal FGF receptor in astrocytes, as proposed by Lai and Lemke[77] and Peters and co-workers.[118] In contrast, FGFR1 appears to be poorly expressed in normal astrocytes, but is abundantly expressed in neurons, as shown by in situ hybridization studies.[51, 118, 159, 160] Despite low to nondetectable levels in normal astrocytes, FGFR1 expression is elevated in human glioblastomas.[101] In this recent study, all glioblastomas evaluated expressed elevated levels of FGFR1 mRNA relative to all non-neoplastic human brain tissue. In addition, frozen sections derived from glioblastoma tissue exhibited intense FGFR1 immunoreactivity, whereas adjacent normal white matter was essentially devoid of FGFR1 immunoreactivity. These results disagree, however, with a recent study reporting no difference in FGFR1 expression between gliomas and normal brain.[149] The variance may reflect the fact that one form of analysis was performed with histologically defined frozen sections of tumor and normal brain, whereas in the other study, tumor biopsies were used that may have contained variable proportions of tumor and normal tissue. Furthermore, only two normal brain specimens were analyzed in the latter study,[149] and these exhibited markedly different levels of FGFR1 expression from each other.

In addition to exhibiting elevated levels of FGFR1 mRNA, glioblastomas appeared to overexpress an alternatively spliced form of the FGFR1 gene.[168] When present in normal brain (gray matter), the α form of FGFR1 predominates over the β form. In this regard the brain is distinct from other tissues, which express nearly equal levels of the α and β forms of FGFR1.[67] When the FGFR1 gene was up-regulated in glioblastomas, a significant shift occurred in the splicing pattern of the gene. The β form represented the predominant transcript in glioblastomas, whereas the α form was predominant in low-grade astrocytic tumors. The shift from α to β was found to correlate with the grade of malignancy in astrocytomas and could eventually provide a useful prognostic indicator for astrocyte-derived tumors. Although the functional consequence of a shift in alternative RNA splicing from the α form (three IgG-like disulfide loops) to the β form (two IgG-like disulfide loops) of the FGFR is not understood, FGFR1β has recently been shown to exhibit a 10-fold greater affinity for FGF1 and FGF2 than for FGFR1α.[137]

FGFR2 expression was also evaluated in human astrocytomas and in normal brain. Surprisingly, the distribution of FGFR2 transcripts in astrocytomas and normal brain was opposite to that observed for FGFR1 expression.[101, 168] Whereas glioblastomas expressed elevated levels of FGFR1, low to nondetectable levels of FGFR2 were observed using the same cDNA samples. Adjacent normal brain obtained from the same tumor specimen expressed low levels of FGFR1 but abundant levels of FGFR2. Low-grade astrocytomas also expressed abundant levels of FGFR2, similar to those of normal brain. Anaplastic astrocytomas expressed variable but higher levels of FGFR2 mRNA than those observed in glioblastomas. The results suggest that the reciprocal loss and gain of FGFR2 and FGFR1, respectively, is associated with malignant progression in astrocytomas from low-grade to high-grade tumors.

The mechanism underlying the loss of FGFR2 expression in glioblastomas is not known. FGFR2 has been localized to the long arm of chromosome 10 (q.26).[85] Approximately 80% of all glioblastomas exhibit a loss of heterozygosity for 10q.[125] The loss of chromosome 10, which is one of the most frequent genetic abnormalities occurring in glioblastomas, has not been associated with lower-grade astrocytic tumors.[60] Although most glioblastomas lose an entire copy of chromosome 10, a subgroup has been shown to exhibit partial loss of chromosome 10. The common region of chromosome 10 deletion extends from 10q24 to 10q26, a region encompassing FGFR2. Although it is not known if FGFR2 is an imprinted gene, it is conceivable that one copy of FGFR2 is lost during the astrocyte transformation process, leaving behind a copy that is transcriptionally inactive. Alternatively, both copies of the FGFR2 gene may be present in glioblastomas, but may be silent following translocation to another chromosome.

In summary, human astrocytomas exhibit several significant changes in FGFR expression that include activation of FGFR1, shifts in alternative RNA splicing of FGFR1, and loss of FGFR2. The presence of FGFR1 in low-grade astrocytomas relative to the lack of FGFR1 in normal white matter suggests that increased FGFR1 expression may be an early event in the genesis of astrocytomas. In contrast, the change in alternative splicing is clearly a late event in the development of astrocytic tumors and may be coupled to the loss of FGFR2 or other genes on chromosome 10. The marked inhibition observed in astrocytoma cell growth following application of FGFR1- but not FGFR2-specific antisense oligonucleotides suggests that these types of receptor alterations may impart a clear growth advantage to glioma cells (Yamada S, Berger MS, Morrison RS: Unpublished observations, 1995).

Transforming Growth Factor-α/ Epidermal Growth Factor Receptor

Epidermal growth factor (EGF) and transforming growth factor-α (TGFA) are small-molecular-weight mitogenic polypeptides. They exhibit a high degree of structural homology (49%), which is shared by other members of the EGF family of proteins. EGF and TGFA interact with a variety of cell types to produce responses suggestive of a broad range of physiologic roles. In addition, both proteins exhibit similar biologic activities and are equally mitogenic for several cell lines. EGF family members initiate biologic responses by binding to the same receptor in most systems tested previously.[10, 84a] The EGF receptor (EGFR) gene product characterized on normal cells is a 170 kD transmembrane glycoprotein. The receptor protein consists of an extracellular binding component, a single transmembrane domain, and an intracellular cytoplasmic region. Binding to the receptor results in activation of the receptor's intracellular tyrosine kinase activity. Sequence analysis has demonstrated a close similarity between the EGFR and the avian erythroblastosis virus (AEV) v-erb B transforming protein. This viral transforming protein contains the transmembrane and the internal tyrosine kinase domains of the avian EGFR. Transformation of cells by AEV leads to the expression of a truncated EGFR lacking the extracellular control domain. Such aberrant control mechanisms clearly have implications for the development and propagation of some astrocytic tumors, which commonly exhibit alterations in the EGFR.

Amplification of the EGFR gene has been documented in approximately 40% of malignant human astrocytomas.[80, 82, 145, 166] Amplification is restricted to malignant astrocytomas and is invariably associated with high levels of EGFR expression.[166] In many of the tumors, amplification is associated with rearrangement of the EGFR gene.[145, 166] Rearrangements involve deletion of most, or more commonly a portion, of the extracellular domain of the EGFR, resulting in the production of truncated receptors. The former type of rearrangement was only observed in one tumor and is most similar to the v-erb B transforming protein. The latter type of rearrangement resulted in the loss of most of the amino-terminal, cysteine-rich domain without involving the EGF/TGFA binding domain. This in-frame deletion also resulted in the generation of a unique junction site that has been used to generate a specific antibody.[59] The antibody detects the mutant protein expressed on glioblastomas but does not react with tumors or normal brain expressing the wild-type EGFR protein. Antibodies specific for mutant or alternatively spliced proteins should provide important reagents for imaging, diagnosis, and therapy of some malignant astrocytic tumors.

The influence of EGFR gene amplification and of rearrangement on the growth of human glioblastomas is not fully understood. A truncation involving most of the extracellular domain, including the binding domain, would produce a receptor whose kinase activity is constitutively active and unregulated. This type of deletion appears to be very infrequent in glial tumors. Deletions in one of the two cysteine-rich domains of the receptor are common, but ligand-binding activity is retained.[58] Nevertheless, these deletions could produce conformational alterations that would result in an abnormally active receptor in the absence of ligand despite the retention of a ligand-binding domain. This is consistent with a report demonstrating that the deletional mutant involving nucleotides 275–1075 has ligand-independent transforming activity.[170] The demonstration that (1) similar deletion mutations are observed in multiple astrocytic tumors, (2) overexpression of the receptor protein is common in malignant astrocytomas, and (3) many malignant astrocytomas simultaneously express the receptor and the ligand TGFA[88] strongly implicates the EGFR transduction pathway in the tumorigenesis of malignant astrocytomas.

Platelet-Derived Growth Factor

Platelet-derived growth factor (PDGF) is a polypeptide mitogen originally purified from platelets, but it is also expressed in a variety of other normal and transformed cell types.[129] It is best characterized for its mitogenic actions on connective tissue cells and glial cells, but it has been found to have neurotrophic actions on CNS neurons.[142] PDGF is composed of two homologous polypeptide chains, A and B, in heterodimeric or homodimeric combinations. The B-chain gene is the normal cellular homologue to the v-*sis* oncogene of simian sarcoma virus. PDGF dimers bind to high-affinity, transmembrane, protein tyrosine kinase receptors. Two receptor types exist for PDGF: the α receptor (PDGFRA), which is capable of binding all three possible dimers, and the β receptor (PDGFRB), which binds the BB homodimer with high affinity and the AB dimer with lower affinity. The specific distribution of receptor types on cells determines the response elicited by the various isoforms.

Indirect evidence implicates PDGF in the development of astrocytomas. Glioma-derived cell lines and tumor biopsies express PDGF growth factor A- and B-chains as well as PDGFRs.[50, 111, 121] PDGFRA and PDGFRB are overexpressed in a subset of glioblastomas.[33] In some cases there is also amplification of the PDGFRA, although this does not appear to be necessary for overexpression.[33, 75] In one instance, an amplified PDGFRA was identified as bearing an 81 amino acid deletion in the immunoglobulin domain of the extracellular region of the receptor.[75] Interestingly, normal cortex adjacent to the tumor expressed the PDGFRA gene amplification but not the deletion. It is not known if this deletion results in autoactivation of the receptor in the absence of ligand or how pervasive this deletion is in malignant astrocytomas.

The cellular targets exhibiting alterations in PDGF and PDGFR expression have been evaluated using in situ hybridization and immunocytochemistry. In situ hybridization analysis for PDGF ligands and receptors in glioblastoma tissue sections demonstrated significant expression of PDGF B-chain and its receptor, and to a lesser extent, PDGF A-chain mRNA in vascular endothelial cells.[50] In marked contrast, tumor cells expressed significantly more mRNA for PDGF A-chain. This is in agreement with another recent report by Plate and co-workers[120] in which PDGF β-receptor mRNA was not detectable in the vessels of normal human brain, but was observed only in the vasculature of low- and high-grade gliomas. Expression was especially pronounced in the endothelial cell proliferations associated with glioblastomas. Extremely low levels of PDGFRB mRNA were associated with tumor cells, irrespective of the histologic grade. These results are also consistent with the demonstration that astrocytoma cells in culture express a PDGF A-chain homodimer, which exhibits a lower mitogenic and chemotactic capacity relative to the PDGF AB-chain heterodimer expressed in platelets.[111]

The results of these studies suggest that there is an upregulation of PDGF A- and B-chain and PDGFRA and PDGFRB in malignant astrocytomas. Up-regulation of PDGF B-chain and PDGFRB occurs in endothelial cells localized specifically within the tumor and suggests that PDGF ligands and receptors may play an important role in the vascularization of malignant astrocytomas. The demonstration that these genes are not activated in normal brain endothelial cells suggests that glioma cell–endothelial cell interactions may activate endothelial cell autocrine growth pathways. The relationship of astrocytoma-derived PDGF A-chain homodimers to direct activation of astrocytoma cell growth remains unclear and will require further study with antisense or other ablation techniques.

Transforming Growth Factor-β

The transforming growth factor-β (TGFB) family of growth factors includes three structurally and functionally related polypeptides, TGFB1, TGFB2, and TGFB3. Although structurally related, each isoform is encoded by a separate gene. The TGFBs exhibit a diverse range of actions and have been shown to influence cell proliferation, differentiation, embryogenesis, and immune function. Biologic activities are transduced after binding to a high-affinity receptor. The type I and II TGFB receptors (TGFBR1 and TGFBR2) appear to express serine-threonine kinase activity. The type III receptor (TGFBR3) contains sites for glycosaminoglycan chains and lacks the kinase signaling domain displayed by TGFBR1 and TGFBR2. The TGFBR3 may act to stabilize TGFBs in the extracellular space to facilitate interactions with extracellular matrix components.

The relationship of the TGFBs to glial cell transformation is emerging, but it is not well defined. Studies utilizing tumor biopsies and cultured astrocytoma cell lines have all demonstrated expression of TGFB1 and TGFB2 mRNA.[65, 83, 87] Evidence has also been presented for the presence of TGFBRs on cultured astrocytoma cell lines.[65] Addition of exogenous TGFB exerts positive or negative effects on growth depending on the degree of anaplasia and karyotypic divergence exhibited by the cultured astrocytoma cells. The ability of TGFB to modulate the growth of some astrocytoma cells may relate to its interactions with other astrocytoma-derived growth factors. A defined role for TGFB as a direct autocrine activator of astrocytoma growth is not fully supported by the available data.

Another mechanism by which TGFB could potentially promote the growth of malignant astrocytomas is by enhancing the angiogenic process in these tumors.[34] Moreover, due to its immunosuppressive actions, TGFB could also contribute to the growth of astrocytomas by inhibiting the activation of B- and T-lymphocytes. This would promote the escape of astrocytes from immunosurveillance, allowing further growth and progression. Clearly, the diverse activities associated with this important family of growth factors warrant continued analysis of its relationship to the development and progression of malignant astrocytomas.

Insulin-like Growth Factors

The insulin-like growth factors (IGFs) are polypeptide hormones belonging to the insulin family of peptides. The IGFs, which express both metabolic and growth promoting properties, have been implicated as autocrine growth factors for a variety of tumor types outside the CNS.[24, 57, 63] Insulin and IGF receptors have been identified in the developing and the mature CNS, which suggests that these proteins may play a role in regulating cellular proliferation in the normal brain. Increasing evidence suggests that IGFs are also expressed in malignant glial cells, and this may contribute to the development of glial tumors. Malignant astrocytoma cells in culture possess specific receptors for the IGFs as determined by competitive binding, affinity labeling, immunoprecipitation, and autophosphorylation studies.[42, 43] Furthermore, IGF1 mRNA and IGF1-immunoreactive protein have also been identified in malignant astrocytomas.[132] IGF1 and IGF2 immunoreactive proteins have also been detected in the cyst fluid from different types of CNS tumors, providing additional evidence for the production of these proteins by CNS tumors.[44]

The simultaneous presence of both IGF1 and the appropriate receptors has suggested that IGF1 expression is coupled to cellular proliferation and tumorigenicity in malignant astrocytomas. This is consistent with results demonstrating that rat C6 glioma cells stably transfected with an IGF1 antisense plasmid lose their tumorigenic properties.[153] The molecular mechanism underlying the loss of tumorigenicity was quite unusual and unexpected: the loss of tumorigenicity appeared to result from a heightened immune response involving infiltration of CD8 + lymphocytes. Interestingly, the injection of IGF1 antisense transfected cells into animals with already-established C6 tumors caused regression of the established tumors.[152] IGF1 expression seems to mask the immunogenicity of C6 glioma cells by a mechanism that is not understood. Blocking IGF1 expression with an antisense plasmid reverses the ability of these cells to evade the immune system. It is not clear how the antisense transfected cells convey this protective effect to parental C6 glioma cells. Nevertheless, the possibility of enhancing astrocytoma cell immunogenicity by modulating growth factor expression

offers an exciting new approach for modulating tumor growth.

ANGIOGENIC FACTORS

Considerable evidence suggests that tumor growth and metastasis are dependent on angiogenesis.[34] The induction of new capillary blood vessels by solid tumors is essential for expansion of a developing tumor mass. In the absence of angiogenesis, tumor growth is restricted to a volume of only a few cubic millimeters. This is due to limitations in the diffusion of nutrients and metabolites both to and from the tumor mass.

The ability of tumors to establish new vasculature is now recognized as a distinct and essential stage of neoplastic progression. The means by which tumors are able to break down or circumvent the mechanisms that normally control angiogenesis are complex. Tumor cells have evolved a number of different means of recruiting new blood vessels (additional details are contained in several excellent reviews).[6, 35–37] One important mechanism includes the production of diffusible factors that directly activate endothelial cell migration and proliferation (angiogenic factors). A number of well-defined angiogenic factors and receptors have recently been identified in human astrocytomas. Other growth factors, discussed in the context of tumor cell activators, may also promote angiogenesis. However, the following discussion is restricted to a growth factor receptor system that may function only during the recruitment of new blood vessels.

Vascular Endothelial Growth Factor

The absence of a classic signal sequence in FGF2 and the inability to document the presence of FGFRs on endothelial cells in vivo led many investigators to search for additional paracrine mediators of endothelial cell growth. In 1983, Senger and co-workers[135] described a factor secreted by line 10 guinea pig hepatocarcinoma cells that induced ascites formation when injected intraperitoneally in animals. The factor was named *vascular permeability factor* (VPF), as it was found to be a potent mediator of microvascular permeability.[135] The VPF cDNA coded for a 189 amino acid polypeptide that was closely related to the B-chain of PDGF.[71] Leung and co-workers[78] simultaneously reported the cloning of a specific endothelial cell mitogen from bovine folliculostellate cells and human HL60 leukemia cells that they named *vascular endothelial growth factor* (VEGF). In addition to its ability to induce endothelial cell proliferation in vitro, it was also able to induce an angiogenic response in chick chorioallantoic membrane. Coincidentally, VEGF had virtually the same nucleotide and amino acid sequences as VPF. Leung and associates[78] also described two other cDNA clones that coded for distinct VEGF isoforms of 121 and 165 amino acids. The same group subsequently described the cloning of a fourth isoform from a fetal liver cDNA library that was composed of 206 amino acids.[55] The 165 amino acid isoform (VEGF$_{165}$) appears to be the most abundantly expressed species in most cells.

VEGF represents a family of polypeptides coded for by a

single gene containing eight exons and seven introns. The four isoforms result from alternative splicing of exons 6 and 7. The $VEGF_{189}$ and $VEGF_{206}$ forms contain both of these exons. The 17 amino acid insertion in $VEGF_{206}$ results from a variant splice donor site in the 5' end of exon 7. If exon 6 is spliced out, $VEGF_{165}$ results. If both exons 6 and 7 are removed, $VEGF_{121}$ is generated.[151]

Unlike other growth factors, such as FGF2, EGF, and PDGF, the mitogenic activity of VEGF appears restricted to vascular endothelial cells. Thus, VEGF may play an important role in the development of blood vessels and in the maintenance of endothelial integrity and permeability in normal tissues. This role is consistent with in situ hybridization studies that demonstrated elevated expression of VEGF in the developing brain and kidney. In adults, however, significant VEGF expression was found only in epithelial cells adjacent to fenestrated endothelium in these organs.[7] Other studies have shown a more widespread distribution of VEGF expression in the adult, including the lungs, adrenal glands, liver, spleen, heart, cardiac myocytes, and vascular smooth muscle cells.[4, 7, 30, 96]

In addition to its role in normal physiology, VEGF may also be involved in a number of pathologic conditions. Of paramount importance is its potential role in stimulating a neovascular response in tumors. The expression and production of VEGF has been demonstrated in numerous human tumors and tumor cell lines, including lymphoma, sarcoma (including AIDS-associated Kaposi's sarcoma), glioblastoma multiforme, adenocarcinoma, and melanoma.[13, 121, 136, 139, 161, 174] In a study of CNS neoplasms, Berkman and coworkers[3] found elevated expression of VEGF mRNA in 22 of 27 tumors that had a high degree of neovascularity and vasogenic cerebral edema. The most significant expression was found in capillary hemangioblastomas, glioblastoma multiforme, and meningiomas. The average level of VEGF mRNA expression in these tumors was sixfold higher than in normal brain.

VEGF expression appears to be related to the histologic grade of astrocytomas.[121] The level of VEGF mRNA transcripts were reportedly found to be 50-fold higher in glioblastomas relative to astrocytomas. In situ hybridization histochemical analysis demonstrated increased VEGF expression in two different subsets of glioblastoma cells. One group consisted of palisading cells adjacent to necrotic areas and the second group consisted of clustered cells without obvious adjacent necrosis. The identification of elevated VEGF expression in palisading glioblastoma cells may help to explain the high density of endothelial cell proliferation in areas of necrosis. The regionalized hypoxia that develops as clusters of malignant astrocytes outgrow their blood supply may serve as a stimulus for increased VEGF expression. Hypoxia has recently been demonstrated to induce the expression of VEGF in a variety of cells. Levels of VEGF mRNA rise rapidly when cells are exposed to hypoxic conditions and return to baseline in the presence of normal oxygen concentrations.[76, 139] The induction of VEGF by hypoxia may require the presence of other cell-derived factors or may be up-regulated independently by other factors.[45]

VEGF Receptors

Three structurally related VEGF receptors have been identified thus far: *flt-1*, *flk-1*, and *flt-4*.[16, 41, 93, 122] The three recep-

tors share similar structural features and have in common seven immunoglobulin-like loops in their extracellular domain, a single transmembrane sequence, and a tyrosine kinase region in their intracellular domain.[86, 114, 138] Although their sequences are very homologous, they are each encoded by separate genes. These three receptors represent a subclass of the *fms* receptor tyrosine kinase family. Other members of this family include the receptors for PDGF and the oncoprotein c-kit.

The expression of these three receptors varies between different tissues and different cells in culture, suggesting that each may play specific and unique physiologic roles. Both *flk-1* and *flt-1* appear to be endothelial cell–specific receptors, and are found in the endothelial cells of a variety of tissues throughout embryogenesis.[16, 93, 122, 138]

The high-affinity VEGF receptors *flt-1* and *flk-1* are specifically induced in the vascular endothelial cells of astrocytomas and glioblastomas. Expression of *flt-1* and *flk-1* was confined to endothelial cells, and little or no expression of these receptors was seen in the endothelial cells of normal brain.[120, 121] In contrast to VEGF, there did not appear to be any difference in the levels of *flt-1* and *flk-1* mRNA between astrocytomas and glioblastomas. These results suggest that tumor angiogenesis in astrocytomas is controlled to a large degree by a paracrine mechanism involving the release of VEGF by malignant astrocytes with its ensuing action on tumor vascular endothelial cells expressing VEGF receptors *flt-1* and *flk-1*. This is consistent with a report describing the use of a retrovirus encoding a dominant-negative mutant of the *flk-1*/VEGF receptor to infect endothelial target cells in a glioblastoma in vivo.[92] Tumor growth was prevented in

TABLE 6–2
MODULATING GROWTH FACTOR ACTIVITY*

Pathways Involved in Growth Factor Action	Currently Available Methods for Modulating Growth Factor Activity
Synthesis	Antisense oligonucleotides/ triplex/tumor suppressors/ transcription factors
Availability	Neutralizing antibodies/inhibitors of protease-mediated release from matrix
Receptor binding	Receptor antagonists
Receptor-mediated signal transduction (tyrosine kinase inhibitors)	Dominant negative mutant receptors/polycyclic organic compounds

*Mechanisms for suppressing growth factor–mediated stimulation of astrocytoma cell growth: A number of potential avenues exist for modulating growth factor effects on astrocytoma cells. (1) Methods are available for suppressing growth factor expression or availability, thereby removing the stimulus. (2) Reagents that neutralize the availability of c growth factor in the extracellular space would limit growth factor signaling. (3) Receptor antagonists would also prevent growth factor–receptor interactions limiting signal transduction. Antagonists could be directed toward a high-affinity receptor or in some instances to companion molecules (such as heparan proteoglycans) that are required for growth factor binding. (4) Agents that prevent receptor dimerization or inhibit tyrosine kinase activity would also limit the transduction pathway. Compounds that prevent the binding of protein kinase receptors with intracellular second messenger complexes, such as phospholipase-Cγ, would also limit the transduction cascade that ultimately impinges on the nucleus. For example, peptides could be directed toward phosphoaminoacids located on receptors and SH2 domains located on secondary transduction complexes required for receptor-complex interactions.

nude mice following infection. These results emphasize the important relationship between angiogenic factors, angiogenesis, and solid tumor growth, and point to the exciting possibility of using retroviruses encoding dominant-negative receptor mutations as a potential modality to curtail tumor progression and metastasis.

SUMMARY

Malignant astrocytomas express a variety of growth factors and growth factor receptors. The utilization of these proteins in various autocrine and paracrine pathways may significantly enhance the ability of transformed astrocytes to proliferate, acquire new vasculature, and escape detection by immune cells. All of these properties would be expected to contribute to the overall growth and progression of astrocytomas. Although the regulatory mechanisms controlling the expression and activity of growth factors and receptors in astrocytes must be better understood, new methods are continually being developed to modulate their expression and activity (Table 6–2). The new reagents will be useful in defining the relationship between growth factor–signaling pathways and aberrant growth in astrocytomas. Thus, growth factors and growth factor receptors may provide new targets for improving tumor diagnosis, prognosis, and, it is hoped, the outcome in patients with malignant astrocytomas.

ACKNOWLEDGMENT

We gratefully acknowledge the help of Margaret Coughlan and Katherine Little in preparing the manuscript.

REFERENCES

1. Agoff SN, Hou J, Linzer DIH, et al: Regulation of the human hsp70 promoter by p53. Science 1993; 259:84–87.
2. Baker SJ, Markowitz S, Fearon ER, et al: Suppression of human colorectal carcinoma cell growth by wild-type p53. Science 1990; 249:912–915.
3. Berkman R, Merrill M, Reinhold W, et al: Expression of the vascular permeability factor/vascular endothelial growth factor gene in central nervous system neoplasms. J Clin Invest 1993; 91:153–159.
4. Berse B, Brown L, Van De Water L, et al: Vascular permeability factor (vascular endothelial growth factor) gene is expressed differentially in normal tissues, macrophages and tumors. Mol Cell Biol 1992; 3:211–220.
5. Blam SB, Mitchell R, Tischer E, et al: Addition of growth hormone secretion signal to basic fibroblast growth factor results in cell transformation and secretion of aberrant forms of the protein. Oncogene 1988; 3:129–136.
6. Bouck N: Angiogenesis: A mechanism by which oncogenes and tumor suppressor genes regulate tumorigenesis. *In* Benz CC, Liu ET (eds): Oncogenes and Tumor Suppressor Genes in Human Malignancies. Boston, Kluwer Academic Publishers, 1993, pp 359–371.
7. Breier G, Albrecht U, Sterrer S, et al: Expression of vascular endothelial growth factor during embryonic angiogenesis and endothelial cell differentiation. Development 1992; 114:521–532.
8. Brem S, Tsanaclis AM, Gately S, et al: Immunolocalization of basic fibroblast growth factor to the microvasculature of human brain tumors. Cancer 1992; 70:2673–2680.
9. Burgess WH, Maciag T: The heparin-binding (fibroblast) growth factor family of proteins. Annu Rev Biochem 1989; 58:575–606.
10. Chalazonitis A, Kessler JA, Twardzik DR, et al: Transforming growth factor α but not epidermal growth factor, promotes the survival of sensory neurons in vitro. J Neurosci 1992; 12:583–594.
11. Chellaiah AT, McEwen DG, Werner S, et al: Fibroblast growth factor receptor (FGFR) 3. J Biol Chem 1994; 269:11620–11627.
12. Chin KV, Ueda K, Pastan I, et al: Modulation of activity of the promoter of the human MDR1 gene by Ras and p53. Science 1992; 255:459–462.
13. Connolly D, Olander J, Heuvelman D, et al: Human vascular permeability factor. J Biol Chem 1989; 265:20017–20024.
14. Dell KR, Williams LT: A novel form of fibroblast growth factor receptor 2. J Biol Chem 1992; 267:21225–21229.
15. Delli-Bovi PD, Curatola AM, Kern FG, et al: An oncogene isolated by transfection of Kaposi's sarcoma DNA encodes a growth factor that is a member of the FGF family. Cell 1987; 50:729–737.
16. De Vries C, Escobedo J, Ueno H, et al: The fms-like tyrosine kinase, a receptor for vascular endothelial growth factor. Science 1992;255:989–991.
17. de Martin R, Haendler B, Hofer-Warbinek R, et al: Complementary DNA for human glioblastoma-derived T cell suppressor factor: A novel member of the transforming growth factor-β gene family. EMBO J 1987; 6:3673–3677.
18. Diller L, Kassel J, Nelson CE, et al: p53 functions as a cell cycle control protein in osteosarcomas. Mol Cell Biol 1990; 10:5772–5781.
19. Dionne CA, Crumley G, Bellot F, et al: Cloning and expression of two distinct high-affinity receptors cross-reacting with acidic and basic fibroblast growth factors. EMBO J 1990; 9:2685–2692.
20. Donehower LA, Harvey M, Slagle BL, et al: Mice deficient for p53 are developmentally normal but susceptible to spontaneous tumours. Nature 1992; 356:215–221.
21. Eckenstein FP, Shipley GD, Nishi R: Acidic and basic fibroblast growth factors in the nervous system: Distribution and differential alteration of levels after injury of central versus peripheral nerve. J Neurosci 1991; 11:412–419.
22. Eguchi J, Nomata K, Kanda S, et al: Gene expression and immunohistochemical localization of basic fibroblast growth factor in renal cell carcinoma. Biochem Biophys Res Commun 1992; 183:937–944.
23. Eisemann A, Ahn JA, Graziani G, et al: Alternative splicing generates at least five different isoforms of the human basic-FGF receptor. Oncogene 1991; 6:1195–1202.
24. El-Badry OM, Romanus JA, Helman LJ, et al: Autonomous growth of a human neuroblastoma cell line is mediated by insulin-like growth factor II. J Clin Invest 1989; 84:829–839.
25. Elde R, Cao Y, Cintra A, et al: Prominent expression of acidic fibroblast growth factor in motor and sensory neurons. Neuron 1991; 7:349–364.
26. El-Deiry WS, Tokino T, Velculescu VE, et al: WAF1, a potential mediator of p53 tumor suppression. Cell 1993; 75:817–825.
27. Eliyahu D, Raz A, Gruss P, et al: Participation of p53 cellular tumor antigen in transformation of normal embryonic cells. Nature 1984; 312:646–649.
28. Fallon JH, Di Salvo J, Loughlin SE, et al: Localization of acidic fibroblast growth factor within the mouse brain using biochemical and immunocytochemical techniques. Growth Factors 1992; 6:139–157.
29. Farmer G, Bargonetti J, Zhu H, et al: Wild-type p53 activates transcription in vitro. Nature 1992; 358:83–86.
30. Ferrara N, Winer J, Burton T: Aortic smooth muscle cells express and secrete vascular endothelial growth factor. Growth Factors 1991; 5:141–148.
31. Finch PW, Rubin JS, Miki T, et al: Human KGF is FGF-related with properties of a paracrine effector of epithelial cell growth. Science 1989; 245:752–755.
32. Finlay CA, Hinds PW, Tan T-H, et al: Activating mutations for transformation by p53 produce a gene product that forms an hsc70-p53 complex with an altered half-life. Mol Cell Biol 1988; 8:531–539.
33. Fleming T, Saxena A, Clark WC, et al: Amplification and/or overexpression of platelet-derived growth factor receptors and epidermal growth factor receptor in human glial tumors. Cancer Res 1992; 52:4550–4553.
34. Folkman J: What is the evidence that tumours are angiogenesis dependent? JNCI 1990; 82:4–6.
35. Folkman J, Hanahan D: Switch to the angiogenic phenotype during tumorigenesis. *In* Harris CC (ed): Multistage Carcinogenesis. Boca Raton, Fla, Japan Scientific Society Press/CRC Press, 1992, pp 339–347.

36. Folkman J, Klagsbrun M: Angiogenic factors. Science 1987; 235:442–447.

37. Folkman J, Shing Y: Angiogenesis. J Biol Chem 1992; 267:10931–10934.

38. Fry DW, Kraker AJ, McMichael A, et al: A specific inhibitor of the epidermal growth factor receptor tyrosine kinase. Science 1994; 265:1093–1095.

39. Fujiwara T, Mukhopadhyay T, Cai DW, et al: Retroviral-mediated transduction of p53 gene increases TGF-b expression in a human glioblastoma cell line. Int J Cancer 1994; 56:834–839.

40. Funk WD, Pak DT, Karas RH, et al: A transcriptionally active DNA-binding site for human p53 protein complexes. Mol Cell Biol 1992; 12:2866–2871.

41. Galland F, Karamysheva A, Pebusque M-J, et al: The FLT4 gene encodes a transmembrane tyrosine kinase related to the vascular endothelial growth factor receptor. Oncogene 1993; 8:1233–1240.

42. Gammeltoft S, Ballotti R, Kowalski A, et al: Expression of two types of receptor for insulin-like growth factors in human malignant glioma. Cancer Res 1988; 48:1233–1237.

43. Glick RP, Gettleman R, Patel K, et al: Insulin and insulin-like growth factor I in brain tumors: Binding and in vitro effects. Neurosurgery 1989; 24:791–797.

44. Glick RP, Unterman TG, Hollis R: Radioimmunoassay of insulin-like growth factors in cyst fluid of central nervous system tumors. J Neurosurg 1991; 74:972–978.

45. Goldman DK, Kim J, Wong WL, et al: Epidermal growth factor stimulates vascular endothelial growth factor production by human malignant glioma cells: A model of glioblastoma multiforme pathophysiology. Mol Biol Cell 1993; 4:121–133.

46. Gomez-Pinilla F, Lee JWK, Cotman CW: Basic FGF in adult rat brain: Cellular distribution and response to entorhinal lesion and fimbria-fornix transection. J Neurosci 1992; 12:345–355.

47. Gross JL, Morrison RS, Eidsvoog K, et al: Basic fibroblast growth factor: A potential autocrine regulator of human glioma cell growth. J Neurosci Res 1990; 27:689–696.

48. Harper JW, Adami GR, Wei N, et al: The p21 cCdk-interacting protein Cip1 is a potent inhibitor of G1 cyclin-dependent kinases. Cell 1993; 75:805–816.

49. Harvey M, Sands AT, Weiss RS, et al: In vitro growth characteristics of embryo fibroblasts isolated from p53-deficient mice. Oncogene 1993; 8:2457–2467.

50. Hermannson M, Nister M, Betsholtz C, et al: Endothelial cell hyperplasia in human glioblastoma: Coexpression of mRNA for platelet-derived growth factor (PDGF) B chain and PDGF receptor suggests autocrine growth stimulation. Proc Natl Acad Sci USA 1988; 85:7748–7752.

51. Heuer JG, Bartheld CS, Kinoshita Y, et al: Alternative phases of FGF receptor and NGF receptor expression in the developing chicken nervous system. Neuron 1990; 5:283–296.

52. Hollstein M, Sidransky D, Vogelstein B, et al: p53 mutation in human cancers. Science 1991; 253:49–53.

53. Hou J, Kan M, McKeehan K, et al: Fibroblast growth factors from liver vary in three structural domains. Science 1991; 251:665–668.

54. Hou J, Kan M, Wang F, et al: Substitution of putative half-cystine residues in heparin-binding fibroblast growth factor receptors. J Biol Chem 1992; 267:17804–17808.

55. Houck K, Ferrara N, Winer J, et al: The vascular endothelial growth factor family: Identification of a fourth molecular species and characterization of alternative splicing of RNA. Mol Endocrinol 1991; 5:1806–1814.

56. Houssaint E, Blanquet PR, Champion-Arnaud P, et al: Related fibroblast growth factor receptor genes exist in the human genome. Proc Natl Acad Sci USA 1990; 87:8180–8184.

57. Huff KK, Kaufman D, Gabbay KH, et al: Secretion of an insulin-like growth factor-I related protein by human breast cancer cells. Cancer Res 1986; 46:4613–4619.

58. Humphrey P, Gangarosa L, Wong A, et al: Deletion-mutant epidermal growth factor receptor in human gliomas: Effect of type II mutation on receptor function. Biochem Biophys Res Commun 1991; 3:1413–1420.

59. Humphrey P, Wong A, Vogelstein B, et al: Anti-synthetic peptide antibody reacting at the fusion junction of deletion-mutant epidermal growth factor receptors in human glioblastoma. Proc Natl Acad Sci USA 1990; 87:4207–4211.

60. James CD, Carlbom E, Dumanski JP, et al: Clonal genomic alterations in glioma malignancy stages. Cancer Res 1988; 48:5546–5551.

61. James CD, Carlbom E, Nordenskjold M, et al: Mitotic recombination of chromosome 17 in astrocytomas. Proc Natl Acad Sci USA 1989; 86:2858–2862.

62. Janet T, Grothe C, Pettmann B, et al: Immunocytochemical demonstration of fibroblast growth factor in cultured chick and rat neurons. J Neurosci Res 1988; 19:195–201.

63. Jaques G, Rotsch M, Wegmann C, et al: Production of immunoreactive insulin-like growth factor IGF-I in small cell lung cancer cell lines. Exp Cell Res 1988; 176:336–343.

64. Jenkins JR, Rudge K, Currie GA: Cellular immortalization by a cDNA clone encoding the transformation-associated phosphoprotein p53. Nature 1984; 312:651–654.

65. Jennings MT, Maciunas RJ, Carver R, et al: HL TGFβ₁ and TGFβ₂ are potential growth regulators for low-grade and malignant gliomas in vitro: Evidence in support of an autocrine hypothesis. Int J Cancer 1991; 49:129–139.

66. Johnson DE, Lu J, Chen H, et al: The human fibroblast growth factor receptor genes: A common structural arrangement underlies the mechanisms for generating receptor forms that differ in their third immunoglobulin domain. Mol Cell Biol 1991; 11:4627–4634.

67. Johnson DE, Williams LT: Structural and functional diversity in FGF receptor multigene family. Adv Cancer Res 1993; 60:1–41.

68. Johnson DE, Lee PL, Lu J, et al: Diverse forms of a receptor for acidic and basic fibroblast growth factors. Mol Cell Biol 1990; 10:4728–4736.

69. Kan M, DiSorbo D, Hou J, et al: High and low affinity binding of heparin-binding growth factor to a 130-kDa receptor correlates with stimulation and inhibition of growth of a differentiated human hepatoma. J Biol Chem 1988; 263:11306–11313.

70. Kan M, Shi E: Fibronectin, not laminin, mediates heparin-dependent heparin-binding growth factor type I binding to substrata and stimulation of endothelial cell growth. In Vitro Cell Dev Biol 1990; 26:1151–1156.

71. Keck P, Hauser S, Krivi G, et al: Vascular permeability factor, an endothelial cell mitogen related to PDGF. Science 1989; 246:1309–1312.

72. Keegan K, Johnson DE, Williams LT, et al: Isolation of additional member of the fibroblast growth factor receptor family, FGFR-3. Proc Natl Acad Sci USA 1991; 88:1095–1099.

73. Kern SE, Kinzler KW, Bruskin A, et al: Identification of p53 as a sequence-specific DNA-binding protein. Science 1991; 252:1708–1711.

74. Kimelman D, Abraham A, Haaparanta T, et al: The presence of fibroblast growth factor in the frog egg: Its role as a natural mesoderm inducer. Science 1988; 242:1053–1056.

75. Kumabe T, Sohma Y, Kayama T, et al: Amplification of α-platelet-derived growth factor receptor gene lacking an exon coding for a portion of the extracellular region in a primary brain tumor of glial origin. Oncogene 1992; 7:627–633.

76. Ladoux A, Frelin C: Hypoxia is a strong inducer of vascular endothelial growth factor mRNA expression in the heart. Biochem Biophys Res Commun 1993; 195:1005–1010.

77. Lai C, Lemke G: An extended family of protein-tyrosine kinase genes differentially expressed in the vertebrate nervous system. Neuron 1991; 6:691–704.

78. Leung D, Cachianes G, Kuang W, et al: Vascular endothelial growth factor is a secreted angiogenic mitogen. Science 1989; 246:306–309.

79. Libermann TA, Friesel R, Jaye M, et al: An angiogenic growth factor is expressed in human glioma cells. EMBO J 1987; 6:1627–1632.

80. Libermann TA, Nusbaum HR, Razon N, et al: Amplification, enhanced expression and possible rearrangement of EGF receptor gene in primary human brain tumours of glial origin. Nature 1985; 313:144–147.

81. Livingstone LR, White A, Sprouse J, et al: Altered cell cycle arrest and gene amplification potential accompany loss of wild-type p53. Cell 1992; 70:923–935.

82. Malden LT, Novak U, Kaye AH, et al: Selective amplification of the cytoplasmic domain of the epidermal growth factor receptor gene in glioblastoma multiforme. Cancer Res 1988; 48:2711–2714.

83. Mapstone TB: Expression of platelet-derived growth factor and transforming growth factor and their correlation with cellular morphology in glial tumors. J Neurosurg 1991; 75:447–451.

84. Marics I, Adelaide J, Raybaud F, et al: Characterization of the HST-related FGF6 gene, a new member of the fibroblast growth factor gene family. Oncogene 1989; 4:335–340.

84a. Massagué J: Epidermal growth factor–like transforming growth factor: Interaction with epidermal growth factor receptors in human placental membranes and A431 cells. J Biol Chem 1983; 258:13614–13620.

85. Mattei M-G, Moreau A, Gesnel M-C, et al: Assignment by in situ hybridization of a fibroblast growth factor receptor gene to human chromosome band 10q26. Hum Genet 1991; 87:84–86.

86. Matthews W, Jordan C, Gavin M, et al: A receptor tyrosine kinase cDNA isolated from a population of enriched primitive hematopoietic cells and exhibiting close genetic linkage to c-kit. Proc Natl Acad Sci USA 1991; 88:9026–9030.

87. Maxwell M, Galanopoulos T, Neville-Golden J, et al: Effect of the expression of transforming growth factor-β 2 in primary human glioblastomas on immunosuppression and loss of immune surveillance. J Neurosurg 1992; 76:799–804.

88. Maxwell M, Nabor SP, Wolfe HJ, et al: Expression of angiogenic growth factor genes in primary human astrocytomas may contribute to their growth and progression. Cancer Res 1991; 51:1345–1351.

89. Mercer WE, Shields MT, Amin M, et al: Negative growth regulation in a glioblastoma tumor cell line that conditionally expresses human wild-type p53. Proc Natl Acad Sci USA 1990; 87:6166–6170.

90. Miki T, Bottaro DP, Fleming TP, et al: Determination of ligand-binding specificity by alternative splicing: Two distinct growth factor receptors encoded by a single gene. Proc Natl Acad Sci USA 1992; 89:246–250.

91. Mikkelsen T, Cairncross JG, Cavenee WK: Genetics of the malignant progression of astrocytoma. J Cell Biochem 1991; 46:3–8.

92. Millauer B, Shawver LK, Plate KH, et al: Glioblastoma growth inhibited in vivo by a dominant-negative Flk-1 mutant. Nature 1994; 367:576–579.

93. Millauer B, Wizigmann-Voos S, Schnurch A, et al: High affinity VEGF binding and developmental expression suggest Flk1 as a major regulator of vasculogenesis and angiogenesis. Cell 1993; 72:835–846.

94. Miyamoto M, Naruo K, Seko C, et al: Molecular cloning of a novel cytokine cDNA encoding the ninth member of the fibroblast growth factor family, which has a unique secretion property. Mol Cell Biol 1993; 13:4251–4259.

95. Miyashita T, Harigai M, Hanada M, et al: Identification of a p53-dependent negative response element in the bcl-2 gene. Cancer Res 1994; 54:3131–3135.

96. Monacci W, Merrill M, Oldfield E: Expression of vascular permeability factor/vascular endothelial growth factor in normal rat tissues. Am J Physiol 1993; 264:C995–C1002.

97. Morrison RS: Suppression of basic fibroblast growth factor expression by antisense oligodeoxynucleotides inhibits the growth of transformed human astrocytes. J Biol Chem 1991; 266:728–734.

98. Morrison RS, Giordano S, Yamaguchi F, et al: Basic fibroblast growth factor expression is required for clonogenic growth of human glioma cells. J Neurosci Res 1993; 34:502–509.

99. Morrison RS, Gross JL, Herblin WF, et al: Basic fibroblast growth factor-like activity and receptors are expressed in a human glioma cell line. Cancer Res 1990; 50:2524–2529.

100. Morrison RS, Sharma A, De Vellis J, et al: Basic fibroblast growth factor supports the survival of cerebral cortical neurons in primary culture. Proc Natl Acad Sci USA 1986; 83:7537–7541.

101. Morrison RS, Yamaguchi F, Bruner J, et al: Fibroblast growth factor receptor gene expression and immunoreactivity are elevated in human glioblastoma multiforme. Cancer Res 1994; 54:2794–2799.

102. Moscatelli D: High and low affinity binding sites for basic fibroblast growth factor on cultured cells: Absence of a role for low affinity binding in the stimulation of plasminogen activator production by bovine capillary endothelial cells. J Cell Physiol 1987; 131:123–130.

103. Murphy PR, Knee RS. Identification and characterization of an antisense RNA transcript (gfg) from the human basic fibroblast growth factor gene. Mol Endocrinol 1994; 8:852–859.

104. Murphy PR, Guo JZ, Friesen HG: Messenger RNA stabilization accounts for elevated basic fibroblast growth factor transcript levels in a human astrocytoma cell line. Mol Endocrinol 1990; 4:196–200.

105. Murphy PR, Sato Y, Knee RS: Phosphorothioate antisense oligonucleotides against basic fibroblast growth factor inhibit anchorage-dependent and anchorage-independent growth of a malignant glioblastoma cell line. Mol Endocrinol 1992; 6:877–884.

106. Naruo K, Seko C, Kuroshima K, et al: Novel secretory heparin-binding factors from human glioma cells (glia-activating factors) involved in glial cell growth. J Biol Chem 1993; 268:2857–2864.

107. Neufeld G, Mitchell R, Ponte P, et al: Expression of human basic fibroblast growth factor cDNA in baby hamster kidney–derived cells results in autonomous cell growth. J Cell Biol 1988; 106:1385–1394.

108. Nguyen M, Strubel NA, Bischoff J: A role for sialyl Lewis-X/A glycoconjugates in capillary morphogenesis. Nature 1993; 365:267–269.

109. Nigro JM, Baker SJ, Preisinger AC, et al: Mutations in the p53 gene occur in diverse human tumor types. Nature 1989; 342:705–708.

110. Nishikawa R, Ji XD, Harmon RC, et al: A mutant epidermal growth factor receptor common in human glioma confers enhanced tumorigenicity. Proc Natl Acad Sci USA 1994; 91:7727–7731.

111. Nister M, Hammacher A, Mellström K: A glioma-derived PDGF A chain homodimer has different functional activities from a PDGF AB heterodimer purified from human platelets. Cell 1988; 52:791–799.

112. Nowell PC: Genetic instability in cancer cells: Relationship to tumor cell heterogeneity. In Owens AH (ed): Tumor Cell Heterogeneity. New York, Academic Press, 1982, pp 351–365.

113. Ohtani H, Nakamura S, Watanabe Y: Immunocytochemical localization of basic fibroblast growth factor in carcinomas and inflammatory lesions of the human digestive tract. Lab Invest 1993; 68:520–527.

114. Pajusola K, Aprelikova O, Korhonen J, et al: FLT 4 receptor tyrosine kinase contains seven immunoglobulin-like loops and is expressed in multiple human tissues and cell lines. Cancer Res 1992; 52:5738–5743.

115. Parada LF, Land H, Weinberg RA, et al: Cooperation between gene encoding p53 tumour antigen and ras in cellular transformation. Nature 1984; 312:649–651.

116. Partanen J, Makela TP, Eerola E, et al: FGFR-4, a novel acidic fibroblast growth factor receptor with a distinct expression pattern. EMBO J 1991; 10:1347–1354.

117. Paulus W, Grothe C, Sensenbrenner M, et al: Localization of basic fibroblast growth factor, a mitogen and angiogenic factor, in human brain tumors. Acta Neuropathol 1990; 79:418–423.

118. Peters KG, Werner S, Chen G, et al: Two FGF receptor genes are differentially expressed in epithelial and mesenchymal tissues during limb formation and organogenesis in the mouse. Development 1992; 114:233–243.

119. Pettmann B, Labourdette G, Weibel M, et al: The brain fibroblast growth factor (FGF) is localized in neurons. Neurosci Lett 1986; 68:175–180.

120. Plate KH, Breier G, Millauer B, et al: Up-regulation of vascular endothelial growth factor and its cognate receptors in a rat glioma model of tumor angiogenesis. Cancer Res 1993; 53:5822–5827.

121. Plate K, Breier G, Weich H, et al: Vascular endothelial growth factor is a potential tumour angiogenesis factor in human gliomas in vivo. Nature 1992; 359:845–848.

122. Quinn T, Peters K, De Vries C, et al: Fetal liver kinase 1 is a receptor for vascular endothelial growth factor and is selectively expressed in vascular endothelium. Proc Natl Acad Sci USA 1993; 90:7533–7537.

123. Rapraeger AC, Krufka A, Olwin BB: Requirement of heparan sulfate for bFGF-mediated fibroblast growth and myoblast differentiation. Science 1991; 252:1705–1708.

124. Rasheed BKA, Bigner SH: Genetic alterations in glioma and medulloblastoma. Cancer Metastasis Rev 1991; 10:289–299.

125. Rasheed BKA, Fuller GN, Friedman AH, et al: Loss of heterozygosity for 10q loci in human gliomas. Genes Chromosom Cancer 1992; 5:75–82.

126. Reid HH, Wilks AF, Bernard O: Two forms of basic fibroblast growth factor receptor-like mRNA are expressed in the developing mouse brain. Proc Natl Acad Sci USA 1990; 87:1596–1600.

127. Rifkin DB, Moscatelli D: Recent developments in the cell biology of basic fibroblast growth factor. J Cell Biol 1989; 109:1–6.

128. Rogelj S, Weinberg RA, Fanning P, et al: Basic fibroblast growth factor fused to a signal peptide transforms cells. Nature 1988; 331:173–175.

129. Ross R, Raines EW, Bowen-Pope DF: The biology of platelet-derived growth factor. Cell 1986; 46:155–169.

130. Rubin JS, Osada H, Finch PW, et al: Purification and characterization of a newly identified growth factor specific for epithelial cells. Proc Natl Acad Sci USA 1989; 86:802–806.

131. Ruta M, Burgess W, Givol D, et al: Receptor for acidic fibroblast

growth factor is related to the tyrosine kinase encoded by the fms-like gene (FLG). Proc Natl Acad Sci USA 1989; 86:8722–8726.

132. Sandberg-Nordqvist A-C, Stahlbom P-A, Reinecke M, et al: Characterization of insulin-like growth factor 1 in human primary brain tumors. Cancer Res 1993; 53:2475–2478.

133. Santhanam U, Ray A, Sehgal PB. Repression of the interleukin 6 gene promoter by p53 and the retinoblastoma susceptibility gene product. Proc Natl Acad Sci USA 1991; 88:7605–7609.

134. Schnurch H, Risau W: Differentiating and mature neurons express the acidic fibroblast growth factor gene during chick neural development. Development 1991; 111:1143–1154.

135. Senger D, Galli S, Dvorak A, et al: Tumor cells secrete a vascular permeability factor that promotes accumulation of ascites fluid. Science 1983; 219:983–985.

136. Senger D, Perruzzi C, Feder J, et al: A highly conserved vascular permeability factor secreted by a variety of human and rodent tumor cell lines. Cancer Res 1986; 46:5629–5632.

137. Shi E, Kan M, Xu J, et al: Control of FGF receptor kinase signal transduction by heterodimerization of combinatorial splice variants. Mol Cell Biol 1993; 13:3907–3918.

138. Shibuya M, Yamaguchi S, Yamane A, et al: Nucleotide sequence and expression of a novel human receptor-type tyrosine kinase gene (flt) closely related to the fms family. Oncogene 1990; 5:519–524.

139. Shweiki D, Itin A, Soffer D, et al: Vascular endothelial growth factor induced by hypoxia may mediate hypoxia-initiated angiogenesis. Nature 1992; 359:843–845.

140. Sidransky D, Mikkelsen T, Schwechheimer K: Clonal expansion of p53 mutant cells is associated with brain tumour progression. Nature 1992; 355:846–847.

141. Smith R, Peters G, Dickson C: Multiple RNAs expressed from the int-2 gene in mouse embryonal carcinoma cell lines encode a protein with homology to fibroblast growth factors. EMBO J 1988; 7:1013–1022.

142. Smits A, Kato M, Westermark B: Neurotrophic activity of platelet-derived growth factor (PDGF): Rat neuronal cells possess PDGF β-type receptors and respond to PDGF. Proc Natl Acad Sci USA 1991; 88:8159–8163.

143. Stefanik DF, Rizakalla LR, Soi A, et al: Acidic and basic fibroblast growth factors are present in glioblastoma multiforme. Cancer Res 1991; 51:5760–5765.

144. Stock A, Kuzis K, Woodward WR, et al: Localization of acidic fibroblast growth factor in specific subcortical neuronal populations. J Neurosci 1992; 12:4688–4700.

145. Sugawa N, Ekstrand AJ, James CD, et al: Identical splicing of aberrant epidermal growth factor receptor transcripts from amplified rearranged genes in human glioblastomas. Proc Natl Acad Sci USA 1990; 87:8602–8606.

146. Taira M, Yoshida T, Miyagawa K, et al: cDNA sequence of human transforming gene hst and identification of the coding sequence required for transforming activity. Proc Natl Acad Sci USA 1987; 84:2980–2984.

147. Takahashi JA, Fukumoto M, Igarashi K, et al: Correlation of basic fibroblast growth factor expression levels with the degree of malignancy and vascularity in human gliomas. J Neurosurg 1992; 76:792–798.

148. Takahashi JA, Mori H, Fukumoto M, et al: Gene expression of fibroblast growth factors in human gliomas and meningiomas: Demonstration of cellular source of basic fibroblast growth factor mRNA and peptide in tumor tissues. Proc Natl Acad Sci USA 1990; 87:5710–5714.

149. Takahashi JA, Suzui H, Yasuda Y, et al: Gene expression of fibroblast growth factor receptors in the tissues of human gliomas and meningiomas. Biochem Biophys Res Commun 1991; 177:1–7.

150. Tanimoto H, Yoshida K, Yokozaki H, et al: Expression of basic fibroblast growth factor in human gastric carcinomas. Virchows Arch B Cell Pathol Incl Mol Pathol 1991; 61:263–267.

151. Tischer E, Mitchell R, Hartman T, et al: The human gene for vascular endothelial growth factor: Multiple protein forms are encoded through alternative axon splicing. J Biol Chem 1991; 266:11947–11954.

152. Trojan J, Johnson TR, Rudin SD, et al: Treatment and prevention of rat glioblastoma by immunogenic C6 cells expressing antisense insulin-like growth factor I RNA. Science 1993; 259:94–96.

153. Trojan J, Blossey BK, Johnson TR, et al: Loss of tumorigenicity of rat glioblastoma directed by episome-based antisense cDNA transcrip-

tion of insulin-like growth factor I. Proc Natl Acad Sci USA 1992; 89:4874–4878.

154. Unger T, Nau MM, Segal S, et al: p53: A transdominant regulator of transcription whose function is ablated by mutations occurring in human cancer. EMBO J 1992; 11:1383–1390.

155. Unsicker K, Reichert-Preibsch H, Schmidt R, et al: Astroglial and fibroblast growth factors have neurotrophic functions and cultured peripheral and central nervous system neurons. Proc Natl Acad Sci USA 1987; 84:5459–5463.

156. Vlodavsky I, Folkman J, Sullivan R, et al: Endothelial cell-derived basic fibroblast growth factor: Synthesis and deposition into subendothelial extra cellular matrix. Proc Natl Acad Sci USA 1987; 84:2292–2296.

157. Vogelstein B, Kinzler KW: p53 function and dysfunction. Cell 1992; 70:523–536.

158. Walicke P, Cowan WM, Ueno N, et al: Fibroblast growth factor promotes survival of dissociated hippocampal neurons and enhances neurite extension. Proc Natl Acad Sci USA 1986; 83:3012–3016.

159. Wanaka A, Johnson EM Jr, Milbrandt J: Localization of FGF receptor mRNA in the adult rat central nervous system by in situ hybridization. Neuron 1990; 5:267–281.

160. Wanaka A, Milbrandt J, Johnson EM Jr: Expression of FGF receptor gene in rat development. Development 1991; 111:455–468.

161. Weindel K, Weich HA: AIDS-associated Kaposi's sarcoma cells in culture express vascular endothelial growth factor. Biochem Biophys Res Commun 1992; 183:1167–1174.

162. Weinert TA, Hartwell LH: The RAD9 gene controls the cell cycle response to DNA damage in *Saccharomyces cerevisiae*. Science 1988; 241:317–322.

163. Weintraub H, Hauschka A, Tapscott SJ: The MCK enhancer contains a p53 responsive element. Proc Natl Acad Sci USA 1991; 88:4570–4574.

164. Werner S, Duan D-SR, de Vries C, et al: Differential splicing in the extracellular region of fibroblast growth factor receptor 1 generates receptor variants with different ligand-binding specificities. Mol Cell Biol 1992; 12:82–88.

165. Wilcox BJ, Unnerstall JR: Expression of acidic fibroblast growth factor mRNA in the developing and adult rat brain. Neuron 1991; 6:397–409.

166. Wong A, Bigner SH, Bigner DD, et al: Increased expression of the epidermal growth factor receptor gene in malignant gliomas is invariably associated with gene amplification. Proc Natl Acad Sci USA 1987; 84:6899–6903.

167. Woodward WR, Nishi R, Meshul CK, et al: Nuclear and cytoplasmic localization of basic fibroblast growth factor in astrocytes and CA2 hippocampal neurons. J Neurosci 1992; 12:142–152.

168. Yamaguchi F, Saya H, Bruner JM, et al: Differential expression of two fibroblast growth factor receptor genes is associated with malignant progression in human astrocytomas. Proc Natl Acad Sci USA 1994; 91:484–488.

169. Yamanaka Y, Friess H, Buchler M, et al: Overexpression of acidic and basic fibroblast growth factors in human pancreatic cancer correlates with advanced tumor stage. Cancer Res 1993; 53:5289–5296.

170. Yamazaki H, Ohba Y, Tamaoki N, et al: A deletion mutation within the ligand binding domain is responsible for activation of epidermal growth factor receptor gene in human brain tumors. Cancer Res 1990; 81:773–779.

171. Yan G, Fukabori Y, McBride G, et al: Exon switching and activation of stromal and embryonic fibroblast growth factor (FGF)-FGF receptor genes in prostate epithelial cells accompany stromal independence and malignancy. Mol Cell Biol 1993; 13:4513–4522.

172. Yayon A, Klagsbrun M, Esko JD, et al: Cell surface, heparin-like molecules are required for binding of basic fibroblast growth factor to its high affinity receptor. Cell 1991; 64:841–848.

173. Yayon A, Zimmer Y, Guo-Hong S, et al: A confined variable region confers ligand specificity on fibroblast growth factor receptors: Implications for the origin of immunoglobulin fold. EMBO J 1992; 11:1885–1890.

174. Yeo K-T, Wang H, Nagy J, et al: Vascular permeability factor (vascular endothelial growth factor) in guinea pig and human tumor and inflammatory effusions. Cancer Res 1993; 53:2912–2918.

175. Yin Y, Tainsky MA, Bischoff FZ, et al: Wild-type p53 restores cell cycle control and inhibits gene amplification in cells with mutant p53 alleles. Cell 1992; 70:937–948.

176. Yu D, Matin A, Hung MC: The retinoblastoma gene product suppresses *neu* oncogene-induced transformation via transcriptional repression of *neu*. J Biol Chem 1992; 267:10203–10206.

177. Zagzag D, Miller DC, Sato Y, et al: Immunohistochemical localization of basic fibroblast growth factor in astrocytomas. Cancer Res 1990; 50:7393–7398.

178. Zambetti GP, Bargonette J, Walker K, et al: Wild-type p53 mediates positive regulation of gene expression through a specific DNA sequence element. Genes Dev 1992; 6:1143–1152.

179. Zhan X, Bates B, Hu X, et al: The human FGF-5 oncogene encodes a novel protein related to fibroblast growth factors. Mol Cell Biol 1988; 8:3487–3495.

ALEXANDER M. SPENCE

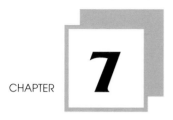

CHAPTER **7**

Glioma Metabolism

The chief reason to investigate glioma metabolism is to improve our understanding of the pathophysiology and response to therapy of these tumors and to use the new knowledge to develop better treatments. This chapter focuses on measurements of several aspects of metabolism in malignant glioma tissue in vivo. Measurement denotes quantitation. To the extent that this can be achieved, quantitation is emphasized. However, imaging of gliomas with radiolabeled tracers, in which the tracer uptake in tumor is higher than in surrounding normal tissue so as to distinguish the former from the latter, is also discussed.

GLUCOSE METABOLISM

To review briefly, glucose metabolism begins with transport from serum through the process of phosphorylation intracellularly to glucose-6-phosphate (G6P), which is catalyzed by hexokinase, one of the most important enzymes in controlling the rate of glucose utilization (Fig. 7–1). G6P is the starting compound for glycogen synthesis, for the Embden-Meyerhof pathway to pyruvate or lactate (glycolysis) and into the tricarboxylic acid (TCA) cycle, and for the pentose shunt (PS). The TCA cycle in turn leads to CO_2 production, some of which leads to pyruvate synthesis via anaplerotic reactions. Glucose serves different functions in glioma tissue than in normal brain tissue, in which maintenance of ionic gradients across cell membranes and electrical impulse transmission are dominant energy-consuming processes. These differences involve not only how much glucose is utilized overall, but also which metabolic pathways are followed. For example, the pentose shunt is utilized more heavily in tumors than in normal tissue and is the route to ribose-5-phosphate (R5P) for nucleic acid synthesis. In this pathway, production of NADPH yields reducing equivalents for biosynthetic reactions important for growth and cell division and for production of glutathione (GSH) for detoxifying reactions. Although malignant brain tumor tissue may show a respiratory quotient as low as 0.70, indicating the use of nonglucose substrates such as fatty acids or amino acids for energy sources,[3, 29, 90] glucose is still the chief source of energy and is also a source for certain amino acids such as alanine for incorporation into new proteins.

Hexokinase and other important enzymes involved in glucose metabolism have been reported by some but not all workers to show increased activity in brain tumors in relation to increased malignancy. These other enzymes, relevant to the pentose shunt, include glucose-6-phosphate dehydrogenase (G6PD) and 6-phosphogluconic acid dehydrogenase (6PGD) (see Fig. 7–1).[22, 49, 56, 86]

Because positron emission tomography (PET) allows estimation of metabolic processes in vivo, PET with [18F]-2-fluoro-2-deoxyglucose (FDG) has been widely applied in both research and clinical settings to assess brain glucose utilization.[32, 67] This approach has grown out of the 2-deoxyglucose (2DG) method with quantitative autoradiography of Sokoloff and co-workers,[80] which is based on the fact that 2DG mimics glucose in its transport across the blood-brain barrier and is phosphorylated by hexokinase to 2DG-6-phosphate (2DG6P). Unlike G6P, 2DG6P is not appreciably further metabolized and accumulates in the tissue proportional to the rate of glucose utilization. The two-compartment model and operational equation that solves for the glucose metabolic rate (MRGlc) contain kinetic constants that describe the processes of transport from plasma to brain and subsequent phosphorylation of 2DG and glucose. A lumped constant (LC) describes the ratio of the 2DG to glucose uptake. These kinetic constants and the LC have been determined in normal rat brain[18, 26, 80] and in normal human brain tissue by Huang and colleagues[37] and Reivich and associates.[70] In normal brain the LC is about 0.50. The determination of these constants and their significance in human pathologic tissues such as tumors remains to be completed.

The LC is a complex constant that contains the Km and Vmax Michaelis-Menten kinetic constants for 2DG and glucose in the hexokinase reaction, the ratios of the volumes of distribution of 2DG and glucose (λ), and a ϕ term, assumed to be 1, for the proportion of glucose that, once phosphorylated, is further metabolized. Mathematically, $LC = (\lambda/\phi)(Km_{Glc} \cdot Vm_{DG}/Km_{DG} \cdot Vm_{Glc})$.[80] It is necessary for calculation of MRGlc from PET with FDG because FDG (or 2DG) and glucose differ in their rates of transport from serum into brain or tumor cells and phosphorylation by hexokinase, and in their respective volumes of distribution in tissues of interest such as normal brain or glioma.

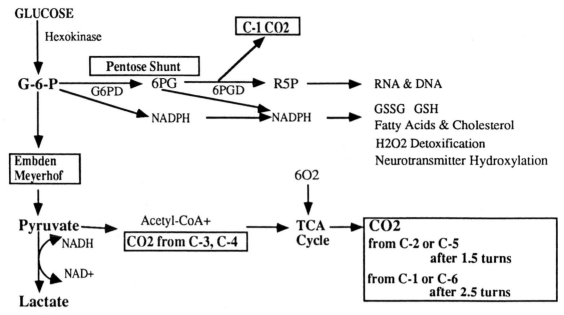

Figure 7–1 The principal metabolic pathways of glucose.

The expression $(Km_{Glc} \cdot Vm_{DG}/Km_{DG} \cdot Vm_{Glc})$ is the phosphorylation ratio (PR) of deoxyglucose relative to glucose. Km_{Glc}, Km_{DG}, Vm_{Glc} and Vm_{DG} can be determined individually in the biochemistry laboratory directly from kinetic experiments on tissue samples from glioma or brain, so that the phosphorylation ratio of gliomas can be compared to that of normal brain. In the rat brain the PR is 0.320, whereas in the 36B10 intracerebral rat glioma it is 0.694.[44] This is an increase of twofold and represents the dominant change in a twofold higher LC in rat glioma compared with normal brain.[44, 81] The phosphorylation ratio for human gliomas can be compared with normal brain values in specimens removed at the time of glioma surgery or temporal lobectomy for intractable epilepsy, respectively.[42] Preliminary results from 18 specimens are consistent with the rat data just given and show that the human glioma PR is roughly 1.5 times higher than that of normal brain.

The PR also equals the ratio of the rate constants for phosphorylation of glucose and FDG, k_{3FDG}/k_{3Glc}, that can be derived by dynamic PET imaging (with 1-[^{11}C]-glucose first, followed by FDG) and by mathematical modeling. In nine patients with glioblastoma multiforme and two with anaplastic astrocytoma, we have analyzed the 1-[^{11}C]-glucose and FDG dynamic tissue data by means of compartmental models and a refined mixture analysis approach which yields estimates of individual kinetic rate constants from pixel-by-pixel parameter optimization.[82] In these cases, the PR for normal brain (PR_N) was 0.36 (0.28 to 0.47, 95% confidence interval) and for gliomas (PR_T) was 0.80 (0.42 to 1.52); $PR_T/PR_N = 2.2$ (1.3 to 3.7) ($P < 0.02$). Because the LC is directly proportional to the phosphorylation ratio, these results collectively underscore the importance of clarifying the relationship of human glioma LC to normal brain LC, for FDG/PET to yield accurate quantitative measurements in vivo.

When patients undergo such imaging studies with dual tracers, the glucose metabolic rate in gliomas can be deter-

mined with radioglucose as well as with FDG. Use of radioglucose obviates the need for an LC in the calculations. However, radioglucose as an agent for measuring glucose metabolism with PET has some disadvantages. It is rapidly processed via several pathways so that the convenience of label trapping provided by FDG is not provided by radioglucose. Additionally, it is difficult to synthesize with the radiocarbon in either the 1- or the 6- position, which allow the longest retention of label in the tissue before production and elimination of radiolabeled CO_2 (see following).

These disadvantages of dynamic PET imaging with 1-[^{11}C]-glucose can be surmounted, as shown by a review of the work of Blomqvist and co-workers.[8] Their estimates of MRGlc with PET and 1-[^{11}C]-glucose in normal human brain have yielded excellent results. After administering 1-[^{11}C]-glucose they collected images with PET and sampled arterial plasma over 24 minutes. These dynamic data were analyzed with a two-compartment model. They additionally sampled jugular venous blood to measure arteriovenous differences for unlabeled O_2, glucose, CO_2, and acidic glucose metabolites, and measured blood flow with [^{11}C]-fluoromethane. Following injection of the 1-[^{11}C]-glucose, plasma metabolites of glucose, including CO_2, increased to approximately 10% of total plasma radioactivity over 24 minutes. In their calculations the researchers made corrections for CO_2 and metabolite loss from the brain tissue and for effects of CO_2 and metabolites on plasma ^{11}C time-activity curves. These corrections yielded a 12% increase in estimated MRGlc from 23.6 ± 0.8 μmol/100 g/minute (uncorrected) to 26.4 ± 0.8 μmol/100 g/minute (corrected). This result was not significantly different from the brain glucose metabolic rate of 28.3 ± 4.3 μmol/100 g/minute that they measured by the Fick principle. Thus, these investigators showed that the error in measurement of normal brain MRGlc from using PET with 1-[^{11}C]-glucose without accounting for CO_2 and metabolites in the tissue and plasma time-activity curves was only about 17%. This is noteworthy in view of the fact

TABLE 7–1
MRGlc, MRFDG, AND LC IN NORMAL BRAIN REGIONS AND
MALIGNANT GLIOMA IN EIGHT PATIENTS

Parameter	Units	Brain Mean ± SD	Glioma Mean ± SD
MRGlc	μmol/100 g/min	21.49 ± 3.09	18.00 ± 3.12
MRFDG*	μmol/100 g/min	10.82 ± 3.01	12.06 ± 3.31
LC†		0.496 ± 0.069	0.716 ± 0.175

*MRFDG = ((K1*k3)/(k2+k3)) (plasma glucose concentration).
†LC glioma/LC brain = 1.54
Abbreviations: MRGlc, glucose metabolic rate; MRFDG, (^{18}F)-2-fluoro-2-deoxyglucose metabolic rate; LC, lumped constant.

TABLE 7–2
MRGlc, MRFDG, AND LC IN THE NORMAL BRAIN REGION AND
MALIGNANT GLIOMA*

Parameter	Units	Brain	Glioma
MRGlc	(μmol/100 g/min)	23.41	20.53
MRFDG†	(μmol/100 g/min)	10.40	14.61
LC		0.444	0.712

*Values for patient in Figures 7–2 and 7–3.
†MRFDG = ((K1*k3)/(k2+k3)) (plasma glucose concentration)
Abbreviations: See Table 7–1 footnote.

that an error as high as 100% in estimation of absolute MRGlc in malignant gliomas could result from an FDG/PET study if the glioma LC is as high as we have previously shown it to be in the rat.[44, 81] These points suggest that quantitation of the glioma MRGlc with 1-[^{11}C]-glucose may be more accurate than FDG/PET studies that utilize an erroneous value for the LC.

In dynamic PET studies in which 1-[^{11}C]-glucose is injected first and FDG is injected 60 to 120 minutes later, the MRGlc and the FDG metabolic rate (MRFDG) can be determined in the same selected tissue regions, either glioma or normal brain, in the same patient in one imaging session. Regional MRGlc and MRFDG are estimated for either glioma or normal brain regions of interest by an optimization program based on two-compartment, four-rate constant models. This permits use of the following relationship to determine the human glioma LC: MRGlc = MRFDG/LC and LC = MRFDG/MRGlc. The LC estimated as MRFDG/MRGlc in tumor-bearing regions in the first eight patients we studied in this fashion ranged up to 0.8, whereas in non–tumor-bearing brain regions it was around 0.496 (Table 7–1).[83] There were seven glioblastomas and one malignant astrocytoma. Three cases were studied prior to radiotherapy and five were studied at the time of recurrence after radiotherapy. Glioma or normal brain tissue regions of interest from one plane were analyzed, and a region of interest from contralateral brain was used for comparison.

The following case represents a good example of these results from sequential PET studies with 1-[^{11}C]-glucose followed by FDG.

□ CASE REPORT

The patient was a 34-year-old man who had a stereotactically biopsied bi-hemispheral and midcallosal glioblastoma multiforme. PET scans were performed after he had received 2 daily fractions of 180 cGy per fraction of whole-brain radiotherapy. Table 7–2 shows data collected as above from 1 plane. The LC in tumor tissue was elevated (namely, 0.712) compared to the patient's normal brain LC of 0.444.

Metabolic images of this patient are shown in Figure 7–2. The FDG image, 1, represents the integrated uptake from 0 to 60 minutes after injection of the tracer; the glucose image, 2, is the integrated uptake from 5 to 25 minutes. The quantitative images, 4, 5, and 6, were produced by the

mixture analysis method.[63] The calculated MRGlc image, 5, shows that the rate of glucose metabolism in the glioma was not higher than that in the cortex, whereas the FDG integrated image, 1, and the calculated MRFDG image, 4, suggest that it was. The ratio image of the regional lumped constant, 6 (LC = MRFDG/MRGlc; image 4 divided by image 5) demonstrates that the lumped constant is higher in the glioma than in normal brain. When image 6 is compared to the integrated FDG uptake image, 1, and the quantitative MRFDG image, 4, these latter two images actually show that the tumor LC, rather than the tumor MRGlc, is elevated.

Figure 7–3 shows a histogram of the frequency of LC values in the normal brain region and in the glioma in this patient. The range is clearly narrower for the normal tissue, with a median of about 0.4, whereas that for the tumor is higher, with a median of about 1.0. There is clearly heterogeneity in the tissues with respect to the range of LC values, and it is decidedly wider-ranging in the glioma.

The data from this case and others strongly suggest that (1) the glioma LC and normal brain LC are not the same, (2) the glioma LC may vary from region to region within the tumor tissue, and (3) quantitation of the glioma MRGlc with FDG requires knowing the LC specific for glioma.

The glucose metabolic rate in malignant gliomas is probably not the quantity that is generally elevated. Rather, as just discussed, it is the phosphorylation ratio that is elevated.[42] A higher phosphorylation ratio suggests that the handling of glucose and FDG in the hexokinase reaction is different in malignant gliomas. This may be due to these substrates having different affinities in the neoplastic tissue. We have found such to be the case in the 36B10 rat glioma model in that a shift occurs from hexokinase I to hexokinases II and III, both of which demonstrate a lower affinity for glucose than does hexokinase I, the predominant form in normal brain tissue.[43]

Consistent with these ideas are several reports that show that cell types with high aerobic glycolysis (e.g., tumor cells) have proportionally higher type II hexokinase levels than the respective normal tissue.[17] This was shown in Rous sarcoma virus–transformed chick embryo fibroblasts,[78] in human T-lymphoblastic leukemia cells,[50] in Ehrlich ascites tumor cells,[53] and in malignant human gliomas.[7] Not only does type II hexokinase have a higher Km (lower affinity) for glucose,[25, 45, 50, 88] it also does for deoxyglucose.[25] It may well

Integrated Uptake Images (units = counts/pixel) and CT

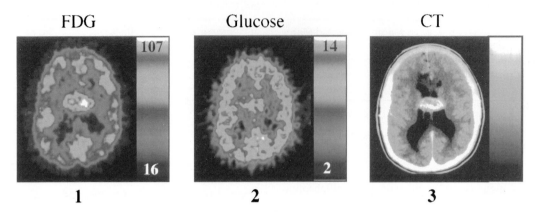

Mixture Analysis Images (units=μmol/100g/min) and LC

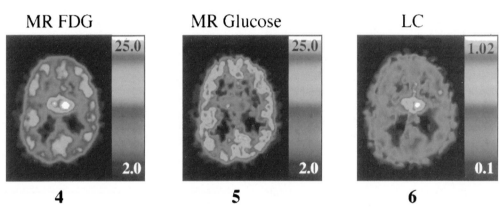

Figure 7–2 FDG and 1-[¹¹C]-glucose images of a butterfly glioblastoma multiforme in a 34-year-old man. See text.

be that a shift to a higher proportion of type II hexokinase in gliomas at least partly explains the higher phosphorylation ratio and LC as well as an overestimation of the MRGlc by the FDG/PET approach based on the normal brain LC.

This chapter has presented the point of view that an understanding of glucose and energy metabolism in malig-

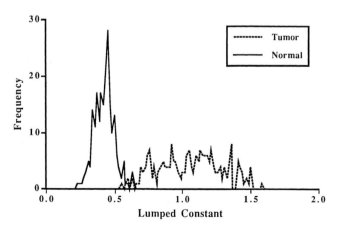

Figure 7–3 Histogram of the frequency of lumped constant values in normal brain and glioma in the same patient as in Figure 7–2.

nant gliomas requires that measurements of glucose metabolism be both quantitative and accurate. Because of the LC problem, FDG/PET imaging probably does not provide quantitative and accurate estimates of glioma MRGlc. This does not detract, in our opinion, from the value of nonquantitative FDG/PET imaging of tumors in general and of gliomas in particular in grading, in distinguishing viable tumor tissue from radionecrosis, or in localizing tumor regions with the highest degree of malignancy.

Di Chiro and co-workers have contributed a series of more that 150 cases of central nervous system (CNS) tumors studied with FDG/PET in which the estimates of MRGlc were calculated with normal tissue rate constants.[13–15] High-grade gliomas, if untreated, contained regions of high glucose utilization (7.3 ± 3.6 mg/100 g/minute; 40.6 ± 20.0 μmole/100 g/minute), and lower-grade gliomas lacked these regions. There was no correlation between CT contrast enhancement and high FDG activity in that high FDG activity could be seen in areas lacking contrast enhancement and vice versa. In 45 patients with grade III or IV astrocytoma, this group of investigators correlated glucose utilization rate, measured by FDG/PET, with survival.[65] Patients with ratios of tumor to contralateral normal brain glucose utilization greater than 1.4:1 had a median survival of 5 months, whereas patients with ratios of less than 1.4:1 showed median survival of 19 months. Most investigators of gliomas with FDG/PET agree with these concepts. However, measurements of glucose metabolism with FDG/PET in gliomas from the Montreal Neurological Institute have shown low but variable rates of glucose metabolism, irrespective of the grade, in untreated cases.[87]

Beyond these considerations is another important question in reference to measurements of glucose metabolism: Are changes in glucose metabolic rate a reliable predictor of the response of tumors to therapeutic interventions (i.e., do glucose metabolic rate measurements in gliomas reveal changes that correlate with lethal injury from treatment? Rasey and others[69] treated C3H mouse RIF-1 sarcomas with 11 Gy of ^{137}Cs in vivo and showed that 24-hour post-irradiation ^{3}H-FDG uptake dropped only 30%, whereas tumor cell survival measured in vitro showed a 70% reduction.[69] These data suggested that FDG uptake post-irradiation may not be a good early indicator of radiation response of tumor cells. On the other hand, Kubota and colleagues[51] examined the radiation response of several tracers in a rat tumor model and found that FDG showed a large change in uptake and a steady response to radiotherapy.

The work of Higashi and colleagues[31] and additional work by Kubota and others[52] provide further insights about the meaning of FDG uptake in tumors imaged with PET. Human ovarian adenocarcinoma cells were assessed in vitro for proliferative rate by DNA flow cytometry and ^{3}H-thymidine incorporation and for ^{3}H-FDG uptake.[31] During lag phase the proliferative rate was highest; it fell significantly in the exponential and plateau phases. In contrast, the uptake of ^{3}H-FDG per cell did not change significantly as the cells went through lag, exponential, and plateau phases. Total ^{3}H-FDG uptake correlated closely with the number of viable cancer cells present ($r = 0.957$), whereas total thymidine uptake underestimated the number of viable cancer cells. These results in vitro suggest that FDG/PET in vivo may reflect the number of viable tumor cells but not be an indicator of the proliferative activity of the tumors.[31]

Kubota and co-workers[52] investigated whether FDG (or ^{3}H-DG) uptake in tumors is solely due to tumor cell metabolism or whether it also distributes to stromal and/or inflammatory cells. C3H/He mice received transplants subcutaneously of FM3A tumors and were examined by microautoradiography and macroautoradiography 1 hour after intravenous injection of ^{18}F-FDG or ^{3}H-DG. They found that granulation tissue around the tumor and macrophages infiltrating areas surrounding necrotic tumor foci showed a higher uptake of ^{18}F-FDG than did the viable tumor cells. These animal tumor data showed that not only tumor cells, but also non-neoplastic cellular elements, contribute to uptake of FDG in tumors. This suggests that some caution is necessary in interpreting human brain tumor FDG images.[52]

Several studies address the potential for FDG/PET to quantify the metabolic response of malignant gliomas to therapeutic interventions. Mineura and others[61] and Ogawa and associates[64] reported seven patients imaged before and after irradiation and chemotherapy and used normal brain kinetic constants and LC in their calculations. All seven patients showed a reduction in tumor glucose metabolic rate by an average of 41%, between pretherapy and 1-month post-therapy FDG scans, indicating a therapeutic effect. This correlated with improvement of clinical symptoms. However, no data were presented on the time to treatment failure, survival, or diminution of tumor size.

Rozental and colleagues[74] studied six previously irradiated patients before and at 1, 7, and 30 days after eight-drugs-in-1-day (8-in-1) chemotherapy (methylprednisolone, vincristine, CCNU, procarbazine, hydroxyurea, cisplatin, cytarabine, dacarbazine) and five patients untreated with chemotherapy at 30-day intervals. They used rate constants and LC from normal brain[66] to calculate a ratio of tumor peak glucose utilization divided by the utilization in contralateral remote white matter (T*/RW). In the chemotherapy-treated patients the ratios increased 20% to 100% 24 hours after chemotherapy and then decreased over the next month to between 22% above and 35% below baseline. In a follow-up report, these authors presented 14 patients, some of whom were in the aforementioned study.[73] Five patients were imaged before and after 8-in-1 chemotherapy, and 9 controls (no chemotherapy) were imaged 30 days after baseline scans. Based on five cases (one in which the patient was alive at the time of the report), the patients with the largest increases in glucose metabolic rate 1 day post-chemotherapy showed the shortest survival times. This suggests that tumors capable of increasing glucose metabolism in response to therapy are resistant to it. In the nine controls, poorer survival correlated with increases in the T*/RW ratio from baseline to 30-day study.

Schifter and co-workers[76] studied 20 patients with gliomas through their clinical course with up to as many as five serial FDG/PET scans. All studies were nonquantitatively visually analyzed. Nevertheless, little change was noted in FDG uptake on serial studies in individual cases, but it was confirmed that patients with high FDG uptake had earlier documented recurrence and shorter survival than patients with lower uptake.

Our preliminary results on the radiation response of malignant gliomas are based on findings in seven adult patients who were imaged within 3 weeks before and 3 weeks after radiotherapy. In each imaging session, patients received a 90-minute study with 1-[^{11}C]-glucose, following which MRGlc was estimated for glioma and normal brain regions of interest by an optimization program based on a two-compartment, four-rate constant model. These preliminary results show that MRGlc measured with ^{11}C-glucose is variable following radiotherapy. Although our results and those of others have begun to raise our level of understanding of metabolic indicators of therapy success or failure, larger series are obviously needed to identify the most sensitive and reliable measurements and to clarify the optimal timing of studies.

PENTOSE SHUNT

G6PD and 6PGD are the initial enzymes of the pentose shunt (see Fig. 7–1). They catalyze the direct production of CO_2 from the C1 carbon of glucose. The pentose shunt converts NADP+ to NADPH for reducing equivalents for biosynthesis and for maintaining glutathione (GSH) in the reduced state.[35, 36] In this pathway glucose yields R5P for nucleic acid synthesis.

Investigations of pentose shunt metabolism stem from an understanding of the fate of the individual carbon atoms of glucose as it is metabolized through several biochemical pathways (see Figs. 7–1 and 7–4).[28] Briefly, in the pentose shunt, the C1 carbon of glucose is directly removed by 6PGDH to produce CO_2 and R5P. In contrast, via the Embden-Meyerhof pathway, neither this carbon nor any of the other carbons yields CO_2 until pyruvate, the chief three-carbon product of glucose breakdown, enters the TCA cycle. C3 and C4 yield CO_2 when pyruvate is converted to acetyl-coenzyme A(CoA). The C2 and C5 carbons do not yield CO_2 until after one-and-a-half turns of the TCA cycle; and C1 and C6 are liberated as CO_2 only after two-and-a-half turns of the TCA cycle. Through glycolysis and the TCA cycle, the C1 and C6 carbons of glucose are processed essentially identically. Therefore, studies of the fate of C1 vs. that of C6 radiolabeled glucose can be used to describe the relative metabolism of glucose in the pentose shunt and the Embden-Meyerhof pathway.[4, 5] When pentose shunt activity is high in a tissue such as glioma, metabolism of C1 radioglucose liberates radioactive CO_2 earlier and at a higher rate than metabolism of C6 radioglucose. Conversely, tissue cells retain radioglucose and its metabolites to a greater degree from metabolism of C6-labeled glucose than from C1-labeled glucose.

Based on this understanding, in normal adult rat brain it has been estimated that the pentose shunt accounts for about 0.5%,[10] 1.4%,[35] 1.5%,[16] 1.4% to 2.9%,[96] or 2.3%[19] of glucose utilization. In isolated perfused brain of monkey, the maximum contribution of the pentose shunt is reported to be 5% to 8%.[34]

In a review of tumor enzymology, Weber reported that flux in the pentose shunt is increased in neoplasms relative to normal tissues.[91, 92] Regarding gliomas, Coleman and Allen[10] presented data from which the pentose shunt fraction of total glucose utilization can be calculated to be 1.9% and 2.2%

in malignant gliomas of the rat spinal cord and brain, respectively. Kingsley-Hickman and co-workers[47] and Ross and colleagues[72] estimated the fraction of pentose shunt glucose metabolism in the rat T-9L gliosarcoma and T-C6 glioma in vitro to be 5.1% and 7.5%, respectively. Lastly, Loreck and associates[55] have estimated the pentose shunt fraction of glucose metabolism in grade IV human astrocytomas to be 4%.

When cultures of glioma cells, explanted slices of glioma, or normal brain cells are fed with glucose labeled with ^{14}C-glucose in either the C1 or the C6 position, the higher the amount of ^{14}C-CO_2 is formed per gram of tissue per hour from 1-[^{14}C]- vs. 6-[^{14}C]-glucose, the greater the relative pentose shunt activity compared to the Embden-Meyerhof pathway/TCA activity. In normal rat brain slices the ratio of CO_2 produced from C1 labeled substrate vs. that from C6 is essentially unity, confirming that pentose shunt activity is low in normal brain.[85] This ratio is as high as 3 as reported by Coleman and Allen[10] and 6 as we have reported[85] in slices of ethylnitrosourea-induced rat gliomas, indicating high pentose shunt activity in these experimental tumors.[10]

We have examined this further in vivo in the rat. Animals bearing 6 to 8 mm diameter grafts of either 36B-10 glioma or C6 glioma at six separate dorsal subcutaneous sites received simultaneous intravenous dual isotope injections of either [1-^{11}C]glucose and [6-^{14}C]glucose, or [1-^{14}C]glucose and [6-^{11}C]glucose.[84] Tumors were successively ligated and sampled every 10 minutes between 5 and 55 minutes post-injection to quantify tumor tissue tracer uptake and retention. Plasma was simultaneously collected to derive an arterial plasma time-activity curve for each isotopic form of glucose so that tumor radioactivity levels could be normalized by plasma radioglucose levels. Uptake and retention of radioglucose in the tumors from C1 relative to C6, namely the C1/C6 ratio, were plotted and compared. The results showed that the curves of the C1/C6 ratios plotted against time of tumor sampling were consistently lower than unity by approximately 6%, indicating that these gliomas do utilize the pentose shunt significantly in vivo (Fig. 7–5).

Additional interesting questions follow from results of this type: (1) Is resistance of tumor cells to radiotherapy or chemotherapy in part due to increased pentose shunt usage for maintenance of glutathione in the reduced state, where it can contribute to detoxification of drugs or free radicals? There is evidence to support this as a potential mechanism for drug resistance, as Gessner and co-workers have shown that there is a two-fold increase in the pentose shunt in P388 daunorubicin-resistant cells compared with that in sensitive cells.[21] (2) Does the pentose shunt increase in tumor or normal tissue in response to therapy?

OXYGEN METABOLISM AND HYPOXIA

Oxygen metabolic rate (MRO_2), blood flow (CBF), oxygen extraction fraction (OEF), and blood volume (CBV) in malignant gliomas have all been examined by several groups.[1, 3, 41, 54, 58, 71, 87, 95] These studies are consistent in showing that oxygen utilization is low relative to normal cortex despite an adequate supply of oxygen at least macroscopically (i.e., blood flow and blood oxygen levels are adequate to meet the

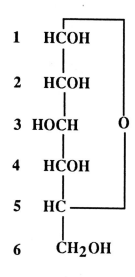

1 HCOH

2 HCOH

3 HOCH   O

4 HCOH

5 HC

6 CH₂OH

α-D-Glucose

Figure 7–4 The structure of glucose, showing the carbon atom numbering.

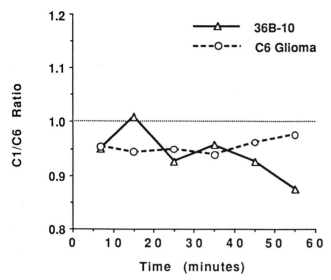

Figure 7–5 The ratio of C1 to C6 radiocarbon retention in the glioma grafts vs. time of tissue sampling after dual tracer administration.

metabolic demands of the tumors). Wise and co-workers[95] in particular noted that both MRO$_2$ and regional oxygen extraction (OER) tend to be lower in malignant gliomas, suggesting the tissue is not macroscopically ischemic or hypoxic. Other major studies agree.[3, 54, 87]

Table 7–3 shows data from seven patients with intermediate- or high-grade gliomas that illustrate the parameters relevant to oxygen metabolism.[71] Note that blood flow in the tumors is the same as in uninvolved brain, whereas MRO$_2$ and OER are roughly half. These results on MRO$_2$ agree with measurements in human adults obtained by the Fick principle.[3]

The utilization of oxygen relative to that of glucose, namely the metabolic ratio, is reduced in malignant gliomas.[71, 87] In normal brain the metabolic ratio is 5.2 mol of oxygen per mole of glucose,[6] whereas in gliomas it is 1.9 mol of oxygen per mole of glucose.[71] A lower than normal metabolic ratio indicates that the tissue is breaking down glucose to lactate (glycolysis) and that nonoxidative metabolism of glucose is occurring. In the presence of adequate blood flow and reduced oxygen extraction in tumors, the reduced metabolic ratio indicates that glycolysis is aerobic rather than anaerobic.[3] Despite adequate oxygenation, lactate production proceeds in tumors, whereas anaerobic conditions lead to this in normal brain.

TABLE 7–3
CBF, MRO$_2$, AND OER FROM GLIOMA AND CONTRALATERAL CORTEX

Function	Units	Tumor	Contralateral Cortex
CBF	mL/100 mL/min	32 ± 9	32 ± 5
MRO$_2$	mL/100 mL/min	1.2 ± 0.6	2.8 ± 0.5
OER		0.21 ± 0.07	0.47 ± 0.05

Abbreviations: CBF, cerebral blood flow; MRO$_2$, oxygen metabolic rate; OER, regional oxygen extraction.
Data from Rhodes CG, Wise RJ, Gibbs JM, et al: In vivo disturbance of the oxidative metabolism of glucose in human cerebral gliomas. Ann Neurol 1983; 14:614–626.

Interpretation of these results on the metabolic ratio depends on the accuracy of the measurements of MRGlc. The difference in metabolic ratio between normal brain and glioma tissue will be overestimated if MRGlc in the gliomas is overestimated, as we suspect it may be, when glucose metabolism in malignant gliomas is measured with the FDG approach as discussed earlier.[83] However, consistent with there being an increase in the metabolic ratio are data from several investigators. Magnetic resonance spectroscopy shows increased lactate in some, but not all, gliomas.[2, 30] Malignant gliomas show increased LDH and a shift of the LDH isozyme pattern toward predominance of the muscle type, indicating that pyruvate reduction to lactate is favored over oxidation via the citric acid cycle.[3, 20, 38] Lastly, data from implanted animal tumors show increased lactate content assessed by a bioluminescence method.[33]

Oxygen metabolism is an especially important function to understand in malignant gliomas because spontaneous necrosis suggests the presence of hypoxic cells that are radioresistant. Such cells may be responsible for repopulation following a course of radiotherapy. Direct measurements of intratumoral oxygen tension by means of polarographic oxygen electrodes have shown that high-grade brain tumors do indeed contain significant regions of hypoxia.[68] Not only can regional oxygen metabolism in malignant tumors be assessed with $^{15}O_2$ tracers, but regional hypoxia can also be evaluated by mapping ^{18}F-fluoromisonidazole uptake and distribution.[48] Three glioma cases have been reported, and tracer uptake consistent with the presence of regional hypoxia may well have occurred in one.[89]

The significance of hypoxia in the response of gliomas to radiotherapy has never been clarified completely. Treatment approaches based on eradication of hypoxic cell populations with radiotherapy either have been unsuccessful, as in the case of hypoxic cell radiosensitizers,[11, 23, 62] or have been too toxic, as in the case of fast neutron therapy.[24]

Data on changes in glioma oxygen metabolic rate in response to therapy are scarce. One series of seven cases in which treatment consisted of radiotherapy plus chemotherapy with ACNU, FT207, and PSK showed a wide range in cerebral metabolic oxygen rates (CMRO$_2$) from a 65% increase before therapy to a 92% decrease after therapy.[64]

PROTEIN METABOLISM

To measure protein synthesis in vivo requires intravenous administration of radiolabeled amino acid (or acids) followed by determination of (1) the arterial time-concentration curve of the amino acid, (2) the exchange from plasma into tumor tissue or brain tissue, (3) the free amino acid pools, and (4) the incorporation in proteins via aminoacyl-tRNA. This is problematic for two reasons. First, the intracellular free amino acid pool receives amino acids from proteolysis in addition to the plasma source, and, second, many amino acids, once in brain or brain tumor tissue, follow several metabolic pathways to compounds other than proteins. For example, methionine functions in transmethylation reactions and tyrosine contributes to synthesis of catecholamines. These two problems together have impeded accurate in vivo measurements of protein synthesis.

Leucine labeled in the C1 position is the most promising amino acid for protein synthesis measurements.[39, 40] It enters brain tissue via the neutral amino acid transport mechanism, and it has a high blood-brain barrier permeability relative to that of other amino acids. From the free amino acid pool in cells, it is channeled into protein synthesis or oxidation via transamination followed by decarboxylation to yield labeled CO_2, which can diffuse out of the tissue for removal by cerebral blood flow.

This notwithstanding, the bulk of the attempts to assess protein synthesis in vivo with labeled amino acids are based on ^{11}C-L-methionine. Bustany and colleagues[9] evaluated 14 patients. The protein synthesis rate estimated by their approach was increased in all gliomas, but the increase was greater in the more anaplastic tumors. Another series of 22 patients was reported by Derlon and co-workers.[12] For each patient they calculated a ratio, R, or the activity in the tumor divided by the activity in the contralateral healthy symmetric brain region, to be used as an "internal standard" in the same patient. The mean values of R were: 1.04 ± 0.27 in grade 2 gliomas (n = 5), 1.68 ± 0.22 in grade 3 gliomas (n = 5), and 2.33 ± 0.86 in grade 4 gliomas (n = 12).[12] Similar findings have been reported by others.[60, 75]

These investigations are clearly supportive of the hypothesis that protein synthesis is increased in malignant gliomas. However, the demonstration of increased uptake per se by an imaging device leaves open the question of whether the uptake is predominantly due to increased protein synthesis or to the additional process involved in uptake, namely, transport. Two arguments that support the idea that transport contributes significantly to uptake stem from the demonstration that the stereoisomers, ^{11}C-methyl-L-methionine and ^{11}C-methyl-D-methionine show similar levels of uptake in gliomas.[77] First, transport is mediated by a carrier of low stereospecificity such that equal accumulation of the stereoisomers in gliomas suggests that uptake is chiefly or solely due to transport. Second, the L isomer of methionine, not the D isomer, is the physiologic substrate for protein synthesis of enzymes. If protein synthesis were increased in gliomas, the L isomer would show higher uptake than would the D isomer. The fact that it does not show such an increase further suggests that uptake is predominantly the result of transport.[57, 77]

Although not based on ^{11}C-L-methionine, the research of Wienhard and associates[94] on the uptake of the amino acid tracer, L-(2-^{18}F)fluorotyrosine (F-Tyr), is highly relevant in clarifying the extent to which amino acid uptake represents transport or protein synthesis. In 15 brain tumor–bearing patients studied with F-Tyr and PET, the researchers performed kinetic analysis of the ^{18}F plasma activity and accumulation in gliomas and in normal brain areas. Although F-Tyr uptake was higher in tumors than in contralateral brain reference regions, this was shown to be the result of a two-fold increase in transport rates into tumors. Measurements of the rate of irreversible incorporation in the tumors (i.e., incorporation in proteins) showed a decreased rate. Interestingly, these workers also showed that the increased F-Tyr transport did not correlate with ^{68}Ga-EDTA uptake in the tumors and therefore could not be a result of disruption of the blood-brain barrier.[94]

The complexity of measuring the protein synthesis rate in vivo was well demonstrated in the prodigious work of Keen and colleagues[46] and Hawkins and associates.[27] In the normal rat brain after intravenous administration of L-[1-^{14}C]-leucine, they measured the time course of change over 35 minutes of plasma levels of (1) labeled leucine and its specific activity; (2) plasma proteins; (3) CO_2; and (4) ketoisocaproate (KIC), the product of transamination of leucine. They also measured brain levels of L-[1-^{14}C]-leucine, L-[1-^{14}C]leucyl-tRNA, and KIC and their specific activities. The main findings were that most of the radiolabel in brain tissue at 10 minutes was in protein, and that at 35 minutes, 90% of the total brain radioactivity was in protein. The specific activity of plasma leucine was greater than that of leucyl-tRNA, which in turn was greater than that of intracellular leucine. This indicated the existence of both (1) free leucine and leucyl-tRNA compartments in the tissue that communicate directly with the plasma and (2) separate free leucine and leucyl-tRNA compartments consisting of endogenous unlabeled leucine derived from proteolysis. The rate of exogenous leucine incorporation in proteins in brain tissue was found to be 3.2 nmol/minute/g of tissue, whereas leucine oxidation was found to be 3.7 nmol/minute/g of tissue.

Widman and others[93] in work on a transplantable rat glioma have presented convincing quantitative evidence that protein synthesis is indeed increased in glioma compared with normal brain tissue. Their approach consisted of administration of ^{14}C-leucine by a programmed infusion rate to achieve steady levels of plasma ^{14}C-leucine and specific activity. Tumor and brain tissues were collected 45 minutes after the onset of the infusion for quantitative autoradiography and for measurements of tissue ^{14}C-leucine, total leucine, and protein levels. This allowed the researchers to approximate the specific activity of ^{14}C-leucyl-tRNA in tissue by the distribution volume, λ, where

$$\lambda = \frac{\text{Tissue }^{14}\text{C-leucine/Total tissue leucine}}{\text{Plasma }^{14}\text{C-leucine/Total plasma leucine}}$$

Leucine incorporation into proteins was then determined using the equation of Smith and co-workers:[79]

$$Ri = \frac{C_i^*(T)}{\lambda \int_o^t (C_p^*/C_p)\,(t)dt}$$

where Ri is the rate of incorporation of leucine into proteins (nmol/g of tissue/minute); C_i^* is tissue radioactivity after removal of free ^{14}C-leucine and ^{14}C metabolites (nCi/g of tissue); and c_p^* (nCi/mL) and c_p (nmol/mL) are the radioactivity of ^{14}C-leucine and the concentration of free leucine in arterial plasma, respectively.[79]

The researchers showed that recycling of endogenous amino acids was 73% of total free leucine pool in brain tumor and 60% to 70% in normal brain tissue. Accounting for endogenous leucine recycling, they showed that leucine incorporation into the tumor was 78.7 ± 16.0 nmol/g of tissue/minute, whereas in the frontal cortex and striatum it was 17.2 ± 4.2 and 9.7 ± 3.3 nmol/g of tissue/minute respectively.[93] These results show that tumor tissue amino acid utilization for protein synthesis is approximately five times normal in this animal model.

Few human glioma cases have been examined before and following therapy to measure changes in amino acid metabolism. (^{11}C-methyl)-L-methionine uptake was examined in six patients following radiotherapy by Mineura and others.[59] Their data suggested that reduction of the uptake of this tracer correlated with a longer period of good neurologic function and improvement in the volume of contrast enhancement on cranial CT scans.

CONCLUSION

A sizeable effort on the part of many investigators has provided insights into several aspects of brain tumor metabolism. Progress to date falls short of providing convenient, clinically available, and reliable quantitative methods for measuring response to therapy for the individual patient's treatment planning. Some of this shortcoming certainly is due to the seriously ineffective treatments of malignant gliomas for which true responses, defined rigorously as disappearance of visible disease by irradiation or chemotherapy, are very uncommon. Measurement of glioma metabolism often can signal that therapy has failed or is failing in individual cases, but in the majority of cases, conventional CT or MRI approaches easily accomplish the same goal. To the extent that metabolic measurements are more or less reliable and clinically useful than CT or MRI remains to be determined in larger series of patients than presently available studies have encompassed.

REFERENCES

1. Ackerman RH: Clinical aspects of positron emission tomography (PET). Radiol Clin North Am 1982; 20:9–14.
2. Alger JR, Frank JA, Bizzi A, et al: Metabolism of human gliomas: Assessment with H-1 MR spectroscopy and F-18 fluorodeoxyglucose PET. Radiology 1990; 177:633–641.
3. Allen N: Respiration and oxidative metabolism of brain tumors. *In* Kirsch WM, Paoletti EG, Paoletti P (eds): The Experimental Biology of Brain Tumors. Springfield, Ill, Charles C Thomas, 1972, pp 243–274.
4. Baquer NZ, Hothersall JS, McLean P: Function and regulation of the pentose phosphate pathway in brain. Curr Top Cell Regul 1988; 29:265–289.
5. Baquer NZ, Hothersall JS, McLean P, et al: Aspects of carbohydrate metabolism in developing brain. Dev Med Child Neurol 1977; 19:81–104.
6. Baron JC, Rougemont D, Soussaline F, et al: Local interrelationships of cerebral oxygen consumption and glucose utilization in normal subjects and in ischemic stroke patients: A positron tomography study. J Cereb Blood Flow Metab 1984; 4:140–149.
7. Bennett MJ, Timperley WR, Taylor CB, et al: Isoenzymes of hexokinase in the developing, normal and neoplastic human brain. Eur J Cancer 1978; 14:189–193.
8. Blomqvist G, Stone-Elander S, Halldin C, et al: Positron emission tomographic measurements of cerebral glucose utilization using [1-11-C]D-glucose. J Cereb Blood Flow Metab 1990; 10:467–483.
9. Bustany P, Chatel M, Derlon JM, et al: Brain tumor protein synthesis and histological grades: A study by positron emission tomography (PET) with C11-L-methionine. J Neurooncol 1986; 3:397–404.
10. Coleman MT, Allen N: The hexose monophosphate pathway in ethylnitrosourea induced tumors of the nervous system. J Neurochem 1978; 30:83–90.
11. Davis LW: Malignant glioma—a nemesis which requires clinical and basic investigation in radiation oncology. Int J Radiat Oncol Biol Phys 1989; 16:1355–1365.
12. Derlon JM, Bourdet C, Bustany P, et al: [^{11}C]L-methionine uptake in gliomas. Neurosurgery 1989; 25:720–728.
13. Di Chiro G: Brain imaging of glucose utilization in cerebral tumors. *In* Sokoloff L (ed): Brain Imaging and Brain Function. New York, Raven Press, 1985, pp 185–197.
14. Di Chiro G: Positron emission tomography using [^{18}F] fluorodeoxyglucose in brain tumors: A powerful diagnostic and prognostic tool. Invest Radiol 1987; 22:360–371.
15. Di Chiro G, DeLaPaz RL, Brooks RA, et al: Glucose utilization of cerebral gliomas measured by [^{18}F] fluorodeoxyglucose and positron emission tomography. Neurology 1982; 32:1323–1329.
16. Domanska-Janik K: Hexose monophosphate pathway activity in normal and hypoxic rat brain. Resuscitation 1988; 16:79–90.
17. Eigenbrodt E, Fister P, Reinacher M: New perspectives on carbohydrate metabolism in tumor cells. *In* Beitner R (ed): Regulation of Carbohydrate Metabolism. Boca Raton, Fla, CRC Press, 1985, pp 141–179.
18. Fuglsang A, Lomholt M, Gjedde A: Blood-brain transfer of glucose and glucose analogs in newborn rats. J Neurochem 1986; 46:1417–1428.
19. Gaitonde MK, Evison E, Evans GM: The rate of utilization of glucose via hexosemonophosphate shunt in brain. J Neurochem 1983; 41:1253–1260.
20. Gerhardt W, Clausen J, Christensen E, et al: Lactate dehydrogenase isoenzymes in the diagnosis of human benign and malignant brain tumors. JNCI 1967; 38:343–357.
21. Gessner T, Vaughan LA, Beehler BC, et al: Elevated pentose cycle and glucuronyltransferase in daunorubicin-resistant P388 cells. Cancer Res 1990; 50:3921–3927.
22. Graham JF, Cummins CJ, Smith BH, et al: Regulation of hexokinase in cultured gliomas. Neurosurgery 1985; 17:537–542.
23. Green SB, Byar DP, Strike TA, et al: Randomized comparisons of BCNU, streptozotocin, radiosensitizer, and fractionation of radiotherapy in the post-operative treatment of malignant glioma. Am Soc Clin Oncol 1984; 3:260.
24. Griffin TW, Davis R, Laramore G, et al: Fast neutron radiation therapy for glioblastoma multiforme: Results of an RTOG study. Am J Clin Oncol 1983; 6:661–667.
25. Grossbard L, Schimke RT: Multiple hexokinases of rat tissues: Purification and comparison of soluble forms. J Biol Chem 1966; 241:3546–3560.
26. Hargreaves RJ, Planas AM, Cremer JE, et al: Studies on the relationship between cerebral glucose transport and phosphorylation using 2-deoxyglucose. J Cereb Blood Flow Metab 1986; 6:708–716.
27. Hawkins RA, Huang SC, Barrio JR, et al: Estimation of local cerebral protein synthesis rates with L-[1-^{11}C]leucine and PET: Methods, model, and results in animals and humans. J Cereb Blood Flow Metab 1989; 9:446–460.
28. Hawkins RA, Mans AM, Davis DW, et al: Cerebral glucose use measured with [^{14}C]glucose labeled in the 1, 2, or 6 position. Am J Physiol 1985; 248(Cell Physiol 17):C170–C176.
29. Heller I, Elliott KAC: The metabolism of normal brain and human gliomas in relation to cell type and density. Canad J Biochem Physiol 1955; 33:395–403.
30. Herholz K, Heindel W, Luyten PR, et al: In vivo imaging of glucose consumption and lactate concentration in human gliomas. Ann Neurol 1992; 31:319–327.
31. Higashi K, Clavo AC, Wahl RL: Does FDG uptake measure proliferative activity of human cancer cells? In vitro comparison with DNA flow cytometry and tritiated thymidine uptake. J Nucl Med 1993; 34:414–419.
32. Hoffman JM, Hanson MW, Coleman RE: Clinical positron emission tomography imaging. Radiol Clin North Am 1993; 31:935–959.
33. Hossmann KA, Mies G, Paschen W, et al: Regional metabolism of experimental brain tumors. Acta Neuropathol 1986; 69:139–147.
34. Hostetler KY, Landau BR, White RJ, et al: Contribution of the pentose cycle to the metabolism of glucose in the isolated, perfused brain of the monkey. J Neurochem 1970; 17:33–39.
35. Hothersall JS, Baquer NZ, McLean P: Pathways of carbohydrate metabolism in peripheral nervous tissue: I. The contribution of alternative routes of glucose utilization in peripheral nerve and brain. Enzyme 1982; 27:259–267.
36. Hotta SS, Seventko JMJ: The hexosemonophosphate shunt and glutathione reduction in guinea pig brain tissue: Changes caused by chlorpromazine, amytal, and malonate. Arch Biochem Biophys 1968; 123:104–108.

37. Huang SC, Phelps ME, Hoffman EJ, et al: Noninvasive determination of local cerebral metabolic rate of glucose in man. Am J Physiol 1980; 238:E69–82.

38. Ikezaki K, Black KL, Conklin SG, et al: Histochemical evaluation of energy metabolism in rat glioma. Neurol Res 1992; 14:289–293.

39. Ishiwata K, Kubota K, Murakami M, et al: Re-evaluation of amino acid PET studies: Can the protein synthesis rates in brain and tumor tissues be measured in vivo? J Nucl Med 1993; 34:1936–1943.

40. Ishiwata K, Kubota K, Murakami M, et al: A comparative study on protein incorporation of L-[methyl-³H]methionine, L-[1-¹⁴C]leucine and L-2-[¹⁸F]fluorotyrosine in tumor bearing mice. Nucl Med Biol 1993; 20:895–899.

41. Ito M, Lammertsma AA, Wise RJ, et al: Measurement of regional cerebral blood flow and oxygen utilisation in patients with cerebral tumours using 15O and positron emission tomography: Analytical techniques and preliminary results. Neuroradiology 1982; 23:63–74.

42. Kapoor R, Spence AM, Graham MM, et al: Measurement of the glucose and deoxyglucose phosphorylation ratio in human brain and gliomas by determining hexokinase Michaelis-Menten kinetics. J Nucl Med 1989; 30:838.

43. Kapoor R, Spence AM, Muzi M, et al: Comparison of the kinetic properties of hexokinase isozymes in normal rat brain and an intracerebrally implanted rat glioma (36B-10) model. 37th Annual Meeting of the Radiation Research Society, Seattle, 1989.

44. Kapoor R, Spence AM, Muzi M, et al: Determination of the deoxyglucose and glucose phosphorylation ratio and the lumped constant in rat brain and a transplantable rat glioma. J Neurochem 1989; 53:37–44.

45. Katzen HM, Schimke RT: Multiple forms of hexokinase in the rat: Tissue distribution, age dependency, and properties. Proc Natl Acad Sci 1965; 54:1218–1225.

46. Keen RE, Barrio JR, Huang SC, et al: In vivo cerebral protein synthesis rates with leucyl-transfer RNA used as a precursor pool: Determination of biochemical parameters to structure tracer kinetic models for positron emission tomography. J Cereb Blood Flow Metab 1989; 9:429–445.

47. Kingsley-Hickman PB, Ross BD, Krick T: Hexose monophosphate shunt measurement in cultured cells with [1-¹³C]glucose: correction for endogenous carbon sources using [6-¹³C] glucose. Anal Biochem 1990; 185:235–237.

48. Koh WJ, Rasey JS, Evans ML, et al: Imaging of hypoxia in human tumors with [F-18]fluoromisonidazole. Int J Radiat Oncol Biol Phys 1992; 22:199–212.

49. Kornblith PL, Cummins CJ, Smith BH, et al: Correlation of experimental and clinical studies of metabolism by PET scanning. Prog Exp Tumor Res 1984; 27:170–178.

50. Kraaijenhagen RJ, Rijksen G, Staal GE: Hexokinase isozyme distribution and regulatory properties in lymphoid cells. Biochim Biophys Acta 1980; 631:402–411.

51. Kubota K, Ishiwata K, Kubota R, et al: Tracer feasibility for monitoring tumor radiotherapy: A quadruple tracer study with fluorine-18-fluorodeoxyglucose or fluorine-18-fluorodeoxyuridine, L-[methyl-14C]methionine, [6-3H]thymidine, and gallium-67. J Nucl Med 1991; 32:2118–2123.

52. Kubota R, Yamada S, Kubota K, et al: Intratumoral distribution of fluorine-18-fluorodeoxyglucose in vivo: High accumulation in macrophages and granulation tissues studied by microautoradiography. J Nucl Med 1992; 33:1972–1980.

53. Kurokawa M, Oda S, Tsubotani E, et al: Characterization of hexokinase isoenzyme types I and II in ascites tumor cells by an interaction with mitochondrial membrane. Mol Cell Biochem 1982; 45:151–157.

54. Lammertsma AA, Wise RJ, Cox TC, et al: Measurement of blood flow, oxygen utilisation, oxygen extraction ratio, and fractional blood volume in human brain tumours and surrounding oedematous tissue. Br J Radiol 1985; 58:725–734.

55. Loreck DJ, Galarraga J, Van der Feen J, et al: Regulation of the pentose phosphate pathway in human astrocytes and gliomas. Metab Brain Dis 1987; 2:31–46.

56. Lowry OH, Berger SJ, Carter JG, et al: Diversity of metabolic patterns in human brain tumors: Enzymes of energy metabolism and related metabolites and cofactors. J Neurochem 1983; 41:994–1010.

57. Meyer GJ, Schober O, Hundeshagen H: Uptake of ¹¹C-L- and D-methionine in brain tumors. Eur J Nucl Med 1985; 10:373–376.

58. Mineura K, Sasajima T, Kowada M, et al: Perfusion and metabolism in predicting the survival of patients with cerebral gliomas. Cancer 1994; 73:2386–2394.

59. Mineura K, Sasajima T, Kowada M, et al: Changes in the (¹¹C-methyl)-L-methionine uptake index in gliomas following radiotherapy. Gan No Rinsho 1989; 35:1101–1104.

60. Mineura K, Sasajima T, Suda Y, et al: Amino acid study of cerebral gliomas using positron emission tomography–analysis of (¹¹C-methyl)-L-methionine uptake index. Neurol Med Chir Tokyo 1990; 30:997–1002.

61. Mineura K, Yasuda T, Kowada M, et al: Positron emission tomographic evaluation of radiochemotherapeutic effect on regional cerebral hemocirculation and metabolism in patients with gliomas. J Neuro-oncol 1987; 5:277–285.

62. Nelson DF, Schoenfeld D, Weinstein AS, et al: A randomized comparison of misonidazole sensitized radiotherapy plus BCNU and radiotherapy plus BCNU for treatment of malignant glioma after surgery: Preliminary results of an RTOG study. Int J Radiat Oncol Biol Phys 1983; 9:1143–1151.

63. O'Sullivan F: Metabolic images from dynamic positron emission tomography studies. Stat Methods Med Res 1994; 3:87–101.

64. Ogawa T, Uemura K, Shishido F, et al: Changes of cerebral blood flow, and oxygen and glucose metabolism following radiochemotherapy of gliomas: A PET study. J Comput Assist Tomogr 1988; 2:290–297.

65. Patronas NJ, Di Chiro G, Kufta C, et al: Prediction of survival in glioma patients by means of positron emission tomography. J Neurosurg 1985; 62:816–822.

66. Phelps ME, Huang SC, Hoffman EJ, et al: Tomographic measurement of local cerebral glucose metabolic rate in humans with (F-18)2-fluoro-2-deoxy-D-glucose: Validation of method. Ann Neurol 1979; 6:371–388.

67. Phelps ME, Mazziotta JC: Positron emission tomography: Human brain function and biochemistry. Science 1985; 228:799–809.

68. Rampling R, Cruickshank G, Lewis AD, et al: Direct measurement of pO₂ distribution and bioreductive enzymes in human malignant brain tumors. Int J Radiat Oncol Biol Phys 1994; 29:427–431.

69. Rasey JS, Krohn KA, Nelson NJ: Biological basis of tumor imaging with radiolabeled glucose analogs. J Nucl Med 1984; 25:P94.

70. Reivich M, Alavi A, Wolf A, et al: Glucose metabolic rate kinetic model parameter determination in humans: The lumped constants and rate constants for [¹⁸F]fluorodeoxyglucose and [¹¹C]deoxyglucose. J Cereb Blood Flow Metab 1985; 5:179–192.

71. Rhodes CG, Wise RJ, Gibbs JM, et al: In vivo disturbance of the oxidative metabolism of glucose in human cerebral gliomas. Ann Neurol 1983; 14:614–626.

72. Ross BD, Higgins RJ, Boggan JE, et al: Carbohydrate metabolism of the rat C6 glioma: An in vivo ¹³C and in vitro ¹H magnetic resonance spectroscopy study. NMR Biomed 1988; 1:20–26.

73. Rozental JM, Levine RL, Nickles RJ: Changes in glucose uptake by malignant gliomas: Preliminary study of prognostic significance. J Neuro-oncol 1991; 10:75–83.

74. Rozental JM, Levine RL, Nickles RJ, et al: Glucose uptake by gliomas after treatment. Arch Neurol 1989; 46:1302–1307.

75. Sato K, Kameyama M, Ishiwata K, et al: Dynamic study of methionine uptake in glioma using positron emission tomography. Eur J Nucl Med 1992; 19:426–430.

76. Schifter T, Hoffman JM, Hanson MW, et al: Serial FDG-PET studies in the prediction of survival in patients with primary brain tumors. J Comput Assist Tomogr 1993; 17:509–516.

77. Schober O, Duden C, Meyer GJ, et al: Non selective transport of [¹¹C-methyl]-L-and D-methionine into a malignant glioma. Eur J Nucl Med 1987; 13:103–105.

78. Singh M, Singh VN, August JT, et al: Transport and phosphorylation of hexoses in normal and Rous sarcoma virus-transformed chick embryo fibroblasts. J Cell Physiol 1978; 97:285–292.

79. Smith CB, Deibler GE, Eng N, et al: Measurement of local cerebral protein synthesis in vivo: Influence of recycling of amino acids derived from protein degradation. Proc Natl Acad Sci USA 1988; 85:9341–9345.

80. Sokoloff L, Reivich M, Kennedy C, et al: The [¹⁴C]deoxyglucose method for the measurement of local cerebral glucose utilization: Theory, procedure, and normal values in the conscious and anesthetized albino rat. J Neurochem 1977; 28:897–916.

81. Spence AM, Graham MM, Muzi M, et al: Deoxyglucose lumped constant estimated in a transplanted rat astrocytic glioma by the hexose utilization index. J Cereb Blood Flow Metab 1990; 10:190–198.

82. Spence AM, Graham MM, Muzi M, et al: Analysis of the fluorode-

oxyglucose phosphorylation ratio in human malignant gliomas and normal brain with PET. J Nucl Med 1995; 36:61P.

83. Spence AM, Muzi M, Graham MM, et al: Analysis of the deoxyglucose lumped constant in human malignant gliomas. Ann Neurol 1991; 30:271–272.

84. Spence AM, Muzi M, Graham MM, et al: Feasibility of imaging pentose shunt glucose metabolism in gliomas with PET: Studies in rat brain tumor models. XVIth International Symposium on Cerebral Blood Flow and Metabolism, Sendai, Japan, 1993.

85. Spence AM, Muzi M, Link JM, et al: Differential use of C1- vs C6-labeled glucose in a rat glioma model. J Nucl Med 1989; 30:911.

86. Timperley WR: Glycolysis in neuroectodermal tumors. *In* Thomas DGT, Graham DI (eds): Brain Tumours, Scientific Basis, Clinical Investigation, and Current Therapy. London, Butterworths, 1980, pp 145–167.

87. Tyler JL, Diksic M, Villemure JG, et al: Metabolic and hemodynamic evaluation of gliomas using positron emission tomography. J Nucl Med 1987; 28:1123–1133.

88. Ureta T: The comparative isozymology of vertebrate hexokinases. Comp Biochem Physiol B 1982; 71:549–555.

89. Valk PE, Mathis CA, Prados MD, et al: Hypoxia in human gliomas: Demonstration by PET with fluorine-18-fluoromisonidazole. J Nucl Med 1992; 33:2133–2137.

90. Victor JV, Wolf A: Metabolism of brain tumors. Res Publ Ass Res Nerv Ment Dis 1937; 16:44–58.

91. Weber G: Enzymology of cancer cells (first of two parts). N Engl J Med 1977; 296:486–492.

92. Weber G: Enzymology of cancer cells (second of two parts). N Engl J Med 1977; 296:541–551.

93. Widmann R, Kocher M, Ernestus RI, et al: Biochemical and autoradiographical determination of protein synthesis in experimental brain tumors of rats. J Neurochem 1992; 59:18–25.

94. Wienhard K, Herholz K, Coenen HH, et al: Increased amino acid transport into brain tumors measured by PET of L-(2-^{18}F)fluorotyrosine. J Nucl Med 1991; 32:1338–1346.

95. Wise RJS, Thomas DGT, Lammertsma AA, et al: PET scanning of human brain tumors. Prog Exp Tumor Res 1984; 27:154–169.

96. Zubairu S, Hothersall JS, El-Hassan A, et al: Alternative pathways of glucose utilization in brain: Changes in the pattern of glucose utilization and of the response of the pentose phosphate pathway to 5-hydroxytryptamine during aging. J Neurochem 1983; 41:76–83.

TOM MIKKELSEN

MARK L. ROSENBLUM

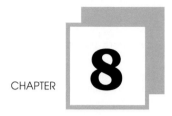

CHAPTER **8**

Tumor Invasiveness

The primary cause of recurrent disease following effective local treatments in the management of malignant gliomas is the insidious infiltration of tumor cells into surrounding normal brain parenchyma adjacent to tumor. Microscopic infiltration of tumor cells makes their removal by gross observation impossible and makes local treatment planning using radiation speculative at best. Inevitably, this results in the pattern of failure that has been described in the clinical literature. If it were possible to interfere with the mechanisms of tumor cell invasion, cell migration could potentially be restrained, making the tumor population more amenable to local therapies, such as surgery or radiation.

This chapter describes the clinical/pathologic and radiologic patterns of tumor growth and progression and discusses the models that have been designed to recapitulate portions of the invasive phenotype of glioma cells. Consideration is given to the specific molecular mechanisms of tumor invasion as well as to efforts intended to approach several of these targets therapeutically.

Brain tumor invasion is a paramount problem that prevents the cure of malignant brain tumors. As better local control is achieved, distant sites of recurrence are becoming more apparent. Tumor cells can invade normal brain structures along a variety of pathways made up of different anatomic and biochemical substrates. Because tumor cells have the capacity to recognize, attach to, and migrate through various normal tissue barriers, an analysis of the clinically relevant pathways should provide direction for research that is likely to have the greatest impact clinically.

The malignant nature of glial tumors is epitomized by the infiltrative nature of their growth. Because of the insidious migration of malignant cells along white matter pathways and perivascular channels away from the tumor mass, surgical management of malignant glioma is rarely, if ever, curative. In fact, attempts at wide local resection up to and including hemispherectomy have been tried with curative intent but without success. The measurement of extent of disease in diagnosis and during the clinical course of malignant glioma is critical to the assessment of clinical remission and, therefore, to the therapeutic response or failure and malignant progression. Studies to assess the regional anatomy of tumor have been carried out clinically with tissue sampling of regions of signal abnormality on magnetic reso-

nance imaging (MRI) and computed tomography (CT) scans, which illustrate that the agreed-on margins of tumor at the enhancing edge are not accurate and that malignant cells can be seen at and even beyond the region of T2 abnormality on MRI. Accurate measurement of the nature of the infiltrating margins of malignant glioma is critical as therapeutic agents ranging from standard radiotherapy and chemotherapy give way to phenotype-specific anti-invasive and anti-angiogenic therapies and molecular genetic therapies that seek to restore normal growth control and cell-to-cell relationships. Current and previous work in our laboratory has addressed the characterization of the molecular nature of malignant progression of glial tumors and the cell biologic characterization of the malignant phenotypes accompanying this progression, including angiogenesis and invasion.

The mechanism of human glioma progression and invasion involves alterations in cellular adhesion, cell motility, and proteolysis of extracellular matrix (ECM) components. We are currently analyzing the expression of several proteolytic enzymes, namely the cysteine protease cathepsin B and the matrix metalloproteases (MMP), in human glial tumors. Current techniques of Northern blot analysis and immunohistochemical analysis performed on frozen samples of primary tumors have shown the expression of these proteases in malignant gliomas. Furthermore, the degree of expression of these proteases appears to be related to their invasive capacity as measured in vitro. The activity of the protease cathepsin B can be inhibited using various strategies. The application of these expression studies and therapeutic approaches to the problem of human glioma invasion requires a well-characterized model system in which the invasion front of infiltrating malignant glioma can be isolated, measured, and followed serially over time.

Such novel molecular therapeutic anti-invasive approaches to the control of malignant glioma depend on accurate quantitation of the process in vivo and the ability to serially assess the process noninvasively. We have developed a novel human tumor model in the nude rat with a method for detecting the presence and detailed three-dimensional (3-D) architecture of human tumor cells on the background of the normal rat brain (unpublished data, 1993). The illustration of patterns of glioma growth, which recapitulate the patterns of tumor invasion in human gliomas, and the sensitivity of the detection method to the single-cell level will allow detailed comparison of this "gold standard" with methods of noninvasive imaging and feature analysis that may be used serially and, on rapid translation, directly in human trials. We believe that the characterization of the natural history of the tumor model using conventional histopathologic techniques and molecular in situ hybridization histochemical techniques, together with imaging techniques, will provide the foundation for the evaluation of a number of innovative therapeutic approaches being developed by our group. Finally, the validation of imaging techniques and invasion feature analyses will warrant their evaluation as measures of response in clinical trials and also in standard clinical practice.

PATHOLOGIC/CLINICAL FEATURES OF MALIGNANT BRAIN TUMORS

Gliomas in general, and more highly anaplastic gliomas in particular, infiltrate and spread great distances in the brain. The regional infiltration during tumor progression has been shown most strikingly in whole-mount studies[1, 2] in which glioblastoma cells appear to arise within a bed of better-differentiated tumor with regional brain infiltration. In histologic sections, most glioblastomas contain a central area of necrosis, a highly cellular rim of tumor, and a peripheral zone of infiltrating cells. Infiltration occurs along white matter tracts, around nerve cells, along blood vessels, and beneath the pia (secondary structures of Scherer). These elegant studies[1, 2] have shown that tumor cells of malignant gliomas have migrated from the primary site by the time of diagnosis in the majority of cases and are responsible for the local recurrence and tumor progression seen clinically. An understanding of the biology of glioma invasion sheds light on the problematic issue of the clinical management of these patients. Specifically targeted anti-invasive therapy would have a profound impact on the management of these tumors and allow effective local therapies, such as surgery and irradiation, to provide local control while limiting the infiltration of the cells beyond the reach of these modalities.

Patterns of Spread and Anatomic Substrates

Clinical recognition of tumor depends on the accuracy of imaging. Tumor cells do extend as far as the most distant area of abnormality seen by prolonged T2 signal.[3] However, using postmortem imaging of formalin-fixed brains, Johnson and co-workers[4] found no tumor cells up to or beyond the MRI-abnormal areas. The nature of these specimens obviously makes clinical correlations difficult.

Burger and colleagues have detailed the clinical appearance of malignant glioma in whole-mount brain sections[5, 6] and their CT correlations.[2, 7] In these studies they described the natural history of malignant glioma by examining untreated cases[8] and anatomic substrates on which tumor cells migrate in the progression of malignancy. The distant spread of tumor cells is not random; it follows distinct fiber pathways, such as the corpus callosum, fornix, anterior and posterior commissures, optic radiations, and association fibers.

Schiffer[9] examined a series of 90 malignant gliomas (85 glioblastomas multiforme, five anaplastic astrocytomas) of which 67 received radiation therapy alone and 18 were untreated. Of the 18 not treated, 12 were not operated on, five underwent surgery only, and one underwent biopsy only. Tumor cell infiltration could be detected histologically at a distance of more than 2 cm from the tumor edge, with fingerlike extensions in the white matter. Foci of infiltrating cells were seen in some cases, whereas mitoses were found in the normal white matter far from the tumor edge in others. Satellitosis was frequently seen as a modality of cortical infiltration, even in the absence of evident infiltration in the underlying white matter. In Schiffer's study,[9] CT could not distinguish edematous areas from underlying lower-grade malignancy or small foci of glioblastoma cells, either in the parenchyma or in subarachnoid deposits. T2-weighted MRI also missed the identification of lower-grade tumors and small foci of tumor cells to some extent.

Pathologically, the patterns of tumor cell spread in the brain indicate which substrates are likely to be critical in the dissemination of tumor cells. Adjacent parenchymal infiltration of tumor cells into normal brain substance, which may occur as single cells or in small cell clusters, would appear to require the dissolution of the cell-cell contacts and scaffolding of the brain matrix. This likely requires the action of proteases. The extension of cells along perivascular basement membrane, such as in Virchow-Robin spaces, and along subpial and subependymal basement membrane presumably requires modulators of cell-cell and cell-substrate adhesion, such as ECM-specific integrins, in addition to motility factors. The widespread infiltration of tumor cells along compact white matter pathways, such as the corpus callosum, the optic radiations, fornix, and association fibers, suggests the involvement of cell-cell and cell-matrix recognition molecules and motility factors. Spread beyond the parenchyma into cerebrospinal fluid (CSF) with leptomeningeal dissemination is also observed, suggesting a breach of the basement membrane.

Patterns of Failure

More than 75% of tumors in clinical series recur radiologically within 2 cm of the original tumor.[10] Multicentric tumors are uncommon, occurring in 1% to 5% of cases, and dissemination throughout the leptomeninges or spinal cord occurs rarely during clinical evolution and is seen in approximately 25% of autopsy cases. Clinical series describing the pattern of therapeutic failure confirm these values and illustrate that recurrence is likely to be local due to the density of residual cells at resection margins (Table 8–1).[10–16] Regional and remote recurrences are less frequent because of a rapid fall-off in the number of tumor cells (Fig. 8–1). Improvement in local control from aggressive surgery and focal irradiation is likely to select for or to allow the occurrence of distant metastasis, which happens beyond the reach of conventional treatment modalities.

Patterns of failure following therapy have been estimated from CT scans. Tsuboi and colleagues[17] estimated doubling

TABLE 8–1
LOCATION OF MALIGNANT GLIOMA RECURRENCE

Study	No. of Patients	Distance From Resection Margins (% of Patients With Recurrence)		
		<2 cm	>2 cm	>4 cm
Hochberg and Pruitt[11]	42	80	20	12
Awad[12]	191	—	—	6
Bashir et al.[13]	62	—	—	5
Wallner et al.[14]	32	78	22	—
Choucair et al.[10]	1,035	—	—	7
Liang et al.[15]	42	67	33	5
Garden et al.[16]	48	—	12	6
Cumulative		75	21	7

times and acquisition of enhancement effect as being indicative of patterns of regrowth. Several studies have confirmed that more than 90% of tumor recurrences take place within the region of the original tumor (see Table 8–1). In the uncommon occurrence of new lesions remote from the original tumor bed, recurrence was almost always accompanied by failure at the original site as well.[17] Improved local control can be expected to result in an increased incidence of remote metastases.

MULTIFOCAL GLIOMAS

Primary multicentric gliomas are uncommon, but a small percentage of recurrent cases demonstrate dissemination of multiple tumor foci that are not anatomically contiguous.[18] Distinction must be made between true multicentric glioma and multiple tumors that occur due to spread along white matter tracts, through adjacent ECM, or through CSF via penetration through the ependymal lining.[19]

We reviewed the imaging studies of a series of 47 patients with malignant gliomas (29 glioblastomas multiforme, 18 highly anaplastic astrocytomas). Of the 47 lesions, 25 (15 glioblastomas multiforme, 10 highly anaplastic astrocytomas) were examined by serial studies. Spread along myelin tracts was observed in 34% of invading tumors (28% involving the corpus callosum, 6% involving other white matter tracts). Among tumors located near the corpus callosum,

T2-weighted studies suggested spread through the corpus callosum in 59% of patients (16/27) at presentation and 82% (14/17) at follow-up. Invasion was noted in 38% of cases through the adjacent ECM and along basement membranes (predominantly subependymal) in 16%. The CSF was the pathway of spread in 6%, and in 6% of cases the pathway of spread was unclassifiable. The most frequent pathways for spread of malignant astrocytomas are the adjacent brain parenchyma and myelin tracts. Adjacent spread could be due to direct tumor cell migration through the glycosaminoglycan- and proteoglycan-containing ECM or along the basement membranes of penetrating blood vessels (histopathologically defined as satellitosis). Migration along subependymal basement membranes made up of laminin, fibronectin, and collagen type IV is also possible. The studies provide the basis for laboratory investigations of brain tumor invasion toward the development of new, clinically relevant anti-tumor strategies.

At onset, malignant brain tumors are predominantly a local disease that requires maximally effective local therapy. The chance of, and sites for, tumor recurrence appear to be dependent on the number and distribution of residual tumor cells. Two different therapeutic strategies should be aimed toward these two distinct compartments, local and remote, that make up malignant gliomas.

EXPERIMENTAL GLIOMA MODELS

In Vitro Models

MATRIGEL BARRIER ASSAY

Various models of glioma invasion have been developed, and several using primary tumor material correlate closely with clinical tumor behavior.[20] Perhaps the most widely used measure of tumor invasiveness is the barrier migration assay. The reconstituted basement membrane Matrigel product[21] has been used as a mechanical barrier through which tumor cells migrate in response to a chemoattractant stimulus (NIH 3T3CM).[22] Migrating cells (i.e., those that are able to pass through the Matrigel-coated barrier filter) are stained and counted. Experience with this assay in human glial tumors

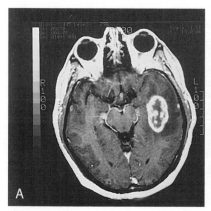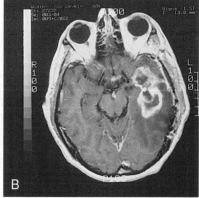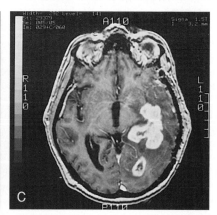

Figure 8–1   Contrast-enhanced T1-weighted MR images in progressive malignant glioma. The patient presented with a left temporal malignant glioma (*A*) and was re-examined 3 months (*B*) and 6 months (*C*) after diagnosis. The images illustrate local progression of the tumor and distal extension posteriorly with the development of a satellite lesion in the occipital lobe superiorly.

is limited.[23] However, use of this assay in the assessment of primary human gliomas is ongoing in our laboratory, and we have found that there does appear to be a relationship between migration through the filter barrier and clinical malignancy (unpublished observations, 1992). This assay is limited in that the dissociated cells are removed from their tissue microenvironment so that there is no cell-cell interaction. Furthermore, the barrier substrate Matrigel consists primarily of laminin, which does not occur in significant amounts in the brain ECM, except for the basement membrane surrounding penetrating blood vessels, the subependyma, and the glia limitans externa. Therefore, we have restricted our use of this invasion model as a screening technique and propose the use of more biologically relevant in vivo invasion models. Some authors have challenged this assay with regard to the validity of the clinical correlation.[24]

SPHEROID CONFRONTATION

The in vitro 3-D tumor-brain spheroid confrontation model was initially developed using syngeneic rat brain and rat glioma cells.[25] Detailed ultrastructural morphology confirmed the differentiated features of the rat brain aggregate.[26] This system preserves tissue architecture, and viable cell-cell interactions are made. Confrontation with human glial tumors provides accurate clinical correlation using primary tissue, primary cultures, and cell lines. Spheroids from well-characterized continuous human glioma cell lines have been tested for invasiveness in this model, which also allows studies of the invasive capacity of glioma cells derived from biopsy material within a week after surgery.[27] The model is an interspecies one, with human-rat confrontation, but the assay has also been performed using human fetal brain aggregates[28] and syngeneic rat tumor lines as targets, with similar results.[29] This system maintains an interactive process between cells, growth factors, proteolytic enzymes, and the ECM, while maintaining access in vitro for manipulation of the culture environment.

Interestingly, confrontation co-culture of glioma and spheroids prepared from leptomeningeal tissue demonstrates the inability of glioma cells to invade this target, whereas metastatic tumor spheroids, from tumor cells metastatic to the brain from breast or lung tumors, are able to invade leptomeningeal spheroids aggressively. Conversely, metastatic tumor spheroids do not invade brain aggregates prepared from brain parenchyma, which glioma spheroids invade readily.[28] This behavior parallels the clinical situation in which glioma tumor cells infiltrate widely within the brain but virtually never disseminate beyond it, whereas metastatic tumors, which breach the vascular basement membrane during metastasis, grow characteristically by expansion and displacement within the brain and do not tend to infiltrate brain parenchyma. Confrontation cultures in 3-D are able to model the processes of single-cell infiltration and parenchymal destruction during the process of glioma invasion.

In Vivo Models

GLIOMA MODELS

In vivo brain tumor models can be classified into several categories. Some animals develop brain tumors spontane-ously.[30–32] In other instances, tumors have been induced by various carcinogenic agents, most commonly by chemical compounds or viruses[33] or, more seldom, by radiation.[34] A major effort toward standardization of in vivo brain tumor research has focused on establishing transplantable brain tumor models. These are either syngeneic or heterogeneic as well as heterotopic or orthotopic. Although large animal models using cats,[35] dogs,[36] and primates[37] are available, these have obvious disadvantages in terms of cost and animal availability. Therefore, rodent models are more commonly used. Syngeneic models, such as the intracerebral 9L gliosarcoma model, have been widely studied[38] and have provided a wealth of information on tumor biology. However, because these tumors are of murine origin and are induced by experimental manipulation, their biologic behavior might be quite different from that of human tumors. Some success with human xenografts has been reported using immunosuppressive treatment regimens in rodents, but these methods are relatively difficult and elaborate.[39, 40] Successful implantation of brain tumors of human origin has been possible, however, since the advent of the nude athymic mouse in the late 1960s. These mice have a genetic deficiency in T-cell–mediated immunity and are limited in their immune response to xenotransplants. Brain tumors have been implanted as both subcutaneous and intracerebral xenografts in nude mice.[41, 42] Cerebral tissue is the most natural environment for these xenografts, but the small size of the nude mouse brain does not allow for a prolonged period of tumor growth nor for detailed examination of the tumor's growth pattern solely within the brain parenchyma. A larger brain, such as the rat brain, obviates this disadvantage. The nude rat, an animal immunodeficient in much the same way as the nude mouse, has been available since about the mid-1960s, but was introduced into biomedical research relatively recently. Reports of intracerebral implantation of human xenografts have appeared sporadically in the literature.[43] Metastatic tumors, medulloblastomas, and gliomas have been used. However, no systematic evaluation of a variety of glial and meningeal cell lines has been done.

Nude rats have been reported to be less efficient than nude mice in allowing establishment and growth of xenografted human tumors, with younger animals being better hosts than older animals. In our experience, the establishment rate has been excellent for several cell lines used, including both established permanent glioma lines and low-passage primary lines, except when small numbers of cells were implanted. In addition, we chose very young animals (weanlings, 8 weeks or younger) as subjects for these implantations.

However, to provide a valid qualitative and quantitative assay of brain parenchyma invasion it is necessary to distinguish each human tumor cell from rodent brain cells. Our group recently developed an assay in the nude mouse that serves to identify, using species-specific genetic markers, the species of cells in the glioma xenograft. To achieve this detection, nonhuman genetic material can be introduced into human tumor cells, such as the gene that encodes β-galactosidase; however, transfection could select subsets of human brain tumor cells or alter their invasiveness. For these reasons, we chose to exploit a cellular element unique and common to human cells only. The Alu DNA repeat elements of the human genome are one of several highly repetitive DNA sequence families dispersed throughout the genome of animals. There are about 500,000 copies per nucleus in human cells, which constitute 3% to 6% of the total human genomic DNA. Human Alu fragments are about 300 bp in length. The murine equivalent is about 130 bp and sufficiently different in structure (about 80% homology) to be differentiated by in situ hybridization techniques.

We reported the use of the Blur-2 human Alu DNA probe to analyze brain tumor growth patterns in the nude mouse brain by in situ hybridization.[44] Three human glioma cell lines were examined: U87MG, U251MGn, and U251MGp. We found that each line could be distinguished by a different pattern of growth in the nude mouse brain: a pushing border without invasion (U87MG), perivascular invasion (U251MGn), and parenchymal infiltration (U251MGp). Significantly, the identification of single tumor cells or clusters was very difficult using standard histochemical stains, which show no species specificity, but the Alu in situ hybridization technique was highly specific with virtually no background (Fig. 8–2). This method allows the identification of single human tumor cells in xenograft with essentially no signal arising from the host rat cells, which makes the discrimination of the infiltrating margins of the tumor highly specific, with essentially single-cell resolution. The implications regarding the use of such high-definition tumor cell resolution for quantitation of the invasion process are readily apparent.

Recently, Pedersen and co-workers[45] demonstrated the growth and spread of lac-Z transfected glioma cells in the CNS. In addition, the migration of developing fetal nervous system cells was shown, which paralleled that of tumor invasion and suggested the emergence of the fetal phenotype in tumor development. Xenografts growing in the complex cytoarchitecture of the adult brain most closely model the human malignant glioma and are directly relevant to clinical phenomena. The ability to accurately model the invasive process with pathologic fidelity lends itself to biologic and therapeutic manipulation and to possible translation to the clinical setting.

Nagano and associates[46] presented morphologic data on the early stage of tumor invasion in the CNS. C6 cells possess the characteristics of high affinity to the endothelial basement membrane and invade along the preexisting blood vessels with brain parenchymal infiltration.

Goldberg and others[47] and Bernstein and colleagues[48] used cortical implantation pockets in adult host rats. By 7 days postinjection a large mass developed that extended above the surface of the brain and invaded the host parenchyma. In addition to the invasion process, grafted C6 cells spread through the host parenchyma by migration. Individual cells migrated into host cortex surrounding the implantation pocket, corpus callosum ventral to the implantation pocket, ipsilateral internal capsule, and bilaterally in the habenula. The preferred routes of migration were on basal lamina and parallel and intersecting nerve fiber bundles. Invasion occurred through gray and white matter.

Bernstein and co-workers[49] showed that cortically homografted C6 glioma-astrocytoma cells both invade the rat host

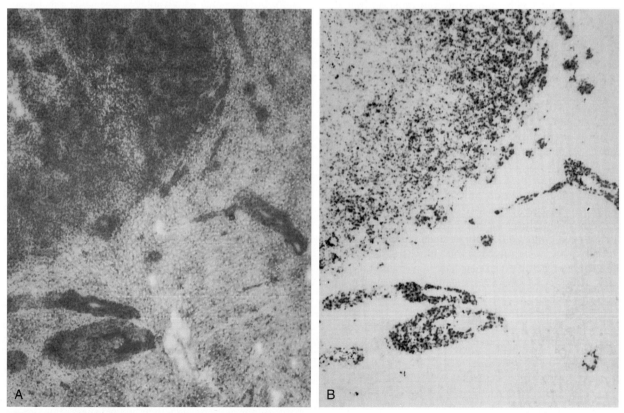

Figure 8–2 Alu in situ hybridization in a human glioma xenograft. The discrimination of human tumor cells xenografted into the nude rat brain is easily made in comparison to a standard section stained with hematoxylin-eosin (*A*) by using a molecular probe to human-specific Alu-repeat sequences on an adjacent section (*B*). Infiltration of single cells into peritumoral host brain and perivascular cuffing of tumor cells can be easily resolved (magnification ×80).

brain as a mass and migrate as individual cells. In contrast, fetal astrocytes derived from homografted whole pieces of fetal cortex migrate only as individual cells throughout the brain of the rat, but they are not capable of invasion. These data indicate that C6 glioma cells, which in vivo appear to be a model for glioblastoma multiforme, migrate primarily as individual cells through artificial basement membrane and form tumor masses secondarily. Progenitor tumor masses form by coalescence of individual C6 cell micropockets or by the division of a single cell in an individual micropocket.

MECHANISMS OF TUMOR CELL INVASION

Proteolytic Enzymes

A role for proteolytic enzymes has been postulated at many stages of malignant progression, including tumor cell infiltration through ECM and endothelial sprouting in the process of angiogenesis. Even the extent of tumor growth is regulated by proteolytic enzymes, as tumors cannot grow beyond about 2 mm in diameter without the development of a blood supply. (For reviews on angiogenesis and cancer, see Kerbel and others.[50]) In the case of angiogenesis, the cells participating in the invasive process are endothelial cells rather than tumor cells. Proteolytic enzymes that have been linked to malignant progression include representatives of each of the four classes of proteases: serine, metalloprotease, cysteine, and aspartic. In evaluating the putative role of these enzymes in cancer, one must recognize the apparent promiscuity in use of proteases by tumors and potential synergistic interactions among the proteases. Specific types of cancers may express high levels of one protease. For example, human breast cancers express high levels of the aspartic protease cathepsin D (for review, see Rochefort and associates[51]) and murine melanomas express high levels of the cysteine protease cathepsin B.[52, 53] In other cancers, high levels of expression of several proteases have been observed. In human breast and colon cancers, the levels of expression of the metalloprotease MMP-2 and the cysteine protease cathepsin B are both increased.[54] In human colorectal adenocarcinoma high levels of expression of both cathepsin B and urokinase define a morphologically and clinically aggressive subset of cases.[55] Such observations suggest the possibility of functional interactions among cathepsin B, MMP-2, and urokinase. Metalloproteinases have been implicated as important factors mediating the tissue migration of a variety of normal and transformed cells. The secretion of a battery of metalloproteinases by astrocytes may be important in facilitating astrocytic migration during development and in pathologic conditions such as inflammation or local invasion of astrocytic neoplasms.[56] Lund-Johansen and co-workers[57] described a continuous rat glioma cell line, BT5C, which causes marked invasion and tissue destruction when co-cultured with fetal rat-brain aggregates. From this cell line they identified a metalloproteinase secreted into the culture medium capable of destroying the neural tissue in a manner morphologically similar to the tissue destruction seen in confrontation co-culture. The report suggests a possible role of metalloproteinases in tissue degradation during brain tumor invasion, as others have suggested.[58–60]

The expression of urokinase[61] has been reported to correlate with the progression of human brain tumors. Expression of plasminogen activator (PA) enzyme activity is believed to be one of the mechanisms by which malignant cells cause pericellular proteolysis of stromal structures during implantation and tissue invasion.[62] Considerable heterogeneity exists among human glioma cells in expression of PA enzymes and inhibitors. The coordinated regulation of these proteins likely determines secreted PA activity and the resultant role of plasminogen activation in tumor implantation and invasion. As an example of the complex regulation involved with the proteolytic cascade of proteases, their inhibitors, and their receptors, Mohanam and associates[63] used anti-urokinase plasminogen activator receptor (uPAR) monoclonal antibody, blocking invasion effectively in a Matrigel assay, by 20% to 57%. These data suggest that the uPARs contribute significantly to the invasive capacity of the cells, possibly by facilitating uPA activity.

Type IV collagenase, a metalloproteinase isolated from rat glioma cell conditioned medium, and PA and plasminogen activator inhibitor (PA-PAI) complexes were identified as being secreted by the same cells.[64] Metalloprotease enzymes can be partially activated by u-PA but not by plasmin in vitro, suggesting a proteolytic cascade in the scheme for the proteolytic degradation of normal brain tissue during tumor invasion. We have examined a series of malignant gliomas with antibodies to metalloproteases and their inhibitors and found high levels of expression (Fig. 8–3) (unpublished observations, 1995).

A single report has described the secretion of cathepsin B by gliomas.[65] We have described the immunolocalization of cathepsin B to glioma cells in tumor core and infiltrating margins in a series of 33 glioblastomas, 33 anaplastic astrocytomas, and 16 astrocytomas.[66] The degree and extent of cathepsin B staining correlated highly with the degree of malignancy. Furthermore, we have also demonstrated staining of neoplastic vascular endothelial cells, implicating cathepsin B in the processes of tumor invasion and angiogenesis (Fig. 8–4). Recently, we have also shown increases in cathepsin B transcript abundance by Northern blot, protein by immunohistochemistry, and enzyme activity and altered subcellular localization correlating with the malignancy grade, histologic invasion, angiogenesis, and clinical invasion as represented by MRI. These data support the hypothesis that cathepsin B plays a role in human glioma progression and invasion.[67]

Human α_2-macroglobulin is a high-molecular-weight plasma proteinase inhibitor capable of binding endopeptidases from all known classes of proteases.[68] Because interactions of proteinases and proteinase-inhibitors appear to influence the migration of metastasizing tumor cells, α_2-macroglobulin expression observed in glioma cells could be involved in tumor cell proliferation and invasion.

Adhesion Molecules

Andersson and colleagues[69] demonstrated that the two cell lines BT4C and BT4Cn differ in their metastatic ability: BT4C cells have a very low capacity for producing experimental metastases, whereas the capacity of BT4Cn cells is

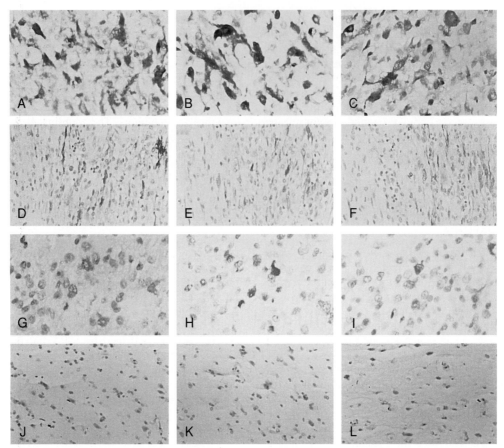

Figure 8–3 Metalloprotease and inhibitor immunohistochemistry. Sections of glioblastoma (*A–C*, magnification ×100), anaplastic astrocytoma (*D–F*, magnification ×40), astrocytoma (*G–I*, magnification ×100), and normal brain (*J–L*, magnification ×60), stained with antibodies to 72-kD collagenase (*A, D, G*, and *J*), 92-kD collagenase (*B, E, H*, and *K*), and metalloprotease tissue inhibitor, type 1 (TIMP-1) (*C, F, I*, and *L*) demonstrating the grade-specific increase in expression of these proteases and an endogenous inhibitor.

high. Conversely, no neural cell adhesion molecule (NCAM) protein synthesis is observed in BT4Cn cells, even though NCAM mRNA is expressed. Thus, development of an increased metastatic capacity is accompanied by the disappearance of NCAM protein expression in this model system. The functional importance of NCAM expression was studied by a cell-substratum binding assay in which the binding of BT4C and BT4Cn cells to NCAM immobilized to glass was assessed. It was found that BT4C cells adhere specifically to NCAM and that adhesion is inhibited by anti-NCAM Fab′-fragments, whereas no specific binding of BT4Cn cells to NCAM was observed. The BT4C and BT4Cn cell lines thus constitute an important new model system for the study of tumor invasion and metastasis and of the role of cell adhesion molecules in these processes.

A cDNA encoding a transmembrane 140 kD isoform of NCAM was transfected into the rat glioma cell line BT4Cn by Edvardsen and colleagues.[70] Transfectants with a homogeneously high expression of NCAM-B showed a decreased capacity for penetration of an artificial basement membrane when compared with cells transfected with expression-vector alone or compared with untransfected cells. However, when injected subcutaneously into nude mice, both NCAM-expressing cells and control cells produced invasive tumors. Nude mice injected with NCAM-positive cells developed

tumors with slower growth rates as compared with those induced by NCAM-negative cells. This implies that NCAM may be involved not only in adhesive and motile behavior of glioma cells, but also in their growth regulation.

Edvardsen and associates[71] have reported that during embryogenesis interactions between cells and ECM play a central role in the modulation of cell motility, growth, and differentiation. Modulation of matrix structure is therefore crucial during development; ECM ligands, their receptors, extracellular proteinases, and proteinase inhibitors all participate in the construction, maintenance, and remodeling of ECM by cells. The NCAM-negative rat glioma cell line BT4Cn secretes substantial amounts of metalloproteinases, as compared with its NCAM-positive mother cell line BT4C. This group has transfected the BT4Cn cell line with cDNAs encoding the human NCAM-B and -C isoforms. The expression of transmembrane NCAM-B, but not of glycosyl-phosphatidylinositol-linked NCAM-C, induces a down-regulation of 92-kD gelatinase (matrix metalloproteinase 9) and interstitial collagenase (matrix metalloproteinase 1), indicating that cellular expression of the recognition molecule NCAM regulates the metabolism of the surrounding matrix.

Basement membrane invasion precedes meningeal dissemination and systemic metastasis of glioma cells. To investigate the invasive ability of glioblastomas and the functional

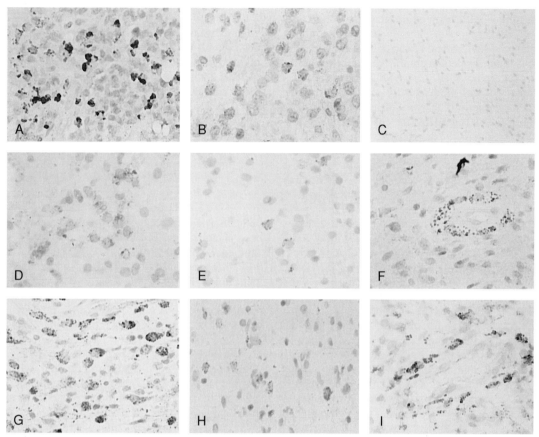

Figure 8–4 Cathepsin B immunohistochemical analysis. Glioblastoma (*A* and *G*, magnification ×100), anaplastic astrocytoma (*B* and *D*, magnification ×100), normal (*C*, magnification ×40), astrocytoma (*E*, magnification ×100), and vascular elements from an anaplastic astrocytoma (*F*, magnification ×100) and glioblastoma (*I*, magnification ×100). *H* (magnification ×80) demonstrates cathepsin B–positive cells in an infiltration zone adjacent to the glioblastoma shown in *G*.

role of ECM receptors, Paulus and Tonn[72] performed in vitro invasion assays in which the number of cells was determined from freshly resected tumors (primary cultures and fifth passages) and from cell lines (U138MG, U373MG, and GaMg) that had migrated through a filter coated with a reconstituted basement membrane (Matrigel). The involvement of integrin adhesion molecules was examined by preincubation of glioma cells with blocking antibodies to specific integrin chains. Cells from all of the glioblastomas had migrated through the Matrigel after 4 to 24 hours; the number of invasive cells was highest in the cell lines. Invasion of U138MG cells was reduced with antibodies to α_7, α_v, β_1, and β_3 integrin chains and markedly increased by anti-α_5, whereas invasion of U373MG cells was reduced by antibodies to α_3, α_v, β_1, and β_3, and increased by anti-α_6. It is concluded that glioma cells are able to penetrate Matrigel, indicating that the basement membrane is not a resistant barrier for infiltrating cells, and that basement membrane invasion is mediated by integrins in a complex manner. Some integrins promote, whereas others inhibit, basement membrane invasion. Furthermore, the integrins involved may differ between various glioma cells.

Growth Factors

In an investigation by Lund-Johansen and others,[73] cultures of fetal rat brain cell aggregates and tumor spheroids from

the human glioma cell line GaMg were treated with epidermal growth factor (EGF), fibroblast growth factor (FGF), or isoforms of platelet-derived growth factor (PDGF-AA or -BB). Radioreceptor binding studies displayed a high binding capacity for EGF and FGF, but not binding of PDGF isoforms in the glioma cells. In serum-free culture, 10 ng/mL of both EGF and FGF caused increased growth and cell shedding in the tumor spheroids, whereas PDGF produced no such effect. Similarly, EGF and FGF stimulated tumor cell migration. EGF increased the proliferation and outgrowth of glial fibrillary acidic protein (GFAP)-positive cells in brain cell aggregates, whereas PDGF-AA and -BB both stimulated the outgrowth of oligodendrocytelike cells, which were negative for GFAP and neuron-specific enolase. FGF stimulated GFAP-positive as well as GFAP-negative cell types. In co-culture experiments using brain aggregates and tumor spheroids, both EGF and FGF treatment caused increased tumor cell invasion. PDGF had no effect on the tumor cells but instead stimulated the proliferation of oligodendrocytelike cells in the brain aggregates. These results indicate that growth factors may facilitate glioma growth as well as invasiveness and cause reactive changes in the surrounding normal tissue.

Lund-Johansen[74] has described the in vitro invasive growth of two continuous human glioma cell lines (D54Mg and GaMg) into aggregates of fetal rat-brain cells. The tumor cells were first cultured as multicellular tumor spheroids and thereafter co-cultured with brain aggregates in medium agar cultures. Two different types of culture media were used for the propagation of spheroids and for co-culture experiments: Dulbecco's modified Eagle's medium, supplemented with 10% newborn calf serum, and Costar SF-X chemically defined hybridoma medium. Both cell lines showed invasive growth into brain tissue in both types of media. Apart from progressive destruction caused by the malignant cells, the brain aggregates maintained characteristics of neural tissue. One cell line (D54Mg) showed reduced invasiveness in chemically defined medium as measured with a grading system to quantify invasion. The co-culture system may represent a basis for studying invasion of human glioma cells in brain tissue under defined chemical conditions.

Pedersen and colleagues[75] studied the effects of five different growth factors (EGF, PDGF-BB, TGF-α [TGFA], basic FGF [FGF2], and IL2) on tumor spheroids obtained from five different human glioma cell lines (U251MG, D263MG, D37MG, D54MG, and GaMG). The expression of EGF and PDGF receptors as well as the endogenous production of TGFA and PDGF was studied by Northern blot analysis. After growth-factor exposure, tumor spheroid volume growth and directional cell migration from the spheroids were studied. In addition, tumor cell invasion was studied in vitro, where fetal rat-brain aggregates were used as a target for the tumor cells. In all the assays EGF was a common stimulator for most of the cell lines. The other growth factors had a more heterogeneous stimulatory effect. Tumor cell invasion, cell growth, and cell migration are biologic properties that are not necessarily related to one another. This may explain why the tumors often responded differently to the growth factors in the various assay systems. Two of the cell lines studied were noninvasive (U251MG, D263MG). These were stimulated in both the directional migration assay and the spheroid-volume-growth assay. However, their noninvasive behavior was not influenced by the growth factors studied.

Motility Factors

Substrate-tumor cell interactions in the CNS and the possible role of ECM components in glioma invasion and migration have been discussed previously, but the nature of the effect of nonpermissive substrates on glioma migration and the relation of matrix components specifically to glioma cell migration make their reiteration in this context relevant.

Direct factors promoting cell motility, such as the autocrine motility factor (AMF), have been described. Autotaxin (ATX) is a potent human motility-stimulating protein that has been identified in the conditioned medium from A2058 melanoma cells.[76] A glioma-derived motility factor (GMF) has also been isolated. In fact, two molecular species of GMF (GMF-I and GMF-II) have been purified to homogeneity from the serum-free conditioned medium of a highly invasive human glioma cell line, T98G.[77] Checkerboard analysis demonstrated that the GMFs had a chemotactic as well as a chemokinetic effect on T98G cells. C6 glioma cells and T98G cells, both of which showed high invasiveness in an in vitro invasion assay with reconstituted basement membrane, Matrigel, migrated to the GMFs with great intensity, whereas

A172 and 9L glioma cells and normal glial cells, all of which weakly infiltrated the Matrigel barrier, migrated to the GMFs with much less intensity. These results indicate that migratory response of glioma cells to the GMFs correlates well with invasiveness, suggesting an important role of the GMFs in the process of glioma cell invasion.

To better understand the cellular mechanism of tumor invasion, the production of a cell motility–stimulating factor by malignant glioma cells was studied in vitro.[78] Serum-free conditioned media from cultures of rat C6 and human T98G cell lines contained a factor that stimulated the locomotion of the producer cells. This factor was termed the *glioma-derived motility factor,* which is a heat-labile protein with a molecular weight greater than 10 kD and a relative stability to acid. The factor showed not only chemotactic activity but also chemokinetic activity in the two types of glioma cells studied. Although GMFs in conditioned media obtained from two different cell origins are likely to be the same, chemokinetic migration of T98G cells to their conditioned medium was much stronger than that of C6 cells to theirs. Co-incubation of cells with cytochalasin B, which disrupts the assembly of cellular actin microfilaments, almost completely inhibited the cell migration stimulated by GMF. Cytochalasin B also induced marked alterations in cell morphology, including cell retraction and arborization, whereas the drug did not affect cell attachment to culture dishes. These results indicate that glioma cells produce a motility factor that may play a role, particularly when tumor cells are detached and migrate away from the original tumor mass, in promoting tumor invasion. Also, glioma cell migration stimulated by the motility factor requires the normal organization of cytoskeletons such as actin microfilaments. Inhibitors of cell motility related to myelin have also been reported[79, 80] and may serve to limit cell traffic.

The metastasis of malignant tumor cells depends on their rapid replication and ability to adhere to the matrix of a biologic barrier, such as basement membrane, to degrade the matrix and to migrate through this more permeable barrier.[81] Secreted enzymes, including the cysteine proteinases cathepsins B and L, are known to degrade basement membrane components. Using a barrier-free substratum, we studied the possible role of cysteine proteinases in influencing the motility per se of metastatic cells. Boike and co-workers[81] found that stefins, the natural inhibitors of cysteine proteinases, markedly decreased the stimulated motility of both human melanoma cells and W256 carcinosarcoma cells at low concentrations (0.5 μM). A stefin also inhibited melanoma cell adherence, but to a lesser extent than it affected motility. Additionally, synthetic inhibitors (E-64, diazomethyl ketones) of cysteine proteinases were found to depress stimulated motility of W256 cells. These results suggest that cysteine proteinases and their inhibitors may have a direct role in the development of a migratory response per se in tumor cells.

DEVELOPMENTAL THERAPEUTICS: ANTIMETASTATIC THERAPEUTIC STRATEGIES

An understanding of the pathogenesis of glioma cell invasion will result in the identification of specific therapeutic targets for use in future therapeutic strategies. With the validation of tumor growth and invasion models, progress in basic science will be translated to clinical application. Protease inhibitors, anti-motility agents, and/or matrix or cell-cell adhesion molecule gene therapy are under investigation. Approaches exploiting the mechanistic targets for anti-protease, anti-angiogenesis, anti-motility, anti–growth factor, and signal transduction inhibition are also under development. CAI, an agent that is known to inhibit G-protein–mediated signal transduction[82] and that down-regulates metalloprotease enzymes, has significant anti-invasive capacity in vitro. We are applying this agent in vivo and hope to have this translational agent available for clinical use in the near future.

REFERENCES

1. Scherer HD: Cerebral astrocytomas and their derivatives. Am J Cancer 1940; 1:159–198.
2. Burger PC, Heinz ER, Shibata T, et al: Topographic anatomy and CT correlations in the untreated glioblastoma multiforme. J Neurosurg 1988; 68:698–704.
3. Kelly PJ, Daumas-Duport C, Scheithauer BW, et al: Stereotactic histologic correlations of computed tomography and magnetic resonance imaging-defined abnormalities in patients with glial neoplasms. Mayo Clin Proc 1987; 62:450–459.
4. Johnson PC, Hunt SJ, Drayer BP: Human cerebral gliomas: Correlation of postmortem MR imaging and neuropathologic findings. Radiology 1989; 170:211–217.
5. Burger PC: The anatomy of astrocytomas. Mayo Clin Proc 1987; 62:527–529.
6. Burger PC, Kleihues P: Cytologic composition of theuntreated glioblastoma with implications for evaluation and needle biopsies. Cancer 1989; 1:2014–2023.
7. Giangaspero F, Burger PC: Correlations between cytologic composition and biologic behavior in the glioblastoma multiforme: A postmortem study of 50 cases. Cancer 1983; 52:2320–2333.
8. Burger PC: Classification, grading, and patterns of spread of malignant gliomas. In Apuzzo MLJ (ed): Malignant Cerebral Glioma. Park Ridge, Ill, American Association of Neurosurgeons, 1990, pp 3–17.
9. Schiffer D: Neuropathology and imaging: The ways in which glioma spreads and varies in its histological aspect. In Walker MD, Thomas DGT (eds): Biology of Brain Tumour. Boston, Nijhoff, 1986, pp 163–172.
10. Choucair AK, Levin VA, Gutin PH, et al: Development of multiple lesions during radiation therapy and chemotherapy in patients with gliomas. J Neurosurg 1986; 65:654–658.
11. Hochberg FH, Pruitt A: Assumptions in the radiotherapy of glioblastoma. Neurology 1980; 30:907–911.
12. Awad IA: Spread of malignant gliomas (letter). J Neurosurg 1987; 66:946–947.
13. Bashir R, Hochberg F, Oot R: Regrowth patterns of glioblastoma multiforme related to planning of interstitial brachytherapy radiation fields. Neurosurgery 1988; 23:27–30.
14. Wallner KE, Galicich JH, Krol G, et al: Patterns of failure following treatment for glioblastoma multiforme and anaplastic astrocytoma. Int J Radiat Oncol Biol Phys 1989; 16:1405–1409.
15. Liang BC, Thornton AF Jr, Sandler HM, et al: Malignant astrocytomas: Focal tumor recurrence after focal external beam radiation therapy. J Neurosurg 1991; 75:559–563.
16. Garden AS, Maor MH, Yung WKA, et al: Outcome and patterns of failure following limited-volume irradiation for malignant astrocytomas. Radiother Oncol 1991; 20:99–110.
17. Tsuboi K, Yoshii Y, Nakagawa K, et al: Regrowth patterns of supratentorial gliomas: Estimation from computed tomographic scans. Neurosurgery 1986; 19:946–951.
18. Heros DO, Renkens K, Kasdon DL, et al: Patterns of recurrence in glioma patients after interstitial irradiation and chemotherapy: Report of three cases. Neurosurgery 1988; 22:474–478.
19. Batzdorf U, Malamud N: The problem of multicentric gliomas. J Neurosurg 1963; 20:122–136.
20. de Ridder L, Calliauw L: Invasion of human brain tumors in vitro: Relationship to clinical evolution. J Neurosurg 1990; 72:589.
21. Kleinman HK, McGarvey ML, Liotta LA, et al: Isolation and characterization of type IV collagen, laminin, and heparin sulfate proteoglycan from the EHS sarcoma. Biochemistry 1982; 21:6188.
22. Terranova VP, Hujanen ES, Loeb DM, et al: Use of a reconstituted basement membrane to measure cell invasiveness and select for highly invasive tumor cells. Proc Natl Acad Sci USA 1986; 83:465.
23. Amar AP, DeArmond SJ, Spencer DR, et al: Development of an in vitro extracellular matrix assay for studies of brain tumor cell invasion. J Neurooncol 1994; 20:1–5.
24. Noel AC, Callé A, Emonard HP, et al: Invasion of reconstituted basement membrane matrix is not correlated to the malignant metastatic cell phenotype. Cancer Res 1991; 51:405.
25. Steinsvaåg SK, Laerum OD, Bjerkvig R: Interaction between rat glioma cells and normal rat brain tissue in organ culture. JNCI 1985; 74:1095–1104.
26. Bjerkvig R, Laerum OD, Mella O: Glioma cell interactions with fetal rat brain aggregates in vitro and with brain tissues in vivo. Cancer Res 1986; 46:4071–4079.
27. Engebraaten O, Bjerkvig R, Lund-Johansen M, et al: Interaction between human brain tumour biopsies and fetal rat brain tissue in vitro. Acta Neuropathol 1990; 81:130–140.
28. Pulliam L, Berens ME, Rosenblum ML: A normal human brain cell aggregate model for neurobiological studies. J Neurosci Res 1988; 21:521–530.
29. Lund-Johansen M, Engebraaten O, Bjerkvig R, et al: Invasive glioma cells in tissue culture. Anticancer Res 1990; 10:1135–1151.
30. Zülch KJ: Brain Tumors: Their Biology and Pathology, ed 3. Berlin, Springer Verlag, 1986.
31. Luginbuhl H, Fankhauser R, McGrath JT: Spontaneous neoplasms of the nervous system in animals. Prog Neurol Surg 1968; 2:86.
32. McGrath JT: Intracranial pathology of the dog. Acta Neuropathol 1962; 1(suppl):3–4.
33. Rabotti GF, Grove AS, Sellers RL, et al: Induction of multiple brain tumors (gliomata and leptomeningeal sarcomata) in dogs. Nature 1966; 209:884–886.
34. McDonald LW: Interaction of Chemical Carcinogens, Radiation and Viruses in the Production of Glial Tumors of the Central Nervous System: Preliminary Report of Induction of Glioma by Ionizing Radiation. Proceedings of the Sixth International Congress of Neuropathology. Paris, Masson, 1970, pp 564–565.
35. Gordon DE, Olson C: Meningiomas and fibroblastic neoplasia in calves induced with the bovine papilloma virus. Cancer Res 1968; 28:2423–2431.
36. Berens ME, Bjotvedt G, Levesque DC, et al: Tumorigenic, invasive, karyotypic, and immunocytochemical characteristics of clonal cell lines derived from a spontaneous canine anaplastic astrocytoma. In Vitro Cell Dev Biol 1993; 29:310–318.
37. Rice JM, Rehm S, Donovan PJ, et al: Comparative transplacental carcinogenesis by directly acting and metabolism-dependent alkylating agents in rodents and nonhuman primates. IARC Sci Publ 1989; 96:17–34.
38. Barker M, Hoshino T, Gurcay O, et al: Development of an animal brain tumor model and its response to therapy with 1,3-bis(2-chloroethyl)-1-nitrosourea. Cancer Res 1973; 33:976–986.
39. Wilson CB, Norrell H Jr, Barker M: Intrathecal injection of methotrexate (NSC-740) in transplanted brain tumors. Cancer Chemother Rep 1967; 51:1–6.
40. Vriesendorp FJ, Peagram C, Bigner DD, et al: Concurrent measurements of blood flow and transcapillary transport in xenotransplanted human gliomas in immunosuppressed rats. JNCI 1987; 79:123–130.
41. Horten BC, Basler GA, Shapiro WR: Xenograft of human malignant glial tumors into brains of nude mice: A histopathological study. J Neuropathol Exp Neurol 1981; 40:493–511.
42. Basler GA, Shapiro WR: Brain tumor research with nude mice. The Nude Mouse in Experimental and Clinical Research 1982; 2:475–490.
43. Bernsen HJJA, Heerschap A, van der Kogel AJ, et al: Image-guided ^{1}H NMR spectroscopical and histological characterization of a human brain tumor model in the nude rat: A new approach to monitor changes in tumor metabolism. J Neurooncol 1992; 13:119–130.
44. DeArmond SJ, Stowring L, Amar A, et al: Development of a non-

selecting, non-perturbing method to study human brain tumor cell invasion in murine brain. J Neurooncol 1994; 20:27–34.

45. Pedersen P-H, Marienhagen K, Mørk S, et al: Migratory pattern of fetal rat brain cells and human glioma cells in the adult rat brain. Cancer Res 1993; 53:5158–5165.

46. Nagano N, Sasaki H, Aoyagi M, et al: Invasion of experimental rat brain tumor: Early morphological changes following microinjection of C6 glioma cells. Acta Neuropathol 1993; 86:117–125.

47. Goldberg WJ, Laws ER Jr, Bernstein JJ: Individual C6 glioma cells migrate in adult rat brain after neural homografting. Int J Dev Neurosci 1991; 9:427–437.

48. Bernstein JJ, Goldberg WJ, Laws ER Jr, et al: C6 glioma cell invasion and migration of rat brain after neural homografting: Ultrastructure. Neurosurgery 1990; 26:622–628.

49. Bernstein JJ, Laws ER Jr, Levine KV, et al: C6 glioma-astrocytoma cell and fetal astrocyte migration into artificial basement membrane: A permissive substrate for neural tumors but not fetal astrocytes. Neurosurgery 1991; 28:652–658.

50. Kerbel R, Greig R, Frost P (eds): Endothelial cells and angiogenic growth factors in cancer growth and metastasis. Cancer Metastasis Rev 1990; 9:171–182.

51. Rochefort H, Capony F, Garcia M: Cathepsin D: A protease involved in breast cancer metastasis. Cancer Metastasis Rev 1990; 9:321–331.

52. Sloane BF, Honn KV, Sadler JG, et al: Cathepsin B activity in B16 melanoma cells: A possible marker for metastatic potential. Cancer Res 1982; 42:980–986.

53. Qian F, Bajkowski AS, Steiner DF, et al: Expression of five cathepsins in murine melanomas of varying metastatic potential and normal tissues. Cancer Res 1989; 49:4870–4875.

54. Buck MR, Roth MJ, Zhuang Z, et al: Increased levels of 72 kilodalton type IV collagenase and cathepsin B in microdissected human breast and colon carcinomas. Proc Am Assoc Cancer Res 1994; 35:59.

55. Visscher DW, Sloane BF, Sakr W, et al: Clinicopathologic significance of cathepsin B and urokinase-type plasminogen activator immmuno-staining in colorectal adenocarcinoma. Int J Surg Pathol 1994; 1:227–234.

56. Apodaca G, Rutka JT, Bouhana K, et al: Expression of metalloproteinases and metalloproteinase inhibitors by fetal astrocytes and glioma cells. Cancer Res 1990; 50:2322–2329.

57. Lund-Johansen M, Rucklidge GJ, Milne G, et al: A metalloproteinase, capable of destroying cultured brain tissue isolated from rat glioma cells. Anticancer Res 1991; 11:1001–1006.

58. Paganetti PA, Caroni P, Schwab ME: Glioblastoma infiltration into central nervous system tissue in vitro: Involvement of a metalloprotease. J Cell Biol 1988; 107:2281–2291.

59. Rao JS, Steck PA, Mohanam S, et al: Elevated levels of Mr 92,000 type IV collagenase in human brain tumors. Cancer Res 1993; 53:2208–2211.

60. Halaka AN, Bunning RA, Bird CC, et al: Production of collagenase and inhibitor (TIMP) by intracranial tumors and dura in vitro. J Neurosurg 1983; 59:461–466.

61. Sawaya R, Ramo OJ, Shi ML, et al: Biological significance of tissue plasminogen activator content in brain tumors. J Neurosurg 1991; 74:480–486.

62. Sitrin RG, Gyetko MR, Kole KL, et al: Expression of heterogeneous profiles of plasminogen activators and plasminogen activator inhibitors by human glioma lines. Cancer Res 1990; 50:4957–4961.

63. Mohanam S, Sawaya R, McCutcheon I, et al: Modulation of in vitro

invasion of human glioblastoma cells by urokinase-type plasminogen activator receptor antibody. Cancer Res 1993; 53:4143–4147.

64. Reith A, Rucklidge GJ: Invasion of brain tissue by primary glioma: Evidence for the involvement of urokinase-type plasminogen activator as an activator of type IV collagenase. Biochem Biophys Res Commun 1992; 186:348–354.

65. McCormick D: Secretion of cathepsin B by human gliomas in vitro. Neuropathol Appl Neurobiol 1993; 19:146–151.

66. Mikkelsen T, Yan P-S, Ho K-L, et al: Immunolocalization of cathepsin B in human glioma: Implications for tumor invasion and angiogenesis. J Neurosurg 1995; 83:285–290.

67. Rempel SA, Rosenblum ML, Mikkelsen T, et al: Cathepsin B expression and localization in glioma progression and invasion. Cancer Res 1994; 54:6027–6031.

68. Businaro R, Fabrizi C, Fumagalli L, et al: Synthesis and secretion of alpha 2-macroglobulin by human glioma established cell lines. Exp Brain Res 1992; 88:213–218.

69. Andersson AM, Moran N, Gaardsvoll H, et al: Characterization of NCAM expression and function in BT4C and BT4Cn glioma cells. Int J Cancer 1991; 47:124–129.

70. Edvardsen K, Brunner N, Spang-Thomsen M, et al: Migratory, invasive and metastatic capacity of NCAM transfected rat glioma cells. Int J Dev Neurosci 1993; 5:681–690.

71. Edvardsen K, Chen W, Rucklidge G, et al: Transmembrane neural cell-adhesion molecule (NCAM), but not glycosyl-phosphatidylinositol-anchored NCAM, down-regulates secretion of matrix metallopro-teinases. Proc Natl Acad Sci USA 1993; 90:11463–11467.

72. Paulus W, Tonn JC: Basement membrane invasion of glioma cells mediated by integrin receptors. J Neurosurg 1994; 80:515–519.

73. Lund-Johansen M, Forsberg K, Bjerkvig R, et al: Effects of growth factors on a human glioma cell line during invasion into rat brain aggregates in culture. Acta Neuropathol 1992; 84:190–197.

74. Lund-Johansen M: Interactions between human glioma cells and fetal rat brain aggregate studied in a chemically defined medium. Invasion Metastasis 1990; 10:113–128.

75. Pedersen PH, Ness GO, Engebraaten O, et al: Heterogeneous response to the growth factors [EGF, PDGF(bb), TGF-alpha, bFGF, IL-2] on glioma spheroid growth, migration and invasion. Int J Cancer 1994; 56:255–261.

76. Stracke ML, Krutzsch HC, Unsworth EJ, et al: Identification, purification, and partial sequence analysis of autotaxin, a novel motility-stimulating protein. J Biol Chem 1992; 267:2524–2529.

77. Ohnishi T, Arita N, Hayakawa T, et al: Purification of motility factor (GMF) from human malignant glioma cells and its biological significance in tumor invasion. Biochem Biophys Res Commun 1993; 193:518–525.

78. Ohnishi T, Arita N, Hayakawa T, et al: Motility factor produced by malignant glioma cells: Role in tumor invasion. J Neurosurg 1990; 73:881–888.

79. Nieto-Sampedro M: Astrocyte mitogen inhibitor related to epidermal growth factor receptor. Science 1988; 240:1784–1786.

80. Caroni P, Schwab ME: Antibody against myelin-associated inhibitor of neurite growth neutralizes nonpermissive substrate properties of CNS white matter. Neuron 1988; 1:85–95.

81. Boike G, Lah T, Sloane BF, et al: A possible role for cysteine proteinase and its inhibitors in motility of malignant melanoma and other tumour cells. Melanoma Res 1992; 1:333–340.

82. Kohn EC, Sandeen MA, Liotta LA: In vivo efficacy of a novel inhibitor of selected signal transduction pathways including calcium, arachidonate, and inositol phosphates. Cancer Res 1992; 52:3208–3212.

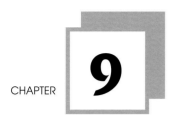

CHAPTER **9**

Angiogenesis

The progressive growth of solid tumors and their metastases is dependent on a dynamic interactive process called *angiogenesis.* This process is characterized by the induction of new microvessels from host tissues and involves a cascade of biochemical events. These processes result in morphologic alterations in the microenvironment around pre-existing microvessels that generate a three-dimensional tumor microcirculation capable of sustaining continued tumor growth. The microvessels of the tumor microcirculation are novel in that they do not resemble normal capillaries, arterioles, or venules and thus possess distinctive morphologic and physiologic characteristics.

This chapter focuses on the biochemical mechanisms of angiogenesis in glial tumors, the consequences of this angiogenesis, and the possible methods for its modulation (angiostatic therapy).

The first concept to clarify is that not all brain tumors are dependent on angiogenesis for their growth. Carcinomatous meningitis, low-grade glial tumors, and some infiltrative tumors such as brain stem gliomas, at least in their early stages, may be predominantly invasive and do not appear to induce new microvessels. Malignant glial tumors are characterized by their angiogenic behavior and the modulation of angiogenesis may be particularly effective in their treatment because (1) malignant cerebral tumors are the most vascular of an extensive group of tumors studied,[1] and (2) malignant cerebral tumors metastasize rarely and control of secondary disease is therefore less of a concern.

TUMOR-ASSOCIATED ANGIOGENESIS

Definitions

Angiogenesis refers to the development of new microvessels. This term can be used to describe vascular development in any form. However, in this chapter it is applied to the development of new microvessels by a process of sprouting from pre-existing vessels. The development of blood vessels during embryogenesis is referred to as *vasculogenesis.* Angiogenesis is a vital component of many physiologic processes, such as wound healing, tissue remodeling, trophoblast implantation, and menstruation. Angiogenesis that occurs during brain tumor growth can be subdivided into three groups:

1. *Tumor-associated angiogenesis,* is the directional sprouting of new microvessels from pre-existing brain microvessels toward a solid tumor.
2. *Tumor-induced vascular modification* occurs when tumor cells infiltrate along and/or in the vicinity of established normal cerebral blood vessels in peritumoral brain tissue and alter their morphologic and functional characteristics.[2] The entrapment and modification of previously normal brain microvessels by the infiltrating glial tumor clearly occurs. However, the proportion of the tumor microcirculation derived from tumor associated angiogenesis or tumor-induced vascular modification in any given glial tumor is unknown.
3. *Vascular expansion* occurs when existing blood vessels predominantly located in normal brain are enlarged and modified to accommodate increased blood flow associated with tumor growth and/or arteriovenous shunting.[3]

The tumor microcirculation of low-grade gliomas is composed predominantly of pre-existing blood vessels surrounded by a variable number of tumor cells. Malignant glial tumors have a complex architectural arrangement involving variable contributions of the three subgroups of angiogenesis described.

Historical Perspective

In 1826, Robert Hooper published a monograph on the morbid anatomy of the human brain. One plate illustrates a solid tumor that Hooper describes as arising "from the medullary substance of the brain" near but not in the ventricle and "covered by a very delicate and highly vascular membrane"[4] (Fig. 9–1). The angiogenic nature of this tumor is clearly demonstrated, and one can speculate that it may be a an exophytic malignant glial tumor.

Bramwell, in 1888, illustrated "the extreme dilations of the blood vessels in a case of glioma" in a number of figures[5] and suggested that these blood vessels were related to the hemorrhage commonly associated with these tumors. The vascular changes associated with the growth and infil-

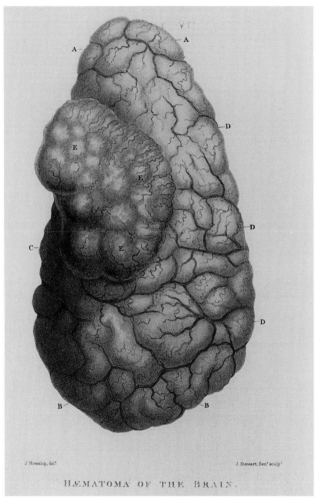

Figure 9–1 Plate X from Hooper, demonstrating an exophytic vascular tumor (*E*), which he called a hematoma of the brain. (From Hooper R: The Morbid Anatomy of the Human Brain Being Illustrations of the Most Frequent and Important Organic Disease to Which That Viscus Is Subject. Birmingham, Classics of Neurology and Neurosurgery Library, 1985.)

tration of malignant glial tumors are well documented in histologic studies in the early 20th century literature.[6–8] Hardman[9] carried out the first systematic studies of the angioarchitecture of malignant human glial tumors and outlined a number of key conclusions related to cerebral tumor angiogenesis: (1) new tumor vessels develop from previously existing vessels; (2) intraluminal endothelial proliferation is common in malignant glial tumors; and (3) necrosis may be secondary to vessel obstruction.

The experimental study of in vivo tumor vessel formation began with the adaptation of the transparent ear chamber model in the rabbit[10] to tumor studies. Algire and Chalkley found that tumor tissue implanted into these ear chambers induced new microvessels whereas normal tissues did not[11] and suggested that continued tumor growth was dependent on the ability of tumor cells to elicit an angiogenic response.[12] The central hypothesis underlying the concept that continued solid tumor growth is dependent on angiogenesis and that the inhibition of angiogenesis (angiostatic therapy) might cause inhibition of tumor growth and metastasis was elaborated on by Folkman.[13, 14] This hypothesis has stimu-

lated extensive research into the biochemical and molecular basis of angiogenesis and has resulted in the development of a number of therapeutic approaches to the treatment of malignant cerebral tumors.

Models of Tumor-Associated Angiogenesis

The intracerebral injection of cultured malignant glial cells is a satisfactory method for reproducible tumor production.[15–19] The intracerebral injection of C6 astrocytoma cells into neonatal Wistar rats results in a tumor with pathologic similarities to glioblastoma multiforme.[16] However, studies of angioarchitecture are difficult in this and other models because many of these tumors are invasive and a well-demarcated interface is not seen.[16] The multicellular tumor spheroid is intermediate in complexity between the two-dimensional monolayer culture in vitro and tumors in vivo.[20] In the absence of blood vessels, C6 astrocytoma spheroids grown in spinner culture begin to demonstrate evidence of central necrosis when they reach a size at which the passive diffusion of oxygen (O_2) and glucose become rate-limiting at a diameter just over 300 μm.[21–23] C6 astrocytoma spheroids continue to grow to maximum diameters of 700 to 800 μm, and at these sizes demonstrate large central areas of necrosis and only a small proliferating outer rim of viable cells.[21–23] These results demonstrate that C6 astrocytoma cells, like most cells, undergo cell death if they are greater that 150 to 200 μm from a source of O_2 and glucose, and this requirement severely restricts the ability to grow large, three-dimensional tumors in vitro. The continued expansion of the initial clone of malignant glial cells in vivo will be crucially dependent on the ability of these cells to either induce an angiogenic response from host tissue or invade host tissues to incorporate preexisting microvessels to supply O_2 and other nutritional requirements for cell division. Local concentrations of O_2 and other metabolites play important roles in the modulation of angiogenesis. Using a combination of in vitro technology to grow avascular spheroids of C6 astrocytoma (400 to 500 μm) and implantation of these spheroids into adult Sprague-Dawley rats, a good model has been developed[24] and used to study angiogenesis-related events. The major advantage of this model is that the implanted tumor grows in a spherical fashion and the brain-tumor interface is readily identified. The implantation of human cell lines and human tumor specimen into the subrenal capsule of nude mice has been used by Martuza and colleagues to study human tumor explant growth and angiogenesis inhibition.[25–28] Angiogenesis has also been assessed in a rabbit model of metastatic adenocarcinoma.[29–31] Unfortunately, none of the in vitro or in vivo models that have been used completely replicate the angiogenic events associated with growth of malignant glial tumor in patients. Information derived from a number of model systems is therefore presented with an appreciation of the limitation of all these approaches.

ANGIOGENESIS CASCADE

One concept that has been particularly useful in the focusing of research in the area of tumor microvessel growth is that of the *angiogenesis cascade.*[2, 32, 33] The idea behind this concept is that angiogenesis occurs via a cascading sequence of events subdivided into initiation, propagation, and termination phases, and that these phases, although interconnected, may be under different biochemical modulation.

Folkman has proposed ten steps of microvessel growth,[32] which forms the foundation of the angiogenesis cascade.[30] The initiation phase of this cascade are the initial five steps which occur in the microenvironment adjacent to a preexisting blood vessel and begin the process of angiogenesis. These steps are as follows:

1. New microvessels usually originate from a postcapillary venule.
2. The key event associated with the initiation phase is the local degradation of the basement membrane, which occurs on the side of the venule closest to the angiogenic stimulus.
3. Endothelial cells begin to elongate and migrate through the opening in the basement membrane.
4. Endothelial cells follow the leading cells, aligning themselves in a bipolar manner resulting in the formation of the initial sprout, which invades the extracellular matrix.
5. Cannulation and lumen formation begins.
6. The leading endothelial cells do not appear to divide, and the propagation phase of the cascade is step 6, in which one can visualize the trailing endothelial cells undergoing mitosis. The division of endothelial cells helps form the lining of the new microvessel, but in glioblastoma multiforme, endothelial proliferation is commonly seen within tumor microvessels. This phenomenon may be considered an abortive propagation phase in which endothelial mitogens result in endothelial division in a situation in which the initiation phase of the angiogenesis cascade has not prepared a suitable receptive microenvironment for microvessel formation.
7. In the termination phase of the angiogenesis cascade, individual sprouts join or anastomose to form loops that continue to converge on the angiogenic target.
8. Intravascular flow begins.
9. Pericytes emerge along the new microvessel.
10. Endothelial cells lay down a new basement membrane. The formation of a new basement membrane appears to signal the termination of the angiogenesis cascade and the beginning of a functional tumor microcirculation. It is unclear if pericytes reappear normally in tumor-associated angiogenesis.

On reviewing the steps of the angiogenesis cascade, a number of dichotomies are striking. The key event in the initiation of angiogenesis is the localized degradation of the vascular basement membrane, whereas the formation of a vascular basement membrane is a crucial event in the termination phase of the cascade. The generation of a new tumor microvessel is crucially dependent on the ability of the migrating endothelial cells of the microvessel sprout to invade the extracellular matrix, whereas the integrity of the tumor microvessel is dependent on the intraluminal endothelial cells remaining quiescent. The degradation of the basement membrane is an essential component of angiogenesis and is crucial to metastatic invasion. Why is it then that the most vascular of all studied human tumors, glioblastoma multiforme, almost never metastasizes? An understanding of the regulation of basement membrane and extracellular matrix degradation by both tumor and endothelial cells would appear to be crucial to the understanding of two closely linked phenomena: cell invasion and angiogenesis.

Structure of Vascular Basement Membrane

The vascular basement membrane is a thin extracellular matrix that separates endothelium from underlying tissue, and in which a number of nonfibrous and fibrous proteins are integrated (Fig. 9–2). Nonfibrous proteins such as integrins and other adhesive molecules, laminin and heparan sulfate proteoglycan (HSPG), are integral components of the normal basement membrane.[34–36] Anchoring proteins associated with type VII collagen, along with a number of other nonfibrous proteins, constitute the basement membrane.[37] Laminin has been identified as the major glycoprotein component of the basement membrane.[36, 37] and it is a potent modulator of cell functions such as cell growth, motility, and differentiation. Heparan sulfate proteoglycans are regularly distributed along the edges of the lamina densa and form a negatively charged field blocking the passage of anionic macromolecules through the membrane. A number of mitogenic growth factors, such as acidic and basic fibroblast growth factor (FGF1 and FGF2) and vascular endothelial growth factor (VEGF), are stored attached to HSPGs as insoluble complexes.[38] The degradation of the basement membrane may release these stored growth factors, resulting in the expression of their biologic activity. The basement membrane is highly insoluble and possesses distinct structured stability against mechanical forces. This is correlated with the presence of a distinct form of collagen, which differs from the fiber-forming interstitial collagens (types I to III) and is referred to as *type IV collagen.* The unique nature of type IV collagen was confirmed by cloning the complete sequences for the constituent α_1 and α_2 (IV) chains.[34] Type IV collagen is the major protein component of the vascular basement membrane and may make up 60% to 90% of the total protein found in both normal cerebral vessels.[34, 35] and microvessels of malignant glial tumors.[39] The degradation and remodeling of basement membranes must involve the coordinated function of a number of different enzymatic nonspecific proteolytic activities that can degrade their nonfibrous proteins as well as collagenase IV activity, which degrades collagen type IV.[40–43]

Mechanisms of Basement Membrane Degradation

Portions of the elements of six distinct pathways that may be involved in the degradation of non-osseous extracellular matrices are outlined in Table 9–1. Basement membrane and interstitial structural macromolecules may be degraded by matrix metalloproteinase (MMP)-dependent, proteasome-dependent, plasmin (Pln)-dependent, polymorphonuclear (PMN) leukocyte serine proteinase–dependent, intracellular lysosomal, and endoglycosidase pathways.[44] The biochemical and molecular characteristics of each pathway are dis-

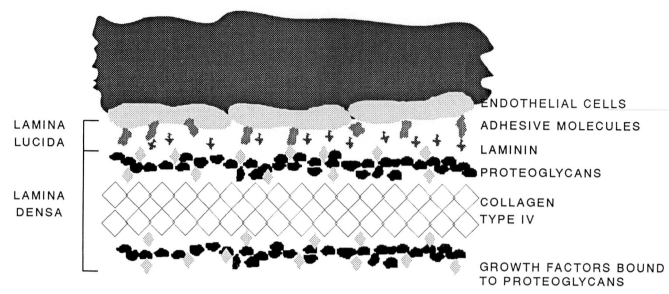

Figure 9–2 Schematic representation of vascular basement membrane structure. Adhesive molecules and laminin are localized to the lamina lucida. Proteoglycans are localized to both edges of the lamina densa, which encloses type IV collagen that is in a reticular pattern. Growth factors are bound to the proteoglycans. (From Vaithilingam IS, McDonald W, Brown NK, et al: Serum proteolytic activity during the growth of C6 astrocytoma. J Neurosurg 1992; 77:595–600.)

cussed individually and an attempt at synthesis of the information pertaining to glial tumors is presented in the form of a conceptual model.

MATRIX METALLOPROTEINASE PATHWAY

Matrix metalloproteinases (MMPs) form a family of at least ten structurally related enzymes that are products of related genes.[40, 44–46] The chief characteristics of the family are as follows: (1) their catalytic mechanisms depend on Zn^{2+} at the active site; (2) they are produced as latent proenzymes; and (3) their activities are inhibited by tissue inhibitors of metalloproteinases (TIMP-1, TIMP-2, and TIMP-3). Four major subclasses of matrix metalloproteinases have been identified[45] (Table 9–2). The enzymes are capable of degrading interstitial collagens (types I to III), basement membrane collagens, and glycoproteins, but they vary in respect to their substrate specificity. A membrane-

type matrix metalloproteinase (MT-MMP) with a potential transmembrane domain and the ability to activate progelatinase A but not progelatinase B has been described.[46] Many interrelationships occur among the family members, and the gelatinase B gene may represent an ancient proteinase gene from which the other metalloproteinases have evolved by the loss of coding sequences[47] (Fig. 9–3). Gelatinase B has seven domains, whereas other family members lack one or more domains. Gelatinase A lacks the type V collagen-like domain,[44, 45] but it is the only other MMP that possesses the fibronectin-like domain, and this domain may facilitate binding of these two enzymes to type IV collagen and gelatins. The crystal structure of the catalytic domain of interstitial collagenase (Int-CI) has been ascertained, and this demonstrates that one calcium and two zinc ions are present, with the second zinc and calcium ions appearing to play a major role in stabilizing the tertiary structure of collagenase.[48]

TABLE 9–1
METABOLIC PATHWAYS FOR DEGRADATION OF BASEMENT MEMBRANE AND EXTRACELLULAR MATRIX

Pathway	Matrix Degraded	Effector Enzymes	Cellular Location
Matrix metalloproteinase	Basement membranes, interstitial connective tissue	Matrix metalloproteinases	Extracellular
Proteasome	Basement membranes, interstitial connective tissue	Proteasome	Intracellular/extracellular
Plasmin-dependent	Interstitial connective tissue, basement membranes	Plasmin	Extracellular
PMN serine proteinase	Interstitial connective tissue, basement membranes	PMN elastase, cathepsin G	Extracellular
Intracellular lysosomal Endoglycosidases	Interstitial connective tissue Interstitial connective tissue	Cathepsins	Intracellular/possibly extracellular
	Hyaluronic acid Heparin sulfate	Hyaluronidase Heparinase	Extracellular

Adapted from Birkedal-Hansen H, Moore WGI, Bodden MK, et al: Matrix metalloproteinases: A review. Crit Rev Oral Biol Med 1993; 4:197–250.

TABLE 9–2
MATRIX METALLOPROTEINASES

Subclass	Enzyme	Abbreviation	Matrix Metalloproteinase	Molecular Weight	Extracellular Matrix Substrates
I	Interstitial collagenase	Int–Cl	MMP–1	57,000/52,000	Collagen I, II, III, VII, VIII, X, gelatin, Pc core protein
II	Neutrophil collagenase	PMN–Cl	MMP–8	75,000	Same as Int–Cl
	Gelatinase B (92 kD type IV gelatinase)		MMP–9	92,000	Gelatin, collagen IV, V, elastin, PG core protein
	Gelatinase A (72 kD type IV gelatinase)		MMP–2	72,000	Gelatin, collagen IV, V, VII, X, XI, elastin, fibronectin, PG core protein
III	Stromelysin-1	SL–1	MMP–3	60,000/55,000	PG core protein, fibronectin, laminin, collagen IV, V, IX, X, elastin, procollagenase
	Stromelysin-2	SL–2	MMP–10	60,000/55,000	Same as SL-1
	Stromelysin-3	SL–3	MMP–11	Not known	Not known
	Macrophage metalloelastase	MME	?	53,000	Elastin
	Matrilysin	MAT	MMP–7	28,000	Fibronectin, laminin, collagen IV, gelatin, procollagenase, PG core protein
IV	Membrane-type metalloproteinase	MT–MMP	?	66,000	Pro-gelatinase A

Adapted from Birkedal-Hansen H, Moore WGI, Bodden MK, et al: Matrix metalloproteinases: A review. Crit Rev Oral Biol Med 1993; 4:197–250.

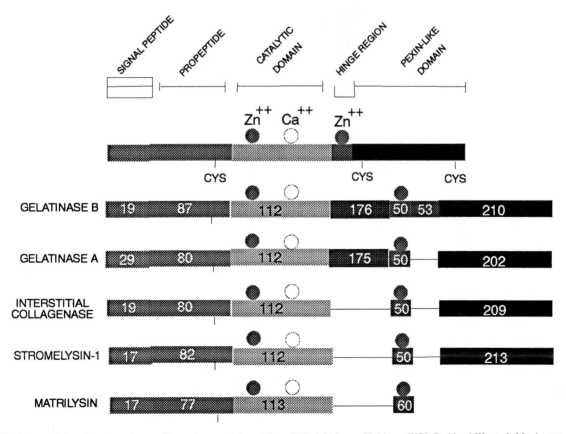

Figure 9–3 Structural domains of matrix metalloproteinases. (Adapted from Birkedal-Hansen H, Moore WGI, Bodden MK, et al: Matrix metalloproteinases: A review. Crit Rev Oral Biol Med 1993; 4:197–250.)

Gelatinases A and B appear to be prime candidates for a role in basement membrane degradation, because of their capacities to degrade collagen type IV, and are the focus of this inquiry into degradative processes. The unique ability of Int-CI and PMN collagenase to cleave interstitial collagens is not shared by other members of the metalloproteinase family, and it suggests that they may play a crucial role in the degradation of macromolecules of the interstitial space.[44] The mechanisms of tumor cell invasion and the role played by metalloproteinases in this process are highlighted in Chapter 8.

REGULATION OF METALLOPROTEINASES

Proteolytic enzymes in vivo are strictly regulated in their synthesis, secretion, and catalytic activity. The reason that the majority of cell lines thus far studied release either gelatinase A or B is not known. Alveolar macrophages,[49] polymorphonuclear leukocytes,[50] and keratinocytes[51] release gelatinase B, and the malignant phenotype of *ras*-transformed NIH/3T3 cells[52] correlates with the release of this enzyme. Gelatinase B levels appear to be elevated in malignant glial tumors.[53] Gelatinase A is perhaps the most widely distributed of all metalloproteinases[44] and has been identified in human fibroblasts,[54] human chondrocytes,[55–57] endothelial cells,[57] human cerebral microvascular endothelium[58] (Costello PC, et al: Unpublished results, 1995) and in a number of malignant cell lines,[44, 54] including C6 astrocytoma.[59] Regulation of these enzymes may occur at the level of gene expression (transcriptional regulation), the activation of these metalloproteinases, and the control of their proteolytic activity.[44, 45]

Transcriptional Regulation   The complete structures of the human genes for gelatinase A[60] and B[47] have been reported, and the main structural difference is the extended 54 amino acid hinge region that occurs in gelatinase B. The regulation of these two genes appears to be quite distinct from other MMPs and distinct from each other.[44, 45] The promoter regions for gelatinase B resemble the promoters of the Int-Cl and stromelysin genes.[47] Gelatinase B has a TATA-like sequence (TTAAA) and two TPA (12-*O*-tetra-decanoylphorbol-13-acetate)–responsive elements (AP-1 binding sites), which are not present in the gelatinase A gene. These findings correlate with the induction of gelatinase B mRNA levels and gelatinase B secretion with TPA stimulation[47] and the lack of response of gelatinase A. Although a *Fos*-binding sequence is present in the gelatinase B gene, transforming growth factor-β (TGFB) does not confer inhibition for reasons that are not apparent.[47] A large number of growth factors, cytokines, and other factors have been shown to stimulate and repress MMP expression[44] at a gene transcriptional level. A synthesis of these data would suggest that at the transcription level MMP genes are modulated in complex patterns and our understanding of how this process pertains to angiogenesis remains rudimentary.

Metalloproteinase Activation   The biologic activation of MMPs is an essential component in the regulation of these enzymes. This knowledge gap may represent the most important obstacle to our understanding of how cells use MMPs to degrade extracellular macromolecules in vivo.[44] A propeptide sequence of amino acids ranging from 77 to 87, which is present on the secreted enzyme, must be cleaved from these enzymes for activation.[44, 45, 61] The vast majority of cells release MMPs as proenzymes, and their activators in vivo are not known. Latency of these proenzymes seems to be at least partially explained by a cysteine-switch model that exposes the Zn^{2+} of active site and displaces the H_2O molecule that is necessary for catalysis[44, 45, 62] (Fig. 9–4). Proteolytic enzymes, conformational alterations, and thiol-reactive agents all may result in an active enzyme, but the relevance of these mechanisms in vivo has been questioned.[44] Three biologic activators of latent MMP proenzymes have been described that may be relevant to cerebral tumor-associated angiogenesis. Weiss and colleagues have described and studied extensively a low-molecular-weight angiogenic compound that has been called *endothelial cell–stimulating angiogenesis factor* (ESAF).[63–70] This nonprotein (approximate molecular weight 600) factor is angiogenic in in vivo assays,[64] activates collagenases,[65] and is capable of reactivating TIMP-inhibited metalloproteinases.[69] It has been found in high concentrations in malignant glial tumors[70] and may be relevant to the angiogenesis that occurs in ocular[67] and non-neural tissues.[66] The presence of ESAF in tissues and serum[71] in an inactive bound form suggests that ESAF may be regulated in biologic tissues. A second factor and/or family of factors, called *collagenase activating factor(s)* (CAFs), has been isolated from the media of C6 astrocytoma cells.[72] The media of C6 astrocytoma cells contains fully activated gelatinase A, which appears to be related to the presence of (approximate molecular weight 1,000) molecule(s), CAF(s). The ability of CAF to activate the latent gelatinase A present in the media of the human malignant glioma cell line U251[72] resulted in its discovery and has provided a useful assay. CAF also activates latent collagenase type IV activity present in specimens from human malignant glial tumors (Del Maestro RF: Unpublished results, 1995). The mechanism by which ESAF and CAF activate latent proenzymes is unknown, but by analogy to other nonphysiological activators it may involve structural alterations (possibly ESAF) and metal-catalyzed (possibly CAF) alterations in the proenzyme amino acid sequence, which results in the exposure of the active Zn^{2+}. The ability of MT-MPP to activate latent gelatinase A suggests that it may play a role in the cell surface activation of gelatinase A,[46] but this begs the questions of what mechanism activates MT-MPP and of how latent gelatinase B is activated. Further information on the physiological activation of latent MMPs appears crucial to the understanding of angiogenesis in malignant glial tumors.

Tissue Inhibitors of Metalloproteinases   A ubiquitous, highly effective metalloproteinase inhibitor family, called TIMPs, are important regulators of metalloproteinase function.[44, 45] Two members of this family have been extensively characterized and a third member, TIMP-3, has been described.[73] TIMP-1 is a 29-kD glycoprotein that preferentially binds to the proenzyme form of gelatinase B.[44, 74, 75] TIMP-2 is a 21-kD, nonglycosylated protein that forms a 1:1 complex with the proenzyme form of gelatinase A.[44, 76–78]

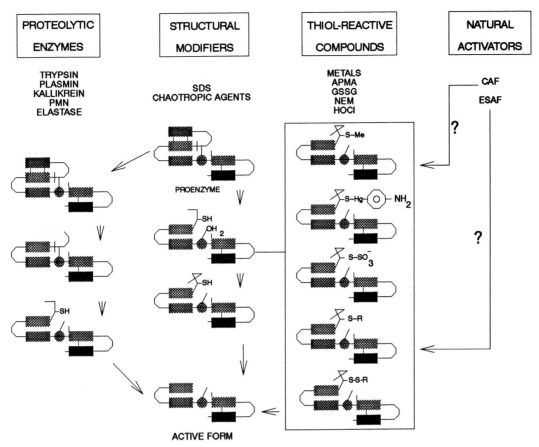

Figure 9–4 Activation of matrix metalloproteinases. The reversible opening of the cysteine switch plays a pivotal role in different activation pathways. Proteolytic enzymes; structural modifiers, such as sodium dodecyl sulfate (SDS) and chaotropic agents; and thiol-reactive compounds, such as metal ions, organomercurials (e.g., aminophenylmercuric acetate) (APMA), oxidized glutathione (GSSG), N-ethylmaleimide (NEM), and hypochlorous acid (HOCl) all can activate metalloproteinases by removal of the propeptide Cys residue. The mechanism of activation by natural activators is unknown. (Adapted from Birkedal-Hansen H, Moore WGI, Bodden MK, et al: Matrix metalloproteinases: A review. Crit Rev Oral Biol Med 1993; 4:197–250.)

The deduced amino acid sequence of TIMP-2 is 65% homologous with that of TIMP-1, and although the crystal structure of compounds has not been ascertained, the presence of cysteines in similar positions suggests that their three-dimensional structures may be quite similar.[44, 78] The active forms of gelatinase A and B are also inhibited by TIMP-1 and TIMP-2, respectively, and TIMP-1 can inhibit all members of the metalloproteinase family.[44] A number of investigators have demonstrated the effectiveness of TIMP-1 and TIMP-2 in a wide range of invasion assays. DeClerck and co-workers[79] have demonstrated the effectiveness of recombinant TIMP-2 (rTIMP-2) on invasion of smooth muscle layers by HT1080 cells and a *ras*-transformed rat embryo fibroblast line. Down-regulation of TIMP-1 mRNA levels via antisense RNA converted a previously non-tumorigenic and non-invasive Swiss 3T3 cell line to a line with invasive and metastatic potential.[80] Halaka and colleagues[81] found an inverse correlation between the levels of TIMP and the invasive potential of human intracranial tumors. However, TIMP has no effect on the spreading of C6 cells on CNS myelin, which calls into question the role of TIMP in glial cell invasion,[82] but a membrane-bound metallo-endoprotease may be involved.[83] The role played by TIMP-1 and TIMP-2 in angiogenesis is also not defined. Bovine aortic endothelial cells produce and release TIMP-1 and TIMP-2.[75] Non-stimulated human umbilical vein and foreskin microvascular endothelial cells express the mRNAs for TIMP-1 and TIMP-2, but the proteins were undetectable or only weakly expressed unless the cells were stimulated with inflammatory mediators such as tumor necrosis factor-α (TNFA) and interleukin 1α (ILIA).[84] The role played by TIMP-1 and TIMP-2 in human glial tumor–associated angiogenesis needs to be further defined.

PROTEASOME PATHWAYS

A number of reports indicate that eukaryotic cells contain large multi-subunit, multicatalytic proteinase complexes called *proteasomes,*[85] which are involved in intracellular protein degradation.[86–89] These subunits are organized in a barrel-shaped complex that, on cross-section, is ring-shaped with a central hole.[87, 90] The digestion of proteins in the barrel of the complex with multicatalytic potential at neutral pH may allow proteolysis to be progressive and extensive while preventing nonspecific proteolytic damage to cell constituents. The rapid removal of abnormal and short-lived regulatory peptides by proteasomes is extralysosomal and at least partially ATP-dependent.[87] Proteasomes are likely to play a critical role in regulating ubiquitin-dependent degradation of regulatory proteins such as cyclins, p53 tumor suppressor, oncogene products, and transcriptional regulators such as MATα$_2$,[90] the proteolytic processing of intracellular antigens for surface antigen presentation[87] and the removal of defective proteins.[87–89] Linkage of these proteins to ubiquitin[87, 91–94] allows their hydrolysis by a very large (26S or 1,500-kD) ATP-dependent proteolytic complex called *26S proteasome*.[93] A component of the 26S complex, 20S proteasome[87] is the major neutral proteolytic activity of mammalian cells.[85–89] The 20S proteasome is found free in eukaryotic cells[93] and contains four to five different peptidase activities,[86] which are neither ATP- nor ubiquitin-dependent.

Regulation of Proteasome Function Complementary DNAs for more than 25 subunits of proteasomes from various eukaryocytes (including eight human cDNAs) have been sequenced.[89] All proteasomal genes examined thus far encode previously unidentified proteins that are evolutionarily related and are called the *proteasome gene family*. Three unique segments, a nuclear translocation signal, and potential tyrosine phosophorylation have been identified on proteasome genes. De Martino and colleagues have identified a series of high-molecular-weight activators (PA28, PA700), inhibitors (P131, P1{x}) and modulators (PA45 enhances PA700 activation) of proteasome function. [90, 95]

Proteasomes, Neoplasia, and Angiogenesis The levels of mRNAs for several subunits of proteasomes were found to be increased in a variety of human hematopoetic and renal tumors.[88, 96, 97] C6 astrocytoma cells release a 1,000-kD extracellular proteasome (EP) with serine-dependent collagenase type IV activity, which is in an active form, and neither ATP, ubiquitin, nor serum is necessary for its activity.[98] The relationship of EP to the intracellular 26S and 20S proteasomes that may be present in these cells is not known, but the 1000-kD size is larger than 20S proteasomes (700-kD). It appears to be composed of three 68- to 70-kD subunits and has collagen type IV and type I degrading activity. Proteasome activity has been detected in human serum, possibly secondary to tumor cell lysis or tissue injury.[99] Activated MMPs and EP in the media of C6 astrocytoma cells each contribute about equally to the degradation of collagen type IV in vitro.[98] The ability of EP to degrade multiple substrates and the extracellular location of EP suggests that EP may play a role in the basement membrane degradation crucial to angiogenesis.

PLASMIN-DEPENDENT PATHWAY

A number of studies have demonstrated that the Pln-dependent pathway plays a role in the remodeling of the extracellular matrix occurring in cell migration, tumor cell invasion, metastasis, and angiogenesis.[44, 100, 101] Plasmin is a broad-spectrum serine proteinase that is generated from an inactive circulatory precursor, plasminogen, to an active form by specific activating enzymes, such as urokinase-type plasminogen activator (uPa) and tissue-type plasminogen activator (tPa). The plasminogen concentration in lymph, interstitial fluids, and plasma is 1 to 2 μM; if activated, this would result in significant tissue destruction.

The role played by the Pln-pathway in tumor-associated angiogenesis is unclear. The formation of capillary tubes from monolayers of bovine endothelial cells in vitro is associated with increased production of uPa activity.[102] Expression of uPa has been associated with angiogenesis in vivo,[103]

and human endothelial cells in monolayer culture are induced to generate uPa by a number of inflammatory mediators such as TNFA and 1L-1A.

Mononuclear leukocytes are encountered at sites of angiogenesis,[44] and their products, such as TNFA, may influence angiogenesis. The degree of overlap between the Pln- and MMP-dependent pathways remains unclear. In vitro MMP activity can be enhanced by plasminogen, which may be related to the ability of plasmin to activate Int-Cl and SL-1.[44] A reluctance has existed in accepting a prominent role for the Pln-pathway in pericellular proteolysis of extracellular macromolecules because (1) the lack of specificity for Pln degradative reactions contrasts sharply with the complex regulatory cascades of highly specific enzymes found in other pathways; (2) certain extracellular components, such as collagen type I and II, are not degraded by the Pln-pathway; and (3) a number of the latent MMPs are not activated by the Pln-pathway.[44]

NEUTROPHIL SERINE PROTEINASE PATHWAY

Polymorphonuclear leukocytes (PMNs) mediate the degradation of extracellular matrix via the release of two serine proteinases secreted from granules, neutrophil elastase and cathepsin G. These proteinases have activity against a wide variety of matrix macromolecules, including collagen type V.[44] This pathway may not play a prominent role in tumor-associated angiogenesis, because there does not appear to be a correlation between the presence of PMNs in experimental in vivo C6 astrocytoma tumors and proteolytic activity (Del Maestro RF: Unpublished results, 1995), and macrophage mediators, such as TNFA, do not alter the release of collagen type IV activity from U251 cells.[104]

INTRACELLULAR LYSOSOMAL PATHWAY

A number of ultrastructural studies have demonstrated intracellular fragments of extracellular matrix associated with lysosomal enzymes.[44] Inhibition studies suggest the involvement of lysosomal cathepsins rather than metalloproteinases in this process.[105] The role played by a lysosomal neutral protease cathepsin B in glial tumors has been studied by Sloane and co-workers.[106, 107] In glial tumors, increases in expression of (mRNA, protein, and activity) and altered trafficking of (localization/secretion) this protease have been found in both human glial tumor and endothelial cells within tumors.[107] A correlation exists between these findings and the grade of glioma, and this information would suggest that alterations in cathepsin B expression and localization may play a role in the preneoplastic to neoplastic transition of malignant tumor cells and their invasive properties.

ENDOGLYCOSIDASE PATHWAYS

These nonproteinase enzymes remove polysaccharide chains (glycosaminoglycans) from proteoglycan core proteins, such as chondroitin sulfate proteoglycans, and degrade hyaluronic acid, major components of the extracellular space of the brain.[108] Heparinase degrades HSPGs, which are important components of the vascular basement membrane, whereas hyaluronidase degrades hyaluronic acid.

Angiogenic Factors

The ability to use cultured endothelial cells, particularly microvessel endothelium, in vitro has resulted in the purification and identification of angiogenic factors that increase endothelial proliferation and/or migration.[3, 109, 110] In certain in vitro conditions, capillary endothelial cells form three-dimensional tube networks that resemble microvascular networks in vivo.[102] Table 9–3 presents a list of some of the angiogenic molecules that may play a role in glial tumors. A detailed explanation of all the factors secreted by normal, tumor, and accessory cells, such as platelets, PMN leukocytes, monocytes, macrophages, lymphocytes, and mast cells, is beyond the scope of this chapter, and a number of reviews are available.[3, 109, 110] This discussion focuses on factors possibly having a role in angiogenesis in glial tumors.

The alternative splicing of vascular endothelial growth factor (VEGF) mRNA transcript results in four polypeptide isoforms, of which $VEGF_{121}$ and $VEGF_{165}$ are secreted and $VEGF_{189}$ and $VEGF_{206}$ are bound to cells and basement membranes.[110, 111] Substantial evidence supporting an important role of VEGF and its receptors VEGFR1 (*flt-1*) and VEGFR2 (*flk-1*) in glial tumor–associated angiogenesis and edema exists.[110–118] This includes the following: (1) that VEGF is produced by malignant glial cell lines;[116, 117] (2) that VEGF mRNA and protein are produced by glioma cells in vivo;[112, 114] (3) that VEGFR1 and VEGFR2 are expressed and up-regulated on the endothelial cells of tumor microvessels and on microvessels at the normal brain tumor interface, but not on normal cerebral capillaries distant from the tumor;[113, 114] (4) that VEGF results in endothelial cell proliferation, migration, and tube formation in vitro;[116] (5) that significant reduction in in vivo tumor growth in nude mice was seen using anti-VEGF monoclonal antibodies, whereas in vitro cell proliferation was unchanged;[118] and (6) that the introduction of a retrovirus encoding a dominant-negative mutant of the *flk-1* (VEGFR2) receptor into cerebral endothelial cells of rats with C6 astrocytoma resulted in inhibition of angiogenesis in vivo.[115] The up-regulation of VEGF but not FGF1, FGF2, and platelet-derived growth factor-β (PDGFB) mRNA in C6 astrocytoma cells in vitro by hypoxia may explain the localization of VEGF to the tumor cells along necrotic areas.[112, 114] VEGF also appears to play a role in the modulation of microvascular permeability in malignant glial tumors.[110, 117]

Transforming growth factor-α and epidermal growth fac-

TABLE 9–3
ANGIOGENIC MOLECULES

| Factor (Isoforms) | Receptor(s) | Endothelial Cell | | | Role in Glial Tumor Angiogenesis | References |
		Proliferation	Migration	Tube Formation		
Vascular endothelial growth factor (VEGF) $VEGF_{121}$ $VEGF_{165}$ $VEGF_{189}$ $VEGF_{206}$	VEGFR1 (*Flt–1*) VEGFR2 (*Flk–1*)	+ +	+ +	+ +	Major role in propagation, permeability change	110–116
Epidermal growth factor (EGF) Transforming growth factor-α (TGFA)	EGFR	+ +	+ +	+ +	No definite correlation between EGFR and ligands with malignant glial tumors, angiogenesis	110, 117, 120
Fibroblast growth factor (7 related peptides) Acidic fibroblast growth factor (FGF1)	Receptors	+	+	0	Low level in tumors	110, 120–122
Basic fibroblast growth factor (FGF2)	Receptors	+ +	+ +	+ +	Major role in propagation	110, 116, 120–126
Platelet-derived growth factor (PDGF) PDGF-AA PDGF-AB PDGF-BB	PDGFRA PDGDRB	+ +	0	+ +	Role for PDGFB/PDGFRB	110, 127–129
Transforming growth factor-β (TGFB) TFG_{B1-5}	Receptors	–ve	–ve	–ve	Role in termination of angiogenesis	110, 130–133
Lipid-derived factors Prostaglandins E_1 and E_2		0	+ +	0	May play role in maintenance of blood flow	134, 135
Endothelial cell–stimulating angiogenesis factor (ESAF)		+ +	+ +	Unknown	Possible basement membrane degradation endothelial proliferation	63, 64
Others Fibrin		0	+ +	0	Facilitates endothelial cell invasion	3, 136

tor (EGF) are the endogenous ligands for the epidermal growth factor receptor (EGFR).[110] This loop stimulates endothelial cell replication, migration, and loop formation in vitro.[119, 120] A correlation does not appear to exist between these ligands and/or their receptor in malignant glial tumor–induced angiogenesis in vivo.[110] EGF increases the production of VEGF by malignant glial cells in vitro, and if this occurs in vivo, there may be a role for this factor in the modulation of VEGF during angiogenesis.[119]

The fibroblast growth factor family is made up of at least seven related polypeptides encoded by separate genes.[121] In glioblastoma multiforme, FGF1 is present in some tumor cells whereas FGF2 is present in the matrix surrounding proliferating blood vessels.[122, 123] Malignant glial cells contain FGF2,[116, 124] but the lack of a signal peptide results in little extracellular secretion.[124] Three mechanisms have been suggested to explain the increased levels of FGF2 seen in the cerebrospinal fluid of glioblastoma patients:[125] (1) cell death, (2) release from extracellular matrix, and (3) secretion by recruited macrophages.[116] The finding that FGF2 plays an important synergistic role with VEGF in the proliferation, elongation, and tube formation of bovine capillary cells in vitro as well as its perivascular location in tumors suggests that FGF2 may play a role in the propagation phase of angiogenesis.[116, 126]

The PDGF family includes three isoforms of disulfide-linked A and B chains (PDGF-AA, PDGF-BB, and PDGF-AB). All three isoforms bind to PDGF receptor-α (PDGFRA), whereas PDGF receptor-β (PDGFRB) binds the B chain exclusively.[110] PDGF-BB has been shown to increase tube formation of endothelial cells in vitro.[127] PDGFB-chain mRNA was found to be predominantly associated with tumor microvessels in malignant gliomas[128] and the PDGFRB receptor is also localized to these microvessels.[128, 129] The PDGFB/PDGFRB paracrine and autocrine loops appear to play a role in the propagation phase of angiogenesis.

Five polypeptides with high structural homology make up the transforming growth factor-β family (TFGB1–5). The in vivo mechanism of activation of the inactive secreted form is unknown. TGFB inhibits endothelial cell propagation, migration, and tube formation in vitro.[130–132] However, low concentrations of TGFB potentiates VEGF- and FGF2-induced tube formation.[132] TGFB2 mRNA is predominantly associated with endothelium surrounding tumor microvessels in glioblastoma multiforme.[133] These results suggest that TGFB may play biphasic roles, increasing angiogenesis at low concentrations and playing a crucial role in termination events at higher concentrations.

A number of other factors may play a role in tumor-induced angiogenesis in glial tumors (see Table 9–3). Inhibition of prostaglandin synthesis in experimental glial tumors results in decreased tumor growth, suggesting a role for such prostaglandins as E_1 and E_2 in tumor-induced angiogenesis.[134, 135] ESAF is an endothelial cell mitogen that is increased in glial tumors.[63, 64] The role of fibrin in facilitating endothelial cell invasion of extracellular matrix has been studied extensively.[136]

In glial tumors, there appears to be a wide overlap and presumed redundancy in the number of angiogenic and motility-enhancing molecules capable of inducing in vitro endo-thelial cell proliferation, migration, and tube formation (see Table 9–3). This may be related to the ability of tumor cells to harness the angiogenesis cascade of the many normal cells that participate in wound healing and tissue repair. These mechanisms are constantly modified and/or augmented, depending on the local microenvironmental concentrations of angiogenic factors, and their available receptor and matrix degradative systems. It appears most appropriate to consider these systems as interactive, nonstatic, heterogeneous, and constantly modulated during the growth of any given tumor.

Conceptual Model

A conceptual model of the angiogenesis cascade in malignant glial tumors is presented. This model is based on the experiments of numerous researchers.

Four problems are evident when considering glial tumor–associated angiogenesis:

1. The compartmentalization of the angiogenesis process is essential to isolate and target a particular basement membrane segment for modification and degradation.
2. A number of different enzyme activities must be involved in the degradation of the vascular basement membrane and extracellular matrix.
3. A coordinated endothelial response to angiogenic and motility factors is necessary if a functional tumor microcirculation is to develop.
4. A number of different cells must be involved in this response, including (1) tumor cells, (2) endothelial cells, (3) inflammatory cells, and (4) a number of normal cells (i.e., pericytes, perivascular glial cells).

NORMAL MICROVESSEL MICROENVIRONMENT

In normal cerebral microvessels, angiogenesis is constitutively repressed by a number of mechanisms (Fig. 9–5A), including the following:

1. *Perivascular pericyte modulation:* These cells produce TGFB, which inhibit endothelial proliferation and thus maintain endothelium in a quiescent state.[130]
2. *Perivascular glial cell modulation:* The perivascular glial cells are not only responsible for the maintenance of specialized endothelial blood brain barrier (BBB) characteristics, but they release diffusible factor(s) that downregulate the release of proteolytic enzymes from endothelial cells (Costello PC: Unpublished results, 1995).
3. *Angiogenic factor receptors:* In normal adult cerebral microvessel endothelium, the receptors for angiogenic factors are down-regulated.
4. *Vascular basement membrane:* The presence of HSPGs in the basement membrane and extracellular matrix may function to sequester and bind growth factors that may down-regulate any aberrant angiogenic stimuli.
5. *Serum proteinase inhibitors:* Endothelial cells are usually bathed in large amounts of inhibitor compounds.[43]

INITIATION

Although the molecular basis of malignant transformation of glial cells is unknown, some of these genetic alterations

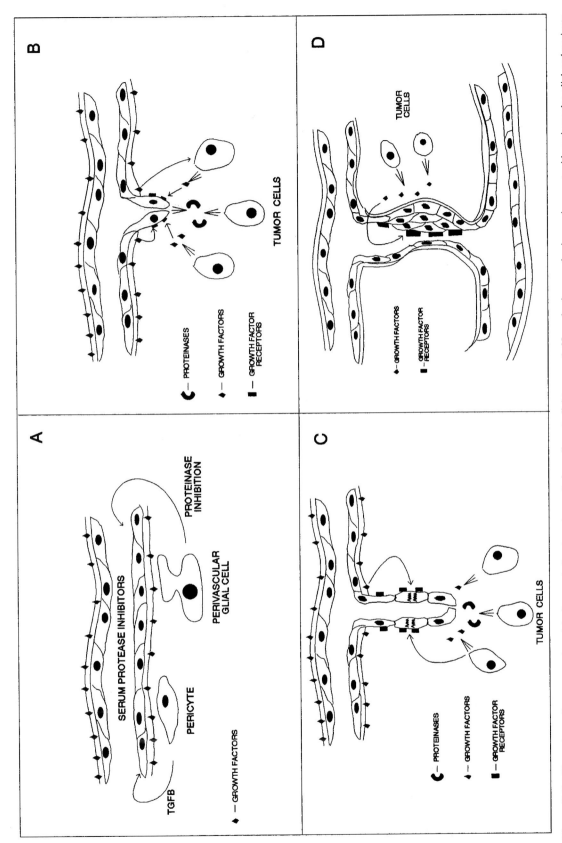

Figure 9-5 Illustrations of a conceptual model of tumor-induced angiogenesis in malignant glial tumors. *A,* Normal microvessel microenvironment with perivascular glial and pericyte modulation of endothelial proteinase release and division, respectively. Basement membrane binding of growth factors, down-regulation of growth factor receptors, and the abundant serum proteinase inhibitors also function to repress angiogenesis. *B,* Initiation of angiogenesis with the localized degradation of basement membrane by proteinases released by both endothelial and tumor cells and the up-regulation of growth factor receptors on endothelial cells. The subsequent elongation of endothelial cells in response to growth and motility factors released by tumor and possibly inflammatory cells. *C,* Propagation of angiogenesis with endothelial mitosis of trailing endothelial cells in response to paracrine loops associated with up-regulation of receptors on endothelial cells and mitogens released from the basement membrane and/or tumor cells. *D,* Termination of angiogenesis with reconstruction of new tumor microvessels and the laying down of new basement membrane. The presence of intravascular endothelial proliferation may be secondary to their continued response to mitogens and/or the absence of pericyte modulation (TGF$_B$) of endothelial division.

up-regulate consitutively repressed angiogenic mechanisms that are present in the endothelial cell–basement membrane–pericyte–perivascular glial cell complex present in normal tissue.[137–140] The balance between activated proteases and their inhibitors in the microenvironment around this complex must be altered by the initial clone of tumor cells in favor of focal proteolytic degradation of the basement membrane.

If information is extrapolated from the secreted collagen type IV degrading activity of C6 cells, then glial cells may use predominantly activated gelatinases and EP to degrade basement membrane macromolecules (Fig. 9–6). The activation of gelatinase A by CAF and/or other activating mechanisms overcomes control mechanisms associated with TIMP-2, whereas EP and other serine proteases may overwhelm local serine inhibitors. The role placed by ESAF in these events is unknown, but its unique ability to activate metalloproteinases bound to TIMPs could play a role. The degradation of the basement membrane results in the local release of growth factors such as VEGF and FGF2, which results in the amplification of the angiogenesis cascade by a number of paracrine loops (see Figs. 9–5B and C). These factors may initiate the transcription and the release of degradative enzymes by local endothelial and tumor cells.[44, 140–141] This amplification system would circumvent the problem of the absence of a signal peptide sequence for FGF2 and its lack of constitutive secretion by most cells. The local release of growth factors by basement membrane undergoing degradation may further aid in the focus and the compartmentalization of the angiogenesis response to a specific microvessel microenvironment. Uncontrolled degradation of the basement membrane would result in hemorrhage, which may explain the hemorrhage seen in malignant glial tumors. Released factors from the basement membrane and local tumor cells may provide the gradient of motility molecules necessary to cause the elongation and directional migration of endothelial cells through the defect in the basement membrane. The exposed laminin of the basement membrane may provide a directional highway into the extracellular matrix. Human cerebral microvascular endothelial cells undergoing elongation and division release gelatinase A (Costello PC:

Unpublished results, 1995). The degradation of the matrix needed for endothelial invasion would be dependent on the local release of enzymatic activities by both endothelial and tumor cells involving the coordinated function of a number of proteinases.

PROPAGATION

Tumor cells in the vicinity of normal microvessels result in the up-regulation of a number of growth factor receptors, VEGFR1, VEGFR2, PDGFRB, and fibroblast growth factor receptors. The up-regulation of the VEGF receptors must occur before significant ischemia is present, because this is seen on tumor microvessel endothelium throughout the tumor and at the tumor–normal tissue interface. The presence of tumor cells in the vicinity of endothelial cells could increase local lactate levels and/or some other metabolites that may be involved in VEGF receptor up-regulation. In tumor regions of incomplete ischemia, VEGF mRNA is induced, resulting in the release of this growth factor from tumor cells and the predominant activation of this paracrine loop. The physical presence of tumor cells may disrupt the relationship of endothelial cells to other members of the complex resulting in a down-regulation of TGFB concentrations and decreased proteinase inhibition. The combination of low levels of TFGB and up-regulated activity in the VEGF, FGFB, PDGFB paracrine loops results in a growth factor microenvironment that is very conducive to endothelial cell proliferation, migration, and tube formation (see Fig. 9–5C).

TERMINATION

The mechanisms by which the endothelial sprouts cannulize and are able to link up with other sprouts in human glial tumors is unknown, but increased TGFB levels may be important in this process. The resulting flow in these microvessels down-regulates endothelial proteolytic enzyme activity by bathing endothelial cells in serum that contains a plethora of serine protease inhibitors.[43] The majority of these inhibitors are targeted against the serine proteases involved

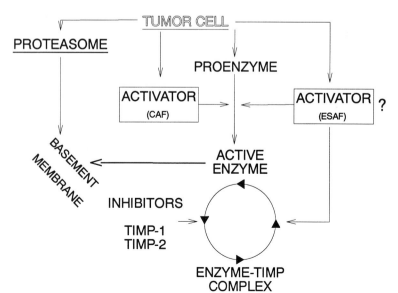

Figure 9–6 Mechanism of basement membrane degradation by glial tumor cells. The tumor cells release the proenzyme of MMPs (gelatinase A), which may be activated by CAF and/or ESAF. ESAF may also play a role in reactivating the proenzyme and active enzyme from their TIMP complexes. The release of extracellular proteasome may also play a crucial role in the basement membrane degradation that is seen.

in coagulation, fibrinolysis, complement activation, and phagocytosis. Anti-proteinases such as α_1-proteinase inhibitor (α_1-antitrypsin), α_1-antichymotrypsin, α_2-macroglobulin, and antithrombin III are the most common of a wide number of antiproteinases that have been studied.[142, 143] The constitution of the basement membrane by the new tumor microvessel endothelium may provide a structural barrier able to bind growth factors that are being secreted by tumor cells and/or that are preventing these substances from reaching endothelial receptors. The finding that endothelial cell proliferation is common within the microvessels of glioblastoma multiforme[9] would suggest that local endothelial mitogen concentrations remain high and/or that the lack of pericytes that decreases TGFB around tumor microvessels allows intravascular endothelial mitosis to continue unabated (see Fig. 9–5D).

THE FUNCTIONAL MICROCIRCULATION OF GLIAL TUMORS

Angioarchitecture

The growth of malignant glial tumors is dependent on both tumor-associated angiogenesis and tumor-induced vascular modification resulting in a tumor angioarchitecture that is both three-dimensionally complex and constantly remodeling. The initial angioarchitecture pattern in the C6 astrocytoma spheroid implantation model involves the development of a heterogeneous group of microvessels that vascularize the avascular spheroid. In larger tumors, two distinct patterns can be ascertained: (1) a peripheral pattern that involves the continuous development of new microvessels and the incorporation of established vessels at the growing edge of the tumor, and (2) a central pattern in which the paucity of tumor microvessels is seen, and this is associated histologically with necrosis (Fig. 9–7). A similar pattern can be seen at times in human glioblastoma multiforme. This is also characterized by a peripheral pattern of large tortuous microvessels, many of which demonstrate intraluminal endothelial proliferation surrounded by tumor cells and a central pattern of necrosis (Fig. 9–8).

Quantitative assessment of brain tumor microvessel angioarchitecture and blood flow before the development of necrosis using the C6 spheroid implantation model has been carried out.[144, 145] The technique used to demonstrate patent vessels in this model was the continuous infusion of Aquablak ink (AQ), whereas the infusion of horseradish peroxidase (HRP) was used to stain only the vessels perfused with blood during the time period when blood flow was measured (30 seconds) with autoradiography. Figure 9–9 provides quantitative information of microvessel diameter, microvessel length, microvessel volume fraction, and microvessel surface area in this tumor model. Tumor angioarchitecture is composed of short microvessels of large diameter, only half of which are being perfused with blood at any given time. The surface area available for exchange at the blood-tumor interface is half that of normal cortex, and tumor functional microcirculation is further reduced by incomplete perfusion.

Tumor Blood Flow

It has been demonstrated both experimentally[18, 144, 146, 147] and clinically[148] that blood flow to malignant gliomas is lower and more heterogeneous than to normal cerebral tissues. Low blood flow in gliomas appears to be related to reduced linear velocity of blood cells in blood vessels coupled with incomplete and/or heterogeneous perfusion.[144] These results suggest that the microcirculation of gliomas is capable of sustaining high flow rates because their angioarchitecture is consistent with a low-resistance, partially perfused network. Tumor microvessels lack arterioles, and this may partially explain low blood flow, because no mechanism for maintaining pressure gradients is available. Jain has suggested that because tumor microvessels are highly permeable and extravasate fluid, local tissue pressures around tumor vessels increase.[149, 150] A balance between decreased intravascular pressure and increased interstitial fluid pressure may result in dynamic alterations of flow in individual vessels and in local flow stasis. This low-flow state, combined with surface alterations on tumor microvessel endothelium,[58] may result in intraluminal platelet deposition and intraluminal thrombosis, which leads to focal areas of necrosis. These intraluminal events may also play a role in tumor-associated hemorrhage.

Microvascular Permeability

The implantation of C6 spheroids into different vascular beds, murine muscle and brain, induces microvessels with endothelial cell morphologic features that are not quantitatively distinguishable.[151] These findings are consistent with previous studies[152] that demonstrate that irrespective of the host tissue from which new tumor microvessels originate, the tumor cells themselves organize the development and the final morphologic features of the microvessels that vascularize them. The leakage of albumin-bound Evans blue into growing C6 astrocytoma tumors parallels the development

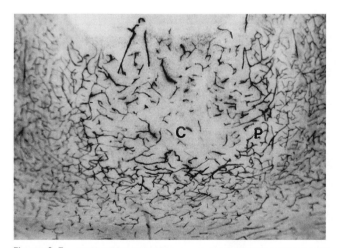

Figure 9–7 Angioarchitecture of tumor microvessels in the C6 spheroid implantation model, stained with alkaline phosphatase, which demonstrates the peripheral (P) and central (C) patterns of microvessel structure.

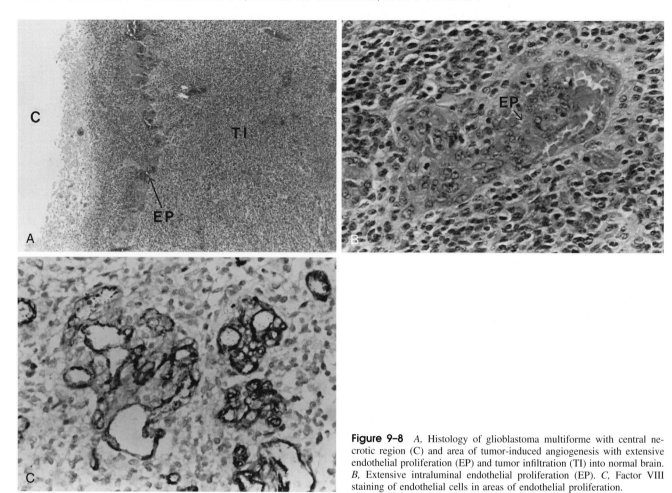

Figure 9–8 *A,* Histology of glioblastoma multiforme with central necrotic region (C) and area of tumor-induced angiogenesis with extensive endothelial proliferation (EP) and tumor infiltration (TI) into normal brain. *B,* Extensive intraluminal endothelial proliferation (EP). *C,* Factor VIII staining of endothelial cells in areas of endothelial proliferation.

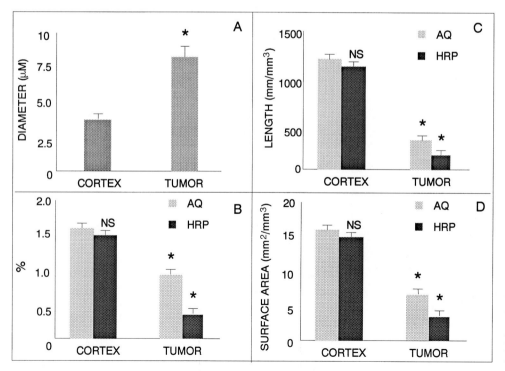

Figure 9–9 Quantitative data on microvessel diameter (*A*), percentage microvessel volume fraction (*B*), microvessel length (*C*), and microvessel surface area (*D*) in the C6 astrocytoma spheroid implantation model. NS indicates *P* > .05; asterisk, *P* < .05.

of the tumor angioarchitecture[24] and may be seen as the contrast-enhanced tumor CT and MRI. No extravasation is seen prior to tumor microvessel ingrowth. An increase in leakage is seen with expanding tumor volume. Significant variability in leakage is found in larger tumors with central necrotic regions. The flux of molecules into the brain is dependent on a functional endothelial barrier having the following three components: (1) a paracellular route through spaces in tight junctional regions, (2) a transcellular route via vesicular transport, and (3) a transcellular route through occasional fenestrae. Stewart and co-workers have carried out a series of quantitative experiments on the endothelial morphology of the tumor microvessels of glioblastoma multiforme[153] and in vivo C6 astrocytoma.[154] These studies demonstrate that the endothelial paracellular routes through abnormal junctions and the occasional presence of a large endothelial gap (fenestra) are the morphologic pathways that result in increased protein and fluid flux seen from tumor microvessels. These larger gaps may be equivalent to the physiologically measured large pore, whereas the endothelial junctional abnormalities may represent the physiologic small pore. The presence of endothelial alterations in human peritumoral microvessels not in direct contact with tumor cells (tumor-induced vascular modification) suggests the action of diffusible factor(s) that act at a distance from the major tumor mass.[155] A number of interacting mechanisms (such as the endothelial abnormalities described) and the action of a number of tumor permeability factors (such as VEGF) combined with immunologic and inflammatory mechanisms may all contribute to the amount and type of endothelial cell dysfunction that is present.[2] Dynamic biophysical factors, such as the flow in peritumoral and tumor microvessels, combined with local interstitial pressure then determine the dynamic flux of fluid and macromolecules across tumor microvessels in any given microenvironment of the tumor.[149]

Serum Proteolytic Activity and Angiogenesis

Protein tumor markers, such as α-fetoprotein and human chorionic gonadotropin, have been found to be increased in intracranial germ cell tumor tissue,[156] CSF,[157] and serum. The presence of two peaks of serum general protease activity and serum type IV collagenase activity associated with the growth of C6 astrocytoma in vivo has suggested that both endothelial cells and tumor cells may contribute to alterations in serum proteolytic activity that may reflect angiogenesis events in vivo.[43] If these data can be extrapolated to human malignant glial tumors, it would predict that a single serum time point of proteolytic activity may not be useful as an assessment of tumor-associated angiogenesis, but that frequent assessments may be of value in monitoring recurrent tumor growth after surgical removal and/or adjuvant therapies.

ANGIOSTATIC THERAPY

Angiostatic therapy may be defined as treatment interventions that are effective in modulating angiogenesis. Concep-

tually, two strategies of angiostatic therapy can be envisioned: acute and chronic treatments. In established tumors, which are at least partially dependent on angiogenesis for their continued growth, acute therapy may be able to limit further growth by inhibiting the angiogenesis cascade and/or causing tumor microvessel regression. A priori acute treatment would not be expected to result in total tumor regression because tumor cells in microenvironments in the vicinity of normal vessels and tumor microvessels not undergoing regression would remain viable. Acute angiostatic therapy may arrest tumor growth, allowing time for other modalities (e.g., radiation and chemotherapy) to be effective. Discontinuation of therapy would result in further tumor growth. Chronic angiostatic therapy would be expected to be beneficial in the following three situations:

1. After the acute therapy of established tumors, chronic treatment may be useful as an adjuvant modality to maintain tumor regression.
2. In low-grade tumors, which frequently undergo malignant transformation to tumors that can induce tumor angiogenesis,[138] chronic treatment may prevent the expression of their new angiogenetic potential and limit tumor growth. In both of these situations, tumor growth by perivascular tumor cell invasion, which results in tumor-induced vascular modification and the incorporation of previously normal blood vessels into the tumor, may continue. Chronic angiostatic therapy combined with therapeutic agents also designed to limit tumor invasiveness would be ideal in these situations. Chronic angiostatic therapy may be of limited efficacy if substantial influences on physiologic angiogenesis, such as occurs in wound healing, menstruation, and vasculogenesis, are encountered.
3. Chronic angiostatic therapy may be useful in the prevention of growth of systemic or CSF metastatic disease. Intravascular tumor cells must adhere to or be trapped on endothelium, degrade the basement membrane, and induce an angiogenic growth response.[3, 158] In carcinomatous meningitis, the growth of large (>1 mm) exophytic lesions is also dependent on the induction of angiogenesis.

Potential angiostatic therapeutic approaches can be divided into those that are effective in the modulation, initiation, propagation, and termination of events. Table 9–4 outlines potential targets of therapeutic intervention, targeted pathways, and therapeutic agents that could be assessed. The serine protease inhibitor Coumadin (warfarin) has been used in a number of human tumors,[159, 160] and a murine model of malignant glioma and appears to have some efficacy.[161] The mechanism of action of this and other serine inhibitors[162] that may have influences on tumor growth is unknown. Potential mechanisms could involve inhibition of the proteasome, Pln-dependent, and PMN serine protease pathways. Consideration of the conceptual model discussed previously would suggest that a ''cocktail'' of inhibitors may need to be used to effectively prevent basement membrane degradation associated with tumor associated angiogenesis. Folkman and co-workers have found that the synthetic analogues of fumagillin, in particular AGM–1470,[163] inhibit angiogenesis and tumor growth. In a number of experiments designed to assess the influence of AGM–1470 on glial tumor growth in

TABLE 9–4
POTENTIAL ANGIOSTATIC THERAPEUTIC APPROACHES

Angiogenesis Cascade	Targets	Pathway	Therapeutic Agents
Initiation	Basement membrane degradation	MMPs	TIMP-1, TIMP-2 Specific MMP inhibitors[48]
		Proteasome	Serine protease inhibitors[161]
		Plasmin-dependent	Serine protease inhibitors
		PMN serine proteinase	Serine protease inhibitors
		Intracellular lysosomal	Cathepsin inhibitors
	Endothelial cell elongation	Adhesion Motility (microtubules)	Prostaglandin inhibition[134, 135]
	Endothelial cell invasion	Same as for basement membrane degradation	
Propagation	Endothelial cell division	Unknown	AGM–1470
	Endothelial cell division	VEGF/VEGFR2	Retrovirus introduction dominant-negative mutant of VEGFR2[115]
	Endothelial cell division	VEGF and other factors	Monoclonal antibodies[118]
Termination	Loop formation	Unknown	None known
Others	Unknown	Copper metabolism	Penicillamine[31] copper depletion
	Unknown	Unknown	Hydrocortisone[26] and heparin

the subrenal model in nude mice, it has been found that this compound suppresses tumor growth and at times regression of tumors is seen.[27, 28] This compound appears to inhibit mitosis of endothelial cells and a wide variety of tumor cells, and it is being assessed in human trials. The mechanism of its action on cell mitosis is not known. Other angiostatic strategies, such as copper depletion,[31] anti-inflammatory agents,[134, 135] steroids and heparin,[26] and monoclonal antibodies,[118] have been assessed for their efficacy in model systems. A systematic approach to the development of angiostatic compounds effective in primary glial tumors has not been carried out. The use of viral vectors to introduce a defective VEGFR protein and the efficacy of this technique in the inhibition of in vivo malignant glial tumor growth open a new door in angiostatic therapy.[115]

The development of effective angiostatic therapeutic approaches to glial and other tumors depends on the unraveling of each of the molecular events associated with the angiogenesis cascade. With this knowledge, strategies can be developed that may involve the use of a number of agents specifically targeted to inhibit components of the tumor-associated angiogenesis cascade but allow physiological angiogenesis to proceed normally.

SUMMARY

The coordinated function of glial tumor and endothelial cells results in a complex angiogenesis cascade with initiation, propagation, and termination steps culminating in a tumor angioarchitecture with a dynamic microcirculation. The functional microcirculation of glial tumors is determined by the angioarchitecture induced by these tumor cells and modulated by local tissue factors such as available microvascular surface area and blood flow. The permeability of the individual microvessels in malignant tumors is high, and some alterations in permeability are also seen in peritumoral tissues; thus, the effectiveness of any chemotherapeutic agent may be crucially dependent on local tumor blood flow rather than on its ability to traverse the blood-brain barrier to

produce therapeutic concentrations in tumors. Angiostatic strategies targeted at tumor angioarchitecture appear to provide novel approaches to tumor modulation.

ACKNOWLEDGMENTS

The author would like to thank his many co-workers who have contributed to research in his laboratory, including Dr. P.A. Stewart, Dr. J.B. Weiss, Dr. I.S. Vaithilingam, Dr. P. Costello, Dr. C.L. Farrell, Dr. J.F. Megyesi, Dr. H.R. Reichman, and especially W. McDonald and E.C. Stroude. I would like to thank Dr. David Ramsay for providing Figure 9–8. Jo-Ann Dunn is thanked for her secretarial assistance.

This work was supported by the Brain Tumor Foundation of Canada, the Royal Arch Masons of Canada "Release a Miracle Donation to Medical Research," and the Victoria Hospital Research Development Fund.

REFERENCES

1. Brem S, Cotran R, Folkman J: Tumor angiogenesis: A quantitative method for histological grading. JNCI 1972; 48:347–356.
2. Del Maestro RF, Megyesi JF, Farrell CL: Mechanisms of tumor-associated edema: A review. Can J Neurol Sci 1990; 17:177–183.
3. Blood CH, Zetter BR: Tumor interactions with the vasculature: Angiogenesis and tumor metastasis. Biochem Biophys Acta 1990; 1032:89–118.
4. Hooper R: The Morbid Anatomy of the Human Brain Being Illustrations of the Most Frequent and Important Organic Diseases to Which That Viscus is Subject. Birmingham, Ala, Classics of Neurology and Neurosurgery Library, 1984.
5. Bramwell B: Intracranial Tumors. Birmingham Ala, Classics of Neurology and Neurosurgery Library, 1988.
6. Carmichael EA: Cerebral gliomata. J Pathol 1928; 31:493–510.
7. Ellesberg CA, Hare CC: The blood supply of the gliomas: Its relation to the tumor growth and its surgical significance. Bull Neurol Inst 1932; 2:210–246.
8. Scherer HJ: The forms of growth in gliomas and their practical significance. Brain 1940; 63:1–35.
9. Hardman J: The angioarchitecture of the gliomata. Brain 1940; 63:91–118.
10. Ide AG, Baker NH, Warren SL: Vascularization of the Brown-Pearce

rabbit epithelioma transplant as seen in the transparent ear chamber. Am J Roentgenol 1939; 42:891–899.

11. Algire GH, Chalkley HW: Vascular reactions of normal malignant tissues in vivo: I. Vascular reactions of mice to wounds and to normal and neoplastic transplants. JNCI 1945/46; 6:73–85.

12. Algire GH: The Biology of Melanomas, vol 4. New York, New York Academy of Science, 1947, pp 159–175.

13. Folkman J: Tumor angiogenesis: Therapeutic implications. N Engl J Med 1971; 285:1182–1186.

14. Folkman J: Anti-angiogenesis: New concept for therapy of solid tumors. Ann Surg 1972; 175:409–416.

15. Bigner DD, Svenberg JA: Experimental Tumors of the Central Nervous System. Kalamazoo, Mich, Upjohn, 1977.

16. Auer R, Del Maestro RF, Anderson R: A simple and reproducible experimental in vivo glioma model. Can J Neurol Sci 1981; 8:325–331.

17. Groothius DR, Fischer JM, Vick NA, et al: Comparative permeability of different glioma models to horseradish peroxidase. Cancer Treat Rep 1981; 65:13–18.

18. Blasberg RG, Molnar PD, Horowitz M, et al: Regional blood flow in RT-9 brain tumors. J Neurosurg 1983; 58:863–873.

19. Hurter T, Mennel HD: Experimental brain tumors and edema in rats. Acta Neuropathol 1981; 55:105–111.

20. Sutherland RM: Cell and environment interactions in tumor microregions: The multicell spheroid model. Science 1988; 240:177–184.

21. Lordo CD, Stroude EC, Del Maestro RF: The effects of diphenylhydantoin on murine astrocytoma radiosensitivity. J Neurooncol 1987; 5:339–350.

22. Lordo CD, Stroude EC, Del Maestro RF: The effects of dexamethasone on C6 astrocytoma radiosensitivity. J Neurosurg 1989; 70:767–773.

23. Megyesi JF, Del Maestro RF: Nuclear magnetic resonance in the investigation of cerebral tumors and cerebral edema: A clue to the cellular alterations that may affect the distribution of water. Biochem Cell Biol 1988; 66:1100–1109.

24. Farrell CL, Stewart PA, Del Maestro RF: A new glioma model in rat: The C6 spheroid implantation technique permeability and vascular characterization. J Neurooncol 1987; 4:403–415.

25. Bodgen AE, Cobb WR, Lepage DJ, et al: Chemotherapy responsiveness of human tumors as first transplant generation xenograft in the normal mouse: Six-day subrenal capsule assay. Cancer 1981; 48:10–20.

26. Lee JK, Choi B, Sobel RA, et al: Inhibition of growth and angiogenesis of human neurofibrosarcoma by heparin and hydrocortisone. J Neurosurg 1990; 73:429–435.

27. Takamiya Y, Friedlander RM, Brem H, et al: Inhibition of angiogenesis and growth of human nerve-sheath tumors by AGM-1470. J Neurosurg 1993; 78:470–476.

28. Takamiya Y, Brem H, Ojeifo J, et al: AGM-1470 inhibits the growth of human glioblastoma cells in vitro and in vivo. Neurosurg 1994; 34:869–875.

29. Zagzag D, Brem S, Robert F: Neovascularization and tumor growth in the rabbit brain: A model for experimental studies of angiogenesis and the blood-brain barrier. Am J Pathol 1988; 131:361–372.

30. Zagzag D, Goldenberg M, Brem S: Angiogenesis and blood-brain barrier breakdown modulate CT contrast enhancement: An experimental study in a rabbit brain-tumor model. AJNR 1989; 153:141–146.

31. Brem SS, Zagzag D, Tranacis AMC, et al: Inhibition of angiogenesis and tumor growth in the brain: Suppression of endothelial cell turnover by penicillamine and the depletion of copper and angiogenic co-factor. Am J Pathol 1990; 137:1121–1142.

32. Folkman J: Angiogenesis: Initiation and modulation. *In* Nicolson GL, Milas L (eds): Cancer Invasion and Metastasis: Biologic and Therapeutic Aspects. New York, Raven Press, 1984, pp 201–208.

33. Folkman J: How is blood vessel growth regulated in normal and neoplastic tissues? Clowes Memorial Award Lecture. Cancer Res 1986; 6:467–473.

34. Stanley JR, Woodley DT, Katz SI, et al: Structure and function of basement membrane. J Invest Dermatol 1982; 79:69–72.

35. Bosman FT, Cluetjens J, Beek C, et al: Basement membrane heterogeneity. Histochem J 1989; 21:629–633.

36. Yurchenco PD, Schittny JC: Molecular architecture of basement membranes. FASEB J 1990; 4:1577–1590.

37. Timpl R: Review: Structure and biological activity of basement membrane proteins. Eur J Biochem 1989; 180:487–502.

38. Klagsbrun M: The affinity of fibroblast growth factors (FGFs) for heparin, FGF-heparin sulfate interactions in cells and extracellular matrix. Curr Opin Cell Biol 1990; 2:857–863.

39. Ogawa K, Oguchi M, Nakashima Y, et al: Distribution of collagen type IV in brain tumors: An immunohistochemical study. J Neurooncol 1989; 7:357–366.

40. Enzyme Nomenclature 1991: Recommendations of the Nomenclature Committee of the International Union of Biochemistry and Molecular Biology on the Nomenclature and Classification of Enzymes. New York, Academic Press, 1992.

41. Vaithilingam IS, Stroude EC, McDonald W, et al: General protease and collagenase (IV) activity in C6 astrocytoma cells, C6 spheroids and implanted C6 spheroids. J Neurooncol 1991; 10:203–212.

42. Vaithilingam IS, McDonald W, Stroude EC, et al: Proteolytic activity during the growth of C6 astrocytoma in the murine spheroid implantation model. Can J Neurol Sci 1992; 19:17–22.

43. Vaithilingam IS, McDonald W, Brown NK, et al: Serum proteolytic activity during the growth of C6 astrocytoma. J Neurosurg 1992; 77:595–600.

44. Birkedal-Hansen H, Moore WGI, Bodden MK, et al: Matrix metalloproteinases: A review. Crit Rev Oral Biol Med 1993; 4:197–250.

45. Woessner JF Jr: Matrix metalloproteinases and their inhibitors in connective tissue remodeling. FASEB J 1991; 5:2145–2154.

46. Sato H, Takino T, Okada Y, et al: A matrix metalloproteinase expressed on the surface of invasive tumor cells. Nature 1994; 370:61–65.

47. Huhtala P, Tuuttila A, Chow LT, et al: Complete structure of the human gene for 92 kDa type IV collagenase: Divergent regulation of expression for the 92- and 72-kilodalton enzyme genes in HT-1080 cells. J Biol Chem 1991; 266:16485–16490.

48. Lovejoy B, Cleasby A, Hassell AM, et al: Structure of the catalytic domain of fibroblast collagenase complexed with an inhibitor. Science 1994; 263:375–377.

49. Senior RM, Griffin GL, Fliszar CG, et al: Human 92- and 72-kilodalton type IV collagenases are elastases. J Biol Chem 1991; 266:7870–7875.

50. Murphy G, Ward R, Hembry RM, et al: Characterization of gelatinase from pig polymorphonuclear leucocytes. Biochem J 1989; 258:463–472.

51. Wihelm SM, Collier IE, Marmer BL, et al: SV40 transformed human lung fibroblasts secrete a 92-kDa type collagenase which is identical to that secreted by normal human macrophages. J Biol Chem 1989; 264:17213–17221.

52. Ballin M, Gomez DE, Sinha CC, et al: Ras oncogene mediated induction of a 92 kDa metalloproteinase: Strong correlation with the malignant phenotype. Biochem Biophys Res Commun 1988; 154:832–838.

53. Rao JS, Steck PA, Mohanam S, et al: Elevated levels of M_r 92,000 type IV collagenase in human brain tumors. Cancer Res 1993; 53:2208–2211.

54. Overall CM, Wrana JL, Sodek J: Independent regulation of collagenase, 72-kDa progelatinase and metalloproteinase inhibitor expression in human fibroblasts by transforming growth factor-β. J Biol Chem 1989; 264:1860–1869.

55. Lefebvre V, Peeters-Joris C, Vaes G: Modulation by interleukin-1 and tumor necrosis factor-α of production of collagenase tissue inhibitor of metalloproteinases and collagen types in differentiated and dedifferentiated articular chondrocytes. Biochim Biophys Acta 1990; 1052:366–378.

56. Lefebvre V, Peeters-Joris C, Vaes G: Production of collagens, collagenase and collagenase inhibitor during the dedifferentiation of articular chondrocytes by serial subculture. Biochim Biophys Acta 1990; 1051:266–275.

57. Kalebic T, Garbisa S, Glaser B, et al: Basement membrane collagen: Degradation by migrating endothelial cells. Science 1983; 221:281–283.

58. Costello P, Del Maestro RF: Human cerebral endothelium: Isolation and characterization of cells derived from microvessels of non-neoplastic and malignant glial tissue. J Neurooncol 1990; 8:231–243.

59. Del Maestro RF, Costello PC, Vaithilingam IS, et al: Gelatinase A activity in human glial tumors. Can J Neurol Sci Suppl 1993; 2:542.

60. Huhtala P, Chow LT, Tryggvason K: Structure of the human type IV collagenase gene. J Biol Chem 1990; 265:11077–11082.

61. Stetler-Stevenson WG, Krutzsch HC, Wacher MP, et al: The activation

of human type IV collagenase proenzyme. J Biol Chem 1989; 264:1353–1356.

62. Springman EB, Angleton EL, Birkedahl-Hansen H, et al: Multiple modes of activation of latent human fibroblast collagenase: Evidence for the role of a cys-73 active site zinc complex in latency and a cysteine switch mechanism for activation. Proc Natl Acad Sci USA 1990; 87:364–368.

63. Weiss JB, Brown RA, Kumar S, et al: An angiogenic factor isolated from tumors: A potent low-molecular weight compound. Br J Cancer 1979; 40:493–496.

64. Schor AM, Schor SL, Weiss JB, et al: Stimulation by a low molecular weight angiogenic factor of capillary endothelial cells in culture. Br J Cancer 1980; 41:790–799.

65. Weiss JB, Hill CR, Davis RJ et al: Activation of procollagenase by a low molecular weight angiogenesis factor. Biosci Rep 1983; 3:171–177.

66. Brown RA, Taylor C, McLaughlin B, et al: Epiphyseal growth plate cartilage and chondrocytes in mineralising cultures produce a low molecular mass angiogenic procollagenase activator. Bone Miner 1987; 3:143–158.

67. Taylor CM, Kissun RD, Schor AM, et al: Endothelial cell-stimulating angiogenesis factor in vitreous from extraretinal neovascularizations. Invest Ophthalmol Vis Sci 1989; 30:2174–2178.

68. Taylor CM, McLaughlin B, Weiss JB, et al: Bovine and human pineal glands contain substantial quantities of endothelial cell stimulating angiogenic factor. J Neural Transm 1988; 71:79–84.

69. McLaughlin B, Cawston T, Weiss JB: Activation of the matrix metalloproteinase inhibitor complex by low molecular weight angiogenic factor. Biochim Biophys Acta 1991; 1073:295–298.

70. Taylor CM, Weiss JB, Lye RH: Raised levels of latent collagenase activating angiogenesis factor (ESAF) are present in actively growing human intracranial tumours. Br J Cancer 1991; 64:164–168.

71. Taylor CM, Weiss JB: Raised endothelial cell stimulating angiogenic factor in diabetic retinopathy. Lancet 1989; 2:1329.

72. Del Maestro RF, Vaithilingam IS, McDonald W, et al: Elevated levels of a collagenase IV activating factor in C6 astrocytoma cells. J Cell Biochem Suppl 1994; 18D:142.

73. Silbiger SM, Jacobsen VL, Cupples RL, et al: Cloning of cDNAs encoding human TIMP-3, a novel member of the tissue inhibitor of metalloproteinase family. Gene 1994; 141:293–297.

74. Welgus HG, Stricklin GP, Eisen AZ, et al: A specific inhibitor of vertebrate collagenase produced by human skin fibroblasts. J Biol Chem 1979; 254:1938–1943.

75. DeClerck YA, Yean TD, Ratzkin BJ, et al: Purification and characterization of two related but distinct metalloproteinase inhibitors secreted by bovine aortic endothelial cells. J Biol Chem 1989; 264:17445–17453.

76. Goldberg GI, Marmer BL, Grant GA, et al: Human 72-kilodalton type IV collagenase forms a complex with a tissue inhibitor of metalloproteinases designated TIMP-2. Proc Natl Acad Sci 1989; 86:8207–8211.

77. Stetler-Stevenson WG, Krutzsch HC, Liotta LA: Tissue inhibitor of metalloproteinase (TIMP-2): A new member of the metalloproteinase inhibitor family. J Biol Chem 1989; 264:17374–17378.

78. Boone TC, Johnson MJ, DeClerck YA, et al: cDNA cloning and expression of a metalloproteinase inhibitor related to tissue inhibitor of metalloproteinases. Proc Natl Acad Sci 1990; 87:2800–2804.

79. DeClerck YA, Yean TD, Chan D, et al: Inhibition of tumor invasion of smooth muscle layers by recombinant human metalloproteinase inhibitor. Cancer Res 1991; 51:2151–2157.

80. Khokha R, Waterhouse P, Yagel S: Antisense RNA-induced reduction in murine TIMP levels confers oncogenicity on Swiss 3T3 cells. Science 1989; 243:947–950.

81. Halaka AN, Bunning RAD, Bird CC: Production of collagenase and inhibitor (TIMP) by intracranial tumors and dura in vitro. J Neurosurg 1983; 59:461–466.

82. Paganetti PA, Caroni P, Schwab ME: Glioblastoma infiltration into central nervous system tissue in vitro: Involvement of a metalloprotease. J Cell Biol 1988; 107:2281–2291.

83. Amberger VR, Paganetti PA, Seulberger N, et al: Characterization of a membrane-bound metalloendoprotease of rat C6 glioblastoma cells. Cancer Res 1994; 54:4017–4025.

84. Hanemaaijer R, Koolwijk P, Le Clercq L, et al: Regulation of matrix metalloproteinase expression in human vein and microvascular endothelial cells. Effects of tumor necrosis factor-α, interleukin-1 and phorbol ester. Biochem J 1993; 296:803–809.

85. Arrigo AP, Tanaka K, Goldberg AL, et al: Identity of the 19S ''prosome'' particle with large multifunctional protease complex of mammalian cells (the proteasome). Nature 1988; 331:192–194.

86. Orlowski M: The multicatalytic proteinase complex, a major extralysosomal proteolytic system. Biochem 1990; 29:10289–10297.

87. Goldberg AL, Rock KL: Proteolysis, proteasomes and antigen presentation. Nature 1992; 357:375–379.

88. Tanaka K, Ichihara A: Proteasomes (multicatalytic proteinase complexes) in eukaryocytic cells. Cell Struct Funct 15:127–132.

89. Tanaka K, Tamura T, Yoshimura T, et al: Proteasomes: Protein and gene structures. The New Biologist 1992; 4:173–187.

90. Gray CW, Slaughter CA, De Martino GN: PA28 activator protein forms regulatory caps on proteasome stacked rings. J Mol Biol 1994; 236:7–15.

91. Hough R, Pratt G, Rechsteiner M: Purification of two high molecular weight proteases from rabbit reticulocyte lysates. J Biol Chem 1987; 262:8303–8313.

92. Eytak E, Ganoth D, Armon A, et al: ATP-dependent incorporation of 20S protease into the 26S complex that degrades proteins conjugated to ubiquin. Proc Natl Acad Sci USA 1989; 86:7751–7755.

93. Kanayama HO, Tamura T, Agai S, et al: Demonstration that a human 26S proteolytic complex consists of a proteasome and multiple associated protein components and hydrolyzes ATP and ubiquitin-ligated proteins by closely linked mechanisms. Eur J Biochem 1992; 206:567–578.

94. Ganoth D, Leshinsky E, Eytan E, et al: A multicomponent system that degrades proteins conjugated to ubiquitin: Resolution of factors and evidence for ATP-dependent complex formation. J Biol Chem 1988; 263:12412–12419.

95. De Martino GN, Slaughter CA: Regulatory proteins of the proteasome. J Cell Biochem Suppl 1994; 18D:119.

96. Kumatori A, Tanaka K, Inamura N, et al: Abnormally high expression of proteasomes in human leukemic cells. Proc Natl Acad Sci USA 1990; 87:7071–7078.

97. Kanayama H, Tanaka K, Aki M, et al: Changes in expressions of proteasomes and ubiquitin genes in human renal cancer cells. Cancer Res 1991; 51:6677–6685.

98. Vaithilingam IS, McDonald W, Malott DW, et al: An extracellular proteasome-like structure from C6 astrocytoma cells with serine collagenase IV activity and metallo-dependent activity on alpha-casein and beta-insulin. J Biol Chem 1995; 270:4588–4593.

99. Wada M, Kosaka M, Saito S, et al: Serum concentration and localization in tumor cells of proteasomes in patients with hematologic malignancy and their pathophysiologic significance. J Lab Clin Med 1993; 121:215–223.

100. Takada A, Takada Y: Physiology of plasminogen: With special reference to activation and degradation. Haemostasis 1988; 18(suppl 1):24–35.

101. Testa JE, Quigley JP: The role of urokinase-type plasminogen activator in aggressive tumor cell behaviour. Cancer Metastat Rev 1990; 9:353–367.

102. Pepper MS, Belin D, Montesano R, et al: Transforming growth factor-beta 1 modulates basic fibroblast growth factor-induced proteolytic and angiogenic properties of endothelial cells in vitro. J Cell Biol 1990; III:743–755.

103. Bacharach E, Itin A, Keshet E: In vivo patterns of expression of urokinase and its inhibitor PAI-1 suggest a concerted role in regulating physiological angiogenesis. Proc Natl Acad Sci USA 1992; 89:10686–10690.

104. Del Maestro RF, Lopez-Torres M, McDonald W, et al: The effect of tumor necrosis factor-α on human malignant glial cells. J Neurosurg 1992; 76:652–659.

105. Everts V, Hembrey RM, Reynolds JJ, et al: Metalloproteinases are not involved in the phagocytosis of collagen fibrils by fibroblasts. Matrix 1989; 9:266–276.

106. Sloane BF, Moin K, Krepla E, et al: Cathepsin B and its endogenous inhibitors: The role in tumor malignancy. Cancer Metastases Rev 1990; 9:333–352.

107. Sloane BF, Sameni M, Berguin IM, et al: Cathepsin B and progression of human tumors. J Cel Biochem Suppl 1994; 18D:121.

108. DeClerck YA, Shimada H, Gonzalez-Gomez I, et al: Tumoral invasion in the central nervous system. J Neurooncol 1994; 18:111–121.

109. Folkman J, Klagsbrun M: Angiogenic factors. Science 1987; 235:442–447.

110. Thorgeirsson UP, Lindsay CK, Cottam DW, et al: Tumor invasion, proteolysis, and angiogenesis. J Neurooncol 1994; 18:89–103.
111. Ferrara N, Houk KA, Jakeman LJ, et al: The vascular endothelial growth factor family of polypeptides. J Cellular Biochem 1992; 47:211–218.
112. Shweiki D, Itin A, Soffer D, et al: Vascular endothelial growth factor induced by hypoxia may mediate hypoxia-initated angiogenesis. Nature 1992; 359:843–845.
113. Plate KH, Breier G, Millauer B, et al: Up-regulation of vascular endothelial growth factor and its cognate receptors in a rat glioma model of tumor angiogenesis. Cancer Res 1993; 53:5822–5827.
114. Plate KH, Breier G, Weich HA, et al: Vascular endothelial growth factor is a potential tumor angiogenesis factor in human gliomas in vivo. Nature 1992; 359:845–848.
115. Millauer B, Shawver LK, Plate KH, et al: Glioblastoma growth inhibited in vivo by dominant-negative Flk-1 mutant. Nature 1994; 267:576–579.
116. Goto F, Goto K, Weindel K, et al: Synergistic effects of vascular endothelial growth factor and basic fibroblast growth factor on the proliferation and cord formation of bovine capillary endothelial cells within collagen gels. Lab Invest 1993; 69:508–517.
117. Goldman CK, Kim J, Wong WL, et al: Epidermal growth factor stimulates vascular endothelial growth factor production by human malignant glioma cells: A model of glioblastoma multiforme pathophysiology. Mol Biol Cell 1993; 4:121–133.
118. Kim KJ, Li B, Winder J, et al: Inhibition of vascular growth factor-induced angiogenesis suppresses tumor growth in vivo. Nature 1993; 362:841–844.
119. Sato Y, Okamura K, Morimoto A, et al: Indispensable role of tissue-type plasminogen activator in growth factor-dependent tube formation of human microvascular endothelial cells in vitro. Exp Cell Res 1993; 204:223–229.
120. Lund-Johansen M, Forsberg K, Bjerkvig R, et al: Effects of growth factors on a human glioma cell line during invasion into rat brain aggregates in culture. Acta Neuropathol 1992; 84:190–197.
121. Klagsbrun M: The fibroblast growth factor family: Structural and biological properties. Prog Growth Factor Res 1989; 4:207–235.
122. Stefanik DF, Rizkalla LR, Soi A, et al: Acidic and basic fibroblast growth factors are present in glioblastoma multiforme. Cancer Res 1991; 51:5760–5765.
123. Brem S, Tsanaclis AMC, Gately S, et al: Immunolocalization of basic fibroblast growth factor to the microvasculature of human brain tumors. Cancer 1992; 70:2673–2680.
124. Okumura N, Takimoto K, Okada M, et al: C6 glioma cells produce basic fibroblast growth factor that can stimulate their own proliferation. J Biochem 1989; 106:904–909.
125. Li V, Watanabe H, Yu C, et al: Cerebrospinal fluid from pediatric brain tumor patients contains a mitogen for capillary endothelial cells. Mol Biol Cell 1992; 3:235.
126. Rogel S, Klagsbrun M, Atzmon R, et al: Basic fibroblast growth factor is an extracellular matrix component required for supporting the proliferation of vascular endothelial cells and the differentiation of PC12 cells. J Cell Biol 1989; 109:823–831.
127. Sato N, Beitz JG, Kato J, et al: Platelet-derived growth factor indirectly stimulates angiogenesis in vitro. Am J Pathol 1992; 142:1119–1130.
128. Hermanson M, Funa K, Hartman M, et al: Platelet-derived growth factor and its receptor in human glioma tissue: Expression of messenger RNA and protein suggests the presence of autocrine and paracrine loops. Cancer Res 1992; 52:3213–3219.
129. Plate KH, Breier G, Farrell CL, et al: Platelet-derived growth factor receptor-B is induced during tumor progression in endothelial cells in human gliomas. Lab Invest 1992; 67:529–534.
130. Antonelli-Orlidge A, Saunders KB, Smith SR, et al: An activated form of transforming growth factor beta is produced by co-cultures of endothelial cells and pericytes. Proc Natl Acad Sci USA 1989; 86:4544–4548.
131. Ray Chadhury A, D'Amore PA: Endothelial cell regulation by transforming growth factor-beta. J Cell Biochem 1991; 47:224–229.
132. Pepper MS, Vassalli JD, Orci L, et al: Biphasic effect of transforming growth factor-β on in vitro angiogenesis. Exp Cell Res 1993; 204:356–363.
133. Bodmer S, Strommer K, Frei K, et al: Immunosuppression and transforming growth factor-β in glioblastoma. J Immunol 1992; 143:3222–3229.
134. Reichman HR, Farrell CL, Del Maestro RF: Effects of steroids and nonsteroidal anti-inflammatory agents on vascular permeability in a rat glioma model. J Neurosurg 1986; 65:233–237.
135. Farrell CL, Megyesi J, Del Maestro RF: Effect of ibuprofen on tumor growth in the C6 spheroid implantation glioma model. J Neurosurg 1988; 68:925–930.
136. Dvorak HF: Tumors: Wounds that do not heal: Similarities between tumor stroma generation and wound healing. N Engl J Med 1986; 315:1650–1659.
137. Maxwell M, Naber SP, Wolfe HJ, et al: Expression of angiogenic growth factor genes in primary human astrocytomas may contribute to their growth and progression. Cancer Res 1991; 51:1345–1351.
138. Folkman J, Watson K, Ingber D, et al: Induction of angiogenesis during the transition from hyperplasia to neoplasia. Nature 1989; 339:58–61.
139. Folkman J: What is the evidence that tumors are angiogenesis dependent? J Natl Cancer Inst 1990; 82:4–6.
140. Pepper MS, Ferrara N, Orci L, et al: Vascular endothelial growth factor (VEGF) induces plasminogen activators and plasminogen activator inhibitor-1 in microvascular endothelial cells. Biochem Biophys Res Commun 1991; 181:902–906.
141. Riordan JF, Vallee BL: Human angiogenin, an organogenic protein. Br J Cancer 1988; 57:587–590.
142. Gebicke-Haerter PJ, Bauer J, Benner A, et al: α2-Macroglobulin synthesis in an astrocyte subpopulation. J Neurochem 1987; 49:1139–1145.
143. Keohane ME, Hall SW, Vandenberg SR, et al: Secretion of α2-macroglobulin, α2-antiplasmin and plasminogen activator inhibitor-1 by glioblastoma multiforme in primary organ culture. J Neurosurg 1990; 73:234–241.
144. Farrell CL, Farrel CR, Stewart PA, et al: The functional microcirculation in a glioma model. Int J Radiation Biol 1991; 60:131–137.
145. Stewart PA, Farrell CL, Del Maestro RF: The effect of cellular microenvironment on vessels in the brain: I. Vessel structure in tumor, peritumor and brain from humans with malignant glioma. Int J Radiat Biol 1991; 60:125–130.
146. Groothuis DR, Molnar P, Blasberg RG: Regional blood flow and blood-to-tissue transport in five brain tumor models. Prog Exp Tumor Res 1984; 7:132–153.
147. Hossmann KA, Niebuhr I, Tamura M: Local cerebral blood flow and glucose consumption of rats with experimental gliomas. J Cereb Blood Flow Metab 1982; 2:25–32.
148. Yeung I, Lee TY, Del Maestro RF, et al: Effects of steroids on lopamidol blood-brain transfer constant and plasma volume in brain tumors measured with x-ray computed tomography. J Neurooncol 1994; 18:53–60.
149. Jain RK: Determinants of tumor blood flow: A review. Cancer Res 1988; 48:2641–2658.
150. Jain RK: Vascular and interstitial barriers to delivery of therapeutic agents in tumors. Cancer Metastasis Rev 1990; 9:253–266.
151. Coomber BL, Stewart PA, Hayakawa EM, et al: A quantitative assessment of microvessels ultrastructure in C6 astrocytoma spheroids transplanted to brain and muscle. J Neuropathol Exp Neurol 1988; 47:29–40.
152. Stewart PA, Wiley MJ: Developing nervous tissue induces formation of blood-brain barrier characteristics in invading endothelial cells: A study using quail-chick transplantation chimeras. Dev Biol 1971; 84:183–192.
153. Coomber BD, Stewart PA, Hayakawa K, et al: Quantitative morphology of human glioblastoma multiforme microvessels: Structural basis of blood-brain barrier defect. J Neurooncol 1987; 5:299–307.
154. Stewart PA, Hayakawa K, Hayakawa E, et al: A quantitative study of blood-brain barrier permeability ultrastructure in a new rat glioma model. Acta Neuropathol 1985; 67:96–102.
155. Stewart PA, Hayakawa K, Farrell CL, et al: Quantitative study of microvessel ultrastructure in human peritumoral brain tissue. J Neurosurg 1987; 67:697–705.
156. Inoue HK, Naganuma H, Ono N: Pathobiology of intracranial germ-cell tumors: Immunochemical immunohistochemical and electron microscopic investigations. J Neurooncol 1987; 5:105–115.
157. Allen JC, Nisselbaum J, Epstein F, et al: Alphafetoprotein and human chorionic gonadotropin determination in cerebrospinal fluid: An aid to the diagnosis and management of intracranial germ-cell tumors. J Neurosurg 1979; 51:368–374.

158. Liotta LA: Tumor invasion and metastases: Role of the extracellular matrix. Rhoads Memorial Award Lecture. Cancer Res 1986; 46:1–7.

159. Zacharski LR, Henderson WG, Rickles FR, et al: Effect of sodium warfarin on survival in small cell carcinoma of the lung. J Am Med Assoc 1981; 145:831–835.

160. Chahinian AP, Ware JH, Zimmer B, et al: Update on anti-coagulation with warfarin and on alternationg chemotherapy in extensive small cell carcinoma of the lung. Proc Am Soc Clin Oncol 1985; 4:191.

161. Del Maestro RF, Vaithilingam IS, McDonald W, et al: Influence of Coumadin on C6 tumor growth. Can J Neurol Sci Suppl 1993; 2:544.

162. Yanamoto H, Kikucki H, Okamoto S, et al: Preventive effect of synthetic serine protease inhibitor FUT-175 on cerebral vasospasm in rabbits. Neurosurg 1992; 30:351–357.

163. Ingber D, Fujita T, Kishimoto S, et al: Synthetic analogues of fumagillin that inhibit angiogenesis and suppress tumor growth. Nature 1990; 348:555–557.

TIMOTHY F. CLOUGHESY

KEITH L. BLACK

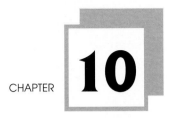

CHAPTER **10**

Peritumoral Edema

DEFINITION

Peritumoral edema (PTE) is defined as an area surrounding a tumor that contains an increase in a plasma ultrafiltrate in the extracellular space. This is due to presence of tumor or tumor growth. Most typically the edema is present immediately surrounding the tumor, but it also can be seen distant to the tumor, seeming to follow white matter tracts (Fig. 10–1). PTE is typically classified as vasogenic, due to the fact that the underlying abnormality is an abnormal blood-tumor barrier accounting for the accumulation of water and protein in the interstitial space.[1] A cytotoxic component may also play a role, as necrosis from ischemia frequently occurs in malignant gliomas, simply as a result of the tumor outgrowing its blood supply.

HISTOLOGY

Microscopic examination shows pallor and abnormal myelin sheaths that are swollen, vacuolated, and bleached. Astrocytes are swollen, and normal-appearing oligodendroglia are present. If persistent, PTE can cause myelin breakdown, leading to formation of cystic spaces in the affected white matter. The gray matter is relatively less affected.[1]

BIOCHEMICAL MAKEUP

The biochemical makeup of PTE has been described in a variety of experimental settings.[2–4] An analysis of electrolyte content in edematous tissue shows an increase in sodium, calcium, and water, with little change in potassium and magnesium, as compared with non-edematous control white matter.[3, 4] Protein content in edematous tissue was also found to be increased in the extracellular space compared with that of control tissue. The amount of protein component in this ultrafiltrate has varied in experimental settings, constituting from 10% to 50% of the plasma protein components.[3, 5] Interestingly, the immunoglobulin-albumin ratio was similar to that found in the serum. The increased water and electrolytes, such as sodium and calcium, are primarily extracellular products, whereas products such as potassium and magne-

sium are primarily intracellular. The ultrafiltrate is consistent in its makeup with extracellular fluid in other systemic organs in the body. These findings help provide clues to the process involved in the transport of the plasma ultrafiltrate. The increase in extracellular ions and water gives credence to a diffusion process that can be due to a leaky blood-brain barrier through an increase in fenestration or a change in the tight junctions. This would limit the content of ultrafiltrate, thus creating a gradient based on molecular weight. Smaller-molecular-weight proteins such as albumin should be seen in higher concentration than immunoglobulins if a diffusion process is employed. But the protein content in PTE has a similar albumin-immunoglobulin ratio to serum; therefore, a bulk flow process such as pinocytosis would be a more likely process.[3]

Metabolic and acid/base changes have also been studied in an animal tumor model.[4] Within the tumor, two metabolic patterns were noted. In regions of high adenosine triphosphate (ATP) content, the pH was alkaline (metabolically active), whereas in regions with low ATP content, the pH was low (energy failure). In this particular tumor model, the two patterns were mixed. In the peritumoral edema region the metabolic findings were more homogeneous: ATP was decreased in conjunction with a relative increase in lactate and a high pH. These findings in the peritumoral edema are thought to be secondary to an increase in the water content of the extracellular space. The pH increases in that setting and lactate is thought to come through bulk flow from the part of the tumor with relative energy failure (increased lactate, decreased ATP, decreased pH). These findings might be useful in the future when using methods such as magnetic resonance (MR) spectroscopy to differentiate tumor from peritumoral edema. Such differentiation is difficult even with present imaging modalities.[6, 7] These findings might be clinically useful in the setting of an infiltrating tumor such as a glioma.

ULTRASTRUCTURAL ANATOMY OF MICROVASCULATURE IN PERITUMORAL EDEMA
Normal Blood-Brain Barrier

Normal blood-brain barrier shows tight junctions between cerebral capillary endothelia that consist of complex folds arranged in such a fashion that the tight junctions are impenetrable to large molecules but are penetrable to smaller molecules. They are without fenestrations, and few pinocytic vesicles are present. A continuous sheath of astrocytic foot processes, little perivascular space, and a high content of mitochondria are also characteristic findings.

Tumor Microvasculature

Tumor microvessels are different than normal microvessels. The endothelial cells are plump with pronounced rough endoplasmic reticulum and free ribosomes. The number of microvilli and pinocytic vesicles is increased. Pinocytosis is a mechanism of transport across vascular endothelial cells.[8] Attenuation of vascular endothelium has been noted and may be responsible for some of the increased permeability. Fenestrated endothelium is seen, but tight junctions are usually not affected.

Peritumoral Microvessels

Most studies have shown no significant changes in the ultrastructural vascular anatomy. One study showed increased pinocytic vesicles located primarily on the luminal side of the endothelial cell. This was thought to be secondary to a resorption process reacting to the increase in extracellular fluid.[8] A higher concentration of pinocytic vesicles can be seen in vessels approximating the tumor.[9]

Summary

PTE seems to be accounted for on the basis of the structural changes in the tumor microvasculature. This creates a functional breakdown of the blood-brain barrier. Important changes in the endothelium include increased pinocytosis, trapping of fluid by long microvillous processes, and attenuation and fenestration of endothelial cells. Changes in tight junctions do not play a role. The content of PTE, a plasma ultrafiltrate, gives credence to the theory that microvascular changes are responsible for the formation of PTE. An understanding of the metabolic makeup of PTE might assist in differentiation of infiltrating tumor from PTE.

BASIC MECHANISMS

Del Maestro and co-workers[10] have conceptualized the basic mechanisms of tumor edema formation as consisting of four dynamic processes: (1) permeability secondary to tumor angiogenesis, (2) permeability due to factors secreted by tumors, (3) immunologic mechanisms, and (4) inflammatory processes. A variety of processes have been implicated as causes of PTE.

Angiogenesis

Angiogenesis is the formation of new capillary blood vessels. Angiogenesis is necessary for continual tumor growth.[11]

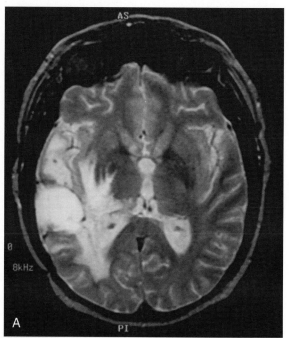
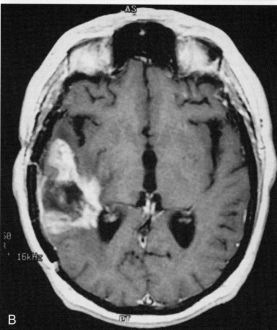

Figure 10–1 Glioblastoma multiforme: MRI T2-weighted axial image (*A*) and T1-weighted axial image with gadolinium enhancement (*B*). *A* demonstrates high-intensity T2 signal area in white matter tracts, distant from the contrast-enhancing lesion, along the extreme external and internal capsule and along the optic radiations. In malignant gliomas, MRI cannot differentiate between the infiltrating tumor and peritumoral edema.

Without angiogenesis, the tumor may be limited to a size of 1 mm.[11] The angiogenic process might be accountable for the ultrastructural changes seen within the tumor vasculature that have been described previously. The angiogenic process is very active in the growing glioblastoma multiforme.[12] Agents that have been studied as angiogenic factors include fibroblast growth factor (FGF), vascular endothelial growth factor (VEGF)/vascular permeability factor (VPF), angiogenin (AGN), tumor necrosis factor-α (TNFA), transforming growth factors-α and -β (TGFA and TGFB), platelet-derived endothelial cell growth factor (PDEGF), platelet-derived growth factor (PDGF), and interleukin-8 (IL-8).

Permeability Factors

VPF is the most well-defined permeability factor; it was identified by concentrating the conditioned medium of guinea pig tumor cells and human histiocytic lymphoma cells.[13] Subsequently it was found in animal glioma cell lines and in human glioblastoma cell lines.[14] When VPF interacts with normal systemic capillaries, it causes a transient hyperpermeability to large proteins. However, VPF has no effect on intact blood-brain barrier, but it does affect the blood-tumor barrier in a fashion similar to its effect on systemic capillaries. The permeability effect on tumor vasculature is of rapid onset, 1 to 5 minutes, and seems to be reversible at 20 to 30 minutes.[15] VPF is a 46-kD dimer of two identical disulfide-linked subunits.[13] VPF messenger RNA (mRNA) is dramatically up-regulated in glioblastoma cells, whereas it is almost absent in normal adult brain.[16] The target site for VPF is the tumor endothelial cell.[17] The VPF receptor was identified as a tyrosine kinase–like receptor. These receptors are in high concentration in the tumor endothelium and are essentially absent in normal brain endothelium.[16] This suggests a paracrine process involving the tumor cell and the tumor endothelium. Studies show the effects of VPF on tumor vasculature to be blocked by dexamethasone; the mechanism of inhibition has not been worked out. VPF also has an effect on angiogenesis and on mitogenesis of the endothelium.[18] VPF may work by creating leaky blood vessels that contribute to a complicated series of events that lead to the formation of the vascular tumor stroma necessary for tumor growth. The increase in extracellular plasma protein provides a favorable substrate for invasion by fibroblasts and blood vessels.[13]

A second tumor permeability factor was also identified in the conditioned medium of animal glioma cell lines and in human gliomas.[19] It has not been as well characterized as VPF. This second factor is a 10-kD molecule that seems to affect both normal and abnormal vessels in brain. It produces a delayed onset of permeability starting at 90 minutes, and it is reversible at 24 hours. Co-incubation with dexamethasone enhances the capillary permeability effect. This factor may trigger the release of lipoxygenase products, such as leukotrienes.[19]

Leukotrienes and Other Mediators of Selective Vascular Permeability

Leukotrienes are biologically active compounds formed from the unsaturated fatty acid arachidonic acid through the 5-lipoxygenase pathway. The conversion of arachidonic acid to leukotrienes is calcium dependent and occurs through the epoxide-intermediated leukotriene A4 (LTA4). Levels of leukotrienes in brain tissue are increased in the setting of postischemic reperfusion,[20] brain tumors,[21] subarachnoid hemorrhage, and concussive brain injury.[22] A positive corre-

lation has been shown between leukotriene C4 (LTC4) levels and brain edema surrounding tumors in humans.[21] Gaetani and others[23] also demonstrated that perilesional brain tissue has significant capacity for an ex vivo synthesis of eicosanoids, and the capacity to synthesize LTC4 correlates significantly with the extent of edema, particularly in cases of neuroepithelial and metastatic tumors. Leukotrienes have also been suggested as biochemical mediators of ischemic brain edema.[24–27] One group hypothesized that macrophages were responsible for the abundance of leukotrienes in brain tumor tissue.[28]

In an earlier study we incorrectly suggested that the intracerebral injection of high doses of leukotrienes in rats increased blood-brain barrier permeability in normal brain.[29, 30] In fact, intracerebral injections of leukotrienes in these studies were not shown to increase permeability in normal brain; however, permeability did increase in the brain tissue immediately under the area where a burr hole had been drilled, suggesting that injury to brain is a prerequisite for leukotrienes to increase permeability.

Subsequently, we have demonstrated that intracarotid infusion of LTC4 selectively increases capillary permeability in tumors and ischemic brain, but not in normal brain.[31, 32] LTC4 also markedly increases vascular permeability in a variety of systemic (non-brain) capillary beds.[33, 34] Normal brain capillaries, unlike systemic capillaries, brain tumor capillaries, or injured brain capillaries, appear to resist the vasoactive increased permeability effects of leukotrienes.

LTC4 is thought to be activated in damaged brain capillary tissue due to the presence of an *enzymatic barrier.* γ-Glutamyl transpeptidase (γGTP) is the enzyme that inactivates LTC4 to leukotriene D4 (LTD4).[35] Both γGTP and dipeptidase, an enzyme that inactivates LTD4 to LTE4, are enzymes that are unique to brain capillaries and that are not present in systemic capillaries.[36] Unlike normal brain capillaries, which are rich in γGTP, tumor capillaries appear to lack γGTP. This knowledge has led us to speculate that normal brain capillaries might use γGTP as an enzymatic barrier to inactivate LTC4 because LTC4 is a potent mediator of vascular permeability in systemic capillaries (capillaries that lack γGTP). Interestingly, LTC4 slightly increased blood-brain barrier permeability in brain adjacent to tumors in which γGTP was also moderately decreased.[31]

It has been demonstrated that inhibitors of 5-lipoxygenase decrease permeability within brain tumors and in brain tissue adjacent to tumors.[37] This suggests that capillary permeability within and adjacent to brain tumors is, at least in part, related to levels of endogenous leukotrienes. After cerebral injury, the leukotriene content is increased.[20, 21] Increased levels of leukotrienes, coupled with increased susceptibility to their vasoactive effects, suggest that leukotrienes might play an important role in vasogenic edema in pathologic lesions.

Unterberg and others have reported that arachidonic acid itself, and not its degeneration products, is responsible for the induction of barrier opening, and they concluded that leukotrienes do not promote brain edema or act as mediators of cerebral edema.[38–42] This conclusion is based mainly on the examination of normal brain tissue in which the enzymatic barrier is intact, protecting brain tissue from the vasoactive effects of leukotrienes. Recently, Unterberg and co-workers[38] also reported that BW755C, a 5-lipoxygenase inhibitor, did not affect brain edema in the cold-induced injury of rabbit brains. Cold-induced injury is a severe form of capillary injury that results in mechanical destruction of brain capillaries. Therefore, cold injury is a poor model to study how biochemical mediators might influence capillary permeability in pathologic conditions such as tumors or ischemia.

Capillary permeability within brain tumors can also be decreased by 5-lipoxygenase inhibitors, suggesting that leukotrienes play a role in the pathogenesis of vasogenic edema surrounding tumors.[37] Recently, an abundance of mRNA for arachidonate 5-lipoxygenase, which is the rate-limiting enzyme in leukotriene synthesis, was determined in a series of human brain tumors.[43] The 5-lipoxygenase transcript is expressed in normal bovine brain and in human brain tumors. The 5-lipoxygenase gene in human brain tumors and in the dimethyl sulfoxide–induced promyelocytic human leukemic HL-60 cells is expressed as a multitranscript family. The abundance of 5-lipoxygenase transcripts, the expression of larger transcripts, and the 5-lipoxygenase/phagocyte–specific oxidase ratio appeared to correlate with tumor malignancy. These findings further support the hypothesis that the 5-lipoxygenase gene product may play a role in human tumor-induced brain edema and provide evidence for tumor-associated expression of high-molecular-weight 5-lipoxygenase transcripts in human brain tumors.

Research is ongoing on the influence of other biologically active compounds released during cerebral insults on barrier permeability. One of the most actively investigated compounds has been arachidonic acid. Chan and others[44] demonstrated that arachidonic acid injected directly into the brain parenchyma increased vascular permeability and resulted in vasogenic edema. Cytotoxic edema was produced when cortical slices were incubated with arachidonic acid.[45] Further, in their studies, arachidonic acid–induced edema could be prevented by pretreatment with dexamethasone but not indomethacin, which is an inhibitor of cyclo-oxygenase.[46] Kontos and colleagues[47] demonstrated structural alterations of the endothelial cells of pial arterioles after superperfusion of the feline cerebral cortex with arachidonic acid. The authors concluded, however, that it was not arachidonic acid itself, but rather it was oxygen-derived free radicals generated from the fatty acid that represented the active principle.

Laboratory investigation has also shown a correlation between tumor plasminogen activator and edema in patients with brain tumors.[48] A role for the kallikrein-kinin system in the formation of brain edema has also been suggested.[49] Interestingly, in addition to the possible direct effects, tumor plasminogen activator is known to activate the kininogen-bradykinin pathway. The brain contains kininogen and kallikrein, the latter of which is the enzyme that converts kininogen to bradykinin. Bradykinin activates phospholipase A2 (PLA2) and releases free arachidonic acid from the membrane phospholipids. Free arachidonic acid released from cell membranes is either reincorporated into membrane phospholipids or oxidized to prostaglandins or leukotrienes. Because intraventricularly infused bradykinin causes brain edema, and because kallikrein- or bradykinin-induced cerebral dilation can be blocked by indomethacin, the possibility exists that tumor plasminogen activator, bradykinin, and arachidonic acid increase blood-brain barrier permeability, at least in part, through their influence on leukotriene formation. It has previously been demonstrated that 5-lipoxygenase inhibitors can decrease arachidonic acid–induced edema.[29] Whether tumor plasminogen activator and bradykinin increase barrier permeability when injected directly into the brain parenchyma and whether tumor plasminogen activator– or bradykinin-induced edema can be decreased by 5-lipoxygenase or PLA2 inhibition remain to be demonstrated.

Intracarotid injection of bradykinin has been shown to transiently increase permeability of the blood-tumor barrier to substances with a variety of molecular weights.[50] It is unclear at this time what mechanism causes this change in permeability and whether it is a significant process in creating peritumoral edema in vivo.

Summary

A variety of molecular biologic processes play a role in the formation of PTE. Although not discussed in this chapter, immunologic and inflammatory processes likely use many of the mediators described herein. No one factor at this time is predominantly responsible for PTE. Future research into the basic mechanisms will provide new clues toward the treatment of PTE and the manipulation of the permeability of the brain tumor vasculature used to aid in the treatment of gliomas.

PERITUMORAL EDEMA FORMATION AND RESOLUTION

Ito and co-workers[51–53] and Reulen and associates[54, 55] have done much work in evaluating patients with regard to the dynamic mechanical aspects of PTE: formation and resolution. This is done by a continuous infusion of intravenous contrast dye and repeated computed tomographic (CT) scans that measure the change in contrast propagation, which allows the dynamic formation of PTE to be shown. These researchers have calculated the formation of the plasma ultrafiltrate from an intracranial tumor to be anywhere from 0.6 to 3.2 mL/hr, 14 to 78 mL in a 24-hour period, or greater.[56] The great variation in the volume of PTE in lesions of similar sizes has led these investigators to consider variations in bulk flow, rather than simple diffusion, to be the predominant source of the plasma filtrate. PTE for the most part maintains a stable volume over several days, although the surrounding brain is confronted with fairly high fluid flow rates. Therefore, mechanisms must be involved in fluid resorption intrinsic to the brain that lead to the equilibration of volume. These resolution mechanisms are thought to include the following: (1) drainage into the CSF, (2) resorption into blood vessels, (3) uptake and phagocytosis of albumin into astrocytes, and (4) removal along perivascular spaces. In the setting of small tumors with PTE and without ventricular contact, the resolution rate of the volume of PTE, an intrinsic property of the tissue, equals the production rate of edema by the tumor. The volume of PTE then becomes a factor of the anatomic placement of the tumor and the intrinsic properties of the surrounding tissue to resorb edema.

A tumor that is located in proximity to the ventricle may have a smaller volume of PTE than a tumor of similar size and ultrafiltrate production that is located at a distance from ventricular structures (Fig. 10–2). Other factors may affect the resorption rate, including increased intracranial pressure, slow venous return, or rheologic parameters.

New techniques offer better methods for examining the effect of drugs on the mechanical aspects of PTE. The same patient can be examined before and after a treatment. The effect of the drug on the production rate, the propagation, the resorption, the total volume, and the extension of the edema can be imaged and measured directly, which can give insight into the mechanism and site of action of a drug.

Using this model, patients have been studied before and after the use of dexamethasone.[51] The primary change noted was a decrease in the formation rate without an effect on resorption. The effect of steroids in this setting is more consistent with a change in vascular permeability as shown in animal models.[57, 58] Not all investigators agree that dexamethasone affects vascular permeability.

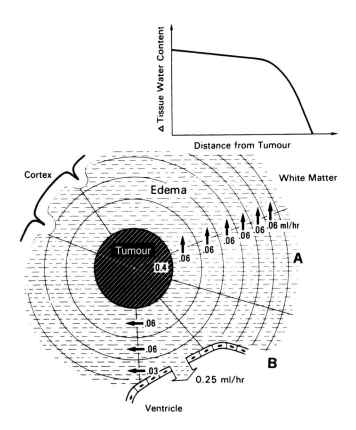

Diameter of Tumour : 36 mm

Production Rate of Edema : 4 ml/hr ≙ 96 ml/day

Figure 10–2 Schematic representation of a spherical model of a brain tumor with extensive peritumoral edema. The spherical model is subdivided in spherical sectors showing the edema extension into the white matter, toward the ventricle, and toward the cortex. In the right upper sector (*A*), the production of edema as well as the edema resorption during tissue passage is demonstrated. In the right lower sector (*B*), the edema resorption during tissue passage and drainage into the ventricular cerebrospinal fluid is shown. (From Reulen HJ, Huber P, Ito U, et al: Peritumoral brain edema. A keynote address. Adv Neurol 1990; 52:307–315.)

BLOOD FLOW AND METABOLIC PARAMETERS

The clinical complications of PTE in brain tumor patients can be devastating. Gaining an understanding of the changes seen in blood flow and metabolic parameters may help to prevent some of these complications.

Hossman and Bloink[59] studied a tumor model in a cat and found a significant decrease in cerebral blood flow in the affected white matter to a level that was 50% of normal. This was explained by a 100% increase in volume of the white matter due to the plasma ultrafiltrate. These researchers showed that the net blood flow per gram of dry tissue had not changed. In the same animal model they also detected no abnormality in autoregulation. They concluded that in the absence of increased intracranial pressure even severe PTE should not cause a clinically significant change in blood flow or flow regulation.[59] Therefore, clinical changes in patients with cerebral edema are likely to be due to increased intracranial pressure with resultant ischemia and possible cytotoxic edema.

Another animal model showed the area of brain with PTE to have a decrease in both local cerebral blood flow and local cerebral glucose utilization. This was reversed with the use of methylprednisolone.[57]

Metabolic and hemodynamic aspects of peritumoral low-density areas on CT scan were evaluated in humans with brain tumors using positron emission tomography to measure regional cerebral blood flow, oxygen utilization, and glucose utilization.[60] Three different tumor types were studied: meningiomas, gliomas, and metastatic tumors. The PTE in the meningioma group showed no changes. However, in the setting of significant mass effect, cerebral blood flow changes were marked. This should be considered to be pure PTE, as the tumor and PTE are clearly demarcated. This is less clear when studying patients with malignant gliomas. Patients showed a decrease in oxygen extraction fraction and regional metabolism rate of oxygen regardless of the mass effect. When mass effect was significant, cerebral blood flow and regional glucose metabolism rate dropped off, such as is seen in the setting of meningiomas with mass effect. An explanation for the differences includes a consideration of a second type of process, such as cytotoxic edema of the low-density area in malignant glioma. However, these metabolic findings may be a reflection of the infiltrating tumor itself rather than of true PTE. Studies have shown similar metabolic changes in glioma tumors that can resemble low-density areas on CT scans.[60]

Summary

It is unclear if PTE without significant increases in intracranial pressure can cause clinically significant changes. In glioma patients, the true clinical effect of PTE is blurred by the fact that modern imaging studies are unable to differentiate between PTE, cytotoxic edema, and infiltrating tumor. Therefore, studies of metabolic factors and blood flow changes in areas defined by modern imaging are difficult to interpret.

TREATMENTS

Corticosteroids

Corticosteroid effect on brain tumors and peritumoral edema has been postulated to consist of multiple mechanisms including (1) vascular permeability, (2) cytotoxic effect, (3) decreased rate of tumor formation, and (4) decreased CSF formation. The clinical and imaging impact has been noted.[61–64] One study showed a mean reduction of edema volume of 31% and tumor volume of 15% when using methylprednisolone in a variety of tumor types.[63] Others found no significant changes in tumor size in malignant gliomas.[62] Typically, a favorable response was usually detected within 24 to 48 hours, with the maximum response occurring by 1 week. A recent study of patients with clinically significant PTE showed that 4 mg of dexamethasone was as effective as 8 or 16 mg in divided daily doses, and it produced fewer side effects according to Karnofsky performance status.[65] The corticosteroid-associated side effects increase in number after more than 3 weeks of drug use. After a therapeutic response is obtained, corticosteroids should be tapered to the lowest effective dose to avoid such adverse effects as steroid diabetes, gastrointestinal hemorrhage, proximal myopathy, or psychiatric disturbances.

A typical starting dose of dexamethasone is 16 mg/day in divided doses. If a good response is seen within 48 hours, that dosage should be continued until any alarming neurologic signs disappear. Then the dosage should be tapered to the lowest possible effective dose. If no significant response is seen, efficacy can be attained by doubling the dose and redoubling it every 48 hours up to a dose of 100 mg/day. Responses can be seen at these higher levels.

Osmotic Dehydration

Mannitol is thought to have three possible mechanisms of action: (1) osmotic effect, (2) rheologic effects, and (3) diuretic effect. The osmotic effect pulls free water out of the extracellular space and into the vasculature, thus decreasing PTE. The rheologic effects allow for increased blood cell deformity and better O_2 delivery to tissue as well as for dilution of hemoglobin and fibrinogen, which lowers the viscosity of blood. This allows for less total cerebral blood volume, yet still meets the nutritional needs of the brain. Less blood volume lowers intracranial pressure. Mannitol is also a diuretic that will cause an eventual negative fluid balance and dehydration of the brain if urine fluid loss is not replenished. Mannitol can also have a "rebound" effect. In brain tumors the blood-brain barrier is not intact in certain regions. Over time, mannitol can accumulate in the extracellular space, causing an osmotic gradient that draws water into the extracellular space. A second possible cause of rebound may be related to dehydration and lowering of systemic blood pressure, which in turn may critically lower cerebral perfusion pressure. This leads to vasodilation, which increases the blood volume in the intracranial cavity and increases intracranial pressure.[66] In general, mannitol should not be considered as a form of definitive treatment of peritumoral brain edema, but it is very readily effective in patients

with critically elevated intracranial pressure and should be instituted while other measures are ongoing to lower intracranial pressure and mass effect. A typical dose of mannitol is 0.25 to 1.0 g/kg every 6 to 12 hours. The goals for osmolality are 310 to 320 mOsm and two-thirds of the diuresed volume should be replaced.

Diuretics

Diuretics such as furosemide have also been used as an adjunct to the treatment of PTE. Furosemide has an additive effect with dexamethasone, which has been shown by measuring water content with CT imaging.[67] Its main mechanism of action in lowering intracranial pressure is most likely secondary to its dehydration effects. In addition, a decrease in CSF production rate could lead to an increased clearance of the interstitial fluid toward the ventricle or other CSF spaces. Acetazolamide can be considered effective by a similar mechanism. Acetazolamide is not traditionally used in the setting of PTE. A typical dose of furosemide is 10 to 20 mg every 6 to 12 hours.

PTE is successfully treated with corticosteroids; however, the side effects are at times intolerable. These side effects have led to an attempt to find other agents that might be as effective in the definitive treatment of PTE.

Nonsteroidal Anti-inflammatory Drugs

Investigators have evaluated the efficacy of nonsteroidal anti-inflammatory drugs (NSAIDs) in the treatment of PTE in terms of their effect on the mediators of inflammation. These agents primarily act as inhibitors of prostaglandin formation through the cyclo-oxygenase pathway. Ibuprofen and indomethacin significantly decrease extravasation of protein in a rat glioma tumor model.[68] Other investigators found no effect of NSAIDs in a similar model.[69] At this time, NSAIDs are not commonly used as treatment for PTE. Blocking the breakdown of arachidonic acid to leukotrienes might be more effective in the treatment of PTE. Animal models have shown the efficacy of a 5-lipoxygenase inhibitor as treatment for PTE.[37]

Lipid Peroxidation Inhibitors

21-Aminosteroids are potent lipid peroxidation inhibitors that have been evaluated in animal models for peritumoral edema.[70, 71] One study showed no effect of these agents,[71] whereas another showed an improvement in neurologic dysfunction when compared with controls.[70] Although no change was evident in tumor vascular permeability, a significant change in tumor size and neurologic dysfunction was noted in the animal model.[70] The mechanism of effect on intracerebral tumors is unknown, and no human studies have been reported to date. These agents have no glucocorticoid effect and could therefore have a significant benefit if they are found to be effective in humans with cerebral PTE.

Summary

Traditional measures for treatment of critically increased intracranial pressure should always be employed. Presently, corticosteroids provide for the majority of the symptomatic treatment of PTE. The development of other agents to treat PTE will help to decrease much of the morbidity associated with the present approaches.

CLINICAL CONDITIONS OF CONCERN IN PATIENTS WITH PTE

Fluid and Electrolyte Balance

Fluid balance is important in patients with PTE. Overhydration can lead to an increase in interstitial fluid accumulation, especially in the setting of hypo-osmolality (e.g., hyponatremia). Identification of the cause of hyponatremia is vital, and appropriate correction will help to prevent clinical deterioration. Hydration during chemotherapy treatment can accentuate PTE, causing clinical deterioration.

Hypertension

Hypertension can also exacerbate PTE. An increase in blood pressure increases the hydrostatic pressure in the capillary bed, especially when the pressures are above the upper limits of autoregulation. This can lead to an increase in the formation rate of PTE through the blood-tumor barrier capillary bed. Clinicians must always keep in mind that adequate cerebral perfusion pressure is imperative to prevention of ischemia in the setting of increased intracranial pressure, but excessive hypertension can cause clinical deterioration.

Seizures

Patients with significant PTE and increased intracranial pressure can show local changes in cerebral blood flow. Seizures create a tremendous metabolic need, which results in increased blood flow. This can increase intracranial pressure from baseline and might cause ischemia, which is manifested as a prolonged or permanent neurologic deficit that might be pathophysiologically different from the short-lived (24 to 48 hours) Todd's phenomenon that occurs in partial epilepsies. Adequate control of seizures is imperative in patients with PTE and increased intracranial pressure.

CONCLUSION

Clearly defining the effect of PTE in patients with malignant gliomas is difficult due to the infiltrating nature of the tumor and the possibility of confounding cytotoxic edema. However, PTE still seems to play an important role in the clinical setting by contributing to many of the symptoms, morbidity, and, at times, mortality of these patients. It is hoped that defining the basic mechanisms will help in development of treatments to lessen the associated clinical problems. In addition, an understanding of the basic mechanisms has led to defining new approaches to the treatment of malignant glioma. Investigators have developed anti-angiogenesis agents as treatment for these tumors. We are attempting to exploit the mediators of vascular permeability to improve delivery of a variety of agents to the tumor.

REFERENCES

1. Klatzo I: Neuropathological aspects of brain edema. J Neuropathol Exp Neurol 1967; 26:1–11.
2. Hwang WZ, Ito H, Hasegawa T, et al: Peritumoral oedema and lipid content. Acta Neurochir 1986; 80:128–130.
3. Hossmann KA, Seo K, Szymas J, et al: Quantitative analysis of experimental peritumoral edema in cats. Adv Neurol 1990; 52:449–458.
4. Okada Y, Kloiber O, Hossmann KA: Regional metabolism in experimental brain tumors in cats: Relationship with acid/base, water, and electrolyte homeostasis. J Neurosurg 1992; 77:917–926.
5. Bothe HW, Bodsch W, Hossmann KA: Relationship between specific gravity, water content and serum protein extravasation in various types of vasogenic brain edema. Acta Neuropathol 1984; 64:37–42.
6. Burger PC, Dubois PJ, Schold SJ, et al: Computerized tomographic and pathologic studies of the untreated, quiescent, and recurrent glioblastoma multiforme. J Neurosurg 1983; 58:159–169.
7. Daumas DC, Monsaingeon V, Blond S, et al: Serial stereotactic biopsies and CT scan in gliomas: Correlative study in 100 astrocytomas, oligo-astrocytomas and oligodendrocytomas. J Neurooncol 1987; 4:317–328.
8. Roy S, Sarkar C: Ultrastructural study of micro-blood vessels in human brain tumors and peritumoral tissue. J Neurooncol 1989; 7:283–292.
9. Petito CK, Schaefer JA, Plum F: Ultrastructural characteristics of the brain and blood-brain barrier in experimental seizures. Brain Res 1977; 127:251–267.
10. Del Maestro RF, Megyesi JF, Farrell CL: Mechanisms of tumor-associated edema: a review. Can J Neurol Sci 1990; 17:177–183.
11. Garretson HD, Shields CB: Angiogenesis in glioblastoma multiforme. Surg Forum 1979; 30:440–441.
12. Brem SS, Cotran RS, Folkman MJ: Angiogenesis in brain tumors: A quantitative histologic study. Surg Forum 1974; 25:462–464.
13. Klasburn M, Soker S: VEGF/VPF: The angiogenesis factor found? Curr Biol 1993; 3:699–702.
14. Bruce JN, Criscuolo GR, Merrill MJ, et al: Vascular permeability induced by protein product of malignant brain tumors: Inhibition by dexamethasone. J Neurosurg 1987; 67:880–884.
15. Criscuolo GR, Merrill MJ, Oldfield EH: Further characterization of malignant glioma-derived vascular permeability factor. J Neurosurg 1988; 69:254–262.
16. Plate KH, Breier G, Weich HA, et al: Vascular endothelial growth factor is a potential tumour angiogenesis factor in human gliomas in vivo. Nature 1992; 359:845–848.
17. Vaisman N, Gospodarowicz D, Neufeld G: Characterization of the receptors for vascular endothelial growth factor. J Biol Chem 1990; 265:19461–19466.
18. Connolly DT, Heuvelman DM, Nelson R, et al: Tumor vascular permeability factor stimulates endothelial cell growth and angiogenesis. J Clin Invest 1989; 84:1470–1478.
19. Ohnishi T, Sher PB, Posner JB, et al: Capillary permeability factor secreted by malignant brain tumor: Role in peritumoral brain edema and possible mechanism for anti-edema effect of glucocorticoids. J Neurosurg 1990; 72:245–251.
20. Moskowitz MA, Kiwak KJ, Hekimian K, et al: Synthesis of compounds with properties of leukotrienes C4 and D4 in gerbil brains after ischemia and reperfusion. Science 1984; 224:886–889.
21. Black KL, Hoff JT, McGillicuddy JE, et al: Increased leukotriene C4 and vasogenic edema surrounding brain tumors in humans. Ann Neurol 1986; 19:592–595.
22. Kiwak KJ, Moskowitz MA, Levine L: Leukotriene production in gerbil brain after ischemic insult, subarachnoid hemorrhage, and concussive injury. J Neurosurg 1985; 62:865–869.
23. Gaetani P, Rodriguez Y, Baena R, et al: "Ex vivo" release of eicosa-

noid from human brain tissue: Its relevance in the development of brain edema. Neurosurgery 1991; 28:853–857.

24. Asano T, Shigeno T, Johshita H, et al: A novel concept on the pathogenetic mechanism underlying ischaemic brain oedema: relevance of free radicals and eicosanoids. Acta Neurochir Suppl 1987; 41:85–96.

25. Dempsey RJ, Roy MW, Cowen DE, et al: Lipoxygenase metabolites of arachidonic acid and the development of ischaemic cerebral oedema. Neurol Res 1986; 8:53–56.

26. Dempsey RJ, Combs DJ, Maley ME, et al: Moderate hypothermia reduces postischemic edema development and leukotriene production. Neurosurgery 1987; 21:177–181.

27. Minamisawa H, Terashi A, Katayama Y, et al: Brain eicosanoid levels in spontaneously hypertensive rats after ischemia with reperfusion: Leukotriene C4 as a possible cause of cerebral edema. Stroke 1988; 19:372–377.

28. Shinonaga M, Chang CC, Kuwabara T: Relation between macrophage infiltrates and peritumoral edema. Adv Neurol 1990; 52:475–481.

29. Black KL, Hoff JT: Leukotrienes increase blood-brain barrier permeability following intraparenchymal injections in rats. Ann Neurol 1985; 18:349–351.

30. Black KL, Hoff JT: Leukotrienes and blood-brain barrier permeability. J Cereb Blood Flow Metab 1985; 5:S263–S264.

31. Black KL, King WA, Ikezaki K: Selective opening of the blood-tumor barrier by intracarotid infusion of leukotriene C4. J Neurosurg 1990; 72:912–916.

32. Baba T, Black KL, Ikezaki K, et al: Intracarotid infusion of leukotriene C4 selectively increases blood-brain barrier permeability after focal ischemia in rats. J Cereb Blood Flow Metab 1991; 11:638–643.

33. Samuelsson B: Leukotrienes: Mediators of immediate hypersensitivity reactions and inflammation. Science 1983; 220:568–575.

34. Ueno A, Tanaka K, Katori M, et al: Species difference in increased vascular permeability by synthetic leukotriene C4 and D4. Prostaglandins 1981; 21:637–648.

35. Aharony D, Dobson P: Discriminative effect of γ-glutamyl transpeptidase inhibitors on metabolism of leukotriene C4 in peritoneal cells. Life Sci 1984; 35:2135–2142.

36. DeBault LE: γ-Glutamyltranspeptidase induction mediated by glial foot process-to endothelium contact in co-culture. Brain Res 1981; 220:432–435.

37. Baba T, Chio CC, Black KL: The effect of 5-lipoxygenase inhibition on blood-brain barrier permeability in experimental brain tumors. J Neurosurg 1992; 77:403–406.

38. Unterberg A, Wahl M, Hammersen F, et al: Permeability and vasomotor response of cerebral vessels during exposure to arachidonic acid. Acta Neuropathol 1987; 73:209–219.

39. Unterberg A, Schmidt W, Polk T, et al: Evidence against leukotrienes as mediators of brain edema. J Cereb Blood Flow Metab 1987; 7:S625.

40. Unterberg A, Schmidt W, Wahl M, et al: Evidence against leukotrienes as mediators of brain edema. J Neurosurg 1991; 74:773–780.

41. Wahl M, Unterberg A, Baethmann A: The effects of free radicals and leukotrienes on blood-brain barrier function. Int J Microcirc Clin Exp 1986; 5:93.

42. Wahl M, Unterberg A, Baethmann A, et al: Mediators of blood-brain barrier dysfunction and formation of vasogenic brain edema. J Cereb Blood Flow Metab 1988; 8:621–634.

43. Boado RJ, Pardridge WM, Vinters HV, et al: Differential expression of 5-lipoxygenase (5-LO) transcripts in human brain tumors. Proc Natl Acad Sci USA 1992; 89:9044–9048.

44. Chan PH, Fishman RA, Caronna J, et al: Induction of brain edema following intracerebral injection of arachidonic acid. Ann Neurol 1983; 13:625–632.

45. Chan PH, Fishman RA: Brain edema: Induction in cortical slices by polyunsaturated fatty acids. Science 1978; 201:358–360.

46. Chan PH, Fishman RA: The role of arachidonic acid in vasogenic brain edema. Fed Proc 1984; 43:210–213.

47. Kontos HA, Wei EP, Povlishoch JT, et al: Cerebral arteriolar damage by arachidonic acid and prostaglandin G_2. Science 1980; 209:1242–1245.

48. Quindlen EA, Bucher AP: Correlation of tumor plasminogen activator with peritumoral cerebral edema: A CT and biochemical study. J Neurosurg 1987; 66:729–733.

49. Unterberg A, Baethmann AJ: The kallikrein-kinin system as mediator in vasogenic brain edema: 1. Cerebral exposure to bradykinin and plasma. J Neurosurg 1984; 61:87–96.

50. Inamura T, Black KL: Bradykinin selectively opens blood-brain barrier in tumors. J Cereb Blood Flow Metab 1994; 14:862–870.

51. Ito U, Tomita H, Tone O, et al: Formation and resolution of white matter oedema in various types of brain tumours. Acta Neurochir Suppl 1990; 51:149–151.

52. Ito U, Reulen HJ, Tomita H, et al: A computed tomography study on formation, propagation, and resolution of edema fluid in metastatic brain tumors. Adv Neurol 1990; 52:459–468.

53. Ito U, Reulen HJ, Tomita H, et al: Formation and propagation of brain oedema fluid around human brain metastases: A CT study. Acta Neurochir 1988; 90:35–41.

54. Reulen HJ, Graber S, Huber P, et al: Factors affecting the extension of peritumoural brain oedema: A CT study. Acta Neurochir 1988; 95:19–24.

55. Reulen HJ, Huber P, Ito U, et al: Peritumoral brain edema: A keynote address. Adv Neurol 1990; 52:307–315.

56. Aaslid R, Groger U, Patlak CS, et al: Fluid flow rates in human peritumoural oedema. Acta Neurochir Suppl 1990; 51:152–154.

57. Yamada K, Ushio Y, Hayakawa T, et al: Effects of methylprednisolone on peritumoral brain edema: A quantitative autoradiographic study. J Neurosurg 1983; 59:612–619.

58. Shapiro WR, Posner JB: Corticosteroid hormones: Effects in an experimental brain tumor. Arch Neurol 1974; 30:217.

59. Hossman KA, Bloink M: Blood flow and regulation of blood flow in experimental peritumoral edema. J Comput Assist Tomogr 1982; 6:586–592.

60. Hino A, Imahori Y, Tenjin H, et al: Metabolic and hemodynamic aspects of peritumoral low-density areas in human brain tumor. Neurosurgery 1990; 26:615–621.

61. Galicich JM, French LA, Melby JC: Use of dexamethasone in the treatment of cerebral edema associated with brain tumors. Lancet 1961; 81:46–53.

62. Hatam A, Yu ZY, Bergstrom M, et al: Effect of dexamethasone treatment on peritumoral brain edema: Evaluation by computed tomography. Acta Neuropathol 1983; 60:223–231.

63. Leiguarda R, Sierra J, Pardal C, et al: Effect of large doses of methylprednisolone on supratentorial intracranial tumors: A clinical and CAT scan evaluation. Eur Neurol 1985; 24:23–32.

64. Andersen C, Haselgrove JC, Doenstrup S, et al: Resorption of peritumoural oedema in cerebral gliomas during dexamethasone treatment evaluated by NMR relaxation time imaging. Acta Neurochir 1993; 122:218–224.

65. Vecht CJ, Hovestadt A, Verbiest HBC: Dose-effect relationship of dexamethasone on Karnofsky performance in metastatic brain tumors: A randomized study of doses of 4, 8, and 16 mg per day. Neurology 1994; 44:675–680.

66. Muizelaar JP, Wei EP, Kontos HA, et al: Mannitol causes compensatory cerebral vasoconstriction and vasodilation in response to blood viscosity changes. J Neurosurg 1983; 59:822–828.

67. Meinig G, Reulen HJ, Simon RS, et al: Clinical, chemical, and CT evaluation of short-term and long-term antiedema therapy with dexamethasone and diuretics. No Shinkei Geka 1980; 8:935–940.

68. Reichman HR, Farrell CL, Del Maestro RF: Effects of steroids and nonsteroid anti-inflammatory agents on vascular permeability in a rat glioma model. J Neurosurg 1986; 65:233–237.

69. Weissman DE, Stewart C: Experimental drug therapy of peritumoral brain edema. J Neurooncol 1988; 6:339–342.

70. King WA, Black KL, Ikezaki K, et al: Novel 21-aminosteroids prevent tumor associated neurological dysfunction. Acta Neurochir 1990; 51:160–162.

71. Megyesi JF, Farrell CL, Del Maestro RF: Investigation of an inhibitor of lipid peroxidation U74006F on tumor growth and protein extravasation in the C6 astrocytoma spheroid implantation glioma model. J Neurooncol 1990; 8:133–137.

HERBERT H. ENGELHARD

DENNIS G. GROOTHUIS

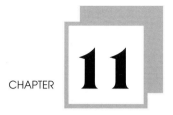

CHAPTER **11**

The Blood-Brain Barrier: Structure, Function, and Response to Neoplasia

The normal blood-brain barrier allows for the maintenance of a protected environment for the unhampered function of the central nervous system (CNS).[1] Normal serum concentrations of many molecules and ions, such as glutamate, glycine, and potassium, are toxic to the brain.[2] Thus, a "barrier" between the bloodstream and the CNS must exist, and is in fact present in the brains of all vertebrates.[3]

The blood-brain barrier has principally been described with anatomic methods (using vital dyes and light microscopy or horseradish peroxidase and electron microscopy) or physiologic models (by tracer methods, which give an estimation of kinetic transport parameters).[3] Anatomically, the blood-brain barrier is composed of a continuous sheet of endothelium that covers the luminal surface of more than 99% of the brain capillaries.[1, 3] It might more accurately be described as the *brain capillary endothelial barrier*. The combined length of capillaries in the human brain is 650 km[3], with the surface area of the human blood-brain barrier being approximately 12 m[2]/g of brain tissue.[4] By way of comparison, the surface area available for exchange at the blood-CSF barrier is 1/5000th that of the blood-brain barrier.[5] Yet, the microvascular endothelial cellular volume is only 0.8 μL/g of brain.[3]

The permeability of the blood-brain barrier has been determined using inert tracers that are not taken up by brain endothelial cell receptors or carrier systems.[2] During development, brain capillaries begin as "leaky" membranes, but they gradually "tighten" and become impermeable.[2] Molecules as small as urea (MW = 60.06) are barred from entry into the brain,[3] a process that has been described as *passive exchange control*. Small, nonpolar, lipid-soluble molecules, such as oxygen, carbon dioxide, and anesthetics, readily cross the blood-brain barrier. The rate of entry of these small molecules parallels their lipophilicity as measured by their oil-water partition coefficients. Ethanol, nicotine, and diazepam are examples of molecules that have high oil-water partition coefficients. Lymphocytes are also known to be transported through the blood-brain barrier.[3]

The first part of this chapter deals with the normal blood-brain barrier, including historical concepts, morphology, function (including transport systems), and cellular interactions. The second part deals with the response of the blood-brain barrier to neoplasia (specifically gliomas), and discusses the effect of neoplasia on blood-brain barrier morphology, vasogenic edema, and results of studies of factors secreted by gliomas that influence the blood-brain barrier. How the blood-brain barrier affects drug delivery and therapeutic methods for "cracking" the barrier are discussed in Chapter 48.

THE NORMAL BLOOD-BRAIN BARRIER

History

The existence of an apparent blood-brain barrier was discovered by Paul Ehrlich in 1885 when he noted that acidic vital dyes injected into the bloodstream of rabbits stained almost every organ except the brain and spinal cord.[3] The concept of the blood-brain barrier continued to develop over the ensuing decades, with contributions being made by numerous investigators including Goldman, Spatz, Walter, Krogh, and Crone.[3, 6] Spatz and Walter, in the early 1930s, suggested the additional existence of a blood-CSF barrier at the endothelial and epithelial lining of the choroid plexus and a brain-CSF barrier at the ependyma.[6] Krogh (1946) focused attention on the active transport processes of the blood-brain barrier.[6] In the 1950s, it was generally believed that glial sheets surrounded the entire surface of the brain capillaries and were instrumental in exerting the barrier function.[6]

In the late 1960s, Reese and Karnofsky[7] and then Brightman and Reese[8] performed a series of experiments in rats using intravenous (IV) injection of the electron-dense marker horseradish peroxidase. Extravasation of this marker was found by electron microscopy to be limited by the cerebrovascular endothelial cells. They concluded that these cells constitute the principal anatomic basis of the blood-brain barrier. The brain capillary endothelium was found to be continuous, with high-resistance tight junctions. A structural basis for the permeability characteristics of the blood-brain barrier was therefore identified.[3, 6] Currently, the blood-brain barrier is envisioned as being a dynamic rather than a rigid barrier. Much of the more recent research focuses on further elucidation of receptor-mediated transport mechanisms,[6] hormonal influences, and regional variability in blood-brain barrier permeability.[9]

Ultrastructure of the Blood-Brain Barrier

Endothelial cells lining blood vessels throughout the body share properties including the production of von Willebrand factor (factor VIII), a nonthrombogenic luminal surface, and an abluminal basement membrane.[2] With respect to their morphology, vascular endothelial cells may be divided into three groups: continuous, fenestrated, or discontinuous.[2] Peripheral endothelial microvessels have fenestrations with a diameter of approximately 50 nm between cells.[6] Within the brain, the endothelial cells have no fenestrations and are continuous, with "epithelial-like" high-resistance tight junctions (zonulae occludentes).[3, 10] Freeze fracture studies show that these "complex" tight junctions are composed of 6 to 8 junctional strands and are pentalaminar in structure.[3, 10]

The high electrical resistance (up to 2000 Ω/cm^2) of the CNS capillary tight junctions distinguishes them from simple tight junctions.[2] CNS tight junctions restrict paracellular diffusion of ions, block movement of proteins, and limit transfer of hydrophilic substances across the capillary wall.[1] Ultrastructural studies of the CNS capillary endothelial cells also show that they contain a very small number of pinocytotic vesicles.[1, 2] The vesicles that are present are not involved in transport functions.[10] CNS capillary endothelial cells contain many mitochondia,[6] indicating the great energy requirements for maintaining the blood-brain barrier. These unique features of the brain capillary endothelial cells are summarized in Table 11–1. The blood-brain barrier has *polarity,* that is, anatomically and functionally, the sides of the brain capillary endothelial cells (luminal vs. abluminal, or toward the brain) are different. An endothelial basement membrane, the basal lamina, abuts the capillary endothelial cells and encloses the pericytes. Abutting the other surface of the basal lamina is the neuropil of the surrounding brain.[10] The perivascular space within the CNS is small and has no collagen and fibroblasts.[10] Ultrastructural studies have shown that the foot processes of astrocytes cover more than 95% of the brain microvascular endothelium, and are therefore interposed between capillaries and the vast majority of CNS neurons.[3, 10] Morphologic differences between peripheral and CNS capillaries are illustrated in Figure 11–1.

In certain areas of the brain (less than 1%), the capillary

TABLE 11–1
UNIQUE FEATURES OF BRAIN CAPILLARIES

Lack of fenestrations
Tight (high-resistance) intercellular junctions
Paucity of pinocytotic vesicles
Abundant mitochondria

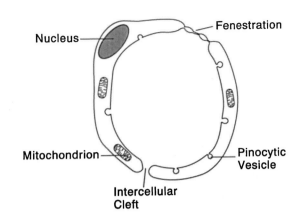

A   **Peripheral Capillary**

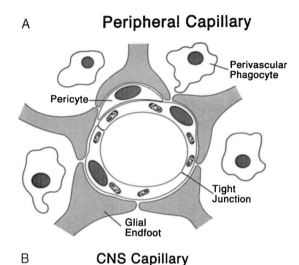

B   **CNS Capillary**

Figure 11–1 Differences in morphology between peripheral *(A)* and CNS *(B)* capillaries. Non-CNS endothelial cells contain pinocytic vesicles and intercellular clefts and fenestrations. CNS endothelial cells have abundant mitochondria and tight junctions. This continuous sheet of capillary endothelium constitutes the morphologic basis for the blood-brain barrier. In addition, the CNS capillary endothelium is covered (95%) by glial foot processes and surrounded by the basal lamina and perivascular phagocytes (including pericytes, microglial cells, and macrophages).

endothelial cells do not have tight junctions but are fenestrated, thereby permitting freer exchange of small molecules. These areas, which are considered gaps in the blood-brain barrier, include (in addition to the choroid plexus) the circumventricular organs (i.e., the pituitary and pineal glands, median eminence, area postrema, subfornical organ, and organum vasculosum of lamina terminalis).[2, 3] Substances that do not readily cross the blood-brain barrier may reach the CNS by means of extravasation at these sites. The blood-CSF barrier of the choroid plexus is represented by fenestrated endothelial cells and by the epithelial cells of the choroid plexus, which have apical tight junctions only.[3]

Functions of the Blood-Brain Barrier

The blood-brain barrier has three major functions: (1) restriction of the free exchange of nutrients and water-soluble substances between the blood and the CNS[1]; (2) selective transport of specific molecules across the cerebral capillary endothelium by means of specialized transport systems[2]; and (3) modification/metabolism of bloodborne and/or brainborne substances.[2]

As mentioned previously, the existence of a physiologic barrier (restriction function) protects the brain from neurotoxic substances in the blood, such as glutamate and glycine (which are neurotransmitters with extracellular levels in the CNS that are 1/1000th those in the blood), and from high potassium levels.[2] Bloodborne proteins enter cerebral endothelial cells rapidly through several mechanisms including bulk phase, adsorptive, and receptor-mediated endocytosis; however, lysosomes within the endothelium degrade the proteins before they can enter the interstitial space of the brain.[11] As a result, the protein in CSF is only 0.4% that in serum. Specific carrier systems that are present in the brain endothelial cells allow control over the exchange of substances between blood and nervous system.[2] This *transport function* is discussed in more detail later. The fact that the brain capillary endothelial cells contain abundant mitochondia has been used to argue that the blood-brain barrier, in addition to its physical barrier properties, may also function as a metabolic barrier (metabolic function).[6]

The concept of special CNS transport systems was first championed by Krogh.[6] The CNS requires many hydrophilic molecules to function; yet the blood-brain barrier limits their transfer across the capillary wall. Transportation of essential hydrophilic substances, including most metabolic substrates and inorganic ions, is therefore performed by carrier-mediated, energy-dependent transport systems.[1, 11] Many CNS transport systems have now been identified, including those for the glucose transporter (glut-1 isoform) and hexoses; monocarboxy acids; amino acids and amines, nucleosides, and purines; insulin; transferrin; and possibly cholesterol (Table 11–2). Other systems transport molecules in the opposite direction, into the bloodstream. An example would be the p-glycoprotein (multidrug resistance) efflux pump.[6] Fig-

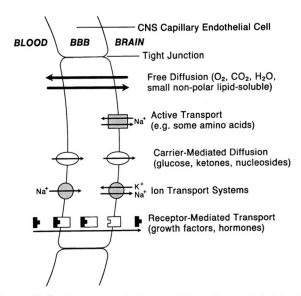

Figure 11-2 Transport mechanisms in CNS capillary endothelial cells: free diffusion, active transport, carrier-mediated diffusion, ion transport systems, and receptor-mediated transport.

ure 11–2 illustrates some of the transport mechanisms present in cerebral endothelium. The brain-type (glut-1) glucose transporter was first described by Mueckler and colleagues.[1] It is insulin-independent and catalyzes the facilitated transport of glucose from blood into brain.[1] The glut-1 protein is present in virtually all brain microvascular endothelium with high-resistance tight junctions; therefore it can be used as a marker for the blood-brain and blood-CSF barriers.[3]

Enzymes contained in other CNS transport systems (such as alkaline phosphatase and γ-glutamyl transpeptidase) have also been used as markers for the brain capillary endothelium.[3] Cerebral endothelial cells and pericytes uniquely contain γ-glutamyl transpeptidase, which is part of an amino acid transport system. The HT7 protein is a cell-surface glycoprotein that is a marker for blood-brain barrier endothelium.[2] A particular marker may be present at the luminal and/or abluminal surface. Knowledge of receptor/carrier systems has been exploited to deliver substances to the brain, including L-dopa, melphalan, and baclofen.[6]

Cellular Interactions

The function and permeability of the brain capillary endothelial cells are greatly influenced by astrocytes and pericytes and even neurons and the basement membrane; complex interactions occur between these components.[1, 6] Astrocytes have been shown to induce blood-brain barrier properties in developing brain and to orchestrate the tissue-specific gene expression of the brain capillary endothelium.[3, 12] Using chick-quail transplantation experiments, Stewart and Wiley were the first to demonstrate unambiguously that blood-brain barrier characteristics could be induced in endothelial cells that had invaded brain transplants.[2, 13] Subsequent experiments by others confirmed that organ-specific characteristics of endothelial cells may be induced and maintained by the

TABLE 11–2
BLOOD-BRAIN BARRIER TRANSPORT SYSTEMS

Transport System	Representative Substrates	V_{max} (nmol/min·g)
Hexose	Glucose	1600
Monocarboxylic acid	Lactate	120
Large neutral amino acid	Phenylalanine, L-dopa, melphalan, baclofen	30
Basic amino acid	Lysine	6
Acidic amino acid	Glutamate	—
Amine	Choline	6
Purine	Adenine	1
Nucleoside	Adenosine	0.7
Thyroid	Triiodothyronine (T_3)	0.1
Thiamine	Thiamine	0.03
Peptides	Dipeptides	NA
Growth factors	Transferrin, insulin	NA
Cholesterol	Cholesterol	NA

NA, not applicable.
Data from Pardridge WM: Advances in cell biology of blood-brain barrier transport. Semin Cell Biol 1991; 2:419–426; and DeBoer AG, Breimer DD: The blood-brain barrier: Clinical implications for drug delivery to the brain. J R Coll Physicians Lond 1994; 28:502–506.

local environment.[2] The fact that morphologic irregularities of the blood-brain barrier in brain tumors (discussed later) correlate with the breakdown of the blood-brain barrier has also led to the hypothesis that healthy astrocytes are necessary for the maintenance of the blood-brain barrier.[2] In vitro model systems have also been used to illustrate that astrocytes can influence the ''tightness'' of the endothelial tight junctions.[14] Pericytes have the capability to contract and have phagocytic activity and an antigen-presenting function.[1, 3] Lymphocytes and pericytes, therefore, may actually be protective of the blood-brain barrier. The blood-brain barrier may also be influenced by hormonal stimuli.[6, 9]

RESPONSE OF THE BLOOD-BRAIN BARRIER TO NEOPLASIA

The progressive growth of a glioma requires the continuing success of many complex processes, including multiplication of tumor cells, destruction of normal brain tissue, and remodeling of the local brain vasculature.[15] Glioma cells infiltrate into the surrounding brain parenchyma, usually along the paths of least resistance. Such paths include white matter tracts and the perivascular Virchow-Robin spaces of blood vessels. Theoretically, proliferation of tumor cells adjacent to small vessels could produce a pressure effect, or directly disrupt vessel integrity. Vascular insufficiency could, in turn, lead to areas of necrosis or hemorrhage within the tumor.[10] With partial capillary disruption, the blood-brain barrier would be ''leaky'' or more permeable, resulting in the formation of vasogenic edema. Formation of vasogenic edema has been studied as the main consequence of the effect of neoplasia on the blood-brain barrier. Exactly how tumors cause edema, however, is still an area of speculation. Clinically, blood-brain barrier permeability is demonstrated by contrast enhancement on computed tomographic (CT) and magnetic resonance imaging (MRI) scans,[16] whereas edema is usually visualized as an area of hypodensity surrounding a region of tumor enhancement on CT scan or as a region of increased T1 or T2 signal surrounding the gadolinium-enhanced area on MRI.[17] Differentiation of tumor-infiltrated cerebral tissue from tumor-associated edema may be difficult in infiltrating malignant tumors and in low-grade gliomas with no enhancement.[17] Vasogenic edema certainly complicates other diseases besides malignancy. However, it is the edema formed in response to CNS malignancy (tumor-associated brain edema) that is so exquisitely responsive to steroid administration. Some investigators have found a relationship between degree of malignancy and degree of barrier opening as assessed by CT scanning with contrast enhancement.[18]

Morphology of the Capillary Endothelium in Gliomas

The capillary endothelium in brain tumors is sometimes referred to as the *blood-tumor barrier*.[10] Raimondi[19] and then Long[20] examined the ultrastructure of capillaries in malignant gliomas by using electron microscopy. Endothelial cells were observed to be hyperplastic, with prominent vesicle

TABLE 11-3
MORPHOLOGIC FEATURES OF CAPILLARIES IN GLIOMAS

Hyperplastic endothelial cells
Frequent fenestrations
Loss of tight intercellular junctions
Prominent intracellular vesicles
Less developed pericapillary sheath formed by the glial foot
   processes

formation. The endothelial surface in tumors was irregular, with deep folds that would facilitate the passage of material through the endothelium.[21] Interendothelial junctions were found to have lost their pentalaminar structure, thus becoming patent to protein passage.[4] Capillaries were observed to have frequent fenestrations and were often surrounded by large collagen-filled extracellular spaces with absent glial processes.[21] These changes are summarized in Table 11–3. Evidence has indicated that an increase in the number of pinocytotic vesicles is characteristic of vasogenic edema.[22] In many brain tumors, the morphologic irregularities of the perivascular ensheathment (enlarged perivascular space, gaps in the basal lamina, and unusual or lacking glial investment) have been found to correlate with the breakdown of the blood-brain barrier.[2]

It is uncertain whether similar changes exist in peritumoral brain tissue.[21] Some studies have shown an increase in open junctions and pinocytotic vesicles in brain adjacent to tumor.[21] Observations regarding the morphology of capillaries around tumors have important implications for explaining the origin, and basis for the increased permeability, of the blood-tumor barrier. The first possibility would be that tumors produce one or more factors that affect the blood-brain barrier (see following). If so, such factors might be able to act at a distance, influencing adjacent brain. Another possibility is that glioma cells, unlike normal brain glial cells, lack the ability to induce the formation of a normal blood-brain barrier. Therefore, any new capillaries growing into the tumor would be like peripheral vessels and, therefore, more permeable.

Gliomas, Vasogenic Edema, and the Blood-Brain Barrier

Brain tumor growth is associated with the development of tumor-associated edema; such edema is responsible for significant patient morbidity.[17] Although various types of cerebral edema have been described, including vasogenic, cytotoxic, hydrostatic, and ischemic, the consensus is that tumors cause vasogenic edema as a result of breakdown of the blood-brain barrier and subsequent damage to the endothelium.[21] The increased vascular permeability results in the extravasation of water, sodium, and other serum components, particularly protein, into the extracellular space within and around the tumor.[21, 22] The precise mechanisms by which brain tumors cause edema remain unclear.[16] An increase in the permeability of the blood-brain barrier is an early event, occurring before the development of brain edema.[22] As with infiltrating tumor cells, edema fluid collects mainly in the extracellular spaces between the white matter fibers, following the anatomic pathway that provides the least resistance.[21] In sharp contrast to the thick network of synapses and junctions in the cortex, no junctions exist between myelin fibers, which are therefore easily split. Cerebral edema influences cerebral blood flow, brain metabolism, and intracranial pressure.[21]

Several mechanisms have been proposed[16, 17] through which malignant gliomas could cause brain edema, including the following: (1) an inflammatory process that involves an increase in phospholipase A2 activity and, therefore, increased arachidonic acid release; this process may also involve leukotrienes and/or prostaglandins[22]; (2) increased microvascular permeability due to the secretion of factors by tumor cells (e.g., *vascular permeability factor* or *capillary permeability factor*); (3) alterations in endothelial enzyme activity; and (4) proliferation of new, permeable microvessels (a "leaky" neovasculature) as a result of tumor angiogenesis. One or more of these mechanisms may be operational. Experiments supporting the various hypotheses have been performed using animal brain tumor models, including the RG-2, C6, 9L, and ENU-induced tumor models.[23] In vitro blood-brain barrier models have also been described.[16, 24, 25]

An important role in the pathogenesis of vasogenic edema is played by degradation of cell membrane phospholipids with subsequent release of arachidonic acid, the main polyunsaturated fatty acid in the brain and its tumors.[21] Release of arachidonic acid is also important in the pathogenesis of the vasogenic and cytotoxic edema caused by ischemia, compression injury, hypoxia, hypoglycemia, and cold injury.[22] The liberation of arachidonic acid in cerebral tumors may trigger a series of events in capillary walls by increasing their permeability and, therefore, increasing the amount of edema.[21] Prostaglandin E and thromboxane B_2 have been found to be vascular permeability factors.[21]

Protein Factors Secreted by Gliomas That May Affect Capillary Endothelial Cells

In recent years, much research has focused on identifying various proteases that are secreted by glioma cells in vitro.[26, 27] Elevated levels of several proteases have also been found in human tumor specimens.[28, 29] Glioma cells secrete the following: (1) urokinase, a serine protease that is a plasminogen activator[15, 30, 32]; (2) matrix metalloproteinases, which include type IV and other collagenases, gelatinases, and stromelysins[29, 31, 33]; and (3) cathepsin B, a cysteine protease.[34] In addition to degrading elements of the brain extracellular matrix, such proteases may act more directly on the tumor and/or brain microvasculature and surrounding structures to affect the blood-tumor and/or blood-brain barrier.

Urokinase and other plasminogen activators, such as tissue plasminogen activator (tPA), convert plasminogen into the active proteolytic enzyme plasmin, which degrades fibrin.[28, 32] Several components of the extracellular matrix, including laminin, fibronectin, and proteoglycans, are also susceptible to plasmin-mediated hydrolysis.[26] Cellular fibrinolytic activity has been found to correlate with brain edema.[35] Urokinase likely plays an important role in glioma

invasion and angiogenesis,[28, 32, 36] whereas tPA is mainly associated with the vascular endothelium.[32] Suramin, a growth factor antagonist, inhibits urokinase activity, endothelial cell migration, and the neovascular response.[37] Upregulation of the urokinase receptor gene in malignant astrocytomas has also been reported.[38, 39] Plasminogen activator inhibitors (PAIs) may determine the level of plasminogen activator activity and thereby strongly influence the ability of tumors (including astrocytomas) to progress.[28, 32, 36]

Matrix metalloproteinases are secreted in zymogen from many cell types in a latent form, which requires activation. They contain a zinc ion and are inhibited by chelating agents.[33] The activity of type IV collagenase and other metalloproteinases has been found to be high in malignant gliomas, metastatic tumors, and some meningiomas.[29, 31] Collagenases would be expected to have higher activity against basement membranes than would plasminogen activators working alone.[40] However, some of these proteases activate other proteases, thereby creating a cascade effect. For example, urokinase activates type IV collagenase[15, 40] and it has been suggested that plasmin (and also the H-*ras* oncogene) activates metalloproteinases in general.[33] As with the plasminogen activators, tissue inhibitors of the metalloproteinases (or TIMPs) may also play important regulatory roles.[29] The cysteine protease cathepsin B has also been found to be overexpressed in gliomas and may play a role in progression and invasion.[34] Cathepsin B is expressed at the invading edge of tumor and around vessels.[34] Cathepsin B has a broad substrate specificity, being able to degrade proteoglycans, laminin, fibronectin, and type IV collagen.[34]

Vascular endothelial growth factor (VEGF), also known as vascular permeability factor (VPF), although not a protease, is a mitogen for endothelial cells and increases microvascular permeability.[41] On a molar basis, it is about 50,000 times more potent than histamine in increasing microvascular permeability.[41] It has been implicated in causing fluid accumulation in solid tumors, promoting tumor angiogenesis, stimulating von Willebrand factor release from endothelial cells, and promoting monocyte migration.[2, 41] VEGF is expressed in malignant gliomas, and its receptor is upregulated in tumor endothelial cells.[42, 43]

Mathematical Modeling of Tumor Capillary Permeability

In the 1980s, a flurry of reports were published about quantitative measurements of brain tumor capillary permeability in animal brain tumor models[44, 45] and in human gliomas.[46, 47] These reports established that capillary permeability in gliomas was regionally variable and that permeability increases of 10 to 30 times that of normal brain were often seen. Transport across the blood-brain barrier can also be studied by positron emission tomography (PET) using tracer analogues of hexoses and amino acids that are not metabolized.[48] Similarly, ^{11}C-methylalbumin can be used to monitor albumin leakage across the blood-brain barrier.[48] PET made it possible to document in patients that the administration of dexamethasone decreased the permeability of tumor capillaries to small hydrophilic molecules.[46]

It was hoped that quantitative information regarding capillary permeability could be used to "rationalize" brain tumor chemotherapy by allowing clinicians to predict the amount of drug that would enter a tumor.[49] However, these hopes have not been realized, and the issue of whether the brain-tumor barrier interferes with delivery of adequate amounts of drug remains controversial.[50] Similar issues about permeability limitations of drug delivery to solid systemic tumors also exist.[51] Among the reasons that these issues have not been resolved are the expense of conducting such studies in humans, the need to use nonmetabolized compounds rather than the chemotherapeutic drugs themselves, and the difficulty of designing studies in which the drug delivery process can be followed to completion. Even a simple model, like that shown in Figure 11–3, which includes influx and efflux constants between the capillary and extracellular fluid (ECF) (k_1 and k_2) and between the cell and ECF (k_3 and k_4), ignores metabolism and movement within the ECF (such as diffusion and bulk flow). Whether quantitative measurements of the movement of drugs into, out of, and through the blood-brain barrier will ultimately be important for therapy has yet to be established.

FUTURE DIRECTIONS

To date, the impact of CT and MRI on the clinical care of brain tumor patients has been profound. In addition to detailed anatomic information, such scans provide an indication of the permeability of the blood-brain barrier in vivo through their detection of edema and by means of enhancement after the injection of protein-bound and water-soluble contrast agents.[11] As with the earlier studies with PET and CT, investigators have attempted to use the movement of gadolinium as seen by MRI to quantitate capillary permeability in brain tumors and to apply this information to tumor classification.[52] Because MRI is a very sensitive method for quantifying accumulation of intracerebral water,[53] further applications can be expected to result from MRI studies of cerebral edema.[54] MRI can also be used to image paramagnetic molecules administered into the CSF.[55] Magnetic resonance spectroscopy (MRS) is being studied as an additional technique for use in tumor diagnosis and grading and has

shown promise in distinguishing recurrent tumor from radiation necrosis.[56] However, because the dominant signal for MRS comes from the hydrogen atom, and because MRS requires millimolar amounts of compound in tissue, it is unlikely that MRS can be used to follow tissue concentrations of drug over time any more successfully than can PET. In the future, it is likely that clinicians will benefit from further improvements in diagnostic techniques, which will provide more information about the integrity of the blood-brain barrier.

REFERENCES

1. Zinke H, Mockel B, Frey A, et al: Blood-brain barrier: A molecular approach to its structural and functional characterization. *In* Ermisch A, Landgraf R, Ruhle HJ (eds): Progress in Brain Research 91. New York, Elsevier Science Publishers, 1992, pp 103–116.
2. Risau W: Molecular biology of blood-brain barrier ontogenesis and function. Acta Neurochir 1994; 60(suppl):109–112.
3. Pardridge WM: Advances in cell biology of blood-brain barrier transport. Semin Cell Biol 1991; 2:419–426.
4. Bradbury MWB: Appraisal of the role of endothelial cells and glia in barrier breakdown. *In* Suckling AJ, Rumsby MG, Bradbury MWB (eds): The Blood-Brain Barrier in Health and Disease. Chichester, England, Ellis Horwood, 1986, pp 128–129.
5. Pardridge WM: Blood-brain barrier transport of nutrients. Fed Proc 1986; 45:2047–2049.
6. DeBoer AG, Breimer DD: The blood-brain barrier: Clinical implications for drug delivery to the brain. J R Coll Physicians Lond 1994; 28:502–506.
7. Reese TS, Karnovsky MJ: Fine structural localization of a blood-brain barrier to exogenous peroxidase. J Cell Biol 1967; 34:207–217.
8. Brightman MW, Reese TS: Junctions between intimately apposed cell membranes in the vertebrate brain. J Cell Biol 1969; 40:648–677.
9. Gross PM, Sposito NM, Pettersen SE, et al: Differences in function and structure of the capillary endothelium in gray matter, white matter and a circumventricular organ of rat brain. Blood Vessels 1986; 23:261–270.
10. Greig NH: Brain tumors and the blood-tumor barrier. *In* Neuwelt EA (ed): Implications of the Blood-Brain Barrier and Its Manipulation, vol. 2. New York, Plenum Medical Book Co, 1989, pp 77–106.
11. Salcman M, Broadwell RD: The blood-brain barrier. *In* Salcman M (ed): Neurobiology of Brain Tumors. Baltimore, Williams & Wilkins, 1991, pp 229–249.
12. Abbott NJ, Revest PA, Romero IA: Astrocyte-endothelial interaction: Physiology and pathology. Neuropathol Appl Neurobiol 1992; 18:424–433.
13. Stewart PA, Wiley MJ: Developing nervous tissue induces formation of blood-brain barrier characteristics in invading endothelial cells: A study using quail-chick transplantation chimeras. Dev Biol 1981; 84:183–192.
14. Tao Cheng JH, Brightman MW: Development of membrane interactions between brain endothelial cells and astrocytes in vitro. Int J Dev Neurosci 1988; 6:25–37.
15. Reith A, Rucklidge GJ: Invasion of brain tissue by primary glioma: Evidence for the involvement of urokinase-type plasminogen activator as an activator of type IV collagenase. Biochem Biophys Res Commun 1992; 186:348–354.
16. Grabb PA, Gilbert MR: Neoplastic and pharmacological influence on the permeability of an in vitro blood-brain barrier. J Neurosurg 1995; 82:1053–1058.
17. Del Maestro RF, Megyesi JF, Farrell CL: Mechanisms of tumor-associated edema: A review. Can J Neurol Sci 1990; 17:177–183.
18. Butler AR, Horii SC, Kricheff II, et al: Computed tomography in astrocytomas: A statistical analysis of the parameters of malignancy and the positive contrast-enhanced CT scan. Radiology 1978; 129:433–439.
19. Raimondi AJ: Localization of radio-labelled serum albumin in human glioma: An electron microscopic study. Arch Neurol 1964; 11:173–184.
20. Long DM. Capillary ultrastructure and the blood-brain barrier in human malignant brain tumors. J Neurosurg 1970; 32:127–144.

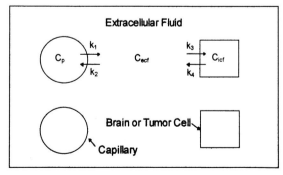

Figure 11–3 Schematic representation of brain or brain tumor. The tissue contains capillaries *(circles)* and cells *(squares)*. Three compartments are shown: the vascular space, extracellular fluid (ecf), and intracellular fluid (icf). The k values are rate constants for movement between either the extracellular fluid and the plasma (k_1 and k_2) or the extracellular fluid and cells (k_3 and k_4).

21. Schiffer D: Brain Tumors: Pathology and Its Biological Correlates. New York, Springer-Verlag, 1993.

22. Chan PH, Fishman RA: The role of arachidonic acid in vasogenic brain edema. Fed Proc 1984; 43:210–213.

23. Groothuis DG, Fischer JM, Lapin G, et al: Permeability of different experimental brain tumor models to horseradish peroxidase. J Neuropathol Exp Neurol 1982; 41:164–185.

24. Arthur FE, Shivers RR, Bowman PD: Astrocyte-mediated induction of tight junctions in brain capillary endothelium: An efficient in vitro model. Dev Brain Res 1987; 36:155–159.

25. Raub TJ, Kuentzel SL, Sawada GA: Permeability of bovine brain microvessel endothelial cells in vitro: Barrier tightening by a factor released from astroglioma cells. Exp Cell Res 1992; 199:330–340.

26. Sitrin RG, Gyetko MR, Kole KL, et al: Expression of heterogenous profiles of plasminogen activators and plasminogen activator inhibitors by human glioma lines. Cancer Res 1990; 50:4957–4961.

27. Bindal AK, Hammoud M, Shi WM, et al: Prognostic significance of proteolytic enzymes in human brain tumors. J Neurooncol 1994; 22:101–110.

28. Landau BJ, Kwaan HC, Verrusio EN, et al: Elevated levels of urokinase-type plasminogen activator and plasminogen activator inhibitor type-1 in malignant human brain tumors. Cancer Res 1994; 54:1105–1108.

29. Nakagawa T, Toshihiko K, Kabuto M, et al: Production of matrix metalloproteinases and tissue inhibitor of metalloproteinases-1 by human brain tumors. J Neurosurg 1994; 81:69–77.

30. Dano K, Dabelsteen E, Nielsen LS, et al: Plasminogen activating enzyme in cultured glioblastoma cells. J Histochem Cytochem 1982; 30:1165–1170.

31. Rao JS, Steck PA, Mohanam S, et al: Elevated levels of Mr 92,000 type IV collagenase in human brain tumors. Cancer Res 1993; 53:2208–2211.

32. Hsu DW, Efird JT, Hedley-Whyte ET: Prognostic role of urokinase-type plasminogen activator in human gliomas. Am J Pathol 1995; 147:114–123.

33. Matrisian LM: Metalloproteinases and their inhibitors in matrix remodeling. Trends Genet 1990; 6:121–125.

34. Rempel SA, Rosenblum ML, Mikkelsen T, et al: Cathepsin B expression and localization in glioma progression and invasion. Cancer Res 1994; 54:6027–6031.

35. Kornblith PL, Walker MD (eds): Advances in Neuro-oncology. Mount Kisco, NY, Futura, 1988, pp 103–135.

36. Yamamoto M, Sawaya R, Mohanam S, et al: Expression and cellular localization of messenger RNA for plasminogen activator inhibitor type 1 in human astrocytomas in vivo. Cancer Res 1994; 54:3329–3332.

37. Takano S, Gately S, Neville ME, et al: Suramin, an anticancer and angiosuppressive agent, inhibits endothelial cell binding of basic fibroblast growth factor, migration, proliferation, and induction of urokinase-type plasminogen activator. Cancer Res 1994; 54:2654–2660.

38. Mohanam S, Sawaya R, Yamamoto M, et al: Proteolysis and invasiveness of brain tumors: Role of urokinase-type plasminogen activator receptor. J Neurooncol 1994; 22:153–160.

39. Gladson CL, Pijuan-Thompson V, Olman MA, et al: Up-regulation of urokinase and urokinase receptor genes in malignant astrocytoma. Am J Pathol 1995; 146:1150–1160.

40. Reich R, Thompson EW, Iwamoto Y, et al: Effects of inhibitors of plasminogen activator, serine proteinases, and collagenase IV on the invasion of basement membranes of metastatic cells. Cancer Res 1988; 48:3307–3312.

41. Berse B, Brown LF, DeWater LV, et al: Vascular permeability factor (vascular endothelial growth factor) gene is expressed differentially in normal tissues, macrophages, and tumors. Mol Biol Cell 1992; 3:211–220.

42. Conn G, Soderman DD, Schaeffer MT, et al: Purification of a glycoprotein vascular endothelial cell mitogen from a rat glioma-derived cell line. Proc Natl Acad Sci USA 1990; 87:1323–1327.

43. Plate KH, Breier G, Weich HA, et al: Vascular endothelial growth-factor is a potential tumor angiogenesis factor in human gliomas in vivo. Nature 1992; 359:845–848.

44. Blasberg RG, Groothuis D, Molnar P: Application of quantitative autoradiographic measurements in experimental brain tumor models. Semin Neurol 1981; 3:203–221.

45. Groothuis DR, Molnar P, Blasberg R: Regional blood flow and blood-to-tissue transport in five brain tumor models: Implications for chemotherapy. In Rosenblum M, Wilson C (eds): Progress in Experimental Brain Tumor Research. S Karger, Basel, 1984, pp 132–153.

46. Jarden JO, Dhawan V, Moeller JR, et al: The time course of steroid action on blood-to-brain and blood-to-tumor transport of 82Rb: A positron emission tomographic study. Ann Neurol 1989; 25:239–245.

47. Groothuis DR, Vriesendorp FJ, Kupfer B, et al: Quantitative measurements of capillary transport in human brain tumors by computed tomography. Ann Neurol 1991; 30:581–588.

48. Brooks DJ: In vivo metabolism of human cerebral tumors. In Thomas DGT (ed): Neuro-oncology: Primary Malignant Brain Tumours. Baltimore, Johns Hopkins University Press, 1990, pp 122–131.

49. Blasberg RG, Groothuis DR: Chemotherapy of brain tumors: Physiological and pharmacokinetic considerations. Semin Oncol 1986; 13:70–83.

50. Stewart DJ: A critique of the role of the blood-brain barrier in the chemotherapy of human brain tumors. J Neurooncol 1994; 20:121–139.

51. Jain RK: Delivery of molecular medicine to solid tumors. Science 1996; 271:1079–1080.

52. Tovi M: MR imaging in cerebral gliomas: Analysis of tumour tissue components. Acta Radiol 1993; 34(suppl 384):1–24.

53. Jolesz FA: Compartmental analysis of brain edema using magnetic resonance imaging. Acta Neurochir 1994; 60 (suppl):179–183.

54. Le Bihan D (ed): Diffusion and Perfusion Magnetic Resonance Imaging: Applications to Functional MRI. New York, Raven, 1995.

55. Engelhard HH, Petruska DA: Movement and imaging of iron oxide-bound antibodies in brain and cerebrospinal fluid. Cancer Biochem Biophys 1992; 13:224–236.

56. Ott D, Hennig J, Ernst T: Human brain tumors: Assessment with in vivo proton MR spectroscopy. Radiology 1993; 186:745–752.

Experimental Therapeutics

PAUL KLEIHUES

OTMAR D. WIESTLER

HIROKO OHGAKI

ADRIANO AGUZZI

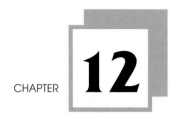

CHAPTER **12**

Animal Models of Tumors of the Nervous System

Because the etiology and genetic basis of human brain tumors are still largely unknown, animal models have been established to study their pathogenesis on the cellular and molecular level and to assess the role of modulating factors, including chemotherapy. Whereas in earlier studies malignant transformation was initiated by treatment with chemical carcinogens and oncogenic viruses, recent approaches directly utilize transformation-associated genes in transgenic mice and retroviral infection of fetal brain cells. This chapter summarizes available animal models and their relationship with human nervous system neoplasms.

CHEMICAL CARCINOGENS

Studies on the induction of neural tumors in experimental animals can be divided into two phases: (1) early studies with polycyclic aromatic hydrocarbons (PAH), which require topical (intracerebral) administration; and (2) studies, which date from 1964, that utilize neurotropic alkylating agents, which induce nervous system neoplasms in rodents after systemic administration.

Polycyclic Aromatic Hydrocarbons

Polycyclic aromatic hydrocarbons (PAHs) were the first carcinogens used to induce brain tumors in experimental animals. Implantation as crystalline PAH powder melted in a porcelain crucible was the technique of choice,[1] but various other methods of pellet administration were subsequently developed.[2] The most efficient PAHs were 3- and 20-methylcholanthrene, benzo[a]pyrene, and 7,12-dimethylbenz[a]anthracene (DMBA). These studies have been reviewed by Bigner and Swenberg.[3] DMBA is the only PAH that produced tumors in the offspring following intravenous injection on day 15.[4, 5] Whole body autoradiographs demonstrated that DMBA crosses the blood-placenta barrier, although labeling of the fetal compartment occurred significantly later

than that of maternal parenchymal tissues, including the central nervous system (CNS).[6] In most laboratories, studies using PAH were discontinued after the discovery that several simple alkylating agents induce brain tumors in rodents after intravenous injection.[7]

N-Nitroso Compounds and Related Alkylating Agents

The chemicals that are most effective in inducing CNS neoplasms in animals are simple alkylating agents. Nitrosourea-derivatives, particularly methylnitrosourea and ethylnitrosourea, cause CNS neoplasms in rats at a high incidence after systemic administration.[8] Dialkylaryltriazenes;[9] azo-, azoxy- and hydrazo- compounds;[10] and 1,2-dialkylhydrazines also induce brain tumors effectively. Ethylnitrosourea and related ethylating agents (1,2-diethylhydrazine, 1-phenyl-3,3-diethyltriazene) are particularly powerful when administered as a single dose transplacentally or shortly after birth.[11] The susceptibility of the rat CNS to the agents begins at the 10th prenatal day (E10), increases gradually, and reaches its maximum at birth, when a single dose is approximately 50 times more effective than in adult rats. The susceptibility of the CNS decreases after birth and reaches that of adult rats at approximately 1 month of age.[11] Procarbazine is a derivative of methylbenzylhydrazine and is widely used in the chemotherapy of human cancer, including brain tumors. It is itself a potent carcinogen and was demonstrated to induce nervous system tumors when administered transplacentally to rats.[12]

N-Nitrosomethylurea and related methylating agents (1,2-dimethylhydrazine, 1-phenyl-3,3-dimethyltriazene) also induce brain tumors transplacentally, although, because of their higher toxicity, to a lesser extent. They have, however, been shown to be very effective neuro-oncogenic agents in adult rats after repetitive administration of small weekly doses.[7, 9, 13]

HISTOGENESIS OF ETHYLNITROSOUREA-INDUCED TUMORS

A general consensus exists that neoplasms of the peripheral nervous system, including cranial nerves, are malignant neurinomas (i.e., of Schwann cell origin).[14] Tumors induced in the CNS have been designated *oligodendrogliomas, astrocytomas,* and *ependymomas,* according to the glial precursor from which they presumably originate.[15, 16] The frequent development of ethylnitrosurea (ENU)-induced neoplasms in the subependymal region of the cerebral hemispheres, the great histopathologic diversity of these neoplasms, and the high incidence of mixed gliomas have led to the hypothesis that the tumors originate from primitive neuroepithelial cells in the subependymal matrix layer of the lateral ventricles. Sequential morphologic studies have shown that neoplastic precursor lesions occur as early as 10 weeks postnatally. They consist of small foci of hyperplastic oligodendrocytes and are located predominantly in the hemispheric white matter.[3, 17] In later stages (after 5 to 6 months) they develop into microtumors, which stain positively with alcian blue. Ultimately, these neoplasms show features of anaplastic oligodendrogliomas. In addition, early neoplastic proliferations appear in the periventricular white matter of 2-month-old rats as single lesions, multiple foci, or a continuous thickening of the subependymal plate.[18] In later stages, they increase in size and develop into astrocytomas, oligodendrogliomas, ependymomas, and, most frequently, mixed gliomas. It was therefore concluded that ENU-induced gliomas originate either from oligodendrocytes or from multipotent precursor cells of the subependymal matrix layer.[17, 18]

This view was supported in an experimental model in which neural tumors were induced in fetal brain transplants. Pregnant rats received a single intravenous (IV) dose of ENU (50 mg/kg) on the 14th day of gestation. One day later, cell suspensions were prepared from the fetal forebrain and stereotactically injected into the caudoputamen of adult rats. After additional exposure to ENU of the host animals 8 days and 9 weeks post-transplantation, brain tumors developed within the neural graft in all rats. Histopathologically, all neoplasms were classified as oligodendrogliomas. Other neoplasms typically induced by ENU transplacentally (astrocytomas, mixed gliomas, ependymomas) were absent. The selective induction of oligodendrogliomas indicates that neoplastic transformation in the nervous system can occur in a differentiated glial cell or a precursor cell committed to oligodendrocytic differentiation, and that transformation of a pluripotent stem cell is not necessary.[19]

It should be mentioned that recent immunohistochemical studies have shown that ENU-induced neoplasms, previously classified as ependymomas, express the neuronal marker synaptophysin and may thus better be termed primitive neuroectodermal tumors with neuronal differentiation.[20] The precursor cells of ENU-induced brain tumors have not yet been identified. The monoclonal antibody gp130RB13-6, generated from immature rat nervous system cells, appears to recognize a subset of neural progenitor cells particularly susceptible to the oncogenic effect of ENU.[112]

ROLE OF DNA MODIFICATIONS AND DNA REPAIR

Malignant transformation by alkylating agents is thought to result from interaction of the ultimate carcinogen (i.e., a methyl or ethyl cation) with cellular DNA.[21] Of the various resulting base modifications produced, nucleophilic substitution at the extranuclear oxygen atoms of guanine, thymine, and cytosine has the greatest mutagenic efficiency and correlates with the carcinogenic potential of the respective chemicals.[22] The major O-alkylated base is O^6-alkylguanine, which during DNA replication mispairs with deoxythymidine, causing GC→AT transition mutations. O^6-methylguanine and O^6-ethylguanine are repaired by the O^6-alkylguanine-DNA alkyltransferase,[23] and this occurs much less efficiently in the brain (i.e. the target tissue) than in the liver and other extraneural tissues.[24, 25] This repair deficiency of the CNS was considered to be the mechanism of preferential induction of nervous system tumors, but comparative studies in mice and gerbils showed that their CNSs are similarly deficient in the repair of O^6-alkylguanines, although ENU and related agents do not have a significant neuro-oncogenic potential in these species.[21] It was concluded that deficient repair of O^6-alkylguanines in rodent brain may be a necessary but not sufficient factor in the malignant transformation of neural cells.

MOLECULAR GENETICS OF CHEMICALLY INDUCED TUMORS IN RODENTS

To date, no transformation-associated gene has been identified as playing a major role in the evolution of ENU- or MNU-induced CNS tumors. In particular, no ras mutations were detected, although these are frequent in mammary tumors induced by the same compounds under similar experimental conditions.[26] Mutations in the p53 tumor suppressor gene have been observed but appear to be rare.[27]

In contrast, the genetic basis of ENU-induced schwannomas has been elucidated. These tumors invariably contain a T:A→A:T transversion at nucleotide 2012 (codon 664; Val→Glu) in the transmembrane domain of the *neu* proto-oncogene, i.e., the rat homolog of the human c-erb-B2 gene.[28, 29] This mutation has been detected as early as 7 days after administration of ethylnitrosourea on postnatal day 1.[30] During early stages of tumor progression, the corresponding normal allele is lost.[30, 31] In vitro, cell lines derived from ENU-induced schwannomas may undergo divergent differentiation with development of a myoblastic phenotype.[32] In ENU-induced neurofibromas of the Syrian hamster, point mutations are typically present in codons 659 and 658 of the neu transmembrane domain; again, the mutation is a T:A→A:T transversion causing a substitution of valine by glutamic acid.[33] No neu mutations are detectable in tumors of the human peripheral nervous system.[34]

ONCOGENIC VIRUSES AND VIRAL ONCOGENES

Several oncogenic viruses induce a high incidence of tumors in rats after postnatal intracerebral injection.[3] In an effort to identify the specific molecular changes responsible for induction of brain tumors, viral oncogenes have been used in transgenic mice and also in a grafting model in which retroviral vectors are used to transfect fetal rat brain cells in vitro: single cell suspensions prepared from fetal rat brains

(E14–E15) are infected with replication-defective retroviral vectors encoding oncogenes and are subsequently injected into the caudoputamen of adult rats using a stereotactic frame.[35]

SV40 Virus

This DNA virus and its transforming gene, large T, exert a broad range of oncogenic effects. At the same time, it is the only oncogenic virus that has been implicated, but not proven to play a role, in the etiology of human brain tumors.

SV40 employs an intriguing mode of transformation. It was shown that the product of its transforming gene, large T, inactivates a variety of growth regulatory nuclear proteins through complex formation. Targets include P53, the p105 RB1 gene product, and a p107 host cell protein.[36] It remains to be shown if the association with these cellular proteins is also responsible for the induction of brain tumors by SV40 large T.

TUMOR INDUCTION BY THE INTACT VIRUS

SV40 was among the earliest oncogenic viruses found to cause cell-specific malignant transformation in the devel-

oping nervous system of rodents. When inoculated intracerebrally in newborn hamsters, it induced choroid plexus papillomas and ependymomas.[37–39] Gliomas resulting from the transplantation of SV40 transfected glial cells into the brain of newborn hamsters show a markedly different extent of invasiveness, and this appears to be associated with distinct viral integration patterns.[40]

EXPRESSION OF SV40 LARGE T ANTIGEN IN TRANSGENIC MICE

Several lines of transgenic mice expressing SV40 large T antigen have been established.[41, 42] Mice expressing SV40 large T antigen typically develop primitive neuroectodermal and endocrine tumors (PNETs), retinoblastomas, or choroid plexus tumors (Table 12–1). The promoter or regulatory sequence used influences the selection of target cells. Under the transcriptional control of rat tyrosine hydroxylase promoter and enhancer, PNETs of the brainstem and adrenal glands developed in transgenic mice expressing SV40 large T antigen,[43] whereas mice regulated by the Moloney murine sarcoma virus (MSV) enhancer developed PNETs of the midbrain and of the endocrine pancreas.[44] Available evidence suggests that in transgenic mice carrying MSV enhancer/ SV40 large T, midbrain tumors originate from the pineal gland, as pinealocytes express the large T and tumors display

TABLE 12–1
TUMORS OF THE NERVOUS SYSTEM IN TRANSGENIC AND KNOCKOUT MICE

Gene	Promoter/Regulatory Sequence	Tumor	Reference
SV40 large T antigen	Rat tyrosine hydroxylase promoter/enhancer	PNET (brainstem)	Sure et al[43]
	MSV enhancer natural promoter of SV40 large T antigen	PNET (pineal gland)	Theuring et al[44]
	Human luteinizing hormone β-subunit promoter	PNET (mesencephalon) Retinoblastoma	Marcus et al,[47] Windle et al[48]
	Human interphotoreceptor retinoid-binding protein promoter	PNET (brain and retina)	Al Ubaidi et al[51]
	GFAP promoter	Choroid plexus hyperplasia and undifferentiated tumors	Danks et al[119]
	IgH intronic enhancer	Choroid plexus tumors	Enjoji et al[120]
	Tryptophan hydroxylase promoter	Pineal tumors	Son et al[113]
	Human phenylethanolamine N-methyltransferase (PNMT) promoter	Retinoblastoma	Hammang et al,[49] Baetge et al[50]
	Olfactory marker protein promoter	Peripheral tumors resembling neuroblastomas	Servenius et al[121]
	LPV enhancer/promoter or SV40 enhancer/promoter	Choroid plexus tumor	Chen & van Dyke[52]
JC virus T antigen	SV40 regulatory region	Choroid plexus papilloma	Ressetar et al[68]
	JC regulatory region	Medulloblastoma/PNET	Krynska et al[122]
Lymphotropic papova virus (LPV) T antigen	LPV enhancer/promoter or SV40 enhancer/promoter	Choroid plexus tumor	Chen & van Dyke[52]
Adenovirus E1A and E1B	MMTV LTR	Neuroblastoma	Koike et al[92]
Polyoma virus middle T antigen	Polyoma early region promoter	Pituitary adenoma	Bautch et al[74]
	Thymidine kinase promoter	Neuroblastoma (rare)	Aguzzi et al[71]
Papilloma virus 16, E6, E7, and ORF	Human β-actin promoter	Ependymoma Pituitary carcinoma Choroid plexus carcinoma	Arbeit et al[93]
v-src	GFAP promoter	Astrocytoma	Weissenberger et al[116]
neu	Myelin basic protein promoter	Oligodendroglioma	Hayes et al[95]
Retinoblastoma Rb		Pituitary adenocarcinoma	Jacks et al[101]
Patched (Ptc)		Medulloblastoma	Goodrich et al[117]
p53		Ependymoma (rare)	Jacks et al[99]

immunoreactivity to S-antigen and rodopsin.[45, 46] Son and others[113] established transgenic mice carrying a construct consisting of 6.1 kb of 5′ flanking region of the tryptophan hydroxylase (TPH) promoter fused to the SV40 T antigen. These animals developed highly invasive pineal tumors and died at age 12 to 15 weeks. Immortalized pinealocyte-derived cell lines from the tumors express TPH and serotonin *N*-acetyltransferase, known to be regulated during circadian cycle. Transgenic mice expressing SV40 large T antigen under the control of a human luteinizing hormone β-subunit promoter developed retinoblastomas, which arise from the inner nuclear layer of the retina. In addition, these mice developed brain tumors, which originated from the subependymal matrix zone of the mesencephalon.[47, 48] Brain tumors were histologically classified as PNETs, and they developed in 19 of 91 animals (21%) between 4 days and 9 months of age.[41, 47] Transgenic mice expressing SV40 large T antigen under transcriptional control of the human *N*-methyltransferase (PNMT) promoter developed retinoblastoma from the inner nuclear and ganglion layers of the retina and pheochromocytoma of the adrenal medulla.[49, 50] Bilateral retinal and brain tumors were observed in transgenic mice expressing SV40 large T antigen under control of the human interphotoreceptor retinoid-binding protein promoter.[51] Histologic examination showed typical PNETs. In some of the bilateral retinal tumors, peculiar rosettes were observed, which were different from the Flexner-Wintersteiner rosettes typically associated with human retinoblastomas.[51]

Using hybrid constructs of SV40 and lymphotropic papovavirus (LPV), Chen and van Dyke[52] analyzed the tissue specificity of tumor development. SV40 and LPV T antigens linked to the same regulatory elements induced similar phenotypes: choroid plexus papillomas developed in transgenic mice carrying a construct of LPV enhancer-promoter/SV40 T antigen coding region and those carrying a construct of LPV enhancer-promoter/LPV T antigen coding region. Those with a construct of SV40 enhancer-promoter/SV40 T antigen coding region and those with a construct of SV40 enhancer-promoter/LPV T antigen coding region manifested choroid plexus papillomas as well as histiocytic lymphoma, thymic hyperplasia, and renal lesions.[52]

Several mutants of SV40 large T antigen, which differ in their ability to form complexes with the tumor suppressors pRB and P53, were tested in transgenic mice. The results showed that binding of T antigen to p53 is not required for induction of choroid plexus tumors. However, tumorigenesis does appear to require the binding of T antigen to the retinoblastoma susceptibility gene product (pRB) and another cellular protein, designated P107.[53]

EXPRESSION OF SV40 LARGE T ANTIGEN IN BRAIN TRANSPLANTS

Rats were transplanted with primary cell suspensions of E14 fetal rat brains infected with a retroviral vector encoding the SV40 large T antigen. Tumors developed in 8 of 14 neural grafts (57%) after latency periods of 176 to 311 days (Table 12–2). This long interval may suggest that sporadic mutations of cellular genes contribute to the formation of the large T–associated tumors. Consistent with the results in transgenic mice, the tumors exhibited features of human PNETs, such as neuroblastic rosettes and immunocytochemical evidence for neuronal and glial differentiation.[54]

TABLE 12–2
BRAIN TUMORS OF THE NEURAL TRANSPLANTS FOLLOWING RETROVIRUS-MEDIATED TRANSFER OF VIRAL ONCOGENE cDNAs

Oncogene	Tumor Type	Latency	Reference
SV40 large T	PNET	5–9 mo	Eibl et al[54]
Polyoma medium T	Hemangioma	2–6 wk	Aguzzi et al[73]
	Anaplastic glioma	9–15 mo	Aguzzi et al[73]
v-Ha-ras	Anaplastic glioma	4–6 mo	Wiestler et al[94]
v-src	Glioma, sarcoma	3–6 mo	Aguzzi et al[73]
v-myc	PNET (rare)		Wiestler et al[94]
v-Ha-ras and v-myc	Anaplastic glioma	2–8 wk	Wiestler et al[94]
v-myc and ENU	Anaplastic glioma	3–6 mo	Brüstle et al[110]

POTENTIAL ROLE OF SV40 IN THE ETIOLOGY OF HUMAN BRAIN TUMORS

Millions of children and adults were treated with SV40-contaminated polio vaccine during 1955 to 1962. A possible association of this treatment with brain tumors has been discussed.[42] However, no conclusive epidemiologic data have been presented to link these vaccinations to an increased risk for brain tumors. Genetic analysis of tumor DNA from scientists working with SV40 virus did not contain SV40 sequences.[55] Recently, natural SV40 strains have been identified in choroid plexus tumors and ependymomas[114] as well as in a variety of gliomas.[115]

JC Virus

JC virus has an extensive nucleotide sequence homology with SV40 and overlapping antigenicity, but the host range is distinctly different. Whereas SV40 does not infect human cells, latent JC infection is very common in human populations, with a serologic prevalence of 40% to 60% in most developed countries. In immunosuppressed patients, JC virus is reactivated and can be detected in the urine. In the brain, it may cause progressive multifocal encephalopathy (PML), which affects up to 5% of patients with terminal AIDS.[57]

TUMOR INDUCTION BY THE INTACT VIRUS

After intracerebral injection in newborn hamsters, JC virus causes brain tumors, mostly consisting of embryonal neoplasms, that is, medulloblastomas (PNETs).[58] Using in situ hybridization, Matsuda and co-workers[59] demonstrated that JC virus primarily infects cells of the external granular layer of the developing cerebellum, which then migrate to the internal granular layer, where incipient medulloblastomas are detectable as early as 30 days after inoculation in newborn golden hamsters.

After intracranial inoculation of newborn rats with JC virus Tokyo-1, a strain isolated from the brain of a patient with PML, more than 70% of animals manifested brain tumors in the forebrain rather than in the cerebellum, as had been the case in hamsters. Immunohistochemical analyses indicated that these tumors were undifferentiated neuroectodermal neoplasms (PNETs), probably originating from the subependymal matrix zones.[60, 61] In an earlier report, two Colombian owl monkeys inoculated with JC polyoma virus derived from human PML cases manifested glial brain tumors after 16 to 25 months.[62] The neoplasms closely resembled human gliomas of astrocytic origin.[63] Glioma cells derived from these tumors produce infectious JC virus in vitro with altered biologic activity.[64]

EXPRESSION OF JC LARGE T ANTIGEN IN TRANSGENIC MICE

Although the JCV, BKV, and SV40 genomes exhibit extensive nucleotide sequence homology, significant differences in their promoter/enhancer regions appear to affect the host cell specificity of these viruses.[65-67] Transgenic mice expressing JC virus T antigen under the control of SV40 regulatory region exhibited extensive pathology, including B-cell lymphoma and osteosarcoma, which contributed to the early death of animals and prevented successful mating. Expression of JCV or SV40 T antigen was demonstrated in the brain, adrenal gland, thymus, intervertebral disks, and lymphoid tissues. Choroid plexus papilloma developed in one mouse at the age of 41 days.[68]

Polyoma Virus

Polyoma virus is a small papova virus whose natural host is the mouse; it can be tumorigenic when inoculated at high titer into newborn mice.[69]

EXPRESSION OF LARGE AND MEDIUM T ANTIGEN IN TRANSGENIC MICE

Transgenic mice carrying polyoma large T antigen linked to polyoma early region promoter developed pituitary adenomas, hyperplasia of the adrenal medulla, and alteration in male reproductive organs at 14 to 22 months of age.[70] In contrast, those carrying polyoma middle T antigen developed hemangiomas arising at multiple sites in the vasculature and with a variable latency of 10 weeks to 12 months.[70]

In one experiment, a transgenic mouse model was established that proved useful in studying the ontogenesis of neuroblastoma, particularly with regard to early preneoplastic lesions.[71] The generation of this model system was serendipitous, since the original goal of these experiments was to study the consequences of deregulated tyrosine kinase activities in vivo. To this end, the middle T antigen (mT), the transforming oncoprotein of polyoma virus, was introduced into the germ line of mice. Although it lacks enzymatic activity on its own, mT forms complexes with intracellular oncogenes such as c-src, c-yes, and c-fyn and increases their tyrosine kinase activity. In the transgenic mouse model, the cDNA of mT was linked to the thymidine kinase (TK) promoter. Because TK is a constitutive housekeeping gene, the transgene was expected to be expressed at low or moderate levels in a wide variety of tissues. Two of four founder mice died perinatally from generalized hemangiomas, which is the typical phenotype induced by mT in vivo.[72, 73] One single transgenic founder animal was established as a transgenic line. This mouse and all of its transgenic offspring manifested multiple neuroblastomas between 2 and 3 months of age. Characteristic preneoplastic lesions in the sympathetic trunk and the adrenal medulla were identified, such as dysplasia, glial and neuronal hyperplasia, and neuroblastoma in situ. At later stages, malignant invasive tumors arose from

these lesions. Eventually, multiple mediastinal and retroperitoneal masses led to clinical symptoms, such as ascites and circulatory and respiratory failure, in the affected mice. Distant hematogenic metastases, however, were seldom observed. These tumors are similar to human neuroblastomas, including typical sites of development. Histologic and ultrastructural examination showed abundant occurrence of neuroblastic rosettes of the Homer-Wright type and expression of diagnostic markers such as synaptophysin. Northern hybridization analysis demonstrated high levels of expression of the N-myc oncogene. However, amplification of the N-myc genomic locus was never detected in primary tumors, nor was it seen in tumors that had been serially transplanted to nude mice. Freshly explanted neuroblastoma cells had a marked tendency toward terminal neuronal differentiation in vitro. Expression of the transgene (determined by tyrosine kinase assays and by in situ hybridization analysis) was restricted to the neurons of the central and peripheral nervous tissue. This pattern of expression suggests a role for the site of integration of the transgene in directing tissue-specific expression. Integration of medium T in this line of mice may have occurred at a locus important for maturation and growth control of sympathetic neuroblasts.

EXPRESSION OF MEDIUM T ANTIGEN IN BRAIN TRANSPLANTS

Rats carrying transplants expressing the polyoma medium T antigen developed endothelial hemangiomas in the graft that led to fatal cerebral hemorrhage within 13 to 50 days after transplantation.[73] This was consistent with the finding that endothelial cells constitute a prime target for the carcinogenic action of mT[72, 74-76] and that tumors of non-endothelial origin probably arise only in situations in which neoplastic transformation of the endothelial compartment is blocked.[71, 77] Transformation of endothelial cells is possible even in mice in which the c-src gene has been inactivated by homologous recombination.[78] This indicates that middle T antigen–induced formation of endothelial hemangiomas is not mediated by the c-src protein tyrosine kinase. Anaplastic gliomas developed after several months in animals who survived the early post-transplantation period. It appears that the rapid induction of hemangiomas is induced by middle T alone, whereas delayed glioma induction requires additional genetic alterations.

Rous Sarcoma Virus (RSV)

Sarcoma viruses were among the first viruses found to have neuro-oncogenic activity.[3, 79] They have long been used in various animal models to assess the efficacy of chemotherapeutic and radiotherapeutic protocols,[80] including interstitial radiation.[81]

TUMOR INDUCTION BY INTACT VIRUS

Intracerebral injection of various strains of RSV produced intracranial neoplasms in hamsters,[82, 83] rats,[84] mice,[85] rabbits,[86] and dogs.[79] The histogenesis of these neoplasms was at first controversial (for review see reference 3), but a consensus now exists that meningothelial and glial cells are the target of malignant transformation. The tumors induced by RSV, dependent on the site of inoculation, are either meningeal sarcomas or malignant astrocytomas. The latter show the typical histopathologic features of astrocytomas and express GFAP.[87] The target cell specificity was independent of the developmental stage; prenatal inoculation also induced astrocytomas and no neuronal neoplasms.[88]

EXPRESSION OF v-src IN TRANSGENIC MICE

Astrocytic tumors of various grades of malignancy were observed in transgenic mice expressing v-src under regulation by the GFAP promoter. Similar to human glioblastomas, some of the neoplasms showed microvascular proliferation and expressed the vascular endothelial growth factor (VEGF).[116]

EXPRESSION OF v-src IN BRAIN TRANSPLANTS

Expression of the v-src gene in fetal brain transplants caused the induction of anaplastic astrocytomas and malignant mesenchymal tumors (sarcomas), with a 70% incidence after latency periods of 2 to 6 months. Thus, the dual neuroectodermal and mesenchymal tropism was similar to that exerted by the intact virus. It was found by in situ hybridization that the retrovirally transduced oncogene was expressed in all major cell types represented in the graft. This indicates that cell-type specific transformation is due to differential susceptibility of the respective target cell to the oncogene rather than to selective integration or expression of the retroviral construct.[73]

Adenovirus

TUMOR INDUCTION BY INTACT VIRUS

Human adenovirus 12 has been shown to induce neuroblastomas and retinoblastomas in mice, rats, and hamsters after intracerebral and intraorbital inoculation.[89] Simian adenovirus (SA7) induced choroid plexus papillomas and medulloblastomas in the hamster.[90, 91]

EXPRESSION OF E1A AND E1B IN TRANSGENIC MICE

Koike and colleagues[92] established transgenic mice expressing the human adenovirus type 12 E1A and E1B genes under the control of the mouse mammary tumor virus long terminal repeat. All 12 homozygous mice that they examined developed tumors in the olfactory sinus and brain between the ages of 6 and 9 months. These tumors were histologically classified as neuroblastomas.

Papilloma Virus

Transgenic mice expressing HPV16 E6 and E7 open reading frames under the trascriptional regulation of a human β-actin promoter developed brain tumors at an incidence of 87/122 (71%) between 2.5 and 10 months of age.[93] The most frequent type of tumor was an anaplastic neuroepithelial tumor associated with the ependyma of the third ventricle, which locally invaded adjacent brain tissue and spread a considerable distance along the ventricular surface. Other types of tumors were well differentiated choroid plexus carcinomas and pituitary carcinomas. In tumor tissues, expression of HPV16 E6 RNA and E7 oncoprotein were demonstrated. Rb and P53 proteins, which are known to bind to HPV16 E6 and E7, were found to be expressed in cell lines derived from brain tumors that developed in these transgenic mice.[93]

Harvey Sarcoma Virus

Rats with neural transplants harboring an activated v-Ha-ras gene developed solid tumors in the graft at an incidence of approximately 50%.[94] The tumors exhibited a spindle cell morphology and a fascicular growth pattern. Immunohistochemically, they expressed the Ca^{2+}-binding protein S100, but they failed to show immunoreactivity for GFAP or neuronal antigens and were tentatively classified as immature gliomas.[94]

OTHER TRANSFORMATION-ASSOCIATED GENES

neu

Transgenic mice harboring an activated neu oncogene under the transcriptional control of the myelin basic protein gene developed a low incidence of brain tumors that express molecular markers specific to oligodendrocytes.[95]

p53

Mutational inactivation in the p53 tumor suppressor gene is one of the most frequent genetic alterations in human astrocytic brain tumors.[96, 97] In addition, patients carrying p53 germline mutations, often within the setting of the Li-Fraumeni syndrome, frequently manifest brain tumors in addition to breast cancer, sarcomas, leukemia, and adrenocortical carcinomas.[96, 98] These findings indicate that loss of function of the p53 gene can play an important role in the evolution of human brain tumors.

Heterozygous p53 knockout mice are considered an animal model for p53 germline mutations. Several lines of p53 knockout mice have recently been established.[99, 100] Heterozygous p53 knockout mice preferentially developed sarcomas and lymphomas and only 1 of 44 heterozygous mice developed an ependymoma. Homozygous p53 knockout mice developed mostly lymphomas and no brain tumors.[99] Malkin[100] pointed out that genetic background affects the target organ specificity in p53 knockout mice. However, none of the three mouse strains with different genetic backgrounds developed brain tumors at an incidence of more than 2%.

Rb

Some heterozygous mice (approximately 25%) with targeted disruption of the retinoblastoma gene (Rb) manifest adenocarcinomas of the pituitary gland but no retinal or CNS neoplasms.[101] Homozygous knockout mice are nonviable and die from extensive developmental defects in neurogenesis and hematopoiesis.[101, 102]

PTC

Germline mutations in the PATCHED (PTC) gene have been identified as the molecular basis of the basal cell nevus syndrome (BCNS). The gene encodes a Sonic hedgehog (Shh) receptor and a tumor suppressor protein. A subset of mice heterozygously expressing a mutated PTC gene developed cerebellar medulloblastomas, a neoplasm that also occurs within the BCNS syndrome.[117]

COOPERATION OF ONCOGENES AND INTERACTION WITH CHEMICAL CARCINOGENS

It is commonly accepted that neoplastic transformation of primary cells proceeds as a multistep process that involves the combined activation and/or inactivation of several genes. A paradigm has been the cooperation of activated ras and myc oncogenes in a variety of cell types and tissues.[103, 104] More recent data demonstrated combined effects of oncogenes and tumor suppressor genes during the formation of various tumor entities including brain tumors.[105–107] Such complementary actions of cancer-related genes can be systematically examined in transgenic animals and gene transfer models.

c-myc and tax

Transgenic mice expressing HTLV-I long terminal repeat (LTR)/c-myc and those expressing immunoglobin promoter/enhancer/tax (HTLV-I transcription activator) did not develop tumors. However, their double transgenic mice developed CD4+ T-cell lymphomas and CNS tumors at 25 to 90 days of age. The brain tumors were composed of small, round nuclei with a diffuse chromatin pattern.[108]

v-Ha-ras and v-myc

Retroviral vectors were used that either encoded a solitary v-Ha-ras or v-gag/myc gene or co-expressed both genes simultaneously from the same retroviral genome for oncogene transfer into brain transplants.[94] The therapeutic gene did not cause any pathologic phenotype in the transplants. On transfer of an activated v-Ha-ras oncogene, approximately 50% of the grafts developed gliomas after latency periods of 6 to 9 months.

Fetal brain transplants harboring both v-Ha-ras and v-myc demonstrated a dramatic cooperative transforming effect of these oncogenes in transforming neural cells in vivo. All recipient animals with vital transplants displayed multiple tumors in the graft within 2 to 6 weeks of stereotactic implantation. These poorly differentiated malignant tumors

most likely originated from glial precursor cells in the fetal CNS preparation, as indicated by the finding of GFAP immunoreactivity in re-transplanted cell lines derived from the neoplasms. The short latency period and the development of multiple tumors indicate that ras and myc can induce transformation of neural precursor cells without the contribution of additional genes.

The co-expression of ras and myc also elicits transformed foci in organotypic CNS cultures in vitro. The short latency period required for focus formation in vitro would be compatible with a single-step transformation event. On cytologic and immunocytochemical analysis, it was shown that these colonies were derived from immature neural cells, without evidence for neuronal or glial differentiation. Thus, neural precursor cells are a major target cell population for ras/myc oncogene cooperation.

Neural grafts exposed to v-Ha-ras and v-myc at later stages of development (E16) gave rise to neoplasms at a much lower incidence. Direct injection of the retroviral vectors into the brains of newborn rats induced a small number of glial and mesenchymal tumors.[109]

v-myc and Ethylnitrosourea

On embryonal day 14 (ED14), pregnant donor animals (F344 rats) received a single intravenous dose of ENU (50 mg/kg). Twenty-four hours later (ED15), the fetal brains were removed, triturated, and incubated with a retroviral vector carrying the v-gag/myc oncogene. Subsequently, these primary cell suspensions were transplanted stereotactically into the caudate-putamen of syngeneic adult recipients. Of ten recipients harboring ED15 fetal brain transplants, five developed macroscopic tumors in the grafts after latency periods of 3 to 6 months. Histologically, all of the tumors were poorly differentiated neuroectodermal tumors.[35, 110] This indicates that ENU has the potential to mutationally activate or inactivate cellular transforming genes, which can cooperate with myc in neurocarcinogenesis. However, the respective target genes of ENU remain unknown. Attempts by transfection assay to identify a transforming gene involved in the induction of CNS gliomas by ENU have failed. This might indicate that ENU-induced carcinogenesis is mediated via a recessive mechanism, for example, inactivation of a tumor suppressor gene.

p53 and Ethylnitrosourea

Although mutations of the *p53* tumor suppressor gene are infrequent in brain tumors induced by ENU and related alkylated agents, recent evidence suggests that the inactivation of this gene can significantly augment the susceptibility of the murine nervous system to chemical neurocarcinogenesis. Ethylnitrosourea administration to *p53*-heterozygous pregnant mice resulted in rapid development of primary brain tumors in 70% of the p53-null offspring. Brain tumors also developed later in 4% of heterozygous mice, but they had lost the wild-type allele. The authors hypothesized that *p53* may protect embryos from DNA damage induced by transplacental exposure to ENU.[118]

SIGNIFICANCE OF ANIMAL MODELS FOR HUMAN NEURO-ONCOGENESIS

Animal models of malignant transformation in the nervous system have two principal objectives: (1) to identify environmental chemicals or biologic agents (viruses) involved in brain tumor etiology and (2) to advance the identification of cellular and genetic alterations associated with the evolution and progression of CNS neoplasms.

Brain Tumor Etiology

Etiology and evolution of human brain tumors are still largely unknown. Analytical epidemiologic studies have revealed an increased risk of human brain tumor development in association with certain occupations,[111] but, with the exception of therapeutic X-irradiation, attempts to identify a specific exposure or causative environmental agent have been unsuccessful. This includes studies specifically aimed at identifying the role of N-nitroso compounds (i.e., powerful neuro-oncogenic agents in rodents). Similarly, no evidence exists that transplacental exposure to alkylating agents plays a role in the etiology of human pediatric brain tumors, although this route of exposure is the most effective model for inducing CNS tumors in animals. So far, none of the many chemicals with neuro-oncogenic properties in animals has been shown to exert similar effects on the human nervous system. This view is supported by the analysis of mutations occurring in sporadic human gliomas. The predominance of G:C→A:T transition mutations at CpG sites points to an endogenous formation (e.g., deamination of 5-methylcytosine) rather than to a causation by chemical carcinogens.[96]

Mice with targeted disruption of tumor suppressor genes may prove invaluable in the identification of a wider range of neurocarcinogens, particularly in view of advancements in tissue-specific gene disruption. Similarly, transgenic mice with nervous system–specific expression of viral or cellular oncogenes may serve to screen additional exposures.

Elucidation of the Multi-step Nature of Neuro-oncogenesis

Carcinogenesis is a multi-step process that is characterized by the sequential acquisition of genetic alterations, including activation of oncogenes and loss or impaired function of tumor-suppressor genes. Although the molecular basis of brain tumor induction in rodents by alkylating agents remains to be identified, significant progress has been made in the identification of genetic alterations associated with the evolution and progression of human astrocytic tumors. Thus, it seems unlikely that animal models of chemical neurocarcinogenesis will contribute significantly to our understanding of brain tumor induction in humans. However, malignant brain tumors (e.g. the glioblastomas multiforme) contain a great number of genetic alterations, and it is difficult to assess their role if they develop in the late stages of tumor progression. Transgenic mice expressing one or several transformation-associated genes or transplants carrying multiple genetic alterations may provide information on the impact of these genes, both alone and in conjunction with other genetic alterations.

REFERENCES

1. Seligman AM, Shear MJ: Studies in carcinogenesis: VIII. Experimental production of brain tumors in mice with methylcholanthrene. Am J Cancer 1939; 37:364–395.
2. Zimmerman HM, Arnold H: Experimental brain tumors: IV. The incidence in different strains of mice. Cancer Res 1944; 4:98–101.
3. Bigner DD, Swenberg JA: Experimental Tumors of the Central Nervous System. Kalamazoo, Mich, Upjohn Company, 1977.
4. Napalkov N, Alexandrov V: Effect of 7,12-dimethyl-benz(a)anthracene in transplacental carcinogenesis. JNCI 1974; 52:1365–1366.
5. Rice J, Joshi S, Shenefelt R, et al: Transplacental carcinogenic activity of 7,12-dimethylbenz[a]anthracene. In Jones PW, Freudenthal RI (eds): Carcinogenesis, vol. 3. New York, Raven Press, 1978, pp 413–422.
6. Kleihues P, Patzschke K, Doerjer G: DNA modification and repair in the experimental induction of nervous system tumors by chemical carcinogens. Ann N Y Acad Sci 1982; 381:290–303.
7. Druckrey H, Ivankovic S, Preussmann R: Selective induction of malignant tumors in the brain and spinal cord of rats with MNU. Z Krebsforsch 1965; 66:389–408.
8. Druckrey H, Preussmann R, Ivankovic S, et al: Organotrope cancerogene Wirkungen bei 65 verschiedenen N-Nitroso-Verbindungen an BD-Ratten. Z Krebsforsch 1967; 69:103–201.
9. Preussmann R, Ivankovic S, Landschütz C, et al: Carcinogene Wirkungen von 13 Aryldialkyltriazenen an Ratten. Z Krebsforsch 1974; 81:285–310.
10. Druckrey H, Ivankovic S, Preussmann R, et al: Transplacental induction of neurogenic malignancies by 1,2-diethylhydrazine, azo-, and azoxyethane in rats. Experientia 1968; 24:561–562.
11. Ivankovic S, Druckrey H: Transplacentare Erzeugung maligner Tumoren des Nervensystems: I. Athyl-nitroso-harnstoff (ANH) an BD IX-Ratten. Z Krebsforsch 1968; 71:320–360.
12. Ivankovic S: Erzeugung von Malignomen bei Ratten nach transplazentarer Einwirkung von N-Isopropyl-a-2-(methyl-hydrazino)-p-toluamid HCl. Arzneimittelforsch 1972; 22:905–907.
13. Swenberg J, Cooper H, Bucheler J: 1,2-Dimethylhydrazine-induced methylation of DNA bases in various rat organs and the effect of pretreatment with disulfiram. Cancer Res 1979; 39:465–467.
14. Swenberg JA, Clendenon N, Denlinger R, et al: Sequential development of ethylnitrosourea-induced neurinomas: Morphology, biochemistry and transplantability. JNCI 1975; 55:147–152.
15. Kleihues P, Lantos PL, Magee PN: Chemical carcinogenesis in the nervous system. Int Rev Exp Pathol 1976; 15:153–232.
16. Wechsler W, Kleihues P, Matsumoto S, et al: Pathology of experimental neurogenic tumors chemically induced during prenatal and postnatal life. Ann NY Acad Sci 1969; 159:360–408.
17. Schiffer D, Giordana MT, Pezzota S, et al: Cerebral tumours induced by transplacental NEU: Study of the different tumoural stages particularly of early proliferations. Acta Neuropathol (Berl) 1978; 41:27–31.
18. Lantos PL, Pilkington GJ: The development of experimental brain tumors: A sequential light and electron microscopic study of the subependymal plate: I. Early lesions (abnormal cell clusters). Acta Neuropathol (Berl) 1979; 45:167–175.
19. Burger PC, Shibata T, Aguzzi A, et al: Selective induction by N-nitrosoethylurea of oligodendrogliomas in fetal forebrain transplants. Cancer Res 1988; 48:2871–2875.
20. Vaquero J, Coca S, Zurita M, et al: Synaptophysin expression in "ependymal tumors" induced by ethylnitrosourea in rats. Am J Pathol 1992; 141:1037–1041.
21. Kleihues P, Rajewsky MF: Chemical neuro-oncogenesis: Role of structural DNA modifications, DNA repair and neural target cell population. Prog Exp Tumor Res 1984; 27:1–16.
22. Singer B, Grunberger D: Molecular Biology of Mutagens and Carcinogens, ed 1. New York, Plenum Press, 1983.
23. Pegg AE: Mammalian O⁶-alkylguanine-DNA alkyltransferase: Regulation and importance in response to alkylating carcinogenic and therapeutic agents. Cancer Res 1990; 50:6119–6129.
24. Goth R, Rajewsky MF: Persistence of O⁶-ethylguanine in rat-brain

DNA: Correlation with nervous system-specific carcinogenesis by ethylnitrosourea. Proc Natl Acad Sci USA 1974; 71:639–643.

25. Margison GP, Kleihues P: Chemical carcinogenesis in the nervous system: Preferential accumulation of O^6-methylguanine in rat brain deoxyribonucleic acid during repetitive administration of N-methyl-N-nitrosourea. Biochem J 1975; 148:521–525.

26. Sukumar S: Ras oncogenes in chemical carcinogenesis. Curr Top Microbiol Immunol 1989; 148:93–114.

27. Calvert R, Hongyo T, Buzard G, et al: Mutations in the p53 gene of transplacentally induced rat gliomas. Proc Am Assoc Cancer Res 1994; 35:1033.

28. Bargmann CI, Hung MC, Weinberg RA: Multiple independent activations of the *neu* oncogene by a point mutation altering the transmembrane domain of p185. Cell 1986; 45:649–657.

29. Perantoni AO, Rice JM, Reed CD, et al: Activated neu oncogene sequences in primary tumors of the peripheral nervous system induced in rats by transplacental exposure to ethylnitrosourea. Proc Natl Acad Sci USA 1987; 84:6317–6321.

30. Nikitin AY, Ballering LAP, Lyons J, et al: Early mutation of the neu(erbB-2) gene during ethylnitrosourea-induced oncogenesis in the rat Schwann cell lineage. Proc Natl Acad Sci USA 1991; 88:9939–9943.

31. Ohgaki H, Vogeley KT, Kleihues P, et al: Neu mutations and loss of normal allele in schwannomas induced by N-ethyl-N-nitrosourea in rats. Cancer Lett 1993; 70:45–50.

32. Nikitin A, Lennartz K, Pozharisski K, et al: Rat model of the human ''Triton'' tumor: Direct genetic evidence for the myogenic differentiation capacity of schwannoma cells using the mutant neu gene as a cell lineage marker. Differentiation 1991; 48:33–42.

33. Nakamura T, Ushijima T, Ishizaka Y, et al: neu proto-oncogene mutation is specific for the neurofibromas in a N-nitroso-N-ethylurea-induced hamster neurofibromatosis model but not for hamster melanomas and human Schwann cell tumors. Cancer Res 1994; 54:976–980.

34. Saya H, Ara S, Lee PS, et al: Direct sequencing analysis of transmembrane region of human Neu gene by polymerase chain reaction. Mol Carcinog 1990; 3:198–201.

35. Wiestler OD, Brüstle O, Eibl RH, et al: Oncogene transfer into the brain. Recent Results Cancer Res 1994; 135:55–66.

36. Green M: When the products of oncogenes and anti-oncogenes meet. Cell 1989; 56:1–3.

37. Duffell D, Hinz R, Nelson E: Neoplasms in hamsters induced by simian virus 40: Light and electron microscopic observations. Am J Pathol 1964; 45:59–73.

38. Eddy BE: Simian virus 40 (SV-40): An oncogenic virus. Prog Exp Tumor Res 1964; 4:1–26.

39. Ikuta F, Ogawa H, Kumanishi T: Experimental DNA virus-induced brain tumors. *In* Kornyey S, Tariska S, Gosztonyi G, (eds): Proceedings of the VIIth International Congress on Neuropathology. Amsterdam, Excerpta Medica, 1975, 1, pp 453–460.

40. Duigou GJ, Walsh JW, Oeltgen J, et al: Alterations in SV40 DNA integration patterns are associated with acquisition of the invasive phenotype in hamster brain tumors. Anticancer Res 1990; 10:1683–1692.

41. Fung K, Trojanowski J: Animal models of medulloblastomas and related primitive neuroectodermal tumors: A review. J Neuropathol Exp Neurol 1995; 54:285–296.

42. Geissler E: SV40 and human brain tumors. Prog Med Virol 1990; 37:211–222.

43. Suri C, Fung BP, Tischler AS, et al: Catecholaminergic cell lines from the brain and adrenal glands of tyrosine hydroxylase-SV40 T antigen transgenic mice. J Neurosci 1993; 13:1280–1291.

44. Theuring F, Götz W, Balling R, et al: Tumorigenesis and eye abnormalities in transgenic mice expressing MSV-SV40 large T-antigen. Oncogene 1990; 5:225–232.

45. Korf HW, Götz W, Herken R, et al: S-antigen and rod-opsin immunoreactions in midline brain neoplasms of transgenic mice: Similarities to pineal cell tumors and certain medulloblastomas in man. J Neuropathol Exp Neurol 1990; 49:424–437.

46. Götz W, Theuring F, Schachenmayr W, et al: Midline brain tumors in MSV-SV 40-transgenic mice originate from the pineal organ. Acta Neuropathol (Berl) 1992; 83:308–314.

47. Marcus DM, Carpenter JL, O'Brien JM, et al: Primitive neuroectodermal tumor of the midbrain in a murine model of retinoblastoma. Invest Ophthalmol Vis Sci 1991; 32:293–301.

48. Windle JJ, Albert DM, O'Brien JM, et al: Retinoblastoma in transgenic mice. Nature 1990; 343:665–669.

49. Hammang JP, Behringer RR, Baetge EE, et al: Oncogene expression in retinal horizontal cells of transgenic mice results in a cascade of neurodegeneration. Neuron 1993; 10:1197–1209.

50. Baetge EE, Behringer RR, Messing A, et al: Transgenic mice express the human phenylethanolamine N-methyltransferase gene in adrenal medulla and retina. Proc Natl Acad Sci USA 1988; 85:3648–3652.

51. al Ubaidi MR, Font RL, Quiambao AB, et al: Bilateral retinal and brain tumors in transgenic mice expressing simian virus 40 large T antigen under control of the human interphotoreceptor retinoid-binding protein promoter. J Cell Biol 1992; 119:1681–1687.

52. Chen JD, van Dyke T: Uniform cell-autonomous tumorigenesis of the choroid plexus by papovavirus large T antigens. Mol Cell Biol 1991; 11:5968–5976.

53. Chen J, Tobin GJ, Pipas JM, et al: T-antigen mutant activities in vivo: Roles of p53 and pRB binding in tumorigenesis of the choroid plexus. Oncogene 1992; 7:1167–1175.

54. Eibl RH, Kleihues P, Jat PS, et al: A model for primitive neuroectodermal tumors in transgenic neural transplants harboring the SV40 large T antigen. Am J Pathol 1994; 144:556–564.

55. Howley PM, Levine AJ, Li FP, et al: Lack of SV40 DNA in tumors from scientists working with SV40 virus. N Engl J Med 1991; 324:494

56. Bergsagel DJ, Finegold MJ, Butel JS, et al: DNA sequences similar to those of simian virus 40 in ependymomas and choroid plexus tumors of childhood. N Engl J Med 1992; 326:988–993.

57. Lang W, Miklossy J, Deruaz JP, et al: Neuropathology of the acquired immune deficiency syndrome (AIDS): A report of 135 consecutive autopsy cases from Switzerland. Acta Neuropathol (Berl) 1989; 77:379–390.

58. Walker D, Padgett B, ZuRhein G, et al: Human papovavirus (JC): Induction of brain tumors in hamsters. Science 1973; 181:674–676.

59. Matsuda M, Yasui K, Nagashima K, et al: Origin of the medulloblastoma experimentally induced by human polyomavirus JC. JNCI 1987; 79:585–591.

60. Ohsumi S, Ikehara I, Motoi M, et al: Induction of undifferentiated brain tumors in rats by a human polyomavirus (JC virus). Jpn J Cancer Res 1985; 76:429–431.

61. Horie Y, Motoi M, Ogawa K: Early stages of development of rat brain tumors induced by JC virus: A sequential histological and immunohistochemical study. Acta Med Okayama 1989; 43:271–279.

62. London WT, Houff SA, Madden DL, et al: Brain tumors in owl monkeys inoculated with human polyomavirus (JC virus). Science 1978; 201:1246–1249.

63. Houff SA, London WT, DiChiro G, et al: Neuroradiological studies of JCV-induced astrocytomas in nonhuman primates. Prog Clin Biol Res 1983; 105:253–259.

64. Major EO, Vacante DA, Traub RG, et al: Owl monkey astrocytoma cells in culture spontaneously produce infectious JC virus which demonstrates altered biological properties. J Virol 1987; 61:1435–1441.

65. Frisque R: Nucleotide sequence of the region encompassing the JC virus origin of DNA replication. J Virol 1983; 46:170–176.

66. Gruss P, Dhar R, Khoury G: The SV40 tandem repeated sequences as an element of the early promotor. Proc Natl Acad Sci USA 1981; 78:943–947.

67. Rosenthal N, Kress M, Gruss P, et al: BK viral enhancer element and a human cellular homolog. Science 1983; 222:749–755.

68. Ressetar HG, Prakash O, Frisque RJ, et al: Expression of viral T-antigen in pathological tissues from transgenic mice carrying JC-SV40 chimeric DNAs. Mol Chem Neuropathol 1993; 20:59–79.

69. Eddy B: Polyomavirus. *In* Foster H, Small J, Fox J, (eds): The Mouse in Biomedical Research. New York, Academic Press, 1982, pp 293–311.

70. Bautch VL: Effect of polyoma virus oncogenes in transgenic mice. Mol Biol Med 1989; 6:309–317.

71. Aguzzi A, Wagner EF, Williams RL, et al: Sympathetic hyperplasia and neuroblastomas in transgenic mice expressing polyoma middle T antigen. New Biol 1990; 2:533–543.

72. Williams RL, Risau W, Zerwes HG, et al: Endothelioma cells expressing the polyoma middle T oncogene induce hemangiomas by host cell recruitment. Cell 1989; 57:1053–1063.

73. Aguzzi A, Kleihues P, Heckl K, et al: Cell type-specific tumor induction in neural transplants by retrovirus-mediated oncogene transfer. Oncogene 1991; 6:113–118.

74. Bautch VL, Toda S, Hassell JA, et al: Endothelial cell tumors develop in transgenic mice carrying polyoma virus middle T oncogene. Cell 1987; 51:529–537.

75. Williams RL, Courtneidge SA, Wagner EF: Embryonic lethalities and endothelial tumors in chimeric mice expressing polyoma virus middle T oncogene. Cell 1988; 52:121–131.

76. Montesano R, Pepper MS, Mohle-Steinlein U, et al: Increased proteolytic activity is responsible for the aberrant morphogenetic behavior of endothelial cells expressing the middle T oncogene. Cell 1990; 62:435–445.

77. Rassoulzadegan M, Courtneidge SA, Loubiere R, et al: A variety of tumours induced by the middle T antigen of polyoma virus in a transgenic mouse family. Oncogene 1990; 5:1507–1510.

78. Thomas JE, Aguzzi A, Soriano P, et al: Induction of tumor formation and cell transformation by polyoma middle T antigen in the absence of Src. Oncogene 1993; 8:2521–2529.

79. Rabotti GF, Grove AS, Sellers RL, et al: Induction of multiple brain tumours (gliomata and leptomeningeal sarcomata) in dogs by Rous sarcoma virus. Nature 1966; 209:884–886.

80. Steinbok P, Mahaley MS, U R, Zinn DC, et al: Synergism between BCNU and irradiation in the treatment of anaplastic gliomas: An in vivo study using the avian sarcoma virus-induced glioma model. J Neurosurg 1979; 51:581–586.

81. Ostertag C, Warnke P, Kleihues P, et al: Iodine-125 interstitial irradiation of virally induced dog brain tumours. Neurol Res 1984; 6:176–180.

82. Rabotti GF, Raine WA: Brain tumours induced in hamsters inoculated intracerebrally at birth with Rous sarcoma virus. Nature 1964; 204:898–899.

83. Bigner D, Odom G, Mahaley MJ, et al: Brain tumors induced in dogs by the Schmidt-Ruppin strain of Rous sarcoma virus: Neuropathological and immunological observations. J Neuropathol Exp Neurol 1969; 28:648–680.

84. Wilfong RF, Bigner DD, Self DJ, et al: Brain tumor types induced by the Schmidt-Ruppin strain of Rous sarcoma virus in inbred Fischer rats. Acta Neuropathol (Berl) 1973; 25:196–206.

85. Kumanishi T, Ikuta F, Yamamoto T: Brain tumors induced by Rous sarcoma virus, Schmidt-Ruppin strain: III. Morphology of brain tumors induced by adult mice. JNCI 1973; 50:95–109.

86. Rabotti GF, Sellers RL, Anderson WR: Leptomeningeal sarcoma and glioma induced in rabbits by Rous sarcoma virus. Nature 1966; 209:524–526.

87. Britt RH, Lyons BE, Eng LF, et al: Immunohistochemical study of glial fibrillary acidic protein in avian sarcoma virus-induced gliomas in dogs. J Neurooncol 1985; 3:53–59.

88. Copeland DD, Bigner DD: Glial-mesenchymal tropism of in vivo avian sarcoma virus neuro-oncogenesis in rats. Acta Neuropathol (Berl) 1978; 41:23–25.

89. Mukai N, Kobayashi S: Primary brain and spinal cord tumors induced by human adenovirus type 12 in hamsters. J Neuropathol Exp Neurol 1973; 32:523–541.

90. Merkow LP, Slifkin M, Pardo M, et al: Pathogenesis of oncogenic simian adenoviruses: VIII. The histopathology and ultrastructure of simian adenovirus 7-induced intracranial neoplasms. Exp Mol Pathol 1970; 12:264–274.

91. Chen T, Mora E, Mealey JJ: Cultivation of medulloblastoma cells derived from simian adenovirus SA7-induced hamster brain tumor. Cancer Res 1975; 35:3566–3570.

92. Koike K, Jay G, Hartley JW, et al: Activation of retrovirus in transgenic mice: Association with development of olfactory neuroblastoma. J Virol 1990; 64:3988–3991.

93. Arbeit JM, Munger K, Howley PM, et al: Neuroepithelial carcinomas in mice transgenic with human papillomavirus type 16 E6/E7 ORFs. Am J Pathol 1993; 142:1187–1197.

94. Wiestler OD, Aguzzi A, Schneemann M, et al: Oncogene complementation in fetal brain transplants. Cancer Res 1992; 52:3760–3767.

95. Hayes C, Kelly D, Murayama S, et al: Expression of the neu oncogene under the transcriptional control of the myelin basic protein gene in transgenic mice: Generation of transformed glial cells. J Neurosci Res 1992; 31:175–187.

96. Ohgaki H, Schäuble B, zur Hausen A, et al: Genetic alterations associated with the evolution and progression of astrocytic brain tumours. Virchows Arch 1995; 427:113–118.

97. Louis DN: The p53 gene and protein in human brain tumors. J Neuropathol Exp Neurol 1994; 53:11–21.

98. Kleihues P, zur Hausen A, Schäuble B, et al: Tumours associated with p53 germline mutations: A synopsis of 75 families. Submitted for publication.

99. Jacks T, Remington L, Williams BO, et al: Tumor spectrum analysis in p53-mutant mice. Curr Biol 1994; 4:1–7.

100. Malkin D: p53 and the Li-Fraumeni syndrome. Biochim Biophys Acta 1994; 1198:197–213.

101. Jacks T, Fazeli A, Schmitt EM, et al: Effects of an Rb mutation in the mouse. Nature 1992; 359:295–300.

102. Lee EYHP, Chang C-Y, Hu N, et al: Mice deficient for Rb are nonviable and show defects in neurogenesis and haematopoiesis. Nature 1992; 359:288–294.

103. Land H, Parada LF, Weinberg RA: Tumorigenic conversion of primary embryo fibroblasts requires at least two cooperating oncogenes. Nature 1983; 304:596–602.

104. Hunter T: Cooperation betweeen oncogenes. Cell 1991; 64:249–270.

105. Vogelstein B, Kinzler KW: The multistep nature of cancer. Trends Genet 1993; 9:138–141.

106. Knudson A: Antioncogenes and human cancer. Proc Natl Acad Sci USA 1993; 90:10914–10921.

107. von Deimling A, Louis DN, Schramm J, et al: Astrocytic gliomas: Characterization on a molecular genetic basis. Recent Results Cancer Res 1994; 135:33–42.

108. Benvenisty N, Ornitz DM, Bennett GL, et al: Brain tumours and lymphomas in transgenic mice that carry HTLV-I LTR/c-myc and Ig/tax genes. Oncogene 1992; 7:2399–2405.

109. Radner H, el Shabrawy Y, Eibl RH, et al: Tumor induction by ras and myc oncogenes in fetal and neonatal brain: Modulating effects of developmental stage and retroviral dose. Acta Neuropathol (Berl) 1993; 86:456–465.

110. Brüstle O, Petersen I, Radner H, et al: Complementary tumor induction in neural grafts exposed to N-ethyl-N-nitrosourea and an activated myc gene. Carcinogenesis 1993; 14:1715–1718.

111. Thomas TL, Waxweiler RJ: Brain tumors and occupational risk factors. Scand J Work Environ Hlth 1986; 12:1–15.

112. Blass-Kampmann S, Bilzer T, Rajewsky MF: gp130RB13-6-Positive neural progenitor cells are susceptible to the oncogenic effect of ethylnitrosourea in pre-natal rat brain. Neuropathol Appl Neurobiol 1998; 24:9–20.

113. Son JH, Chung JH, Huh SO, et al: Immortalization of neuroendocrine pinealocytes from transgenic mice by targeted tumorigenesis using the tryptophan hydroxylase promoter. Brain Res Mol Brain Res 1996; 37:32–40.

114. Lednicky JA, Garcea RL, Bergsagel DJ, et al: Natural simian virus 40 strains are present in human choroid plexus and ependymoma tumors. Virology 1995; 212:710–717.

115. Martini F, Iaccheri L, Lazzarin L, et al: SV40 early region and large T antigen in human brain tumors, peripheral blood cells, and sperm fluids from healthy individuals. Cancer Res 1996; 56:4820–4825.

116. Weissenberer J, Steinbach JP, Malin G, et al: Development and malignant progression of astrocytomas in GFAP-v-src transgenic mice. Oncogene 1997; 14:2005–2013.

117. Goodrich LV, Milenkovitch L, Higgins KM, et al: Altered neural fates and medulloblastoma in mouse patched mutants. Science 1997; 277:1109–1113.

118. Oda H, Zhang S, Tsurutani N, et al: Loss of p53 is an early event in induction of brain tumors in mice by transplacental carcinogen exposure. Cancer Res 1997; 57:646–650.

119. Danks RA, Orian JM, Gonzales MF, et al: Transformation of astrocytes in transgenic mice expressing SV40 T antigen under the transcriptional control of the glial fibrillary acidic protein promoter. Cancer Res 1995; 55:4302–4310.

120. Enjoji M, Iwaki T, Nawata H, et al: IgH intronic enhancer element HE2 (mu B) functions as a cis-activator in choroid plexus cells at the cellular level as well as in transgenic mice. J Neurochem 1995; 64:961–966.

121. Servenius B, Vernachio J, Price J, et al: Metastasizing neuroblastomas in mice transgenic for simian virus 40 large T (SV40T) under the olfactory marker protein gene promoter. Cancer Res 1994: 54:5198–5205.

122. Krynska B, Otte J, Franks R, et al: Human ubiquitous JCV.CY T-antigen gene induces brain tumors in experimental animals. Oncogene (in press).

123. Rovigatti U, Afanasyeva T, Brandner S, et al: Transgenic mice as research tools in neurocarcinogenesis. J Neurovirol 1998; 4:159–174.

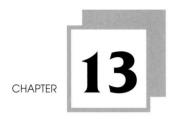

13

Human Glioma Cultures and In Vitro Analysis of Therapeutic Response

Since the pioneering works of Kredel[54] and Buckley,[27] significant advances have been made in the science and technology of in vitro culture of human and animal gliomas, particularly during the period leading up to the early 1970s, when major developments in basic culture techniques were accomplished.[16, 24, 48, 49, 59, 60, 62–64, 74, 75, 84, 85, 108] In vitro culture models have been indispensable in advancing our understanding of the cellular and molecular mechanisms underlying the biology and clinical behavior of human normal brain and of glial neoplasms[11, 17, 20, 29, 31, 55, 92, 94, 106, 109] and have also served as powerful preclinical models in the screening of new agents and in the evaluation of novel therapeutic strategies.[15, 36, 50, 82, 86, 99] This chapter reviews current advances in the culture and characterization of human glial tumors and the use of these systems in pharmacologic studies and in pretherapeutic determination of tumor sensitivity and/or resistance to chemotherapeutic agents.

ESTABLISHING HUMAN GLIOMAS IN CULTURE

With current techniques, the majority of human malignant gliomas, particularly astrocytomas, can be successfully established in culture.[3, 31, 35, 56] This is largely a reflection of the methodological progress that has been accomplished, particularly in the development of enzymatic techniques for dissociating primary specimens into single cells.[81, 91, 97] Single cell suspensions of gliomas not only facilitate the successful establishment of in vitro cultures, but the resulting cultures, compared with the earlier methods of "organ" culture and tissue explants, are more representative of the cellular composition of the tumors. Furthermore, single cell suspensions are a prerequisite for quantitative cell biologic studies, such as clonogenic assays and glioma cell growth kinetic analysis.[47]

The basic method of obtaining single cell suspensions from primary gliomas involves treating the minced tumor specimen with an enzyme cocktail consisting of DNase type I (2,000 units/mg), neutral protease (1 unit/mg), and type Ia collagenase (125 units/mg) in Ca^{2+}/Mg^{2+}–free Hank's balanced salt solution (CMF-HBSS) for a period of up to 1 hour at 37 °C. The resulting cell suspension is sieved through a 60-μm mesh nylon sieve, the cells are washed twice by centrifugation at $300 \times g$ for 10 minutes, and the cell pellet is resuspended in fresh Dulbecco's minimum essential medium (DMEM). Primary cultures are then established from this cell suspension by plating at 1 to 5×10^5 cells/mL in DMEM containing fetal calf serum (FCS) that had been heat-inactivated at 65 °C for 1 hour. Under these conditions, human glioma cells grow as monolayers; when confluent, they are passaged by treating the monolayers for 1 to 3 minutes with a solution of 0.125 mg/mL of trypsin and 0.02 mg/mL of Na_2EDTA in CMF-HBSS. To avoid contamination, it is an absolute requirement that aseptic technique be used throughout the initiation and passage of cultures and that all materials and solutions be sterile.

CELLULAR, BIOCHEMICAL, AND MOLECULAR CHARACTERIZATION OF CULTURED GLIOMA CELLS

Despite the relative ease of culturing human gliomas, their inherent high degree of cellular and biologic heterogeneity[20, 56, 76, 93, 100] make them complex biologic systems to study. It is thus critical that once they are established glioma cultures are well characterized with respect to their glial and neoplastic nature and to other phenotypic and genotypic characteristics relevant to the question being studied. The earliest and most frequently used technique for characterizing glial tumors in culture is cytomorphology.[20, 40, 73, 83] This is performed by phase-contrast microscopy of live cells or by bright-field microscopic examination of formalin-fixed and hematoxylin-eosin stained cultures. Figure 13–1 shows representative hematoxylin-eosin stained cultures of human gliomas of varying malignancies and, in contrast, cultures of nonglial brain tumors: meningioma and medulloblastoma.

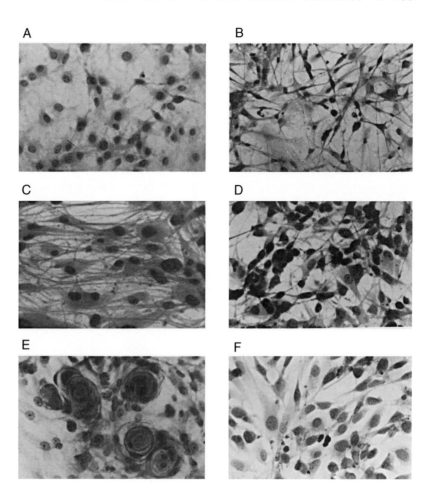

Figure 13–1 Hematoxylin-eosin staining of cultures of human malignant gliomas and non-glial brain tumors: *A,* normal reactive astrocytes; *B,* astrocytoma; *C,* anaplastic astrocytoma; *D,* glioblastoma multiforme; *E,* meningioma; and *F,* medulloblastoma. Notice the cellular pleomorphism of the malignant astrocytoma cultures and the whorl formation that is characteristic of meningothelial cells in meningioma.

Human glioma cells grown in two-dimensional in vitro culture fall into one of three main morphologic types, or variations thereof, namely: (1) fibroblastic, bipolar cells; (2) small polygonal cells with multiple processes; and (3) large epithelioid cells with little to no process formation. Most tumors, particularly in early in vitro culture, consist of mixtures of these different cell types, and the predominance of one or another cell type imparts a unique growth pattern to the culture.[20] As shown in Figure 13–1, cells of highly malignant astrocytomas are typically highly pleomorphic in shape and size and in the number, size, and shape of nuclei and nucleoli. Significant intercellular variability in nuclear and cytoplastic staining also occurs, and little to no contact inhibition takes place, resulting in the "piling up" of cells as they proliferate.

Ultrastructural morphology, examined by both transmission and scanning electron microscopy, offers an additional method of characterization of glioma cells in culture.[95] Figure 13–2A shows a scanning electron micrograph of a cell of a human glioblastoma multiforme in in vitro culture.

Immunologic techniques are also commonly used in the characterization of cultured glioma cells. This can be performed either by immunocytochemistry, immunofluorescence or western blotting. The antibodies used include those against glial cell specific proteins, such as glial fibrillary acidic protein (GFAP) for astrocytes,[18, 19, 33] or galactocerebroside for oligodendroglial cells[77] and against other nervous system or brain tumor antigens.[42, 44, 46, 104] Figure 13–2B shows malignant astrocytoma cultures of different cytomorphological cell types stained for GFAP with the avidin-biotin immunoperoxidase method.

Molecular analyses, including determining the level and pattern of gene expression with techniques of polymerase chain reaction, in situ hybridization, Northern blotting, and functional protein assays are powerful tools for characterizing cultured glioma cells. Structural alterations in specific genes, such as amplifications, rearrangements, and deletions and losses of oncogenes, suppressor genes, and growth factor genes, are also used to characterize glial tumor cells in culture. Finally, biologic parameters, such as cytogenetics, growth kinetics, cell-cycle phase distribution, and pattern of response to anticancer agents and radiation are useful for characterizing glioma cultures in specific cases.

The utility of in vitro glioma cultures for cellular and molecular studies often depends on the preservation, during culture, of the phenotypic and/or genotypic traits of interest. Generally, however, many of these features are unstable in culture and evolve rapidly after culture initiation.[22, 70, 79, 84, 93] It is thus critical that the cells be monitored with respect to the phenotype and/or genotype being studied at regular intervals during in vitro culture. One striking example of in vitro–induced changes is the loss of some of the cellular complexity and characteristic pleomorphism that often characterize early cultures of malignant gliomas. These changes

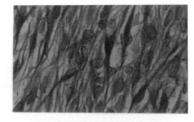

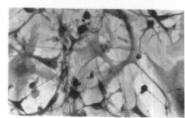

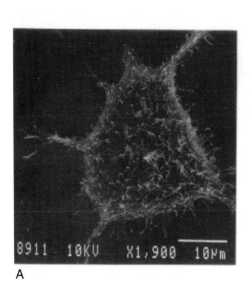

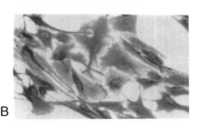

Figure 13–2 Characterization of cultured malignant glioma cells. *A,* Scanning electron micrograph of a glioblastoma multiforme cell in culture. Note the extensive process formation. *B,* Avidin-biotin immunoperoxidase staining for GFAP in cells of glioblastoma multiforme (*top* and *center*) and anaplastic astrocytoma (*bottom*). Note the positive GFAP reactivity of cells of different shapes and sizes.

in cultured glioma cells over time reflect, in part, the inherent genetic instability of human gliomas, but they also reflect the epigenetic pressures resulting from factors such as lack of interaction with other cell types, the two-dimensional monolayer growth on plastic, and/or selective growth advantage of specific subpopulations of cells that have the highest in vitro growth rates and/or that adapt most readily to in vitro growth conditions.

The molecular genetics and cytogenetics of gliomas have been discussed extensively in other sections of this book. These aspects of glioma cells also undergo significant changes in extended in vitro culture, leading to altered gene expression with accompanying changes in phenotype.[22] Cytogenetic changes that have been observed during long-term glioma cultures include the gain and/or loss of whole chromosomes, changes in karyotype, and acquisition of new chromosomal markers.[22, 70, 92] Figure 13–3 shows karyotypes of three glioblastoma cell lines established in the author's laboratory. Recently, evidence from different laboratories has shown that in comparison to primary specimens, glioma cell lines have a significantly higher level of deletions in the newly discovered p16 putative tumor suppressor gene, which encodes an inhibitor of the cyclin-dependent kinase, CdK4, and is involved in cell cycle regulation.[28, 98] This high level of p16 gene deletions in cell lines could be an artifact of in vitro culture or could represent the selective in vitro growth of cells with this genetic abnormality.

CLONING OF HUMAN GLIOMA STEM CELLS

Human tumor cell cloning is based on the concept that tumors are biologic self-renewing systems that contain sub-

populations of tumor stem cells with a high proliferative capacity, also referred to as *clonogenic cells.*[34, 71] Conceptually, therefore, tumor stem cells are responsible for the expansion of the tumor burden and for tumor response to therapy. Tumor stem cells can be quantified in vitro by cloning them in a semi-solid matrix, such as agar, plasma clot, or methylcellulose, or on plastic tissue culture surfaces.[45, 66, 87, 89] Such clonogenic assays are powerful tools for screening for new anticancer agents, for testing new therapeutic modalities, and for pretherapeutic determination of tumor response to therapy. Clonogenic assays are also invaluable in studies of the effect of protein inhibitors, growth factors, antisense oligodeoxynucleotides, and regulators of cell growth and differentiation. A variety of cell cloning techniques have been adapted for cloning human glioma stem cells.[8, 81, 87] Because of their selectivity for malignant cells, however, anchorage-independent assays are biologically more appropriate for cloning of glial tumor cells, and they generally will not support the clonal growth of normal and/or reactive astrocytes and other normal cells that are usually present in the tumor. In the author's laboratory, a specific variant of the tumor clonogenic cell assay, one that utilizes glass capillaries,[5, 66] has been developed. The capillary glioma clonogenic cell assay requires as little as a tenth the amount of cells and materials, has higher plating efficiencies, and yields higher rates of cloning success than other clonogenic assays.[10, 101] The basic technique of the capillary tumor stem cell assay for gliomas is relatively simple; it has been described in detail.[3] It consists of the preparation of a cloning mixture containing glioma cells at 5×10^4 cells/mL in an enriched DMEM cloning medium containing 0.2% low–melting-point agarose. Drugs, test agents, or additives are then added to the desired final concentrations, and after thorough mixing, 50 µL of the

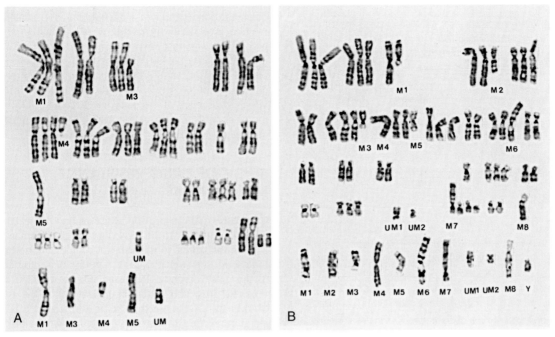

Figure 13–3 *A* and *B,* Karyotypes of cells of two glioblastoma multiformes in culture. The cells had undergone nine in vitro passages prior to analysis. Marker chromosomes are noted in each case.

cloning mixture is drawn in triplicate into sterile glass micro-capillary tubes; it is then allowed to solidify on a cold surface and is incubated at 37 °C for approximately 2 to 3 weeks. The capillary contents are then flushed onto glass slides, and colonies approximately 60 μm in diameter are counted under inverted phase microscopy. Using this method, the cloning success rate in the author's laboratory is approximately 75% for malignant gliomas. Figure 13–3C shows typical colonies of an anaplastic astrocytoma under indirect illumination.

DETERMINATION OF DRUG SENSITIVITY OF GLIOMA CELLS

One of the best studied applications of tumor cell cultures and clonogenic cell assays is for the determination of the inherent tumor sensitivity and/or resistance to anticancer agents.[26, 50, 51, 69, 82, 88, 90, 99] Such information has been used both retrospectively and prospectively to analyze patient response to specific anticancer agents or to a combination of agents, and to prospectively design chemotherapy for individual patients.[4, 53, 87, 89, 103] It should be emphasized, however, that the ultimate response of a glioma patient to therapy is dependent on a complex variety of many different factors, some of which are tumor-related and others of which are not. Among the latter are the blood-brain barrier, the degree of tumor vascularization, drug metabolism and pharmacokinetics, drug delivery, and the degree of hypoxia in the tumor. Significant interpatient and intertumoral differences also exist with respect to these factors. It is thus difficult to quantitatively assess many of these factors and their relative contribution to patient response. The inherent drug sensitivity of the tumor cells, on the other hand, is

largely a result of the inherent biology of the tumor cells and is quantifiable with clonogenic assays; in some cases, in vivo parameters can be mimicked in these assays. For example, pharmacokinetic principles and drug metabolism using hepatic microsomal activating systems[58] have been successfully incorporated into tumor clonogenic assays.

A large number of retrospective and prospective clinical correlative trials have been reported that show that tumor clonogenic cell assays are capable of predicting patient response to therapy, often with a higher degree of accuracy for resistance than for sensitivity.[4, 51, 87, 89, 103, 105] In ovarian carcinoma, therapy directed by a clonogenic assay has been shown to result in a higher rate of complete and partial remissions and fewer failures than standard therapy or the physician's best choice of therapy.[105] Using the capillary clonogenic cell assay in a prospective clinical study[4] of brain tumors in 19 patients, 17 of which were gliomas, my colleagues and I have shown a true-positive prediction of 67% for patients who responded to therapy and a 100% accuracy in predicting patients who failed to respond. Although the number of patients was small, the study clearly demonstrated the potential of these types of analyses and suggested that their appropriate use could play an important role in the management of the brain tumor patient. In another study,[6] my colleagues and I used the clonogenic assay to determine cross-resistance patterns of 12 carmustine-resistant primary malignant gliomas (anaplastic astrocytomas and glioblastomas multiforme) to different anticancer agents that have been used, alone or in combination with other agents, in the treatment of human gliomas. The results, summarized in Table 13–1, showed that of the nine drugs tested, cisplatin had the lowest degree of cross-resistance with carmustine, and procarbazine had the highest level. These data suggest that cisplatin might be a useful agent to combine with

TABLE 13–1

CROSS-RESISTANCE PATTERN OF CARMUSTINE-RESISTANT HUMAN PRIMARY MALIGNANT ASTROCYTOMAS TO ANTICANCER AGENTS USED IN CLINICAL BRAIN TUMOR CHEMOTHERAPY*

Anticancer Agents Tested	No. of Tumors Tested	% Carmustine Cross-Resistance†
Cis-dichlordiammineplatinum II	16	40
Etoposide	12	73
Procarbazine	16	87
Dianhydrogalactitol	16	67
Methotrexate	12	81
Hydroxyurea	16	73
Fluorouracil	12	60
Thioguanine	16	67
Vincristine	14	69

*Drug sensitivity was determined by the capillary clonogenic cell assay.

†Percent carmustine (BCNU) cross-resistance (%CR) of a given drug is defined as follows:

$$\%CR = (N_{drug}/N_{BCNU}) \times 100$$

where N_{BCNU} is the total number of carmustine-resistant tumors and N_{drug} is the number of tumors resistant to the drug.

carmustine in glioma treatment protocols or, alternatively, that cisplatin will be a useful second-line agent in the therapy of carmustine-resistant gliomas.

An important consideration in the use of clonogenic assays to predict glioma patient response to therapy relates to the drug concentrations to which the tumor cells are exposed.[2, 9] It is critical that these drug concentrations and the duration to which the tumor cells are exposed to them are clinically relevant. In the planning of such predictive assays, clinically relevant drug exposure parameters, namely, drug concentrations, exposure times, and areas under the curve (AUCs), can be determined from in vitro drug decay kinetics, as previously described,[8] using the following equations:

$$k = 0.693/t_{1/2}$$

where k is the in vitro drug decay rate constant and $t_{1/2}$ is the drug half-life under the in vitro assay conditions, and

$$AUC = C_o/k$$

where C_o is the drug concentration to which the cells are exposed in vitro to achieve the specific drug exposure, or AUC.

By setting the in vitro AUC to be equal to that achievable in the patient (available from published phase I clinical trials), the appropriate drug concentration to which tumor cells should be exposed for any given time can be computed easily.

The prediction of patient response to therapy also requires that a sensitivity index is established from the dose-response data. This can be determined by plotting the clonogenic surviving fractions of the tumor cells against increasing drug concentrations and by computing from the resulting dose-response curve the level of clonogenic cell kill achieved at the predetermined clinically relevant concentration of drug.[68] Generally, a reduction of clonogenic survival by 70% at this

concentration correlates well with in vivo sensitivity. This method is particularly useful when applied to single drugs being tested against several tumors. However, for determining the relative sensitivities of multiple drugs on a single patient's tumor, an alternative method has been proposed for determination of sensitivity indices that takes into consideration differences in the pharmacokinetics of the drugs and the shape of the dose-response curves obtained with the different drugs.[9]

STUDY OF DRUG RESISTANCE MECHANISMS

Clinically, malignant gliomas are among the least responsive of human tumors to therapy, and for the anaplastic gliomas and glioblastoma multiformes, complete remissions and/or long-term survival is rare.[43, 57] A major factor contributing to this poor outcome in human glioma therapy is the high inherent drug and radiation resistance of the tumor cells. Significant efforts are thus being directed at a better understanding of the cellular and molecular parameters and mechanisms underlying the ability of glioma cells to circumvent the toxic actions of chemotherapeutic agents. This research is critically dependent on the availability of in vitro culture models of human gliomas in which the drug resistance profile has been well characterized (e.g., with clonogenic assays) to allow tumors with different degrees of drug resistance to be selected for further analysis of drug resistance mechanisms. This strategy has facilitated the identification of a number of potential mechanisms of glioma drug resistance, including the repair of DNA monoadducts of 2-chloroethylnitrosoureas,[1] DNA interstrand cross-link repair,[10, 13] glutathione and glutathione S-transferases.[13, 14, 37, 96] Recently, using glioma cell lines, colleagues and I demonstrated that human gliomas are capable of significant repair of drug-induced DNA interstrand cross-links, and showed that this repair, more than the absolute level of cross-linking, is the critical determinant of sensitivity or resistance to carmustine and cisplatin.[7] We have also used tumor cells from a malignant oligodendroglioma obtained from a patient before treatment and at time of remission to show that the acquisition of clinical cisplatin resistance is associated with increased DNA repair capacity and with an up-regulation of the DNA repair–associated proteins DNA polymerase α and DNA ligase in the tumor cells.[10] Other studies with xenografts[38] have also shown up-regulation of DNA polymerases and topoisomerase II activities in melphalan and topotecan resistance of human gliomas.

An important aspect of in vitro glioma culture systems and clonogenic assays in the study of drug resistance is that they offer a means of evaluating strategies to overcome such resistance. The best characterized of these strategies is one that is based on the inhibition of O[6]-alkylguanine DNA alkyltransferase[32, 39, 41] and is currently being investigated clinically with the specific inhibitor, O[6]-benzylguanine. Other promising strategies include the suppression of the repair of drug-induced DNA damage by inhibitors of DNA topoisomerase II and DNA polymerases, the inhibition of glutathione S-transferases, and the depletion of glutathione.[7, 37, 96]

In conclusion, although in vitro cultures and clonogenic assays have significantly advanced the field of brain tumor biology and therapy, their role in these areas and in the development of novel therapeutic strategies for human gliomas are likely to become even more important in the future, as novel approaches such as gene replacement therapy, downregulation of gene expression with antisense oligodeoxyribonucleotides, and the rational design of protein inhibitors are being explored for the treatment of human gliomas.

ACKNOWLEDGMENT

The author is grateful to Ms. Patricia Richter for excellent secretarial assistance in the preparation of the manuscript. Some of the work for this chapter was supported by grants CA 55835 and CA 55261 to the author from the National Cancer Institute, National Institutes of Health, Bethesda, Md.

REFERENCES

1. Aida T, Cheitlin RA, Bodell WJ: Inhibition of O⁶-alkylguanine-DNA alkyltransferase activity potentiates cytotoxicity and induction of SCE's in human glioma cells resistant to 1,3-bis(2-chloroethyl)-1-nitrosourea. Carcinogenesis 1987; 8:1219–1223.
2. Alberts DS, Chen GH-S, Salmon SE: Tabular summary of pharmacokinetic parameters relevant to in vitro drug assay. In Salmon SE (ed): Cloning of Human Tumor Stem Cells. New York, Alan R. Liss, 1980, pp 197–207.
3. Ali-Osman F: Culture of human normal brain and malignant brain tumors for cellular, molecular, and pharmacological studies, In Jones GE (ed): Methods in Molecular Medicine: Human Cell Culture Protocols. Totowa, New Jersey, Humana Press, 1996, p 63.
4. Ali-Osman F: Prediction of clinical response to therapy of adult and pediatric brain tumor patients by chemosensitivity testing in the capillary brain tumor clonogenic cell assay. In Bleyer AW, Packer R, Pochedly C (eds): New Trends in Pediatric Neuro-Oncology, vol 3. Switzerland, Harwood Academic Publisher, 1991, pp 220.
5. Ali-Osman F, Beltz PA: Optimization and characterization of the capillary human tumor clonogenic cell assay. Cancer Res 1988; 48:715–724.
6. Ali-Osman F, Berger MS, Livingston RB, et al: Cross-resistance patterns of human malignant gliomas to chemotherapeutic agents. Proc Am Assoc Clin Oncol 1989; 8:337.
7. Ali-Osman F, Berger MS, Rairkar A, et al: Enhanced repair of a cisplatin-damaged reporter chloroamphenicol-O-acetyltransferase gene and altered activities of DNA polymerases α and β, and DNA ligase in cells in human malignant glioma following in vivo cisplatin therapy. J Cell Biochem 1994; 54:11–19.
8. Ali-Osman F, Giblin J, Dougherty D, et al: Application of in vivo and in vitro pharmacokinetics for physiologically relevant drug exposure in a human tumor clonogenic cell assay. Cancer Res 1987; 47:3718–3724.
9. Ali-Osman F, Maurer HR, Bier J: In vitro cytostatic drug sensitivity testing in the human tumor stem cell assay: A modified method for the determination of the sensitivity index. Tumor Diagn Ther 1983; 4:1–6.
10. Ali-Osman F, Rairkar A, Young P: Formation and repair of 1,3-bis-(2-chloroethyl)-1-nitrosourea and cisplatin induced total genomic DNA interstrand crosslinks in human glioma cells. Cancer Biochem Biophys 1995; 14:213–214.
11. Ali-Osman F, Schofield D: Cellular and molecular studies in brain and nervous system oncology. Curr Opin Oncol 1990; 2:655–665.
12. Ali-Osman F, Srivenugopal K, Berger MS, et al: DNA interstrand crosslinking and strand break repair in human glioma cell lines of varying [1,3-bis(2-chloroethyl)-1-nitrosourea] resistance. Anticancer Res 1990; 10:677–682.
13. Ali-Osman F, Stein DE, Renwick A: Glutathione content and glutathione-S-transferase expression in 1,3-bis(2-chloroethyl)-nitrosourea-re-

14. sistant human malignant astrocytoma cell lines. Cancer Res 1990; 50:6976–6980.
14. Allalunus-Turner MJ, Day RS III, McKean JDS, et al: Glutathione levels and chemosensitizing effects of buthionine sulfoximine in human malignant glioma cells. J Neurooncol 1991; 11:157–164.
15. Barker M, Hoshino T, Gurcay O, et al: Development of an animal brain tumor model and its response to therapy with 1,3-bis(2-chloroethyl)-1-nitrosourea. Cancer Res 1973; 33:916–986.
16. Barker M, Wilson CB, Hoshino T: Tissue culture of human brain tumors. In Kirsch WM, Grossi-Paoletti E, Paoletti P (eds): The Experimental Biology of Brain Tumors. Springfield, Ill, Charles C. Thomas, 1972, p 57.
17. Baumann N: Brain cultures: A tool in neurobiology. Dev Neurosci 1985; 7:5–6.
18. Bignami A, Dahl D: Astrocyte-specific protein and neuroglial differentiation: An immunofluorescence study with antibodies to the glial fibrillary acidic protein. J Comp Neurol 1974; 153:27.
19. Bignami A, Eng LF, Dahl D, et al: Localization of the glial fibrillary acid protein in astrocytes by immunofluorescence. Brain Res 1972; 43:429.
20. Bigner DD, Bigner SH, Ponten J, et al: Heterogeneity of genotypic and phenotypic characteristics of 15 permanent cell lines derived from human gliomas. J Neuropathol Exp Neurol 1981; 40:201–229.
21. Bigner SH, Friedman HS, Biegel JA, et al: Specific chromosomal abnormalities characterize four established cell lines derived from malignant human gliomas. Acta Neuropathol 1986; 72:86–97.
22. Bigner SH, Mark J, Bigner DD: Chromosomal progression of malignant human gliomas from biopsy to establishment as permanent lines in vitro. Cancer Genet Cytogenet 1987; 24:163–176.
23. Bigner SH, Wong AJ, Mark J, et al: Relationship between gene amplification and chromosomal deviations in malignant human gliomas. Cancer Genet Cytogenet 1987; 28:165–170.
24. Bland J: Tissue culture of gliomata. J Anat 1936; 71:149.
25. Bodell WJ, Aida T, Berger MS, et al: Increased repair of O⁶-alkylguanine DNA adducts in glioma-derived human cells resistant to the cytotoxic and cytogenetic effects of 1,3,-bis(2-chloroethyl)-1-nitrosourea. Carcinogenesis 1986; 7:879–993.
26. Bogdahn U, Rupniak HTR, Ali-Osman F, et al: Comparison of a colony-forming assay with a proliferation-microassay for the determination of chemosensitivity of malignant human brain tumors. Int J Cell Cloning 1983; 1:295.
27. Buckley RC: Tissue culture studies of the glioblastoma multiforme. Am J Pathol 1929; 5:467–472.
28. Cairns P, Mao L, Merlo A, et al: Rates of p16 (MTS1) mutations in primary tumors with 9p loss. Science 1994; 265:415–417.
29. Canady KS, Ali-Osman F, Rubel EW: Extracellular potassium influences DNA and protein syntheses and glial fibrillary acidic protein expression in cultured glial cells. Glia 1990; 3:368–374.
30. Canti RG, Bland JOW, Russell DS: Tissue culture in gliomata: Cinematograph demonstration. Res Pub Assist Nerv Ment Dis 1937; 16:1.
31. Collins VP: Cultured human glial and glioma cells. Int Rev Exp Pathol 1983; 24:135–202.
32. Dolan ME, Stine L, Mitchell RB, et al: Modulation of mammalian O⁶-alkylguanine-DNA alkyltransferase in vivo by O⁶-benzylguanine and its effect on the sensitivity of a human glioma tumor to 1-(2-chloroethyl)-3-(4-methylcyclohexyl)-1-nitrosourea. Cancer Commun 1990; 2:371–377.
33. Eng LF, deArmand SJ: Immunocytochemistry of the glial fibrillary acidic protein. Prog Neuropathol 1983; 5:19–39.
34. Fialkow P: The origin and development of human tumors studied with cell markers. N Engl J Med 1974; 291:260–265.
35. Freshney RI: Tissue culture of gliomas. In Thomas DGT, Graham DI (eds): Brain Tumors: Scientific Basis, Clinical Investigation and Current Therapy. London, Butterworths, 1980, pp 21–50.
36. Friedman HS, Bigner SH, Schold SC, et al: The use of experimental models of human 27 medulloblastoma in the design of rational therapy. In Walker MD, Thomas DGT (eds): Biology of Brain Tumors. Boston, Martinus Nijhoff, 1986, pp 405–409.
37. Friedman HS, Colvin OM, Griffith OW, et al: Increased melphalan activity in intracranial human medulloblastoma and glioma xenografts following buthionine-sulfoximine mediated glutathione depletion. JNCI 1989; 81:524–527.
38. Friedman HS, Dolan ME, Kaufmann SH, et al: Elevated DNA polymerase α, DNA polymerase β, and DNA topoisomerase II in a

melphalan-resistant rhabdomyosarcoma xenograft that is cross-resistant to nitrosoureas and topotecan. Cancer Res 1994; 54:3487–3493.

39. Friedman HS, Dolan ME, Moschel RC, et al: Enhancement of nitrosourea activity in medulloblastoma and glioblastoma multiforme. JNCI 1991; 84:1926–1931.

40. Froelich JS, Lapham LW: Tissue culture studies of gliomas: I. Intranuclear inclusions in glial cells. Am J Pathol 1965; 47:147.

41. Gerson SL, Trey JE, Miller K: Potentiation of nitrosourea cytotoxicity in human leukemic cells by inactivation of O⁶-alkylguanine-DNA alkyltransferase. Cancer Res 1988; 48:1521–1527.

42. Graham DR, Thomas DGT, Brown I: Nervous system antigens. Histopathology 1983; 37:1–21.

43. Grossman SA: Chemotherapy of brain tumors. In Salcman M (ed): Neurobiology of Brain Tumors: Concepts in Neurosurgery, vol 4. Baltimore, Williams & Wilkins, 1991, pp 321–340.

44. Haglid K, Carisson CA, Starvou D: An immunological study of human brain tumors concerning the brain specific proteins S-100 and 14.3.2. Acta Neuropathol 1973; 24:187–196.

45. Hamburger AW, Salmon SE: Primary bioassay of human myeloma stem cells. J Clin Invest 1977; 60:846–854.

46. Hash EA, Boss BD, Cowan WM: Production and characterization of monoclonal antibodies against the ''brain-specific'' proteins 14.3.2 and S-100. Proc Natl Acad Sci USA 1982; 78:7585–7589.

47. Hoshino T, Barker M, Wilson CB: The kinetics of cultured human glioma cells. Acta Neuropathol 1975; 32:235.

48. Kersting G: Die Gewebszuchtung menschlicher Hirngeschwulste. Berlin, Springer-Verlag, 1961.

49. Kersting G: Tissue culture of human gliomas. Prog Neurol Surg 1968; 2:165–202.

50. Kimmel DW, Shapiro JR, Shapiro WK: In vitro drug sensitivity testing in human gliomas. J Neurosurg 1987; 66:161–171.

51. Kornblith PL, Smith BH, Leonard LA: Response of cultured human brain tumors to nitrosoureas: Correlation with clinical data. Cancer 1981; 47:225–265.

52. Kornblith PL, Szypko PE: Variations in response of human brain tumors to BCNU in vitro. J Neurosurg 1978; 48:580.

53. Kovach JS: In vitro models as guides to clinical chemotherapy. Adv Biosci 1986; 58:49–57.

54. Kredel FE: Intracranial tumors in tissue culture. Arch Surg 1929; 18:2008–2018.

55. Laerum OD, Steinvag S, Bjerkvig R: Cell and tissue culture of the central nervous system: Recent developments and current applications. Acta Neurol Scand 1985; 72:529–549.

56. Lee Y, Wikstrand CJ, Humphrey PA, et al: In vitro growth of brain tumors. In Salcman M (ed): Neurobiology of Brain Tumors: Concepts in Neurosurgery, vol 4. Baltimore, Williams & Wilkins, 1991, pp 163–183.

57. Levin VA: Chemotherapy of primary brain tumors. Neurol Clin 1985; 3:855–866.

58. Lieber MM, Ames MM, Powis G, et al: Anticancer drug testing in vitro: Use of an activating system with the human tumor stem cell assay. Life Sci 1981; 28:287–293.

59. Liss L: Glial and parenchymal neoplasms in tissue culture. In Scharenberg K, Liss L (eds): Neuroectodermal Tumors of the Central and Peripheral Nervous System. Baltimore, Williams & Wilkins, 1969, p 183.

60. Lumsden CE: The study by tissue culture of tumours of the nervous system. In Russell DS, Rubinstein LJ (eds): Pathology of Tumours of the Nervous System. London, Edward Arnold, 1971, p 334.

61. Lumsden CE: Tissue culture of brain tumours. In Vinken PJ, Bruyn GW (eds): Handbook of Clinical Neurology. Amsterdam, North-Holland Publishing Co, 1971.

62. Lumsden CE, Pomerat CM: Normal oligodendrocytes in tissue culture: A preliminary report on the pulsatile glial cells in tissue cultures from the corpus callosum of the normal adult rat brain. Exp Cell Res 1951; 2:103.

63. Mackillop WJ, Blundell J, Steele P: Short term culture of pediatric brain tumors. Child Nerv Syst 1985; 1:163–168.

64. Manuelidis EE: Long-term lines of tissue cultures of intracranial tumors. J Neurosurg 1965; 22:368.

65. Mark J, Westermark B, Ponten J: Banding patterns in human glioma cell lines. Hereditas 1977; 87:243–260.

66. Maurer HR, Ali-Osman F: Tumor stem cell cloning in agar-contorimic capillaries. Naturwissenschaften 1981; 67:381–383.

67. Mitchell RB, Moschel RC, Dolan ME: Effect of O⁶-benzylguanine on the sensitivity of human tumor xenografts to 1,3-bis(2-chloroethyl)-1-nitrosourea and on DNA interstrand cross-link formation. Cancer Res 1992; 52:1171–1175.

68. Moon PE: Quantitative and statistical analysis of the association between in vitro and in vivo studies. In Salmon SE (ed): Cloning of Human Tumor Stem Cells. New York, Alan R. Liss, 1980, pp 209–221.

69. Morgan D, Freshney RI, Thomas DGT, et al: Screening samples of human astrocytoma for drug sensitivity by scintillation autofluorography. Br J Cancer 1978; 37:476.

70. Nister M, Wodell B, Betsholtz C, et al: Evidence for progressional changes in the human malignant glioma line U-343 MOa: Analysis of karyotype and expression of genes encoding the subunit chains of platelet derived growth factor. Cancer Res 1987; 47:4953–4960.

71. Nowell PC: The clonal evolution of tumor cell populations. Science 1976; 1194:23–28.

72. Pegg AE: Mammalian O⁶-alkylguanine-DNA alkyltransferase: Regulation and importance in response to alkylating carcinogenic and therapeutic agents. Cancer Res 1990; 50:6119–6129.

73. Pomerat CM, Crue BL, Kasten F: Observations on the cytology of an oligodendroglioma cultivated in vitro. JNCI 1964; 33:517.

74. Ponten J: Neoplastic human glia cells in culture. In Fogh J (ed): Human Tumor Cells In Vitro. New York, Plenum, 1975, p 175.

75. Ponten J, MacIntyre EH: Long-term culture of normal and neoplastic human glia. Acta Pathol Microbiol Scand 1968; 74:465.

76. Raff MC, Miller RH, Noole M: A glial progenitor cell that develops in vitro into an astrocyte or an oligodendrocyte depending on culture medium. Nature 1983; 303:390–396.

77. Raff MC, Mirsky R, Fields KF, et al: Galactocerebroside: A specific cell surface antigenic marker for oligodendrocytes in culture. Nature 1978; 274:813–816.

78. Raimondi AJ, Mullan S, Evans JP: Human brain tumors (an electron-microscope study). J Neurosurg 1962; 19:731.

79. Ray JA, Bello MJ, Campos JM, et al: Cytogenetic follow-up from direct preparation to advanced in vitro passages of a human malignant glioma. Cancer Genet Cytogenet 1989; 41:175–183.

80. Rosenblum ML: Chemosensitivity testing for human brain tumors. In Salmon SE (ed): Cloning of Human Tumor Stem Cells. New York, Alan R. Liss, 1980, pp 259–276.

81. Rosenblum ML, Vasquez DA, Hoshino T, et al: Development of a clonogenic cell assay for human brain tumors. Cancer 1978; 41:2305–2314.

82. Rosenblum ML, Wheeler KT, Wilson CB, et al: In vitro evaluation of in vivo brain tumour chemotherapy with 1,3-bis(2-chloroethyl)-1-nitrosourea. Cancer Res 1975; 35:1387.

83. Rubenstein LJ, Herman MM: Studies on the differentiation of human and experimental gliomas in organ culture systems. Cancer Res 1975; 51:35.

84. Rubenstein LJ, Herman MM, Foley VL: In vitro characteristics of human glioblastomas maintained in organ culture systems: Light microscopy observations. Am J Pathol 1973; 71:61.

85. Russell DS, Bland JOW: A study of gliomas by the method of tissue culture. J Pathol Bacteriol 1933; 36:273–283.

86. Saez RJ, Campbell RJ, Laws ER: Chemotherapeutic trials on human malignant astrocytomas in organ culture. J Neurosurg 1977; 46:320.

87. Salmon SE (ed): Cloning of Human Tumor Stem Cells. New York, Alan R. Liss, 1980.

88. Salmon SE, Hamburger AW, Soehnlen B, et al: Quantitation of differential sensitivity of human tumor stem cells to anticancer drugs. N Eng J Med 1978; 298:1321.

89. Salmon SE, Trent JE: Human Tumor Cloning. Orlando, Grune & Stratton, 1984.

90. Salmon SE, Von Hoff DD: In vitro evaluation of anticancer drugs with the human tumor stem cell assay. Semin Oncol 1988; 8:4, 377–385.

91. Sanford KK, Earle WR, Likely GD: The growth in vitro of single isolated tissue cells. JNCI 1948; 9:229–246.

92. Shapiro JR: Biology of gliomas: Heterogeneity, oncogenes and growth factors. Semin Oncol 1986; 1:14–15.

93. Shapiro JR, Yung WKA, Shapiro WR: Isolation, karyotype, and clonal growth of heterogeneous subpopulations of human malignant gliomas. Cancer Res 1981; 41:2349–2359.

94. Silbergeld DL, Ali-Osman F, Winn HR: Induction of transformational changes in normal endothelial cell by cultured human astrocytoma cells. J Neurosurg 1991; 75:604–612.

95. Sipe JC, Herman MM, Rubinstein LJ: Electron microscopic observations on human glioblastomas and astrocytomas maintained in organ culture systems. Am J Pathol 1973; 73:589.
96. Skapek SX, Colvin OM, Griffith OW, et al: Buthionine sulfoximine-mediated depletion of glutathione in intracranial human glioma-derived xenografts. Biochem Pharmacol 1988; 37:4313–4317.
97. Slocum HK, Powelic ZP, Rustum YM: An enzymatic method for the disaggregation of human solid tumors for studies of clonogenicity and biochemical determinants of drug action. *In* Salmon SE (ed): Cloning of Human Tumor Stem Cells. New York, Alan R. Liss, 1980, pp 339–343.
98. Spruck CH III, Gonzalez-Zulueta M, Shibata A, et al: p16 Gene in uncultured tumours. Nature 1994; 370:183–184.
99. Thomas DOT, Darling JL, Paul EA, et al: Assay of anti-cancer drugs in tissue culture relationship of relapse free interval (RFI) and in vitro chemosensitivity in patients with malignant cerebral glioma. Br J Cancer 1985; 51:525–532.
100. Vaheri A, Ruoslahti E, Westermark B, et al: A common cell-type specific surface antigen in cultured human glial cells and fibroblasts: Loss in malignant cells. J Exp Med 1976; 143:64.
101. Von Hoff DD: He's not going to talk about in vitro predictive assays again, is he? JNCI 1990; 82:96–101.
102. Von Hoff DD, Clark GM, Stogdill BJ, et al: Prospective clinical trial of a human tumor cloning system. Cancer Res 1983; 43:1926–1931.
103. Von Hoff DD, Forseth BJ, Huong M, et al: Improved plating efficiencies for human tumors cloned in capillary tubes versus petri dishes. Cancer Res 1986; 46:4012–4017.
104. Wahlstrom T, Linder E, Saksela E, et al: Tumour-specific surface antigens in established cell lines from gliomas. Cancer 1974; 34:272.
105. Welander CE, Homesley HD, Jobson VW: Multiple agent chemotherapy prospectively selected by the human tumor clonogenic assay (HTCA) for advanced ovarian cancers. Int J Cell Cloning 1983; 1:290–291.
106. Westermark B: Growth regulatory interactions between stationary human glia-like cells and normal neoplastic cells in culture. Exp Cell Res 1973; 81:195.
107. Wiestler O, Kleihues P, Pegg AE: O^6-Alkylguanine-DNA alkyltransferase activity in human brain and brain tumors. Carcinogenesis 1984; 5:121–124.
108. Wilson CB, Barker M, Slagel DE: Tumors of the central nervous system in monolayer culture. Arch Neurol 1966; 15:275.
109. Zulch KJ: Brain Tumors: Their Biology and Pathology. Berlin, Springer-Verlag, 1986.

JOHN R. SILBER

MICHAEL S. BOBOLA

A. BLANK

DOUGLAS D. KOLSTOE

MITCHEL S. BERGER

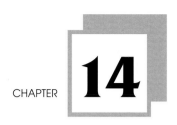

CHAPTER **14**

DNA Repair–Mediated Resistance to Alkylating Agents

A major goal of our laboratory is to increase the effectiveness of alkylating agent chemotherapy for primary and recurrent malignant brain tumors by suppressing DNA repair-mediated resistance. Chloroethylnitrosoureas (CENUs), such as BCNU [1,3-bis(2-chloroethyl)-1-nitrosourea] and CCNU [1-(2-chloroethyl)-3-cyclohexyl-1-nitrosourea]; methylating nitrosoureas, such as procarbazine; and imidazotetrazines, such as temozolomide, are chemotherapeutic agents used in treatment of brain tumors. Unfortunately, intrinsic and acquired resistance to these alkylating agents limits their utility. This chapter reviews information relating to the cytotoxicity of alkylating agents and the contribution of the DNA repair protein O^6-methylguanine-DNA methyltransferase (MGMT) to resistance. The hypothesis that repair of abasic sites by base excision repair is an important determinant of resistance to both CENUs and methylating agents is also examined. Finally, other DNA repair and DNA damage tolerance mechanisms that may increase resistance are briefly discussed.

ALKYLATING AGENTS AND BRAIN TUMOR CHEMOTHERAPY

CENUs

CENUs are central to chemotherapy of brain tumors. Clinical trials have established the effectiveness of CENUs in single-agent and combination chemotherapy protocols for primary and recurrent malignant gliomas. No single anti-tumor drug has proved more effective than have CENUs, leading to their continued widespread use at initial diagnosis and at recurrence. When given after surgery and postoperative radiotherapy, BCNU and CCNU modestly improve response rates and survival times.[1–6] Other studies have demonstrated the efficacy of CENUs in the treatment of medulloblastoma,[7] a common pediatric malignant brain tumor.[8] Yet CENU-based therapy has limited efficacy, due in part to intrinsic and acquired resistance. For example, malignant gliomas constitute the majority of newly diagnosed malignant brain tumors. Some of these tumors do not respond to CENUs, and for those that do, responses are generally of short duration (24 to 44 weeks).[6] The poor prognosis for malignant brain tumors (2-year survival rates less than 20%) has generated intense interest in the mechanisms of CENU resistance and strategies to combat them.[5, 9]

Methylating Agents

Methylating agents are used in chemotherapy of brain tumors. The methylating agent procarbazine has been used alone or in combination chemotherapy for malignant gliomas.[2, 5, 10] Results of a clinical trial[3] have shown a slight advantage of postradiation adjuvant therapy with CCNU, procarbazine, and vincristine over BCNU for anaplastic gliomas. The potential importance of methylating agents for glioma therapy is emphasized by promising initial results with temozolomide. This agent has recently been reported to be active in patients with newly diagnosed and recurrent high-grade gliomas.[11, 12] The current significance of procarbazine and temozolomide for brain tumor therapy underscores the need to consider mechanisms of methylating agent resistance.

ALKYLATING AGENT–INDUCED DNA DAMAGE

CENUs

The full spectrum of DNA lesions contributing to CENU cytotoxicity is unknown. CENUs are bifunctional alkylating agents that carry both N^1-chloroethyl and N^1-nitrosourea groups, and differ in their substituents at the N^3 position.[13] CENUs decompose in aqueous solution, yielding alkylating species that react at nucleophilic sites in DNA to produce a large number of diverse purine and pyrimidine derivatives.[14]

143

The major site of base alkylation is the N^7 atom of guanine, although substituents can probably be attached to any of the nucleophilic sites. The cytotoxic effects of CENUs are related to base modifications, three types of which have been characterized: monosubstituted bases, exocyclic ethano derivatives, and intrastrand and interstrand cross-links.

The number and identity of cytotoxic lesions caused by CENUs is incompletely established. Because CENUs introduce a multitude of modifications in DNA, it is difficult to assign lethality to any particular one. Moreover, not all CENU-induced lesions have been characterized, quantitatively minor products may have large biologic effects,[15] and some lethal lesions may be unstable to manipulations in vitro. Therefore, to consider CENU cytotoxicity exclusively in light of the few modifications presently associated with lethality would be an oversimplification.

CROSS-LINKS

CENU cytotoxicity is associated with the interstrand cross-link 1-(3-cytosinyl)-2-(1-guanyl)ethane,[16] whose monoadduct precursor is O^6-chloroethylguanine.[14] The O^6-chloroethyl monoadduct rearranges by internal cyclization to form the reactive exocyclic derivative O^6,N^1-ethanoguanine, which then forms an ethane bridge with the opposite, complementary cytosine to produce the cross-link. Formation of the monoadduct in DNA occurs within minutes, but cross-link formation is slow, requiring up to 10 hours to complete. A role for interstrand cross-links in CENU-induced killing of brain tumors is suggested by the observation that increased CENU sensitivity of human brain tumor–derived cell lines is accompanied by elevated levels of cross-links.[17]

Intrastrand cross-links between adjacent guanosine residues are implicated in the cytotoxicity of the anti-tumor drug cisplatin, suggesting that the CENU-induced intrastrand cross-link 1,2-bis-(7-guanyl)-ethane may also be lethal.[22]

ABASIC SITES

Abasic sites, generated by spontaneous depurination/depyrimidination or the action of DNA glycosylases,[23–25] are the most common DNA lesions in cells.[15, 26] Alkylation of the N^3 or N^7 atoms of purines can increase the lability of the N-glycosylic bond in deoxynucleosides by orders of magnitude,[27] thereby promoting formation of abasic sites. For example, at neutral pH and 37 °C, the half-life of the N-glycosylic linkage of N^7-methyldeoxyguanosine in DNA is 144 hours, compared with 6.4×10^6 hours for unmodified deoxyguanosine. The lethality of abasic sites is manifested in the hypersensitivity to alkylating agents of bacterial[24] and yeast[28] mutants deficient in apurinic/apyrimidinic endonuclease (Ap endonuclease) activity. Abasic sites have several effects that may confer lethality, including blocking DNA replication.[29–31]

Abasic sites most likely contribute to the cytotoxicity of CENUs. N^7-Chloroethylguanine and its derivative N^7-hydroxyethylguanine, which constitute the majority of monosubstituted bases produced in DNA by CENUs,[17, 32] destabilize the N-glycosylic linkage in guanosine.[33] Treatment of plasmid DNA with chloroethylnitrosourea (CNU) produces depurination at GG sequences within 30 minutes and at GT sequences after 1 hour.[34] This finding, together with the observation that haloethylation of DNA by exposure to 3-(2-haloethyl)aryltriazenes yields lesions that are substrates for Ap endonuclease,[35] indicates that the predominant base monoadducts produced by CENUs are precursors of abasic sites.

UNCHARACTERIZED CYTOTOXIC LESIONS

Studies with a series of 1-aryl-3-alkyltriazenes and alkyltriazenylimidazoles, including chloroethylating species, have shown that differences in sensitivity of human colon carcinoma- and fibroblast-derived cell lines are detectable in the absence of cross-link formation.[36, 37] These results indicate that O^6-chloroethylguanine adducts and/or their derivatives, such as the imidazole ring-open forms,[38] are lethal in their own right.

Other studies have shown that polyamine deprivation prior to exposure to CENUs increases the killing of MGMT-proficient (Mer$^+$), but not MGMT-deficient (Mer$^-$), human tumor cell lines.[39] This killing is not the result of an increase in cross-link formation.[40, 41] It is proposed that Mer$^-$ cells are killed by their inability to remove cross-link precursors, whereas Mer$^+$ cells, which are able to prevent formation of all detectable cross-links, are killed by inability to repair an as yet unidentified lesion(s).

Several unidentified adducts, which have chromatographic properties similar to but different from those of the major monoadducts 7-chloroethylguanine and 7-hydroxyethylguanine, are implicated in CENU cytotoxicity by virtue of their reduced abundance in resistant vs. sensitive human glioma cell lines.[17] Although the CENU-induced derivatives have not been studied, N-alkylpurines, especially N^3-alkyladenines, are toxic to mammalian cells.[15, 22]

Methylating Agents

Methylating agents react at numerous sites in purine and pyrimidine bases.[42] The N^7 and O^6 positions of guanine and the N^3 position of adenine are predominant sites of base methylation, but more than a dozen other sites have been identified.[42, 43] The relative abundance of N- and O-alkylation products depends on the methylating agent. For example, N-nitroso compounds produce a greater yield of O-methyl derivatives than do methyl sulfates or methylmethane sulfonates.[42] Notably, the yield of N-methyl adducts is invariably at least 10-fold greater than that of O-methyl derivatives.[42, 43]

Although many methyl adducts have been characterized chemically, the cytotoxicity of most is unknown. As in the case of CENUs, assigning lethality to any one adduct is difficult because of the multiplicity of lesions produced. In addition to abasic sites (see earlier discussion), two base adducts have been demonstrated to be lethal.

O^6-METHYLGUANINE

The cytotoxicity of O^6-methylguanine in DNA has been documented in studies showing that the hypersensitivity of cell lines deficient in MGMT, a DNA repair protein that catalyzes the removal of alkyl groups from the O^6 position of guanine,[18, 19] can be abolished by expression of bacterial or human MGMT. Recent evidence indicates that the lethality of O^6-methylguanine is due, at least in part, to its inability to form a complementary base pair with any nucleotide.[43] Following DNA replication, the mispaired nucleotide incorporated opposite O^6-methylguanine is excised by post-replication mismatch repair.[43] However, because O^6-methylguanine remains in the template strand, another mismatch is formed during DNA synthesis to fill the gap resulting from excision of the non-complementary nucleotide. Reiterative attempts to remove the mispair are believed to be the mechanism responsible for the cytotoxicity of O^6-methylguanine.

N^3-METHYLADENINE

N^3-Methyladenine in DNA is cytotoxic in *Escherichia coli*[24] and in the eukaryote *Saccharomyces cerevisiae*.[45] Importantly, expression of bacterial or mammalian 3-methyladenine glycosylase, an enzyme that excises N^3-methyladenine from DNA, confers resistance to methylating agents in a number of mammalian cell lines.[46, 47] It has been concluded that repair of N^3-methyladenine can be a limiting factor in resistance of mammalian cells to alkylating agents.[22]

CONTRIBUTION OF O^6-METHYLGUANINE–DNA METHYLTRANSFERASE (MGMT) TO RESISTANCE

MGMT: Function and Gene Structure

Human MGMT is a monomeric 22 kD protein that catalyzes the transfer of small alkyl adducts from the O^6 position of guanine in DNA to an internal cysteine, yielding *S*-alkylcysteine and guanine.[18, 19] Because the alkyl receptor is not regenerated, the number of O^6-alkylguanine adducts that can be removed from DNA in vivo is limited by the number of MGMT molecules and the rate of resynthesis of the protein. This ''suicide'' mechanism is shared by all prokaryotic and eukaryotic MGMTs examined. The preferred substrate of mammalian MGMT is O^6-methylguanine in double-stranded DNA. Alkyl groups as large as *n*-butyl are removed at progressively slower rates, and branched alkyl groups are removed even more slowly. Indirect evidence indicates that MGMT can remove chloroethyl groups from the O^6 atom of guanine.[17, 47] In addition, MGMT reacts in vitro with O^6, N^1-ethanoguanine in DNA, the precursor of CENU-induced interstrand cross-links.[48] MGMT opens the exocyclic ethano ring, becoming covalently linked via an ethyl group to the N^1 atom of guanine. Whether this reaction occurs in vivo and what effect it would have on CENU sensitivity remain to be determined.

Full-length cDNAs for MGMT from bacteria, yeast, rodents, and man have been isolated.[19] Homology between bacterial, yeast, and mammalian MGMT is high, especially at the alkyl acceptor site, which is defined by the pentapeptide sequence PCHRV. The human gene has been mapped to the distal end of the long arm of chromosome 10.[51] The complete genomic sequence has been obtained, revealing a greater than 170 kb gene consisting of 5 exons,[49] the first of which is untranslated.[50] The 5′ upstream region is GC-rich and lacks consensus sequences such as TATA and CAAT boxes. To our knowledge, no evidence has been found of differential splicing of human MGMT mRNA or isoforms of the protein. Fully active human MGMT has been expressed in *E. coli*, suggesting that post-translational modification may not be required for activity.[51, 52]

Regulation of MGMT Expression in Human Brain and Brain Tumor-Derived Cell Lines

Approximately 20% of cell lines derived from human tumors and 50% of virally transformed cell lines are devoid of detectable MGMT activity[18, 19] and are designated Mer⁻ (*Me*thyl *r*epair deficient) or Mex⁻ (*Me*thyl *ex*cision deficient). Mer⁻ human tumor–derived cell lines examined to date have neither detectable MGMT protein nor mRNA, but they do have an intact MGMT gene,[53–55] suggesting that MGMT gene expression is controlled transcriptionally. A growing body of evidence suggests that MGMT expression is regulated by methylation of CpG dinucleotides in the promoter and body of the gene. In cell lines derived from a variety of human tumors, including gliomas, promoter sequences of the MGMT gene are hypomethylated in Mer⁻ lines vs. Mer⁺ lines.[54, 55] Moreover, demethylation of a Mer⁺ human colon carcinoma line by long-term exposure to 5-azacytidine abolished MGMT expression.[54] A study of human glioma-derived cell lines reports that promoter methylation is inversely correlated with expression, whereas methylation of the gene body is directly correlated with expression.[50] The authors conclude that graded expression of MGMT is associated with the level of methylation of both the body and promoter of the gene. Although overall hypomethylation of the MGMT promoter is associated with Mer⁻ status, a single SmaI restriction site 69 nucleotide 5′ from the transcription start site has been found to be methylated in all three Mer⁻, but not in four Mer⁺, human rhabdomyosarcoma cell and xenograft lines.[56] Methylation of the SmaI site was also observed in two Mer⁻ glioma-derived cell lines, but not in four Mer⁺ brain tumors or one Mer⁺ normal brain specimen.[57] The apparent epigenetic control of MGMT expression provides an explanation for the high frequency of Mer⁻ cell lines and the observation that Mer⁻ lines can spontaneously revert to Mer⁺ phenotype.[58–60]

MGMT Content of Neoplastic and Normal Human Brain

MGMT content varies widely among tissues, and large interindividual variation has been observed in both normal and neoplastic tissues.[61–65] A varying proportion of samples (around 5% to 57% in various studies) has been reported to lack detectable activity. Early studies of brain[61–64] did not reveal the full extent or patterns of variability of MGMT expression because of small sample size. The putative importance of MGMT in brain tumor alkylating agent resistance led us to quantitate the MGMT content of 60 newly operated and recurrent tumors.[65] This study revealed a greater than 200-fold variation in MGMT content among tumors and an

8-fold difference in mean MGMT levels between tumor types. These differences, however, were not statistically significant due to heterogeneity within each group. Notably, 27% of specimens had no detectable activity ($\leq$0.5 fmol/10^6 cells, $\leq$300 molecules/cell), and were designated Mer$^-$. Mean MGMT level did not differ between males and females but was higher for patients younger than 20 years than for those older than 20 years (13.2 $\pm$ 4.3 vs. 5.2 $\pm$ 1.3 fmol/10^6 cells, P = 0.058). We also assayed MGMT content in histologically normal brain from 25 patients. The range of detectable activity was comparable to that of tumors; however, a larger proportion of the normal brain specimens (52%) was Mer$^-$. For 60% of the 25 tumor/normal pairs, tumor activity was 2-fold to more than 38-fold greater than that of normal brain, demonstrating that elevation of MGMT content occurs frequently during tumorigenesis.

We have expanded our original study and, to date, have compiled data for 123 tumors, as summarized in Figure 14–1. Of special relevance to alkylating agent resistance is the large inter-individual variation in MGMT content within all diagnostic groups. For 91 Mer$^+$ tumors ($\geq$0.5 fmol/10^6 cells, i.e., $\geq$300 molecules/cell), MGMT activity ranged 300-fold. Variability was 80-fold to 300-fold within the three astrocytic glioma subgroups that constitute the majority of human brain tumors, and 150-fold for medulloblastoma. Mean MGMT content differed as much as 6-fold between diagnostic groups, but the differences are not statistically significant due to heterogeneity within each group. The wide inter-individual variability in MGMT content is potentially significant because, as has been noted,[5] brain tumors vary in intrinsic sensitivity to CENU therapy and the mechanisms by which many eventually become refractory are not known. The inter-individual variability is not uniquely large. We have observed comparable heterogeneity between individuals and diagnostic groups for urokinase and tissue plasminogen activator and plasminogen activator inhibitor-1 in human brain tumors.[66] Of potential clinical importance is the absence of detectable MGMT activity in 35 (28%) of the 123 tumors. All diagnostic groups contain Mer$^-$ samples, with medulloblastoma having the lowest incidence and ependymoma the highest.

The wide variation in MGMT content observed within all tumor groups will facilitate assessment of the importance of MGMT level for response to alkylating agent therapy. It will be of paramount interest to determine if Mer$^-$ status is associated with a more favorable response, and, conversely, if tumors with high MGMT levels are associated with poorer outcome. We are currently collecting outcome data (time to tumor progression) for patients receiving alkylating agent chemotherapy and are analyzing additional tumors to amass the requisite data base to assess correlation of MGMT level with clinical outcome.

MGMT Contributes to Resistance in Human Brain Tumor Cells in Vitro

OVERVIEW

Two kinds of evidence implicate MGMT in alkylating agent resistance in human glioma and medulloblastoma cells grown in culture or as nude mouse xenografts. The first kind is indirect and correlative: Greater sensitivity to chloroethylating agents has been associated with low or absent MGMT activity.[17, 47, 67] The second kind is direct and mechanistic: Depletion of MGMT with the substrate analog O^6-benzylguanine[68] reduces resistance to chloroethylating and methylating agents.[69–79] Notably, the greater CENU sensitivity of MGMT-deficient cells is accompanied by elevated levels of interstrand cross-links,[73] a finding that implicates the role of cross-links in CENU-induced lethality and indicates that the contribution of MGMT to CENU resistance is mediated, at least in part, by prevention of interstrand cross-link formation.

VARIABLE CONTRIBUTION OF MGMT

To approach the question of whether the contribution of MGMT to alkylating agent resistance varies among tumors, we quantitated the contribution of MGMT to MNNG and BCNU sensitivity in six medulloblastoma-derived and eight astrocytic glioma–derived human cell lines.[78, 79] To do this, we determined the effect on survival of ablating MGMT activity with the substrate analog O^6-benzylguanine (O^6-BG).[68, 74] MGMT was assayed by quantitating the transfer of radioactivity from DNA containing O^6-[^{3}H]methylguanine to protein.[65] We verified this assay for extracts prepared from cultured cells by demonstrating that (1) the increase in radioactivity transferred to protein is linear over a 5-fold range of added extract; (2) transfer of radioactivity is prevented by O^6-BG; (3) transferred radioactivity is sensitive to protease digestion; and (4) transferred radioactivity migrates on an SDS-polyacrylamide gel with a relative molecular mass (M_r) of 22,000, identical to that reported for MGMT.[80] Reduction of MGMT to undetectable levels (no counts per minute [cpm] above that of an unincubated control) was verified for each cell line in at least three separate experiments.

We employed four different cytotoxicity assays and thereby discovered that an important variable is whether cells are exposed to alkylating agent while adherent to a plastic substratum or while suspended in medium. Drug sensitivity was determined by analysis of survival curves (log-surviving fraction vs. dose) using standard methods.[81] A curve-fitting program (Graph III, Computer Associates, Islandia, NY) was used to generate a survival curve for each cell line in each cytotoxicity assay from a minimum of three independent experiments (i.e., a minimum of nine determinations per drug concentration) in the absence or presence of O^6-BG. Of the several survival parameters analyzed, only LD_{10}, or the dose that reduces survival to 10%, is discussed here. As an internal standard, either the human colon carcinoma cell line HT29 or the medulloblastoma line UW228–1 was always assayed concurrently when determining the sensitivity of other lines. LD_{10} for these internal standards varied no more than 20%, establishing the precision of independent assays. Examples of survival curves are shown in Figure 14–2.

ANALYSIS OF CELLS ALKYLATED WHILE PROLIFERATING ON A PLASTIC SUBSTRATUM

The survival of 12 cell lines treated with MNNG or BCNU while growing as adherent monolayers, together with

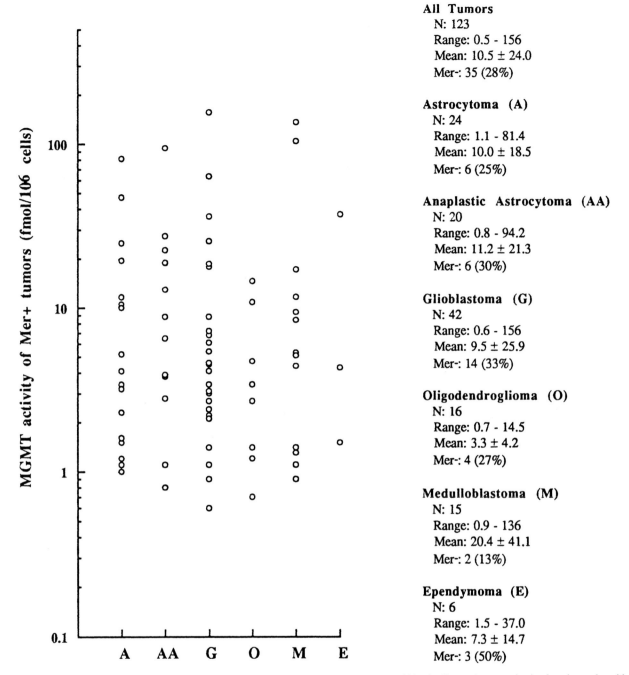

All Tumors
N: 123
Range: 0.5 - 156
Mean: 10.5 ± 24.0
Mer-: 35 (28%)

Astrocytoma (A)
N: 24
Range: 1.1 - 81.4
Mean: 10.0 ± 18.5
Mer-: 6 (25%)

Anaplastic Astrocytoma (AA)
N: 20
Range: 0.8 - 94.2
Mean: 11.2 ± 21.3
Mer-: 6 (30%)

Glioblastoma (G)
N: 42
Range: 0.6 - 156
Mean: 9.5 ± 25.9
Mer-: 14 (33%)

Oligodendroglioma (O)
N: 16
Range: 0.7 - 14.5
Mean: 3.3 ± 4.2
Mer-: 4 (27%)

Medulloblastoma (M)
N: 15
Range: 0.9 - 136
Mean: 20.4 ± 41.1
Mer-: 2 (13%)

Ependymoma (E)
N: 6
Range: 1.5 - 37.0
Mean: 7.3 ± 14.7
Mer-: 3 (50%)

Figure 14–1 MGMT content of 123 brain tumors. The MGMT activity of 91 Mer$^+$ tumors within six diagnostic categories is plotted on a logarithmic scale. The number of specimens (N), range of activity, mean and SD of activity, and fraction of Mer$^-$ specimens (those with activity below the limit of detection, i.e., ≤0.5 fmol/10^6 cells or ≤300 molecules/cell are listed for each diagnostic category. Mer$^-$ specimens were assigned a value of 0.25 fmol/10^6 cells when calculating mean MGMT activities.

MGMT content, is summarized in Table 14–1. Survival is reported as LD_{10} in the absence or presence of O^6-BG; the contribution of MGMT to resistance is reported as the fold-change in LD_{10}. Major results are as follows:

1. Measurable MGMT activity ranged from 10 to 119 fmol/10^6 cells. Only the glioblastoma-derived line SNB19 had no detectable activity. Mean MGMT content was compa-

rable between glioma- and medulloblastoma-derived lines (59 ± 42 vs. 59 ± 39 fmol/10^6 cells).

2. The cell lines differ in intrinsic sensitivity to alkylating agents. The LD_{10} in the absence of O^6-BG varied 28-fold for MNNG (column 3) and 7.5-fold for BCNU (column 6). The Mer$^-$ line SNB19 showed the greatest sensitivity to both agents.

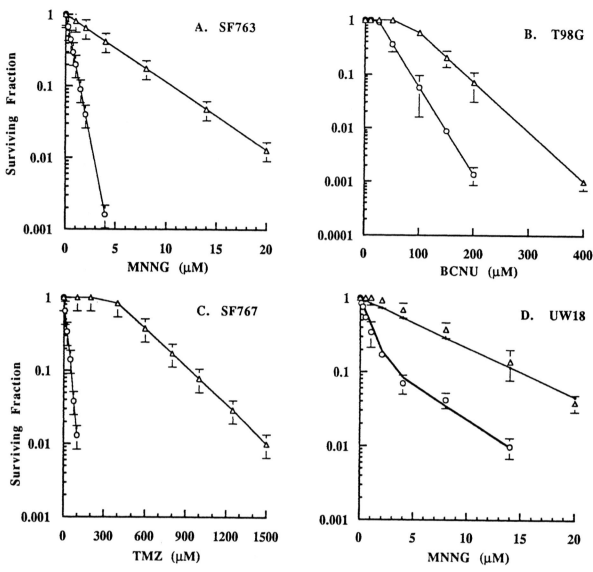

Figure 14–2 Alkylating agent survival of human brain tumor cell lines in the presence (*triangles*) or absence (*circles*) of O^6-benzylguanine (O^6-BG). *A*, Glioma line SF763 displays linear survival curves when exposed to MNNG in the absence or presence of O^6-BG. Linearity is indicative of uniform response throughout the cell population. *B*, Glioma line T98G exposed to BCNU shows a linear survival curve with a shoulder (threshold dose). O^6-BG increases BCNU sensitivity by decreasing the threshold dose and slightly increasing the rate of killing on the exponential portion of the curve (D37). Reduction of the threshold dose indicates that removal of O^6-chloroethylguanine by MGMT is responsible, in part, for prevention of lethality at low BCNU concentrations. *C*, Glioma line SF767 exposed to temozolomide shows a linear survival curve with a shoulder. O^6-BG increases sensitivity by increasing the rate of killing and eliminating the shoulder. Elimination of the shoulder shows that removal of O^6-methylguanine by MGMT is responsible for prevention of lethality at low doses. *D*, Glioma line UW18 exposed to MNNG displays a linear response. O^6-BG increases sensitivity by increasing the rate of killing sixfold in a subpopulation (80%) of cells. The remaining subpopulation (20%) of cells is less responsive to O^6-benzylguanine as evidenced by a twofold decrease in the rate of killing.

3. The contribution of MGMT to MNNG resistance differs widely among the lines, as shown by the 31-fold range in reduction of LD_{10} effected by O^6-BG (column 5). As expected, the Mer⁻ line SNB19 showed no potentiation of killing. The average reduction of LD_{10} in the Mer⁺ lines was 10-fold and the maximum reduction was 31-fold. We have obtained similar results for six lines with a different methylating agent, temozolomide (Table 14–2).

4. The contribution of MGMT to BCNU resistance is much smaller than to MNNG resistance. The average reduction

in LD_{10} for BCNU in the Mer⁺ lines was 2.1-fold, the maximum reduction being 3.4-fold (see Table 14–1, column 8). Again, the Mer⁻ line SNB19 showed no potentiation. Notably, two Mer⁺ lines U373MG and U138MG also showed no potentiation. SF763, SF767 and the human colon carcinoma line HT29 displayed potentiation comparable to that observed by others.[69, 73, 82]

5. Importantly, alkylating agent resistance differs among the lines *even after ablation of MGMT*. Thus, LD_{10} in the presence of O^6-BG varied 20-fold for MNNG (see Table

TABLE 14–1
EFFECT OF ABLATING MGMT WITH O^6-BENZYLGUANINE ON BCNU AND MNNG SENSITIVITY OF HUMAN GLIOMA- AND MEDULLOBLASTOMA-DERIVED CELL LINES: ALKYLATION OF PROLIFERATING MONOLAYERS*

Line	MGMT	LD$_{10}$MNNG			LD$_{10}$BCNU		
		$-O^6$-BG	$+O^6$-BG	Change	$-O^6$-BG	$+O^6$-BG	Change
		Glioma-Derived Lines					
SNB19	<0.5	0.8 ± 0.2	0.8 ± 0.2	1.0	49 ± 8	46 ± 7	1.1
U373MG	11 ± 2	9.9 ± 1.1	0.7 ± 0.03	14.1	84 ± 8	63 ± 6	1.2
UW455	30 ± 11	4.6 ± 0.2	0.7 ± 0.04	6.6	84 ± 6	55 ± 5	1.5
SF767	61 ± 12	9.4 ± 1.0	0.3 ± 0.06	31.3	129 ± 12	46 ± 10	2.8
U138MG	71 ± 23	19 ± 1.0	1.4 ± 0.05	13.6	141 ± 16	119 ± 12	1.2
UW18	74 ± 20	15 ± 1.6	3.2 ± 1.6	4.7	97 ± 15	99 ± 10	2.0
T98G	104 ± 14	5.6 ± 1.0	0.8 ± 0.09	7.0	184 ± 22	84 ± 10	2.2
SF763	119 ± 19	11 ± 1.4	1.4 ± 0.2	7.9	366 ± 24	184 ± 20	2.0
HT29	71 ± 15	11 ± 1.0	1.3 ± 0.1	8.5	284 ± 20	48 ± 10	4.8
		Medulloblastoma-Derived Lines					
UW443	10 ± 3	7.7 ± 0.5	2.4 ± 0.1	3.2	138 ± 7	41 ± 3	3.4
UW228-2	82 ± 15	19 ± 2.0	5.2 ± 0.8	3.7	117 ± 15	85 ± 9	1.4
UW228-1	91 ± 15	22 ± 2.0	6.1 ± 1.4	3.6	197 ± 20	85 ± 8	2.3
UW228-3	99 ± 7	17 ± 1.7	1.1 ± 0.1	15.5	213 ± 61	74 ± 6	2.9

*The MNNG and BCNU sensitivity of cells treated as monolayers was assayed as survival of colony-forming ability on a plastic substratum. LD$_{10}$ (μM) was estimated from survival curves (e.g., Fig. 14–2) and represents the mean and SD of at least three independent experiments (at least nine determinations for each dose) in the absence or presence of O^6-benzylguanine (O^6-BG). MGMT content (fmol/10^6 cells) is the mean and SD of at least ten independent determinations. A full description of methods and a detailed analysis of survival curves is presented in references 78 and 79. Change refers to LD$_{10}$($-O^6$-BG)/LD$_{10}$ ($+O^6$-BG). Changes ≥1.3 are statistically significant at $P \le 0.05$, assessed by Student's t statistic.

14–1, column 4), 9-fold for temozolomide (see Table 14–2, column 4) and 4-fold for BCNU (see Table 14–1, column 7).

CONCLUSIONS FOR CELLS ALKYLATED WHILE ADHERENT TO A PLASTIC SUBSTRATUM

1. MGMT contributes to MNNG resistance in all Mer$^+$ lines (3-fold or greater decrease of LD$_{10}$), and is a major determinant of resistance in four lines (10-fold or greater decrease in LD$_{10}$).

2. In contrast, MGMT affords only limited resistance to BCNU (less than 3-fold decreases in LD$_{10}$ in all Mer$^+$ lines save one).

3. The variation in LD$_{10}$ that persists in the presence of O^6-BG (item 5 in the preceding list) demonstrates that

TABLE 14–2
POTENTIATION OF TEMOZOLOMIDE CYTOTOXICITY BY O^6-BENZYLGUANINE*

Cell Line	MGMT	LD$_{10}$ Temozolomide (μM)		
		$-O^6$-BG	$+O^6$-BG	Change
SNB19	<0.5	406	377	1.1
SF767	61 ± 12	930	45	20.7
UW18	74 ± 20	1061	297	3.6
T98G	104 ± 14	980	400	2.2
SF763	119 ± 19	915	212	4.3
UW228-1	91 ± 15	1036	140	7.4

*Cytotoxicity was assessed from survival curves as described in the legend to Table 14–1.

alkylating agent resistance depends on a mechanism in addition to MGMT.

RESULTS AND CONCLUSIONS FOR CELLS TREATED WITH ALKYLATING AGENTS WHILE SUSPENDED IN GROWTH MEDIUM

Concomitant detailed analysis of ten lines corroborated the results described for adherent cells, and revealed important further complexity (Table 14–3). Both variability in resistance and dependence of resistance on MGMT are smaller when cells are treated with alkylating agents in suspension. In the case of BCNU, most lines were unresponsive to O^6-BG or contained an unresponsive subpopulation. The smaller contribution of MGMT to resistance is exemplified in average potentiations of LD$_{10}$ of 4.8-fold for MNNG and 1.2-fold for BCNU in 11 Mer$^+$ lines. The basis of the reduced alkylating agent susceptibility and reduced dependence on MGMT is not known, though our observation that incorporation of thymidine ceases on release of cells into suspension suggests that a proliferative state is involved.

CLINICAL IMPLICATIONS

1. Our data support the presumption that the approximately one-quarter of primary malignant brain tumors[65] that are Mer$^-$ could have heightened sensitivity to methylating agents when compared with the three-quarters of tumors that are Mer$^+$.

2. If O^6-BG can be used clinically, it may be more effective in conjunction with a methylating agent than a CENU. At estimated clinically achievable doses of BCNU (25 to 30 μM),[83] the effect of O^6-BG on survival of our cell lines was negligible.

TABLE 14–3
EFFECT OF ABLATION OF MGMT WITH O^6-BENZYLGUANINE ON BCNU AND MNNG SENSITIVITY OF HUMAN GLIOMA- AND MEDULLOBLASTOMA-DERIVED CELL LINES: ALKYLATION OF CELLS IN SUSPENSION*

Line	MGMT	LD_{10}MNNG			LD_{10}BCNU		
		$-O^6$-BG	$+O^6$-BG	Change	$-O^6$-BG	$+O^6$-BG	Change
Glioma-Derived Lines							
SNB19	<0.5	24 ± 3.0	24 ± 4.0	1.0	222 ± 12	222 ± 15	1.0
SF767	61 ± 12	34 ± 5.6	3.3 ± 0.4	10.3	214 ± 20	129 ± 25	1.7
U138MG	71 ± 23	59 ± 11	4.7 ± 0.3	12.6	160 ± 13	164 ± 14	1.0
UW18	74 ± 20	31 ± 4.0	11 ± 2.0	2.8	92 ± 19	197 ± 15	1.0
T98G	104 ± 14	37 ± 3.4	4.7 ± 1.8	7.9	480 ± 33	440 ± 35	1.1
SF763	119 ± 19	65 ± 5.0	69 ± 4.0	0.9	414 ± 29	401 ± 25	1.0
HT29	71 ± 15	11 ± 1.0	1.3 ± 0.1	8.5	286 ± 23	114 ± 32	2.5
Medulloblastoma-Derived Lines							
UW443	10 ± 3	32 ± 3.0	29 ± 3.0	1.1	301 ± 25	242 ± 32	1.2
UW228-2	82 ± 15	24 ± 3.0	14 ± 2.0	1.6	198 ± 48	142 ± 28	1.4
UW228-1	91 ± 15	26 ± 3.0	14 ± 2.0	1.9	309 ± 65	223 ± 40	1.4
UW228-3	99 ± 7	25 ± 1.0	6.7 ± 1.0	3.7	228 ± 18	176 ± 32	1.3

*The MNNG and BCNU sensitivity of cells alkylated in suspension was assayed as survival of soft agar colony-forming ability. LD_{10} (μM) was estimated from survival curves (see Fig. 14–2) and represents the mean and SD of at least three independent experiments (at least nine determinations for each dose) in the absence or presence of O^6-benzylguanine (O^6-BG). MGMT content (fmol/10^6 cells) is the mean and SD of at least 10 independent determinations. A full description of methods and a detailed analysis of survival curves is presented in references 78 and 79. Change refers to LD_{10} ($-O^6$-BG)/LD_{10} ($+O^6$-BG). Changes ≥ 1.3 are statistically significant at $P \leq 0.05$, assessed by Student's t statistic.

3. That cells are less susceptible to alkylating agent killing when suspended in growth medium, and less dependent on MGMT for survival, may be unfavorable. The presence in tumors of a resistant subpopulation akin to those seen in our experiments—whether genetically determined and/or cell cycle–dependent—would be expected to increase the number of tumor cells that survive therapy. In fact, it has been shown that a resistant minority subpopulation caused regrowth of a heterogeneous human tumor xenograft in nude mice after initial response to BCNU treatment.[84] These results were interpreted to suggest that the magnitude of clinical response may reflect the relative proportions of sensitive and resistant subpopulations, and that the duration of remission may reflect the growth characteristics of the resistant subpopulation(s).

4. Resistance to CENUs and methylating agents is multifactorial, MGMT being one probable determinant. It is now necessary to identify other resistance mechanisms and to devise strategies to surmount them while pursuing a phase I or II study, or both, with an MGMT inhibitor.

BASE EXCISION REPAIR CONTRIBUTES TO CENU RESISTANCE: A STRONG HYPOTHESIS

That MGMT has a role in BCNU resistance, albeit small, establishes that DNA damage is at least partly responsible for cytotoxicity and that DNA repair affects resistance. Importantly, our results indicate that resistance to BCNU, and to MNNG, is multifactorial in human brain tumor cell lines. In view of the diversity of potentially cytotoxic derivatives produced by CENUs, this conclusion is predictable. We propose that another major DNA repair mechanism, namely base excision repair, contributes to CENU resistance of brain tumors.

Base Excision Repair Pathways Are Known

Base excision repair is a ubiquitous defense against DNA damage that has been conserved from bacteria to man. It is responsible for removing a plethora of adducted bases from DNA, including those produced by alkylation. Base excision repair is initiated by one of many DNA glycosylases having different substrate specificities, and proceeds through an abasic site intermediate.[22–25] In the five-step major pathway observed in human cell extracts, steps subsequent to glycosylase action are catalyzed by apurinic/apyrimidinic endonuclease (Ap endonuclease), which cleaves the DNA backbone 5′ to the abasic site, and DNA deoxyribophosphodiesterase, which excises the 5′-terminal sugar phosphate to generate a single nucleotide gap. The gap is filled by DNA polymerase β and sealed by DNA ligase.[85]

That unrepaired abasic sites are lethal is confirmed by the alkylating agent hypersensitivity of bacterial and yeast mutants deficient in Ap endonuclease activity.[24, 28] Single-strand DNA gaps arising as a consequence of DNA repair in alkylating agent-treated cells are also lethal when not repaired, as evidenced by the hypersensitivity of bacterial[86] and yeast[87] mutants deficient in DNA polymerase activity, and of permeabilized human fibroblasts treated with DNA polymerase inhibitors.[88]

Characterization of Human Base Excision Repair Enzymes

3-METHYLADENINE DNA GLYCOSYLASE

3-Methyladenine DNA glycosylases from diverse sources, including man, have been characterized. When expressed in glycosylase-deficient *E. coli*, recombinant human 3-methyl-adenine DNA glycosylase (3-MAG) rescues bacteria from killing by the methylating agent methylmethane sulfonate (MMS).[89] Yeast 3-MAG removes CENU-induced N^7-chloro-ethylguanine and N^7-hydroxyethylguanine from DNA and protects cells against CENU cytotoxicity.[90] The bacterial enzyme has been shown to excise these two derivatives, as well as the CENU-induced intrastrand cross-link 1,2-bis(7-guanyl)ethane.[91, 92] Whether human 3-MAG[93, 94] or other DNA glycosylases[95] also act on these DNA modifications, and whether such activity contributes to CENU resistance remains to be determined. Interestingly, initial studies indicate that a human glioma line (SF188) that is resistant to 1-(2-chloroethyl)-1-nitrosourea has elevated 3-methyladenine DNA glycosylase activity relative to a sensitive line (SF126).[96]

APURINIC/APYRIMIDINIC ENDONUCLEASE

The major human Ap endonuclease[97–99] cleaves the phosphodiester bond 5' to abasic sites, yielding 5'-phosphoryl and 3'-hydroxyl ends, and is structurally and functionally related to the major Ap endonucleases of *E. coli*,[100] *S. cerevisiae*,[101] *Drosophila*,[102] and other mammals.[103, 104] The yeast[28] and bacterial[24] enzymes protect cells against the cytotoxicity of alkylating agents. Expression of the human enzyme in Ap endonuclease-deficient *E. coli* confers resistance to killing by methylmethane sulfonate.[98] The nucleotide sequence of the entire human gene, together with 0.5 kb of upstream sequence, has been determined,[105] revealing four small introns and five exons, the first of which is untranslated.

DNA POLYMERASE β

Mammalian DNA polymerase β has long been considered a primary catalyst for DNA repair synthesis, particularly short-patch repair.[106, 107] A nucleoside triphosphate analog inhibitor of DNA polymerase β sensitizes permeabilized human fibroblasts to the lethal effects of MNNG.[88] Recently, human DNA polymerase β has been implicated in base excision repair in extracts of HeLa cells.[85] Mechanistically, it is relevant that expression of DNA polymerase β in *E. coli* rescues the alkylating agent sensitivity caused by mutation in the host DNA polymerase I.[108] Apparently, DNA polymerase β can fill repair gaps in a heterologous bacterial host as well as in mammalian cells. The sequence of the entire human DNA polymerase β gene, consisting of 13 exons, is known[109] together with flanking sequence required for functional promoter activity.[110] In the last year, crystal structures have been reported from two laboratories.[111–113] An explicit impetus for determination of the three-dimensional structure[111] is that it may facilitate design of structure-based inhibitors that could increase the efficacy of anti-tumor radiation and chemotherapy.

Base Excision Repair Protects Cells Against CENU Killing

A direct in vivo demonstration that base excision repair protects against CENU cytotoxicity is available in the model eukaryote *S. cerevisiae*. In *S. cerevisiae*, disruption of the gene for 3-MAG renders cells hypersensitive to killing by CENU. Moreover, when yeast 3-MAG is expressed in glycosylase-deficient *E. coli*, the yeast glycosylase increases survival of CENU-treated bacteria.[90] The ability of a eukaryotic DNA glycosylase to protect bacteria against CENU-induced lethality suggests that base excision repair protects human cells from CENU cytotoxicity. If human 3-MAG or other glycosylase activity protects against CENU cytotoxicity, it follows that varying levels of glycosylase activity may contribute to the differing sensitivity of brain tumors to CENUs that is observed clinically. Fragmentary data are consistent with this idea. Extracts of the CENU-resistant human glioma line SF188 have two to three times more 3-MAG activity than the sensitive line SF126.[96] Following CENU treatment, DNA from resistant SF188 is depleted relative to DNA from sensitive SF126, in several as yet uncharacterized lesions that have chromatographic properties of 7-substituted guanines, but are not either of the major adducts N^7-chloroethylguanine or N^7-hydroxyethylguanine. It is possible that at least some of these lesions are cytotoxic and are removed by human glycosylase activity because they are substrates for the bacterial 3-MAG.[91, 92]

Base Excision Repair Protects Against Methylating Agent Cytotoxicity

A strong case, based on the nature of the DNA alkylation products and extensive experimental evidence, can be made for a role for base excision repair in resistance to methylating agent chemotherapy. It has been shown directly that base excision repair protects against methylating agent cytotoxicity in genetically tractable organisms. For example, in *E. coli* and in *S. cerevisiae*, mutants deficient in 3-methyladenine DNA glycosylase,[24, 45] Ap endonuclease[24, 28] and DNA repair polymerase activities[86, 87] are hypersensitive to methylating agents. Comparable mutants of mammalian cells are not available. However, it should be emphasized that the conservation of major DNA repair mechanisms from bacteria to man,[22] encompassing homology in base excision repair enzymes, makes it highly likely that base excision repair protects human cells from killing by methylating agents.

Base Excision Repair Enzymes in Neoplastic and Normal Brain

We have conducted an initial survey of Ap endonuclease and DNA polymerase β activities together with MGMT in 12 tumors and adjacent histologically normal brain (Table 14–4). DNA polymerase β and MGMT activities vary 50-fold among the tumors, whereas Ap endonuclease activity varies 4-fold. None of the specimens lacks DNA polymerase β or Ap endonuclease activity, although four tumor and five normal brain specimens lack measurable MGMT. The small sample reveals no statistically significant relationship between levels of the three activities in tumor or normal brain, indicating that they are not expressed coordinately. A majority of tumors show elevation of at least one repair activity relative to adjacent normal brain, but no consistent

TABLE 14–4
DNA REPAIR ACTIVITIES IN TUMORS AND ADJACENT NORMAL BRAIN*

Patient, Age (Yr)/Sex/ Diagnosis†	DNA Polymerase β‡			Ap Endonuclease§			MGMT		
	Tumor	Normal	T/N	Tumor	Normal	T/N	Tumor	Normal	T/N
5/F/A	0.11	0.10	1.1	216	199	1.1	Mer⁻	5.7	<0.09
20/F/A	0.13	0.053	2.4	233	56	4.2	10	3.5	2.9
33/F/O	0.42	0.31	1.4	316	151	2.1	14.5	3.5	4.1
34/F/G	0.25	0.11	2.3	116	40	2.9	2.4	Mer⁻	>4.8
35/F/A	0.065	0.090	0.72	199	183	1.1	19.5	Mer⁻	>39.0
38/F/AA	0.30	0.40	0.75	216	75	2.9	Mer⁻	1.6	<0.3
40/M/G	0.29	0.084	2.4	131	60	2.2	7.2	3.9	1.8
41/M/G	3.1	0.26	12.1	199	233	0.85	25.6	22.6	1.1
43/F/O	0.12	0.073	1.6	136	171	0.80	4.7	3.2	1.5
44/M/G	1.3	0.13	10.0	211	47	4.5	4.5	Mer⁻	>9.0
47/M/G	0.44	0.15	2.9	71	146	0.49	Mer⁻	Mer⁻	—
72/M/G	0.25	0.16	1.6	183	166	1.1	Mer⁻	Mer⁻	—

*Activities are expressed as pg/10^6 cells for DNA polymerase β, pmol Ap sites nicked/10^6 cells/min for Ap endonuclease, and fmol/10^6 cells for MGMT. Values for DNA polymerase β and Ap endonuclease are the average of duplicate determinations, whereas MGMT levels are the mean of five or more determinations. SDs for MGMT content are 20% or less of the mean.

†*Abbreviations:* A, astrocytoma; AA, anaplastic astrocytoma; G, glioblastoma; O, oligodendroglioma.

‡DNA polymerase β: Cells isolated from tissue,[65] as well as the DNA polymerase β standard, were dissolved in sample buffer, heated, and applied to a 12.5% SDS-polyacrylamide gel cast with gapped DNA in the matrix. After electrophoresis, the enzyme was renatured in situ and activity was detected by incorporation of α-^{32}P-labeled dTTP.[114, 115] Activity was visualized by autoradiography and quantitated by phosphor imaging. Activity of cells is normalized to the DNA polymerase β standard.

§Ap endonuclease: A high-speed supernatant of sonicated cells was incubated with acid-treated pUC19 plasmid DNA, after which supercoiled and nicked DNA was resolved in an agarose gel.[116] The gel was stained with ethidium bromide, photographed, and scanned using Adobe Photoshop 2.5. Band density of the scanned image was quantitated using NIH Image Version 1.55. Activity is calculated from the fraction of nicked molecules.[117]

pattern of elevation is seen among the three activities. Apparently, tumorigenesis in brain promotes enhanced expression of DNA repair activities that could contribute to alkylating agent resistance.

Future assay of a large number of specimens will allow us to discern patterns of variability, if any, in tumor repair activities. Low or absent activities could provide a rationale for treatment with a specific class of DNA damaging agent in order to exploit apparent deficits in repair capability and for concomitant suppression of the remaining activities with anti-resistance therapies.

CONTRIBUTION OF OTHER DNA REPAIR MECHANISMS AND DNA DAMAGE TOLERANCE TO RESISTANCE

Nucleotide Excision Repair

Nucleotide excision repair (NER) mediates the removal of large helix-distorting lesions such as UV-induced dipyrimidine dimers and cisplatin-induced damage.[118] A role for NER in monofunctional alkylating agent resistance is demonstrated by the ethylating and methylating agent hypersensitivity[119, 120] of fibroblast cell lines derived from patients with xeroderma pigmentosum, an autosomal recessive disease characterized by defective NER and increased sensitivity to UV and UV-mimetic drugs,[121, 122] relative to fibroblast lines from normal individuals. The greater sensitivity to ethylnitrosourea of one xeroderma pigmentosum line was associated with a reduced rate of removal of O^6-ethylguanine.[123] Indirect evidence suggests that NER may also participate in the removal of O^6-methylguanine.[124]

NER contributes to CENU resistance in bacteria[125] and

can be a major determinant of CENU resistance in mammalian cells as evidenced by the 20-fold greater sensitivity of NER-deficient CHO cell lines.[126, 127] In human cells, NER may act in concert with MGMT to remove chloroethyl adducts from the O^6 position of guanine as has been demonstrated for ethyl adducts.[131, 132] We have recently reported elevated levels in brain tumors relative to adjacent, histologically normal brain of mRNA for ERCC1, a NER protein that participates in DNA strand incision.[128] This finding is significant because elevated levels of tumor ERCC1 mRNA are associated with resistance to platinum-based therapy of ovarian cancer.[129]

Recombination

Recombination may contribute to CENU resistance, as evidenced by the CENU hypersensitivity of recombination-deficient bacteria[125] and yeast.[130] Recombination may act on a variety of lesions implicated in CENU cytotoxicity. For example, differential CENU resistance of two human glioma lines is accompanied by lesser abundance of the intrastrand cross-link 1,2-(diguan-7-yl)-ethane and the adducts 3-(2-hydroxyethyl)deoxyuridine, 1-(2-hydroxyethyl)deoxyguanosine, and 7-(2-chloroethyl)deoxyguanosine in the more resistant line.[17] These lesions may be substrates for NER, as well.

Mismatch Repair (MMR)

Tolerance of the cytotoxic effects of O^6-methylguanine resulting from inactivation of MMR may also reduce sensitivity to methylating agents.[43] MMR corrects DNA polymerase insertion errors that have escaped proofreading.[43, 133, 134] Although the mechanism is best understood in *E. coli*, four human proteins homologous to bacterial and yeast MMR proteins have been identified. *hMSH2* is a homolog of the bacterial mutS gene and apparently codes for a protein that recognizes and binds mismatches. *hMLH1*, *hPMS1*, and *hPMS2* are homologs of mutL. In bacteria, the MutL protein forms a complex with MutS that activates a mismatch-excising endonuclease activity encoded by mutH. The function of the human homologs of mutL remains to be defined.

Importantly, Mer⁻ status has been observed to lead to loss of mismatch repair.[43] Revertants of Mer⁻ cell lines that have become insensitive to the cytotoxicity of persistent O^6-methylguanine lesions sometimes retain their Mer⁻ status. The methylation-tolerant phenotype of these revertants results from loss of MMR and can be explained as follows. Because O^6-methylguanine cannot form a Watson-Crick base pair, replication opposite this adduct invariably forms a substrate for mismatch repair. Persistence of O^6-methylguanine in the template strand guarantees formation of another mismatch during DNA synthesis to fill the gap resulting from excision of the non-complementary nucleotide. Repeated attempts to remove the mispair are thought to be responsible for the lethality of O^6-methylguanine. Defects in MMR render cells insensitive to O^6-methylguanine lethality at the cost of greatly elevated rates (as much as 100-fold) of G to A transitions.[43]

In addition to acting at single base mispairs, MMR also removes small, extrahelical loops that can arise at reiterative and short tandem repeat sequences (microsatellite sequences) during DNA replication.[43] Thus, defects in MMR predispose to frameshift mutations in these sequences.[135, 136] The potential clinical significance of MMR for brain tumors is underscored by the finding of microsatellite instability in human astrocytic gliomas. Seventeen microsatellite loci on seven chromosomes have been analyzed in ten glioblastomas and in six lower-grade astrocytomas.[136] Five tumors (31%), all of them glioblastomas, displayed frameshifts at one or more loci. These results suggest that loss of MMR may be a frequent late event in the progression of human astrocytic gliomas.[136]

It has been suggested that loss of MMR may confer a selective advantage in Mer⁻ cells by mitigating the lethality of O^6-methylguanine.[43] It will therefore be of interest to examine the incidence of microsatellite instability among Mer⁺ and Mer⁻ brain tumors (see Fig. 14–1), especially tumors that have recurred following chemotherapy with a methylating agent.

SUMMARY AND PERSPECTIVE

We have presented a synopsis of evidence implicating DNA repair in human brain tumor resistance to alkylating agents. Several laboratories, including our own, have demonstrated a role for MGMT in promoting resistance to methylating and chloroethylating agents. However, it is of cardinal importance that our data also show alkylating agent resistance to be multifactorial. The diversity of alkylation-induced DNA damage, together with studies in bacteria, yeast, and non–brain tumor-derived mammalian cell lines, implicate base excision repair, nucleotide excision repair, recombina-tion, and loss of mismatch repair as potential resistance mechanisms. Because the prognosis for malignant gliomas in adults and children remains dismal, the contribution of repair mechanisms in addition to MGMT should be documented, and strategies to overcome DNA repair-mediated resistance to known clinically useful agents should be meticulously developed and carefully evaluated.

ACKNOWLEDGMENTS

This work was funded by grants from the American Cancer Society (EDT-53 and Professor of Clinical Oncology 071) and NIH (T32CA-09437 and OIG-R35-CA39903). Additional support was provided by the Neuro-oncology Research Endowment and Jessie's Perfect Peach Gift Fund of Childrens' Hospital and Medical Center of Seattle, and the John Gallagher Fund of the Department of Neurological Surgery, University of Washington, Seattle. We thank Lawrence Loeb for his interest and support.

REFERENCES

1. Kornblith PL, Walker MJ: Chemotherapy for malignant brain tumors. J Neurosurg 1988; 68:1–17.
2. Stewart DJ: The role of chemotherapy in the treatment of gliomas in adults. Cancer Treatment Rev 1989; 16:129–160.
3. Levin VA, Silver P, Hannigan A, et al: Superiority of post-radiother-apy adjuvant chemotherapy with CCNU, procarbazine and vincristine (PVC) over BCNU for anaplastic gliomas: NCOG 6G61 final report. Int J Radiat Oncol Biol Phys 1990; 18:321–324.
4. Yung WKA: Chemotherapy for malignant brain tumors. Curr Opinion Oncol 1990; 2:673–678.
5. Berger MS, Spence AM, Stelzer KJ: Brain tumors. *In* Brain MC, Carbone PP (eds): Current Therapy in Hematology/Oncology. St Louis, Mosby–Year Book, 1994.
6. Rostomily RC, Spence AM, Duong D, et al: Multimodality manage-ment of recurrent adult malignant gliomas: Results of a phase II multiagent chemotherapy study and analysis of cytoreductive surgery. Neurosurgery 1994; 35:378–388.
7. Packer RJ, Siegel KA, Sutton LN, et al: Efficacy of adjuvant chemo-therapy of patients with poor-risk medulloblastoma: A preliminary report. Ann Neurol 1988; 24:503–558.
8. Friedman HS, Oakes WJ, Bigner SH, et al: Medulloblastoma: Tumor biological and clinical perspectives. J Neurooncol 1991; 11:1–15.
9. McVie JG: The therapeutic challenge of gliomas. Eur J Cancer 1993; 29A:936–939.
10. Levin VA, Prados MD: Treatment of recurrent gliomas and metastatic brain tumors with a polydrug protocol designed to combat nitrosourea resistance. J Clin Oncol 1992; 10:766–777.
11. Newlands ES, Blackledge G, Slack JA, et al: Phase I trial of temozo-lomide (CCRG 8 1045: M&B 39831: NSC 362856). Br J Cancer 1992; 65:287–291.
12. O'Reilly SM, Newlands ES, Glaser MG, et al: Temozolomide: A new oral cytotoxic chemotherapeutic agent with promising activity against primary brain tumors. Eur J Cancer 1993; 29A:940–942.
13. McCormick JE, McElhinney RS: Nitrosoureas from chemist to physi-cian: Classification and recent approaches to drug design. Eur J Cancer 1990; 26:207–221.
14. Ludlum DB: DNA alkylation by the haloethylnitrosoureas: Nature of modifications produced and their enzymatic repair or removal. Mutat Res 1990; 233:117–126.
15. Lindahl T: Instability and decay of the primary structure of DNA. Nature 1993; 362:709–715.
16. Kohn KW, Erickson LC, Laurent G, et al: DNA crosslinking and the origin of sensitivity to chloroethylnitrosoureas. *In* Prestayko AW, Cooke ST, Baker LH, et al (eds): Nitrosoureas: Current Status and New Developments. New York, Academic Press, 1981.

17. Bodell WJ, Tokuda K, Ludlum DB: Differences in DNA alkylation products formed in sensitive and resistant human glioma cells treated with N-(2-chloroethyl)-N-nitrosourea. Cancer Res 1988; 48:4489–4492.

18. Pegg AE: Mammalian O^6-alkylguanine-DNA alkyltransferase: Regulation and importance in response to alkylating carcinogenic and therapeutic agents. Cancer Res 1990; 50:6119–6129.

19. Pegg AE, Byers TL: Repair of DNA containing O^6-alkylguanine. FASEB J 1992; 6:2303–2310.

20. Brent TP, Remack JS: Formation of covalent complexes between human O^6-alkylguanine-DNA alkyltransferase and BCNU-treated defined length synthetic oligonucleotides. Nucleic Acids Res 1988; 16:6779–6788.

21. Gonzaga PE, Brent TP: Affinity purification and characterization of human O^6-alkylguanine-DNA alkyltransferase complexed with BCNU-treated synthetic oligonucleotide. Nucleic Acids Res 1989; 17:6581–6590.

22. Barnes DE, Lindahl T, Sedgwick B: DNA repair. Curr Opin Cell Biol 1993; 5:424–433.

23. Lindahl T, Sedgwick B, Sekiguchi M, et al: Regulation and expression of the adaptive response to alkylating agents. Annu Rev Biochem 1988; 57:133–157.

24. Sancar A, Sancar GB: DNA repair enzymes. Annu Rev Biochem 1988; 57:29–67.

25. Volkert MR: Adaptive response of Escherichia coli to alkylation damage. Environ Mol Mutagen 1988; 11:241–255.

26. Lindahl T, Nyberg B: Rate of depurination of native deoxyribonucleic acid. Biochemistry 1972; 11:3610–3618.

27. Loeb LA, Preston BD: Mutagenesis by apurinic/apyrimidinic sites. Annu Rev Genet 1986; 20:201–230.

28. Ramotar D, Popoff SC, Gralla EB, et al: Cellular role of yeast APN1 apurinic endonuclease/3′-diesterase: Repair of oxidative and alkylation DNA damage and control of spontaneous mutation. Mol Cell Biol 1991; 11:4537–4544.

29. Sagher D, Strauss B: Insertion of nucleosides opposite apurinic/apyrimidinic sites in deoxyribonucleic acid during in vivo synthesis: Uniqueness of adenine nucleotides. Biochemistry 1983; 22:4518–4526.

30. Schaaper RM, Kunkel TA, Loeb LA: Infidelity of DNA synthesis associated with bypass of apurinic sites. Proc Natl Acad Sci USA 1983; 80:487–491.

31. Gentil A, Margot A, Saracin A: Apurinic sites cause mutations in simian virus 40. Mutat Res 1984; 236:173–201.

32. Tong WP, Kohn KW, Ludlum DB: Modifications of DNA by different haloethylnitrosoureas. Cancer Res 1982; 42:4460–4464.

33. Muller N, Eisenbrand G: The influence of the N^7 substituents on the stability of N^7-alkylated guanosines. Chem Biol Interact 1985; 53:173–181.

34. Prakash AS, Gibson NW: Sequence-selective depurination, DNA interstrand cross-linking and DNA strand break formation associated with alkylated DNA. Carcinogenesis 1992; 13:425–431.

35. Lown JW, Singh R: Mechanism of the action of anti-tumor 3-(2-haloethyl)aryltriazenes in deoxyribonucleic acid. Biochem Pharmacol 1982; 31:1257–1266.

36. Gibson N, Zlotogorski C, Erickson LC: Specific DNA repair mechanisms may protect some human tumor cells from DNA interstrand crosslinking by chloroethylnitrosoureas but not from crosslinking by other anti-tumor alkylating agents. Carcinogenesis 1985; 6:445–450.

37. Gibson NW, Hartley JA, LaFrance RJ, et al: Differential cytotoxicity and DNA-damaging effects produced in human cells of the Mer+ and Mer− phenotypes by a series of alkyltriazenylimidazoles. Carcinogenesis 1986; 7:259–265.

38. Laval F, Lopes F, Madelmont JC, et al: Excision of imidazole ring-opened N^7-hydroxyethylguanine from chloroethylnitrosourea-treated DNA by Escherichia coli formamidopyrimidine-DNA glycosylase. IARC Sci Publ 1991; 105:412–416.

39. Seidenfeld J, Sprague WS: Comparisons between sensitive and resistant human tumor cell lines regarding effects of polyamine depletion on chloroethylnitrosourea efficacy. Cancer Res 1990; 50:521–526.

40. Ducore J: α-Difluoromethylornithine effects on nitrosourea-induced cytotoxicity and crosslinking in a methylation excision repair positive (Mer+) human cell line. Biochem Pharmacol 1987; 36:2169–2174.

41. Seidenfeld J, Barnes D, Block AL, et al: Comparison of DNA interstrand cross-linking and strand breakage by 1,3-bis(2-chloroethyl)-1-nitrosourea in polyamine-depleted and control human adenocarcinoma cells. Cancer Res 1987; 47:4538–4543.

42. Saffhill R, Margison GP, O'Conner PJ: Mechanisms of carcinogenesis induced by alkylating agents. Biochim Biophys Acta 1985; 823:111–145.

43. Karran P, Bignami M: DNA damage tolerance, mismatch repair and genomic instability. BioEssays 1994; 16:833–839.

44. Chen J, Derfler B, Samson L: Saccharomyces cerevisiae 3-methyladenine DNA glycosylase has homology to the AlkA glycosylase of E. coli and is induced in response to DNA alkylation damage. EMBO J 1990; 9:4569–4575.

45. Klungland A, Fairbairn L, Watson AJ, et al: Expression of the E. coli 3-methyladenine DNA glycosylase 1 gene in mammalian cells reduces the toxic and mutagenic effects of methylating agents. EMBO J 1992; 11:4439–4444.

46. Harbraken Y, Laval F: Increased resistance of the Chinese hamster mutant irs1 cells to monofunctional alkylating agents by transfection of the E. coli or mammalian N3-methyladenine-DNA glycosylase gene. Mutat Res 1993; 293:187–195.

47. Bodell WJ, Aida T, Berger MS, et al: Increased repair of O^6-alkylguanine DNA adducts in glioma-derived human cells resistant to the cytotoxic and cytogenetic effects of 1,3-bis(2-chloroethyl)-1-nitrosourea. Carcinogenesis 1986; 7:879–883.

48. Gonzaga PE, Potter PM, Niu T, et al: Identification of the cross-link between human O^6-methylguanine-DNA methyltransferase and chloroethylnitrosourea-treated DNA. Cancer Res 1992; 52:6052–6058.

49. Nakatsu Y, Hattori K, Hayakawa H, et al: Organization and expression of the human gene O^6-methylguanine-DNA methyltransferase. Mutat Res 1993; 293:119–132.

50. Costello JF, Futscher BW, Tano K, et al: Graded methylation in the promoter and body of the O^6-methylguanine-DNA methyltransferase (MGMT) gene correlates with MGMT expression in human glioma cells. J Biol Chem 1994; 269:17228–17237.

51. Rydberg B, Spurr N, Karran P: cDNA cloning and chromosome assignment of the human O^6-methylguanine-DNA methyltransferase. J Biol Chem 1990; 265:9563–9569.

52. von Wronski MA, Shiota S, Tano K, et al: Structural and immunological comparison of indigenous human O^6-methylguanine-DNA methyltransferase with that encoded by a cloned cDNA. J Biol Chem 1991; 266:1064–1070.

53. Tano K, Shiota S, Collier J, et al: Isolation and structural characterization of a cDNA clone encoding the human repair protein for O^6-alkylguanine. Proc Natl Acad Sci USA 1990; 87:686–690.

54. Pieper RO, Costello JF, Kroes RA, et al: Direct correlation between methylation status and expression of the human O^6-methylguanine-DNA methyltransferase gene. Cancer Comm 1991; 3:241–253.

55. Wang Y, Kato T, Ayaki H, et al: Correlation between DNA methylation and expression of O^6-methylguanine-DNA methyltransferase gene in cultured human tumor cells. Mutat Res 1992; 273:221–230.

56. von Wronski MA, Harris LC, Tano K, et al: Cytosine methylation and suppression of O^6-methylguanine-DNA methyltransferase expression in human rhabdomyosarcoma cell lines and xenografts. Oncol Res 1992; 4:167–174.

57. von Wronski MA, Brent TP: Effect of 5-azacytidine on expression of the human DNA repair enzyme O^6-methylguanine-DNA methyltransferase. Carcinogenesis 1994; 15:577–582.

58. Arita I, Tatsumi K, Tachibana A, et al: Instability of the Mex− phenotype in human lymphoblastoid cell lines. Mutat Res 1988; 280:167–172.

59. Arita I, Fujimori A, Takebe H, et al: Evidence for the spontaneous conversion of Mex− to Mex+ in human lymphoblastoid lines. Carcinogenesis 1990; 11:1733–1738.

60. Strauss B: The control of O^6-methylguanine-DNA methyltransferase (MGMT) activity in mammalian cell: A pre-molecular view. Mutat Res 1990; 233:139–150.

61. Yarosh DB: The role of O^6-methylguanine-DNA methyltransferase in cell survival, mutagenesis and carcinogenesis. Mutat Res 1985; 145:1–16.

62. Gerson SL, Trey JE, Miller K, et al: Comparison of O^6-alkylguanine-DNA alkyltransferase activity based on DNA content in human, rat and mouse tissues. Carcinogenesis 1986; 7:745–749.

63. Frosina G, Rossi O, Arena G, et al: O^6-alkylguanine-DNA alkyltransferase activity in human brain tumors. Cancer Lett 1990; 55:153–158.

64. Citron M, Decker R, Chen S, et al: O^6-methylguanine-DNA methyl-

transferase in human normal and tumor tissue from brain, lung and ovary. Cancer Res 1991; 51:4131–4134.

65. Silber JR, Mueller BA, Ewers TG, et al: Comparison of O^6-methylguanine-DNA methyltransferase activity in brain tumors and adjacent normal brain. Cancer Res 1993; 53:3416–3420.

67. Bodell WJ, Aida T, Berger MS, et al: Repair of O^6-(2-chloroethyl)guanine mediates the biological effects of chloroethylnitrosoureas. Environment Health Perspect 1985; 62:119–126.

68. Dolan ME, Moschel RC, Pegg AE: Depletion of mammalian O^6-alkylguanine DNA alkyltransferase provides a means to evaluate the role of this protein in protection against carcinogenic and therapeutic alkylating agents. Proc Natl Acad Sci USA 1990; 87:5368–5372.

69. Dolan ME, Stine L, Mitchell RB, et al: Modulation of mammalian O^6-alkylguanine-DNA alkyltransferase in vivo by O^6-benzylguanine and its effects on the sensitivity of a human glioma tumor to 1-(2-chloroethyl)-3-(4-methyl cyclohexyl)-1-nitrosourea. Cancer Comm 1990; 2:371–377.

70. Dolan ME, Mitchell RB, Mummert C, et al: Effect of O^6-benzylguanine analogues on sensitivity of human tumor cells to the cytotoxic effects of alkylating agents. Cancer Res 1991; 51:3367–3372.

71. He X, Ostrowski LE, von Wronski MA, et al: Expression of O^6-methylguanine-DNA methyltransferase in six human medulloblastoma cell lines. Carcinogenesis 1991; 12:1739–1744.

72. Friedman HS, Dolan ME, Moschel RC, et al: Enhancement of nitrosourea activity in medulloblastoma and glioblastoma multiforme. JNCI 1992; 84:1926–1931.

73. Mitchell RB, Moschel RC, Dolan ME: Effect of O^6-benzylguanine on the sensitivity of human tumor xenografts to 1,3-bis(2-chloroethyl)-1-nitrosourea and on DNA interstrand cross-link formation. Cancer Res 1992; 52:1171–1175.

74. Silber JR, Bobola MS, Ewers TG, et al: O^6-alkylguanine-DNA alkyltransferase is not a major determinant of sensitivity to 1,3-bis(2-chloroethyl)-1-nitrosourea in four medulloblastoma cell lines. Oncol Res 1992; 4:241–248.

75. Felker GM, Friedman HS, Dolan ME, et al: Treatment of subcutaneous and intracranial brain tumor xenografts with O^6-benzylguanine and 1,3-bis(2-chloroethyl)-1-nitrosourea. Cancer Chemother Pharmacol 1993; 32:471–476.

76. Sarkar A, Dolan ME, Gonazola GG, et al: The effects of O^6-benzylguanine and hypoxia on the cytotoxicity of 1,3-bis(2-chloroethyl)-1-nitrosourea in nitrosourea-resistant SF-173 cells. Cancer Chemother Pharmacol 1993; 32:477–481.

77. Hotta T, Saito Y, Mikami T, et al: Interrelationship between O^6-alkylguanine-DNA alkyltransferase activity and susceptibility to chloroethylnitrosoureas in several glioma cell lines. J Neurooncol 1993; 17:1–8.

78. Bobola MS, Blank A, Berger MS, et al: Contribution of O^6-methylguanine-DNA methyltransferase to monofunctional alkylating agent resistance in human brain tumor-derived cell lines. Mol Carcinog 1995; 13:70–80.

79. Bobola MS, Berger MS, Silber JR: Contribution of O^6-methylguanine-DNA methyltransferase to resistance to 1,3-bis(2-chloroethyl)-1-nitrosourea in human brain tumor-derived cell lines. Mol Carcinog 1995; 13:81–88.

80. Major GN, Gardner EJ, Lawley PP: Direct assay for O^6-methylguanine-DNA methyltransferase and comparison of detection methods for the methylated enzyme in polyacrylamide gels and electroblots. Biochem J 1991; 277:87–96.

81. Harm W: Biological Effects of Ultraviolet Radiation. Cambridge, England, Cambridge University Press, 1980.

82. Marathi UK, Kroes RA, Dolan ME, et al: Prolonged depletion of O^6-methylguanine-DNA methyltransferase activity following exposure to O^6-benzylguanine with or without streptozotocin enhances 1,3-bis(2-chloroethyl)-1-nitrosourea sensitivity in vitro. Cancer Res 1993; 53:4281–4286.

83. Ali-Osman F, Giblin J, Dougherty D, et al: Application of in vivo and in vitro pharmacokinetics for physiologically relevant drug exposure in a human clonogenic cell assay. Cancer Res 1987; 47:3718–3724.

84. Aabo K, Roed H, Vindelo LL, et al: A dominated and resistance subpopulation causes regrowth after response to 1,3-bis(2-chloroethyl)-1-nitrosourea treatment of a heterogeneous small cell lung cancer xenograft in nude mice. Cancer Res 1994; 54:3295–3299.

85. Dianov G, Price A, Lindahl T: Generation of single-nucleotide repair patches following excision of uracil residues from DNA. Mol Cell Biol 1992; 12:1605–1612.

86. Kornberg A, Baker TA: DNA Replication. New York, Freeman, 1992.

87. Blank A, Kim B, Loeb LA: DNA polymerase δ is required for base excision repair of DNA methylation damage in Saccharomyces cerevisiae. Proc Natl Acad Sci USA 1994; 91:9047–9051.

88. Hammond RA, McClung JK, Miller MR: Effect of DNA polymerase inhibitors on DNA repair in intact and permeable human fibroblasts: Evidence that DNA polymerases delta and epsilon are involved in DNA repair synthesis induced by N-methyl-N′-nitro-N-nitrosoguanidine. Biochemistry 1990; 29:286–291.

89. Samson L, Derfler B, Boosalis M, et al: Cloning and characterization of a 3-methyladenine cDNA from human cells whose gene maps to chromosome 16. Proc Natl Acad Sci USA 1991; 88:9127–9131.

90. Matijasevic Z, Boosalis M, Mackay W, et al: Protection against chloroethylnitrosourea cytotoxicity by eukaryotic 3-methyladenine DNA glycosylase. Proc Natl Acad Sci USA 1993; 90:11855–11859.

91. Carter CA, Habraken Y, Ludlum DB: Release of 7-alkylguanines from haloethylnitrosourea-treated DNA by E. coli 3-methyladenine glycosylase II. Biochem Biophys Res Commun 1988; 155:1261–1265.

92. Habraken Y, Carter CA, Kirk MC, et al: Release of 7-alkylguanines from N-(2-chloroethyl)-N′-cyclohexyl-N-nitrosourea modified DNA by 3-methyladenine glycosylase II. Cancer Res 1991; 51:499–503.

93. Saparbaev M, Laval J: Excision of hypoxanthine from DNA containing dIMP residues by the Escherichia coli, yeast, rat and human alkylpurine DNA glycosylases. Proc Natl Acad Sci USA 1994; 91:5873–5877.

94. Dosanjh MK, Chenna A, Kim E, et al: All four known cyclic adducts formed in DNA by the vinyl chloride metabolite chloroacetaldehyde are released by a human DNA glycosylase. Proc Natl Acad Sci USA 1994; 91:1024–1028.

95. Bessho T, Roy R, Yamamoto K, et al: Repair of 8-hydroxyguanine in DNA by mammalian N-methylpurine-DNA glycosylase. Proc Natl Acad Sci USA 1993; 90:8901–8904.

96. Matijasevic Z, Bodell WJ, Ludlum DB: 3-Methyladenine DNA glycosylase activity in a glial cell line sensitive to the haloethylnitrosoureas in comparison with a resistant cell line. Cancer Res 1991; 51:1568–1570.

97. Kane CM, Linn S: Purification and characterization of an apurinic/apyrimidinic endonuclease from HeLa cells. J Biol Chem 1981; 256:3405–3415.

98. Demple B, Herman T, Chen DS: Cloning and expression of APE, the cDNA encoding the major human apurinic endonuclease: Definition of a family of DNA repair enzymes. Proc Natl Acad Sci USA 1991; 88:11450–11454.

99. Robson CN, Hickson ID: Isolation of cDNA clones encoding a human apurinic/apyrimidinic endonuclease that corrects DNA repair and mutagenesis defects in E. coli xth (exonuclease III) mutants. Nucleic Acids Res 1991; 19:5519–5523.

100. Cunningham RP, Saporito SM, Spitzer SG, et al: Endonuclease IV (nfo) mutant of Escherichia coli. J Bacteriol 1986; 168:1120–1127.

101. Popoff SC, Spira AS, Johnson AW, et al: The yeast structural gene (APN1) for the major apurinic endonuclease: homology to E. coli endonuclease IV. Proc Natl Acad Sci USA 1990; 87:4193–4197.

102. Nugent M, Huang S-M, Sander M: Characterization of the apurinic endonuclease activity of Drosophila Rrp 1. Biochemistry 1993; 32:11445–11452.

103. Seki S, Akiyama S, Watanabe M, et al: cDNA and deduced amino acid sequence of a mouse DNA repair enzyme (APEX nuclease) with homology to Escherichia coli exonuclease III. J Biol Chem 1991; 266:20797–20802.

104. Robson CN, Milne AM, Pappin DJC, et al: Isolation of cDNA clones encoding an enzyme from bovine cells that repairs oxidative DNA damage in vitro: Homology with bacterial repair enzymes. Nucleic Acids Res 1991; 19:1087–1092.

105. Harrison L, Ascione G, Menninger JC, et al: Human apurinic endonuclease gene (APE): Structure and genomic mapping (chromosome 14q11.2–12). Hum Mol Genet 1992; 1:677–680.

106. Fry M, Loeb LA: Animal Cell DNA Polymerases. Boca Raton, Fla, CRC Press, 1986.

107. Singhal RK, Wilson SH: Short gap-filling synthesis by DNA polymerase β is processive. J Biol Chem 1993; 268:15906–15911.

108. Sweasy JB, Loeb LA: Detection and characterization of mammalian DNA polymerase β mutants by functional complementation in Escherichia coli. Proc Natl Acad Sci USA 1993; 90:4626–4630.

109. Chyan Y-J, Ackerman S, Shepherd NS, et al: The human DNA

polymerase β gene structure: Evidence of alternative splicing in gene expression. Nucleic Acids Res 1994; 22:2719–2725.

110. Widen SG, Kedar P, Wilson SH: Human beta polymerase gene: Structure of the 5′-flanking region and active promoter. J Biol Chem 1988; 263:16992–16998.

111. Davies JF, Almassy RJ, Hostomsky Z, et al: 2.3 Å crystal structure of the catalytic domain of DNA polymerase beta. Cell 1994; 76:1123–1133.

112. Pelletier H, Sawaya MR, Kumar A, et al: Structure of tertiary complexes of rat DNA polymerase β, a DNA template-primer and ddCTP. Science 1994; 264:1891–1893.

113. Sawaya MR, Pelletier H, Kumar A, et al: Crystal structure of rat DNA polymerase β: evidence for a common polymerase mechanism. Science 1994; 264:1930–1935.

114. Blank A, Silber JR, Thelen MP, et al: Detection of enzymatic activities in sodium dodecyl-sulfate-polyacrylamide gels: DNA polymerases as model enzymes. Anal Biochem 1983; 135:423–430.

115. Longley MJ, Mosbaugh DW: Simultaneous in situ detection of DNA polymerase and associated exonuclease following SDS-polyacrylamide gel electrophoresis. Methods Mol Cell Biol 1989; 1:79–94.

116. Chen DS, Herman T, Demple B: Two distinct human DNA diesterases that hydrolyze 3′-blocking fragments from oxidized DNA. Nucleic Acids Res 1992; 19:5907–5914.

117. Warner HR, Demple BF, Deutsch WA, et al: Apurinic/apyrimidinic endonucleases in repair of pyrimidine dimers and other lesions in DNA. Proc Natl Acad Sci USA 1980; 77:4602–4606.

118. Sancar A: Mechanisms of DNA excision repair. Science 1994; 266:1954–1956.

119. Simon L, Hazard RM, Maher V, et al: Enhanced cell killing and mutagenesis by ethylnitrosourea in xeroderma pigmentosum cells. Carcinogenesis 1981; 2:567–570.

120. Teo IA, Arlett CF: The response of a variety of human fibroblast cell strains to the lethal effects of alkylating agents. Carcinogenesis 1983; 3:33–37.

121. Hanawalt PC, Sarasin A: Cancer-prone hereditary diseases with DNA processing abnormalities. Trends Genet 1986; 2:124–129.

122. McCormick J, Kateley-Kohler S, Watanabe M, et al: Abnormal sensitivity of human fibroblasts from xeroderma pigmentosum variants to transformation to anchorage independence by ultraviolet radiation. Cancer Res 1986; 46:489–492.

123. Bodell WJ, Singer B, Thomas GH, et al: Evidence for removal at different rates of O-ethyl pyrimidines and ethylphosphotriesters in two human fibroblast lines. Nucleic Acids Res 1979; 6:2819–2829.

124. Huang J-C, Hsu DS, Kazantsev A, et al: Substrate spectrum of human exinuclease: Repair of abasic sites, methylated bases, mismatches and bulky adducts. Proc Natl Acad Sci USA 1994; 91:12213–12217.

125. Kacinski BM, Rupp WD, Ludlum DB: Repair of haloethylnitrosourea-induced DNA damage in mutant and adapted bacteria. Cancer Res 1985; 45:6471–6474.

126. Wu Z, Chan C-L, Eastman A, et al: Expression of human O⁶-methylguanine DNA methyltransferase in a DNA excision repair-deficient Chinese hamster ovary line and its response to certain alkylating agents. Cancer Res 1992; 52:32–35.

127. Hata H, Numata M, Tohda H, et al: Isolation of two chloroethylnitrosourea-sensitive Chinese hamster cell lines. Cancer Res 1991; 51:195–198.

128. Dabholkar MD, Berger MS, Vionnet JA, et al: Malignant and nonmalignant brain tissues differ in their messenger RNA expression patterns for ERCC1 and ERCC2. Cancer Res 1995; 55:1261–1266.

129. Dabholkar MD, Bostick-Bruton F, Weber C, et al: ERCC1 and ERCC2 expression in malignant tissues from ovarian cancer patients. JNCI 1992; 84:1512–1517.

130. Ferguson LR: Mutagenic and recombinogenic consequences of treatment with 1,3-bis(2-chloroethyl)-1-nitrosourea in *Saccharomyces cerevisiae*. Mutation Res 1990; 241:369–377.

131. Bronstein SM, Cochrane JE, Craft TR, et al: Toxicity, mutagenicity and mutational spectra of N-ethyl-N-nitrosourea in human cell lines with different repair phenotypes. Cancer Res 1991; 51:5188–5197.

132. Bronstein SM, Hooth MJ, Swenber JA, et al: Efficient repair of O⁶-ethylguanine, but not O⁴-ethylthymine or O²-ethylthymine, is dependent upon O⁶-alkylguanine-DNA alkyltransferase and nucleotide excision repair activities in human cells. Cancer Res 1992; 52:3851–3856.

133. Modrich P: Mechanisms and biological effects of mismatch repair. Ann Rev Genet 1991; 25:229–253.

134. Modrich P: Mismatch repair, genetic stability and cancer. Science 1994; 266:1959–1960.

135. Parsons R, Li GM, Longley MJ, et al: Hypermutability and mismatch deficiency in MER⁺ tumor cells. Cell 1993; 75:1227–1236.

136. Dams E, Van de Kelft EJZ, Martin JJ, et al: Instability of microsatellites in human gliomas. Cancer Res 1995; 55:1547–1549.

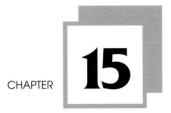

ZVI RAM

EDWARD H. OLDFIELD

CHAPTER **15**

Gene Therapy for Malignant Brain Tumors

As a result of the great strides in the understanding of the molecular basis of biology that have occurred since the early 1980s, biologic approaches to cancer treatment are now possible. Several approaches attempt to use immune enhancement to prompt the immune system to eradicate malignancy specifically. In most human cancers, however, these experimental approaches have not been successful, and new biologic approaches to cancer treatment are being pursued. The recognition that specific molecular events (e.g., inherited or acquired chromosomal aberrations, including gene mutation and gene loss leading to activation of oncogenes and inhibition of tumor suppressor genes) underlie the pathogenesis of tumors also provides new molecular targets for therapy. Advances in knowledge and technique in virology and molecular biology now furnish the necessary tools for investigation of gene therapy. Gene therapy is the transfer of genetic material into the host's cells for treatment. It has the potential of providing new therapy that is more specific and more effective than current approaches for several categories of disease of the nervous system, including various types of tumors, vascular disorders, degenerative disorders (particularly those that affect defined regions of the brain, such as Parkinson's disease), inborn errors of metabolism, and (by the development of new vaccines and regulatory control of gene expression) various infectious and inflammatory disorders. Advances in the past few years have led to considerable enthusiasm for gene therapy, which has increased the amount of research and the number of published reports in this area. Genetic vectors can be used to replace defective or missing genes or to introduce a new function to recipient cells. These approaches include the transfer of new genetic material and its regulatory elements and the use of genetic material, such as oligonucleotides, ribozymes, or naked DNA, to directly regulate gene expression in the treated tissue. Gene transfer can be used to modify a tumor to enhance its immunogenicity and to allow effective immune-mediated anti-tumor effects or to specifically target tumor cells for transfer of a gene whose product will provide selective toxicity to recipient tumor cells. Approaches that use genetically modified viruses to target their intrinsic cytopathic effects selectively to tumor cells are also considered to be gene therapy.

In this chapter, some of the concepts of genetic therapy for brain tumors are briefly reviewed and a selection of preclinical and clinical approaches that are being investigated are summarized.

PRINCIPLES UNDERLYING GENE THERAPY FOR TUMORS AND PRECLINICAL STUDIES

Methods for gene transfer can be broadly categorized as in vitro and in vivo techniques. In the in vitro approach, the genetically modified cells are reimplanted after gene transfer into the body to bring about the therapeutic effect. Because of difficulties with gene transfer in vivo, most of the early efforts with gene therapy, such as treatment of adenosine deaminase deficiency[1] and studies to monitor the trafficking of tumor-infiltrating lymphocytes,[2] used in vitro genetic transduction. Similarly, for disorders of the central nervous system (CNS), grafting of genetically modified cells was examined as a means of replacing deficient neurotransmitters in experimental Parkinson's disease.[3] For tumors, one approach to overcome the current limitations of gene transfer in solid tissues is to genetically transduce tumor cells in vitro to convert them into a "vaccine." Peripheral implantation of genetically modified brain tumor cells, which had been made immunogenic by inhibiting expression of the local immunosuppressor insulin-like growth factor 1 (IGF1) to generate a systemic immune response against the rat C6 glioma, was described by Trojan and colleagues.[4, 5] Interruption of IGF1 expression by transfecting the tumor cells ex vivo with antisense (cDNA) for IGF1 not only caused the tumor cells to lose their tumorigenicity, but subcutaneous injection of the modified tumor cells prevented formation of implanted brain tumors and induced cell-mediated immune regression of established C6 gliomas in the brain. A clinical investigation of this approach has been undertaken. A similar approach has been developed based on the suppression of transforming growth factor-β (TGFB), another peptide that suppresses cell-mediated immunity and that has been shown to be effective in animals with experimental brain tumors.

In contrast to these approaches, most approaches that attempt to use gene therapy for brain tumors use in vivo methods to transfer the therapeutic gene to the tumor cells in situ. A variety of vectors, viral and nonviral, have been examined. These include retroviruses, adenoviruses, adeno-associated virus, adenoviral-protein conjugates, and cationic liposomes. The characteristics and the advantages and disadvantages of these vectors have been reviewed by several authors.[6–10] Only the principal vectors now used for genetic transduction of somatic cells in situ in experimental and clinical studies are described in this chapter.

Retroviral Vectors

Retroviruses, which are ribonucleic acid (RNA) viruses that can be genetically modified to contain a gene at the expense of losing the capacity to replicate, only transduce dividing cells. They integrate into the host cell genome randomly along the chromosomes.[11] This random integration into the host cell genome is the basis for one potential complication of retrovirus-mediated gene transfer. That is, the integrated gene may inactivate regulatory genes (such as tumor suppressor genes) or activate oncogenes to induce tumor formation, a process known as *insertional mutagenesis*. An additional hazard of retroviruses is their potential recombination into a replication-competent retrovirus and uncontrolled replication in the host. To minimize this hazard, the genes encoding proteins that are required for replication are deleted from the vector and introduced into packaging cells (cells that continually produce the replication-incompetent retroviral vector).[12] The capacity of retroviral vectors to transduce only replicating cells allows their use in selectively targeting tumors in the brain, where the tumor cells are the predominant cell type undergoing deoxyribonucleic acid (DNA) synthesis.

Most experimental studies using retrovirus-mediated gene transfer for the treatment of brain tumors have used the gene for herpes simplex type I thymidine kinase (HStk) gene as the therapeutic gene.[13–17] In this approach, first proposed and used by Moolten and others,[18, 19] cells expressing HStk are sensitized to the antiviral drug ganciclovir. Ganciclovir is preferentially metabolized by HStk-transduced tumor cells to the nucleoside analog ganciclovir phosphate, which functions as a chain terminator and inhibitor of DNA polymerase to mediate cytotoxicity.

Because retroviral vectors have a very short half-life (hours) at 37 °C, and because at any given time the fraction of tumor cells that are replicating (those required for retroviral gene integration) is low, local delivery of the vector is provided by the use of genetically engineered vector-producer cells (VPC) that continuously produce and shed the retroviral vector particles. The VPC are derived from the murine 3T3 fibroblast cell line. They are implanted into the tumor to provide a continuous source of the retroviral vector

for several days, enhancing the fraction of the tumor cells that are transduced.

Significant tumor regression of established brain tumors in animals can be achieved by intratumoral implantation of HStk VPC and ganciclovir therapy (Fig. 15–1).[13–15, 20, 21] In animal studies the antitumor effects are not associated with significant toxic effects, even after repeated intracerebral implantation of producer cells and ganciclovir administration.[22] A unique and important feature of the HStk-ganciclovir approach is that even if only a small fraction of the tumor cells receive the therapeutic gene, significant antitumor activity can still be achieved (Fig. 15–2).[14, 20, 23, 24] This "bystander effect" results principally from transfer of toxic phosphorylated forms of ganciclovir to non-transduced cells via gap junctions.[24] Additional bystander mechanisms that enhance tumor regression include targeting of mitotically active endothelial cells in tumor vessels (Fig. 15–3) and of zones of tumor infarction after their destruction when ganciclovir is administered,[25] and immune-associated antitumor effects.[21]

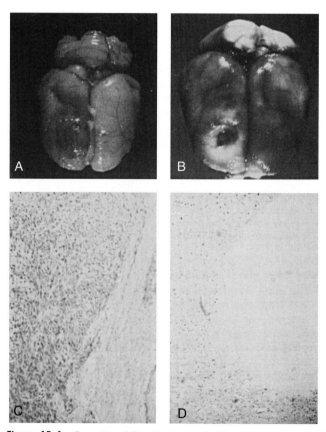

Figure 15–1 Gross *(A and B)* and microscopic *(C and D)* morphology of rat brains containing a 9L glioma after stereotactic injection with control *(A and C)* or HS-tk retroviral vector-producer cells (VPC) that were producing and shedding a replication-incompetent retrovirus that contained the gene for the herpes simplex type of thymidine kinase *(B and D)*, followed by treatment with ganciclovir beginning 5 days later. Treatment with the producer cells and ganciclovir eliminated the noninvasive tumor without injuring the surrounding brain *(D)*, whereas saline infusion produced no response of the tumor in the control animals. (From Culver K, Ram Z, Walbridge S, et al: In vivo gene transfer with retroviral vector-producer cells for treatment of experimental brain tumors. Science 1992; 256:1550–1552.)

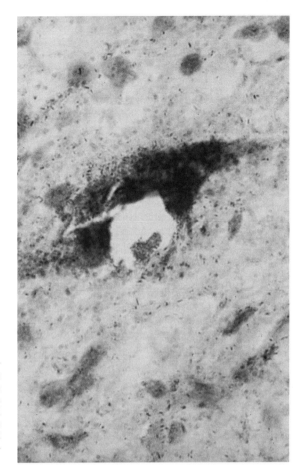

Figure 15–2 Endothelial cells in a capillary next to a 9L tumor are transduced after intratumoral placement of a retroviral vector containing the lacZ gene for *Escherichia coli* β-galactosidase. The vector producer cells (NIH 3T# fibroblasts, engineered to continuously produce and shed a replication-incompetent retroviral vector) were injected into the glioma 7 days after tumor implantation and the animal was sacrificed 9 days later. Transduced cells expressing β-galactosidase appear dark blue with the X-Gal stain. (From Ram Z, Culver K, Walbridge S, et al: In situ retroviral-mediated gene transfer for the treatment of brain tumors in rats. Cancer Res 1986; 46:5276–5281.)

To enhance the efficacy of this approach, Takamiya and co-workers[26, 27] achieved increased anti-tumor activity by using HStk vector-producer cells in the presence of a replication-competent wild-type retrovirus. Enhanced sensitivity of the tumor cells to ganciclovir with a potent "bystander effect" was found. The authors hypothesized that infection with wild-type retrovirus enhanced the sensitivity of tumor cells to ganciclovir and that pseudotyping (packaging of the HStk gene by retroviral envelope) increased the number of available therapeutic vectors and enhanced transduction efficiency. However, the presence of replication-competent retrovirus also increases the possibility of insertional mutagenesis. Further, the enhanced anti-tumor effect that occurred in the presence of replication-competent retrovirus

Figure 15–3 The genomic organization of the type 5 adenovirus *(top)* and the structure of a replication-incompetent adenoviral vector expressing the *Escherichia coli* lacZ gene (Av1LacZ4) are shown. The Av1-LacZ4 vector contains a deletion in the E1 region from 1.1 to 9.2 map units (mu) and in the E3 region from 78.5 to 84.7 mu. The E1 deletion is replaced by an expression cassette containing the Rous sarcoma virus (RSV) promoter/Ad5 tripartite leader combined with a nucleus-targeted β-galactosidase gene and a poly A signal from SV40 with a residual portion of the E1b gene. ITR, inverted terminal repeat. (From Viola J, Ram Z, Walbridge S, et al: Adenovirus-mediated gene transfer into experimental solid brain tumors and leptomeningeal cancer. J Neurosurg 1995; 82:70–76.)

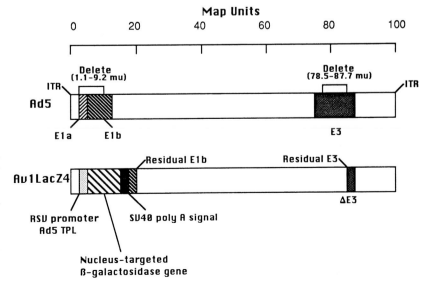

was not observed in a different model of malignancy (lepto-meningeal neoplasia) in rats, suggesting that it may be tumor-type or model specific.[28]

Adenoviral Vectors

Adenoviruses, whose natural target is the respiratory epithelium, are non-enveloped regular icosahedrons with a genome of approximately 35 kbp. The genome consists of linear, double-stranded DNA that can be manipulated to produce replication-deficient vectors capable of accommodating foreign genes (Fig. 15–3). Insertion of the foreign genetic material is most commonly done at the E1A early region of the virus. Up to 7.5 kbp can be inserted without reducing infectivity.[29] Several features of adenoviruses make them an attractive option as a vehicle to transfer genes into CNS neoplasms. They have low pathogenicity in humans and are not neurotoxic. In addition, very high titers of the virus can be achieved, which allows higher levels of gene expression in treated tissues than the levels achieved using other vector delivery systems.[30] Furthermore, the adenovirus DNA does not integrate into the host cell genome, but assumes an episomal position, thus avoiding the potential risks of insertional mutagenesis at the expense of achieving only transient gene expression. However, with the prodrug gene therapy approach using HStk with ganciclovir, and with certain other genes with similar function, only transient gene expression is necessary, as the activity of the expressed therapeutic gene is only needed during administration of the drug to be converted (e.g., ganciclovir with adenovector containing HStk).

Several reports suggest the feasibility of using adenovirus vectors containing HStk to treat solid and leptomeningeal cancer in experimental animal models.[31, 32] High transduction efficiency and levels of gene expression were observed after direct injection of the adenoviral vector into cerebral tumors and into the CSF in an animal model of leptomeningeal neoplasia.[32] Potent therapeutic efficacy of adenovirus-mediated HStk gene transduction of rat C6 glioma cells followed by ganciclovir administration was demonstrated by Chen and colleagues[31] in nude mice; the tumor volume in treated animals was reduced 500-fold compared with that in control animals. Efficacy has also been demonstrated in rats with implanted cerebral 9L gliosarcomas, in whom tumors were eliminated, and long-term survival occurred in most animals (Fig. 15–4).[33] In addition to the bystander effects achieved with the use of HStk and ganciclovir, tumor response associated with the HStk-containing adenoviral vectors and ganciclovir is associated with the development of an immune response that is itself sufficient to eliminate distant, untreated tumors. However, the highly immunogenic nature of adenovirus is the basis for concerns about the safety of its use in humans.

Viral-Mediated Cytotoxicity

Another type of biologic therapy considered as gene therapy is the use of viral-mediated cytotoxicity to selectively target and kill brain tumor cells. Pathogenic viruses have the poten-

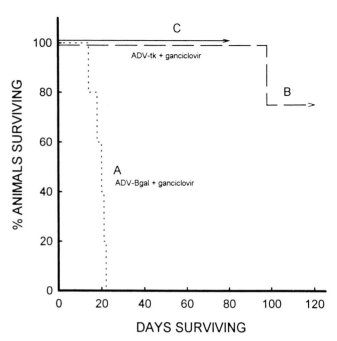

Figure 15–4 Survival of rats with cerebral 9L gliomas treated with intratumoral injection of an adenoviral vector containing either the gene for the *Escherichia coli* β-galactosidase gene (ADV-Bgal) *(A)* or the gene for HStk (ADV-tk) *(B and C)*. All groups received ganciclovir. Almost all animals treated with ADV-tk and ganciclovir had remission of preexisting tumors. (From Perez-Cruet M, Trask T, Chen S, et al: Adenovirus-mediated gene therapy of experimental gliomas. J Neuroscr Res 1994; 39:506–511.)

tial to be genetically altered so that they will selectively target their toxic effects to a desired population of cells. Examples examined by Martuza and co-workers[34] are mutants of the herpes simplex virus that are defective in certain genes, such as the gene that encodes HStk.[34] Because thymidine kinase is necessary for viral replication, and because nondividing mammalian cells (e.g., neurons, glia) express little thymidine kinase, viral replication in viruses without thymidine kinase is limited in normal cells, and neurovirulence is attenuated. In contrast, replicating tumor cells express higher levels of thymidine kinase, which permits viral replication and consequent cell lysis to occur only in the dividing tumor cells. When the engineered virus was used in the presence of a brain tumor in experimental animal models, preferential infection of tumor cells was achieved and the lytic action of the herpes virus destroyed tumor cells, whereas the surrounding normal tissue was affected less severely (Fig. 15–5).[34] In another development, a replication-competent herpes simplex virus was engineered that retains its thymidine kinase gene, but in which the gene for ribonucleotide reductase (an enzyme required for viral replication that is expressed preferentially in tumor cells compared to normal cells) is defective.[35] In this system the virus replicates preferentially in tumor cells, but not in postmitotic cells, which enhances the level of expression of HStk in the tumor cells and provides selective anti-tumor activity when ganciclovir is administered. In these experiments long-term survival of 48% of treated rats harboring 9L gliosarcoma was achieved.

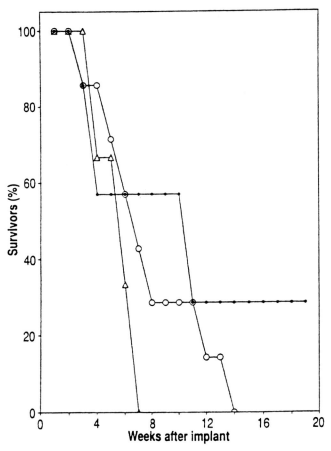

Figure 15–5 Treatment of human intracranial U87 gliomas in nude mice with intratumoral inoculation with a thymidine kinase–negative mutant of herpes simplex virus-1 (*dls*ptk). The tumors were treated with either 10^3 pfu of *dls*ptk *(open circles)*, 10^5 pfu of *dls*ptk *(solid circles)*, or medium alone *(triangles)*. By week 7 all control animals were dead, whereas 3 of 7 in the 10^3 pfu group and 4 of 7 in the 10^5 pfu group were alive ($P<0.05$ vs. controls). Two animals in the 10^5 pfu group were alive at week 19, at which point no microscopic tumor could be found in their brains. (From Martuza RL, Malick A, Markert JM, et al: Experimental therapy of human glioma by means of a genetically engineered virus mutant. Science 1991; 252:854–856.)

Technical Limitations of Gene Delivery into Solid Tumors

Significant technical limitations to the successful delivery and distribution of genetic material to solid tissues restrict the available approaches of gene therapy that can be used to treat brain tumors. In most studies the genetic vector has been injected directly into the tumor, and distribution of the vector is achieved by evenly spacing the injection tracts in the tumor. Another potential route for delivery of genes into tumors of the CNS is via the vasculature. Genetic vectors administered intravascularly are unlikely to penetrate the blood-brain barrier and to transfer the gene into the brain parenchyma. Although distribution of small (20 nm) iron oxide particles in brain tissue has been described after blood-brain barrier disruption with intra-arterial mannitol and intravascular infusion of the particles,[36] the size of these particles is significantly smaller than that of all currently used viral genetic vectors except the adeno-associated virus. It may

also be possible to intra-arterially deliver vectors that selectively target endothelial cells of the tumor vessels and elicit antitumor effects by selectively injuring the tumor vasculature. Transduction of endothelial cells after intratumoral implantation of murine vector-producer cells for continuous release of retroviral vectors carrying the HStk gene contributed to tumor regression after ganciclovir therapy, probably by inducing local ischemia within the tumor.[25]

CLINICAL STUDIES OF GENE THERAPY FOR BRAIN TUMORS

Fifteen patients were enrolled in a study designed to evaluate the safety and efficacy of intratumoral implantation of HStk vector-producer cells plus ganciclovir administration in patients with malignant brain tumors.[37] To allow magnetic resonance imaging (MRI) assessment of anti-tumor activity, only the enhancing portion of the tumor was targeted for injection of the cells. Multiple linear tracts were used to homogeneously distribute the vector-producer cells within the tumor volume. Intravenous ganciclovir was started 7 days after intratumoral injection of the vector-producer cells and was administered for 14 days at 5 mg/kg, twice daily.

Local loss of contrast-enhancement on MRI, which was considered to represent an anti-tumor effect, never occurred during the week after producer-cell injection alone, but it became evident only after ganciclovir administration. Some patients had at least a 50% reduction in the contrast-enhancing tumor volume. Tumors that showed more than 50% decrease in contrast-enhancing volume tended to be smaller than tumors that did not respond, suggesting that the density of distribution of the vector in the tumor is important for antitumor activity.

To determine in vivo gene transfer, resected tumor specimens that had been injected with HStk vector-producer cells 7 days earlier were evaluated. In situ hybridization of the specimens using an antisense oligonucleotide probe for the thymidine kinase mRNA demonstrated deposits of HStk-expressing cells within the tumor. Some of the HStk-staining cells stained positive for glial fibrillary acid protein (GFAP), which indicated that in vivo gene transfer into tumor cells had occurred. However, semiquantitative molecular analysis of the resected tissues indicated that the transduction efficiency was extremely limited. The low rate of gene transfer and the limited mononuclear cellular infiltrate that was present 1 week after placement of the producer cells suggested that the bystander effect must have been the principal contributor to the observed anti-tumor effects.

The results of this study indicate the feasibility and safety of in vivo, retrovirus-mediated transfer of genes into tumors using intratumoral implantation of xenogeneic vector-producer cells. They also indicate that anti-tumor activity against human brain tumors in situ occurs in some patients. However, the results also suggest that new delivery techniques will be necessary to enhance the efficiency and success of therapeutic gene transfer in solid tissues. In addition, identification of possible response-modifiers, such as enhancement of the bystander effect, optimization of producer cells and vectors, and exploitation of additional mechanisms involving the immune system need to be investigated further to enhance the activity of this therapeutic approach.

SUMMARY

Combining the unlimited versatility of protein design inherent in recombinant DNA technology, the strides being made in the understanding of the basic biologic mechanisms of regulation of cell growth and immunology, and the capacity to harness the cell targeting and distribution functions intrinsic to viruses provides the potential for the development of new therapeutic approaches using gene therapy. However, the development of gene therapy is in its infancy and limitations to its successful clinical use are considerable.

Progress will require the use of animal models that are analogous to human disease. Yet the rapidly replicating tumors that are commonly used for animal studies often have doubling times of less than 24 hours. Further, they are very small tumors, have no necrosis, and have a maximum diameter that is usually no more than 2 to 4 mm when they are treated. Genetic transduction, particularly with retroviral vectors (the efficacy of which depends on the rate of replication and the distribution of the vector in the tumor), and the bystander effect occur to a much greater extent than is expected in much larger, more slowly progressing necrotic tumors in patients. Furthermore, the immune approaches, such as the antisense approaches using vectors that suppress IGF1 or TGFB production, or the use of adenovirus that contains a therapeutic vector, depend greatly on cell-mediated immunity, and as most of the tumor lines that are commonly used in brain tumor laboratories are no longer truly syngeneic, the results in clinical trials may not be as striking as they are in the laboratory.

Depending on the disorder, effective gene therapy will require successful delivery and distribution of an appropriate genetic vector in the target tissue with selective targeting of specific tissues or anatomic regions for genetic transduction and gene expression. Many diseases, such as Parkinson's disease, will require long-term and stable integration of the therapeutic gene into the genome of the target cells. For most disorders it will also require appropriate regulation of the therapeutic gene. These are complex issues. We are only now beginning to understand most of them, such as regulation of gene expression, in the most basic biological systems. The difficulties with, for example, delivery and distribution of genetic vectors, efficient gene transfer in situ, and integration of genetic vectors into the host cell genome of nonreplicating cells, are being overcome gradually by systematic and stepwise advances. These advances in gene therapy demonstrate the rapid progress that is now occurring in the application of basic science to treat human disease, and which offers very much in the years ahead.

REFERENCES

1. Culver KW, Osborne WR, Miller AD, et al: Correction of ADA deficiency in human T lymphocytes using retroviral-mediated gene transfer. Transplant Proc 1991; 23:170–171.
2. Rosenberg SA: Gene therapy of cancer. Important Adv Oncol 1992; 17–38.
3. Gage FH, Fisher LJ, Jinnah HA, et al: Grafting genetically modified cells to the brain: Conceptual and technical issues. Prog Brain Res 1990; 82:1–10.
4. Trojan J, Blossey BK, Johnson TR, et al: Loss of tumorigenicity of rat glioblastoma directed by episome-based antisense cDNA transcription of insulin-like growth factor I. Proc Natl Acad Sci USA 1992; 89:4874–4878.
5. Trojan J, Johnson TR, Rudin SD, et al: Treatment and prevention of rat glioblastoma by immunogenic C6 cells expressing antisense insulin-like growth factor I RNA. Science 1993; 259:94–97.
6. Anderson WF: Human gene therapy. Science 1992; 256:808–813.
7. Gutierrez AA, Lemoine NR, Sikora K: Gene therapy for cancer. Lancet 1992; 339:715–721.
8. Russell SJ: Gene therapy for cancer (letter). Lancet 1992; 339:1109–1110.
9. Verma IM: Gene therapy. Sci Am 1990; 263:68–72.
10. Miller A: Human gene therapy comes of age. Nature 1992; 357:455–460.
11. Miller DG, Adam MA, Miller AD: Gene transfer by retroviral vectors occurs only in cells that are actively replicating at the time of infection. Mol Cell Biol 1990; 10:4239–4242.
12. Danos O, Mulligan RC: Safe and efficient generation of recombinant retroviruses with amphotropic and ecotropic host ranges. Proc Natl Acad Sci USA 1988; 85:6460–6464.
13. Barba D, Hardin J, Ray J, et al: Thymidine kinase-mediated killing of rat brain tumors. J Neurosurg 1993; 79:729–735.
14. Culver KW, Ram Z, Walbridge S, et al: In vivo gene transfer with retroviral vector-producer cells for treatment of experimental brain tumors. Science 1992; 256:1550–1552.
15. Ezzeddine ZD, Martuza RL, Platika D, et al: Selective killing of glioma cells in culture and in vivo by retrovirus transfer of the herpes simplex virus thymidine kinase gene. New Biol 1991; 3:608–614.
16. Ram Z, Culver KW, Oshiro EM, et al: Gene therapy for malignant brain tumors: Preliminary results of a clinical study using retroviral-mediated in situ transduction with the herpes thymidine kinase gene. 43rd Annual Meeting of the Congress of Neurosurgery, Vancouver, British Columbia, 1993.
17. Takamiya Y, Friedlander RM, Brem H, et al: Inhibition of angiogenesis and growth of human nerve-sheath tumors by AGM-1470. J Neurosurg 1993; 78:470–476.
18. Moolten FL: Tumor chemosensitivity conferred by inserted herpes thymidine kinase genes: paradigm for a prospective cancer control strategy. Cancer Res 1986; 46:5276–5281.
19. Moolten FL, Wells JM: Curability of tumors bearing herpes thymidine kinase genes transferred by retroviral vectors. J Natl Cancer Inst 1990; 82:297–300.
20. Ram Z, Culver K, Walbridge S, et al: In situ retroviral-mediated gene transfer for the treatment of brain tumors in rats. Cancer Res 1993; 53:83–88.
21. Barba D, Hardin J, Sadelain M, et al: Development of anti-tumor immunity following thymidine kinase-mediated killing of experimental brain tumors. Proc Natl Acad Sci USA 1994; 91:4348–4352.
22. Ram Z, Culver KW, Walbridge S, et al: Toxicity studies of retroviral-mediated gene transfer for the treatment of brain tumors. J Neurosurg 1993; 79:400–407.
23. Caruso M, Panis Y, Gagandeep S, et al: Regression of established macroscopic liver metastases after in situ transduction of a suicide gene. Proc Natl Acad Sci USA 1993; 90:7024–7028.
24. Freeman SM, Abboud CN, Whartenby KA, et al: The bystander effect: Tumor regression when a fraction of the tumor mass is genetically modified. Cancer Res 1993; 53:5274–5283.
25. Ram Z, Walbridge S, Shawker T, et al: The effect on tumoral vasculature and growth of thymidine kinase-transduced, ganciclovir-treated 9L gliomas in rats. J Neurosurg 1994; 81:256–260.
26. Takamiya Y, Short MP, Ezzeddine ZD, et al: Gene therapy of malignant brain tumors: A rat glioma line bearing the herpes simplex virus type 1-thymidine kinase gene and wild type retrovirus kills other tumor cells. J Neurosci Res 1992; 33:493–503.
27. Takamiya Y, Short MP, Moolten FL, et al: An experimental model of retrovirus gene therapy for malignant brain tumors. J Neurosurg 1993; 79:104–110.
28. Ram Z, Walbridge S, Oshiro EM, et al: Intrathecal gene therapy for malignant leptomeningeal neoplasia. Cancer Res 1994; 54:2141–2145.
29. Stratford-Perricaudet L, Perricaudet M: In Cohen-Haguenauer O,

Boiron M, Libbey J (eds): Human Gene Transfer. London, Eurotext, 1991, pp 51–61.

30. Lemarchand P, Jaffe H, Danel C, et al: Adenovirus-mediated transfer of a recombinant human alpha1-antitrypsin cDNA to human endothelial cells. Proc Natl Acad Sci USA 1992; 89:6482–6486.

31. Chen SH, Shine HD, Goodman JC, et al: Gene therapy for brain tumors: Regression of experimental gliomas by adenovirus-mediated gene transfer in vivo. Proc Natl Acad Sci USA 1994; 91:3054–3057.

32. Viola JJ, Ram Z, Walbridge S, et al: Adenovirus-mediated gene transfer into experimental solid brain tumors and leptomeningeal cancer. J Neurosurg 1995; 82:70–76.

33. Perez-Cruet M, Trask T, Chen S, et al. Adenovirus-mediated gene therapy of experimental gliomas. J Neurosci Res 1994; 39:506–511.

34. Martuza RL, Malick A, Markert JM, et al: Experimental therapy of human glioma by means of a genetically engineered virus mutant. Science 1991; 252:854–856.

35. Boviatsis E, Park J, Sena-Esteves M, et al: Long-term survival of rats harboring brain neoplasms treated with ganciclovir and a herpes simplex virus vector that retains an intact thymidine kinase gene. Cancer Res 1994; 15:5745–5751.

36. Neuwelt E, Weissleder R, Nilaver G, et al: Delivery of virus-sized iron oxide particles to rodent CNS neurons. Neurosurgery 1994; 34:777–784.

37. Oldfield EH, Ram Z, Culver KW, et al: Gene therapy for the treatment of brain tumors using intra-tumoral transduction with the thymidine kinase gene and intravenous ganciclovir. Hum Gene Ther 1993; 4:39–69.

WALTER A. HALL

ERIC P. FLORES

WALTER C. LOW

CHAPTER **16**

Antisense Oligonucleotide Targets

The conventional treatment of primary malignant tumors of the central nervous system (CNS) that includes surgery, radiation therapy, and chemotherapy has not significantly extended survival for this disease.[1] Both radiation therapy and systemic chemotherapy lack specificity for malignant cells that can lead to dose-limiting side effects and unacceptable CNS toxicity. Two novel types of therapy are currently being developed by investigators for clinical utilization that have increased specificity for cancer cells compared with normal neural tissue. The first therapeutic modality is targeted toxins, which are monoclonal antibodies or other carrier ligands covalently bound to protein toxins directed against tumor-associated antigens; they possess exquisite cell-type selectivity and extraordinary potency.[1] The second therapeutic approach to malignant CNS tumor cells involves the use of molecular biology to inhibit either DNA transcription or messenger RNA (mRNA) translation by inserting or blocking specific nucleotide sequences. Viral vectors can be used to insert a specific gene (e.g., thymidine kinase) into the genetic material of replicating cells, which can then be inhibited by systemically administering an antiviral agent (e.g., ganciclovir). Technical difficulties associated with vector production and tumor cell transfection currently limit the efficacy of this form of gene therapy. Another innovative method for specifically turning off or down-regulating individual gene expression involves the use of antisense oligodeoxynucleotides, which are the focus of this chapter.

The antisense concept, whereby mRNA translation can be regulated by chemically synthesized complementary oligodeoxynucleotides or oligomers, was first realized as early as 1967.[2] Since the mid-1970s, advances in synthetic chemistry and molecular biology have stimulated an interest in developing antisense oligonucleotides as potential therapeutic agents for clinical use.[3] Although investigators have appreciated for some time that gene expression can be regulated by complementary RNA, this technology has only recently been applied to the CNS. The initial use of antisense oligonucleotides in the CNS has been primarily directed toward the inhibition of malignant brain tumor cell proliferation.

CHEMICAL STRUCTURE

Antisense oligo(deoxy)nucleotides or oligomer analogs represent a sequence of 15 to 21 nucleotide base pairs in length,
with the order of the nucleotides providing the molecule with the specificity to target complementary genetic material. In order to specifically recognize a unique mammalian gene sequence, it has been estimated that an oligomer must be at least 14 bases long.[4] Shorter oligonucleotides are less likely to hybridize with complementary sequences.[4] These short nucleotide sequences can be synthesized to be complementary to messenger RNA or to a specific gene.[5] Although the exact cost for those quantities necessary for clinical use have not been determined, automated technology has enhanced the ease with which antisense oligonucleotides can be produced with a resultant decrease in the cost of their synthesis.

The stability and subsequent half-life ($t_{1/2}$) of these compounds is largely determined by whether they have been chemically modified. Unmodified phosphodiester antisense oligonucleotides and certain modified antisense oligonucleotides are sensitive to rapid degradation by endonucleases and exonucleases, mainly 3′-exonucleases.[2, 5] In serum, the half-life of phosphodiester antisense oligonucleotides is only a few hours, and in some instances no more than 15 minutes.[6] Chemical modification (Table 16–1) can affect the internucleotidic phosphate backbone (e.g., methylphosphonates and phosphorothioates), the sugar configuration (e.g., α-oligomers and 2′-O-methyl oligomers), or the 3′ end.[2] Phosphorothioate-, phosphorodithioate-, methylphosphonate-, phosphoramidate-, 2′-O-methyl- and α-anomer–modified oligomers are considered resistant to degradation by nucleases.[5] A nontoxic dose of phosphorothioate antisense oligonucleotides administered to mice is excreted in the urine over 2 to 3 days, or more rapidly in the case of phosphodiester antisense oligonucleotides.[6] For injected phosphorothioates ($t_{1/2} \sim$ 20 to 40 hours), the urinary excretion rate in mice and rats is much slower than that of methylphosphonates ($t_{1/2} <$ 1 hour), which suggests that the former may be more efficacious in vivo.[5] Very few antisense oligonucleotides are excreted in fecal matter.[6] Ribozymes are small oligoribonucleotides that have natural self-splicing activity and a specific base sequence.[6]

Antisense oligodeoxynucleotides that target double-stranded DNA form a *triple-helix* through Hoogsteen base pairing and are considered anti-gene agents.[6] Triple-helix formation occurs between homopurine and homopyrimidine sequences in the target DNA. Triple-strand formation is

TABLE 16–1
CHEMICAL STRUCTURE OF ANTISENSE OLIGONUCLEOTIDES

Nuclease sensitive
Phosphodiester
Ribozyme
Nuclease resistant
Phosphorothioate
Phosphorodithioate
Phosphoramidate
Methylphosphonate
α-Oligomer
2'-O-Methyl oligomer

sensitive to pH conditions and is rapidly destabilized by DNA transcription, replication, and repair.[6]

MECHANISM OF ACTION AND CELL DELIVERY

Antisense oligodeoxynucleotides cause down-regulation of a dominant oncogene or the interruption of an autocrine or paracrine signaling loop in a cytostatic manner, which implies that repeated or continuous administration will be necessary for tumor suppression.[6] Mechanisms of action for antisense oligonucleotides (Table 16–2) are considered passive, reactive, or activating.[3, 6] Passive inhibition of function occurs by steric hindrance whereby mRNA cannot either pass from the nucleus to the cytoplasm or effectively interact with ribosomes.[6] Reactive processes occur when antisense oligonucleotides bind directly to a target sequence and either block its action or cause its cleavage.[3, 6] Cleavage of the target RNA by the endogenous enzyme RNase H is an activating process.[3, 6] Following cleavage of the target RNA, the oligomer will be released intact to recycle and to bind to other target sequences.[3] Irrespective of the point of antisense attachment, the activation of RNase H will result in digestion of the target mRNA.

These oligomers will block gene transcription by binding to target DNA, or they can bind to mRNA to interrupt translation and to inhibit protein synthesis. In cell-free translation systems, the best sites for binding to mRNA are at the 5' end (around the initiator AUG codon) and at sites for ribosome complex assembly.[6] Phosphodiester antisense oligonucleotides hybridize very efficiently to complementary RNA sequences to block translation, but they also recruit

the enzyme RNase H to cleave the RNA component of the RNA/DNA duplex.[5, 6] Methylphosphonate antisense oligonucleotides are highly stable, with low toxicity to cells, but they hybridize poorly and do not induce RNase H activity.[6] Although phosphorothioate antisense oligonucleotides hybridize efficiently and induce RNase in a concentration-dependent fashion, they have nonspecific toxicity in some systems and are not well internalized by cells.[6] α-Oligodeoxynucleotides form parallel rather than anti-parallel duplexes with complementary DNA or RNA strands and hybridize as efficiently as phosphorothioates, but they do not induce RNase H.[3, 6] Ribozymes or catalytic RNAs have a mode of action different from that of other antisense oligonucleotides and are particularly sensitive to nuclease degradation.[6] Ribozymes can be directed against any RNA target by including an antisense sequence in their structure.[6] Properties considered ideal for antisense oligonucleotides are listed in Table 16–3.

After binding to cell surface antigens, antisense oligonucleotides enter cells by pinocytosis and/or by receptor-mediated endocytosis.[2] Charged oligomers enter cells by endocytosis, and uncharged oligomers enter by passive diffusion.[4] Long-term sequestration of antisense oligonucleotides in lysosomes or endosomes has raised concern regarding their intracellular availability and stability.[4] Methods for increasing the intracellular uptake of antisense oligonucleotides have included their conjugation to a synthetic polypeptide poly(L-lysine) tail that may or may not be bound to transferrin.[2, 3, 5–7] Conjugation of antisense oligonucleotides to cholesterol or their encapsidation in cationic or antibody-targeted liposomes can increase cellular uptake and biologic efficacy.[2, 3, 9] Cholesterol attachment can increase retention time in plasma 10-fold.[3] A major drawback of employing liposomes for nucleic acid delivery is their poor encapsulation efficiency (~3%).[2] Once inside the cell, antisense oligonucleotides are thought to diffuse through nuclear pores to accumulate in the nucleus, supporting the existence of nuclear binding proteins.[2]

IN VITRO STUDIES

Few studies have been performed using antisense oligonucleotides in vitro to inhibit the growth of malignant brain tumor cells.[10, 11, 22] Two glioblastoma-derived cell lines, HTZ-146 and HTZ-17, were screened for the expression of platelet-derived growth factor-α (PDGFA) and -β (PDGFB) polypeptides and for basic fibroblast growth factor (FGF2) expression by Northern blotting and by immunochemical methods.[10] Cell proliferation was inhibited in both cell lines using 14-mer phosphorothioate oligodeoxynucleotides targeted against PDGFA mRNA, PDGFB mRNA, and FGF2 mRNA

TABLE 16–2
MECHANISM OF ACTION OF ANTISENSE OLIGONUCLEOTIDES

Inhibit DNA transcription
  Triple-helix formation
Inhibit mRNA translation
  Passive inhibition
    Steric hindrance of RNA interaction with ribosomes
    Inability of RNA to pass from nucleus to cytoplasm
  Reactive inhibition
    Direct binding to target sequence blocks its action
    Direct binding to target sequence causes its cleavage
  Activating inhibition
    Cleavage of target RNA by RNase H

TABLE 16–3
IDEAL PROPERTIES OF ANTISENSE OLIGONUCLEOTIDES

Nuclease resistant	Rapid nuclear entry
Hybridizes efficiently	No nonspecific binding
Aqueous soluble	Activates RNase H
Rapid cell entry	

(Table 16–4). Basic FGF mRNA-specific antisense molecules inhibited HTZ-146 cell proliferation by 50% but had no effect on HTZ-17 cell proliferation. PDGFA mRNA antisense molecules inhibited HTZ-17 cells by 55% but had no effect on HTZ-146 cell growth. Neither cell line was inhibited by antisense molecules to PDGFB mRNA.[10]

The c-*sis* oncogene encodes for the β-polypeptide chain of PDGF. In the A172 glioblastoma cell line, an 18-base pair antisense oligonucleotide complementary to the ATG initiation codon of mRNA of c-*sis* was examined for its effect on cellular growth.[11] Using the polymerase chain reaction, mRNA transcripts of c-*sis* were detected in three of four glioma cell lines and in two of five glioblastoma multiforme tissue samples. The antisense oligonucleotides complementary to c-*sis* mRNA were efficiently incorporated in A172 cells, with the maximum uptake occurring after a 48-hour incubation period. Antisense oligonucleotides complementary to the first initiation codon of c-*sis* inhibited cell proliferation in a time- and dose-dependent fashion.[11] By flow cytometric analysis, antisense oligonucleotides were shown to block the de novo synthesis of intracellular c-*sis* protein in A172 cells.[11] Corresponding sense oligonucleotides did not inhibit c-*sis* protein synthesis or glioma cell growth.[11]

Using reverse transcription-polymerase chain reaction, U87 glioblastoma-derived cells were shown to express mRNA for both FGF2 and the FGF2 receptor.[12] The addition of FGF2-specific antisense oligonucleotide to the U87 cell line significantly inhibited the growth rate of these cells within 48 hours and blocked proliferation beyond 2 days.[12] The effect of FGF2-specific antisense on U87 cells was dose dependent, with the greatest effect seen with a concentration of 20 μM. Antisense oligonucleotides significantly inhibited U87 colony formation in soft agar. The addition of oligonucleotides in the sense configuration was without effect.[12] Using 50 μM of FGF2-specific antisense primer, the growth of the human glioma cell line SNB19 was inhibited by 80%.[13] The effects seen were specific and saturable. Antisense primers to two different sites on the FGF2 mRNA inhibited growth of the SNB19 glioma cell line whereas sense primer was ineffective.[13] No effect was seen after treating normal glia with either antisense or sense primers to FGF2 mRNA.[13] Rat C6 astrocytoma cells transfected with antisense FGF2 complementary DNA (cDNA) had reduced levels of immunologically detectable intracellular and extracellular FGF2 and diminished growth in vitro, whereas transfection with FGF2 cDNA in the sense configuration had the opposite effect.[14]

To investigate the function of glial fibrillary acidic protein (GFAP), the U251 astrocytoma cell line was investigated.[15] Expression of GFAP was suppressed by transfecting U251 cells with an antisense GFAP construct.[15] When U251 cells were grown in culture with neurons, the average increase in process length for transfected cells was 14% compared with 400% for nontransfected cells.[15] Other neuron-induced astrocytic responses, such as proliferative arrest, were not affected in these cells.[15]

To determine whether type 1 insulin-like growth factor (IGF1) expression was coupled to glioma tumorigenicity, antisense RNA for IGF1 was employed in vitro and in vivo.[16] Using an antisense IGF1 expression vector that incorporates Epstein-Barr virus replicative signals and the ZnSO₄-inducible metallothionein I transcriptional promoter, stable rat C6 glioma transfectants were derived that constitutively express IGF1.[16] Transfected C6 cells were shown to express high levels of IGF1 mRNA by in situ hybridization and high levels of IGF1 protein by immunohistochemistry, in the absence of $ZnSO_4$.[16] Elevated levels of antisense transcript accumulated in the cells and the levels of endogenous IGF1 mRNA and IGF1 protein decreased dramatically after addition of $ZnSO_4$ to the culture medium.[16]

IGF1-mediated growth of C6 glioma cells in monolayers and clonogenicity in soft agar was inhibited by antisense IGF1-receptor oligodeoxynucleotides and stable transfection with a plasmid expressing an antisense IGF1-receptor RNA.[17] Sense oligodeoxynucleotides or sense-expressing plasmid did not affect growth in monolayers and clonogenicity in soft agar. Tyrosine-phosphorylated IGF1 receptors were not detectable in stable antisense transfectants but were easily detected in wild-type cells.[17]

The U87 human glioblastoma cell line was stably transfected with the antisense cDNA encoding protein kinase C-α (PKCA).[18] U87 cells and two other glioma cell lines expressed high levels of PKCA. Clonal isolates of transfected U87 cells expressing antisense PKCA cDNA did not express PKCA antigen by immunoblotting with a PKCA polyclonal antibody.[18] A 95% reduction in total Ca^{2+}/phosphatidylserine-dependent PKC activity was seen in U87 cells stably transfected with the antisense PKCA cDNA.[18] An increase in doubling time in vitro, less serum-dependent growth, and reduced sensitivity to a selective PKC inhibitor was seen in U87 cells expressing antisense PKCA.[18]

Only one study has examined the effects of antisense oligonucleotides to the c-*myb* oncogene on brain tumor cells to date. Raschella and colleagues[19] found that c-*myb* antisense down-regulated Myb protein expression and inhibited the proliferation of the LAN-5 neuroblastoma cell line. Neuroblastoma cells treated with antisense to the N-*myc* oncogene ATG initiation site demonstrated inhibition of expression for mRNA of both N-*myc* and Ki-67, a proliferation-associated antigen.[3]

Cellular *myb* Oncogene Studies

The proto-oncogene c-*myb* is the normal cellular homolog of the avian myeloblastosis virus–transforming gene v-*myb*.[7]

TABLE 16–4
ANTISENSE OLIGONUCLEOTIDE TARGETS IN BRAIN TUMORS

Target	References
Growth factors	
PDGFA	10
PDGFB	10
FGF2	10, 12–14
IGF1	16, 22
Growth factor receptors	
IGF1 receptor	17
Intracellular proteins	
c-*sis* Proto-oncogene encoded protein	11
c-*myb* Proto-oncogene encoded protein Myb	19, 21
Glial fibrillary acidic protein	15
PKCA isoform	18

c-*myb* encodes for the nuclear protein Myb, which acts as a sequence-specific DNA transcription factor.[7] c-*myb* is preferentially expressed in immature hematopoietic cells and its expression declines as cells differentiate terminally.[7] Because of the poorly differentiated nature of glioblastoma multiforme cells, the c-*myb* oncogene is amplified 10-fold as determined by densitometry.[20]

In our laboratory we have suppressed proliferation of T98, U87, and U373 glioma and DAOY medulloblastoma-derived cells as measured by tritiated (^{3}H)-thymidine incorporation after the addition of phosphorothioate antisense oligonucleotides either to the 5' cap initiator region or to the transactivation sequence of c-*myb*.[21] Mean proliferation after 48 hours of incubation with antisense oligonucleotides to the 5' cap region of c-*myb* was 20%, 52%, 53%, and 53% of controls for U87, U373, T98, and DAOY cells, respectively.[21] Antisense oligonucleotides to the transactivation sequence inhibited cell proliferation to 25%, 76%, 61%, and 45% of controls, respectively, for U87, U373, T98, and DAOY cells.[21] The c-*myb* sense configuration oligonucleotides did not show significant differences in proliferative activity when compared with controls. A single antisense oligonucleotide treatment inhibited cell proliferation within 6 hours; the inhibition was sustained for 36 hours. The mechanism by which growth inhibition occurred is not known, but it may be mediated through cell surface growth factor receptor expression. In vivo studies are in progress to determine the effect of antisense oligonucleotides to c-*myb* administered directly into a nude mouse human glioma flank tumor.

IN VIVO STUDIES

The initial in vivo application of antisense oligonucleotide technology to CNS tumors was performed in a rodent C6 glioma flank tumor model.[16] In this animal model, antisense RNA for IGF1 was used to determine whether IGF1 expression was coupled to tumorigenicity of C6 glioma cells. An antisense IGF1 construct was assembled in an expression vector that incorporated Epstein-Barr virus replicative signals with the $ZnSO_4$-inducible metallothionein I transcriptional promoter. Subcutaneous injection in rats of either nontransfected C6 cells or the injection of transfected C6 cells without IGF1 sequences yielded large tumors after 2 weeks. Rats injected with transfected C6 cells did not have tumor development after 40 weeks. Large tumors developed after 2 weeks in rats injected with transfected or nontransfected B-104 neuroblastoma cells that did not express IGF1.[16] The mechanism by which animals had no tumor development was thought to be immune-mediated because histologic examination showed a few glioma cells infiltrated by a large number of mononuclear cells.[16] No infiltration of mononuclear cells was seen in the flank tumors that resulted from the injection of nontransfected cells.[16] Rats injected with IGF1 antisense transfected C6 cells did not have brain tumor development induced by nontransfected C6 cells.[22] Subcutaneous injection of IGF1 antisense transfected C6 cells into rats bearing intracerebral C6 gliomas at a point distal to the tumor resulted in intracranial tumor regression.[22] The anti-tumor effect was felt to be mediated by a glioma-specific immune response involving CD8+ lymphocytes.[22]

The subcutaneous injection of wild-type C6 glioma cells into syngeneic immunocompetent rats yields a tumor within 1 week. When rats were injected with C6 cells stably transfected with plasmids that expressed antisense RNA to IGF1 receptor RNA, tumors did not develop, and antisense IGF1 receptor RNA was overexpressed.[17] Rats injected with C6 IGF1 receptor antisense cells had prevention of subsequent tumor formation when wild-type C6 cells were injected 1 to 3 weeks later into the opposite flank.[17] Rats with established wild-type C6 flank tumors had complete tumor regression within 2 weeks after injection of C6 IGF1 receptor antisense cells into the opposite flank.[17] The mechanism by which these tumors regressed is unknown.

In nude mice given subcutaneous transplantation of U87 cells stably transfected with the antisense cDNA encoding PKCA, tumor development did not occur by 70 days.[18] Measurable tumors developed in mice 7 to 50 days after subcutaneous transplantation of nontransfected U87 cells.[18]

CLINICAL STUDIES

The clinical application of antisense oligonucleotides is currently limited and does not involve the CNS. Ex vivo autologous antisense oligonucleotide–purged bone marrow transplantation after standard chemotherapy and radiotherapy has been proposed as a phase I to II clinical trial for patients with chronic myelogenous leukemia.[23] For patients with chemotherapy-refractory acute myelogenous leukemia, phase I clinical trials are planned using phosphorothioate antisense oligonucleotides complementary to p53 mRNA.[23] The treatment of AIDS represents another area of potential application for antisense oligonucleotides. Phosphorothioate analogs can cause dose-dependent inhibition of human immunodeficiency virus, type 1 (HIV-1) replication at concentrations less than 10 μM.[4] The mechanism of action may be due to inhibition of HIV-1 reverse transcriptase or through surface binding inhibition of the virus.[4] One potential application of antisense oligonucleotides to CNS disease may be in the treatment of malignant primary brain tumors. The ability to inhibit glioma cell growth after the addition of c-*myb* antisense oligonucleotides suggests that this oncogene may be an appropriate target for future clinical trials. Because antisense oligonucleotides have a static mechanism of action, their clinical utility is uncertain and the co-administration of cidal chemotherapeutic agents or targeted toxins may be necessary to obtain a significant therapeutic effect. Although their overall size is small, the most effective route for delivery of antisense oligonucleotides to malignant glial neoplasms has not been determined. Delivery of specific antisense oligonucleotide sequences to brain tumors may be possible with the convection-enhanced infusion system that is currently used to administer intratumoral immunotoxin therapy in phase I clinical trials. Another possible method for antisense oligonucleotide delivery to intraparenchymal neoplastic disease may be via blood-brain barrier disruption, which has been used to successfully treat CNS lymphoma, germ cell tumors, primitive neuroectodermal tumors, and glioblastomas multiforme. This technique has been used to administer chemotherapy, monoclonal antibodies, viruses, and other molecules much larger than antisense oligonucleotides. Future investigation of antisense oligonucleotides should include these various drug delivery techniques to maximize clinical utility.

CONCLUSION

The poor prognosis associated with malignant primary brain tumors has led investigators to seek and develop new, innovative treatment modalities. Current adjuvant therapies lack tumor specificity, which can lead to toxic CNS side effects. Advances in molecular biology now allow specific gene sequences to be inserted or targeted in the malignant cell genome. Antisense oligodeoxynucleotides represent complementary nucleic acid sequences that can recognize and bind to target genes, resulting in the arrest of DNA transcription or translation of mRNA. Chemical modification of these agents has decreased their susceptibility to degradation by nucleases. These molecules enter cells by simple diffusion or active endocytosis and temporarily inhibit glioma cell proliferation in a time- and dose-dependent fashion. Although few in vivo studies have evaluated the efficacy of antisense oligonucleotides in animal models, complete tumor regression has been reported by mechanisms that are not yet fully understood. Because of the encouraging preliminary results in CNS tumors, investigators are developing this unique form of gene therapy for future clinical application. By combining static antisense oligonucleotides with more potent cidal chemotherapeutic drugs or immunotoxins, the therapeutic efficacy of the latter for the treatment of malignant brain tumors may increase, accompanied by a consequent decrease in dose-limiting systemic toxic effects. The ability of antisense oligonucleotides to recognize specific gene sequences and to down-regulate gene expression make them ideal agents for use in targeting oncogenes that are overexpressed in CNS neoplasms.

REFERENCES

1. Hall WA, Fodstad Ø: Immunotoxins and central nervous system neoplasia. J Neurosurg 1992; 76:1.
2. Leonetti JP, Degols G, Clarenc P, et al: Cell delivery and mechanisms of action of antisense oligonucleotides. Prog Nucleic Acid Res Mol Biol 1993; 44:143.
3. Rothenberg M, Johnson G, Laughlin C, et al: Oligodeoxynucleotides as anti-sense inhibitors of gene expression: Therapeutic implications. JNCI 1989; 81:1539.
4. Cohen JS: Biochemical therapy: Antisense compounds. *In* Devita VT Jr, Hellman S, Rosenberg SA (eds): Biologic Therapy of Cancer. Philadelphia, JB Lippincott, 1991, pp 763–775.
5. Calabretta B, Skorski T, Szczylik C, et al: Prospects for gene-directed therapy with antisense oligodeoxynucleotides. Cancer Treat Rev 1993; 19:169.
6. Carter G, Lemoine NR: Antisense technology for cancer therapy: Does it make sense? Br J Cancer 1993; 67:869.
7. Calabretta B, Skorski T, Zon G: Antisense oligonucleotides. Cancer Biol 1992; 3:391.
8. Citro G, Perrotti D, Cucco C, et al: Inhibition of leukemia cell proliferation by receptor-mediated uptake of c-*myb* antisense oligodeoxynucleotides. Proc Natl Acad Sci USA 1992; 89:7031.
9. Yu ACH, Lee YL, Eng LF: Inhibition of GFAP synthesis by antisense RNA in astrocytes. J Neurosci Res 1991; 30:72.
10. Behl C, Winkler J, Bogdhan U, et al: Autocrine growth regulation in neuroectodermal tumors as detected with oligodeoxynucleotide antisense molecules. Neurosurgery 1993; 33:679.
11. Nitta T, Sato K: Specific inhibition of c-*sis* protein synthesis and cell proliferation with antisense oligodeoxynucleotides in human glioma cells. Neurosurgery 1994; 34:309.
12. Murphy PR, Sato Y, Knee RS: Phosphorothioate antisense oligonucleotides against basic fibroblast growth factor inhibit anchorage-dependent and anchorage-independent growth of a malignant glioblastoma cell line. Mol Endocrinol 1992; 6:877.
13. Morrison RS: Suppression of basic fibroblast growth factor expression by antisense oligodeoxynucleotides inhibits the growth of transformed human astrocytes. J Biol Chem 1991; 266:728.
14. Redekop GJ, Naus CCG: Transfection with bFGF sense and antisense cDNA resulting in modification of malignant glioma growth. J Neurosurg 1995; 82:83.
15. Weinstein DE, Shelanski ML, Liem RKH: Suppression by antisense mRNA demonstrates a requirement for the glial fibrillary acidic protein in the formation of stable astrocytic processes in response to neurons. J Cell Biol 1991; 112:1205.
16. Trojan J, Blossey BK, Johnson TR, et al: Loss of tumorigenicity of rat glioblastoma directed by episome-based antisense cDNA transcription of insulin-like growth factor I. Proc Natl Acad Sci USA 1992; 89:4874.
17. Resnicoff M, Sell C, Rubini M, et al: Rat glioblastoma cells expressing an antisense RNA to the insulin-like growth factor-1 (IGF-1) receptor are nontumorigenic and induce regression of wild-type tumors. Cancer Res 1994; 54:2218.
18. Ahmed S, Mineta T, Martuza RL, et al: Antisense expression of protein kinase C-alpha inhibits the growth and tumorigenicity of human glioblastoma cells. Neurosurgery 1994; 35:904.
19. Raschella G, Negroni A, Skorski T, et al: Inhibition of proliferation by c-*myb* antisense RNA and oligodeoxynucleotides in transformed neuroectodermal cell lines. Cancer Res 1992; 52:4221.
20. Welter C, Henn W, Theisinger B, et al: The cellular *myb* oncogene is amplified, rearranged and activated in human glioblastoma cell lines. Cancer Lett 1990; 52:57.
21. Flores EP, Chiang L, Wen DYK, et al: Suppression of human medulloblastoma cell proliferation with antisense oligonucleotides to the c-*myb* oncogene. Soc Neurosci Abstracts 1994; 20:835.
22. Trojan J, Johnson TR, Rudin SD, et al: Treatment and prevention of rat glioblastoma by immunogenic C6 cells expressing antisense insulin-like growth factor I RNA. Science 1993; 259:94.
23. Stein CA, Cheng Y-C: Antisense oligonucleotides as therapeutic agents: Is the bullet really magical? Science 1993; 261:1004.

Pathology

SCOTT R. VANDENBERG

MARIA BEATRIZ SAMPAIO LOPES

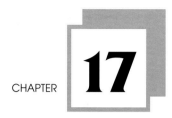

CHAPTER **17**

Classification

During the last decade, the pathologic diagnosis of gliomas has been remarkably affected by the application of immuno-histochemical and molecular biologic studies. These techniques have extended our understanding of the diversity of tumor cell differentiation, with particular emphasis on expression of cytoskeletal and membrane proteins, production and secretion of growth factors, kinetics of cell proliferation, and molecular cytogenetics. Such insights have contributed substantially to both the classification of gliomas and the grading of their malignant potential. New experimental models that enable the study of gliogenesis from primitive progenitors and the effects of extrinsic factors on the proliferation and maturation of specific glial lineages will lead to a better understanding of the biologic diversity and differentiation of neoplastic glial populations.[1] In these models, molecular biologic strategies combined with morphologic techniques will better define two fundamental biologic aspects of glial neoplasia: (1) the progenitor cells/glial lineages and diverse glial phenotypes that are distinct targets for transformation; and (2) the genetic alterations and epigenetic processes that are selectively altered by neoplastic transformation and malignant progression in specific glial genotypes. Such advances will progressively and dramatically change the diagnostic tableau for gliomas.

Advances in neuroimaging techniques and the expanded use of stereotactic biopsies have dramatically affected clinical neuro-oncology. These diagnostic approaches have been a major impetus to better understanding the earlier stages of glioma formation with detection of smaller lesions and tumors in the setting of other neurologic disorders. Stereotactic guidance of biopsies and limited resections in these clinical settings have challenged contemporary neuropathologists to effectively optimize data from minute tissue specimens to better assess heterogeneous tumors and adjacent brain. Part of this optimization necessarily involves a strong integration of neuroimaging techniques and histopathologic approaches to appropriately address the complex issues of tumor biology and tumor-brain interactions.

ASTROCYTIC TUMORS

The astrocytic tumors are divided into two major classes, which are based on the overall pattern of growth with respect

to a capacity for brain invasion and the progressive malignant potential.[2] The more common class of astrocytic tumor is designated by the general term *astrocytoma* (diffuse astrocytic tumors). This group of tumors is generally characterized by a significant potential to undergo anaplastic progression and a high capacity for brain invasion with diffuse tumor cell infiltration beyond the macroscopic tumor-brain interface. The grading of anaplasia and malignant growth potential in astrocytomas is a salient aspect of their histopathologic classification. These tumors are, accordingly, designated as astrocytoma (WHO grade II), anaplastic astrocytoma (WHO grade III), and glioblastoma (astrocytoma, WHO grade IV). Despite the apparently fixed classification of the astrocytomas into three subtypes, the astrocytoma group may be more appropriately envisioned as a biologic continuum on which three major subsets, defined by a limited collection of histopathologic features, have been empirically arranged. Although not strictly related to anaplasia or malignant potential, cytoarchitectural variants of astrocytoma cells are usually recognized as fibrillary, gemistocytic, and protoplasmic forms.

The second, smaller class of astrocytic tumors is composed of three relatively dissimilar neoplasms (pilocytic astrocytoma, pleomorphic xanthoastrocytoma, and subependymal giant cell astrocytoma). The distinctive histopathologic features of these tumors preclude the direct application of the same histologic indices of anaplasia that are generally applied to the more diffuse astrocytomas. In addition to their distinctive clinicopathologic features, two properties are shared among the tumors in this group that, in combination, generally result in a more favorable prognosis than for the group of diffuse astrocytomas. These are (1) a more circumscribed growth pattern, with limited microscopic infiltration of adjacent brain; and (2) a diminished malignant potential with infrequent anaplastic progression.

Astrocytoma Group

HISTOPATHOLOGIC VARIANTS AND ASTROCYTIC DIVERSITY

Three major histopathologic variants of diffusely infiltrating astrocytomas are recognized: *fibrillary*, *gemistocytic*, and *protoplasmic.* This subclassification of astrocytic tumors tends to correlate the morphologic characteristics of the neoplastic astrocytes to the classic astroglial forms present in normal and reactive brain (i.e., fibrillary, protoplasmic, and gemistocytic astrocytes). Although the designated variant is based on the predominant "cell type" present in a given tumor, most astrocytomas are often variable mixtures of the astroglial cell types. Among these variants, the *fibrillary astrocytic* tumors are the most common (Fig. 17–1). *Gemistocytic astrocytoma* is usually defined as a tumor with greater than 60% of gemistocytes[3] and is the second most common variant, constituting a range of approximately 10% to 20% of astrocytomas in most series.[3] Gemistocytic cells are discernible as round to slightly angulated polygonal cells with abundant, well-defined eosinophilic cytoplasm and eccentric nuclei (Fig. 17–2). The tumor cells often have shorter, less conspicuous processes compared with the prominent radiating processes of reactive astrocytes. In one well-documented compilation of cases, tumors composed of more than 20% gemistocytes appeared to have a more aggressive biologic behavior than the more fibrillary tumors of similar grade.[3] However, cells with gemistocytic characteristics can be observed in astrocytomas of all grades. Tumors that can be regarded as *protoplasmic astrocytomas* are rarely observed, representing fewer than 1% of the astrocytomas.[4] Protoplasmic astrocytomas have a matrix composed of poorly fibrillated processes, and the tumor cells tend to have a more stellate geometry with short, delicate processes (Fig. 17–3).

In *fibrillary astrocytomas,* the elongated glial processes can be highlighted on phosphotungstic acid hematoxylin (PTAH) stain, but for diagnostic purposes the far more specific immunohistochemical demonstration of glial fibrillary acidic protein (GFAP) is in more common use. GFAP is the major constituent of intermediate filaments in normal, reactive, and neoplastic astrocytes. Immature oligodendrocytes and anaplastic oligodendrogliomas, reactive and neo-

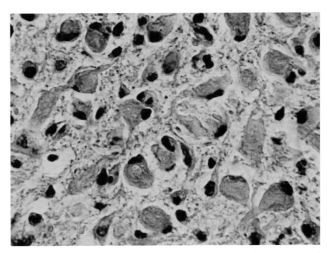

Figure 17–2 Gemistocytic astrocytoma (WHO grade II) cells are typically polygonal with prominent eosinophilic cytoplasm and eccentric hyperchromatic nuclei. The fibrillary quality of the intercellular matrix tends to be modest, whereas more stout and blunted glial processes are readily observed. Cellular pleomorphism and nuclear atypia are mild in this grade II astrocytoma (hematoxylin-eosin stain).

plastic ependymal cells, and choroid plexus epithelium may also show variable GFAP immunoreactivity. The relatively frequent expression of this intermediate filament protein has diagnostic implications in that it serves as a marker of glial differentiation. In astrocytomas, the relative expression of GFAP appears to be related to cellular differentiation and to proliferative potential in vitro.[5] An exception is the protoplasmic astrocytoma, which demonstrates minimal or no GFAP immunoreactivity.[4, 6]

Studies of the multiple glial lineages from the developing and mature mammalian brain suggest that the current histopathologic subclassifications of astroglial neoplasms may not accurately encompass the regional differences in physiologic properties that could profoundly affect tumor biology.[7–25] This diversity is most likely to be developmentally regulated in a stage-specific manner such that region-associated prop-

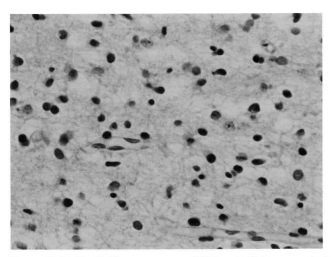

Figure 17–1 The fibrillary astrocytoma (WHO grade II) is composed of tumor cells with thin, often tapering, cytoplasmic processes that constitute a relatively conspicuous fibrillary matrix. Note that the grade II neoplasm displays a mild to moderate degree of nuclear pleomorphism without conspicuous cytologic pleomorphism, mitoses, or a high degree of cellularity (hematoxylin-eosin stain).

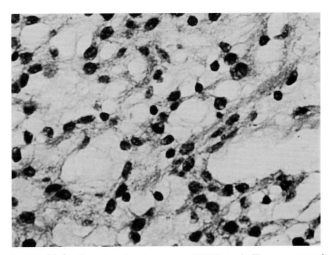

Figure 17–3 Protoplasmic astrocytomas (WHO grade II) are composed of cells with attenuated, relatively inconspicuous processes in a lacy webwork that is punctuated by multiple microcysts. Note the mild cellular pleomorphism (hematoxylin-eosin stain).

erties would be preserved after neoplastic transformation. Such regional properties include distinct extracellular matrix domains, intercellular electrical (and ionic) coupling, specific neuronal-glial interactions, and differences in cell surface receptors and in receptor-mediated gene expression. Therefore the neoplastic astroglial biology modified by these regional properties could include infiltrative/invasive capacity into the adjacent brain, cellular interactions with surrounding reactive glia and neurons, and a variety of membrane receptors coupled to second messenger systems that affect cell proliferation and differentiation.

CRITERIA FOR GRADING MALIGNANT POTENTIAL

Histopathologic Features The process of evaluating histologic features to ascertain the malignant potential of tumors imposes a static and correlative histopathologic designation for a variable, dynamic growth process. Grading in the astrocytoma group should therefore conceptually define histopathologic features that may be predictive of the following: (1) the nature of brain invasion at the tumor-brain interface, (2) the potential for rapid growth, and (3) the capacity to infiltrate brain for distant spread in the neuraxis. Historically, the initial approaches focused more on tumor histogenesis and were too complex to be applied uniformly. Both a comparative historical review[26] and an updated discussion relevant to the current World Health Organization (WHO) tumor classification[27] are informative commentaries on the salient histopathologic features for the classifying and grading of gliomas. From the first formulation of Kernohan and Sayre's scheme in the early 1950s[28] to the contemporary "simplified" systems (see following), two practical points must be carefully considered. First, the conventional histologic criteria that are used to indicate an increased growth potential in astrocytomas are relatively insensitive (e.g., mitotic figures to indicate the proliferative cell pool) or are only indirect manifestations of neoplastic physiology (e.g., cellular pleomorphism, necrosis, and microvascular hyperplasia).

The second caveat to any grading system for astrocytomas is the major limitation of tumor heterogeneity. This is an inherent property of gliomas in particular.[29-33] In a thorough postmortem study of 18 glioblastomas, both the degrees of cellularity and the topographic distribution of cytoarchitectural pleomorphism were significantly heterogeneous.[30] In a large clinicopathologic review of 241 gliomas with postmortem data, 7.5% of the glioblastomas appeared multicentric and 2.5% had such divergent histopathologic features in the different foci as to suggest different astrocytic tumors.[31] A combination of immunohistochemical proliferative indices (Ki-67 epitope) and histopathologic evaluation of multiple regions in a series of 14 astrocytic tumors demonstrated significant independent regional heterogeneity of both cell proliferation and histopathologic features.[33] This heterogeneity, combined with limited sampling, especially within border zones, can result in grading inaccuracies due to the nonrandom distribution of necrosis[34] and microvascular hyperplasia. The importance of combining magnetic resonance imaging (MRI) with stereotactic techniques to improve overall accuracy has been proposed.[32] The multiple sampling of targets in conjunction with stereotactic techniques signifi-

cantly increases the precision of the St. Anne-Mayo grading system, described in the following text.[35]

Most current approaches to grading have essentially evolved into three-tiered systems, corresponding to the WHO designations of astrocytoma (WHO grade II), anaplastic astrocytoma (WHO grade III), and glioblastoma (WHO grade IV). Separation of the diffuse astrocytic tumors into three groups is generally supported by clinical survival data,[36-39] even though the specific histopathologic criteria, their weighting, and the lines of division still vary among laboratories.[26] The histopathologic features include magnitude of cellularity, degree of cellular pleomorphism (cytoplasmic and/or nuclear), mitotic activity, and presence and/or prominence of microvascular endothelial and/or pericytic proliferation and necrosis. These have been described in detail elsewhere.[40]

Large studies using this three-tiered approach have been described previously.[26, 41, 42] For all systems, a combination of features designating both cellular atypia and anaplasia is used. Aside from tumor necrosis and endothelial proliferation, most of these features have a significant subjective quality that is highly influenced by previous experience. For separating the intermediate group (anaplastic astrocytoma, WHO grade III) from the lowest-grade group (astrocytoma, WHO grade II), most schemes use intermediate degrees of cellularity combined with various scales of cellular atypia (as reflected by nuclear and/or cytoplasmic ratios and nuclear and/or cytoplasmic pleomorphism) in the continuum between glioblastoma multiforme and astrocytoma (WHO grade II).

The division between glioblastoma and anaplastic astrocytoma is usually set selectively on the basis of tumor necrosis and/or microvascular endothelial proliferation as the highly weighted features, accompanied by features of increased cellular atypia. Another approach[26] differs in that it does not define necrosis as an important variable but highly weights multiple parameters of cellular atypia in addition to vascular endothelial proliferation. The group of glioblastomas that are designated by these criteria appears to have a proliferative index (bromodeoxyuridine [BUdR] labeling, see following text) comparable to that of the glioblastomas, defined by the combined features of necrosis and endothelial proliferation.[37, 38]

Daumas-Duport and co-workers[43] described a conceptual four-tiered numeric grading system for astrocytomas. Currently denoted as the St. Anne-Mayo system, it differs from previously published three-tiered systems by noting simply the presence or absence of nuclear atypia, mitoses, endothelial proliferation, and necrosis, without rating the intensity or ranking the significance of particular combinations. According to this scheme, tumors with none of these features are grade 1, those with one feature are grade 2, those with two features are grade 3, and those with three or four features are grade 4. The application of the St. Anne-Mayo system demonstrated strong interobserver reproducibility and a high degree of correlation between the histologic ranking and survival curves in two large series.[36, 43]

Despite the lack of an implicit hierarchy in the St. Anne-Mayo system, the criteria make their appearance in a largely predictable order. Grade 2 tumors exhibit nuclear atypia, grade 3 lesions show the addition of mitoses, and grade 4 tumors further show endothelial proliferation and/or necrosis. Therefore, in very small biopsies, the presence of atypia combined with endothelial/pericytic proliferation without any observed mitoses or necrosis would still be highly suggestive of a grade IV astrocytoma. This is justified by the observation that necrosis and endothelial proliferation do appear to function independently as significant predictors of patient survival.[36] The three highest grades correspond roughly to astrocytoma, anaplastic or malignant astrocytoma, and glioblastoma of three-tiered systems. The grade 1 astrocytoma of the St. Anne-Mayo scheme is so uncommon (~1%) that the system is essentially three-tiered. The WHO grading system basically represents a simplification of the St. Anne-Mayo system wherein the grade designation is determined by combinations of the same morphologic criteria (atypia, mitoses, endothelial proliferation, necrosis). Accordingly, tumors with a single feature (usually nuclear or cytoplasmic atypia) are designated WHO grade II, those with two criteria (usually atypia and mitotic activity) are WHO grade III, and those with three or four features are WHO grade IV. No implicit hierarchy of grading features exists within this grading system.

Estimation of Growth Potential The use of mitotic activity as a significant grading criterion emphasizes the importance of evaluating the proliferative fraction of cells in astrocytomas. Special techniques that provide the advantage of a more reproducible and sensitive index of evaluating proliferative activity therefore provide a useful complement to routine neuropathologic evaluation. A number of approaches have been described, including nuclear silver-stained nucleolar organizer region labeling and several immunohistochemical techniques. The most suitable appear to be the detection of proliferation-associated proteins or BUdR/DNA epitopes (see Lopes and VandenBerg[44] for a review). The first is the immunohistochemical detection of an epitope, designated Ki-67, that defines a family of nuclear proteins necessary for the maintenance of the proliferative state.[45] The expression of Ki-67 is tightly regulated during the cell cycle, and its expression occurs during the G1, S, G2, and M phases of the cell cycle but is absent in the G0 phase.[46, 47] Recent cell cycle studies show minimal expression of Ki-67 epitope in late G1/early S phase and accumulation in S phase, with an increasing rate during the last half.[48] Pertinent to its use as a marker for cycling cells, Ki-67 epitope appears to disappear rapidly from postmitotic cells, with a half-life less than 16% of the G1 phase.[48]

A significant limitation of the early immunodetection of Ki-67 was the necessity of using frozen tissue specimens; however, a commercial monoclonal antibody (MIB-1) is now available that reacts with the Ki-67 epitope in routinely processed, paraffin-embedded material.[49–52] Due the simplicity of the procedure and the highly reliable staining results, the application of MIB-1 staining is rapidly becoming the most common method for determining tumor proliferative indices in neuropathology laboratories. The number of actively proliferating cells identified by Ki-67 immunohistochemistry appears to correlate well with the histopathologic grade of astrocytomas in a number of series.[52–58] Nonetheless, the innate heterogeneity of astrocytomas can produce

false interpretation of labeling results when limited samples are analyzed.[59]

The second method for the evaluation of growth fraction in astrocytomas is the in vivo (perioperative) labeling of cells in S phase with BUdR.[60–63] Its incorporation with subsequent immunohistochemical labeling of BUdR-containing cells in the resected tumor specimen permits an accurate assessment of cells in the S phase at the time of tumor resection. The only limitation is that this in situ method is applicable only in centers with appropriate resources that are committed to the technique. A recent study from the University of California at San Francisco, a center well recognized for the development of this technique, compared MIB-1 immunohistochemistry for Ki-67 and BUdR labeling indices and showed a significant correlation between the two techniques in each grade of astrocytoma.[64] Although a few studies with in vitro BUdR labeling of resected tumor tissue[61] suggest that this method may be potentially helpful in diagnostic assessment, the feasibility of this approach for routine use has yet to be established.

Molecular Cytogenetic Alterations in Astrocytomas and Tumor Subtypes The process of anaplastic progression in astrocytic tumors is reflected in genetic events. Mutations of the tumor suppressor gene p53 seem generally to represent one of the earliest detectable genetic alterations that occur in the adult astrocytoma group.[65–67] Indeed, one pathway for anaplastic progression to glioblastoma may be related to a clonal expansion of cells carrying a p53 mutation[68] (see following). Such cells can be identified in approximately 30% of astrocytomas of all grades. Loss of heterozygosity on chromosome 17p occurs in approximately 30% of astrocytomas, independent of tumor grade; it is frequently associated with point mutations in the p53 tumor suppressor gene.[65, 69, 70] In contrast to astrocytomas arising in the adult brain, pediatric astrocytomas appear to have an overall lower incidence of p53 mutations, suggesting a different trend for oncogenetic mechanisms in these tumors.[71–73] However, one study of malignant brainstem tumors suggests that this distinction may not be as definitive in high-grade lesions.[74] Genetic abnormalities other than those that selectively affect the p53 gene are found in diffusely infiltrating astrocytomas. Allelic deletions have been demonstrated on chromosomes 9p, 10, 13, 17p, 19q, and 22q (see Collins and James[75] for a review). Chromosome 10 deletions are found primarily in anaplastic astrocytoma and glioblastoma.[69] Genetic amplifications occur on chromosomes 7 (including the epidermal growth factor receptor [EGFR] locus, with or without rearrangements), 9, and 12 (including the MDM2 gene locus)[76, 77]; they also occur with a higher frequency in higher-grade neoplasms.

In an attempt to relate molecular cytogenetic abnormalities to oncogenesis and anaplastic progression, tentative subclassifications of glioblastomas have been proposed.[73, 78] One subtype appears to have deletions on the short arm of chromosome 17 and/or a p53 gene mutation without deletions on chromosome 10 and/or EGFR gene amplification. This type of glioblastoma occurs primarily in younger patients and may develop with anaplastic progression from lower-grade astrocytomas. Early p53 mutations may enhance genetic instability and lead to the accumulation of genetic alterations that culminate with malignant progression. This may be an oversimplification, as the p53 gene product has multiple interrelated functions associated with cell cycle stop points and/or checkpoints, transcriptional activation, and programmed cell death, or apoptosis.[79] A second subset of glioblastoma that shows early deletions on chromosome 10 and EGFR gene amplification without apparent deletions on chromosome 17 may develop as a de novo tumor in an older patient population. Consistent with age as a significant prognostic factor in the astrocytoma group, the first subset tends to have better survival than the second. Other molecular cytogenetic features that appear to correlate with tumor prognosis and that may constitute additional subgroups are those seen in younger patients with microsatellite instability[80, 81] and with aneuploidy.[82]

ASTROCYTOMA (WHO GRADE II)

The macroscopic consistency of astrocytomas depends on the predominant component of the tumor (see Figs. 17–1 through 17–3). A high proportion of fibrillary astrocytic differentiation confers firmness to the tumor specimen. In contrast, protoplasmic astrocytomas appear as gelatinous masses due to the frequent presence of microcystic degeneration. Intraoperative smears of the well-differentiated astrocytomas readily demonstrate the astrocytic nature of the tumors, with a variably abundant fibrillary matrix formed by cytoplasmic processes. The cytoarchitecture may range from a barely discernible perinuclear rim of cytoplasm to more fusiform or markedly elongated forms. Regardless of the predominant cell type, grade II astrocytomas exhibit only mild cellular atypia, and cellularity varies from near normal to mild, with focally moderate increases. By definition, mitoses, endothelial proliferation, and necrosis are lacking. Such tumors are equivalent to grade 2 astrocytomas in the St. Anne-Mayo scheme.

ANAPLASTIC ASTROCYTOMA (WHO GRADE III)

All types of diffusely infiltrating astrocytomas, among which fibrillary tumors are most frequent, have a variable capacity for progression to anaplastic astrocytomas. Although anaplastic progression is anticipated in up to 80% of such tumors,[4, 83] the latent period to progression is quite variable. In recurrent astrocytomas, the frequency of progression to a higher grade than the original tumor is approximately 50% to 75%.[4] Anaplastic astrocytomas may also arise de novo, without an intermediate phase of anaplastic progression from a lower tumor grade. As do grade II astrocytomas, anaplastic astrocytomas exhibit considerable variation in cellularity as well as in morphologic heterogeneity. As a rule, cellularity is greater, atypia is more conspicuous, and mitotic figures are present (Figs. 17–4 and 17–5). Such tumors are equivalent to those of St. Anne-Mayo grade 3.

GLIOBLASTOMA MULTIFORME (WHO GRADE IV)

Glioblastomas represent 15% to 20% of all intracranial tumors and approximately 50% of gliomas in adults.[84] In most series, a significant number of these arise from anaplastic progression in astrocytomas and anaplastic astrocyto-

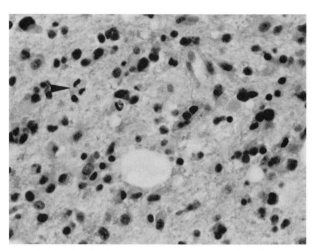

Figure 17–4 Anaplastic astrocytoma (WHO grade III): the neoplastic astrocytes demonstrate a moderate to high degree of cellular pleomorphism with greater numbers of enlarged, hyperchromatic nuclei. Mitotic activity is readily observed (*arrowhead*). Note the sparse but delicate microvasculature and lack of necrosis (hematoxylin-eosin stain).

mas.[85–87] A particular subgroup of glioblastomas, one with mutations in the conserved region of the p53 gene, appears to selectively affect women and young adults.[67] Less frequently, glioblastomas arise de novo, without evidence for an antecedent lower-grade lesion. Consistent with the de novo appearance of glioblastomas, a clinicopathologic study of gliomas less than 2 cm in the largest dimension revealed that approximately 20% are glioblastomas, even at the earliest stages.[88] Glioblastomas may also occur in the pediatric group,[89] but these tumors appear to have different molecular cytogenetic features.[71, 72]

Glioblastomas have neuroimaging and macroscopic features that reflect the aggressive nature of the lesion. Salient features include an expansive lesion on computed tomography (CT) or MRI, with vascular contrast enhancement that is variably diminished in the center of the lesion. Whereas

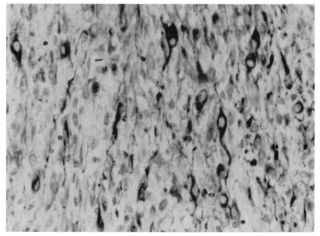

Figure 17–5 Anaplastic astrocytoma (WHO grade III): GFAP immunohistochemistry highlights the conspicuous cellular pleomorphism in this anaplastic astrocytoma. Note the high degree of cellularity but the overall astroglial nature of the cytoarchitecture (GFAP-ABC immunoperoxidase with hematoxylin counterstain).

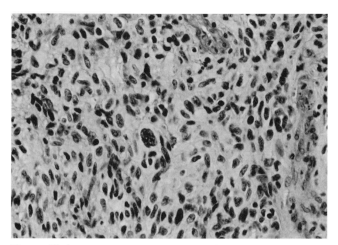

Figure 17–6 Glioblastoma multiforme (WHO grade IV): the intense anaplasia that is a typical histopathologic feature of glioblastomas results from a combination of extensive cytoplasmic and nuclear pleomorphism. Note the focus of multilayered microvascular hyperplasia (hematoxylin-eosin stain).

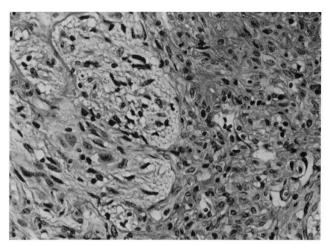

Figure 17–8 Glioblastoma multiforme (WHO grade IV): microvascular hyperplasia denoted as ''endothelial proliferation'' is a hallmark feature of glioblastomas that, as in this field (*right*), can be quite exuberant (hematoxylin-eosin stain).

the latter represents necrosis, the zone of enhancement corresponds to hypercellular—often solid—tumor with neovascularization.[90] The often heterogeneous signal noted on T2-weighted MRI correlates with areas of hypocellularity and vascularity alternating with regions of necrosis and/or lower cellularity. Despite the rather circumscribed neuroimaging and macroscopic appearance of the glioblastomas, diffuse infiltration of the surrounding brain parenchyma by isolated single cells or small clusters of neoplastic cells is almost invariable. The extent of parenchymal infiltration is highly variable, as has been demonstrated by detailed mapping studies of glioblastomas.[91] Indeed, it may range from a few millimeters to many centimeters. Spreading of the tumor cells along fiber tracts may be particularly extensive, with the classic example of extension across the corpus callosum to the opposite hemisphere (''butterfly'' pattern).

The histopathologic characteristics of glioblastomas are marked by conspicuous cellular heterogeneity (Fig. 17–6), ranging from closely packed, small cells with scant cytoplasm and round to oval variably hyperchromatic nuclei to bizarre, multinucleated giant cells. Most tumors exhibit a mixed pattern. Mitotic figures, including atypical forms, are often readily identified, but these vary considerably within different portions of the tumor. Immunohistochemical indices of cellular proliferation likewise vary, but they tend to be significantly elevated (Fig. 17–7). Previous studies have set the Ki-67 (MIB-1) indices in the range of 23.9 ± 13.5.[64] Endothelial proliferation (Fig. 17–8) and necrosis (Fig. 17–9) are equivalent features in distinguishing glioblastomas from astrocytomas of grade III (WHO grading and St. Anne-Mayo systems). Either micronecrosis or broad geographic zones of necrosis (see Fig. 17–9), when surrounded by dense palisades of tumor cells, generally reflect true tumor necrosis. In comparison, radiation necrosis is not usually associated with cellular palisading. In recurrent tumors, the presence of

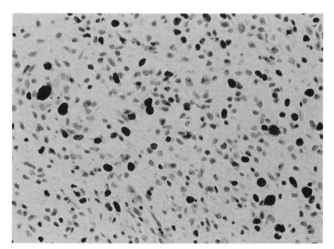

Figure 17–7 Glioblastoma multiforme (WHO grade IV): the numerous proliferative cells in glioblastomas are readily detected as Ki-67 immunoreactive nuclei (MIB-1–ABC immunoperoxidase with hematoxylin counterstain).

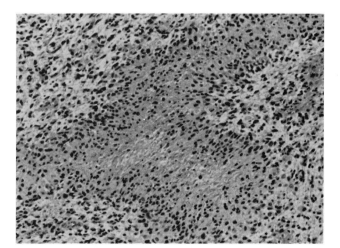

Figure 17–9 Glioblastoma multiforme (WHO grade IV): geographic necrosis with peripheral palisades of tumor cells is the typical form of cellular necrosis in glioblastomas and is dissimilar from the commonplace manifestation of radionecrosis (hematoxylin-eosin stain).

intrinsic tumoral necrosis and microvascular alterations should be distinguished from prior radiation therapy. As distinct histopathologic features, endothelial proliferation and necrosis need not be specifically related; they may be present in the same microscopic field or they may be widely dispersed. Microvascular hyperplasia may be present in locations that are remote from the tumor mass.[92] As defined in the present WHO scheme, glioblastomas correspond to astrocytomas of St. Anne-Mayo grade 4. Other histopathologic features that may be present in glioblastomas are cytoplasmic lipidization, stromal mucin accumulation, myxoid change, and desmoplasia in areas of meningeal—particularly dural—invasion.[4, 93] It is important to emphasize that the biology of glioblastomas is complex and that the aggressive growth and spread of these tumors is not simply a direct relationship to cell proliferation. A recent study of 98 primary and recurrent glioblastomas showed that there was no significant association between the levels of BUdR-labeling indices and patient survival.[94]

Two distinct histopathologic subvariants of glioblastomas are recognized in the WHO classification. The first of these, *giant cell glioblastoma*, appears to have distinctive neuroradiologic and, to a lesser extent, clinical features. This lesion has a slight predilection for the temporal lobe[95] and gives an impression of having more circumscribed borders with neuroimaging and on gross examination. Affected patients may frequently exceed the median survival time for those with more ordinary glioblastomas.[4, 95] Histologically, giant cell glioblastomas in large part are composed of bizarre, multinucleated giant cells with abundant eosinophilic cytoplasm and large vesicular nuclei. The initial impression of these tumors often brings to mind metastatic carcinoma, but there is always a less conspicuous population of fibrillary cells or small astrocytes that confirms the astrocytic nature of these malignant tumors. A variable histologic feature is an increase in reticulin fibers, one most conspicuous in relation to blood vessels and areas of necrosis. Whereas the giant cells are immunoreactive for S-100 protein, they often lack significant immunoreactivity for GFAP, the latter being more prominent in the more astrocytic fusiform cells.

Gliosarcoma is the second principal variant of glioblastoma. The derivation of the sarcomatous element is usually attributed to malignant transformation of either the mesenchymal elements associated with hyperplastic microvasculature or those within adjacent meningeal membranes. Although endothelial and pericytic proliferation is a significant feature of all glioblastomas, the frequency of sarcomatous transformation in these tumors ranges from only 2% to 8%.[96, 97] Immunohistochemical and ultrastructural studies suggest that the sarcomatous elements are derived from vascular mesenchymal cells with a capacity for differentiation along endothelial, smooth muscle, and pericytic cell types.[98–102] However, this concept regarding the histogenesis of gliosarcomas may be an oversimplification about a heterogeneous group of tumors. Neoplastic astrocytes have the capacity to produce basal lamina and to elaborate extracellular matrix associated with mesenchymal phenoytpes. The molecular cytogenetic relationship between the ''sarcomatous'' and the glial elements in some tumors suggests a common cellular origin.[103–105]

The ratio of two types of cell populations is highly variable, both within individual tumors and in the group as a whole. The relative proportions of the two cell populations is such that the glial component tends over time to become minor. As a result, the lesion may eventuate in a primarily sarcomatous proliferation. As a rule, the two components can readily be distinguished on the basis of their morphologic features as evidenced by special stains, such as reticulin and PTAH preparations, and by immunohistochemistry for GFAP, which is reactive in the neoplastic glial component. Reticulin and collagen stains serve to highlight the sarcomatous component, which in most cases resembles either fibrosarcoma or malignant fibrous histiocytoma. Osteocartilagenous and rhabdomyoblastic elements may also rarely be present.[106, 107]

Special Types of Astrocytic Tumors

PILOCYTIC ASTROCYTOMA

Pilocytic astrocytomas occur most frequently in children and in young adults, with a peak incidence in the second decade. In adult patients, these tumors tend to appear one decade earlier (mean age, 22 years) than do those in the diffusely infiltrating astrocytoma group.[108] Pilocytic astrocytomas arise at all levels of the neuraxis; however, these tumors are typically located in the midline structures (e.g., cerebellum, third ventricular region, optic pathways, brainstem, and spinal cord). Although supratentorial pilocytic astrocytomas tend to have a predilection for the temporoparietal region, thalamus, hypothalamus, or third ventricle, they may also arise in the frontoparietal lobes.[109] Pilocytic astrocytomas also constitute a large proportion (58%) of spinal gliomas; these lesions tend to occur in an older population, as compared with intracranial pilocytic tumors.[110] Compared with the diffusely infiltrating astrocytoma group (see preceding text), pilocytic astrocytomas are less biologically aggressive, relatively well-circumscribed tumors that displace—rather than infiltrate—the surrounding brain. As a result, they have a more favorable prognosis,[109, 111] with a designation of WHO grade I.

Although pilocytic astrocytomas are often macroscopically circumscribed, some degree of parenchymal infiltration can occur. The most striking aspect of the nonparenchymal spread of pilocytic astrocytomas is a propensity to invade the leptomeninges, which is particularly common in cerebellar examples.[112] Even distant cerebrospinal metastases have been reported,[113] but such behavior does not indicate any anaplastic progression.[114] Despite the rather indolent behavior and low proliferative potential of pilocytic astrocytomas, these tumors do recur, particularly after incomplete resection.[115]

Macroscopic features common to these tumors are variably sized cyst formation with a solid mural nodule. Microscopically, pilocytic astrocytomas typically show a biphasic pattern of growth consisting of bipolar highly fibrillated or piloid cells accompanied by Rosenthal fibers, and a loosely knit microcystic component made up of stellate cells resembling protoplasmic astrocytes (Fig. 17–10). The latter cell type is often associated with the typical ''granular bodies'' or protein droplets. GFAP immunoreactivity highlights the dense fibrillated cell populations that are often juxtaposed to the prominent microvasculature, whereas this is highly vari-

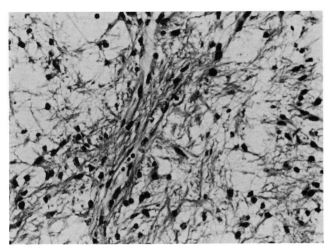

Figure 17-10 Pilocytic astrocytoma (WHO grade I): the common biphasic growth pattern of pilocytic astrocytomas is a combination of piloid cells forming fibrillary fascicles admixed with more loosely arranged stellate astrocytes. Rosenthal's fibers are commonly present in these tumors (hematoxylin-eosin stain).

able in the microcystic areas. In contrast, vimentin immunoreactivity is equally conspicuous in both types of cellular patterns.[116] Cellular atypia and pleomorphism, including multinucleated cells, may be present and are considered to be degenerative features not associated with anaplastic progression in these tumors. Microvascular proliferation may be present and sometimes simulates the glomeruloid type of hyperplasia in glioblastomas, but this does not connote malignant transformation. Brisk mitotic activity may portend recurrence with anaplastic progression, a process that is rarely documented in these tumors.[117] In a recent series of 107 pilocytic astrocytomas of the cerebellum,[112] anaplastic progression occurred in only 0.9% of cases; these tumors had relatively high fractions of S-phase cells on DNA flow cytometry. The prognosis of such tumors is still favorable relative to that of anaplastic astrocytomas.[112]

PLEOMORPHIC XANTHOASTROCYTOMA

The pleomorphic xanthoastrocytoma is a relatively rare glioma of the central nervous system (CNS) with distinctive clinicopathologic features. These tumors constitute fewer than 1% of all astrocytic tumors and typically arise, without predilection for gender, in children and young adults (usually ranging in age from the first to the third decades) with a longstanding history of seizures. Tumors that occur in older patients (after the fourth decade) are exceptional.[118–120]

Most pleomorphic xanthoastrocytomas arise in the cerebrum, with a proclivity for the temporal lobe. Although the overlying leptomeninges are commonly involved, dural infiltration is exceptional.[121–124] Tumors resembling pleomorphic xanthoastrocytomas do occasionally develop in other locations, including the cerebellum and spinal cord,[118, 125] but the biologic behavior of the tumors at other sites may not be comparable to that of the supratentorial tumors.[118] Regardless of site, the neoplasms are commonly a combination of cystic and solid portions and frequently include a conspicuous cystic component.

The striking histopathologic feature of these tumors is the high degree of astrocytic pleomorphism. Tumor cells vary from small round forms to fusiform and polygonal cells, usually arranged in fascicular patterns; the nuclei are commonly hyperchromatic with variable pleomorphism (Fig. 17–11). Multinucleated cells and lipidized giant cells with bizarre, often hyperchromatic nuclei, are common. The predominant cytoarchitectural forms can vary between regions in the same tumor and between different tumors. GFAP immunoreactivity highlights the pleomorphic glial cells, which include stout polygonal cells without conspicuous processes and interlacing bundles of the more fusiform cells within a variably fibrillated matrix. Cellularity is usually moderate, but areas of high cellular density are not uncommon. Mitoses, when present, are in low numbers, and cytofluorometry shows an extremely low fraction of S-phase cells.[126] Cytoplasmic lipidization, especially notable in the polygonal and giant cells, can be a prominent, although inconsistent, feature. Variable perivascular lymphocytic infiltration is usually present, but it has no specific histopathologic significance.

The tumors commonly have a prominent reticulin-positive stroma that is most conspicuous in the areas adjacent to leptomeningeal involvement, often in association with a prominent microvascular component. This is usually considered to be a hallmark (Fig. 17–12), although a small number of cases with otherwise typical features of pleomorphic xanthoastrocytoma do not evidence this prominent stroma.[124] In typical cases, it delineates fascicles of cells, and it is variably distributed between single tumor cells. Ultrastructural studies typically demonstrate a basal lamina-like deposition of extracellular matrix around the cell borders,[127, 128] a feature that the neoplastic astrocytes share with subpial astrocytes.[129] This stroma may be present in any portion of the tumor and can be quite variable among tumors. The prominence of the reticulin-positive stroma may also change with the astroglial features between initial and recurrent tumors. In one case from our institutional files in which there was no malignant

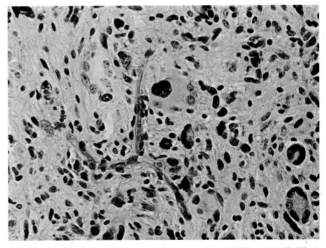

Figure 17-11 Pleomorphic xanthoastrocytoma (WHO grade II–III): a heterogeneous mixture of astroglial cell morphologies consisting of small polygonal and more elongated forms is typical of a pleomorphic xanthoastroctyoma. Mitotic figures, although present, are not conspicuous. Note the absence of necrosis and "endothelial proliferation," which distinguishes these tumors from glioblastomas (hematoxylin-eosin stain).

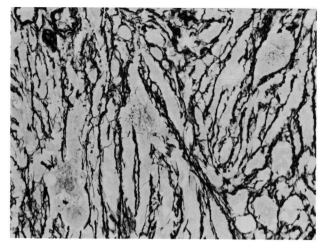

Figure 17–12 Pleomorphic xanthoastrocytoma (WHO grade II–III): the intercellular reticulin network around individual cells and cell clusters is often a prominent feature in pleomorphic xanthoastrocytomas (Wilder's reticulin stain).

transformation after a 20-year interval between the first and second resections, the reticulin-positive stroma and the fibrillary astrocytic components of the two specimens varied considerably. Although the exuberant stroma tends to form a well-defined macroscopic border with the adjacent brain, portions of the tumor do show microinfiltration of the surrounding brain and penetration into the adjacent perivascular spaces. In these areas, there may not be a well-defined plane of dissection. The involvement of the superficial Virchow-Robin spaces may be quite striking in otherwise very indolent tumors.

In approximately five cases, the co-existence of atypical ganglionic cells admixed with otherwise typical pleomorphic xanthoastrocytomas has been documented.[125, 130–133] The proportion of the neuronal and glial components appears to vary from clusters of possibly entrapped neuronal elements to tumors in which the pleomorphic xanthoastrocytoma represents the glial portion of a ganglioglioma.[125, 130] The histogenic relationship between these rare cases and other desmoplastic glioneuronal neoplasms is presently unclear.

Most pleomorphic xanthoastrocytomas have relatively indolent clinical behavior, with long-term survival of the patient after tumor resection; however, there is a risk of tumor recurrence and malignant progression. This shift in biologic behavior can occur either after a relatively short postoperative course or after a long interval of many years. There are presently no histopathologic criteria for the prospective identification of higher-grade biologic potential in this type of astrocytic tumor, and the WHO grade II–III designation reflects this uncertainty.[2] The histopathologic character of the infiltrating margin may be important with respect to evaluating the potential for both tumor recurrence and anaplastic progression.[127, 128, 134]

The number of reported cases is yet too limited to determine either a definitive frequency of recurrence or the histopathologic criteria to define this biologic potential. In the group with recurrence there appears to be a significant incidence of malignant progression, reaching about 50% in recurrent tumors. As inferred from these cases, the presence of either abundant mitoses, necrosis, and/or vascular endothelial/pericytic proliferation should be considered to be clear evidence of malignant transformation in pleomorphic xanthoastrocytomas.[127, 128, 134] Increased mitotic rates may be associated with tumor recurrence,[135] and proliferative indices may therefore be a useful parameter for estimating the potential for recurrence but not necessarily for estimating that of malignant progression. The average interval to recurrence in cases without histologic evidence of malignant transformation appears to be slightly longer than in those with transformation.[121, 127, 128, 135, 136] This relationship is not necessarily a strict one, as a malignant recurrence after an interval of 15 years has been documented.[128]

SUBEPENDYMAL GIANT CELL ASTROCYTOMA

Subependymal giant cell tumors develop as part of the constellation of hamartomatous lesions in the tuberous sclerosis complex; they show no gender predilection. The clinical signs usually become apparent within the first two decades of life (range, 1 to 31 years; median age, ~13 years).[137, 138] In about one third of the cases, symptoms referable to the tumor may be the first manifestation of tuberous sclerosis[137]; but in most cases, patients have long-standing antecedent seizures due to disease-related cortical glioneuronal hamartomas (tubers) and white matter heterotopias. In a large series of 345 well-documented cases of tuberous sclerosis complex,[138] subependymal giant cell tumors that could be confirmed by histopathologic analysis were clinically evident in about 6% of cases. Their actual incidence as a component of the tuberous sclerosis complex may reach 14%,[137] as not all tumors may acquire sufficient size to warrant surgical intervention or definitive histologic diagnosis. Although tumors rarely appear to arise without subsequent evidence of a phakomatosis,[4, 139] the subependymal giant cell tumor should be considered as a distinct clinicopathologic component of the tuberous sclerosis complex.

The most common location of subependymal giant cell tumors is in the wall of the lateral ventricle near the foramen of Monro. As these well-demarcated tumors grow and impinge on the foramen, signs of elevated intracranial pressure are the usual initial clinical manifestation; however, this may also be a result of acute hemorrhage from the conspicuous tumor vasculature. Aside from the prominent vessels, the heterogeneous macroscopic appearance of the tumor mass is partly due to the nodular and multicystic pattern of growth, which is punctuated by variable calcification.

The histologic appearance of subependymal giant cell astrocytomas is characterized by an admixture of heterogeneous cell populations. Three major types of cytoarchitecture are present in a variably fibrillated astroglial matrix: (1) small spindle-shaped or elongated cells, (2) intermediate size polygonal or "gemistocytic" cells, and (3) globoid cells (Fig. 17–13). The nuclei are usually pleomorphic, are round to oval, and contain a finely granular chromatin with distinct—sometimes prominent—nucleoli. Polygonal cells may be quite conspicuous and may contain eccentric nuclei, and the enlarged globoid cells often have an eosinophilic, homogeneous cytoplasm. Giant pyramidal cells with a "ganglion cell–like" appearance (see Fig. 17–13, *inset*) are not

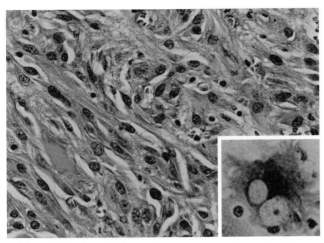

Figure 17–13 Subependymal giant cell astrocytoma (WHO grade I): heterogeneity of cytoarchitecture is typical for subependymal giant cell astrocytomas. Polygonal cells are admixed with broad, spindle-shaped, and smaller fibrillated astrocytes (hematoxylin-eosin stain). *Inset,* Ganglion-like cells, sometimes binucleate, are not uncommon. Some demonstrate immunoreactivity for neuron-associated (class III) β-tubulin.

uncommon, and multinucleated cells can usually be found in most specimens. The tumor microvasculature is often prominent, and it not uncommonly forms dilated channels with either thin or hyalinized walls that may hemorrhage, either spontaneously or after surgical manipulation. Apart from the operative morbidity, these tumors have a uniformly favorable prognosis despite the occasional presence of moderate atypia, mitoses, micronecrosis, and even rare vascular hyperplasia. Despite the exceptional recurrence even after an extended postoperative interval of 47 years, no malignant transformations have been reported.[139]

In the subependymal giant cell tumors, GFAP immunoreactivity is readily demonstrated in cellular processes as well as in the cytoplasm of spindle, polygonal, and ganglion-like cells. The distribution of GFAP-immunoreactive cells can vary from small clusters to widespread populations. Similar distribution and intensity of S-100 immunoreactivity can also be demonstrated, although the protein is more localized to cell bodies than to cellular processes. Immunoreactivity for certain neuron-associated cytoskeletal proteins can also be demonstrated to a more variable, less abundant extent. In a recent study of 20 cases,[140] immunoreactivity for class III β-tubulin (TUJ1), a neuron-associated β-tubulin, was found in the large majority of the cases (~85%). Staining for TUJ1 could be found in the cytoplasm of most cytoarchitectural types; however, it was most apparent in the polygonal and ganglion-like cells. Epitopes for the medium- and high-molecular-weight neurofilament proteins (NF-M/H) were usually less readily demonstrable; nevertheless, the patterns of the various phosphorylation-dependent epitopes in the cell bodies and processes were consistent with the expected distribution for mature neurons. Synaptophysin immunoreactivity, however, is not readily demonstrated. Although both glial and neuron-associated proteins may be identified in similar types of tumor cells, co-localization is limited to a small fraction of these cells.

The histogenesis of this subependymal giant cell tumor, as reflected in the differentiation of its heterogeneous cell populations, is poorly understood. Despite the WHO designation of the subependymal giant cell tumor as a special type of well-circumscribed astrocytoma,[4] these uncommon tumors—when subjected to systematic immunohistochemical and ultrastructural analyses—suggest a more mixed glial-neuronal differentiation.[140, 141] Although multiple studies have reported variable glial (astrocytic/ependymal), neuronal, or mixed glial-neuronal differentiation on the basis of ultrastructural and immunohistochemical features, with few exceptions,[140, 141] most have been limited to isolated cases or small series.[139, 142–155] In contrast to astrocytic differentiation, which is readily apparent in these tumors, evidence for neuronal phenotypes is present in a smaller fraction of cells. Immunohistochemistry, as described previously, and the ultrastructural features of large cells with secretory granules and the rare presence of synapse-like structures[141, 145, 149] have provided additional supportive data.

The mixed glial-neuronal differentiation in subependymal giant cell tumors suggests the presence of cellular lineages with a variable capacity to display divergent phenotypes, including neuroendocrine differentiation.[140, 141] The degree of variation and/or the overlap of divergent glial-neuronal differentiation within populations of morphologically similar cells differs from the spectrum of mixed cell populations within other glial-neuronal neoplasms, such as the dysembryoplastic neuroepithelial tumor and the gangliogliomas. The subependymal giant cell tumor may be the neoplastic manifestation of the malformative processes that occur in tuberous sclerosis, in which case these tumors may result from selective transformation of the cell lineages that give rise to the subependymal nodules.[156, 157]

OLIGODENDROGLIAL TUMORS

Oligodendrogliomas

Oligodendrogliomas generally account for about 5% of all intracranial neoplasms and about 10% to 17% of all intracranial gliomas.[158–160] Within the group of low-grade tumors, oligodendrogliomas account for a higher percentage of tumors, ranging from 19% to 25% of gliomas, with higher incidences in centers for the surgical treatment of epilepsy.[161, 162] The majority of tumors affect adults, with a peak incidence between the fourth and fifth decades.[158, 159, 163] These tumors can also arise within the first two decades (≤6% of oligodendrogliomas),[158, 163] with a mean age for the onset of clinical symptoms of approximately 10 years.[164] Both sexes are affected in all age groups, but a variable male predominance is seen, ranging from slightly over 1.0 to 2.0.[158, 163, 165]

Oligodendrogliomas most frequently occur in the cerebral hemispheres, particularly in the frontotemporal region. The size of the tumor can vary considerably at the time of clinical presentation, but 20% of tumors were 5 cm or greater in a recently reported series.[163] In large series of cases at referral centers,[158, 159, 163, 165] primary involvement of the frontal lobes occurred in about 17% to 38%. In adults, the neoplasms involve multiple lobes in about 50% of cases, with bilateral tumors presenting in about 20%. In tumors that arise in the pediatric/adolescent age group, in which the mean size at presentation is about 3.5 cm, confinement to one lobe (temporal more often than frontal) appears to be more the rule.[164] Although the cerebellum, brainstem (including the fourth ventricle), and spinal cord are affected infrequently,[166–168] tumors may arise anywhere in the neuraxis, wherein the regional frequency is determined in part by the volume of white matter. Tumors that arise or grow in close proximity to the ventricular system, particularly the lateral and fourth ventricles, may seed and disseminate in the CSF with meningeal gliomatosis as a delayed process not associated with the initial clinical presentation.[167, 169, 170] Oligodendrogliomas may also spread along subpial zones and show focal leptomeningeal infiltration without necessarily displaying histologic atypia.

Oligodendrogliomas are soft, gelatinous masses that have relatively well-defined macroscopic margins with the adjacent brain. Calcification, which is readily detected by neuroimaging, can variably confer a gritty texture that may be noted on preparation of unfixed tissue smears. When such tumors span from the white to the gray matter, the lesion typically obliterates the gray-white junction and has a tendency to focally infiltrate leptomeninges. Areas of cystic degeneration may be seen in large tumors, but macroscopic necrosis is limited only to malignant tumors. Oligodendrogliomas are well vascularized, and occasional cases of spontaneous hemorrhage have been reported.

Although the microscopic appearance of most oligodendrogliomas is highly distinctive, these tumors may present a wide variety of histologic patterns. In optimally fixed specimens, the tumor cells have scant but distinct cytoplasm and are distributed within a delicately fibrillated matrix. The nuclei are characteristically round and relatively uniform, whereas increases in nuclear size and/or nuclear hyperchromatism is usually more common after anaplastic progression. Cells may be arranged in either a diffuse or a pseudolobulated pattern, the latter resulting from subdivision of the tumor into smooth, contoured groups surrounded by the geometry of delicate branching vessels (Fig. 17–14). This highly characteristic vascular geometry is often described as a "chicken-wire" pattern. Other cellular arrangements include the following: (1) sheets of cells interrupted by numerous microcysts with the formation of ill-defined, patternless nodules; (2) parallel rows of cells with somewhat fusiform nuclear outlines arranged in palisades[171]; and (3) a rare, more angiocentric pattern in which the tumor cells are arranged around small blood vessels as papillary pseudorosettes of small polygonal to broadly fusiform cells.

Mucin deposition, often erroneously interpreted as a degenerative feature, may be present in oligodendrogliomas, particularly in low-grade examples. Reactive, hypertrophic astrocytes are often found scattered throughout the tumor (Fig. 17–15), commonly as a component of the gliovascular stroma. The cellular proliferative activity in oligodendrogliomas is not high, but a low number of mitotic figures may be observed without other histopathologic evidence of malignant transformation. Oligodendrogliomas often diffusely infiltrate the cerebral cortex in a characteristic pattern of perineuronal satellitosis, and they may spread along subpial zones.

The histopathologic characterization of the oligodendroglial phenotype in oligodendrogliomas has primarily relied

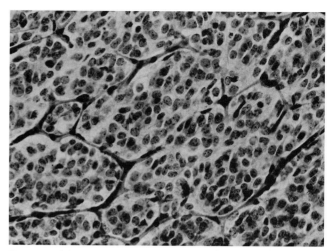

Figure 17–14 Oligodendroglioma (WHO grade II): these display a relatively uniform cell population with regular, round-oval nuclei that contain moderately coarse chromatin and small chromocenters. In this particular case, perinuclear halos are not present because of optimal processing. The delicate microvasculature with an arcuate branching pattern that incompletely segregates clusters of tumor cells is a typical feature (hematoxylin-eosin stain).

on combined recognition of the few salient morphologic features noted earlier, complemented by immunohistochemical and ultrastructural studies that alone are not particularly specific for these tumors. Although a number of candidate epitopes, in association with membrane proteoglycans, glycolipids, and polypeptides, arise during the development and cellular maturation of nontransformed oligodendroglial cell lineages, none has proven to be especially useful to the immunohistochemical characterization of oligodendrogliomas. The majority are either inconstantly expressed by the tumor cells[172, 173] or cannot withstand routine histologic processing. Conflicting results have also been reported in studies analyzing the expression of galactocerebroside (GalC), a putative oligodendrocyte-specific lipid,[174] in neoplastic oligodendrocytes.[172, 175] It is notable that when GalC immunore-

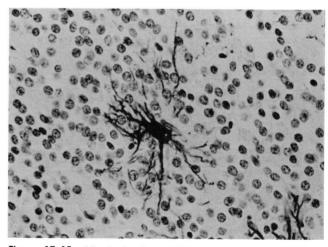

Figure 17–15 Oligodendroglioma (WHO grade II): the reactive astrocytes, often associated with the delicate vascular stroma, are not uncommon in oligodendrogliomas and are readily highlighted by GFAP immunohistochemistry (GFAP-ABC immunoperoxidase with hematoxylin counterstain).

activity was present in most oligodendrogliomas of one series,[175] it was also observed in both the oligodendroglial and the astrocytic populations in all mixed oligoastrocytomas; likewise, variable numbers of cultured astrocytomas can have GalC immunoreactivity.[172]

The progressive differentiation of oligodendroglial progenitor lineages may be associated, in part, with selective expression and interaction of specific cell surface proteoglycans and the extracellular matrix. From this perspective, lectin labeling of specific carbohydrate moieties, including those enriched in D-galactose, *N*-acetyl-galactosamine, may have potential utility in characterizing the cytologic maturation of oligodendroglial tumor cells.[176] However, technical standardization, including divalent cation concentrations and pH, is necessary in larger numbers of cases to determine the routine diagnostic utility of this approach. Other antigens that are associated with CNS myelin, including myelin basic protein (MBP), proteolipid protein (PLP), myelin-associated glycoprotein (MAG), and Leu-7 (carbohydrate epitope of myelin), can be variably demonstrated in oligodendrogliomas; however, inconsistent results and a significant degree of nonselectivity preclude routine diagnostic use.

The expression of intermediate filaments in neoplastic glial cells appears to discriminate reasonably between astrocytomas and oligodendrogliomas. Vimentin, an intermediate filament protein with a relatively wide cellular distribution, is not expressed in the majority of oligodendrogliomas.[177] Vimentin, however, is expressed in normal and neoplastic astrocytes and in ependymal cells, and this expression is useful in discriminating between oligodendrogliomas and astrocytomas or ependymomas. Anaplastic oligodendrogliomas, on the other hand, are more likely to have vimentin immunoreactivity.[178]

Although ultrastructural features do not definitively distinguish oligodendrogliomas from other gliomas, two features may be considered as more typical for oligodendroglial tumor cells. The first is the paucity of the compact bundles of cytoplasmic intermediate glial filaments that are common in astrocytes. Any condensed stacking of intermediate filaments appears to be only a focal phenomenon. Second, variable laminar arrangements of overlapping cellular processes may form abbreviated concentric sheaths, but these arrangements are not particularly common or restricted to oligodendrogliomas.[179–181] "Gliofibrillary oligodendrocytes" and "mini-gemistocytes," as the neoplastic oligodendrocytes[182–185] that commonly have relatively intense glial fibrillary acidic protein (GFAP) immunoreactivity,[185, 186] contain skeins or whorls of intermediate filaments within their cytoplasm. This pattern differs from the random distribution of short intermediate filaments noted in classic gemistocytes in astrocytic tumors.[185]

ANAPLASTIC OLIGODENDROGLIOMAS

A subset of oligodendrogliomas with aggressive biologic behavior constitutes a minority of oligodendroglial tumors, accounting for fewer than 5% of newly diagnosed malignant gliomas in one series.[187] Anaplastic oligodendrogliomas, analogous to high-grade astrocytomas, appear either to evolve from well-differentiated oligodendrogliomas or to develop de novo. Retrospective studies of survival data have variously suggested that high cellularity, nuclear atypia and pleomorphism with marked cellularity, brisk mitotic activity,

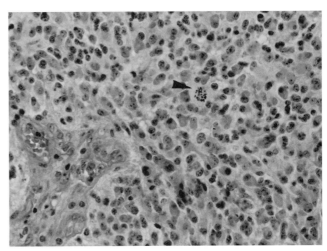

Figure 17–16 Anaplastic oligodendroglioma: cellular pleomorphism with prominent nuclear atypia, increased mitotic activity (*arrowhead*), and "endothelial/pericytic proliferation" are a combination of features indicative of anaplastic progression of oligodendrogliomas (hematoxylin-eosin stain).

microvascular hyperplasia, and necrosis[158, 163, 188, 189] are salient features of anaplastic oligodendrogliomas with significantly more aggressive clinical behavior (Fig. 17–16). These "malignant" tumors are currently diagnosed on the combined basis of clinical, neuroimaging, and general histopathologic features of cellular anaplasia (see Fig. 17–16), as neither a standardized grading system nor a consensus exists regarding the key histologic features. The nosology is further complicated by a general tendency for an increased prominence of GFAP-immunoreactive cells in malignant oligodendrogliomas.[182, 186] This prominence of GFAP-immunoreactive gliofibrillary oligodendrocytes (mini-gemistocytes) further blurs the histopathologic criteria for distinguishing the malignant mixed gliomas that are composed of more poorly differentiated oligodendroglial and astrocytic cellular phenotypes. Some authors recognize more conventional parameters, such as mitotic activity (Fig. 17–17) and necrosis, to

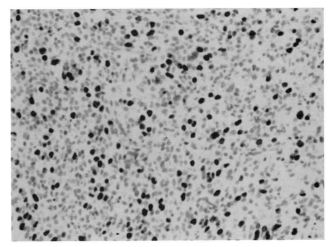

Figure 17–17 Anaplastic oligodendroglioma: elevated numbers of MIB-1 (Ki-67) immunoreactive nuclei is an important prognostic feature associated with anaplastic progression of oligodendrogliomas (MIB-1-ABC immunoperoxidase with hematoxylin counterstain).

be the most important prognostic indicators.[189] DNA flow cytometric studies have demonstrated that although ploidy per se may have limited value for predicting the biologic behavior of oligodendrogliomas,[190, 191] proliferative activity assessed by S-phase fraction appears to be strongly associated with survival.[191]

MOLECULAR CYTOGENETIC ALTERATIONS IN OLIGODENDROGLIOMAS

The overall incidence of point mutations of the p53 tumor suppressor gene in oligodendrogliomas appears to be significantly lower than for the astrocytomas,[67, 69, 70, 192, 193] which suggests a fundamental difference in the molecular cytogenetic alterations between these two groups of gliomas. Allelic deletions on chromosome 19 (19q) are present in more than 60% of cases in some series of oligodendrogliomas and oligoastrocytomas,[65, 194–196] and alterations on chromosome 1p are also more common[194–197] than in the astrocytoma group. In one study of 12 oligodendroglial tumors and 3 oligoastrocytomas, all low-grade oligodendrogliomas, more than 80% of the anaplastic oligodendrogliomas, and more than two thirds of the oligoastrocytomas had 1p deletions.[197] In another series of 37 oligodendrogliomas and mixed oligoastrocytomas, more than 75% of the tumors with allelic loss on 19q also had a deletion on 1p,[193] and this high proportion of both 19q and 1p allelic losses was confirmed by a subsequent study of 47 oligodendrogliomas and oligoastrocytomas.[196] Thus, increasing data strongly suggest that the early genomic events that occur during the development of oligodendrogliomas may be quite distinct from the development of astrocytomas. Chromosome Y[194] and chromosome 22 deletions, as well as a complete loss of chromosome 22, also have been described in a small number of cases.[198]

Despite the apparently different molecular genetic events that accompany early oligodendroglial and astrocytic transformation, malignant progression in oligodendrogliomas may be accompanied by 9p and 10 deletions, similar to anaplastic astrocytomas and glioblastomas.[69, 199, 200] Highlighting this trend, allelic losses on chromosome 10 were detected in a histologically well-differentiated oligodendroglioma, which thereafter progressed to a more aggressive tumor.[201] Thus, the finding of chromosome 10 deletion may indicate common modes of malignant tumor progression between oligodendrogliomas and astrocytomas and may have diagnostic relevance, serving to identify potentially aggressive oligodendrogliomas.

EPENDYMAL TUMORS

Ependymoma

Ependymomas represent approximately 10% of brain tumors and 6% of intracranial gliomas,[4] and they generally consitute a higher percentage of the gliomas in children and adolescents than in adults.[202] The tumors typically develop in the vicinity of the ventricular system, with the fourth ventricle being the most frequent site, followed by the aqueduct and the spinal cord. In children and adolescents, ependymomas tend to be intracranial, and a high proportion of tumors arise in the fourth ventricle, whereas in adults they represent more than 60% of spinal cord gliomas.[203]

Ependymomas are well demarcated by macroscopic "pushing borders," which often permit a plane for neurosurgical resection. Despite the more circumscribed nature of these neoplasms, a small proportion do gain access to the ventricular space, with subsequent subarachnoid spread. This is particularly true of fourth ventricular ependymomas that show a tendency to expand into the surrounding cisterns, with a capacity to encase the cervical cord. Macroscopic cystic degeneration and calcifications are common features. A microscopic hallmark of ependymomas is the "neuroepithelial" nature of the tumor cells with a proclivity to form polarized arrangements around a lumen of extracellular space (*ependymal rosette/tubules*) or around the microvasculature (*pseudorosettes*), with a centripedal radiation of cell processes (Fig. 17–18). Ultrastructural features of ependymal tumors also reflect this cellular polarity with the formation of microlumina (microrosettes), juxtaluminal intercellular junctions composed primarily of zonulae adherentes, and the elaboration of microvilli and cilia that may extend into extracellular rosettes.[204–206] Between the ependymal rosettes and pseudorosettes, tumor cells usually form relatively amorphous sheets with a variably fibrillated matrix. The elongate cell processes that contribute to the fibrillary matrix can be highlighted by PTAH staining or by immunostains for GFAP or vimentin. Cellularity varies, but most ependymomas are moderately cellular, apart from the rosettes. The often clustered nuclei vary in appearance from ones with delicate "open" chromatin to ones that are somewhat hyperchromatic. Distinct nucleoli are a helpful diagnostic feature of ependymomas. Nuclear atypia and even small foci of necrosis may be present without indicating anaplastic change (see following). Mitoses can be observed but are usually infrequent.

The WHO classification recognizes three histologic variants of ependymomas: *cellular*, *papillary*, and *clear cell*.

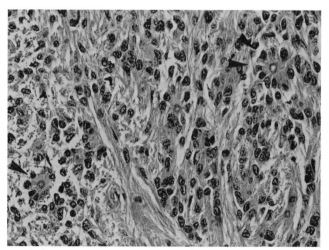

Figure 17–18 Ependymoma: A hallmark feature of ependymomas is the tendency of the tumor cells to form true rosettes (*arrowheads*), ependymal tubules, and perivascular pseudorosettes interspersed within a variably fibrillated matrix. Note that the nuclear chromatin is irregularly distributed in delicate nodes, which produces an "open" pattern.

The clinical outcome of these tumors is basically the same, but their recognition as variants of ependymoma is important in distinguishing them from anaplastic gliomas, choroid plexus tumors, and oligodendrogliomas, respectively. *Cellular* ependymomas vary considerably in pattern and cytologic features. Some are patternless and exhibit little in the way of rosetting. In the *papillary* variant, the cellular sheets tend to be replaced by the formation of multiple epithelial ribbons and papillae, somewhat mimicking choroid plexus tumors. The ependymal nature of such tumors is most easily confirmed by immunoreactivity for GFAP and vimentin, with a relative lack of cytokeratin staining. The *clear cell* variant shows a distinct honeycomb appearance due to perinuclear halo formation within the crowded cells.[207] Such tumors may present a problem in differential diagnosis with oligodendrogliomas. The proper diagnosis is suggested by other clinicopathologic features, such as sharp demarcation, contrast enhancement on CT and MRI, and ultrastructural features.

ANAPLASTIC EPENDYMOMA

Anaplastic progression of ependymomas can occur in tumors at most sites, but it is very uncommon in ependymomas of the spinal cord.[4] Anaplastic ependymomas are histologically recognized by their increased cellularity, varying degree of cellular/nuclear atypia, and brisk mitotic activity, and by the frequent presence of microvascular hyperplasia in the form of "endothelial proliferation" (Fig. 17–19). The correlation between histopathologic features of such tumors and the clinical outcome of patients with anaplastic ependymomas is not well defined. One prognostic factor of particular significance in supratentorial examples is the mitotic index,[208] and this observation is consistent with proliferative indices, either by BUdR uptake[209] or Ki-67 immunohistochemistry.[210] High indices correlate with high histologic grade and early tumor recurrence. A recent study of pediatric ependymomas suggests that the clinical progression relates closely to a set of clinicopathologic parameters, particularly age, DNA ploidy, and histologic grade.[211]

An important distinction should be drawn between the

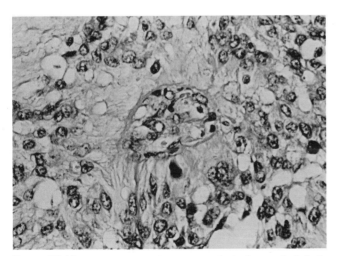

Figure 17–19 Anaplastic ependymoma: anaplastic features include increased cellularity, increased mitotic rate, and conspicuous "endothelial/pericytic" hyperplasia. Note the presence of this microvascular hyperplasia within the center of a pseudorosette (hematoxylin-eosin stain).

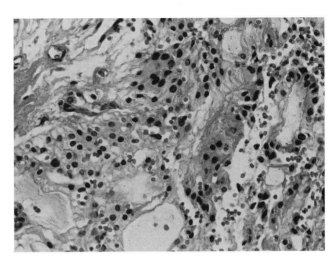

Figure 17–20 Myxopapillary ependymoma: in this variant of ependymoma, palisading and cuboidal epithelial arrangements of neoplastic cells with long, fibrillated processes are arranged around hyalinized blood vessels. Extracellular mucin may be focally conspicuous (hematoxylin-eosin stain).

anaplastic ependymomas and the ependymoblastomas. The latter, an embryonal neoplasm, represents a highly malignant, often bulky tumor, which usually arises in the supratentorial region in infants and children younger than 5 years. In contrast to ependymomas, ependymoblastomas aggressively invade surrounding structures and show a distinct tendency for early craniospinal seeding.

MYXOPAPILLARY EPENDYMOMA

The myxopapillary ependymoma is a slow-growing, distinct clinicopathologic variant of ependymoma most commonly occurring in the cauda equina of adults.[212–214] At the initial clinical presentation, these tumors either are discrete, sausage-shaped masses that arise from the filum terminale or compress spinal nerve roots of the cauda equina or are lesions that demonstrate local dissemination beyond a single mass. Myxopapillary ependymomas present infrequently as extradural lesions in the presacral space or in retrosacral soft tissue. Such ectopic tumors probably arise from ependymal rests.[212, 214] Although the majority of the tumors are biologically benign and are slow growing, local recurrences are common. Spreading within the neuraxis is far more common than are rare extraneural metastases.[213, 215, 216] The prognosis of this unique ependymoma variant is related to successful resection. These tumors should be resected intact; puncture or fragmented removal of the tumor in situ appears to facilitate recurrence and to diminish the likelihood of cure.[213]

The histologic pattern of most myxopapillary ependymomas consists in part of papillary arrangements of variably elongated, sometimes fibrillary cells with processes that extend radially to blood vessels. These conspicuous vascular elements display variable mural hyalinization. The perivascular stroma typically has a mucinous character, and mucin may also accompany neoplastic cells that are not in contact with vessels (Fig. 17–20). Electron microscopy has confirmed the ependymal nature of these lesions and has revealed cytoplasmic intermediate filaments, pockets of microvilli often associated with numerous cellular interdigitations, and abundant basal lamina.[217, 218] The presence of glial fibrils, verified by PTAH stain and immunohistochemistry for GFAP, distinguishes this tumor from schwannomas and paragangliomas, which also occur in this region.[213]

Subependymoma

Subependymomas are well-circumscribed, generally asymptomatic nodules that are located in the walls of the fourth and lateral ventricles; nearly two thirds are associated with the fourth ventricle.[219, 220] The septum pellucidum, foramen of Monro, and, less commonly, spinal cord may also be affected by these tumors.[221] Although the majority are incidental discoveries at postmortem examination, symptomatic subependymomas do present with either increased intracranial pressure due to obstruction of CSF flow or to spontaneous tumoral hemorrhage, usually in older adults.

The histologic features of subependymomas reflect both an ependymal and an astrocytic differentiation. The tumor is characteristically hypocellular and composed of a dense fibrillary matrix, and its low-power architecture is characterized by clusters of cells surrounded by skeins of fibrillar processes (Fig. 17–21). Ependymal features such as pseudorosettes are not uncommon, whereas true rosettes are rare. Astrocytic-appearing cells, elongated to somewhat gemistocytic, may also be present focally. The association of astrocytic and ependymal features has also been confirmed by electron microscopic and tissue culture studies.[222, 223] Microcystic degeneration and microcalcification are common, as is vascular hyalinization and hemosiderin deposition suggestive of previous, often subclinical, hemorrhage. Nuclear atypia and limited mitotic activity may be present, but these are of no prognostic significance. The most important prognostic factors are tumor location and surgical factors relative to the degree of attempted resection, particularly with respect to tumors situated on the floor of the fourth ventricle.[220]

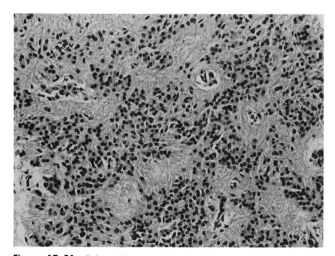

Figure 17–21 Subependymoma: arrays and clusters of tumor cell nuclei are enmeshed in a densely fibrillary matrix of cell processes. The cytologic features of the cells recall both ependymal and astrocytic properties (hematoxylin-eosin stain).

MIXED GLIOMAS

The definition of what constitutes the "mixed" gliomas has been a longstanding problem. Tumors composed of admixtures of neoplastic glial elements are, therefore, one of the challenges of diagnostic neuropathology in the 1990s. Techniques developed since the early 1970s, particularly electron microscopy and immunohistochemistry, have brought about a notion that such tumors (usually ones composed of astrocytes and oligodendroglia and, less frequently, ones with ependymal components) are not rare. Their recognition and proper classification are, however, problematic. There is at present no accepted definition of mixed gliomas; even the percentage of the various cellular components varies among different laboratories. Furthermore, the principal cells comprising such lesions, particularly neoplastic oligodendroglia, vary considerably in terms of their morphology. Not only does the relative proportion of the different cells pose a problem, but their relationship within any one tumor varies from diffuse admixtures to geographically discrete populations. Attempting to set guidelines, some workers have defined mixed tumors as gliomas in which the minor cell type exceeds 30%.[224] Tumor heterogeneity also frustrates the diagnosis of mixed gliomas in that adequate tissue sampling is necessary. Thus, the array of special techniques currently available for the study of mixed tumors often cannot be applied, particularly to nonrepresentative or to stereotactic biopsies. Last, the features that indicate anaplastic progression vary among different components of gliomas, with certain cells (e.g., gemistocytic astrocytes) being more likely to undergo anaplastic transformation. This aspect is especially significant in oligoastrocytomas, in which the morphologic criteria for anaplasia are not equivalent in the two glial populations. Progression also alters the histopathologic character of the tumor from one point to another.

Mixed Oligoastrocytoma

These mixed gliomas are composed of oligodendrocytes and a significant population of neoplastic astrocytes. The predominant component is often oligodendroglial,[225] but proportions do vary considerably. The two neoplastic cell populations may be focally or diffusely distributed. Mixed oligoastrocytomas must be distinguished from oligodendrogliomas, which contain varying numbers of reactive astrocytes. This is especially problematic for the oligodendrogliomas that contain large numbers of gliofibrillary and mini-gemistocytic cells. The mixed oligodendroglioma-astrocytomas (oligoastrocytomas) are lesions with a less favorable prognosis.[185, 187]

The histogenesis of mixed oligoastrocytomas remains unclear. They may arise from "transitional" cells, which have characteristics that are intermediate between mature oligodendrocytes and astrocytes,[182] or from transformed precursor cells analogous to the O-2A progenitor cells described in the rodent optic nerve.[226] Recent experimental studies have demonstrated the presence of such true progenitor cells that generate both oligodendrocytes and type 2 astrocytes in the adult rat brain[227] and O-2A–like progenitor cells in the human cerebrum.[228] Although most data on the development of dual glial lineages are derived principally from rodent tissue in culture,[226, 229] a better understanding of these progenitor cells in the human adult nervous system may shed light on the histogenesis of oligodendrogliomas and mixed oligoastrocytomas.[228, 230] The close relationship between the oligodendrogliomas and mixed oligoastrocytomas in contrast with the astrocytic tumors is also implied by the molecular cytogenetic alterations in oligoastrocytomas.[194–197] The possibility that one glial cell type induces neoplastic transformation in a second, distinct glial lineage cannot be excluded but is less probable.

Malignant Oligoastrocytoma

The frequency with which oligoastrocytomas undergo anaplastic progression is unknown. It is generally agreed that the astrocytic component is more susceptible to anaplastic change.[4, 85] The histopathologic features of the anaplastic elements of these tumors are similar to those previously described for anaplastic astrocytomas and oligodendrogliomas.

REFERENCES

1. VandenBerg SR: The developing brain and cellular targets for neoplastic transformation. *In* Kaye AH, Laws ER Jr (eds): Brain Tumors: An Encyclopedic Approach. Edinburgh, Churchill Livingstone, 1995, p 9.
2. Kleihues P, Burger PC, Scheithauer BW: Histological Typing of Tumours of the Central Nervous System, ed 2. Berlin, Springer-Verlag, 1993.
3. Krouwer HGJ, Davis RL, Silver R, et al: Gemistocytic astrocytomas: A reappraisal. J Neurosurg 1991; 74:399.
4. Russell DS, Rubinstein LJ: Pathology of Tumours of the Nervous System, ed 5. London, Edward Arnold, 1989.
5. Rutka JT, Smith SL: Transfection of human astrocytoma cells with glial fibrillary acidic protein complementary DNA: Analysis of expression, proliferation and tumorigenicity. Cancer Res 1993; 53:3624.
6. Perentes E, Rubinstein LJ: Recent applications of immunoperoxidase histochemistry in human neuro-oncology. Arch Pathol Lab Med 1987; 111:796.
7. Denis-Donini S, Glowinski J, Prochiantz A: Glial heterogeneity may define the three-dimensional shape of mouse mesencephalic dopaminergic neurones. Nature 1984; 307:641.
8. Hansson E: Astroglia from defined brain regions as studied with primary cultures. Prog Neurobiol 1988; 30:369.
9. Butt AM: Macroglial cell types, lineage, and morphology in the CNS. Ann NY Acad Sci 1991; 633:90.
10. Miller RH, Szigeti V: Clonal analysis of astrocyte diversity in neonatal rat spinal cord cultures. Development 1991; 113:353.
11. Ransom BR: Vertebrate glial classification, lineage, and heterogeneity. Ann NY Acad Sci 1991; 633:19.
12. Young JZ: The concept of neuroglia. Ann NY Acad Sci 1991; 633:1.
13. Noble M, Wren D, Wolswijk G: The O2-A adult progenitor cell: A glial stem cell of the adult central nervous system. Semin Cell Biol 1992; 3:413.
14. Vayasse PJJ, Goldman JE: A distinct type of GD3+, flat astrocyte in rat CNS cultures. J Neurosci 1992; 12:330.
15. Levison SW, Goldman JE: Astrocyte origins. *In* Murphy S (ed): Astrocytes: Pharmacology and Function. San Diego, Academic Press, 1992, p 1.
16. Steindler DA: Glial boundaries in the developing nervous system. Annu Rev Neurosci 1993; 16:445.
17. Levine JM, Stincone F, Lee Y-S: Development and differentiation of glial precursor cells in the rat cerebellum. Glia 1993; 7:307.
18. Marriott DR, Wilkin GP: Substance p receptors on O-2A progenitor cells and type-astrocytes in vitro. J Neurochem 1993; 61:826.
19. Chamak BA, Fellows J, Glowinski J, et al: MAP2 expression and neurite outgrowth and branching are co-regulated through region-specific neuro-astroglial interactions. J Neurosci 1987; 7:3163.
20. Beyer C, Epp B, Fassberg J, et al: Region- and sex-related differences in maturation of astrocytes in dissociated cell cultures of embryonic rat brain. Glia 1990; 3:55.
21. Cockram CS: Growth factors, astrocytes and astrocytomas. Semin Dev Biol 1990; 1:421.
22. Gillaspy GE, Mapstone TB, Samols D, et al: Transcriptional patterns of growth factors and proto-oncogenes in human glioblastomas and normal glial cells. Cancer Lett 1992; 65:55.
23. Ma YJ, Berg-von der Emde K, Moholt-Siebert M, et al: Region-specific regulation of transforming growth factor (TGF) gene expression in astrocytes of the neuroendocrine brain. J Neurosci 1994; 14:5644.
24. Eddleston M, Mucke L: Molecular profile of reactive astrocytes: Implications for their role in neurologic disease. Neuroscience 1993; 54:15.
25. Hatton JD, Nguyen MH, U HS: Differential migration of astrocytes grafted into the developing rat brain. Glia 1993; 9:113.
26. Davis R: Grading of gliomas. *In* Fields WS (ed): Primary Brain Tumors: A Review of Histologic Classification. New York, Springer-Verlag, 1989, p 150.
27. Kleihues P, Burger PC, Scheithauer BW: The new WHO classification of brain tumours. Brain Pathol 1993; 3:255.
28. Kernohan JW, Sayre GP: Tumors of the central nervous system, fascicle 35. *In* Atlas of Tumor Pathology. Washington, DC, Armed Forces Institute of Pathology, 1952.
29. Shapiro JR, Shapiro WR: Clonal tumor cell heterogeneity. Prog Exp Tumor Res 1984; 27:49.
30. Burger PC, Kleihues P: Cytologic composition of the untreated glioblastoma with implications for evaluation of needle biopsies. Cancer 1989; 63:2014.
31. Barnard RO, Geddes JF: The incidence of multifocal cerebral gliomas: A histologic study of large hemisphere sections. Cancer 1987; 60:1519.
32. Roselli R, Iacoangeli M, Scerrati M, et al: Natural history of neuroepithelial tumours: Contribution of stereotactic biopsy. Acta Neurochir 1989; 46(suppl):79.
33. Coons SW, Johnson PC: Regional heterogeneity in the Ki67 labelling indices of gliomas. J Neuropathol Exp Neurol 1992; 51:331.
34. Glantz MJ, Burger PC, Herndon JE II, et al: Influence of the type of surgery on the histologic diagnosis in patients with anaplastic gliomas. Neurology 1991; 41:1741.
35. Daumas-Duport C: Histological grading of gliomas. Curr Opin Neurol Neurosurg 1992; 5:924.
36. Kim TS, Halliday AL, Hedley-Whyte ET, et al: Correlates of survival and the Daumas-Duport grading system for astrocytomas. J Neurosurg 1991; 74:27.
37. Hoshino T, Prados M, Wilson CB, et al: Prognostic implications of the bromodeoxyuridine labeling index of human gliomas. J Neurosurg 1989; 71:335.
38. Fujimaki T, Matsutani M, Nakamura O, et al: Correlation between bromodeoxyuridine-labeling indices and patient prognosis in cerebral astrocytic tumors of adults. Cancer 1991; 67:1629.
39. Salmon I, Kiss R, Dewitte O, et al: Histopathologic grading and DNA ploidy in relation to survival among 206 adult astrocytic tumor patients. Cancer 1992; 70:538.
40. Burger PC, Green SB: Patient age, histologic features, and length of survival in patients with glioblastoma multiforme. Cancer 1987; 59:1617.
41. Nelson JS, Tsukada Y, Schoenfeld D, et al: Necrosis as a prognostic criterion in malignant supratentorial, astrocytic gliomas. Cancer 1983; 52:550.
42. Burger PC, Vogel FS, Green SB, et al: Glioblastoma multiforme and anaplastic astrocytoma: Pathologic criteria and prognostic implications. Cancer 1985; 56:1106.
43. Daumas-Duport C, Scheithauer B, O'Fallon J, et al: Grading of astrocytomas. A simple and reproducible method. Cancer 1988; 62:2152.
44. Lopes MBS, VandenBerg SR: Tumors of the central nervous system. *In* Fletcher CDM (ed): Diagnostic Histopathology of Tumors. Edinburgh, Churchill Livingstone, 1995, p 1161.
45. Schlüter C, Duchrow M, Wohlenberg C, et al: The cell proliferation-associated antigen of antibody Ki-67: A very large, ubiquitous nuclear

protein with numerous repeated elements, representing a new kind of cell cycle-maintaining proteins. J Cell Biol 1993; 123:513.

46. Gerdes J, Schwab U, Lemke H, et al: Production of a mouse monoclonal antibody reactive with a human nuclear antigen associated with cell proliferation. Int J Cancer 1983; 31:13.

47. Gerdes J, Lemke H, Wacker HH, et al: Cell cycle analysis of a cell proliferation-associated human nuclear antigen defined by the monoclonal antibody Ki-67. J Immunol 1984; 133:1710.

48. Bruno S, Darzynkiewicz Z: Cell cycle dependent expression and stability of the nuclear protein detected by Ki-67 antibody in HL-60 cells. Cell Prolif 1992; 25:31.

49. Cattoretti G, Becker MHG, Key G, et al: Monoclonal antibodies against recombinant parts of the Ki-67 antigen (MIB 1 and MIB 3) detect proliferating cells in microwave-processed formalin-fixed paraffin sections. J Pathol 1992; 168:357.

50. Sawhney N, Hall PA: Ki67: Structure, function and new antibodies (editorial). J Pathol 1992; 168:161.

51. Gerdes J, Becker MHG, Key G, et al: Immunohistochemical detection of tumour growth fraction (Ki-67 antigen) in formalin-fixed and routinely processed tissues. J Pathol 1992; 168:85.

52. Karamitopoulou E, Perentes E, Diamantis I, et al: Ki-67 immunoreactivity in human central nervous system tumors: A study with MIB 1 monoclonal antibody on archival material. Acta Neuropathol 1994; 87:47.

53. Giangaspero F, Doglioni C, Rivano MT, et al: Growth factor in human brain tumors defined by the monoclonal antibody Ki-67. Acta Neuropathol 1987; 74:179.

54. Burger PC, Shibata T, Kleihues P: The use of the monoclonal antibody Ki-67 in the identification of proliferating cells: Application to surgical neuropathology. Am J Surg Pathol 1986; 10:611.

55. Patsouris E, Stocker U, Kallmeyer V, et al: Relationship between Ki-67 positive cells, growth rate and histological type of human intracranial tumors. Anticancer Res 1988; 8:537.

56. Reifenberger G, Prior R, Deckert M, et al: Epidermal growth factor receptor expression and growth fraction in human tumours of the nervous system. Virchows Arch A Pathol Anat Histopathol 1989; 414:147.

57. Louis DN, Edgerton S, Thor AD, et al: Proliferating cell nuclear antigen and Ki-67 immunohistochemistry in brain tumors: A comparative study. Acta Neuropathol 1991; 81:675.

58. Schroder R, Bien K, Kott R, et al: The relationship between Ki-67 labeling and mitotic index in gliomas and meningiomas: Demonstration of the variability of the intermitotic cycle time. Acta Neuropathol 1991; 82:389.

59. Coons SW, Johnson PC: Regional heterogeneity in the proliferative activity of human gliomas as measured by the Ki-67 labeling index. J Neuropathol Exp Neurol 1993; 52:609.

60. Hoshino T, Rodriguez LA, Cho KG, et al: Prognostic implications of the proliferative potential of low-grade astrocytomas. J Neurosurg 1988; 69:839.

61. Nishizaki T, Orita T, Saiki M, et al: Cell kinetics studies of human brain tumors by in vitro labeling using anti-BUdR monoclonal antibody. J Neurosurg 1988; 69:371.

62. Nishizaki T, Orita T, Furutani Y, et al: Flow-cytometric DNA analysis and immunohistochemical measurement of Ki-67 and BUdR labeling indices in human brain tumors. J Neurosurg 1989; 70:379.

63. Labrousse F, Daumas-Duport C, Batorski L, et al: Histological grading and bromodeoxyuridine labeling index of astrocytomas. Comparative study in a series of 60 cases. J Neurosurg 1991; 75:202.

64. Onda KO, Davis RL, Shibuya M, et al: Correlation between the bromodeoxyuridine labeling index and the MIB-1 and Ki-67 proliferating cell indices in cerebral gliomas. Cancer 1994; 74:1921.

65. von Deimling A, Louis DN, von Ammon K, et al: Evidence for a tumour suppressor gene on chromosome 19q associated with human astrocytomas, oligodendrogliomas, and mixed gliomas. Cancer Res 1992; 52:4277.

66. von Deimling A, Louis DN, von Ammon K, et al: Association of epidermal growth factor receptor gene amplification with loss of chromosome 10 in human glioblastoma multiforme. J Neurosurg 1992; 77:295.

67. Louis DN, von Deimling A, Chung RY, et al: Comparative study of p53 gene and protein alterations in human astrocytic tumors. J Neuropathol Exp Neurol 1993; 52:31.

68. Sidranski D, Mikkelsen T, Schwechheimer K, et al: Clonal expansion

of p53 mutant cells is associated with brain tumour progression. Nature 1992; 355:846.

69. Fults D, Brockmeyer D, Tullous MW, et al: p53 mutation and loss of heterozygosity on chromosome 17 and 10 during human astrocytoma progression. Cancer Res 1992; 52:674.

70. Frankel RH, Bayonna W, Koslow M, et al: p53 mutations in human malignant gliomas: Comparison of loss of heterozygosity with mutation frequency. Cancer Res 1992; 52:1427.

71. Ahmed Rasheed BK, McLendon RE, Herndon JE, et al: Alterations of the TP53 gene in human gliomas. Cancer Res 1994; 54:1324.

72. Litofsky NS, Hinton D, Raffel C: The lack of a role for p53 in astrocytomas in pediatric patients. Neurosurgery 1994; 34:967.

73. Lang FF, Miller DC, Koslow M, et al: Pathways leading to glioblastoma multiforme: A molecular analysis of genetic alterations in 65 astrocytic tumors. J Neurosurg 1994; 81:427.

74. Louis DN, Rubio MP, Correa KM, et al: Molecular genetics of pediatric brain stem gliomas: Application of PCR techniques to small and archival brain tumor specimens. J Neuropathol Exp Neurol 1993; 52:507.

75. Collins VP, James CD: Gene and chromosomal alterations associated with the development of human gliomas. FASEB J 1993; 7:926.

76. Fischer U, Wullich B, Sattler HP, et al: DNA amplifications on chromosomes 7, 9 and 12 in glioblastoma detected by reverse chromosome painting. Eur J Cancer 1994; 30A:1124.

77. Reifenberger G, Reifenberger J, Ichimura K, et al: Amplification of multiple genes from chromosomal region 12q13–14 in human malignant gliomas: Preliminary mapping of the amplicons shows preferential involvement of CDK4, SAS, and MDM2. Cancer Res 1994; 54:4299.

78. von Deimling A, von Ammon K, Schoenfeld A, et al: Subsets of glioblastoma multiforme defined by molecular genetic analysis. Brain Pathol 1993; 3:19.

79. Louis DN: The p53 gene and protein in human brain tumors. J Neuropathol Exp Neurol 1994; 53:11.

80. Gibbons MC, Rosenberg J, Jedlicka AE, et al: Microsatellite instability in gliomas. J Neuropathol Exp Neurol 1995; 54:420.

81. Hamilton SR, Liu B, Parsons RE, et al: The molecular basis of Turcot's syndrome. N Engl J Med 1995; 332:839.

82. Ganju V, Jenkins RB, O'Fallon JR, et al: Prognostic factors in gliomas. Cancer 1994; 74:920.

83. Scherer HJ: Cerebral astrocytomas and their derivatives. Am J Cancer 1940; 40:159.

84. Burger PC, Scheithauer BW, Vogel FS: Surgical Pathology of the Nervous System and Its Coverings, ed 3. New York, Churchill Livingstone, 1991.

85. Muller W, Afra D, Schroder R: Supratentorial recurrences of gliomas: Morphological studies in relation to time intervals with 544 astrocytomas. Acta Neurochir 1977; 37:75.

86. Laws ER Jr, Taylor WF, Clifton MB, et al: Neurosurgical management of low-grade astrocytoma of the cerebral hemispheres. J Neurosurg 1984; 61:665.

87. Dropcho EJ, Wisoff JH, Walker RW, et al: Supratentorial malignant gliomas in childhood: A review of 50 cases. Ann Neurol 1987; 22:355.

88. Tamura M, Ono N, Zama A, et al: Small gliomas: Clinicopathological study. Neurol Med Chir (Tokyo) 1993; 33:425.

89. Itoh Y, Kowada M, Mineura K, et al: Congenital glioblastoma of the cerebellum with cytofluorometric deoxyribonucleic acid analysis. Surg Neurol 1987; 27:163.

90. Earnest F IV, Kelly PJ, Scheithauer BW, et al: Cerebral astrocytomas: Histopathologic correlation of MR and CT contrast enhancement with stereotactic biopsy. Radiology 1988; 166:823.

91. Burger PC, Kleihues P: Cytologic composition of the untreated glioblastoma with implications for evaluation of needle biopsies. Cancer 1989; 63:2014.

92. Romberger CF, Wollman RL, Wainer BH: Distant angiogenesis in a patient with glioblastoma multiforme. Clin Neuropathol 1990; 9:97.

93. Kepes JJ, Rubinstein LJ, Chiang H: The role of astrocytes in the formation of cartilage in gliomas: An immunohistochemical study of four cases. Am J Pathol 1984; 117:471.

94. Ritter AM, Sawaya R, Hess KR, et al: Prognostic significance of bromodeoxyuridine labeling in primary and recurrent glioblastoma multiforme. Neurosurgery 1994; 35:192.

95. Margetts JC, Kalyan-Raman UP: Giant-celled glioblastoma of brain: A clinico-pathological and radiological study of ten cases (including immunohistochemistry and ultrastructure). Cancer 1989; 63:524.

96. Morantz RA, Feigin I, Ransohoff J III: Clinical and pathological study of 24 cases of gliosarcoma. J Neurosurg 1976; 45:398.
97. Meis JM, Martz KL, Nelson JS: Mixed glioblastoma multiforme and sarcoma: A clinicopathologic study of 26 Radiation Therapy Oncology Group cases. Cancer 1991; 67:2342.
98. Grant JW, Steart PV, Aguzzi A, et al: Gliosarcoma: An immunohistochemical study. Acta Neuropathol 1989; 79:305.
99. Ho K-L: Histogenesis of sarcomatous component of the gliosarcoma: An ultrastructural study. Acta Neuropathol 1990; 81:178.
100. Ng THK, Poon WS: Gliosarcoma of the posterior fossa with features of a malignant fibrous histiocytoma. Cancer 1990; 65:1161.
101. Miller LL, Ostrow PT, Chau R: Characterization of gliosarcomas by image analysis of superimposed serial sections (abstract). J Neuropathol Exp Neurol 1991; 50:365.
102. Haddad SF, Moore SA, Schelper RL, et al: Smooth muscle can comprise the sarcomatous component of gliosarcomas. J Neuropathol Exp Neurol 1992; 51:493.
103. Jones H, Steart PV, Weller RO: Spindle cell glioblastoma or gliosarcoma? Neuropathol Appl Neurobiol 1991; 17:177.
104. Paulus W, Bayas A, Ott G, et al: Interphase cytogenetics of glioblastoma and gliosarcoma. Acta Neuropathol 1994; 88:420.
105. Parekh HC, O'Donovan DG, Sharma RR, et al: Primary cerebral gliosarcoma: Report of 17 cases. Br J Neurosurg 1995; 9:171.
106. Barnard RO, Bradford R, Scott T, et al: Gliomyosarcoma: Report of a case of rhabdomyosarcoma arising in a malignant glioma. Acta Neuropathol 1986; 69:23.
107. Hayashi H, Ohara N, Jeon HJ, et al: Gliosarcoma with features of chondroblastic osteosarcoma. Cancer 1993; 72:850.
108. Garcia DM, Fulling KH: Juvenile pilocytic astrocytoma of the cerebrum in adults: A distinctive neoplasm with favorable prognosis. J Neurosurg 1985; 63:382.
109. Forsyth PA, Shaw EG, Scheithauer BW, et al: Supratentorial pilocytic astrocytomas: A clinicopathologic, prognostic and flow cytometric study of 51 patients. Cancer 1993; 72:1335.
110. Minehan K, Scheithauer B, Shaw E, et al: Astrocytic tumors of the spinal cord (abstract). J Neuropathol Exp Neurol 1993; 52:289.
111. Clark GB, Henry JM, McKeever PE: Cerebral pilocytic astrocytoma. Cancer 1985; 56:1128.
112. Tomlinson FH, Scheithauer BW, Hayostek CH, et al: The significance of atypia and histologic malignancy in pilocytic astrocytoma of the cerebellum: A clinicopathologic and flow cytometric study. J Child Neurol 1994; 9:301.
113. Obana WG, Cogen PH, Davis RL, et al: Metastatic juvenile pilocytic astrocytoma. J Neurosurg 1991; 75:972.
114. Mishima K, Nakamura M, Nakamura H, et al: Leptomeningeal dissemination of cerebellar pilocytic astrocytoma. J Neurosurg 1992; 77:788.
115. Brown MT, Friedman HS, Oakes J, et al: Chemotherapy for pilocytic astrocytoma. Cancer 1992; 71:3165.
116. Schiffer D, Giordana MT, Mauro A, et al: Immunohistochemical demonstration of vimentin in human cerebral tumors. Acta Neuropathol 1986; 70:209.
117. Schwartz AN, Ghatak NR: Malignant transformation of benign cerebellar astrocytoma. Cancer 1990; 56:333.
118. Herpers MJHM, Freling G, Beuls EAM: Pleomorphic xanthoastrocytoma in the spinal cord: Case report. J Neurosurg 1994; 80:564.
119. Mackenzie J: Pleomorphic xanthoastrocytoma in a 62-year-old male. Neuropathol Appl Neurobiol 1987; 13:481.
120. Nishio S, Takeshita I, Fujii K, et al: Supratentorial astrocytic tumours of childhood: A clinicopathologic study of 41 cases. Acta Neurochir 1989; 101:3.
121. Kepes JJ, Rubinstein LJ, Eng LF: Pleomorphic xanthoastrocytoma: A distinctive meningocerebral glioma of young subjects with relatively favorable prognosis. Cancer 1979; 44:1839.
122. Strom EH, Skullerud K: Pleomorphic xanthoastrocytoma: Report of 5 cases. Clin Neuropathol 1983; 2:188.
123. Pasquier B, Kojder I, Labat F, et al: Le xanthoastrocytome du sujet jeune: Revue de la littérature à propos de deux observations d'évolution discordante. Ann Pathol 1985; 5:29.
124. Kawano N: Pleomorphic xanthoastrocytoma (PXA) in Japan: Its clinico-pathologic features and diagnostic clues. Noshuyo Byori 1991; 8:5.
125. Lindboe C, Cappelen J, Kepes J: Pleomorphic xanthoastrocytoma as a component of a cerebellar ganglioglioma: Case report. Neurosurgery 1992; 31:353.
126. Hosokawa Y, Tsuchihashi Y, Okabe H, et al: Pleomorphic xanthoastrocytoma: Ultrastructural, immunohistochemical, and DNA cytofluorometric study of a case. Cancer 1991; 68:853.
127. Weldon-Linne GM, Victor TA, Groothuis DR, et al: Pleomorphic xanthoastrocytoma: Ultrastructural and immunohistochemical study of a case with a rapidly fatal outcome following surgery. Cancer 1983; 52:2055.
128. Kepes JJ, Rubinstein LJ, Ansbacher L, et al: Histopathological features of recurrent pleomorphic xanthoastrocytomas: Further corroboration of the glial nature of this neoplasm: A study of three cases. Acta Neuropathol 1989; 78:585.
129. Whittle IR, Gordon A, Misra BK, et al: Pleomorphic xanthoastrocytoma: Report of four cases. J Neurosurg 1989; 70:463.
130. Furuta A, Takahashi H, Ikuta F, et al: Temporal lobe tumor demonstrating ganglioglioma and pleomorphic xanthoastrocytoma components: Case report. J Neurosurg 1992; 77:143.
131. Maleki M, Robitaille Y, Bertrand G: Atypical xanthoastrocytoma presenting as a meningioma. Surg Neurol 1983; 20:235.
132. Kros JM, Vecht ChJ, Stefanko SZ: The pleomorphic xanthoastrocytoma and its differential diagnosis: A study of five cases. Hum Pathol 1991; 22:1128.
133. Kordek R, Wojciech B, Wojciech S, et al: Pleomorphic xanthoastrocytoma with a gangliomatous component, an immunohistochemical and ultrastructural study. Acta Neuropathol 1995; 89:194.
134. Daita G, Yonemasu Y, Muraoka S, et al: A case of anaplastic astrocytoma transformed from pleomorphic xanthoastrocytoma. Noshuyo Byori 1991; 8:63.
135. Macaulay R, Jay V, Hoffman H, et al: Increased mitotic activity as a negative prognostic indicator in pleomorphic xanthoastrocytoma. J Neurosurg 1993; 79:761.
136. Zorzi F, Facchettti F, Baronchelli C, et al: Pleomorphic xanthoastrocytoma: An immunohistochemical study of three cases. Histopathology 1992; 20:267.
137. Kingsley DP, Kendall BE, Fitz CR: Tuberous sclerosis: A clinicoradiological evaluation of 110 cases with particular reference to atypical presentation. Neuroradiology 1986; 28:38.
138. Shepherd CW, Scheithauer BW, Gomez MR, et al: Subependymal giant cell astrocytoma: A clinical, pathological, and flow cytometric study. Neurosurgery 1991; 28:864.
139. Halmagyi GM, Bignold LP, Allsop JL: Recurrent subependymal giant-cell astrocytoma in the absence of tuberous sclerosis. J Neurosurg 1979; 50:106.
140. Lopes MBS, Altermatt HJ, Scheithauer BW, et al: Immunohistochemical characterization of subependymal giant cell astrocytomas. Acta Neuropathol (in press).
141. Hirose T, Scheithauer BW, Lopes MBS, et al: Tuber and subependymal giant cell astrocytoma associated with tuberous sclerosis: An immunohistochemical, ultrastructural, and immunoelectron microscopic study. Acta Neuropathol 1995; 90:387.
142. Ribideau-Dumas JL, Poirier J, Escourolle R: Étude ultrastructurale des lésions cérébrales de la sclérose tubéreuse de Bourneville chez un premature. Acta Neuropathol 1973; 25:259.
143. Sima AAF, Robertson DM: Subependymal giant-cell astrocytoma: Case report with ultrastructural study. J Neurosurg 1979; 50:240.
144. De Chadarévian J-P, Hollenberg RD: Subependymal giant cell tumor of tuberous sclerosis: A light and ultrastructural study. J Neuropathol Exp Neurol 1979; 38:419.
145. Bender BL, Yunis EJ: Central nervous system pathology of tuberous sclerosis in children. Ultrastruct Pathol 1980; 1:287.
146. Stefansson K, Wollmann RL: Distribution of glial fibrillary acidic protein in central nervous system lesion of tuberous sclerosis. Acta Neuropathol 1980; 52:135.
147. Trombley IK, Mirra SS: Ultrastructure of tuberous sclerosis: Cortical tuber and subependymal tumor. Ann Neurol 1981; 9:174.
148. Stefansson K, Wollmann RL: Distribution of neuronal specific protein, 14-3-2, in central nervous system lesions of tuberous sclerosis. Acta Neuropathol 1981; 53:113.
149. Nakamura Y, Becker LE: Subependymal giant-cell tumor: Astrocytic or neuronal? Acta Neuropathol 1983; 60:271.
150. Bonnin JM, Rubinstein LJ, Papasozomenos SC, et al: Subependymal giant cell astrocytoma: Significance and possible cytogenetic implications of an immunohistochemical study. Acta Neuropathol 1984; 62:185.
151. Nakamura S, Tsubokawa T: Ultrastructure of subependymal giant cell

astrocytoma associated with tuberous sclerosis. J Clin Electron Microsc 1987; 20:5.

152. Chou TM, Chou SM: Tuberous sclerosis in the premature infant: A report of a case with immunohistochemistry on the CNS. Clin Neuropathol 1989; 8:45.

153. Bancel B, Belin MF, Meiniel A, et al: Contribution à l'étude de l'histogenèse des gliomes sous-épendymaires de la sclérose tubéreuse de Bourneville. Ann Pathol 1990; 10:109.

154. Ho YS: Subependymal giant cell astrocytoma with tuberous sclerosis: Significance and possible cytogenetic implications on an immunohistochemical study. Acta Histochem Cytochem 1990; 23:703.

155. Iwasaki Y, Yoshikawa H, Sasaki M, et al: Clinical and immunohistochemical studies of subependymal giant cell astrocytomas associated with tuberous sclerosis. No To Hattatsu 1990; 12:478.

156. Morimoto K, Mogami H: Sequential CT study of giant cell-astrocytoma associated with tuberous sclerosis. J Neurosurg 1986; 65:874.

157. Fujiwara S, Takaki T, Hikita T, et al: Subependymal giant-cell astrocytoma associated with tuberous sclerosis: Do subependymal nodules grow? Childs Nerv Syst 1989; 5:43.

158. Mørk SJ, Lindegaad K-F, Halvorsen TB, et al: Oligodendroglioma: Incidence and biological behavior in a defined population. J Neurosurg 1985; 63:881.

159. Zülch KJ: Brain Tumours: Their Biology and Pathology, ed 3. Berlin, Springer-Verlag, 1986.

160. Tola MR, Casetta I, Granieri E, et al: Intracranial gliomas in Ferrara, Italy, 1976 to 1991. Acta Neurol Scand 1994; 90:312.

161. Morris HH, Estes ML, Gilmore R, et al: Chronic intractable epilepsy as the only symptom of primary brain tumor. Epilepsia 1993; 34:1038.

162. Sjors K, Blennow G, Lantz G: Seizures as the presenting symptom of brain tumors in children. Acta Paediatr 1993; 82:66.

163. Shaw EG, Scheithauer BW, O'Fallon JR, et al: Oligodendrogliomas: The Mayo Clinic experience. J Neurosurg 1992; 76:428.

164. Tice H, Barnes PD, Goumnerova L, et al: Pediatric and adolescent oligodendrogliomas. Am J Neuroradiol 1993; 14:1293.

165. Kros JM, Pieterman H, van Eden CG, et al: Oligodendroglioma: The Rotterdam-Dijkzigt experience. Neurosurgery 1994; 34:959.

166. Greenwood J Jr, Otenasek FJ, Yelin FS: Oligodendrogliomas of the fourth ventricle: Report of two cases. J Neurol Neurosurg Psychiatry 1969; 32:226.

167. Pitt MA, Jones AW, Reeve RS, et al: Oligodendroglioma of the fourth ventricle with intracranial and spinal oligodendrogliomatosis: A case report. Br J Neurosurg 1992; 6:371.

168. Fortuna A, Celli P, Palma L: Oligodendrogliomas of the spinal cord. Acta Neurochir 1980; 52:305.

169. Natelson SE, Dyer ML, Harp DL: Delayed CSF seeding of benign oligodendroglioma. South Med J 1992; 85:1011.

170. Grant R, Naylor B, Junck L, et al: Clinical outcome in aggressively treated meningeal gliomatosis. Neurology 1992; 42:252.

171. Schiffer D, Cravioto H, Giordana MT, et al: Is polar spongioblastoma a tumour entity? J Neurosurg 1993; 78:587.

172. Kennedy PGE, Watkins BA, Thomas DGT, et al: Antigenic expression by cells derived from human gliomas does not correlate with morphological classification. Neuropathol Appl Neurobiol 1987; 13:327.

173. Noble M, Ataliotis P, Barnett SC, et al: Development, regeneration and neoplasia of glial cells in the central nervous system. Ann NY Acad Sci 1991; 633:35.

174. Norton WT, Cammer W: Isolation and characterization of myelin. In Morell P (ed): Myelin, ed 2. New York, Plenum Press, 1984, p 147.

175. de la Monte SM: Uniform lineage of oligodendrogliomas. Am J Pathol 1989; 153:529.

176. Figols J, Cervos-Navarro J, Cruz-Sanchez FF: Lectins: Reliable differentiation markers in human oligodendrogliomas. Noshuyo Byori 1993; 10:1.

177. Jagadha V, Halliday WC, Becker LE: Glial fibrillary acidic protein (GFAP) in oligodendrogliomas: A reflection of transient GFAP expression by immature oligodendroglia. Can J Neurol Sci 1986; 13:307.

178. Cruz-Sanchez FF, Rossi ML, Buller JR, et al: Oligodendrogliomas: A clinical, histological, immunocytochemical and lectin-binding study. Histopathology 1991; 19:361.

179. Hossmann K-A, Wechsler W: Ultrastructural cytopathology of human cerebral gliomas. Oncology 1971; 25:455.

180. Baloyannis S: The fine structure of the isomorphic oligodendroglioma. Anticancer Res 1981; 1:243.

181. Min KW, Scheithauer BW: Oligodendroglioma: The ultrastructural spectrum. Ultrastruct Pathol 1994; 18:47.

182. Herpers MJHM, Budka H: Glial fibrillary acidic protein (GFAP) in oligodendroglial tumours: Gliofibrillary oligodendroglioma and transitional oligoastrocytoma as subtypes of oligodendroglioma. Acta Neuropathol 1984; 64:265.

183. Nakagawa Y, Perentes E, Rubinstein LJ: Immunohistochemical characterization of oligodendrogliomas: An analysis of multiple markers. Acta Neuropathol 1986; 72:15.

184. Wondrusch E, Huemer M, Budka H: Production of glial fibrillary acidic protein (GFAP) by neoplastic oligodendrocytes: Gliofibrillary oligodendroglioma and transitional oligoastrocytoma revisited. Noshuyo Byori 1991; 8:11.

185. Kros JM, de Jong AA, van der Kwast ThH: Ultrastructural characterization of transitional cells in oligodendrogliomas. J Neuropathol Exp Neurol 1992; 51:186.

186. Kros JM, Van Eden CG, Stefanko SZ, et al: Prognostic implications of glial fibrillary acidic protein containing cell types in oligodendrogliomas. Cancer 1990; 66:1204.

187. Cairncross JG, Macdonald DR, Ramsay DA: Aggressive oligodendroglioma: A chemosensitive tumour. Neurosurgery 1992; 31:78.

188. Smith MT, Ludwig CL, Godfrey AD, et al: Grading of oligodendrogliomas. Cancer 1983; 52:2107.

189. Burger PC: The grading of astrocytomas and oligodendrogliomas. In Fields WS (ed): Primary Brain Tumours. A Review of Histologic Classification. New York, Springer-Verlag, 1989, p 171.

190. Kros JM, van Eden CG, Vissers CJ, et al: Prognostic relevance of DNA flow cytometry in oligodendroglioma. Cancer 1992; 69:1791.

191. Coons SW, Johnson PC, Pearl DK, et al: Prognostic significance of flow cytometry deoxyribonucleic acid analysis of human oligodendrogliomas. Neurosurgery 1994; 34:680.

192. Ohgaki H, Eibl RH, Wiestler OD, et al: p53 mutations in nonastrocytic human brain tumours. Cancer Res 1991; 51:6202.

193. Reifenberger J, Reifenberger G, Liu L, et al: Molecular genetic analysis of oligodendroglial tumors shows preferential allelic deletions on 19q and 1p. Am J Pathol 1994; 145:1175.

194. Jenkins RB, Kimmel DW, Moertel CA, et al: A cytogenetic study of 53 human gliomas. Cancer Genet Cytogenet 1989; 39:253.

195. Ransom DT, Ritland SR, Kimmel DW, et al: Cytogenetic and loss of heterozygosity studies in ependymomas, pilocytic astrocytomas, and oligodendrogliomas. Genes Chromosom Cancer 1992; 5:348.

196. Kraus JA, Koopman J, Kaskel P, et al: Shared allelic losses on chromosomes 1p and 19q suggest a common origin of oligodendroglioma and oligoastrocytoma. J Neuropathol Exp Neurol 1995; 54:91.

197. Bello MJ, Vaquero J, de Campos JM, et al: Molecular analysis of chromosome 1 abnormalities in human gliomas reveals frequent loss of 1p in oligodendroglial tumors. Int J Cancer 1994; 57:172.

198. Thiel G, Losanowa T, Kintzel D, et al: Karyotypes in 90 human gliomas. Cancer Genet Cytogenet 1992; 58:109.

199. Watanabe K, Nagai M, Wakai S, et al: Loss of constitutional heterozygosity in chromosome 10 in human glioblastoma. Acta Neuropathol 1990; 80:251.

200. Fults D, Pedone CA, Thomas GA, et al: Allelotype of human malignant astrocytoma. Cancer Res 1990; 50:5784.

201. Wu JK, Folkerth RD, Ye A, et al: Aggressive oligodendroglioma predicted by chromosome 10 restriction fragment polymorphism analysis: Case study. J Neurooncol 1992; 15:29.

202. Yates AJ, Becker LE, Sachs LA: Brain tumors in childhood. Childs Brain 1979; 5:31.

203. Salazar OM, Castro-Vita H, VanHoutte P, et al: Improved survival in cases of intracranial ependymoma after radiation therapy: Late report and recommendations. J Neurosurg 1983; 59:652.

204. Ho KL: Abnormal cilia in a fourth ventricular ependymoma. Acta Neuropathol 1986; 70:30.

205. Sara A, Bruner JM, Mackay B: Ultrastructure of ependymoma. Ultrastruct Pathol 1994; 18:33.

206. Guccion JG, Saini N: Ependymoma: Ultrastructural studies of two cases. Ultrastruct Pathol 1991; 15:159.

207. Kawano N, Yada K, Yagishita S: Clear cell ependymoma: A histological variant with diagnostic implications. Virchows Arch A Pathol Anat Histopathol 1989; 415:467.

208. Schiffer D, Chiò A, Giordana MT, et al: Histologic prognostic factors in ependymoma. Childs Nerv Syst 1991; 7:177.

209. Asai A, Hoshino T, Edwards MSB, et al: Predicting the recurrence of ependymomas from the bromodeoxyuridine labeling index. Childs Nerv Syst 1992; 8:273.

210. Schröder R, Ploner C, Ernestus RI: The growth potential of ependymomas with varying grades of malignancy measured by the Ki-67 labelling index and mitotic index. Neurosurg Rev 1993; 16:145.
211. Keating G, Scheithauer BW, Groover RV, et al: Pediatric ependymomas: The relation of histologic and flow cytometric parameters to prognosis (abstract). Mod Pathol 1993; 6:128.
212. Morantz RA, Kepes JJ, Batnitzky S, et al: Extraspinal ependymomas: Report of three cases. J Neurosurg 1979; 51:383.
213. Sonneland PRL, Scheithauer BW, Onofrio BM: Myxopapillary ependymoma: A clinicopathologic and immunocytochemical study of 77 cases. Cancer 1985; 56:883.
214. Pulitzer DR, Martin PC, Collins PC, et al: Subcutaneous sacrococcygeal (''myxopapillary'') ependymal rests. Am J Surg Pathol 1988; 12:672.
215. Patternson RH Jr, Campbell WG Jr, Parsons H: Ependymoma of the cauda equina with multiple visceral metastases: Report of a case. J Neurosurg 1961; 18:145.
216. Rubinstein LJ, Logan WJ: Extraneural metastases in ependymoma of the cauda equina. J Neurol Neurosurg Psychiatry 1970; 33:763.
217. Rawlinson DG, Herman MM, Rubinstein LJ: The fine structure of a myxopapillary ependymoma of the filum terminale. Acta Neuropathol 1973; 25:1.
218. Specht CS, Smith TW, DeGirolami U, et al: Myxo-papillary ependymoma of the filum terminale: A light and electron microscopic study. Cancer 1986; 58:310.
219. Scheithauer BW: Symptomatic subependymoma: Report of 21 cases with review of the literature. J Neurosurg 1978; 49:689.
220. Lombardi D, Scheithauer BW, Meyer FB, et al: Symptomatic subependymoma: A clinicopathological and flow cytometric study. J Neurosurg 1991; 75:583.
221. Pagni CA, Canavero S, Giordana MT, et al: Spinal intramedullary subependymomas: Case report and review of the literature. Neurosurgery 1992; 30:115.
222. Fu Y-S, Chen ATL, Kay S, et al: Is subependymoma (subependymal glomerate astrocytoma) an astrocytoma or ependymoma? A comparative ultrastructural and tissue culture study. Cancer 1974; 34:1992.
223. Azzarelli B, Rekate HL, Roessman U: Subependymoma: A case report with ultrastructural study. Acta Neuropathol 1977; 40:279.
224. Hurtt MR, Moosy J, Donovan-Peluso M, et al: Amplification of epidermal growth factor receptor gene in gliomas: Histopathology and prognosis. J Neuropathol Exp Neurol 1992; 51:84.
225. Rubinstein LJ: Tumors of the central nervous system, fascicle 6. *In* Atlas of Tumor Pathology. Washington, DC, Armed Forces Institute of Pathology, 1972.
226. Miller RH, French-Constant C, Raff MC: The macroglial cells of the rat optic nerve. Annu Rev Neurosci 1989; 12:517.
227. Wren D, Wolwijk G, Noble M: In vitro analysis of the origin and maintenance of O-2A^{adult} progenitor cells. J Cell Biol 1992; 116:167.
228. Scolding NJ, Rayner PJ, Sussman J, et al: A proliferative adult human oligodendrocyte progenitor. Neuroreport 1995; 6:441.
229. Lillien LE, Raff MC: Differentiation signals in the CNS: Type-2 astrocyte development in vitro as a model system. Neuron 1990; 5:111.
230. Bishop M, de la Monte SM: Dual lineage of astrocytomas. Am J Pathol 1989; 135:517.

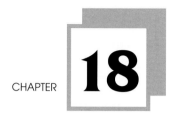

DAVIDE SCHIFFER

MARIA TERESA GIORDANA

CHAPTER **18**

Immunologic Cell Markers

The possibility of revealing the occurrence of cell-specific antigens in brain tumors greatly contributed not only to the improvement of histologic diagnosis but also to a better understanding of cytogenesis and anaplasia of cerebral oncotypes.

Some of the immunologic markers employed in the diagnosis and investigation of gliomas, such as S–100 protein, glial fibrillary acidic protein (GFAP), and myelin basic protein (MBP), are mainly expressed in the nervous system. Others are not neural cell-specific and are expressed by astrocytes (vimentin and glutamine synthetase), ependymal cells (vimentin), and oligodendrocytes (carbonic anhydrase). The recognition of antigens specifically expressed by cells of the neuronal line is of great help to the histologic diagnosis of brain tumors; neuronal markers of practical use are proteins of the neuronal cytoskeleton (neurofilaments, τ-protein, and microtubule-associated proteins) and cytoplasmic proteins (synaptophysin, ubiquitin, β-protein precursor, and neuron-specific enolase). Neovascularization and endothelial proliferation are characteristic phenomena of many glial tumors; therefore, the demonstration of vessel cell markers (factor VIII–related antigen [factor VIII/RAg], fibronectin, type IV collagen, laminin, α-actin, and tenascin) provides further reliable information about glioma biology and prognosis.

The demonstration of these antigens on tissue sections is obtained by immunohistochemical procedures employing immune sera or monoclonal antibodies, the latter being more specific and generally less sensitive than the former.[50] The demonstration involves many technical problems, starting with that of fixation. All fixatives affect the molecular structure of antigens, to a greater or lesser degree, either by destroying the antigenic sites or by masking the epitopes or making them inaccessible to the antibody.[7, 84, 89, 116] An enzymatic predigestion of the tissue is sometimes required.[7, 84, 86, 89] Many antigens, especially surface antigens, do not tolerate fixation, and must be demonstrated on frozen tissue sections. The wide possibility of artifactual staining[31] suggests great care in interpreting immunohistochemical results in brain tumors.

The subcellular localization of cell-specific antigens, obtained by immune electron microscopy, is helpful both in confirming the antigen specificity and in giving insight into the biology of tumor cells.[91, 92]

The expression of some cell-specific antigens is related to the differentiation stage of the cell; neoplastic transformation modifies the cell phenotype, usually toward less mature or more atypical features. Therefore, by the positive-negative rate of antigen expression in a tumor cell population it is possible to evaluate anaplasia, and the prognostic value of the histologic diagnosis increases.

GLIAL MARKERS

The first and most important marker in astrocytic tumors is GFAP. Originally purified from plaques of multiple sclerosis[26] and from normal white matter,[14] it is a 50-kD protein representing the chemical subunit characteristic of gliofilaments. These are a subclass of intermediate filaments (IF) with a diameter of approximately 10 nm. Polyclonal and monoclonal antibodies are available. GFAP is present in normal astrocytes of the gray and white matter and Bergmann's glia, in reactive astrocytes (Fig. 18–1A), and in every cell with fibrillogenetic capacity. Electron microscopy confirms that the antigen is localized on the glial intermediate filaments; the amount of antigen usually correlates with the number of filaments.[5]

Vimentin is the 57-kD protein of another IF; it is the earliest IF protein to appear during development in all cytotypes, but in adult cells it is usually replaced by the IF characteristic of each cell type. In mature astrocytes it is co-expressed with GFAP[137]; during development of the nervous tissue its appearance precedes that of GFAP.[15, 25] Tanycytes co-express vimentin and cytokeratin.[137] Vimentin is the only IF protein of mature endothelial cells, fibroblasts, macrophages, chondrocytes, and lymphocytes. The proteins of different IFs share some amino acid sequences,[33, 115] so that in tissue sections some antisera and monoclonal antibodies may react with more than one IF. Actually, a cross-reaction for GFAP and vimentin occurs when using any commercially available antibody.[115, 119]

S–100 protein, a dimeric calcium-binding protein composed of two variously combined subunits, was first isolated in the nervous system. It was considered specific for the

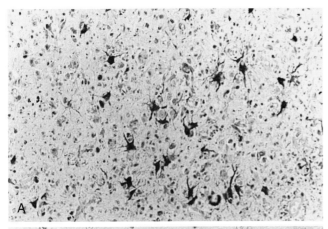

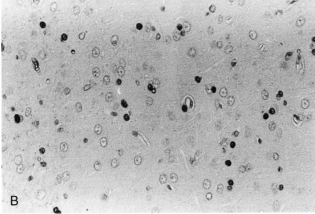

Figure 18–1 *A,* GFAP in reactive astrocytes (PAP-DAB, ×200). *B,* Carbonic anhydrase marks normal rat oligodendrocytes (PAP-DAB, ×400).

nervous tissue, but it has been found in many non–nervous system cells: chondrocytes, adipocytes, myoepithelial cells, Langerhans cells, and melanocytes. In nervous system tissue it is considered more a glial than a neuronal marker, and it is demonstrable in astrocytes, oligodendrocytes, and ependymal cells.[57, 80, 83, 98]

Glutamine synthetase (GS) is an enzyme localized in glia and retinal cells.[103, 104] It has been considered to be a specific marker for rat astrocytes.[104] GS is of limited value for diagnostic purposes in brain tumors, because of its lack of tight specificity; it is expressed by other cells, such as hepatocytes.[111] Carbonic anhydrase is expressed in all animal cells as two isoenzymes; in neural tissue the isoenzyme C is present, and it is localized in oligodendroglia (see Fig. 18–1B)[74] and in Müller's retinal cells.

MBP is present in the rat myelin by the 10th day of extrauterine life. It has been immunohistochemically demonstrated in the cell body and processes of oligodendrocytes in the newborn rat.[146, 147] It is also expressed by human immature oligodendrocytes, but never in the human adult oligodendroglia.[59]

Myelin-associated glycoprotein (MAG) is present in central and peripheral myelin, in Schwann cells, and in immature oligodendroglia. The monoclonal antibody anti-Leu-7, which can specifically detect human natural killer (HNK) cells, has been found to identify normal and neoplastic oligodendrocytes,[95] and has consequently been considered to

be a useful marker for oligodendrocytes. Anti-Leu-7 also recognizes an epitope of MAG.[102]

VESSEL CELL AND VESSEL WALL MARKERS

The antigen correlated with factor VIII of coagulation (factor VIII/RAg) is the most widely employed endothelial marker. It is a component of the anti-hemophilia factor (factor VIII); it is produced by endothelial cells and megakaryocytes. In extra–nervous system tumors factor VIII is a marker of endothelial proliferation.[96] The *Ulex europaeus* lectin is a nonimmunologic endothelial cell marker. Fibronectin, laminin, and type IV collagen are markers of basement membrane.[76] Fibronectin is the major noncollagenous component of the connective tissue matrix[152]; in vitro, the best producers of fibronectin are endothelial cells and fibroblasts.[45] Although in vitro cultures of astrocytic cells immunoreact with fibronectin, astrocytes in histologic sections do not. Laminin is a specific glycoprotein of basement membrane.[150] In the central nervous system (CNS), the immunohistochemical distribution of laminin corresponds to endothelial, glial, and pial basement membrane[35]; the whole vascular network, including capillaries, is sharply visualized[35] (Fig. 18–2). Type IV collagen is a typical marker of basement membranes, whereas type III collagen is produced mainly by fibroblasts.[76] Monoclonal antibodies against muscle-specific α-actin (MSA) and smooth muscle–specific α-actin (SMSA) recognize vascular smooth muscle cells and pericytes,[47, 142, 151] which are also present in the CNS.[42]

Tenascin is a polymorphic extracellular matrix glycoprotein of high molecular mass.[141] It has recently been demonstrated that tenascin is the same protein as glioma-associated extracellular matrix (ECM) antigen.[4] The tissue distribution of tenascin is much more restricted than that of fibronectin and laminin.[27] During embryogenesis, tenascin is transiently present in the mesenchyme surrounding the developing CNS[6]; its expression is believed to correlate with cell proliferation and migration and with remodeling of the ECM.[27]

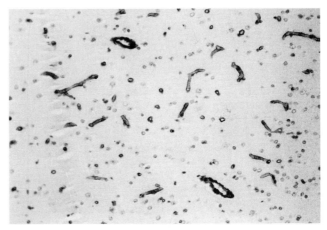

Figure 18–2 Laminin in the capillary network of normal cerebral cortex (PAP-DAB, ×100).

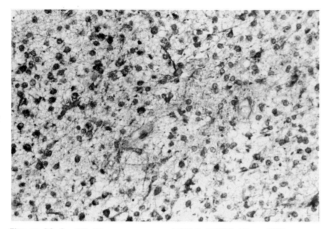

Figure 18–3 Fibrillary astrocytoma (GFAP, PAP-DAB, ×200).

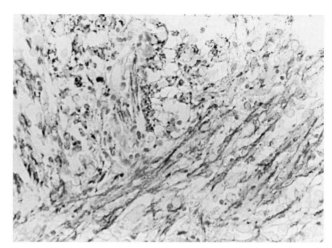

Figure 18–5 Pilocytic astrocytoma (GFAP, PAP-DAB, ×200).

ASTROCYTIC TUMORS

In fibrillary astrocytoma GFAP is expressed in the delicate astrocytic processes (Fig. 18–3), which are easily distinguishable from the larger and thicker processes of reactive astrocytes.[22] It is also positive in the cytoplasms and short processes of protoplasmic and gemistocytic (Fig. 18–4) variants and in the elongated, bipolar cells of pilocytic astrocytoma (Fig. 18–5). The expression of GFAP by tumor cells of astrocytomas indicates that neoplastic transformation has almost not modified the phenotype in comparison with the normal astrocytes.

In vitro observations[118] demonstrate two distinct lines of glial development, one giving rise to type 1 astrocytes and the other (O2A) to type 2 astrocytes and to oligodendrocytes. A2B5, a monoclonal antibody to a ganglioside, decorates O2A cells as well as type 2 astrocytes, which correspond to fibrillary astrocytes predominating in the white matter; type 1 astrocytes correspond to protoplasmic astrocytes of the cortex. The largest part of astrocytomas do not contain A2B5-positive cells; this would indicate an origin from type 1 astrocytes. Tumors possibly derived from type 2 lineage (because they show A2B5-positive cells) are less common and have a better prognosis than tumors deriving from type 1 lineage.[1] Astrocytic tumors arising from the white matter contain more A2B5-positive cells and show shorter preoperative periods than do cortically based low-grade astrocytomas[112]; the site of tumor involvement may be an important variable that correlates with antigen expression.

In astrocytomas, vimentin distributes like GFAP[49, 135] and the co-expression of the two markers has prompted conclusions on the maturation stage of tumor astrocytes (Fig. 18–6). Because vimentin precedes GFAP in the maturation of glia cells in the rat and mouse,[15, 137] its presence in glioma cells might indicate immaturity.[163] However, this conclusion seems to be oversimplified. First of all, the appearance of GFAP during development does not coincide with the disappearance of vimentin in the same cells,[113, 137] and, second, vimentin appears only at a certain stage of maturity of the neural tube, as a marker of differentiation.[56] Whereas GFAP is a glia-specific marker, and its expression, therefore, indicates the astroglial nature of cells, the same is not true for vimentin.

Glutamine synthetase is positive in differentiated astrocytomas, but the enzyme cannot be considered specific, as it is also positive in other cells.[111] S–100 protein is positive in differentiated astrocytomas[44, 100, 149, 158] and also in malignant astrocytomas without any correlation with the degree of differentiation.[101]

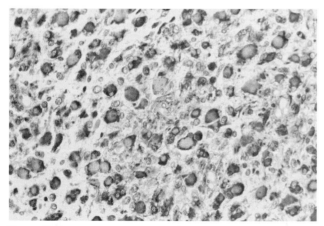

Figure 18–4 Gemistocytic astrocytoma (GFAP, PAP-DAB, ×200).

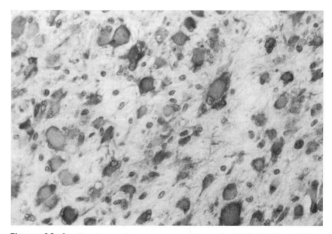

Figure 18–6 Gemistocytic astrocytoma (vimentin, PAP-DAB, ×200).

GFAP staining is intense in bipolar cells and variable in stellate cells of pilocytic astrocytomas; both cell types have a conspicuous vimentin immunoreactivity. It has been suggested that the differential GFAP and vimentin immunoreactivity may imply the origin of pilocytic astrocytoma as being radial glia.[154]

The pathologic hallmark of pilocytic astrocytomas are Rosenthal's fibers, which are composed of masses of degenerated glial filaments[28, 39, 55] that arise from an accumulation of osmiophilic material in tumor cells followed by a fragmentation of filaments.[136] The fundamental ultrastructural elements are then osmiophilic masses and filaments.[40] Usually, Rosenthal's fibers are GFAP-negative or -positive only in a thin peripheral rim (Fig. 18–7), depending on the quantity of the amorphous granular osmiophilic material. When it is scarce, as in early Rosenthal's fibers, GFAP is diffusely positive.[82, 144] This proves that amorphous material, centrally placed, derives from degenerating gliofilaments. By immunoelectron microscopy, GFAP antibody is also seen to be localized on amorphous material.[20] The granular electron-dense masses of the Rosenthal's fibers represent a rare example of GFAP immunopositivity without filamental appearance.[5] It is interesting to note that the peripheral part of Rosenthal's fibers and the compact GFAP-positive bundles are positive for ubiquitin (Fig. 18–8).[79] This means either that the GFAP-positive material is represented by abnormal proteins, which are then destined to proteolysis with overloading of the ubiquitin-dependent proteolytic system, or that ubiquitin acts like a cytoprotective agent in isolating the abnormal proteins.[21]

In pleomorphic xanthoastrocytoma, tumor cells are strongly but variably positive for GFAP and vimentin. The positivity of GFAP in bizarre giant cells (Fig. 18–9), surrounded by delicate reticulin fibers, and in heavily lipidized cells has contributed to the recognition of this tumor entity.[64] Reticulin fibers represent basal lamina of neoplastic astrocytes.[72] A detailed immunohistochemical study has demonstrated that all of the cells—spindle-shaped, gemistocytic, xanthomatous—are positive for GFAP, vimentin, α_1-antitrypsin, and α_1-antichymotrypsin.[71] The positivity for the two monohistiocytic markers, together with the undeniable mesenchymal aspect of the tumor, were an argument against

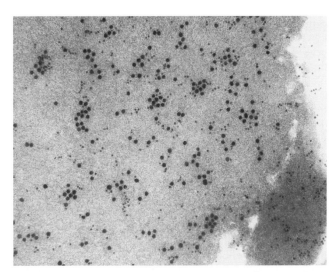

Figure 18–8 Rosenthal's fibers: immunogold electron microscopy. Large granules decorate ubiquitin; small granules, GFAP ($\times 40{,}000$).

the glial nature of the neoplasia, wherein the GFAP-positive cells could be considered as being limited to the cortical areas of infiltration or as migrating astrocytes. These findings could be consistent with the interpretation of the tumor as a fibroxanthoma of the meninges,[107, 108] in line with the original interpretation.[63] The solution of this problem is not easy, although in case of malignant transformation the evolution is always toward glioblastoma and not sarcoma.[62] In one case,[71] neoplastic neuronal cells that expressed neurofilament proteins and synaptophysin were found, which made the distinction and differential diagnosis from desmoplastic infantile ganglioglioma[155] very difficult. The expression of neurofilament proteins by a pleomorphic xanthoastrocytoma leads to the hypothesis of a dysgenetic origin of the tumor.[53]

In subependymal giant cell astrocytoma, giant cells and bundles of processes are GFAP-positive. Doubts, however, had arisen that the large cells could be neuronal in origin,[37] and they have even been found to be positive for neuron-specific enolase (NSE).[145] Moreover, GFAP was found to be positive in some cells only[156] or in the peripheral rim of the

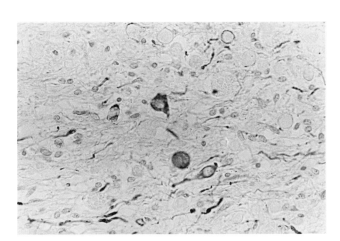

Figure 18–7 Rosenthal's fibers express GFAP in a thin peripheral rim (PAP-DAB, ×400).

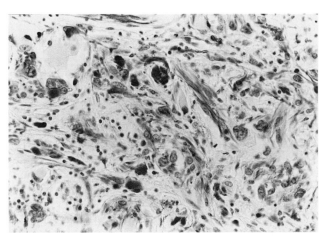

Figure 18–9 Pleomorphic xanthoastrocytoma: bizarre GFAP-positive astrocytes (PAP-DAB, ×400).

cells,[24] or it was even found to be absent.[99] It was then ascertained that the tumor is characterized by GFAP-positive cells when it is not associated with tuberous sclerosis. In this case, a positivity for 68-kD neurofilaments (NF) and NSE was observed.[3] A possible conclusion is that giant cells are dysgenetic, with a bi-directional differentiation that never reaches a full neuronal stage. It is important to note that dense core vesicles have been described,[120, 123] even in the glial component.[140]

In anaplastic astrocytomas the expression of GFAP decreases with the increasing extent of anaplasia (Fig. 18–10); this is consistent with the increasing phenotypic heterogeneity due to the genotypic heterogeneity that accompanies glioma progression. In gliomas, GFAP expression is inversely correlated with the degree of anaplasia,[25, 153, 156] being absent in too-primitive and in anaplastic cells. This is even more evident in glioblastoma, in which the small hyperchromatic cells, which proliferate rapidly[54] and are responsible for tumor invasion and growth,[34] are GFAP-negative.[156] The appearance of anaplasia in astrocytoma and the active cell proliferation in glioblastoma are sustained by the progressive increase of a cell population that is rich in mitoses, with isomorphic nuclei, and that is negative for GFAP.[75, 131]

GLIOBLASTOMA AND GLIOSARCOMA

Unlike astrocytoma, glioblastoma elicits a strong glial reaction both in the cortex and in the white matter, which is revealed by strongly GFAP-positive reactive astrocytes with stubby and long processes. Reactive astrocytes may be included in the advancing tumor and remain visible amongst GFAP-negative tumor cells (Figs. 18–11 and 18–12).[134] This may lead to wrong interpretation of the degree of malignancy when such areas are examined alone for diagnosis. Cytokeratin expression was reported in glioblastomas and was related to the occurrence of epithelium-like areas.[94] The immunohistochemical expression of non-glial intermediate filaments in gliomas of various histologic grades of malignancy has been studied with a panel of commercially available antibodies[53]; the occurrence of high-molecular-weight cytokeratins in glioma cells may reflect the close relationship between nervous

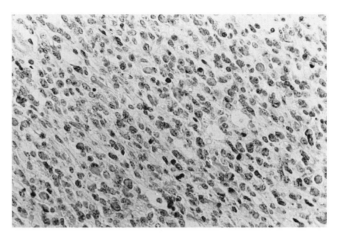

Figure 18–11 Glioblastoma: no cell expresses GFAP (PAP-DAB, ×200).

system and epidermis in ontogenesis; a cross-reaction of desmin polyclonal antibody with GFAP and vimentin may occur and depends on the high antigenic homology among the three IF proteins; rare, malignant glioma cells are immunoreactive for neurofilament antibodies.[53]

In the giant cell variant of glioblastoma, however, a diffuse GFAP positivity is seen in tumor cells, which creates some difficulty in differentiating this tumor from other oncotypes, such as pleomorphic xanthoastrocytoma. In malignant gliomas, especially in glioblastomas, the stromal component (i.e., the proliferative response of endothelial or vessel cells) has become a crucial problem that has been studied mainly by means of immunologic markers, in relation to the general problem of angiogenesis. Endothelial proliferation is a pathologic hallmark of glioblastoma, but it is not synonymous with angiogenesis.[130] Endothelial cells of blood vessels in glioblastoma increase in number, acquire immature features (e.g., a paucity in organelles and a high nucleocytoplasmic ratio[160]), feature mitoses, and modify the blood vessels, which become tortuous and glomeruloid.[130] Many sproutings are formed. Proliferating endothelial cells are rich in Weibel-

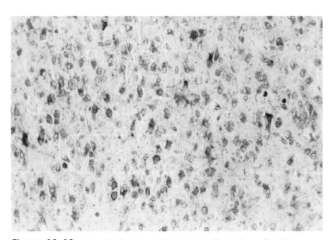

Figure 18–10 Anaplastic astrocytoma: a small number of cells express GFAP (PAP-DAB, ×200).

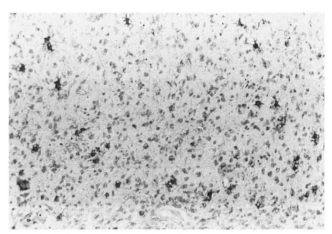

Figure 18–12 Glioblastoma: GFAP-positive reactive astrocytes dispersed in a GFAP-negative cell population (PAP-DAB, ×200). (From Schiffer D, Giordana MT, Mauro A, et al: Glial fibrillary acidic protein (GFAP), FVIII/RAg, laminin, and fibronectin in gliosarcomas: An immunohistochemical study. Acta Neuropathol 1984; 63:108.)

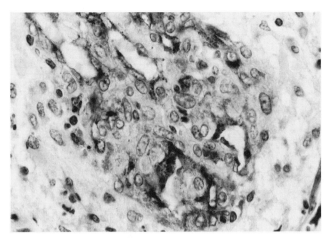

Figure 18–13 Factor VIII/RAg decorates the cells facing the lumen of glomeruloid structures in glioblastoma (PAP-DAB, ×400).

Palade bodies[73] and are positive for factor VIII/RAg. The immunoreactivity for factor VIII is found in Weibel-Palade bodies and in intracytoplasmic vacuoles discharging into the vessel lumen. In glomeruloid formations of glioblastoma, factor VIII marks only the cells lining the vessel lumen (Fig. 18–13) and not those far from it,[86, 93, 133, 159] although factor VIII/RAg has been found, by immunoelectron microscopy employing colloidal gold, in Weibel-Palade bodies of cells that do not line the vessel lumen.[91] It is generally assumed that glomeruloid formations of glioblastoma arise from the proliferation of vascular endothelium; however, increasing evidence suggests that not all the cells are of endothelial origin. It has been suggested that factor VIII-negative cells of glomeruloid structures may be pericytes.[87, 159] SMSA has been detected in some of the adventitial cells of the glomerular structures (Fig. 18–14).[130] It has been shown that the MSA and SMSA cells outnumber the negative cells in the glomeruloid formations, and it has been hypothesized that the vascular proliferation resulting in glomeruloid structures is due in large measure to pericytes and/or smooth muscle hyperplasia.[42, 161] A paracrine influence of neoplastic astrocytes on pericytes and/or smooth muscle cells through growth factors (insulin-like growth factors [IGF], platelet-

derived growth factors [PDGF]) may underlie this hyperplasia.[42]

In the small vessels of astrocytoma and oligodendroglioma, the laminin immunostaining is thicker than in capillaries of normal tissue.[35] In glioblastoma, laminin antiserum decorates two distinct basement membranes around glomeruloid formation: the external glial basement membrane is continuous and delimits the vascular structures from the tumor cells; the inner endothelial membrane is frequently thickened and multiplied, so that the endothelial cells appear to be immersed in a net of laminin (Fig. 18–15). The immunoreaction of fibronectin is diffuse in the vessel wall and is more intense at the basement membrane position.[133] Fibronectin might play an important role in glioma cell invasion; human malignant glioma cells migrate in response to in vitro stimulation by fibronectin and express fibronectin receptors.[51]

The immunohistochemical distribution of tenascin has been comparatively studied with that of fibronectin and GFAP in human malignant gliomas.[52] Tenascin was localized in the basement membrane zone of tumor vessels and, occasionally, in the extracellular space around tumor cells. The intensity of the stain for tenascin correlated well with the degree of endothelial proliferation. The expression of tenascin and fibronectin in the vessel walls was mutually exclusive; moreover, most tenascin-positive tumor vessels were surrounded by GFAP-negative tumor cells. Anaplastic glioma cells may produce tenascin or induce the tumor vessels to express it; it has been suggested that the expression of tenascin may play a role in the promotion of angiogenesis in malignant gliomas,[52] through the looser adhesion of endothelial cells to tenascin than to fibronectin.[78]

Circumscribed necroses are usually associated with glomeruloid formations in glioblastoma. Perhaps necroses release fibroblast growth factor (FGF), a potent mitogenic and angiogenetic factor, which stimulates tumor cells and endothelial cells to proliferate. This may be one explanation of pseudopalisading and endothelial hyperplasia.[105] Another possibility is that FGF leaks extracellularly from dying astrocytes and from the extracellular location affects smooth muscle cells,[162] which in some cases represent the majority

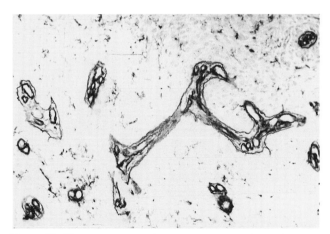

Figure 18–15 Glioblastoma: thickened basement membranes in glomeruli (laminin, PAP-DAB, ×150). (From Schiffer D, Giordana MT, Mauro A, et al: Glial fibrillary acidic protein (GFAP), FVIII/RAg, laminin, and fibronectin in gliosarcomas: An immunohistochemical study. Acta Neuropathol 1986; 63:108.)

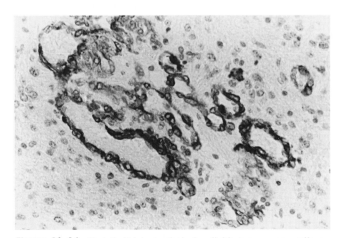

Figure 18–14 Endothelial hyperplasia in glioblastoma: many cells express α-actin (SMSA, PAP-DAB, ×400).

of the cells of glomeruloid formations in glioblastomas.[42] Also, PDGF may stimulate both endothelial cells[46, 121] and smooth muscle cells.[11, 126, 138] It is also possible that necroses develop as a result of the inadequacy of the vessel tree to support tumor cells, because of its deformation by endothelial hyperplasia.[130] Other observations suggest different interpretations. It has been shown that vascular endothelial growth factor (VEGF), which has a structural homology to PDGF, has a role in angiogenesis,[114] and its mRNA is strongly expressed by in situ hybridization in anaplastic cells of perinecrotic pseudopalisading of glioblastoma. The VEGF receptor is strongly expressed after in situ hybridization in endothelial cells of glioblastoma. The VEGF antibody strongly immunostains endothelial tumor cells.[114] The most important remark is that VEGF mRNA is up-regulated in a subset of malignant glioma cells during the transition from astrocytoma to glioblastoma. VEGF can be induced by hypoxia.[139]

Gliosarcoma actually owes its recognition as a tumor entity to immunologic differentiation markers. The tumor has two cell components: glial and mesodermic. The first is easily recognizable for its GFAP positivity (Fig. 18–16A), even when it is composed of a few cells dispersed in a large mesodermic environment (see Fig. 18–16B). Sometimes GFAP-positive cells appear as ribbons or show adenoid features and simulate cells of adenocarcinoma,[65] except for their GFAP. Foci of epithelial metaplasia may develop from the glial component, as also happens in glioblastoma, and

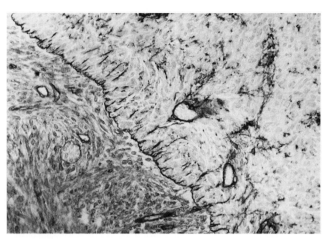

Figure 18–17 Gliosarcoma: a basement membrane evidenced by laminin separates the two components (PAP-DAB, ×200). (From Schiffer D, Giordana MT, Mauro A, et al: Glial fibrillary acidic protein (GFAP), FVIII/RAg, laminin, and fibronectin in gliosarcomas: An immunohistochemical study. Acta Neuropathol 1986; 63:108.)

appear as cytokeratin-positive squamous cells and keratin pearls.[94] The two components are sharply demarcated by a basement membrane that is easily evidenced by the demonstration of laminin (Fig. 18–17).[35]

The main problem concerning gliosarcoma is the cell type of the mesodermal component; immunohistochemistry has greatly contributed to the solution of this problem. The sarcomatous component of gliosarcoma originates from the malignant transformation of the vascular hyperplasia seen in glioblastoma. The first observation is that factor VIII/RAg, which is positive in the cells lining the vessel lumina in glomeruloid formations of glioblastoma, is negative in the fibrosarcomatous cell population of gliosarcoma. This finding speaks against the sarcomatous component's originating from proliferating endothelial cells of glioblastoma,[30] unless in the process of neoplastic transformation endothelial cells lose the capacity to express factor VIII/RAg. The observation of transitional features between factor VIII/RAg–positive endothelial cells of glomeruli and the negative cells of the fibrosarcomatous proliferation could support this hypothesis.[133, 143] Because histiocytic markers, such as α₁-antichymotrypsin, lysozyme, and α₁-antitrypsin, are positive in the mesodermic component, the adventitial histiocytes have been suggested as the source of the fibrosarcomatous proliferation.[68] Histiocytes are concentrated around the vessels and are positive for fibronectin,[13] which in turn diffusely decorates the mesodermic component (Fig. 18–18).[85, 133] Histiocytes may promote the proliferation of fibroblasts or endothelial cells.[68] Fibroblasts and undifferentiated mesenchymal elements have been considered to be the source of the mesodermic component of gliosarcoma.[38]

In some experiences, spindle or polygonal GFAP-negative cells of the mesodermic component have been found to express MSA and SMSA, which suggests vascular smooth muscle and/or pericytes as the origin of the malignant mesenchymal component.[41, 43] It can be deduced that malignant glia induces smooth muscle and/or pericyte proliferation and malignant transformation in a paracrine fashion.[43] The factors that mediate such an event can be PDGF, IGF, or

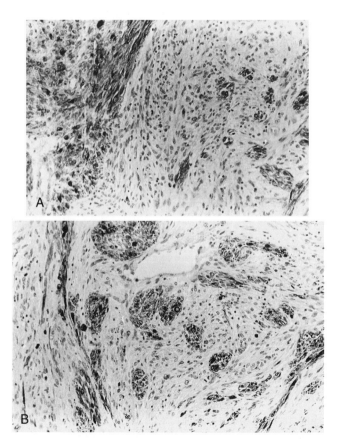

Figure 18–16 Gliosarcoma. GFAP decorates the glial component. Clear-cut demarcation toward mesodermic component (A) and islets (B) of tumoral glial cells (PAP-DAB, ×200).

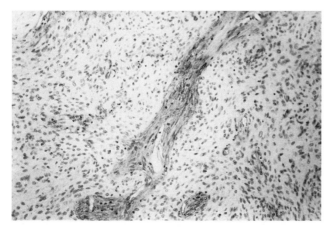

Figure 18–18   Gliosarcoma: the mesodermic proliferation is fibronectin-positive (PAP-DAB, ×150).

FGF.[58, 105] Immunohistochemistry of MSA and SMSA cannot distinguish between pericytes and vascular smooth muscle cells. On the one hand, both cell types represent contractile elements,[43] but on the other hand, no resemblance exists between gliosarcoma and hemangiopericytoma, which is composed of pericytes.[128] Spindle cells of the mesodermic component may even show a co-expression of SMSA and GFAP; the tumor may be considered to be of total glial origin and is therefore called *desmoplastic spindle-cell glioblastoma*.[60] An interesting debate has arisen on this point, because according to some[106] the reported tumors were actually different from those called *gliosarcoma,* which display a definite sarcomatous appearance. The possibility that tumor glial cells lose GFAP expression and appear to be non-glial in origin[60] further complicates this unresolved problem.

OLIGODENDROGLIOMA

Although astrocytes have a specific and sensitive marker, GFAP, which is helpful and reliable in the histologic diagnosis of tumor type, no specific marker exists for oligodendroglioma tumor cells.

Carbonic anhydrase C does not mark human and experimental oligodendroglioma cells.[36] Also, myelin basic protein has not been evidenced in oligodendroglial tumors.[2, 16] Negative results have also been obtained for MAG.[125] Anti-Leu-7 Mab is positive in a high percentage of oligodendrogliomas, in the cytoplasmic membranes and processes.[97] It seems to be reliable as a diagnostic marker of oligodendroglioma[95]; in positive cases it is demonstrable in more than half of the tumor cells,[109] but not all cases are positive. However, it cannot be considered as an oligodendroglioma cell-specific marker, because it has strong affinity for reactive and neoplastic astroglia, normal and neoplastic ependymal cells, and choroid plexus cells.[77, 109] It has been proposed, therefore, as a marker when the differential diagnosis is a choice between neuroepithelial and non-neuroepithelial tumors.[109]

The main problem concerning the immunologic markers of oligodendroglioma is the occasional expression of GFAP. Apart from reactive astrocytes, GFAP can be expressed by neoplastic astrocytes,[97] which belong to the astrocytic component of mixed oligoastrocytomas or by cells with an oligodendroglial appearance.[17, 88, 132, 153] The oligoastrocytomas are defined as glial tumors with separate areas or mixtures of two cell types. Although oligodendrogliomas consist predominantly of neoplastic oligodendrocytes, cells with astrocytic differentiation are commonly observed. GFAP-positive tumoral oligodendrocytes have been interpreted either as being small gemistocytic astrocytes, "mini-gemistocytes" (Fig. 18–19), or as being oligodendrocytes expressing GFAP *gliofibrillary oligodendrocytes*; they might be transitional cells between oligodendrocytes and astrocytes.[48, 117, 153] Oligodendrogliomas with GFAP-positive cells were called *transitional gliomas*.[48] GFAP immunopositivity was related to the presence of IF in the cell cytoplasm[69]; occasionally it was revealed not only on IF, but also on patchy electron-dense cytoplasmic corpuscles.[5] The discussion on these cells has not yet been concluded, and different interpretations are presented continuously. For example, it has been suggested that GFAP-positive astrocytes may even form halos, thus resembling oligodendrocytes.[61] It is also important to consider that in oligodendrogliomas, large, classic gemistocytes may occur.[70]

Oligodendrogliomas immunoreact with antibody to A2B5, which is consistent with the derivation of their cells from the A2B5-positive progenitor. In mixed oligoastrocytomas, cells occur that are positive both for A2B5 and GFAP.[18] The problem is whether the expression of GFAP is evidence that oligodendrocytes belong to the astrocytic lineage. In developing brain tissue, oligoglial and astroglial cells are believed to derive from a common precursor cell. In vitro studies have shown the potential for developing glial cells to express astrocytic and oligodendroglial markers simultaneously.[66] Moreover, during development, myelin-forming glia transiently expresses GFAP.[9] The immunohistochemical studies of tumors provide some circumstantial evidence for conversion potency of neoplastic oligodendroglia to astrocytic lineage.[69]

In anaplastic oligodendrogliomas, small GFAP-positive mini-gemistocytes seem to be characteristic.[8] They contain intermediate filaments.[127] However, no clearcut relationship between GFAP expression and malignancy grade has been found. The only GFAP-positive cells associated with shorter survival are gemistocytes.[70]

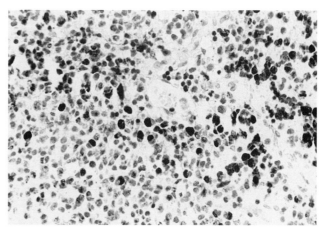

Figure 18–19   Oligodendroglioma with GFAP-positive mini-gemistocytes (PAP-DAB, ×200).

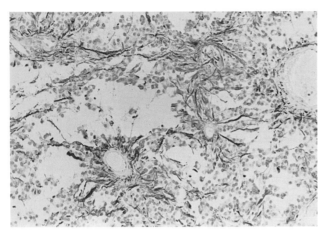

Figure 18–20 Ependymoma: perivascular pseudorosettes with GFAP-positive cell processes (PAP-DAB, ×200).

EPENDYMAL TUMORS

In ependymomas, the most important feature from the immunohistochemical point of view is the expression of GFAP in some cells. These may be either reactive astrocytes or tumor cells belonging to the perivascular pseudorosettes (Fig. 18–20), or cells with multipolar or gemistocytic aspects, located in the intervascular tissue (Fig. 18–21). In canals and rosettes, the mesenchymal pole of the cells may be GFAP-positive, and positive and negative cells may alternate in papillae (Fig. 18–22), as occurs in tanycytes of the third ventricle. GFAP positivity in ependymomas inspired the discussion on the cells of origin. According to some authors, the scarcity of GFAP-positive cells among vessels means that tanycytes, which may be GFAP-positive and are possible progenitors of GFAP-positive cells,[19] contribute only partially to the cell population of ependymoma.[23] The debate started with the observation that normal and neoplastic ependymocytes contain intracytoplasmic filaments,[32, 110, 124] which in culture are similar to the astrocytic filaments[157]; but adult ependymocytes do not express GFAP. In neoplastic conditions, however, they revert to more immature stages and express GFAP.[122] During development, GFAP appears in

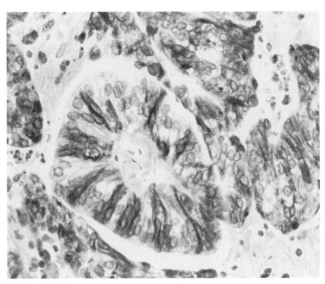

Figure 18–22 Ependymoma: GFAP immunoreactivity of papillae (PAP-DAB, ×400). (From Schiffer D, Giordana MT, Mauro A, et al: Immunohistochemical demonstration of vimentin in human cerebral tumors. Acta Neuropathol 1986; 70:209.)

ependymocytes when mitotic activity decreases, as a sign of differentiation[122]; but in the adult, GFAP is not produced in such quantity as to be visible on immunohistochemical analysis. Tanycytes contain GFAP during development, but not all become negative in adult life. Vimentin[135] and S–100 protein[67, 148] show the same distribution as GFAP.

Cytokeratin may also be demonstrated in ependymomas,[81] contrary to previous observations[10, 90]; this could be a sign of transition toward papilloma of the choroid plexus. Epithelial membrane antigen (EMA) has been shown to be positive on the cell surfaces in papillary structures and in ependymal epithelium, especially on the pole facing the lumina of rosettes. The expression of EMA by ependymomas was found to be directly related to the degree of differentiation: "malignant" ependymomas were negative for EMA.[12] In subependymoma, GFAP is positive both in the fibrous bundles and in cells of astrocytic type.[23, 153]

In the anaplastic variant of ependymoma, as identified according to the prognostic factors put in evidence by multivariate analysis,[129] GFAP expression decreases as the cell density and the number of mitoses increase, and the aspect of perivascular pseudorosettes is simplified and incomplete.

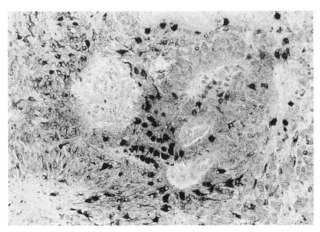

Figure 18–21 Ependymoma: GFAP-positive gemistocytic astrocytes (PAP-DAB, ×200).

REFERENCES

1. Bishop MB, de la Monte SM: Dual lineage of astrocytomas. Am J Pathol 1989; 135:517.
2. Bonnin JM, Rubinstein LJ: Immunohistochemistry of the central nervous system tumors: Its contributions to neurosurgical diagnosis. J Neurosurg 1984; 60:121.
3. Bonnin JM, Rubinstein LJ, Papasozomenos S, et al: Subependymal giant cell astrocytoma: Significance and possible cytogenetic implications of an immunohistochemical study. Acta Neuropathol 1984; 62:185.
4. Bourdon MA, Wikstrand CJ, Furthmayr H, et al: Human glioma-mesenchymal extracellular matrix antigen defined by monoclonal antibody. Cancer Res 1983; 43:2796.
5. Bozóky B, Krenács T, Rázga ZS, et al: Ultrastructural characterization

of glial fibrillary acidic protein expression in epoxy resin-embedded human brain tumors. Acta Neuropathol 1993; 86:295.

6. Bronner-Fraser M: Distribution and function of tenascin during cranial neural crest development in the chick. J Neurosci Res 1988; 21:135.

7. Brozman M: Immunohistochemical analysis of formaldehyde and trypsin-treated material. Acta Histochem 1978; 63:251.

8. Burger PC, Scheithauer BW, Vogel FS: Surgical Pathology of the Nervous System and its Coverings, ed 3. New York, Churchill Livingstone, 1991.

9. Choi BH, Kim RC: Expression of glial fibrillary acidic protein in immature oligodendroglia. Science 1984; 223:407.

10. Coakham HB, Garson JA, Allan PA: Immunohistological diagnosis of central nervous system tumors using a monoclonal antibody panel. J Clin Pathol 1985; 38:165.

11. Corjay MH, Blank RS, Owens GK: Platelet-derived growth factor–induced destabilization of smooth muscle alpha-actin mRNA. J Cell Physiol 1990; 145:391.

12. Cruz-Sanchez FF, Rossi ML, Esiri MM, et al: Epithelial membrane antigen expression in ependymomas. Neuropathol Appl Neurobiol 1988; 14:197.

13. D'Ardenne AJ, Kirkpatrick P, Sykes BC: Distribution of laminin, fibronectin and interstitial collagen type III in soft tissue tumors. J Clin Pathol 1984; 37:815.

14. Dahl D, Bignami A: Glial fibrillary acidic protein from normal human brain, purification and properties. Brain Res 1973; 57:343.

15. Dahl D, Rueger DC, Bignami A: Vimentin, the 57.000 molecular weight protein of fibroblast filaments, is the major cytoskeletal component in immature glia. Eur J Cell Biol 1981; 24:191.

16. De Armond SJ, Eng LF: Immunohistochemistry: Techniques and application to neurooncology. In Rosenblum ML, Wilson CB (eds): Brain Tumor Biology. Prog Exp Tumor Res 1984; 27:92.

17. De Armond SJ, Eng LF, Rubinstein LJ: The application of glial fibrillary acidic (GFA) protein immunohistochemistry in neurooncology: A progress report. Pathol Res Pract 1980; 168:374.

18. De la Monte SM: Uniform lineage of oligodendroglioma. Am J Pathol 1989; 135:529.

19. Deck JHN, Eng L, Bigbee J, et al: The role of glial fibrillary acidic protein in the diagnosis of central nervous system tumors. Acta Neuropathol 1978; 42:183.

20. Dinda AK, Sarkar C, Roy S: Rosenthal's fibres: An immunohistochemical, ultrastructural and immunoelectron microscopic study. Acta Neuropathol 1990; 79:456.

21. Doherty FJ, Wassell JA, Mayer RJ: A putative protein sequestration site involving intermediate filaments for protein degradation by autophagy: Studies with micro-injected glycolytic enzymes. Biochem J 1987; 241:793.

22. Duffy PE: Astrocytes: Normal, Reactive and Neoplastic. New York, Raven Press, 1983.

23. Duffy PE, Graf L, Huang YY, et al: Glial fibrillary acidic protein in ependymomas and other brain tumors: Distribution, diagnostic criteria, and relation to formation of processes. J Neurol Sci 1979; 40:133.

24. Duffy PE, Huang YY, Graf L: Glial fibrillary acidic protein in giant cell tumors of brain and other gliomas. Acta Neuropathol 1980; 52:51.

25. Eng LF, Rubinstein LF: Contribution of immunohistochemistry to diagnostic problems of human cerebral tumors. J Histochem Cytochem 1978; 26:513.

26. Eng LF, Vanderhaeghen JJ, Bignami A, et al: An acidic protein isolated from fibrous astrocytes. Brain Res 1971; 28:351.

27. Erickson HP, Bourdon MA: Tenascin: An extracellular matrix protein prominent in specialized embryonic tissue and tumors. Annu Rev Cell Biol 1989; 5:71.

28. Escourolle R, Poirier J: Étude en microscopie èlectronique des tumeurs du système nerveux. Neurochir 1971; 25:1.

29. Fedoroff S, White R, Neal J, et al: Astrocyte cell lineage: II Mouse fibrous astrocytes and reactive astrocytes in cultures have vimentin and GFAP containing intermediate filaments. Dev Brain Res 1983; 7:303.

30. Feigin I, Allen LB, Lipkin L, et al: The endothelial hyperplasia of the cerebral blood vessels with brain tumors and its sarcomatous transformation. Cancer 1958; 11:264.

31. Franke FE, Schachenmayr W, Osborn M, et al: Unexpected immunoreactivities of intermediate filament antibodies in human brain and brain tumors. Am J Pathol 1991; 139:67.

32. Friede RL, Pollack A: The cytogenetic basis for classifying ependymomas. J Neuropathol Exp Neurol 1978; 37:103.

33. Geisler N, Plessmann U, Weber K: Related amino acid sequences in neurofilament and non-neuronal intermediate filaments. Nature 1982; 296:448.

34. Giangaspero F, Burger PC: Correlations between cytologic composition and biological behavior in the glioblastoma multiforme: A postmortem study of 50 cases. Cancer 1983; 52:2320.

35. Giordana MT, Germano I, Giaccone G, et al: The distribution of laminin in human brain tumors: An immunohistochemical study. Acta Neuropathol 1985; 67:51.

36. Giordana MT, Schiffer D, Mauro A, et al: Transplacental ENU tumors of the rat: Immunohistochemical contribution to the recognition of cell types. In Walker MD, Thomas DGT (eds): Biology of Brain Tumor. Boston, Nijhoff, 1986, p 121.

37. Globus JH: Malformations in the central nervous system. In Penfield W (ed): Cytology and Cellular Pathology of the Nervous System. New York, Hoeffer, 1932.

38. Grant JW, Steart PV, Aguzzi A, et al: Gliosarcoma: An immunohistochemical study. Acta Neuropathol 1989; 79:305.

39. Gullotta F: Kleinhirngeschwülste des Kindesalters (eine vergleichende elektronen-optische und Gewebekulturuntersuchung). Verh Dtsch Ges Pathol 1971; 55:315.

40. Gullotta F, Fliedner E: Spongioblastomas, astrocytomas and Rosenthal fibres: Ultrastructural, tissue culture and enzyme histochemical investigations. Acta Neuropathol 1972; 22:68.

41. Haddad SF, Moore SA, Schelper RL, et al: Smooth muscle cells can comprise the sarcomatous component of gliosarcoma. J Neuropathol Exp Neurol 1991; 50:1036.

42. Haddad SF, Moore SA, Schelper RL, et al: Vascular smooth muscle hyperplasia underlies the formation of glomeruloid vascular structures of glioblastoma multiforme. J Neuropathol Exp Neurol 1992; 51:488.

43. Haddad SF, Moore SA, Schelper RL, et al: Smooth muscle can comprise the sarcomatous component of gliosarcomas. J Neuropathol Exp Neurol 1992; 51:493.

44. Haglid K, Carlsson CA, Stavrou D: An immunological study of human brain tumors concerning the brain specific proteins S-100 and 14.3.2. Acta Neuropathol 1973; 24:187.

45. Hay ED: Extracellular matrix. J Cell Biol 1981; 91:205s.

46. Heldin CH, Westermark B, Wasteson A: Specific receptors for platelet-derived growth factor on cell derived from connective tissue and glial. Proc Natl Acad Sci USA 1981;78:3664.

47. Herman IM, D'Amore PA: Microvascular pericytes contain muscle and non-muscle actins. J Cell Biol 1985; 101:42.

48. Herpers MJHM, Budka H: Glial fibrillary acidic protein (GFAP) in oligodendroglial tumors: Gliofibrillary oligodendroglioma and transitional oligoastrocytoma as subtypes of oligodendroglioma. Acta Neuropathol 1984; 64:265.

49. Herpers MJHM, Ramaekers FCS, Aldeweireldt J, et al: Co-expression of glial fibrillary acidic protein and vimentin-type intermediate filaments in human astrocytomas. Acta Neuropathol 1986; 70:333.

50. Hickey WF, Lee V, Trojanowski JQ, et al: Immunohistochemical application of monoclonal antibodies against myelin basic protein and neurofilament triplet protein subunits: Advantage over antisera and technical limitations. J Histochem Cytochem 1983; 31:1126.

51. Higuchi M, Ohnishi T, Arita N, et al: Immunohistochemical localization of fibronectin, laminin and fibronectin-receptor in human malignant gliomas: In relation to tumor invasion. Brain Nerve 1991; 43:17.

52. Higuchi M, Ohnishi T, Arita N, et al: Expression of tenascin in human gliomas: Its relation to histological malignancy, tumor dedifferentiation and angiogenesis. Acta Neuropathol 1993; 85:481.

53. Hirato J, Nakazato Y, Ogawa A: Expression of non-glial intermediate filament in gliomas. Clin Neuropathol 1994; 13:1.

54. Hoshino T: Cellular aspects of human brain tumors (gliomas). Neurobiology 1981; 2:167.

55. Hossmann KA, Wechsler W: Zur Feinstruktur menschlicher Spongioblastome. Dtsch Ztschr Nervenheilk 1965; 187:327.

56. Houle J, Fedoroff S: Temporal relationship between the appearance of vimentin and neural tube development. Dev Brain Res 1983; 9:189.

57. Hydén H, McEwen B: A glial protein specific for the nervous system. Proc Natl Acad Sci USA 1986; 55:354.

58. Ikeda U, Ikeda M, Oohara T, et al: Mitogenic action of interleukin-1a on vascular smooth muscle cells mediated by PDGF. Atherosclerosis 1990; 84:183.

59. Itoyama Y, Sternberger NH, Kies MW, et al: Immunocytochemical method to identify myelin basic protein in oligodendroglia and myelin sheaths of the human nervous system. Ann Neurol 1980; 7:157.

60. Jones H, Steart PV, Weller RO: Spindle-cell glioblastoma or gliosarcoma? Neuropathol Appl Neurobiol 1991; 17:177.

61. Kamitani H, Masuzawa H, Sato J, et al: Mixed oligodendroglioma and astrocytoma: Fine structural and immunohistochemical studies of four cases. J Neurol Sci 1988; 83:219.

62. Kepes JJ: Pleomorphic xanthoastrocytoma: The birth of a diagnosis and a concept. Brain Pathol 1993; 3:269.

63. Kepes JJ, Kepes M, Slowik F: Fibrous xanthomas and xanthosarcomas of the meninges and the brain. Acta Neuropathol 1973; 23:187.

64. Kepes JJ, Rubinstein LJ, Eng LF: Meningocerebral xanthoastrocytoma: A distinctive glioma of young subjects presumably originating from subpial astrocytes, with relatively favorable prognosis: A study of ten cases. Proceedings of the 8th International Congress on Neuropathology, Washington, DC, 1978, p 641.

65. Kepes JJ, Fulling KH, Garcia JH: The clinical significance of ''adenoid'' formations of neoplastic astrocytes, imitating metastatic carcinoma, in gliosarcomas: A review of five cases. Clin Neuropathol 1982; 1:139.

66. Kim SU: Antigen expression by glial cells grown in culture. J Neuroimmunol 1985; 8:255.

67. Kimura N, Sasano N, Ishioka K: Use of formaldehyde-induced fluorescence for cytological diagnosis of pheochromocytoma. Acta Pathol Japan 1986; 36:1049.

68. Kochi N, Budka H: Contribution of histiocytic cells to sarcomatous development of the gliosarcoma. Acta Neuropathol 1987; 73:124.

69. Kros JM, De Jono AAW, Van der Kwast THH: Ultrastructural characterization of transitional cells in oligodendrogliomas. J Neuropathol Exp Neurol 1992; 51:186.

70. Kros JM, van Eden CG, Stefanko SZ, et al: Prognostic implications of glial fibrillary acidic protein containing cell types in oligodendrogliomas. Cancer 1991; 66:1204.

71. Kros JM, Vecht CJ, Stefanko SZ: The pleomorphic xanthoastrocytoma and its differential diagnosis: A study of five cases. Hum Pathol 1991; 22:1128.

72. Kuhajda FP, Mendelsohn G, Taxy JB: Pleomorphic xanthoastrocytoma: Report of a case with light and electron microscopy. Ultrastruct Pathol 1981; 2:25.

73. Kumar P, Kumar S, Marsden HB, et al: Weibel-Palade bodies in endothelial cells as a marker for angiogenesis in brain tumors. Cancer Res 1980; 40:2010.

74. Kumpulainen T, Korhonen LK: Immunohistochemical localization of carbonic anhydrase isoenzyme C in central and peripheral nervous system of the mouse. J Histochem Cytochem 1982; 30:283.

75. Kunz J, Gottschalk J, Jänisch W, et al: Zellproliferation und Expression des säuren Gliafaserproteins (GFAP) in Hirntumoren. Acta Histochem 1986; 80:53.

76. Laurie GW, Leblond CP, Martin GR: Localization of type IV collagen, laminin, heparan sulfate proteoglycan and fibronectin to the basal lamina of basement membrane. J Cell Biol 1982; 95:340.

77. Lipinski M, Braham K, Cailland J-M, et al: The HNK-1 antibody detects an antigen expressed on neuroectodermal cells. J Exp Med 1983; 158:1773.

78. Lotz MM, Burdsal CA, Erickson HP, et al: Cell adhesion to fibronectin and tenascin: Quantitative measurements of initial binding and subsequent strengthening response. J Cell Biol 1989; 109:1795.

79. Lowe J, Morrell K, Lennox G, et al: Rosenthal fibres are based on the ubiquitination of glial filaments. Neuropathol Appl Neurobiol 1989; 15:45.

80. Ludwin SK, Kosek JC, Eng LF: The topographical distribution of S-100 and GFAP proteins in the adult rat brain: An immunohistochemical study using horseradish peroxidase-labeled antibodies. J Comp Neurol 1976; 165:197.

81. Mannoji H, Becker LE: Ependymal and choroid plexus tumors: Cytokeratin and GFAP expression. Cancer 1988; 61:1377.

82. Marsden HB, Kumar S, Kahn J, et al: A study of glial fibrillary brain tumours. Int J Cancer 1983; 31:439.

83. Matus A, Mughal S: Immunohistochemical localization of S-100 protein in brain. Nature 1975; 258:746.

84. Mauro A, Bertolotto A, Germano I, et al: Collagenase in the immunohistochemical demonstration of laminin, fibronectin and Factor VIII/RAg in nervous tissue after fixation. Histochemistry 1984; 80:157.

85. McComb RD, Moul JM, Bigner DD: Distribution of type VI collagen in human gliomas: Comparison with fibronectin and glioma-mesenchymal matric glycoprotein. J Neuropathol Exp Neurol 1987; 46:623.

86. McComb RD, Jones TR, Pizzo SV, et al: Specificity and sensitivity of immunohistochemical detection of factor VIII/von Willebrand factor antigen in formalin-fixed paraffin-embedded tissue. J Histochem Cytochem 1982; 30:371.

87. McComb RD, Jones TR, Pizzo SV, et al: Immunohistochemical detection of factor VIII/von Willebrand factor in hyperplastic endothelial cells in glioblastoma multiforme and mixed glioma sarcoma. J Neuropathol Exp Neurol 1982; 41:479.

88. Meneses AC, Kepes JJ, Sternberger NH: Astrocytic differentiation of neoplastic oligodendrocytes. J Neuropathol Exp Neurol 1982; 41:368.

89. Mepham BL, Frater W, Mitchell RS: The use of proteolytic enzymes to improve immunoglobulin staining by the PAP technique. Histochem J 1979; 11:345.

90. Miettinen M, Clark R, Virtanen I: Intermediate filament proteins in choroid plexus and ependyma and their tumors. Am J Pathol 1986; 123:231.

91. Migheli A, Attanasio A, Mocellini C, et al: Ultrastructural localization of factor VIII-related antigen in endothelial proliferations of malignant gliomas. Neuropathol Appl Neurobiol 1991; 17:11.

92. Migheli A, Mocellini C: Ultrastructural immunocytochemistry in glial tumors. J Neurosurg Sci 1990; 34:219.

93. Miyagami M, Smith BH, McKeever PE, et al: Immunocytochemical localization of factor VIII-related antigen in tumors of the central nervous system. J Neurooncol 1987; 4:269.

94. Mörk SJ, Rubinstein LJ, Kepes JJ, et al: Patterns of epithelial metaplasia in malignant gliomas: II. Squamous differentiation of epithelial-like formation in gliosarcomas and glioblastomas. J Neuropathol Exp Neurol 1988; 47:101.

95. Motoi M, Yoshino T, Hayashi K, et al: Immunohistochemical studies on human brain tumors using anti-Leu7 monoclonal antibody in paraffin-embedded specimens. Acta Neuropathol 1985; 66:75.

96. Mukai K, Rosai J: Factor VIII-related antigen: An endothelial marker. In De Lellis RA (ed): Advances in Immunohistochemistry. New York, Masson, 1984, p 253.

97. Nakagawa Y, Perentes E, Rubinstein LJ: Immunohistochemical characterization of oligodendrogliomas: An analysis of multiple markers. Acta Neuropathol 1986; 72:15.

98. Nakajima T, Kameya T, Watanabe S, et al: S-100 protein distribution in normal and neoplastic tissues. In De Lellis RA (ed): Advances in Immunohistochemistry. New York, Masson, 1984, p 141.

99. Nakamura Y, Becker LE: Subependymal giant-cell tumor: Astrocytic or neuronal? Acta Neuropathol 1983; 60:271.

100. Nakamura Y, Becker LE, Marks A: Distribution of immunoreactive S-100 protein in pediatric brain tumors. J Neuropathol Exp Neurol 1983; 43:136.

101. Nakopoulou L, Kerezoudi E, Thomaiodes T, et al: An immunocytochemical comparison of glial fibrillary acidic protein, S-100p and vimentin in human glial tumors. J Neurooncol 1990; 8:33.

102. Nobile-Orazio E, Hays AP, Laton N, et al: Specificity of mouse and human monoclonal antibodies to myelin-associated glycoprotein. Neurology 1984; 34:1336.

103. Norenberg MD: The distribution of glutamine synthetase in the rat central nervous system. J Histochem Cytochem 1979; 27:756.

104. Norenberg MD, Martinez-Hernandez A: Fine structural localization of glutamine synthetase in astrocytes of rat brain. Brain Res 1979; 161:303.

105. Paulus W, Grothe C, Sensenbrenner M: Localization of basic fibroblastic growth factor, a mitogen and angiogenic factor, in human brain tumors. Acta Neuropathol 1990; 79:418.

106. Paulus W, Jellinger K: Desmoplastic spindle-cell glioblastoma or gliosarcoma? (letter to the editor). Neuropathol Appl Neurobiol 1992; 18:207.

107. Paulus W, Peiffer J: Does the pleomorphic xanthoastrocytoma exist? Problems in the application of immunological techniques to the classification of brain tumors. Acta Neuropathol 1988; 76:245.

108. Paulus W, Peiffer J: History, histology, histochemistry and histiocytic histogenesis of the pleomorphic xanthoastrocytoma. Noshuyo Byori 1991; 8:67.

109. Perentes E, Rubinstein LJ: Immunohistochemical recognition of human neuroepithelial tumors by anti-Leu-7 (HNK-1) monoclonal antibody. Acta Neuropathol 1986; 69:227.

110. Peters A, Palay SL, Webster HD: The fine structure of the nervous system: The neurons and supporting cells. Philadelphia, WB Saunders, 1976.

111. Pilkington GJ, Lantos PL: The role of glutamine synthetase in the diagnosis of cerebral tumours. Neuropathol Appl Neurobiol 1982; 8:227.

112. Pipmeier JM, Fried I, Makuch R: Low-grade astrocytomas may arise from different astrocyte lineages. Neurosurgery 1993; 33:627.

113. Pixley SK, de Vellis J: Transition between immature radial glia and mature astrocytes studied with a monoclonal antibody to vimentin. Dev Brain Res 1984; 15:201.

114. Plate KH, Breier G, Weich HA, et al: Vascular endothelial growth factor is a potential tumour angiogenesis factor in human gliomas in vivo. Nature 1992; 359:845.

115. Pruss RM, Mirsky R, Raff MC: All classes of intermediate filaments share a common antigenic determinant defined by a monoclonal antibody. Cell 1981; 27:419.

116. Puchtler H, Meloan SN: On the chemistry of formaldehyde fixation and its effects on immunohistochemical reactions. Histochemistry 1985; 82:201.

117. Raff MC: Glial cell diversification in the rat optic nerve. Science 1989; 243:1450.

118. Raff MC, Abney ER, Miller RH: Two glial cell lineages diverge prenatally in rat optic nerve. Dev Biol 1984; 106:53.

119. Ramaekers FCS, Puts JJG, Kant A, et al: Antibodies to intermediate filaments as a tool in tumor diagnosis. Cell Biol Int Rep 1983; 6:652.

120. Robertson DM, Hendry WS, Vogel FS: Central ganglioneuroma: A case study using electron microscopy. J Neuropathol Exp Neurol 1964; 23:692.

121. Robinson RA, Teneyck CJ, Hart MN: Growth control in cerebral microvessels-derived endothelial cells. Brain Res 1986; 384:114.

122. Roessmann U, Velasco ME, Sindely SD, et al: Glial fibrillary acidic protein (GFAP) in ependymal cells during development: An immunohistochemical study. Brain Res 1980; 200:13.

123. Rubinstein LJ, Herman MM: A light- and electron microscopic study of a temporal-lobe ganglioglioma. J Neurol Sci 1972; 16:27.

124. Russell DS, Rubinstein LJ: Pathology of Tumours of the Nervous System, ed 4. London, Arnold, 1977.

125. Russell DS, Rubinstein LJ: Pathology of Tumours of the Nervous System, ed 5. London, Arnold, 1989.

126. Sachinidis A, Locher R, Vetter W, et al: Different effects of platelet-derived growth factor isoforms on rat vascular smooth muscle cells. J Biol Chem 1990; 265:10238.

127. Sarkar C, Roy S, Tandon PN: Oligodendroglial tumors: An immunohistochemical and electron microscopic study. Cancer 1988; 61:1862.

128. Schiffer D: Brain Tumors: Pathology and its Biological Correlates. Berlin, Springer-Verlag, 1993.

129. Schiffer D, Chiò A, Cravioto H, et al: Ependymoma: Internal correlations among pathologic signs and the anaplastic variant. Neurosurgery 1991; 29:206.

130. Schiffer D, Chiò A, Giordana MT, et al: The vascular response to tumor infiltration in malignant gliomas: Morphometric and reconstruction study. Acta Neuropathol 1989; 77:369.

131. Schiffer D, Giordana MT, Germano I, et al: Anaplasia and heterogeneity of GFAP expression in gliomas. Tumori 1986; 72:163.

132. Schiffer D, Giordana MT, Mauro A, et al: Glial fibrillary acidic protein (GFAP) in human cerebral tumors: An immunohistochemical study. Tumori 1983; 69:95.

133. Schiffer D, Giordana MT, Mauro A, et al: GFAP, FVIII/RAg, laminin, and fibronectin in gliosarcomas: An immunohistochemical study. Acta Neuropathol 1984; 63:108.

134. Schiffer D, Giordana MT, Mauro A, et al: Reactive astrocytes in the morphologic composition of peripheral areas of gliomas. Tumori 1988; 74:411.

135. Schiffer D, Giordana MT, Mauro A, et al: Immunohistochemical demonstration of vimentin in human cerebral tumors. Acta Neuropathol 1986; 70:209.

136. Schlote W: Behaviour of blastomatous astrocytes in the human cerebral white matter: An electron microscopic study. J Neuropathol Exp Neurol 1966; 25:173.

137. Schnitzer J, Franke WW, Schachner M: Immunocytochemical demonstration of vimentin in astrocytes and ependymal cells of developing and adult mouse nervous system. J Cell Biol 1981; 90:435.

138. Schwartz SM, Campbell GR, Campbell JH: Replication of smooth muscle cells in vascular disease. Circ Res 1986; 58:427.

139. Shweiki D, Itin A, Soffer D, et al: Vascular endothelial growth factor induced by hypoxia may mediate hypoxia-initiated angiogenesis. Nature 1992; 359:843.

140. Sima AAF, Robertson DM: Subependymal giant-cell astrocytoma: Case report with ultrastructural study. J Neurosurg 1979; 50:240.

141. Siri A, Carnemolla B, Saginati M, et al: Human tenascin: Primary structure, pre-mRNA splicing patterns and localization of the epitopes recognized by two monoclonal antibodies. Nucleic Acids Res 1991; 19:525.

142. Skalli O, Ropraz P, Trzeciak A, et al: A monoclonal antibody against a-smooth muscle actin: A new probe for muscle differentiation. J Cell Biol 1986; 103:2787.

143. Slowik F, Jellinger K, Gaszo L, et al: Gliosarcomas: Histological, immunohistochemical, ultrastructural, and tissue culture studies. Acta Neuropathol 1985; 67:201.

144. Smith DA, Lantos PL: Immunocytochemistry of cerebellar astrocytomas: With a special note on Rosenthal fibres. Acta Neuropathol 1985; 66:155.

145. Stefansson K, Wolmann R: Distribution of the neuronal specific protein, 14-3-2, in central nervous system lesions of tuberous sclerosis. Acta Neuropathol 1981; 53:113.

146. Sternberger NH, Itoyama Y, Kies MW, et al: Immunocytochemical method to identify basic protein in myelin-forming oligodendrocytes of newborn rat CNS. J Neurocytol 1978; 7:251.

147. Sternberger NH, Itoyama Y, Kies MW, et al: Myelin basic protein demonstrated immunocytochemically in oligodendroglia prior to myelin sheath formation. Proc Natl Acad Sci USA 1978; 75:2521.

148. Tabuchi K, Moriya J, Furuta T, et al: S 100 protein in human glial tumours: Qualitative and quantitative study. Acta Neurochir 1982; 65:239.

149. Takahashi K, Isobe T, Ohtsuki Y, et al: Immunohistochemical study of the distribution of α e β subunits of S-100 protein in human neoplasms and normal tissues. Virchows Arch B Cell Pathol 1984; 45:385.

150. Timpl R, Rohde H, Robey PG, et al: Laminin: A glycoprotein from basement membranes. J Biol Chem 1979; 254:9933.

151. Tsukada T, Tippens D, Gordon D, et al: HHF35, a muscle-actin-specific monoclonal antibody: I. Immunocytochemical and biochemical characterization. Am J Pathol 1986; 126:51.

152. Vaheri A, Mosher DF: High molecular weight, cell surface-associated glycoprotein (fibronectin) lost in malignant transformation. Biochem Biophys Acta 1978; 516:1.

153. Van der Meulen JD, Houthoff HJ, Ebels EJ: Glial fibrillary acidic protein in human gliomas. Neuropathol Appl Neurobiol 1978; 4:177.

154. VandenBerg SR: Current diagnostic concepts of astrocytic tumors. J Neuropathol Exp Neurol 1992; 51:664.

155. VandenBerg SR, May EE, Rubinstein LJ, et al: Desmoplastic supratentorial neuroepithelial tumors of infancy with divergent differentiation potential ('desmoplastic infantile gangliogliomas'): Report on 11 cases of a distinctive embryonal tumor with favorable prognosis. J Neurosurg 1987; 66:58.

156. Velasco ME, Dahl D, Roessmann U, et al: Immunohistochemical localization of glial fibrillary acidic protein in human glial neoplasms. Cancer 1980; 45:484.

157. Vraa-Jensen J, Herman MNM, Rubinstein LJ, et al: In vitro characteristics of a fourth ventricle ependymoma maintained in organ culture systems: Light and electron microscopic observations. Neuropathol Appl Neurobiol 1976; 2:349.

158. Weiss SW, Langloss JM, Enzinger FM: Value of S-100 protein in the diagnosis of soft tissue tumors with particular reference to benign and malignant Schwann cell tumors. Lab Invest 1983; 49:299.

159. Weller RO, Davis BE, Wilson POG, et al: Capillary proliferation in cerebral infarction, gliomas, angioblastic meningiomas, and hemangioblastomas. In Cervòs-Navarro J, Fritschka E (eds): Cerebral Microcirculation and Metabolism. New York, Raven, 1979, p 41.

160. Weller RO, Foy M, Cox S: The development and ultrastructure of the microvasculature in malignant gliomas. Neuropathol Appl Neurobiol 1977; 3:303.

161. Wesseling P, Vandersteenhoven JJ, Downey BT, et al: Cellular components of microvascular proliferation in human glial and metastatic brain neoplasms. Acta Neuropathol 1993; 85:508.

162. Westphal M, Herrmann HD: Growth factor biology and oncogene activation in human gliomas and their implications for specific therapeutic concepts. Neurosurgery 1989; 25:681.

163. Yung WKA, Luna M, Borit A: Vimentin and glial fibrillary acidic protein (GFAP) in human brain tumors. J Neurooncol 1985; 3:35.

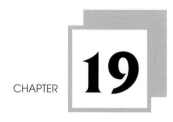

CHAPTER **19**

Cell Kinetics

The mixed nature of the cellular components of human gliomas and their morphologic complexity are well documented. This heterogeneity encompasses chromosomal abnormalities, variability in proliferation kinetics, and variations in DNA content.

Since the concept of a cell cycle was introduced by Howard and Pelc[1] in 1953, many investigators have sought to determine the cell kinetics of normally and abnormally proliferating tissues in vivo and in vitro. The synthesis of tritiated (^{3}H)-thymidine led to the development of many sophisticated approaches to define the rate and pattern of cellular proliferation. The *labeling index* (LI), which is the proportion of tumor cells engaged in DNA synthesis (S phase) in preparation for mitosis, and which can be obtained by autoradiography of tumor tissue exposed to a pulse of ^{3}H-thymidine, have helped in understanding the malignancy and the proliferative activity of gliomas. Flow cytometry has made it possible to efficiently and accurately quantitate multiple cell populations in terms of DNA content from fresh specimens of gliomas. The development of a monoclonal antibody against bromodeoxyuridine was a breakthrough for quantitating the proliferative potential of individual tumors without time-consuming procedures or ethical problems, as occurred in the study using ^{3}H-thymidine.

This chapter describes some theoretical background of cell kinetics, and introduces basic and clinical data for gliomas obtained by the three methods just mentioned. Most of the analyses were performed by Hoshino, a great pioneer in the field on neuro-oncology, and his study group.

PHASES OF THE CELL CYCLE

Each proliferating cell passes through four separate stages, defined on the basis of nuclear DNA content (Fig. 19–1). The most easily identifiable stage (by light microscopy) is the mitotic phase (M phase), during which the previously duplicated chromosomes are distributed to the two daughter cells. These daughter cells then enter the postmitotic gap (pre-DNA synthetic or G1 phase), during which they synthesize RNA, enzymes, and proteins in preparation for the beginning of DNA syntheses. From the G1 phase, cells progress into the DNA synthetic phase (S phase), in which

they replicate DNA. When exogenous thymidine, or thymidine analog (bromodeoxyuridine or iododeoxyuridine) is available to a population of proliferating cells, only the cells in the S phase can incorporate them into their nuclear DNA. Chromosomal duplication is completed by the end of the S phase. Following the S phase, another gap (post-DNA synthetic, premitotic, or G2 phase) occurs, during which RNA and proteins are made in preparation for the ensuing mitosis and the completion of the cell cycle. Cell cycle time, therefore, is a sum of the duration of these four phases.

Cells in the G1, S, and G2 phases are called *intermitotic cells*, in contrast to cells in the mitotic phase. In the G1 phase, the amount of DNA in the nucleus, which is normally 2C (representing a diploid amount of DNA), increases during the S phase to 4C (a tetraploid complement of DNA) at the completion of DNA synthesis. The DNA complement remains 4C throughout the G2 phase.

In many cell populations, a non-proliferating group of cells, designated as G0 cells, leave the cell cycle as G1 cells instead of progressing into the S phase, and therefore carry a 2C DNA complement. Other G0 cells leave the cell cycle in the G2 phase and carry double the normal DNA complement (4C) in their nuclei. These resting, or G0, cells may remain viable but reproductively inactive for extended periods. Physical crowding and nutrient depletion are conditions that encourage the movement of cells into the non-proliferating compartment, and the majority of cells in large tumors may reside there. Not all G0 cells are sterile, and they can re-enter the proliferating pool of cycling cells and proceed through the G1, S, G2, and M phases in a normal manner.

Growth fraction is a ratio of proliferating cells to the entire population. Growth fraction is less than 1.0 in most tumors, and tumor population doubling time invariably exceeds cell cycle time. Cells in the proliferating pool must divide more than once to double the total population because non-proliferating cells contribute nothing and, further, because cell death acts to reduce the population.

Cell loss in a tumor is recognized by the presence of individual dead cells, massive or focal necrosis, and exfoliation of cells from the tumor mass, although quantitative estimation of the rate of loss is difficult. To express the magnitude of cell loss, Steel[2] defined the *cell loss factor*

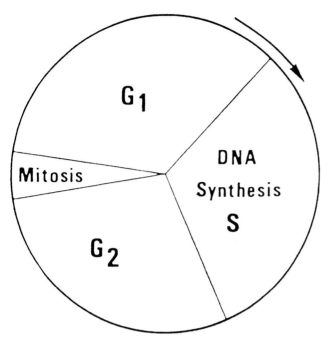

Figure 19–1 Diagram of a cell cycle.

(CLF) as a fraction of the rate at which cells are added to the total population by mitoses. Thus, a CLF of 1.0 (or 100%) indicates that cell loss is counterbalanced by cell production, with neither growth nor regression of tumor (i.e., the total cell population remains constant). At the other extreme, a CLF of 0 implies exponential growth without cell loss. A value between these two indicates that the fraction of newborn cells that are offset by concurrent loss of cells results in greater cell loss, smaller growth fraction, and longer doubling time.

³H-THYMIDINE AUTORADIOGRAPHY

The cells in the S phase are labeled by a pulse of ³H-thymidine, and the fraction of labeled cells (LI) has been used to estimate the approximate proliferative ability of the tissue investigated.

The growth fraction (GF) was calculated from a ratio of the observed LI to the theoretical LI. The theoretical LI, representing the number of cells in S phase compared with the total number of cells in the proliferating pool, could be calculated from the ratio of the number of labeled mitoses of total mitoses, as developed by Mendelsohn.[3] By injecting ³H-thymidine prior to mitostatic agent (vincristine or vinblastine), a modification of stathmokinetic analysis, it becomes possible to estimate the cell cycle time (Tc).[4] The equation is as follows:

$$Tc = t \log 2 / \log (1 + Mt(t)/GF$$

Hoshino and Wilson[4] administered 5 to 10 mCi (millicuries) of ³H-thymidine to 28 patients with gliomas, and counted the number of labeled cells on the autoradiographs. They also made a stathmokinetic study, mentioned earlier. All glioblastomas except one had an LI of more than 5%;

most anaplastic astrocytomas had an LI of 1% to 4%; and well-differentiated gliomas exhibited an LI of less than 1%. Average LIs were 9.3% for all glioblastomas, 4.0% for anaplastic astrocytomas, and 1% for differentiated gliomas. The GFs of malignant gliomas varied from 0.14 to 0.44 (mean, 0.31). Tc values calculated for eight cases of malignant gliomas were within a range of 2 to 3 days, with two exceptions. Tc appears to have little relationship to the LI or GF of any tumor type. By plotting the value of GF against the corresponding LI, a linear correlation between the two was demonstrated, with an equation of GF = 1.22 × (LI)[0.6]. These researchers concluded that the main factor that predicted biologic malignancy was GF, and that this GF could be estimated fairly accurately from the LI of individual tumors.

When patients died who had been given ³H-thymidine before surgery for cell kinetic studies, the second autoradiography of autopsied materials provided more important information. Hoshino and colleagues[5] estimated the LIs of nine autopsied gliomas (five glioblastoma, three anaplastic astrocytoma, and one mixed glioma). It was found that two of the glioblastomas and one of the anaplastic astrocytomas diluted out the labeling in the 2- to 4-month interval between labeling and autopsy, whereas three other glioblastomas, the two anaplastic astrocytomas, and one mixed glioma, retained labeled neoplastic cells at autopsy, after intervals of from 3 weeks to 7 years following labeling. This indicates that some cells stop dividing, even in a favorable environment. Truly malignant cells (those with an unlimited capacity to proliferate) do not stop dividing. The presence of a few labeled cells in these tumors establishes that differentiating tumor cells can survive for as long as 7 years with only a few divisions. Most patients whose tumors demonstrated foci of labeled cells at autopsy survived longer (1.5 to 7 years).

Cell kinetic parameters are also estimated by measuring actual tumor growth clinically. Matsutani and Hoshino[6] analyzed seven glioblastoma patients who underwent macroscopic total removal of a glioblastoma and who experienced recurrence at a later date. Assuming a GF of approximately 0.3, they calculated a cell cycle time in the range of 1.4 to 2.4 days, not unlike the estimated times previously calculated by Mendelsohn.[3] Tsuboi and others[7] calculated the tumor doubling time in 27 gliomas from the change in volume of enhanced and low-density areas on CT scans; it was 43.8 ± 7.6 days in malignant astrocytomas and 31.2 ± 7.7 days in glioblastomas.

FLOW CYTOMETRY

The development of flow cytometry has made it possible to obtain a measurement similar to the autoradiographic LI by quantifying the intensity of DNA fluorescence in individual tumor cells.[8, 9] The technique, which relies on the quantification of fluorescence emitted by a DNA-bound dye as tumor cell nuclei rapidly flow past a high-intensity laser beam, permits the construction of peaks showing the relative frequency of cell populations with diploid and multiploid karyotypes; from those peaks may be derived the relative percentage of cells in DNA synthesis.

The first peak (2C-area) represents postmitotic or presynthetic (G1) cell nuclei as well as non-proliferating G0 cell nuclei (Fig. 19–2). In this area also irreversible postmitotic and dead cells with diploid DNA content will be found. The second (4C) peak already indicates a certain amount of proliferative activity. This area contains cell in premitotic G2 or M phase. The intermediate slope between the 2C and 4C peaks and the hyperploid peaks, respectively, contain cell nuclei in the S phase. Theoretically, it will increase at a growing proliferative activity and show a relative prolongation of the S phase in cell cycle.

Malignant human gliomas have a highly variable distribution of cell nuclei, consisting of diploid and/or other populations in terms of nuclear DNA content.[8, 10] Hohsino and others[11] studied in vitro clonogenicity of each population detected by flow cytometry. The colony-formation efficiencies of the individual populations sorted according to DNA content were similar within individual tumors. These results suggest not only that malignant gliomas are composed of multiple populations in terms of DNA content, but also that each of these populations contains clonogenic cells. The morphologic structure of cells within and among colonies did not appear to relate to DNA content.

Vavruch and associates,[12] using flow cytometry, compared the DNA index and the S-phase measurement of fresh cells with those of fixed paraffin-embedded specimens from 33 astrocytic tumors; they demonstrated a significant correlation between the two specimens regarding the S phase and the DNA index.

BROMODEOXYURIDINE LABELING

Gratzner[13] developed a monoclonal antibody against bromodeoxyuridine and iododeoxyuridine, which are thymidine analogs that can be detected by direct conjugation of fluorescein isothiocyanate (FITC) to the antibody, by indirect conjugation of FITC using an FITC-tagged secondary antibody, or by immunoperoxidase methods. The immunoperoxidase method is based on the immunoperoxidase demonstration of bromodeoxyuridine, which is incorporated into the nuclear DNA of cells in S phase after intravenous injection at the time of craniotomy.[14] Compared with autoradiography, the technique has the advantages of speed and of avoiding possible radiation hazard and myelotoxicity. The results of Hoshino and colleagues[15] indicate that the LI provided by this procedure are closely similar to those obtained with the much more laborious technique of autoradiography.

Hoshino and others[16] studied bromodeoxyuridine LIs of 127 primary gliomas and 55 recurrent gliomas with immunohistochemical method. The mean and median bromodeoxyuridine LIs of primary tumors were 8.6% in glioblastomas, 4.6% in highly anaplastic astrocytomas, and 1.2% in moderately anaplastic astrocytomas. Highly anaplastic and moderately anaplastic astrocytomas from patients older than 50 years had significantly higher LIs than those from younger patients, whereas no age-related difference in LIs was seen in the glioblastomas. A follow-up study of the patients revealed that the probability of survival was higher in patients with tumor LIs less than 1% than in those with LIs greater than 5%, and that patients with tumor LIs of 1% to 5% had an intermediate probability of survival.

Fujimaki and associates[17] estimated bromodeoxyuridine LIs of 50 consecutive adult patients with cerebral astrocytic tumors (10 differentiated astrocytomas, 12 anaplastic astrocytomas, and 28 glioblastomas). The obtained LIs distributed continuously in a broad range from 0% to 19%, with well-differentiated tumor cells having the lowest LI and poorly differentiated ones having the highest (Fig. 19–3). These findings indicate the continuity of astrocytic tumors from the point of view of their proliferative potential, although the World Health Organization classification,[18] and others proposed by Nelson and others[19] and Burger and colleagues,[20] divides astrocytic tumors roughly into three groups, disregarding their continuity. The mean LIs were 8.5% in glioblastomas, 4.2% in anaplastic astrocytomas, and 1.2% in well-differentiated astrocytomas. When patients were subdivided into three groups according to their LI (i.e., more than 5%, 3% to 5%, and less than 3%), the median recurrence-free period was 9.0 months, 14.7 months, and more than 36.0 months, respectively. The difference among three groups was significantly different.

In both studies reported by Hoshino and co-workers[16] and Fujimaki and colleagues,[17] the average LI of each glioma was similar and was significantly different between the three tumor types, suggesting that the LI reflects histologic malignancy.

The optimal radiation dose for glioblastoma cells was

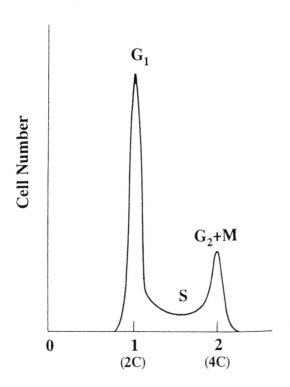

Relative Fluorescence Intensity

Figure 19–2 A flow cytometric profile of a growing cell. The relative fluorescence intensity values of 1 and 2 correspond to the position of nuclei with a 2C and a 4C DNA content, respectively. Cells in the first peak are in the G1 phase and those that have a fully replicated component of DNA are in the G2 or the M phase. Cells with an intermediate DNA are in the S phase.

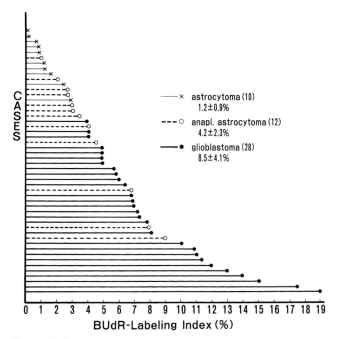

Figure 19–3 The labeling index obtained from astrocytic tumors distributed continuously in a wide range from 1% or less to 19%; this distribution parallels the degree of tumor differentiation. Abbreviation: anapl., anaplastic. (From Fujimaki T, Matsutani M, Nakamura O, et al: Correlation between bromodeoxyuridine-labeling indices and patient prognosis in cerebral astrocytic tumors of adults. Cancer 1991; 67:1629–1634.)

analyzed by bromodeoxyuridine-LI study in 47 adult patients with cerebral glioblastomas.[21] Comparing the LIs at initial surgery and those after radiation therapy, it was demonstrated that the mean LI fell from 8.2% to 3.8% after radiation therapy, and that the lowest LI, less than 0.1%, was obtained in cases treated with a dose of 70 Gy or more. The patients with LIs of less than 1% after radiation therapy showed significantly longer survival and time to recurrence than those with LIs of more than 5%. At least 70 Gy irradiation was recommended for glioblastoma to obtain the lowest LI of less than 0.1%.

The proliferative potential reflected by the bromodeoxyuridine LI is surely a good clinical indicator for predicting the rate of tumor growth in cerebral astrocytic tumors. Nagashima and associates[22] compared bromodeoxyuridine LI obtained from tissue sections and flow cytometry. The LIs determined by flow cytometry also correlated well with the LIs determined by immunohistochemistry, despite the difference in values between them.

By continuous exposure of a cell population to ³H-thymidine or bromodeoxyuridine for a period lasting at least as long as the cell cycle time, it is possible to approximate the GF. All cycling cells will pass through the S phase during that period and will incorporate ³H-thymidine or bromodeoxyuridine. Cells that fail to incorporate them are considered to be noncycling (or G0) cells. Yoshii and others[23] administered bromodeoxyuridine intravenously every 8 hours for 3 days before surgery to 25 patients with brain tumors, and estimated the GF as ranging from 9.1% to 46.5% in malignant gliomas, and 2.0% to 6.7% in low-grade gliomas. The estimated cell cycle time was 5 to 12 days in most malignant gliomas; however, the actual cell cycle time should be substantially shorter because cell loss was not considered in the calculation. These results confirm that the faster-growing tumors contain a larger population of proliferating cells. In addition, the growth fractions of malignant gliomas in this study are quite similar to those reported by Tym[24] and by Mendelsohn,[3] who used a different method to estimate the GF in gliomas.

DOUBLE LABELING OF BROMODEOXYURIDINE AND IODODEOXYURIDINE

The development of a new monoclonal antibody against bromodeoxyuridine (BR-3) provided more information about cell kinetics. Unlike earlier anti-bromodeoxyuridine monoclonal antibody[13] which reacted with bromodeoxyuridine and with iododeoxyuridine, which is another thymidine analog, the new antibody reacts only with bromodeoxyuridine.[25] Double-labeling studies with these two thymidine analogs administered sequentially at proper intervals before surgery made it possible to estimate S-phase duration.[26] When iododeoxyuridine is administered at time "0", all cells in the S phase will be labeled with iododeoxyuridine. Subsequently, some iododeoxyuridine-labeled cells will complete DNA synthesis and move into the G2 (premitotic gap) phase. When bromodeoxyuridine is administered after an interval of time "t", the iododeoxyuridine-labeled G2 cells will not incorporate bromodeoxyuridine. Thus, the proportion of cells that have left the S phase to those that are in the S phase can be determined, and the S phase duration can be estimated by dividing time "t" by this proportion. The potential doubling time (the time required for the tumor cell population to double in the absence of cell loss) can be calculated by dividing the S-phase duration by the S-phase fraction, or LI, as each fraction of labeled cells will proceed to mitosis and will eventually double in number.

Shibuya and associates,[27] using this double-labeling method, calculated the duration of the S phase (Ts) and the potential doubling time (Tp) from biopsy specimens of 66 gliomas. Ts was fairly uniform (mean, 9.2 ± 2.1 hours), but Tp varied from 1 day to more than 2 months among different histologic subtypes (Table 19–1). Although the actual doubling time (aTd) of a tumor may be substantially longer owing to considerable cell loss, the potential doubling time provides a quantitative estimate of how fast the tumor could proliferate. The Tp values correlated closely with the bromodeoxyuridine LI, or S-phase fraction, and can be calculated from the equation: $Tp = 26.9/LI^{1.02}$. Hoshino[28] summarized the tentative cell kinetic parameters of glial tumors with the double-labeling study. A tumor with an LI of 1%, for example, has a GF of 0.08, a Tc of 2.5 days, a Tp of 23 days, and a probable aTd of 4 months, assuming a cell loss factor of 0.8. Similarly, a tumor with an LI of 5% may have a Tc of 1.2 days, a Tp of 5 days, and an aTd of 25 days; a tumor with a LI of 10% may show a larger GF (0.31) and the other three parameters may be shorter (Tc, 0.9 days; Tp, 2.7 days; aTd, 14 days).

TABLE 19–1
RESULTS OF DOUBLE-LABELING STUDY OF GLIOMAS

Pathologic Lesion (No.)	BUdR LI (%)	Ts (Hr)	Tp (Days)
Glioblastoma multiforme (21)	8.0 ± 5.5	9.1 ± 2.5	5.9 ± 6.3
Primary (13)	8.8 ± 6.0	9.3 ± 2.6	4.2 ± 2.3
Recurrent (8)	6.6 ± 4.5	8.8 ± 2.3	8.6 ± 9.5
Anaplastic astrocytoma (18)	3.8 ± 5.7	8.9 ± 2.3	17.5 ± 14.6
Primary (6)	2.8 ± 3.7	9.7 ± 2.7	24.5 ± 20.7
Recurrent (12)	4.2 ± 6.6	8.6 ± 2.2	14.0 ± 9.7
Mixed malignant glioma (11)	1.9 ± 1.6	9.5 ± 2.0	24.4 ± 16.0
Low-grade glioma (16)	1.6 ± 2.2	8.9 ± 1.6	35.9 ± 26.5

Abbreviations: BUdR LI, bromodeoxyuridine labeling index; Ts, S-phase duration; Tp, potential doubling time.
Data from Shibuya M, Ito S, Davis R, et al: A new method for analyzing the cell kinetics of human brain tumors by double labeling with bromodeoxyuridine in situ and with iododeoxyuridine in vitro. Cancer 1993; 71:3109–3113.

CONCLUSION

The cell kinetic studies of gliomas using ^{3}H-thymidine autoradiography, flow cytometry, and bromodeoxyuridine labeling have provided a valuable fundamental knowledge of their proliferative activity for understanding biologic malignancy of individual tumors. The classification of brain tumors is important, but the knowledge of the biologic characteristics of a tumor is as important as, or more important than, its histologic expression. Whether or not we depend on cell kinetic analysis with bromodeoxyuridine/iododeoxyuridine or other markers, such as proliferating cell nuclear antigen or cyclin,[29] thymidine synthase,[30] Ki-67 or MIB-1,[31] or nuclear organizing region,[32] cell kinetic information obtained by these methods in routine clinical practice is needed.

REFERENCES

1. Howard A, Pelc SR: Synthesis of deoxyribonucleic acid in normal and irradiated cells and its relation to chromosomal breakage. Heredity 1953; (suppl)6:261–273.
2. Steel GG: Cell loss from experimental tumors. Cell Tissue Kinet 1968; 1:193–207.
3. Mendelsohn ML: Autoradiographic analysis of cell proliferation in spontaneous breast cancer of C3H mouse: III. The growth fraction. JNCI 1962; 28:1015–1029.
4. Hoshino T, Wilson CB: Cell kinetic analysis of human malignant brain tumors (gliomas). Cancer 1979; 44:956–962.
5. Hoshino T, Townsend JJ, Muraoka I, et al: An autoradiographic study of human gliomas: Growth kinetics of anaplastic astrocytoma and glioblastoma multiforme. Brain 1980; 103:967–984.
6. Matsutani M, Hoshino T: Analysis of tumor growth in recurrent malignant gliomas (in Japanese). Brain Nerve 1985; 27:274–276.
7. Tsuboi K, Yoshii Y, Nakagawa K, et al: Regrowth patterns of supratentorial gliomas: Estimation from computed tomographic scans. Neurosurgery 1986; 19:946–951.
8. Hoshino T, Nomura K, Wilson CB, et al: The distribution of nuclear DNA from human brain tumor cells: Flow cytometric studies. J Neurosurg 1978; 49:13–21.
9. Frederiksen P, Reske-Nielsen E, Bichel P: DNA content of meningiomas. Acta Neuropathol 1979; 46:65–68.
10. Kawamoto K, Herz F, Wolley RC, et al: Flow cytometric analysis of the DNA distribution in human brain tumors. Acta Neuropathol 1979; 46:39–44.
11. Hoshino T, Knebel KD, Rosenblun ML, et al: Clonogenicity of multiple populations of human glioma cells sorted by DNA content. Cancer 1982; 50:997–1002.
12. Vavruch L, Enestrom S, Carstensen J, et al: DNA index and S-phase in primary brain tumors: A comparison between fresh and deparaffined specimens studied by flow cytometry. J Neurosurg 1994; 80:85–89.
13. Gratzner HG: Monoclonal antibody of 5-bromo- and 5-iododeoxyuridine: A new reagent for detection of DNA replication. Science 1982; 218:474–476.
14. Nagashima T, DeArmond SJ, Murovic J, et al: Immunocytochemical demonstration of S-phase cells by anti-bromodeoxyuridine monoclonal antibody in human brain tumor tissues. Acta Neuropathol 1985; 67:155–159.
15. Hoshino T, Nagashima T, Murovic JA, et al: In situ cell kinetics studies on human neuroectodermal tumors with bromodeoxyuridine labeling. J Neurosurg 1986; 64:453–459.
16. Hoshino T, Prados M, Wilson CB, et al: Prognostic implications of the bromodeoxyuridine labeling index of human gliomas. J Neurosurg 1989; 71:335–341.
17. Fujimaki T, Matsutani M, Nakamura O, et al: Correlation between bromodeoxyuridine-labeling indices and patient prognosis in cerebral astrocytic tumors of adults. Cancer 1991; 67:1629–1634.
18. Kleihues P, Burger PC, Scheithauer BW: Histological Typing of Tumours of the Central Nervous System, ed 2. Berlin, Springer-Verlag, 1993.
19. Nelson JS, Tsukada Y, Schoenfeld D, et al: Necrosis as a prognostic criterion in malignant supratentorial, astrocytic gliomas. Cancer 1983; 52:550–554.
20. Burger PC, Vogel FS, Green SB, et al: Glioblastoma multiforme and anaplastic astrocytoma: Pathologic criteria and prognostic implications. Cancer 1985; 56:1106–1111.
21. Fujimaki T, Matsutani M, Takakura K: Analysis of BUdR (bromodeoxyuridine) labeling indices of cerebral glioblastomas after radiation therapy (in Japanese). J Jpn Soc Ther Radiol Oncol 1990; 2:263–273.
22. Nagashima T, Hoshino T, Cho KG, et al: Comparison of bromodeoxyuridine labeling indices obtained from tissue sections and flow cytometry of brain tumors. J Neurosurg 1988; 68:388–392.
23. Yoshii Y, Maki Y, Tsuboi K, et al: Estimation of growth fraction with bromodeoxyuridine in human central nervous system tumors. J Neurosurg 1986; 65:659–663.
24. Tym R: Distribution of cell doubling times in in vivo human cerebral tumors. Surg Forum 1969; 20:445–447.
25. Dolbeare F, Kuo WL, Vanderlaan M, et al: Cell cycle analysis by flow cytometric analysis of the incorporation of iododeoxyuridine (IdUrd) and bromodeoxyuridine (BrdUrd) (abstract). Proc Am Assoc Cancer Res 1988; 29:477.
26. Shibui S, Hoshino T, Vanderlaan M, et al: Double labeling with iodo- and bromodeoxyuridine for cell kinetic studies. J Histochem Cytochem 1989; 37:1007–1011.
27. Shibuya M, Ito S, Davis R, et al: A new method for analyzing the cell kinetics of human brain tumors by double labeling with bromodeoxyuri-

dine in situ and with iododeoxyuridine in vitro. Cancer 1993; 71:3109–3113.

28. Hoshino T: Cell kinetics of glial tumors. Rev Neurol 1992; 148:396–401.

29. Tabuchi K, Honda C, Nakane P: Demonstration of proliferating cell nuclear antigen (PCNU/Cyclin) in glioma cells. Neurol Med Chir 1987; 27:1–5.

30. Shibui S, Hoshino T, Iwasaki K, et al: Cell cycle phase dependent emergence of thymidylate synthase studied by monoclonal antibody (M-TS-4). Cell Tissue Kinet 1989; 22:259–268.

31. Gerdes J, Schwab U, Lemke H, et al: Production of a mouse monoclonal antibody reactive with a human nuclear antigen associated with cell proliferation. Int J Cancer 1983; 31:13–20.

32. Kajiwara K, Nishizaki T, Orita T, et al: Silver colloid staining technique for analysis of glioma malignancy. J Neurosurg 1990; 73:113–117.

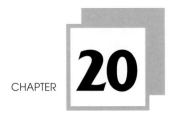

CHAPTER **20**

Anatomy and Growth Patterns of Diffuse Gliomas

Any discussion of glioma growth and anatomy should begin with an acknowledgment of the fundamental work of Scherer, whose detailed descriptions of the growth patterns of untreated gliomas remain the standard and form a major foundation for this chapter. These studies are valuable resources both for their elegant anatomic descriptions and for their historical perspective, insight, and philosophy regarding the pathologic analysis of gliomas.[43–45]

This said, the question of the need for a new chapter on glioma growth and anatomy arises. Early studies of tumor anatomy were based on untreated end-stage tumors at autopsy. Imaging methods and surgical techniques have now allowed pathologic studies on earlier stages in glioma growth. The terminology of older studies does not reflect the current understanding of glioma histogenesis and tumor progression. In particular, the relationship of glioblastoma multiforme (GBM) as a derivative of astrocytoma was not well recognized historically. Similarly, recent insight into tumor grading and classification, particularly in regard to greater recognition of the prevalence of oligodendroglial tumors, warrants reassessment of the older concepts of growth patterns. Analyses of treatment effects and patterns of glioma recurrence also provide insight about the growth of primary gliomas that was unavailable before the era of therapy and chemotherapy. Finally, variation in histologic features in different areas of the tumor is a well-recognized phenomenon in gliomas, and such regional heterogeneity has been identified at the molecular and genetic levels as well. Studies of molecular and genetic heterogeneity reveal clues to an underlying structure that is fundamental to the growth and development of gliomas. An appreciation of this "molecular anatomy" is essential to understanding the anatomy of gliomas and to forming a rational basis for their treatment.

This chapter addresses the growth patterns of *diffuse* supratentorial gliomas, which are tumors whose infiltrative growth creates ill-defined margins, both grossly and microscopically; they usually, therefore, defy complete surgical extirpation. Astrocytomas and oligodendrogliomas are the focus of discussion; reference is made to other gliomas, primarily for comparison. Astrocytomas and oligodendrogliomas share many morphologic features, but specific significant differences are noted. The misleading terms *benign* and *malignant* are avoided in reference to the degree of malignancy in gliomas; instead, specific diagnoses (e.g., GBM, or relative terms such as low-grade and high-grade) are used. Anatomic issues are emphasized as they relate to a rationale for treatment and include a review of both gross and histologic anatomy as well as a correlation with imaging studies. The growth of recurrent tumors is considered as it provides insight into the morphology and biology of primary tumor growth. Issues raised by recent studies of regional heterogeneity as well as molecular and genetic analyses of gliomas are reviewed.

GENERAL MACROSCOPIC AND MICROSCOPIC ANALYSIS

Scherer[44] observed that brain tumors demonstrate a variable combination of two patterns of growth and spread: *infiltrative* and *expansive*. Based on similar observations, Daumas-Duport and co-workers[20, 21] defined three patterns of glioma growth based on mass formation and tumor cell infiltration. Type I tumors correspond to purely expansive growth; they are composed of a locally destructive cellular core that is sharply circumscribed, with little invasion of adjacent brain. Type II tumors have a mixed expansive-infiltrative growth pattern and combine a cellular core with a variable, often extensive, corona or rim of individual infiltrating tumor cells. Type III tumors correspond to the purely infiltrative type and are diffusely infiltrative, without a cellular core.

Expansive Growth

In expansive growth, the tumor enlarges as a discrete, cohesive mass, pushing aside the surrounding brain parenchyma. As a result, this growth pattern is characterized by a broad

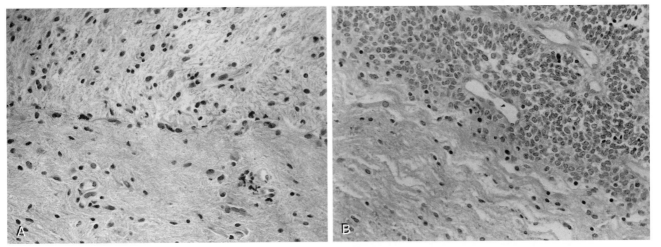

Figure 20–1 Expansive growth *A*, Pilocytic astrocytoma. The border between the neoplasm and surrounding gliotic brain is sharply circumscribed, with only a few infiltrating tumor cells extending away from the main tumor mass. *B*, Anaplastic ependymoma. The tumor has a broad expansive margin without infiltration of individual tumor cells into the surrounding brain (hematoxylin-eosin; original magnification ×250).

interface with the adjacent brain. The gross tumor margins are defined sharply and often present an apparent cleavage plane between the tumor and uninvolved brain tissue. A similar sharp circumscription usually is seen at the microscopic level. This growth pattern is characteristic of metastatic carcinoma and both primary and metastatic sarcomas. Among the gliomas, ependymomas,[44] and the (related) rarely invasive malignant choroid plexus tumors[13] consistently grow in this manner (Fig. 20–1). Pilocytic astrocytomas often are circumscribed on gross inspection, but microscopically they usually have limited local infiltration.[13, 44] However, unlike other astrocytomas, the narrow zone of infiltration is a characteristic feature that reflects a biologic difference between the pilocytic and the infiltrative astrocytomas. Daumas-Duport and colleagues[21] reported that minimally infiltrative tumors comprised 25% of astrocytomas, but the majority were pilocytic astrocytomas. Ordinary astrocytomas and GBM with this growth pattern are rare.[9, 21, 44]

Infiltrative Growth

By definition, purely infiltrative tumors lack a defined tumor core. Depending on the density and distribution of tumor cells, they may merely expand the infiltrated parenchyma without producing a mass, or they may have an obvious, if ill-defined, mass on macroscopic examination (Figs. 20–2 to 20–4). A yellowish discoloration is often present, which reflects protein-rich edema fluid.[45] As a result, not only are tumor margins poorly defined, but it is occasionally impossible to define the abnormality as neoplastic on gross examination alone. Degenerative changes,[45] in particular microcystic change, may produce macroscopic and textural changes that create a false tumor border. In oligodendrogliomas, such changes correspond to regions of tumor that are readily removed by suction. Microscopic examination of such areas as well of as adjacent normal-appearing tissue often show mucopolysaccharide-rich stroma in the soft area and more obvious parenchymal preservation in the "normal" areas; however, difference in tumor cell density is often little to

nonexistent. Tumor cell density in low-grade gliomas is typically two to four times that of normal brain.[45] Microscopic analysis shows infiltrating tumor cells and edema to be present in variable (and grossly unpredictable) proportions, with sparing of brain parenchyma. Autopsy studies of untreated gliomas have identified this growth pattern in as many as 25% of tumors.[44] Daumas-Duport and associates[20, 21] identified this pattern in 15% of cases. Purely infiltrative

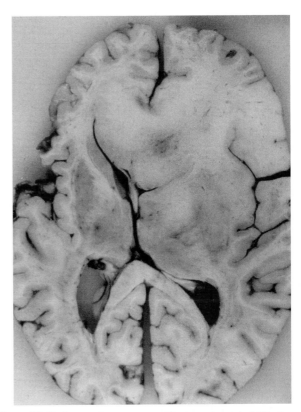

Figure 20–2 Low-grade astrocytoma. The tumor is purely infiltrative and lacks a cellular core. It expands the right frontal white matter, crosses the corpus callosum, and infiltrates the left frontal white matter.

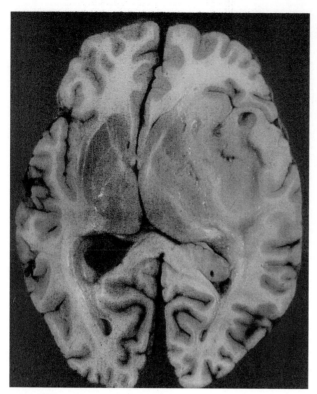

Figure 20–3 Oligodendroglioma, grade 2. The tumor expands and infiltrates the right frontotemporal white matter. It lacks a cellular core and has ill-defined margins. Note the thickening of the cortex and blurring of the gray-white junction, which is indicative of permeation of the gray matter by the tumor.

fuse and usually bilateral involvement of the cerebral hemispheres, is the ultimate manifestation of this form of growth (see Fig. 20–4). The rarity of this pattern indicates that most diffuse gliomas produce symptoms when they are smaller or, more commonly, when they progress to higher-grade tumors. Interestingly, Scherer[44] found contralateral infiltration to be more common in low-grade tumors than in high-grade tumors. Currently, imaging evidence of "crossing the midline" is interpreted as being indicative of a high-grade tumor. Presumably, we now identify and treat most low-grade tumors prior to such spread.

That extensive infiltrative growth may occur with little or no destruction of pre-existing parenchyma creates a therapeutic dilemma. This growth pattern is a particular problem in oligodendrogliomas, in which residual axons often are identifiable even in a highly cellular tumor. This pattern of growth also creates a diagnostic delay. Because the involved parenchyma may be functional, the tumor may be extensive before clinical manifestations lead to a diagnosis. Clinical indication of the presence of a tumor may occur when parenchymal irritation produces seizure activity with mass effect from a large tumor or with malignant progression to a high-grade destructive neoplasm.

Oligodendrogliomas are often superficial.[44] This characteristic relates to a much greater tendency for permeation of gray matter by lower-grade oligodendroglial tumors than by astrocytomas, in which extensive gray matter involvement usually reflects destructive lesions of high-grade tumors. With cortical involvement, the gray matter becomes pale and thickened and the gray-white matter border becomes

growth is characteristic of low-grade astrocytomas, especially oligodendrogliomas. Scherer[44] included all low-grade gliomas in this category, noting only rare examples of GBM without circumscribed masses. Thus, the formation of a circumscribed destructive mass may be a property of high-grade gliomas and an element of tumor progression. Recent analyses have elucidated several of the cytogenetic and molecular changes associated with tumor progression. However, the mechanism that prompts a tumor to form a localized mass remains unknown.

At autopsy, untreated diffuse low-grade gliomas involve a larger portion of the brain than do mass-forming high-grade tumors.[9, 44, 45] Whether this observation reflects the relative invasiveness of the tumor grades is unclear. As a result of their locally destructive growth and more severe associated edema, high-grade gliomas, such as GBM, typically become symptomatic at a smaller size than do lower-grade gliomas. Also, the high proliferative activity of many high-grade tumors may result in overgrowth of the infiltrating corona, creating an appearance of expansive growth and masking the extent of infiltration. In contrast, structural and functional parenchymal sparing and the lack of associated massive edema often allow infiltrative low-grade tumors to attain a large size without producing significant symptoms.[44] Parenchymal destruction may be limited, even after many years and irrespective of high cellularity.[44] As a result, most low-grade gliomas involve more than one lobe, and contralateral extension is typical.[45] Gliomatosis cerebri, with dif-

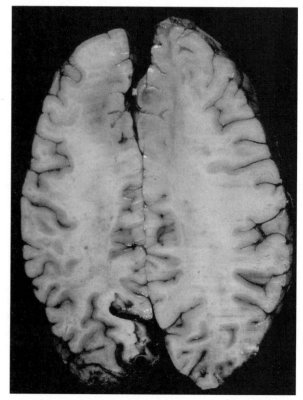

Figure 20–4 Gliomatosis cerebri. There is diffuse expansion of white matter throughout the right hemisphere without a defined cellular core.

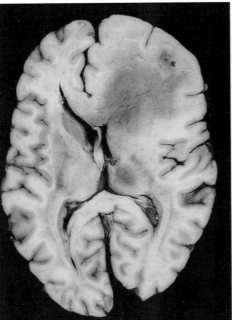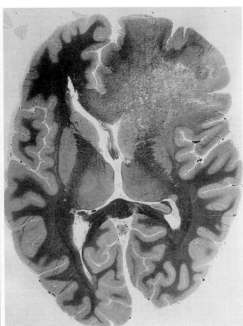

Figure 20–5 Anaplastic astrocytoma. *A,* The tumor has mixed expansive-infiltrative growth. The central dark discoloration represents the cellular core. The infiltrating margins of the tumor are indistinct. *B,* Whole brain section demonstrating that expansion and growth of tumor is confined primarily to white matter, with the gray matter serving as a barrier to tumor growth (Weil's stain).

indistinct,[45] features that are most commonly seen in oligodendroglial tumors (see Fig. 20–3). The older literature notes that many lower-grade astrocytomas lack fibrillary differentiation, particularly those with extensive cortical involvement. Scherer[45] attributed this phenomenon to phenotypic changes induced by microenvironmental differences between gray and white matter. Based on current definitions, it is likely that many of the afibrillary cortical neoplasms were in fact oligodendroglial tumors.[18] Older studies report that oligodendroglial tumors comprise only 10% to 15% of gliomas.[13] However, a recent study has suggested that oligodendroglial tumors are more common than previously thought, comprising up to 25% of supratentorial gliomas.[18]

Scherer[44] and Burger and co-workers[13] describe oligodendrogliomas as frequently having a narrow zone of infiltration in the white matter. However, many oligodendroglial tumors have extensive growth beyond their hypercellular centers, which testifies to their significant infiltrative capacity. In my experience, a grossly circumscribed hypercellular area, often with myxoid degeneration, is surrounded by variably infiltrated parenchyma. The tumor infiltration may extend for a great distance, with a gross appearance of only expanded white matter with an abnormally firm texture that merges with normal-appearing tissue.

Mixed Expansive-Infiltrative Growth

Some gliomas, such as ependymomas and pilocytic astrocytomas, tend to be purely expansive, but most combine an expansive central mass with diffusely infiltrative margins (Daumas-Duport type II). This pattern may be seen in low-grade tumors, but it is characteristic of high-grade gliomas (Figs. 20–5 and 20–6). The distribution of cells in this growth pattern is highly variable, and microscopic examination invariably reveals more extensive tumor than the macroscopic examination would predict.

Whereas lower-grade gliomas may have fairly uniform morphology throughout the tumor mass, the appearance of a high-grade tumor may be quite pleomorphic at both the gross and microscopic levels. As exemplified by the GBM, high-grade gliomas have a highly cellular compact zone of tumor cells, the density of which may be many times that of normal brain. The cellular core tends to have smooth or

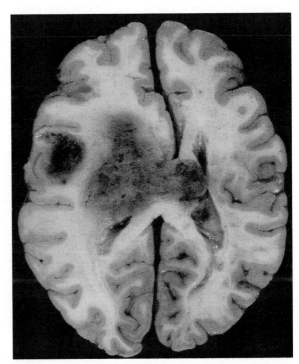

Figure 20–6 Glioblastoma multiforme. The tumor has a mixed expansive-infiltrative growth pattern. The cellular core is focally destructive of gray matter, but the tumor generally infiltrates through white matter. Note the apparent multicentricity with focal central and peripheral expansive lesions.

rounded contours, which suggests expansive growth but probably reflects an infiltrating tumor with a proliferative capacity that exceeds its invasive capacity. Within the cellular core, non-neoplastic elements are destroyed almost completely. Rapidly proliferating tumors may outgrow their blood supply, resulting in foci of tumor necrosis. Microthrombi often are associated with tumor necrosis, which suggests a role for vascular injury in the production of necrosis. The necrotic foci vary from scattered microscopic islands to large areas that may compose the majority of the tumor mass. The necrotic areas are associated with edema and reactive glial changes. Hemorrhage is a frequent but variable feature of high-grade gliomas. Thus, the morphology of a high-grade glioma reflects a combination of proliferating tumor cells, necrosis, and hemorrhage, as well the reactive responses of the injured brain (edema, gliosis, macrophages, and inflammation).

Surrounding the core is a corona of infiltrative tumor that extends irregularly and asymmetrically into the surrounding brain. Although the infiltrating tumor is variably destructive, the infiltrated parenchyma is usually preserved less than in purely infiltrative low-grade tumors.[44] The transition from tumor core to infiltrating corona is often abrupt, but it may be gradual. The gradient of decrease in tumor cell density at the periphery of a tumor is unpredictable, so that the extent of infiltrating corona also is highly variable. Scherer[44] observed that as many as 20% of high-grade astrocytomas had very abrupt borders with minimal zones of infiltration (Fig. 20–7). Burger[9] found these circumscribed gliomas to be less common but reported a GBM with only a 2-mm margin of identifiable tumor cells around the cellular core at autopsy. For such tumors, the gross tumor margin corresponds closely to the actual extent of tumor. Far more commonly, gliomas have a more gradual decrease in cellularity as infiltrating tumor cells mingle with the surrounding normal and reactive glia (Fig. 20–8). The infiltrating edge typically extends 1 or 2 cm, but it may infiltrate for many centimeters and far exceed the gross tumor limit.[9–11, 24, 44] Daumas-Duport and colleagues[21] observed that the infiltrative portion of a tumor typically occupied a volume 2 to 3 times larger than the

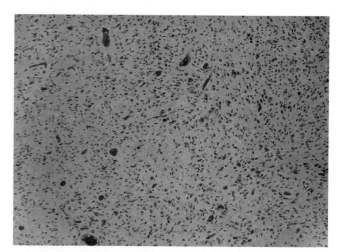

Figure 20–8 Glioblastoma multiforme. This tumor demonstrates a gradual decrease in cell density from the central core as it infiltrates the surrounding parenchyma (hematoxylin-eosin; original magnification ×100).

solid core. Although a tendency exists to attribute a high degree of invasiveness to high-grade tumors, many studies, from those of Scherer[44] to Burger and associates,[9, 10] have found greater areas of infiltrating tumor in low-grade tumors. Burger[9] noted that infiltrating tumor comprised only 25% of GBM, compared to 67% of lower-grade tumors. It is unclear whether this finding reflects differing degrees of invasiveness or more rapid overgrowth and mass formation by the higher-grade tumors. Small anaplastic cells, which may be present in primary tumors and which are often preponderant in recurrent GBM, appear to be highly invasive.

Consistent with Scherer's observations,[44] Burger and colleagues[11] found no correlation between the growth pattern and degree of malignancy, except that all high-grade tumors had a cellular core. The cellular portions of tumors were localized unilaterally or in a single vascular distribution in just 7 of 15 cases. When the infiltrating corona was included, only 3 of 15 tumors were so restricted.[11]

In their autopsy studies of untreated gliomas, neither Scherer[44] nor Burger and associates[11] found a persistent zone of low-grade astrocytoma around the cellular core of mixed expansive-infiltrative high-grade gliomas to be common. Some of the tumors consist purely of high-grade elements, with invasion by the cells that compose the cellular mass. However, the infiltrative areas of most of the tumors include lower-grade elements, so that the high-grade compact zone coexists with lower-grade diffusely infiltrative tumor cells. In untreated GBM, Burger and co-workers[11] found that the infiltrating corona was composed primarily of small anaplastic cells or a combination of small anaplastic cells and better differentiated astrocytes. In the presumed basis for this pattern, the cellular core is indicative of malignant progression of a preexisting lower-grade tumor. In lesions with coexisting low- and high-grade tumor, the cellular core of high-grade tumor often is sharply circumscribed, both on macroscopic and microscopic examination.[45] Scherer[44, 45] found this pattern less frequently than did others who studied surgical specimens[17, 24, 40] (and in which studies tumors often were identified at earlier stages). Both of my studies,[16, 17] and those of Paulus[40] found that areas of low-grade tumor

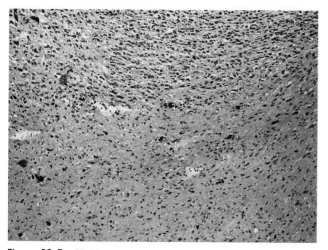

Figure 20–7 Glioblastoma multiforme. The cellular core of this tumor is relatively circumscribed with a limited degree of infiltration into the surrounding brain (hematoxylin-eosin; original magnification ×100).

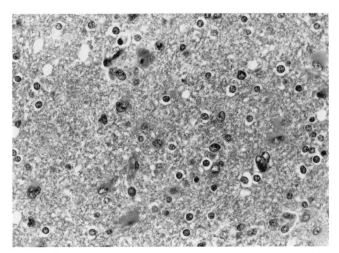

Figure 20–9 Individual tumor cells (ITC). Scattered ITC are recognizable by their large, irregular nuclei (hematoxylin-eosin; original magnification ×400).

are found in most high-grade gliomas and comprise approximately 20% of the tumor. This finding suggests that in end-stage gliomas, the transformed cells often overrun and obscure the preexisting tumor from which they evolved.

Interpretation of these studies on the distribution of infiltrating tumor cells must consider the problem of their identification. The individual infiltrating tumor cells tend to have irregular, elongated, and hyperchromatic nuclei, often with little appreciable cytoplasm. When sufficiently atypical, the tumor cells are recognizable among the preponderant nonneoplastic elements. However, their cytologic features also can be similar to those of reactive astrocytes or of migrating microglia (monocytes, rod cells) (Fig. 20–9). Also, as the density of infiltrating tumor cells decreases, their presence may not be documented due to sampling error, particularly in studies that rely on biopsies.[31, 32] Consequently, certain identification becomes impossible, resulting in a tumor margin that is not defined accurately. The lack of a definable margin and the propensity to infiltrate some distance into functional parenchyma are central problems of glioma management.

Cytologic Correlates of Tumor Growth

No growth pattern is specific to a cytologic subtype, and cytologically similar tumors have different growth patterns, which indicates that cytology alone is insufficient to characterize a neoplasm. Also, the invasiveness of a tumor typically is not correlated with the cytologic features of the tumor cells. The one cytologic subtype that has been correlated with invasiveness is controversial. Scherer[44] observed that GBM composed primarily of small cells tend to be less invasive than other cytologic types. In contrast, Burger and others[10] and Giangaspero and Burger[24] found that small anaplastic and small fibrillated astrocytes were highly invasive, particularly in recurrent tumors (Fig. 20–10). The difference may at least partly reflect the different growth patterns between primary and recurrent tumors. The small cells are

highly proliferative, and their rapid growth may have masked their invasive potential in Scherer's studies.

Interaction of Tumor and Brain in Determining Glioma Morphology

To this point, tumor growth has been considered only in regard to the intrinsic properties of the tumor per se. In fact, the overall morphology of a glioma is partially determined by the balance between proliferative and invasive forces of the tumor itself as well as by the interaction of the infiltrating tumor cells with the adjacent brain. In a uniform environment, both expansive and infiltrative tumors would develop as enlarging spheres. However, diffuse gliomas grow in an environment that offers both desirable pathways and almost inviolate barriers to spread. The result is a complicated gross morphology.

Gliomas tend to infiltrate via white matter pathways, and the tumor periphery typically follows the shape of the adjacent white matter. Consequently, an irregular contour develops between the cortical convolutions and the deep diencephalic nuclei.[43, 44] The pattern of spread in white matter is not random: tumors tend to infiltrate *along* white matter tracts in such a way that intersecting white matter tracts are somewhat inhibitory to invasion (Fig. 20–11). In a review of 100 high-grade gliomas at autopsy, Matsukado and colleagues[36] confirmed that glioma infiltration tends to follow major white matter pathways, such as the the corpus callosum and internal capsule. Thus, access to these pathways often directs and predicts tumor spread. In particular, there is a predilection for bilateral spread of frontal tumors via the corpus callosum.[36] The diffuse connections of the corona radiata and the superior longitudinal fasciculus provide parietal tumors with pathways for extensive interlobar spread anteriorly and posteriorly, whereas the diencephalic nuclei and peripheral cortex prevent lateral expansion.[36] Frontotemporal spread via the uncinate fasciculus and occipital spread via the optic radiations are also common.

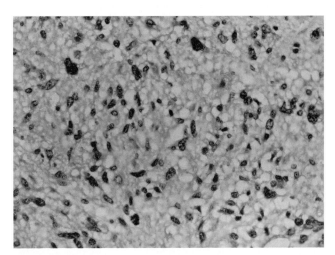

Figure 20–10 Glioblastoma multiforme (GBM). Small anaplastic and small fibrillated cells with small, irregular nuclei and poorly developed processes are typically present in GBM and are preponderant in recurrent tumors (hematoxylin-eosin; original magnification ×400).

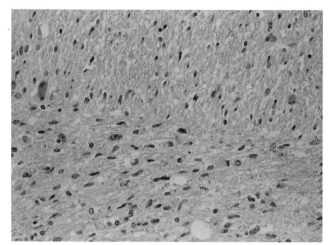

Figure 20-11 Glioblastoma multiforme. Tract-specific white matter infiltration is seen. The white matter tract in the upper portion of the figure has a course perpendicular to the tract in the lower area. The lower tract is extensively infiltrated by tumor cells that are characterized by large, elongated nuclei. The upper tract contains few, if any, recognizable tumor cells (hematoxylin-eosin, original magnification ×250).

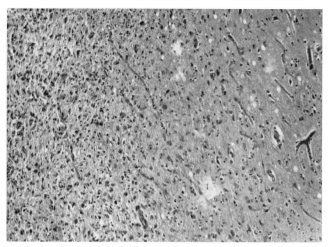

Figure 20-12 Glioblastoma multiforme. The gray matter serves as a barrier to the infiltrating neoplasm. Despite extensive infiltration of the adjacent white matter, few cells are present in the cortex (hematoxylin-eosin; original magnification ×100).

The predilection for tract-specific spread may reflect that parallel axons provide both directional guidance and little resistance to cell migration.[35] Tumor cell infiltration consistently is accompanied by edema, a feature that permits the close correlation between the histologic tumor margins and the margins predicted by magnetic resonance imaging (MRI).[30] The edema develops as a reactive response to the presence of the tumor, as a result of the vascular injury it produces, and from abnormal tumor vasculature. The basis for the relationship between peritumoral edema and infiltrating tumor cells remains unclear. Edema expands the extracellular space, spreading axons apart, and may thus further facilitate migration of tumor cells.[38] The edema associated with the white matter around tumors also limits identification of the gross margins of gliomas.

Scherer described "secondary structures" associated with glioma growth in addition to the solid core and the advancing edge.[43, 44] The development of these structures depends on preexisting tissue elements.[43] Included in this category are the observations of spread along white matter tracts and the barrier properties of gray matter (discussed later). Additional features include perineuronal clustering (satellitosis), perivascular growth, and clustering around nerve fibers (perifascicular and intrafascicular growth). Less common patterns of infiltration include subpial spread in the cortical molecular layer. These structures often appear adjacent to uninvaded parenchyma and may herald massive invasion.

Astrocytomas often spread great distances through white matter with minimal extension of tumor cells into gray matter. Particularly for astrocytomas, the gray matter, including both cortex and deep nuclei, forms a barrier against tumor infiltration (see Figs. 20-5, 20-6, and 20-12).[36, 44] Locally, this barrier can create the misleading appearance of circumscribed growth. The basis for this barrier property is unclear, but the feltwork distribution of fibers in gray matter is a distinct contrast to the parallel "highways" provided by white matter, and gray matter does not develop vasogenic edema.

Based on their frequently extensive, nondestructive involvement of superficial cortex, low-grade oligodendrogliomas appear much more capable of developing in gray matter than their astrocytoma counterparts, which rarely show such a pattern (see Figs. 20-3, 20-13). Such prominent nondestructive expansion in gray matter or on MRI is a helpful diagnostic feature of oligodendroglial lineage tumors. This finding suggests that gray matter is not a formidable barrier to oligodendroglial growth. Nevertheless, gray matter involvement is usually a local phenomenon, and distant spread of oligodendrogliomas occurs through the white matter.

Although subarachnoid invasion is common, the pia also appears to resist the spread of tumor.[44] Despite pial contact, many tumors do not invade the meninges. When the subarachnoid membrane is invaded, growth is usually limited to the areas in contact with the tumor and is rarely extensive.

The ependyma also serves as a barrier to glioma invasion.

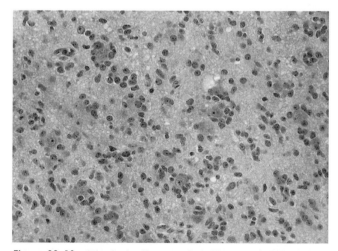

Figure 20-13 Oligodendroglioma, grade 2. The tumor is diffusely invasive of gray matter. Perineuronal satellitosis is readily identified (hematoxylin-eosin; original magnification ×250).

However, subependymal spread is common. When it has occurred, extension into the ventricles has not reflected histologic subtype or malignancy. Once in the ventricles, gliomas may spread extensively and diffusely along the surfaces or they may grow in a circumscribed, expansive manner. After intraventricular spread, the choroid plexus is often invaded.[44] Gliomas also demonstrate other important patterns of spread. Subependymal spread may result in microscopic or minimal gross disease along the surfaces of the ventricles, or it may present as obstructive ventricular masses.

Involvement of the ventricles or subarachnoid space provides access to the cerebrospinal fluid (CSF), and metastasis through CSF pathways can lead to tumor growth at distant intracranial and spinal sites. Although relatively common in primitive neuroectodermal tumors, such as medulloblastomas, spread through CSF pathways is considered rare in gliomas; it occurs in an estimated 1.5% of cases.[15] However, one autopsy study found CSF spread in 14 of 51 gliomas (27%), which suggests that asymptomatic or unrecognized CSF spread may be more common than initially appreciated.[39]

In contrast to non-CNS malignancies, primary untreated gliomas almost never produce systemic metastases. The blood vessels appear to pose an impenetrable barrier to glioma cells. Alternatively, glioma cells that penetrate blood vessels may fail to become established at sites outside the CNS. Despite the resistance of blood vessels per se to invasion by glioma cells, spread along perivascular pathways is common, particularly in high-grade tumors, in which it may result in apparently discrete and separate tumor foci.

Approximately 4% to 10% of gliomas appear to be multicentric (i.e., to have more than one ''central'' mass on macroscopic examination) (see Figs. 20–6 and 20–14).[29, 36, 44] Often, multicentric tumors have grossly obvious connections. Even when the gross connection is inapparent or inconclusive, a careful microscopic examination often reveals a trail of infiltrating tumor cells extending between the apparently discrete masses. Secondary formation of compact zones at distant sites of white matter infiltration is the major cause of multicentricity. The barrier property of gray matter is another mechanism that can cause apparent multicentricity when curving white matter bundles connect tumor masses separated by gray matter structures. The connections also may be related to spread of subependymal tumor deposits. Less commonly, no cellular trail is identifiable; in such cases, multifocality may develop via perivascular subpial spread. Current views on the genesis of gliomas from local clonal expansion argue against true multifocal origin.[7, 37]

CORRELATION OF TUMOR MORPHOLOGY WITH IMAGING STUDIES

The anatomy described thus far primarily has been defined by studying untreated tumors at autopsy. These analyses provide elegant descriptions of the natural history of gliomas and of end-stage glioma morphology. However, the few cases in which gliomas were present in patients who were dying of unrelated causes do not provide an adequate basis to assess the morphology of less mature tumors. For example,

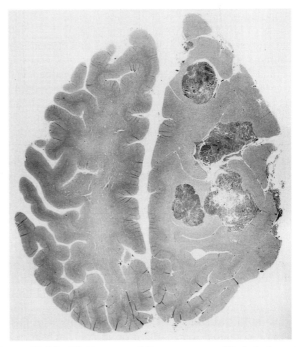

Figure 20–14 Glioblastoma multiforme, recurrent. Whole brain section showing multicentric expansive lesions. These highly cellular nodules of small anaplastic cells did not infiltrate the surrounding parenchyma (hematoxylin-eosin).

Scherer[44] described 20% of GBM as comparatively small tumors, measuring about 120 cm³. Today, this would be considered a fairly large tumor, because computed tomography (CT) and MRI permit diagnosis before tumors reach this size. This is particularly true for oligodendrogliomas, which MRI can detect years sooner than would have been the case with older diagnostic methods, including CT. As a result, treatment now intervenes at a potentially much earlier stage in glioma development.

Because of the importance of defining the extent of a tumor in planning treatment, attempts have been made to correlate pathologic findings with CT and MRI studies. These studies have correlated premortem and preoperative imaging studies with autopsy and biopsy pathologic analyses, respectively, to determine the histologic correlates of contrast enhancement and other imaging abnormalities.[9–11, 20, 21, 29, 31, 32, 57] These studies, as well as postmortem MRI and whole-brain section studies,[30] have evaluated the relationship between edema and the extent of infiltrating tumor.

Contrast enhancement on CT or MRI consistently correlates with a highly cellular tumor core.[9–11, 20, 21, 29, 32] As such, the enhancing margin often correlates with the macroscopic margin. Because enhancement depends on the breakdown of the blood-brain barrier, an association with tumor vasculature has also been sought and identified. The principal vascular alterations in enhancing tumors include microvascular or endothelial proliferation (the abnormal thickening of blood vessel walls that characterizes high-grade gliomas), fibrin microthrombi, and neovascularization, characterized by thin-walled blood vessels with prominent endothelial cells. Enhancement may be solid or may manifest as a ring around a hypodense center. The center of such ring-enhancing lesions is composed primarily of necrotic tumor but also may contain nests of histologically viable tumor cells.[10, 11, 20, 21] Selker and co-workers[47] reported similar findings in recurrent irradiated tumors, in which central radiation necrosis was hypodense and the surrounding enhancing rim contained viable high-grade tumor. However, postradiation enhancement may reflect only vascular injury in non-neoplastic tissue.[22] Neither CT nor MRI can distinguish the core of a nonenhancing low-grade tumor from infiltrating tumor cells.[32]

The distribution of tumor cells in non-enhancing areas of tumor is more variable, but it is of fundamental importance. On CT, these areas are hypodense,[20, 21] whereas on MRI their increased water content creates high signal intensity on T2-weighted images. As suggested by histologic studies, the area of low density or edema tends to follow white matter tracts. Studies correlating the extent of CT abnormalities with histologic findings of untreated gliomas at biopsy[20, 21, 31, 47] and autopsy[9, 10, 29] frequently found tumor cells throughout the area of abnormality. Tumor cells have been found as far as 3 cm from the enhancing areas.[10] Hochberg and Pruitt[29] found a good correlation between CT and histologic tumor margins in 16 treated and 19 untreated patients with GBM. The most common source of error in the delineation of tumor was in patients with ventricular seeding. Also, involvement of deep gray matter structures created error. In 15 patients with untreated GBM and autopsy correlation of CT findings, approximately half had infiltrating tumor cells confined to the area of low density, whereas half had more extensive tumor infiltration.[11] Occasionally, CT may overestimate tumor extent, but it more frequently provides underestimations. Using stereotactic biopsies, Kelly and co-workers[31, 32] correlated the distribution of tumor cells in the areas of high signal intensity on T2-weighted images. As on CT, these areas included both highly cellular areas of tumor, which lacked significant vascular changes (particularly in oligodendrogliomas) as well as areas of necrosis or edema. Peripheral low attenuation on CT and high signal intensity on T2-weighted images corresponded to areas of edema with or without tumor cells. However, MRI more accurately identified both the extent of edema and tumor infiltration. MRI consistently identified a greater volume of edematous parenchyma and areas that contained infiltrating tumor cells with high T2-weighted signal intensity but normal CT density. Neither imaging method allowed prediction of the density or distribution of tumor cells in the edematous areas. In some but not all cases, tumor cells were present at the far edge of the area defined by high T2-weighted signal intensity, which indicates that tumor cells may be present wherever edema is present.

The area of edema defined by the T2-weighted signal merely identifies the minimum area that is *likely* to contain tumor in untreated tumors. In a limited number of biopsies from normal areas adjacent to areas of high signal intensity on T2-weighted images, infiltrating tumor cells were present 40% of the time. This finding actually may underestimate the frequency because of the difficulty of identifying infiltrating tumor cells. In a study that combined MRI with open resections and needle biopsies, Watanabe and associates[57] also found that tumor infiltration typically extended as far as, and often beyond, the area of T2-weighted images. Similar results were obtained in autopsy studies that correlated postmortem MRIs with whole-brain sections. Among a total of six untreated patients, infiltrating tumor cells were present at the edge of the T2-weighted abnormality in three cases, and they extended beyond the T2-weighted abnormality in three cases.[30, 55]

MRI is most effective in predicting the extent of solid tumor and the extent of tumor infiltration of white matter. In contrast, Johnson and colleagues[30] found that MRI could not accurately identify subarachnoid invasion or gray matter infiltration adjacent to white matter tracts. These observations relate to the nature of MRI. Abnormalities on T2-weighted images reflect only the increased water content—edema—in the white matter surrounding cellular areas of gliomas. Thus, the identification of infiltrating tumor by MRI is based on the high correlation between edema and the presence of infiltrating tumor cells. Because gray matter and the subarachnoid space do not demonstrate similar disturbances in water content, infiltrating tumor cells in these locations escape detection by MRI.

These studies have all primarily addressed astrocytomas. No series have specifically correlated imaging with histologic anatomy of oligodendrogliomas. An imaging study of 35 oligodendrogliomas found that approximately half had sharp margins on CT and 75% had them on MRI.[33] As was the case for astrocytomas, MRI more reliably detected edema.

GLIOMA RECURRENCE

Thus far the discussion has been limited to primary untreated tumors. However, more recent studies of glioma growth patterns have included both primary and recurrent tumors. As newer approaches to treatment improve local control and patient survival, the growth and anatomy of the recurring tumor become increasingly important. Although an extensive discussion of the growth of recurrent gliomas is beyond the scope of this chapter, features with implications for the anatomy and treatment of primary tumors are considered.

Morphologic studies of recurrent gliomas address a mixed group of cases. Although the cause of death for most glioma patients is tumor related, a significant number die even though little tumor is identified at autopsy. Giangaspero and Burger[24] described significant tumor mass or infiltration of vital structures in 50% to 60% of 50 cases reviewed at autopsy. In a similar study, Johnson and others[30] found tumor resulting in potentially lethal herniation in only about 25% of 25 patients. Instead of tumor, lethal mass effects often were a consequence of treatment-induced necrosis, massive edema, or a combination of factors. This observation has great implications for treatment as well as for the interpretation of patient survival data. This finding was seen more often in patients treated with stereotactic implants who did not undergo a second resection. Many glioma patients die from disability-related processes, such as pneumonia, or from unrelated events, such as coronary artery disease. Consequently, tumors in autopsy studies are at widely variable stages of development. This variability has the advantage of allowing the pattern of recurrent tumor growth to be pieced together.

Typically, tumor recurrence is defined as the growth of

clinically significant tumor after treatment. Although tumor may recur from distant white matter spread or CSF dissemination, the initial site of recurrence is within 2 cm of the original (enhancing) tumor core in almost all cases.[5, 9–11, 23, 26, 29, 34, 51, 56] In addition, these histologic and imaging studies indicate that most of the compact enhancing tumor is contained within a similar boundary. Although the principal recurrent mass develops locally, recurrent GBM are often characterized by wide dissemination, particularly by small anaplastic tumor cells (Fig. 20–15).[10, 24, 43] Studies evaluated recurrence patterns in patients treated with different approaches to radiotherapy, including whole-brain[23, 56] and limited-volume (tumor plus a 2- to 3-cm margin)[28, 34] external beam radiation, and external beam radiation plus interstitial implant boost to the tumor.[26, 51] Many patients also received a variety of chemotherapy agents. The striking consistency among the results of the studies strongly suggests that the pattern of recurrence of these tumors is intrinsic and unrelated to therapy. Understanding the basis for this recurrence pattern is fundamental to designing new treatment strategies.

Several possible mechanisms for the development of recurrent tumor have been proposed, and it is likely that all play a role in recurrence. The infiltrative growth of gliomas, combined with studies showing mixed results regarding the survival benefits of aggressively pursuing gross total removal of the tumor core,[46] has led to the following view: recurrence results from proliferation of individual tumor cells that escape the surgeon and infiltrate beyond the standard radiation treatment volume (i.e., 2 to 3 cm beyond the area of contrast enhancement). Because the neurologic cost of more aggressive surgery or radiotherapy usually precludes complete ex-

tirpation, therapists often conclude that they are engaged in a losing battle of chasing the tumor from behind. However, these studies relied on the surgeons' estimates of residual tumor. Studies by Forsting and associates[22] and Albert and co-workers[1] documented that early postoperative MRI more accurately predicted tumor margins and frequently identified residual enhancing tumor when none was grossly apparent. Moreover, the progression-free interval and rate of tumor recurrence were highly correlated with the presence or absence of residual enhancing tumor on postoperative MRI. The presence of residual enhancement was associated with clinically significant regrowth in 98% of cases,[1] and the site of recurrence corresponded to the area of residual contrast enhancement.[22] Yoshida and others[58] also found increased survival in patients who underwent total resection of gliomas, as judged by MRI criteria. A similar CT study by Ammirati and colleagues[3] also found significantly longer survival in patients with gross total resection as judged by postoperative CT. Thus, increasing evidence suggests that the tumor core, and not infiltrating tumor cells, is the principal culprit in recurrence, particularly early recurrence in gliomas. These studies neither preclude a role for infiltrating tumor cells in recurrence nor suggest that the elimination of contrast-enhancing tumor was curative. Although recurrence was delayed, tumor did recur in the absence of residual contrast enhancement.

When a combination of surgery and radiation therapy achieves good initial local control, a characteristic pattern of recurrence often develops. A period of remission often exists before active regrowth, during which cellular foci are small, if present (Fig. 20–16). The treated area consists primarily of

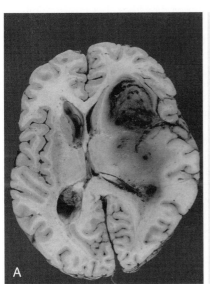
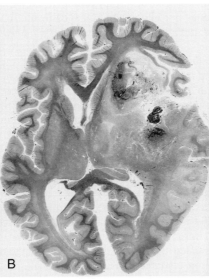
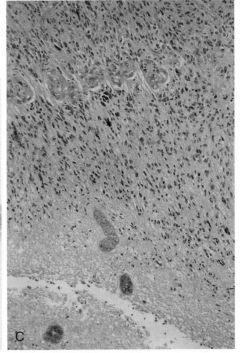

Figure 20–15 Glioblastoma multiforme (GBM), recurrent. *A,* Gross specimen showing typical appearance of recurrent GBM. Expansive cellular foci and infiltrating tumor are admixed with radiation necrosis and hemorrhage. *B,* Whole brain section showing extensive tumor infiltration. Infiltrating tumor extended throughout surrounding edematous areas, which are identified by their pallor (Weil's stain). *C,* Highly cellular foci of small anaplastic astrocytes are seen adjacent to areas of radiation necrosis and vascular injury (hematoxylin-eosin; original magnification ×100).

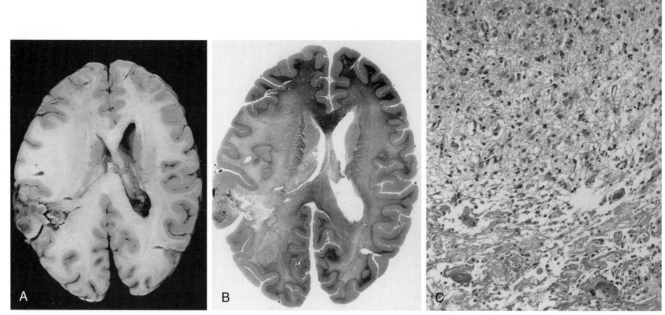

Figure 20–16 Glioblastoma multiforme, remission. *A,* Variegated appearance of lesion is similar to that seen in recurrence, with areas representing radiation necrosis, gliosis, and edema. However, expansive cellular foci are not identified. *B,* Whole brain section. Unlike the recurrent tumor, no recognizable tumor cells were seen in the extensive area of edema, which extends throughout the hemisphere (Weil's stain). *C,* In remission, radiation necrosis, gliosis, and edema predominate. Scattered atypical cells, often with bizarre nuclei, are seen. Whether these represent radiation damage, reactive astrocytes, or residual tumor cells cannot be determined. Cellular tumor foci are lacking (hematoxylin-eosin; original magnification × 100).

radiation-induced changes, including vascular abnormalities, necrosis, and scattered cells with cytologic atypia, which make it difficult to distinguish reactive astrocytes from residual neoplastic cells. The clinical potential of these cells is unclear; however, they have little proliferative activity and do not grow well in cell culture, which suggests that they may be damaged, end-stage cells.[4] CT scans during remission show low-density areas that corresponded to chronic edema containing variable numbers of infiltrating tumor cells and reactive astrocytes histologically.[10] In this stage, the MRI appearance of tumors is confusing and does not allow reliable distinction between viable tumor and radiation effects. Early tumor recurrence after remission is heralded microscopically by the appearance of highly cellular clusters of small, poorly differentiated cells that develop in the radiation-damaged areas. Rapid proliferation leads to coalescence of the microscopic foci and emergence of a new tumor mass (see Fig. 20–15).

The development of recurrent tumor in the absence of residual cellular foci indicates that even "effectively" treated tumor harbors isolated cells capable of producing a recurrence. These findings question the ability of radiation therapy to provide consistent local control of gliomas. Cytogenetic studies of irradiated gliomas support this view. After effectively delivered radiation therapy, cells did not remain viable in culture, which suggests that they were lethally injured by the treatment.[4] However, some irradiated tumors sampled from the site of interstitial implantation contained cells that were viable in culture, which indicates that they had not been treated adequately. That external beam radiation does not kill all of the targeted tumor cells is expected on the basis of dosage limitations. This study, however,

indicates that even interstitial radiation does not reliably and lethally injure all of the tumor cells in the treatment volume.

Irrespective of the mechanism by which the recurrent mass develops, subsequent unchecked growth typically results in extensive multilobar ipsilateral or contralateral spread. For unknown reasons, recurrent high-grade gliomas appear to be more invasive than their primary counterparts. However, their pattern of spread is similar to that of primary tumors: the infiltrating cells spread along white matter tracts, primarily in anteroposterior directions, but also through the corpus callosum and down the internal capsule into the brainstem.[30, 54] MRI estimates of the extent of infiltrating recurrent tumor are unreliable. The abnormal signal intensity on T2-weighted images has underestimated the extent of tumor 30% of the time, correlated well 45% of the time, and overestimated tumor extent 25% of the time.[30] As was the case for primary tumors, gray matter involvement was poorly predicted, but distant white matter involvement beyond the area of abnormality on T2-weighted images also occurred.

Small anaplastic or small fibrillated astrocytes are often the predominant tumor cell type, particularly in late tumor recurrence.[10, 11, 24, 30, 54] In addition to their proliferative capacity, these cells are highly infiltrative and, consequently, may be remarkably widely disseminated. Cytogenetic studies have identified a cell that appears to correspond to the small anaplastic astrocyte. These cells have a similar poorly differentiated cytologic appearance and share the rapid growth and migrational characteristics found in vivo. Of particular interest are cytogenetic studies comparing pairs of primary and recurrent tumors. Whereas the small anaplastic cells often dominate in recurrent tumors, they usually are only a minor, often hard-to-detect subpopulation in primary tumors. Their increase relative to other tumor cell populations presumably reflects a selective growth advantage, the basis of which is unknown. Cytogenetic studies have shown increased resistance to radiation and chemotherapy in such cells.[2]

The foregoing introduces the issue of the evolution of multiple populations within a tumor. The presence of significant histologic variation within gliomas is well known, and recent studies have documented similar heterogeneity in a variety of genotypic and molecular phenotypic features. Recent studies suggest that the relationships of these varied tumor populations are of great clinical importance as discussed below.

TUMOR HETEROGENEITY AND CLONAL ANATOMY

Tumor heterogeneity may be defined as cellular variation in genotype and/or phenotype within a tumor. The differential expression of these cellular features may occur on a diffuse, cell-to-cell basis or may have a regional distribution. In regional heterogeneity, individual cells tend to be similar to their immediate neighbors, whereas more distant cells have different characteristics.

The histologic heterogeneity of gliomas has been well documented for more than 50 years.[11, 12, 17, 24, 44] Typically, gliomas are composed of cells with different cytologic features (e.g., fibrillary, gemistocytic, small anaplastic). These different cell types may be diffusely admixed or spatially separate. After histologic grading systems were developed, autopsy studies on whole-brain sections also documented the variability of diagnostically important histologic features in gliomas, including cytologic atypia, mitotic activity, tumor necrosis, and microvascular proliferation.[12, 24] These features may have a limited distribution, creating the potential for diagnostic sampling errors. Sampling errors related to heterogeneity are influenced by biopsy location and size. Modern imaging modalities help in the first regard, and some reports suggest that multiple properly directed needle biopsies are at least as effective as open biopsies.[14, 20] However, small sample size and localized sample sites limit the chance of identifying a regionally distributed feature.

Recent studies provide compelling evidence of the diagnostic importance of regional heterogeneity and the essential need for broad sampling to enhance diagnostic accuracy. Glantz and co-workers[25] found a much lower rate of diagnosis of GBM in needle biopsies compared to larger open biopsies. GBM was diagnosed in 82% and anaplastic astrocytomas in 18% of open biopsies. In contrast, needle biopsies yielded 49% GBM and 51% anaplastic astrocytomas. Paulus and Peiffer[40] provided quantitative confirmation of the great potential for diagnostic errors. Multiple small samples from 50 large resection specimens of astrocytic and oligodendroglial tumors were reviewed as a model for needle biopsies. Twenty-two percent of the samples from overall high-grade tumors had only low-grade histologic features. Different grades were present in 82% of tumors, and 62% had both low-grade (grade 2) and higher-grade areas.[40] The coexistence of low- and high-grade tumor elements has already been noted.[10, 11, 16, 17, 44] This study points out a contrast

between tumors at the time of biopsy and at autopsy: Scherer[44] found a much lower frequency of low-grade tumors in his series of untreated cases at autopsy.

Gliomas also demonstrate heterogeneity in karyotype[7, 8, 19, 49] and deoxyribonucleic acid (DNA) ploidy,[16, 19] in proliferative activity, in the expression of growth factors[41, 42] and their receptors,[53] in oncogene expression,[50] in a number of glioma-associated antigens,[52] and in intrinsic resistance to chemotherapy and radiotherapy.[2, 6, 48] Regional heterogeneity appears to be a ubiquitous feature of gliomas, which must be addressed as new methods for evaluating gliomas are developed. In addition, glioma heterogeneity is a barrier to the development of target-specific therapies.

Consideration of the genetic evolution of tumors provides insight into glioma growth and anatomy and into the development of heterogeneity. Most tumors, including gliomas, are believed to have monoclonal origins. This contention is supported by a study of X chromosome gene inactivation and genetic loss in chromosomes 10 and 17, which are known to be related to astrocytoma progression.[7] The presence of identical genetic losses throughout a tumor provides strong evidence for a monoclonal origin. Malignant tumor progression reflects a series of mutations in the original monoclonal tumor that promote the ability to proliferate, infiltrate, and otherwise compete more successfully for resources in a hostile environment, which includes both natural defenses and therapeutic factors, such as radiation and chemotherapy. This process is thought to result from the clonal expansion of single mutant cells.[37] Continued proliferation of a successful mutant clone is followed by further clonal evolution until the tumor contains many diverse but related populations. The process of progression is not necessarily linear or restricted to the evolution of a single population. More than one successful mutation can develop in a tumor, and the development of competing clones creates additional genotypic differences. Because each specific individual mutation is a local phenomenon, the expansion of successful clonal populations creates regional genetic differences within a tumor. The result is the development of multiple competing clones with various degrees of spatial overlap.

Molecular and genetic studies of glioma heterogeneity support this model of glioma evolution. Recent detailed cytogenetic analyses provide insight into the expression and development of cellular heterogeneity, particularly in regard to the spatial distribution of evolving clonal populations as they may relate to tumor progression. My colleagues and I[19] studied 38 regions from an evolving low-grade glioma (Fig. 20–17). The spatial relationships of the four unrelated clonal subpopulations were of particular interest. Three clonal populations had limited distributions, each being present in only a few regions. The regions in which a karyotypic deviation was observed were usually contiguous, and little or no overlap was seen between these regions. Each karyotypically distinct clonal subpopulation was spatially separated from the other clonal microfoci. Thus, each subpopulation appeared to result from the expansion of a successful mutant cell. The clone with the largest representation (47,Xy, + 7) was widely distributed throughout the tumor. As was true of the other clones, the regions containing the 47,Xy, + 7 karyotype were contiguous. Because of its extensive distribution, it shared some regions of the tumor with the three

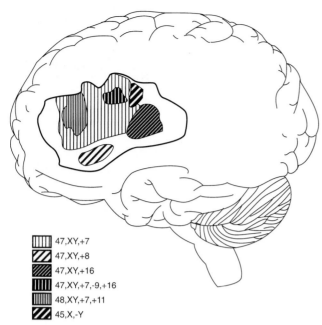

47,XY,+7
47,XY,+8
47,XY,+16
47,XY,+7,-9,+16
48,XY,+7,+11
45,X,-Y

Figure 20–17 Anatomic model of evolution and expansion. Note the development of spatially isolated clonal populations within the overall tumor. Subsequent generations of the mutation/clonal expansion cycle demonstrate similar spatial properties. The primary and derivative subpopulations with trisomy 7 are indicated by the regions with *vertical stripes.* The areas with *diagonal stripes* indicate unrelated populations.

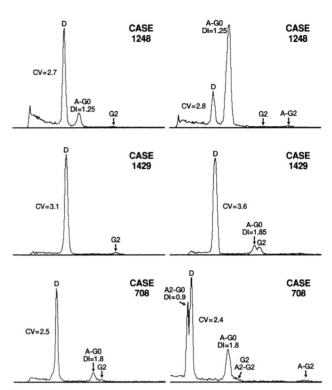

Figure 20–18 Histograms demonstrating different patterns of heterogeneity in DNA ploidy. *Top,* Variation in the relative percentages of near diploid and aneuploid tumor populations. *Center,* Different regions of tumors may be diploid or aneuploid. *Bottom,* Different numbers of aneuploid peaks may be seen in aneuploid tumors.

other clonal subpopulations. However, the regions with the greatest concentration of the karyotype were separate from the other microfoci, which suggests a spatially separate origin with subsequent infiltrative migration. The analyses also indicated that the 47,Xy, + 7 cell line underwent additional karyotypic evolution and generated a number of sideline populations. Each of these sideline populations was present as a spatially isolated focus within the area occupied by the parent 47,Xy, + 7 clone. Thus, each sideline population also exhibited spatial localization similar to that of the first-generation clonal populations.

Flow cytometry studies of regional heterogeneity in DNA ploidy also demonstrate that populations may have varied distributions within a tumor (Fig. 20–18). Regions with the highest percentages of an aneuploid population often cluster (Fig. 20–19). In studies of proliferative activity using flow cytometry S-phase measurements and Ki-67 immunohistochemistry, heterogeneity in proliferative activity is seen (Fig. 20–20), and the most highly proliferative regions have a similar pattern of clustering. Regions with similar proliferative activity tend to cluster, with a gradient of proliferative activity that decreases as one moves away from the most active area (Fig. 20–21). Both observations indicate the presence of a population of tumor cells that are expanding and infiltrating within the overall structure of the tumor. In particular, the kinetic data are indicative of expansive infiltration of a more aggressive cell line.

These analyses strongly support a tumor progression model in which a local successful mutation is followed by clonal expansion. Continued expansion is associated with successive generations of the mutation-expansion cycle.[37] Such a model actually predicts the juxtaposition and overlap

Aneuploid Peak DNA Index=1.85

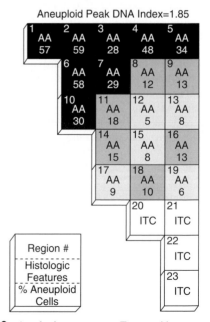

Figure 20–19 Anaplastic astrocytoma. Topographic representation showing distribution of an aneuploid population in histologically similar areas of an anaplastic astrocytoma. The regions with the highest concentration of aneuploid cells are clustered, with a gradual decrease in the percentage of aneuploid cells extending away from this area. Abbreviations: ITC, individual tumor cells; AA, anaplastic astrocytoma.

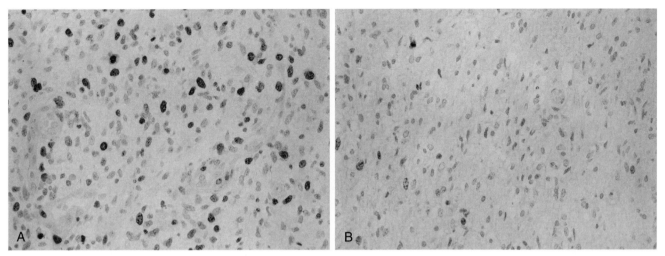

Figure 20–20 Anaplastic astrocytoma. Marked variability in tumor proliferative activity as measured by the Ki-67 labeling index (LI) may be seen in different areas of a tumor. *A*, LI = 22%. *B*, LI = 3%. (MIB–1 immunohistochemistry with hematoxylin counterstain; original magnification ×250.)

of competing clones that, when coupled with microenvironmental differences, produce the genotypic and phenotypic variety observed in gliomas. Thus, the heterogeneity in gliomas is an expected result of tumor progression and reflects the genetic instability that is a fundamental property of gliomas and is central to their evolution. Because most mutations are unsuccessful, a high rate of mutation presumably increases the likelihood of producing successful clones. Thus, it is not surprising that glioma heterogeneity consistently increases with grade.[16, 17]

Local clonal expansion also explains the coexistence of low- and high-grade areas in gliomas. A high-grade clone

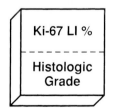

5.0 AA-R	4.7 AA-R	4.6 AA-R	2.4 AA-R
4.4 AA-R	3.3 AA-R	1.1 AA-R	0.2 AA-R
5.4 AA-R	3.1 AA-R	2.2 AA-R	1.1 AA-R

Ki-67 LI %

Histologic Grade

Figure 20–21 Anaplastic astrocytoma, recurrent (AA-R). Topographic representation of Ki-67 labeling index/heterogeneity. *Shading* highlights regions of similar labeling index. There is a decrease in grading of proliferative activity away from the regions with the highest labeling index, which are clustered.

grows not only into the surrounding brain but also into preexisting low-grade tumor. The mixed expansive-infiltrative growth of high-grade gliomas juxtaposes low- and high-grade cells on both a regional and individual cell-to-cell basis. Given enough time, high-grade clones completely overgrow preexisting lower-grade tumor. This advantage explains the relative rarity of coexisting low- and high-grade tumor in untreated gliomas at autopsy[44] compared to those seen earlier in their development.[17, 40] The analysis of recurrent tumors supports the idea of emergence of more aggressive clones. Just as histologic studies have demonstrated that small anaplastic astrocytes frequently constitute the principal population in recurrent astrocytomas, molecular and cytogenetic studies have made similar observations. Flow cytometry DNA and cytogenetic studies of a recurrent tumor have shown the emergence of a dominant aneuploid population that was present as only a minor population in the primary tumor.[16, 48]

The anatomy and morphology of gliomas must be considered beyond just the relationships of histologic features and patterns of infiltration and spread. Tumors have an underlying structure that is related to the evolution and competition of different populations, and this clonal anatomy has important implications for treatment. The diffusely infiltrative nature of gliomas precludes cure by available therapies.[27] However, a recent review of surgical treatment of GBM concluded that radical tumor removal offers the potential for long-term survival.[46] In addition, imaging studies that have found delayed recurrence and/or prolonged survival in patients with no residual enhancing tumor suggest that removal of high-grade elements can prolong survival.[1, 3, 22, 57, 58] The observations regarding tumor heterogeneity and clonal anatomy may provide an explanation. High-grade gliomas typically have a somewhat circumscribed cellular core and often appear to be expansive rather than infiltrative. Scherer[44] and Selby[46] have argued that high-grade tumors may be more readily resectable than low-grade tumors because of this apparent difference in invasiveness. Although this view disregards the overall diffuse growth of gliomas that usually makes them unresectable, it shows insight regarding the

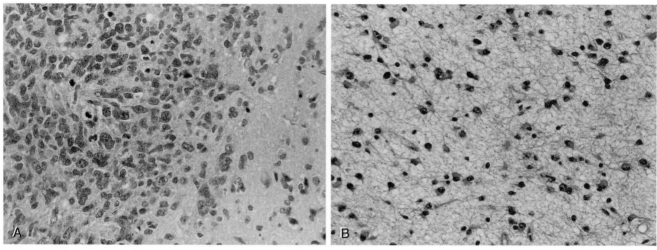

Figure 20–22 Primary glioblastoma multiforme with subsequent recurrence as low-grade astrocytoma. *A,* Primary glioblastoma multiforme. The initial resection demonstrated a highly pleomorphic and proliferative neoplasm with areas of tumor necrosis (not shown). *B,* Recurrent low-grade astrocytoma. The tumor is composed of infiltrating, well-differentiated fibrillary astrocytes.

potentially limited distribution of high-grade elements within a tumor. Because tumor progression is a local phenomenon, the distribution of the transformed cells initially is restricted. Thus, high-grade tumor may be spatially distinct within the fabric of a low-grade tumor. Such localization of high-grade elements may permit their complete surgical extirpation. As a whole, the tumor would not be cured, but theoretically it would be converted back to its lower-grade phase.

My colleagues and I have described a patient who had subtotal resection of a typical GBM (Fig. 20–22*A*).[59] Regional mapping studies demonstrated that the tumor was highly proliferative, with the Ki-67 labeling index (LI) averaging 19%. Similarly, the tumor showed loss of *DCC* (deleted in colon cancer) and RPTPβ (receptor protein tyrosine phosphatase β) gene expression, which has been associated with aggressive, high-grade astrocytomas. Cytogenetic studies showed a near-diploid tumor with numerous marker chromosomes. The patient underwent a second extensive resection 6 months later. Similar regional analyses disclosed a diffusely low-grade astrocytoma (Fig. 20–22*B*). The Ki-67 LI of the recurrent/residual tumor was only 3.6%. Similarly, expression of DCC and RPTPβ and decreased marker chromosomes increased, which is consistent with a lower-grade tumor. The patient survived 4 years from the original diagnosis. Thus, histologic, molecular, and clinical evidence was shown for ''conversion'' of a GBM to a low-grade astrocytoma by aggressive surgical management.

Experience teaches us that such a fortuitous outcome is rare. Such a result is only possible when the high-grade tumor elements are localized. Although current views on tumor progression indicate that most tumors go through a period of such localization, the window of opportunity before the more aggressive tumor cells permeate the tumor may be small. Furthermore, no direct means exists of ascertaining if the high-grade tumor was completely removed. Laboratory studies can only address the tumor that is removed, and not that which remains in the patient. Irrespective of the likelihood of such an outcome, the anatomic issues related to tumor progression, regional heterogeneity, and clonal anatomy must be considered in the management of individual patients and in the design of clinical trials.

REFERENCES

1. Albert FK, Forsting M, Sartor K, et al: Early postoperative magnetic resonance imaging after resection of malignant glioma: Objective evaluation of residual tumor and its influence on regrowth and prognosis. Neurosurgery 1994; 34:45.
2. Allam A, Taghian A, Gioioso D, et al: Intratumoral heterogeneity of malignant gliomas measured in vitro. Int J Radiat Oncol Biol Phys 1993; 27:303.
3. Ammirati M, Vick N, Liao Y, et al: Effect of the extent of surgical resection on survival and quality of life in patients with supratentorial glioblastomas and anaplastic astrocytomas. Neurosurgery 1987; 21:201.
4. Arbit E, Shapiro JR, Fiola M, et al: The significance of morphologically viable glioma cells found at the time of operation after interstitial brachytherapy. Neurosurgery 1993; 32:105.
5. Bashir R, Hochberg F, Oot R: Regrowth patterns of glioblastoma multiforme related to planning of interstitial brachytherapy radiation fields. Neurosurgery 1988; 23:27.
6. Benediktsson G, Blomquist E, Carlsson J: Heterogeneity in cell loss and frequency of slow growing colonies of human glioma cell lines: Some effects of radiation. Anticancer Res 1989; 9:1483.
7. Berkman RA, Clark WC, Saxena A, et al: Clonal composition of glioblastoma multiforme. J Neurosurg 1992; 77:432.
8. Bigner DD: Biology of gliomas: Potential clinical implications of glioma cellular heterogeneity. Neurosurgery 1981; 9:320.
9. Burger PC: Pathologic anatomy and CT correlations in the glioblastoma multiforme. Appl Neurophysiol 1983; 46:180.
10. Burger PC, Dubois PJ, Schold SC, Jr, et al: Computerized tomographic and pathologic studies of the untreated, quiescent, and recurrent glioblastoma multiforme. J Neurosurg 1983; 58:159.
11. Burger PC, Heinz ER, Shibata T, et al: Topographic anatomy and CT correlations in the untreated glioblastoma multiforme. J Neurosurg 1988; 68:698.
12. Burger PC, Kleihues P: Cytologic composition of the untreated glioblastoma with implications for evaluation of needle biopsies. Cancer 1989; 63:2014.
13. Burger PC, Scheithauer BW, Vogel FS: Surgical Pathology of the Nervous System and its Coverings. New York, Churchill Livingstone, 1991, pp 193–437.
14. Chandrasoma PT, Smith MM, Apuzzo MLJ: Stereotactic biopsy in the diagnosis of brain masses: Comparison of results of biopsy and resected surgical specimen. Neurosurgery 1989; 24:160.

15. Choucair AK, Levin VA, Gutin PH, et al: Development of multiple lesions during radiation therapy and chemotherapy in patients with gliomas. J Neurosurg 1986; 65:654.

16. Coons SW, Johnson PC: Regional heterogeneity in the DNA content of human gliomas. Cancer 1993; 72:3052.

17. Coons SW, Johnson PC: Regional heterogeneity in the proliferative activity of human gliomas as measured by the Ki-67 labeling index. J Neuropathol Exp Neurol 1993; 52:609.

18. Coons SW, Johnson PC, Scheithauer BW, et al: Improving interobserver correlation in the classification and grading of gliomas. J Neuropathol Exp Neurol 1993; 52:288.

19. Coons SW, Johnson PC, Shapiro JR: Cytogenetic and flow cytometry DNA analysis of regional heterogeneity in a low grade human glioma. Cancer Res 1995; 55:1569.

20. Daumas-Duport C, Monsaingeon V, N'Guyen JP, et al: Some correlations between histological and CT aspects of cerebral gliomas contributing to the choice of significant trajectories for stereotactic biopsies. Acta Neurochirurgica Suppl 1984; 33:185.

21. Daumas-Duport C, Monsaingeon V, Szenthe L, et al: Serial stereotactic biopsies: A double histological code of gliomas according to malignancy and 3-D configuration, as an aid to therapeutic decision and assessment of results. Appl Neurophysiol 1982; 45:431.

22. Forsting M, Albert FK, Kunze S, et al: Extirpation of glioblastomas: MR and CT follow-up of residual tumor and regrowth patterns. AJNR 1993; 14:77.

23. Gaspar LE, Fisher BJ, Macdonald DR, et al: Supratentorial malignant glioma: Patterns of recurrence and implications for external beam local treatment. Int J Radiat Oncol Biol Phys 1992; 24:55.

24. Giangaspero F, Burger PC: Correlations between cytologic composition and biologic behavior in the glioblastoma multiforme. Cancer 1983; 52:2320.

25. Glantz MJ, Burger PC, Herndon JE II, et al: Influence of the type of surgery on the histologic diagnosis in patients with anaplastic gliomas. Neurology 1991; 41:1741.

26. Gutin PH, Leibel SA, Wara WM, et al: Recurrent malignant gliomas: Survival following interstitial brachytherapy with high-activity iodine-125 sources. J Neurosurg 1987; 67:864.

27. Halperin EC, Burger PC, Bullard DE: The fallacy of the localized supratentorial malignant glioma. Int J Radiat Oncol Biol Phys 1988; 15:505.

28. Hess CF, Schaaf JC, Kortmann RD, et al: Malignant glioma: Patterns of failure following individually tailored limited volume irradiation. Radiother Oncol 1994; 30:146.

29. Hochberg FH, Pruitt A: Assumptions in the radiotherapy of glioblastoma. Neurology 1980; 30:907.

30. Johnson PC, Hunt SJ, Drayer BP: Human cerebral gliomas: Correlation of postmortem MR imaging and neuropathologic findings. Radiology 1989; 170:211.

31. Kelly PJ, Daumas-Duport C, Kispert DB, et al: Imaging-based stereotaxic serial biopsies in untreated intracranial glial neoplasms. J Neurosurg 1987; 66:865.

32. Kelly PJ, Daumas-Duport C, Scheithauer BW, et al: Stereotactic histologic correlations of computed tomography– and magnetic resonance imaging–defined abnormalities in patients with glial neoplasms. Mayo Clin Proc 1987; 62:450.

33. Lee Y-Y, Van Tassel P: Intracranial oligodendrogliomas: Imaging findings in 35 untreated cases. AJNR 1989; 152:361.

34. Liang BC, Thornton AF Jr, Sandler HM, et al: Malignant astrocytomas: Focal tumor recurrence after focal external beam radiation therapy. J Neurosurg 1991; 75:559.

35. Maria BL, Eskin TA, Quisling RG: Brainstem and other malignant gliomas: II. Possible mechanisms of brain infiltration by tumor cells. J Child Neurol 1993; 8:292.

36. Matsukado Y, MacCarty CS, Kernohan JW: The growth of glioblastoma multiforme (astrocytomas, grades 3 and 4) in neurosurgical practice. J Neurosurg 1961; 18:636.

37. Nowell PC: The clonal evolution of tumor cell populations. Science 1976; 194:23.

38. Ohnishi T, Arita N, Hayakawa T, et al: Motility factor produced by malignant glioma cells: Role in tumor invasion. J Neurosurg 1990; 73:881.

39. Onda K, Tanaka R, Takahashi H, et al: Cerebral glioblastoma with cerebrospinal fluid dissemination: A clinicopathological study of 14 cases examined by complete autopsy. Neurosurgery 1989; 25:533.

40. Paulus W, Peiffer J: Intratumoral histologic heterogeneity of gliomas: A quantitative study. Cancer 1989; 64:442.

41. Reifenberger G, Deckert M, Wechsler W: Immunohistochemical determination of protein kinase C expression and proliferative activity in human brain tumors. Acta Neuropathol 1989; 78:166.

42. Scheck AC, Beikman MK, Korn MC, et al: Regional analysis of genes potentially involved in resistance to BCNU in human malignant gliomas. Proc Am Assoc Cancer Res 1991; 32:358.

43. Scherer HJ: Structural development in gliomas. Am J Cancer 1938; 34:333.

44. Scherer HJ: The forms of growth in gliomas and their practical significance. Brain 1940; 63:1.

45. Scherer HJ: Cerebral astrocytomas and their derivatives. Am J Cancer 1940; 40:159.

46. Selby R: The surgical treatment of cerebral glioblastoma multiforme: An historical review. J Neurooncol 1994; 18:175.

47. Selker RG, Mendelow H, Walker M, et al: Pathological correlation of CT ring in recurrent, previously treated gliomas. Surg Neurol 1982; 17:251.

48. Shapiro JR, Scheck AC, Mehta BM, et al: Minor subpopulation of intrinsically chemoresistant and radioresistant cells in primary gliomas become the dominant population in recurrent tumors. J Cancer Res Clin Oncol 1990; 116:1135.

49. Shapiro JR, Shapiro WR: The subpopulations and isolated cell types of freshly resected high grade human gliomas: Their influence on the tumor's evolution in vivo and behavior and therapy in vitro (review). Cancer Metastasis Rev 1985; 4:107.

50. Sidransky D, Mikkelsen T, Schwechheimer K, et al: Clonal expansion of p53 mutant cells is associated with brain tumour progression. Nature 1995; 355:846.

51. Sneed PK, Gutin PH, Larson DA, et al: Patterns of recurrence of glioblastoma multiforme after external irradiation followed by implant boost. Int J Radiat Oncol Biol Phys 1994; 29:719.

52. Stavrou D, Bise K, Groeneveld J, et al: Antigenic heterogeneity of human brain tumors defined by monoclonal antibodies. Anticancer Res 1989; 9:1489.

53. Strommer K, Hamou MF, Diggelmann H, et al: Cellular and tumoural heterogeneity of EGFR gene amplification in human malignant gliomas. Acta Neurochir (Wien) 1990; 107:82.

54. Tamura M, Ohye C, Nakazato Y: Pathological anatomy of autopsy brain with malignant glioma. Neurol Med Chir (Tokyo) 1993; 33:77.

55. Tovi M, Hartman M, Lilja A, et al: MR imaging in cerebral gliomas: Tissue component analysis in correlation with histopathology of whole-brain specimens. Acta Radiologica 1994; 35:495.

56. Wallner KE, Galicich JH, Krol G, et al: Patterns of failure following treatment for glioblastoma multiforme and anaplastic astrocytoma. Int J Radiat Oncol Biol Phys 1989; 16:1405.

57. Watanabe M, Tanaka R, Takeda N: Magnetic resonance imaging and histopathology of cerebral gliomas. Neuroradiology 1992; 34:463.

58. Yoshida J, Kajita Y, Wakabayashi T, et al: Long-term follow-up results of 175 patients with malignant glioma: Importance of radical tumour resection and postoperative adjuvant therapy with interferon, ACNU and radiation. Acta Neurochir (Wien) 1994; 127:55.

59. Scheck AC, Shapiro JR, Coons SW, Norman SA, et al: Biological and molecular analysis of a low grade recurrence of a glioblastoma multiforme. Clin Cancer Res 1996; 2:187.

DONG H. KIM

GAYATRY MOHAPATRA

BURT G. FEUERSTEIN

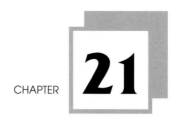

CHAPTER **21**

Tumor Markers in Gliomas

The diagnosis of malignancy by molecules related to the presence of tumor was first described over 150 years ago. The discovery occurred when most physicians still believed that disease was a manifestation of humoral disorders, a system of pathology promulgated in the 2nd century by the School of Galen. In 1845, Henry Bence Jones and William MacIntyre detected a protein in urine from a patient with severe bone pain and edema who on autopsy had soft bones and abnormal marrow but no renal disease.[1, 2] Multiple myeloma was described in 1873,[3] and in 1889 Otto Kahler[4] related the disease to Bence Jones proteinuria. It is remarkable that this marker is still used for diagnosis of multiple myeloma. In this chapter, we discuss definitions and simple theory of markers, the present status of markers in glioma diagnosis and prognosis, and probable directions for marker development in this disease.

WHAT IS A TUMOR MARKER?

A marker is a variable that describes a patient and accurately predicts an outcome.[5, 6] For neoplastic disease, outcomes are the incidence of disease, recurrence, progression, or death. The marker is useful as information to predict the outcome of therapeutic intervention or to simply help the patient in personal planning. However, a truly effective marker eventually ensures that the intervention triggered by the test translates to improved survival or rates of cure.

To determine if a marker predicts an outcome, the assay must be reliable and its prevalence in clinical material should be known. The clinical utility is initially tested in pilot studies, then confirmed in an unselected patient sample, and finally validated in larger populations.

Objective studies of survival are not easy to perform and they are subject to bias. In *lead time bias,* the differences in time of diagnosis might change the apparent survival. For example, a screening test might diagnose a disease before onset of clinical symptoms. This apparent change in survival time may simply reflect early diagnosis without actually benefiting the individual. In *length bias,* cases diagnosed at screening may behave differently from those diagnosed when symptoms appear. For example, the average patient who receives a diagnosis earlier in the clinical course might

have a better prognosis than a patient whose diagnosis is made later. In *selection bias,* a self-selected cohort entering into a screening trial may have a different probability of developing a disease than the population at large. For example, individuals with a positive family history of a disease may be more motivated to enter a screening trial than individuals with no family history. Thus, statistical methods should ensure that bias emanating from selection or treatment is minimized. Study design must also ensure that the power of the study (i.e., the number of patients enrolled) is adequate to answer the question, and that the study ends at the right time: the outcome must be achieved in enough of the study population for a conclusion to be reached.

Single tumor markers may assess the risk, diagnosis, or prognosis of malignant disease. *Risk* is the propensity for developing malignant disease at some future time. *Diagnosis* means that the marker is an absolute predictor of malignant disease. A risk factor or a group of risk factors that predict that a patient is certain to develop malignant disease at some point in the future are called *preclinical diagnostic factors.* Because patients who have preclinical diagnostic factors do not yet have malignant disease, they are good candidates for preventive therapy. *Clinical diagnostic factors* occur in patients who actually have asymptomatic or symptomatic malignant disease. These patients need therapy to treat the malignancy. Clinical diagnostic markers may be useful for monitoring the results of therapy or the recurrence of disease.

Both preclinical and clinical diagnostic factors are invaluable for monitoring progression of disease. We need the ability to detect the potential for neoplastic progression, to predict individual risk of neoplasia, and to develop strategies to reduce the risk. We also may be able to intervene when malignant disease is already evident, to delay progression.

Prognostic factors occur in patients with malignant disease and they predict outcome. Endpoints that measure prognosis include survival, recurrence, time to progression, and response to therapy. Prognostic factors may predict the natural history of disease. Prognostic value may depend on the context within the disease process, and it may change when treatment alters the natural history of disease. Above all, prognostic factors must be significant (occur rarely by chance), independent (retain prognostic value with addition

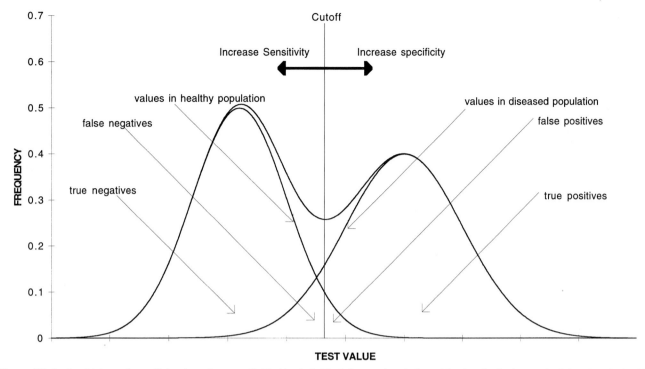

Figure 21–1 Sensitivity and specificity depend on cutoff. Healthy individuals have values indicated by the distribution to the *left* (values in healthy population), and diseased individuals have values indicated by the distribution to the *right* (values in diseased population). The curve above indicates the sum of frequencies in both populations at each test value. The cutoff is indicated by the vertical line. Values below the cutoff indicate health and those above the cutoff indicate disease. As the cutoff moves higher, the number of false-positive results decreases, increasing specificity. As the cutoff moves lower, the number of false-negative results decreases, increasing sensitivity.

of other prognostic factors), and clinically important (have an impact on patient management and outcome).

TESTING THEORY

The foundation for a statistical approach to the evaluation of test results derives from a treatise published in the 18th century.[7] The medical incarnation of the treatise is the model of sensitivity and specificity. This model hinges on the value that discriminates between people with disease and people without disease. Because overlap often occurs in the marker status of these two populations, there will be people who are healthy but who have a positive test (false positives) and people who have the disease but who have a negative test (false negatives). Determining whether a test identifies an acceptable number of false positives or false negatives requires a large number of measurements in matched control and diseased populations.

Sensitivity (SE) measures how well a test can diagnose disease by giving a positive result. In a group with the disease, it is the percentage of individuals that have positive results.

$$SE = \frac{\text{True positives}}{\text{True positives} + \text{false negatives}}$$

Specificity (SP) measures how well a test classifies a person as disease free. In a group that is disease free, specificity is the percentage with a negative test result.

$$SP = \frac{\text{True negatives}}{\text{True negatives} + \text{false positives}}$$

The sensitivity and the specificity of a test is determined by the value that one chooses to indicate disease (Fig. 21–1). If the cutoff moves (higher) toward values that indicate disease, there will be fewer false-positive results but more false-negative results. If the cutoff moves (lower) toward values that indicate health, there will be more false-positive results and fewer false-negative results.

To optimize the sensitivity and specificity of the test, one has to take the consequences of results into account. For example, if a good therapy does not exist or if the chance for a cure in a patient is not very good, maintaining high specificity is reasonable. However, if the disease is serious but should not be missed because effective therapy is available, high sensitivity should be emphasized.

How Good Is a Test?

If a test is random, a positive result has an equal chance of being false or true. Thus, in a random test, the percentage of true positives in the group with disease is equal to the percentage of false positives in the group without disease. If prevalence (P) is the number of affected individuals per 100,000 of the population, then (P)(SE)/P is the percentage of true positives in the group with disease, and (1 − P)(1 − SP)/(1 − P) is the percentage of false positives in the group without disease. Setting the two equal as follows,

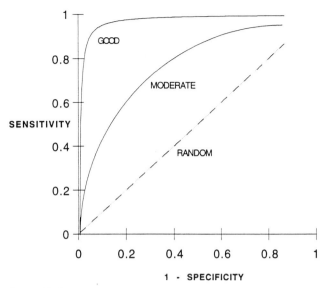

Figure 21–2 Plots of the receiver operating characteristic (ROC). If high sensitivity is maintained over nearly all specificities and high specificity is maintained over nearly all sensitivities, the test is "well behaved." However, as the sum of sensitivity and specificity approaches 1, the test approaches randomness.

$$\frac{(P)(SE)}{P} = \frac{(1 - P)(1 - SP)}{(1 - P)}$$

we find that

$$SE = 1 - SP$$

Thus, in a random test

$$SE + SP = 1$$

When sensitivity is plotted as a function of $1 - SP$, a graph called the *receiver operating characteristic* (ROC) plot is obtained. A random test will give a straight line at 45 degrees to the axes, whereas a highly discriminatory test will show high sensitivity even at high specificity (Fig. 21–2).[8–12]

Testing in a Population

Although high sensitivity and specificity are essential ingredients, a good test's usefulness within a population also depends on the prevalence of disease. Bayes' theorem and its application to medical testing allows one to calculate the probability of disease in a patient with a positive test result.[7, 13] If prevalence is P, then $(P)(SE)$ are the true positives in a population and $(1 - P)(1 - SP)$ are the false positives. The positive predictive value (PPV) is

$$PPV = \frac{\text{True positives}}{\text{True positives } + \text{ false positives}}$$

or, substituting,

$$PPV = \frac{(P)(SE)}{(P)(SE) + (1 - P)(1 - SP)}$$

The benefit of this value to a requesting clinician is obvious:

if a test has a 99% PPV, then a patient with a positive test has a 99% chance of having the disease.

For example, a test with 99% specificity and 99% sensitivity might appear to be excellent. If the incidence of glioma is approximately 20/100,000, the test would identify 99% of those patients: all 20. However, it would also identify the 1% false positives: 1,000 people without disease. Thus, a positive result would indicate that the person has a 0.2% chance of being disease positive. However, if one could identify a high-risk group for glioma in which the prevalence is increased to 10%, false positives would remain at 1,000, but the true positives would increase to 10,000, and the PPV would increase to greater than 90%. Thus, effective screening for groups with disease needing antineoplastic therapy or with high risk who require prevention demands the identification of a population with high enough prevalence to keep down the relative number of false-positive results.

Known groups of patients at increased risk for glioma may be particularly amenable to screening. These include patients with tuberous sclerosis,[14–16] Li-Fraumeni syndrome,[17, 18] von Recklinghausen's neurofibromatosis (types 1 and 2),[19–22] and Turcot syndrome.[23–25] Possible high-risk groups that deserve more study are families of patients with brain tumors[26–33] and those that are exposed to certain environmental toxins, electromagnetic fields, or radiation.[34–42]

GLIOMA PATHOGENESIS AND MARKER DEVELOPMENT

Little is known about the details of initiation and progression in malignant gliomas. It is believed that they mirror the pathogenesis of other tumors, arising from normal glial cells or glial precursors through a stepwise selective process that is predicated on genetic instability.[43–45] The process results in the formation of malignant cells that grow and survive without proper control.[46–48] Further selection results in progressively aggressive phenotypes that invade normal structures and disrupt physiologic function.

The process of tumor initiation and progression can be related to gains and losses of cellular function that occur in the context of glial cells in the central nervous system. For example, normal growth is a balance of positive and negative forces that incline a cell toward or away from DNA synthesis. Selection may exaggerate the function of a growth stimulatory pathway in a glioma precursor cell by increasing activity at a positive regulatory step (an oncogene function) or by decreasing activity at a negative regulatory step (a tumor suppressor function). Either of these events tends to strip the normal regulatory apparatus from the growth process. Repeated selections of cells that grow more quickly result in a population of cells growing out of control (see later discussion on growth).

Similar selections could occur in pathways that regulate other processes that define malignant transformation or progression. For example, unregulated cell division in a tumor might cause it to outstrip its nutritional resources. Selection might then occur in pathways that regulate cell-cell interactions, resulting in tumor cells that can move into regions with more nutritional resources by invading normal parenchyma (see later discussion on invasion).

Evidence that losses and gains in function are related to the genome is contained in studies of chromosomal material in tumor cells. These experiments find that particular losses and gains of genetic material recur in gliomas, that they are associated with histologic grade, and that their number increases as tumors progress[46, 49-53] (see later discussion on genetic losses and gains).

The diagnosis of glioma does not yet reflect the preceding hypothesis. Diagnosis is based on history, physical examination, and imaging studies, as well as on the tumor's anatomy, histology, and expression of lineage and differentiation markers. General markers of proliferation are often assayed as well, but specific regions of the genome responsible for the growth phenotype are not yet generally useful (see later discussions of markers of growth and of genetic loss and gain). If a tumor presents in the CNS, diagnosis is arranged to distinguish metastatic lesions from primary CNS tumors; to establish whether a primary is of glial, neuronal, or other lineage; and to determine whether a glial tumor is of high or low grade: these findings determine the therapeutic approach.

Grading of gliomas has long been debated. Histologic approaches to grading relate a tumor's cytologic appearance to normal cells at different stages of neural development,[54] and to degree of anaplasia.[55-57] Unfortunately, histologic criteria used to classify glioma grade are often subjective, which leads to diagnostic variability. The fact that no universal scheme exists for grading gliomas has led to confusion in interpreting prognostic and therapeutic trials, because tumors are not always placed in uniform or comparable categories.[58, 59] The field awaits both advances in the understanding of normal CNS development to provide better markers of lineage and of differentiation and a better understanding of malignant transformation to provide specific indicators of anaplasia.

Despite its present failings, histologic grading is an important prognostic factor for patients with gliomas.[56] Tumor-related factors such as subependymal spread, invasion into the midline commisural fibers, and gliomatosis cerebri also predict outcome.[60] Together with patient age and performance status at diagnosis,[61, 62] these factors constitute most of the present prognostic armamentarium for treatment of gliomas. Thus, therapeutic trials must be tailored to groups of patients defined by these factors. Obviously, markers that can be evaluated objectively and that correlate with clinical outcome or biologic behavior will help provide an improved classification system for these tumors and aid in proposing and assessing therapeutic regimens.

Even taking these facts into account, it is surprising how much variability exists in the clinical and biologic behavior of gliomas that is not a result of known prognostic factors. For example, some patients with anaplastic astrocytoma respond well to a combination of radiation and chemotherapy, whereas others do not.[63, 64] Indeed, patients with ''uniformly fatal'' glioblastoma multiforme can occasionally survive over the long term.[65] These facts are strong evidence that factors unrelated to the present grading system can determine the clinical course of glioma.

One other important consideration in the development and utilization of prognostic markers for gliomas is the effect of regional heterogeneity on the accuracy of the measurement.

Heterogeneity in histologic grading of gliomas is a well-known problem, and adequate sampling is an important part of histologic diagnosis. The implication is that heterogeneity and adequate sampling are significant variables to consider in the evaluation and use of tumor markers in gliomas.[66-68] Further, because pathogenesis is believed to be predicated on genetic instability and selection, genetic heterogeneity that bears on tumor biology is likely to occur from cell to cell in clinical material. Thus, methods that evaluate markers in biopsy material on a single-cell basis are likely to be invaluable.

In summary, the glioma markers that are presently useful assay the histogenesis of tissue, the degree of anaplasia, and the general state of proliferation. Various clinical considerations such as patient age, performance status, and tumor-related factors are important to the prognosis of disease, but the mechanisms that underlie their effects are unknown.[69] Furthermore, it is evident that other unknown factors also affect the outcome of disease. Finally, heterogeneity in these tumors constitutes a significant problem and makes the evaluation of subpopulations an important consideration. Better descriptions of glioma biology and clinical outcome, as well as new therapies, will result both from the discovery of genes that are responsible for initiation and progression and from better descriptors of the tissue of origin.

GLIOMA MARKERS

We have somewhat arbitrarily divided glioma markers into four main groups. *Markers of lineage and differentiation* identify the tumor tissue or cell of origin. *Markers of growth* and *markers of invasion* represent general phenotypes that are or may be selected during glioma pathogenesis. Markers that depend on *loss or gain of genetic material* represent pathogenetic mechanisms that rely on alterations in gene copy number or function to provide tumor cells with a survival advantage.

Lineage and Differentiation

Markers of lineage and differentiation consist of RNA, proteins, or other products of cellular metabolism that are expressed in tissues of interest, and they can help in diagnosis of cases for which light and electron microscopy are equivocal or for which adequate material is not available. Their use is based on the idea that tumor cells are derived from cells of a particular lineage at a particular state of differentiation. In a general way, the biology of the tumor—and thus its response to therapy—is believed to reflect how the functions obtained through genetic instability and selection interact with the functional state of the cell of origin. However, because gene expression in neoplastic cells is disordered, differentiation and lineage markers may not always reflect the cell of origin. Thus, diagnosis based on these markers requires care and experience. The elucidation of molecules that unambiguously identify both the cell of origin and the events of neoplastic initiation and progression will eventually provide a more meaningful description of glial tumors.

GLIAL PROTEINS

Glial proteins are markers that help to distinguish between glial and nonglial tumors, especially when morphologic features and routine staining cannot establish the diagnosis, to identify astrocytic areas of mixed tumors, and to establish the glial origin of neoplastic cells in tumors metastatic to organs outside of the CNS. They are not yet used for grading.

The most widely used immunochemical diagnostic marker for glial neoplasms is glial fibrillary acidic protein (GFAP). It is a 55 kD class III intermediate filament (IF),[70, 71] a major component of the normal glial cytoskeleton, and it is usually present in perikaryon and cytoplasmic processes. It is used to identify astrocytes and tumors of astrocytic origin. However, caveats should be observed in conjunction with its use. GFAP expression in glia is linked to the functional and developmental state of the cell and thus is dependent on environment.[72–75] In addition, GFAP can be found in developing, reactive, and neoplastic ependymal cells,[76, 77] in developing and neoplastic oligodendroglia,[78, 79] and in a variety of primary CNS tumors that are not glial in origin.[80–83] It has even been found in the peripheral nervous system and in extraneural tissues.[84–89]

Other IFs are also expressed in specific mature tissues. However, because some are expressed as part of normal development in the CNS, they are likely candidates for glioma markers.[90–96] Keratins are class I and II IFs expressed in mature epithelial cells and in cells of primordial neuroectoderm. As neural tube development proceeds, they are replaced in CNS by the class III IF vimentin (most often associated with mesenchymal cells and their products). GFAP expression occurs with further astrocytic differentiation. Each of these IFs is expressed in a proportion of gliomas.

Nestin is a class VI intermediate filament that is specifically expressed in the developing CNS. As neural and glial cells differentiate, it is down-regulated, and other type-specific intermediate filaments are expressed. Biopsies and cell lines derived from a number of primary CNS tumors express the protein; it may also prove to be an important lineage determinant.[90, 92]

The IF-associated proteins (IFAP)[97] are a group of proteins that include those associated with keratins, vimentin, GFAP, and neurofilaments. Among others, the vimentin-associated IFAP (300 kD) may be specific for glial tumors and IFAP-70 (280 kD) may be more specific for reactive processes.[94] Other proteins that have been touted as glioma markers, such as S-100 protein, are apparently involved in GFAP assembly.[98, 99]

NONGLIAL PHENOTYPES

Markers that help to distinguish neuronal, epithelial, mesenchymal, or other phenotypes are helpful in the diagnosis of glial tumors. Synaptophysin,[100–102] class III β-tubulin,[103] neurofilaments,[91, 104] and the microtubule-associated proteins MAP2 and τ-protein[105–107] are examples of neuronal proteins that may help distinguish neuronal elements of neoplastic and normal tissue.[108]

Other useful markers include those that distinguish the macrophage or histiocyte lineage, such as factor XIII and HAM (human alveolar macrophage)-56. These HAM-56 antibodies help to distinguish processes that may mimic gliomas, such as malignant fibrous histiocytoma primary to the CNS or Krabbe's globoid cell dystrophy.

GLYCOLIPIDS

These molecules are sugar-containing lipids. Specific types are present in high concentrations in the CNS and mark development and differentiation of specific glial lineages.[109–117] Involvement in signal transduction may form the basis for the ability of these molecules to mark growth and neoplastic progression.[118–127] Particular glycolipids of interest include those of the ganglio 1b and neolacto series gangliosides. Both grade and survival are correlated with the amount of 1b, and the amount of neolacto series compounds adds significance to the data.

Growth

The ability of a cell to reproduce provides an important selective force in the process of neoplastic transformation. Macroscopic tumor growth results from the relative proportion of cells in three populations of cells: proliferating, quiescent, and dying. Thus, the duration of the cell cycle, the size of the growth fraction, and the fraction of cells lost determine the rate of tumor growth. Because most primary intracranial neoplasms do not metastasize, and because intracranial volume is limited by the skull, a reasonable hypothesis is that the simple act of occupying space is an important prognostic factor for glial tumors. The faster the growth, the more quickly space is appropriated and intracranial pressure increases: this implies that survival should be related to the rate of growth. A great deal of effort has been expended in evaluating markers of proliferation in gliomas to determine the fraction of cycling cells. Quiescent and dying cells have been less well studied. We discuss methods that are currently utilized to evaluate tumor growth.

DNA DISTRIBUTION IN ASYNCHRONOUS CELLS

The relationship of DNA distribution to cell proliferation lies in the fact that cellular DNA content indicates the cell cycle phase. Normal human cells in G1 phase have diploid DNA content. In S phase, the cells continuously increase their DNA content until they reach the G2 and M phases, where they have twice the DNA content as G1 phase cells. Thus, an accounting of the amount of DNA in each cell within a population estimates the fraction of cells in each phase of the cell cycle. Because normal cells in S or G2/M are proliferating, their percentage is related to the total percentage of cells actually in cycle.[128]

Although the content of DNA in a population of diploid cells is related to proliferation, populations of tumor cells present special difficulties. Tumor cells may be diploid or aneuploid, and a single tumor may have a number of cells that are diploid and multiple populations of cells that are aneuploid. This makes it difficult to pigeonhole a cell as being in G1, S, or G2/M phase. Furthermore, cells with a DNA content that describes them as being in S phase may or may not be synthesizing DNA, because genetic instability in tumor cells may result in cell death or cell cycle arrest. These problems illustrate the utility of assays that measure the proliferating fraction more directly.[67]

DNA LABELING

The incorporation of thymidine analogs into DNA is a direct measure of DNA synthesis. Radiolabeled thymidine, bromodeoxyuridine (BUdR), and iododeoxyuridine have all been used. For in vivo labeling, the patient receives an intravenous infusion of an analog preoperatively. BUdR and iododeoxyuridine both have activity as radiation sensitizers, which strengthens the rationale for their use. Labeling can also be accomplished in vitro on primary explants.[129, 130]

The BUdR labeling index is the percentage of cells in a sample that incorporates a standard dose of thymidine analog over a period of time. It generally correlates with the histologic grade of a glioma.[131-133] It is an independent predictor of survival in adult low-grade and anaplastic astrocytomas[134, 135] and in mixed tumors,[136] but not in glioblastoma multiforme[135, 137] or juvenile pilocytic astrocytoma.[138] Preliminary results for pediatric tumors are similar to those in adults: the labeling index is strongly prognostic for low-grade and anaplastic astrocytomas but is less prognostic for glioblastoma multiforme.[139] Thus, direct measurements suggest that the aggressiveness of lower-grade astrocytic tumors is dependent on the fraction of cells synthesizing DNA, but that other factors are involved in glioblastoma multiforme.

OTHER MEASURES OF PROLIFERATION

Several indirect measures of proliferation have been developed. Ki-67/MIB-1 and proliferating cell nuclear antigen (PCNA) assays detect proteins that are associated with proliferation. Nucleolar organizer region–associated argyrophilic protein (AgNOR) measures silver staining proteins associated with the loops of ribosomal DNA present in nucleoli. These measurements are attractive because they measure proteins already present in tumor tissue and thereby avoid infusions of possibly toxic thymidine analogs.

Ki-67 is a monoclonal antibody that selectively reacts with nuclei of proliferating cells.[140] It is expressed in active phases of the cell cycle and may be necessary for maintaining cell proliferation,[141] but it is absent in resting cells[142, 143] and in cells undergoing DNA repair.[144] MIB-1 is a monoclonal antibody directed against another epitope of the same molecule.[145]

In normal human cells, PCNA is a key regulator of DNA synthesis and repair. It complexes with a cyclin, a cyclin-dependent kinase (CDK), and p21, a CDK regulator, to function in regulation of normal DNA synthesis; in transformed cells, these complexes are often disrupted.[146-151] PCNA also functions in DNA nucleotide excision repair.[152-157]

AgNOR reflects the ''nucleolar activity'' of the cell; this is related to the degree of ribosomal RNA synthesis.[158] Nucleolar organizer regions contain loops of DNA with many copies of ribosomal DNA in tandem. Silver binds to and stains several proteins associated with these structures, including B23 and C23.[159-161] An advantage of this technique is its ease and quickness.

Ki-67, PCNA, and AgNOR are promising markers for glioma diagnosis. Ki-67 and PCNA both clearly correlate with grade,[66, 162-166] as well as with each other and with BUdR labeling index.[68, 163, 167, 168] It is not yet certain whether the same is true for AgNOR.[68, 163, 164, 167-169] In pilot studies, PCNA was prognostic in low-[170] but not in high-grade tumors,[171] which bears out the results derived using the BUdR labeling index. AgNOR may help to distinguish low-grade gliomas and gliosis.[172] However, because large trials have not yet been conducted, the clinical usefulness of Ki-67, PCNA, and AgNOR has not yet been well established for glioma.

POTENTIAL DOUBLING TIME

Potential doubling time (t_{pot}) is the doubling time of a tumor in the absence of cell loss. It can be calculated by estimating the duration of the cell cycle and the growth fraction. This has been accomplished by measuring the percent of labeled mitoses at various times after administration of labeled thymidine.[173-175] It can also be appraised by labeling cells with thymidine analog and estimating the rate of increase in DNA concentration[174, 176] or by sequential labeling with two different thymidine analogs (e.g., BUdR followed by iododeoxyuridine).[177, 178] It is unclear whether this parameter will be clinically useful; studies need to be performed.

CELL LOSS/CELL DEATH

Cell loss is difficult to evaluate in a patient. In model systems, one measures how a tumor actually grows and compares it with the t_{pot}. The ratio between the actual and the expected rate of growth is a measure of cell loss.[179] Cell loss can be both variable and substantial: values greater than 40% have been reported.[67, 180] Indirect indicators of cell loss or actual assays for pathways involved in cell loss, such as apoptosis[181-183] may eventually help to evaluate this factor more easily in the clinic.

SUMMARY

Clinical trials indicate that the labeling index is an independent predictor of clinical outcome in glial tumors and that it complements conventional pathologic examination of glial tumors. Although most studies suggest that BUdR is safe, evidence shows that this compound does have potential side effects, because it is a mutagen and a carcinogen in some experimental systems.[184] A number of alternative assays for growth have been developed based on an increased understanding of cell and molecular biology. However, until these approaches are better characterized, the clinical application of bromodeoxyuridine will continue to play an important role in predicting the clinical behavior of many CNS tumors.

Invasion

The ability of glioma cells to infiltrate adjacent structures may mark the grade of tumor and provide a target for intervention.[185] Receptors for extracellular matrix,[186-191] including integrins, various lectins, and other adhesion molecules such as NCAM (neural cell adhesion molecules), are associated with neoplastic and normal glial cells and may permit cells to enter privileged environments. Proteinases and their inhibitors may hasten invasion by modifying brain parenchyma.[192] In pilot studies, the presence of the cysteine protease cathepsin B,[193–195] urokinase plasminogen activator receptor,[196, 197] urokinase plasminogen activator,[196, 198–200] and the absence of tissue plasminogen activator[201, 202] each correlate directly with grade; the latter two also correlate with survival.[203] Larger unselected studies are needed to confirm and extend these findings.

Loss or Gain in Genetic Material

The ability of a cell to alter its genetic material is strictly regulated in normal cells. This regulation is lost in tumor cells, and the amount of genetic material in tumor cells often differs from the amount in normal cells. Once the genome becomes unstable, selection can take place, and as the cell divides, genetic material that codes for growth promotion can accumulate, whereas genetic material that codes for growth control can be lost.

Cells may alter their genome through a variety of mechanisms. For example, cells may go through the S phase of the cell cycle but fail to divide. This leaves them with double the amount of genetic material, but does not select particular pieces of DNA for their tumorigenic properties. Another mechanism may involve a malfunctioning mitotic spindle, leading to losses or gains of whole chromosomes in postmitotic cells. Smaller lesions may result from recombination events or from DNA damage and repair events that result in deletions, translocations, or duplications of DNA.

The gains and losses of DNA that result from genetic instability can be maintained in progeny due to selective pressures. In amplification, particular pieces of genetic material that include genes that code for growth-promoting functions (oncogenes) may accumulate. In deletion, pieces of genetic material with genes that code for growth-inhibiting functions (tumor suppressor genes) may be lost. Thus, pieces of the genome that are gained or lost may be signposts for genes that encode or regulate functions acquired by the tumor.

PLOIDY

DNA content is often utilized to estimate tumor ploidy, which has been studied as a candidate marker in glioma. DNA index (DI) is calculated by dividing the modal DNA content of the population being studied by the DNA content of corresponding normal cells. Thus, samples with a DNA content equal to that of normal cells have a DI equal to 1. Most normal human cells are diploid (2N) because they have two homologous copies of each chromosome (except for the sex chromosomes). Aneuploid cells have extra or missing chromosomal material, and they may be triploid (3N), tetraploid (4N), or intermediate (i.e., 3.4N would be hypertriploid).

Pilot studies in 1979 and 1980 found that aneuploidy was associated with higher tumor grade.[204–206] The data linking aneuploidy and tumor aggressiveness was confirmed in other kinds of cancer,[207] and a study of 153 patients confirmed that aneuploid glial tumors were of higher grade and had

shorter survival times.[208] However, the clinical value of DNA quantitation was later questioned[209] and results from a series of 78 gliomas in 1989 found that of 78 gliomas,[210] more than 60% of tumors were diploid. Simple categorization as aneuploid or diploid did not correlate with histologic grade and did not predict survival or response to therapy. Recent studies of several large series of astrocytic tumors classified them as diploid, hyperdiploid, triploid, hypertriploid, tetraploid, or polymorphic.[211–214] Most tumors were diploid, and the only significant clinical prognosticator was better survival in the small hypertriploid group. In 85 cases of oligodendroglioma, ploidy did not correlate with either survival or tumor grade.[215] Similarly, flow cytometric analysis did not add independent prognostic information for 51 patients with pilocytic astrocytoma.[216] Thus, despite the long history of ploidy measurements in gliomas, and although data links DNA content to prognosis and to grade, the data are conflicting, and a definitive study has not addressed the clinical utility of ploidy measurement.

GENETIC ABERRATIONS, ONCOGENES, AND TUMOR SUPPRESSOR GENES

Because the genome is the ultimate target for selections that will be passed on in progeny, and because genetic aberrations are the products of that selection in tumors, recurring genetic aberrations must harbor the genes that drive tumor initiation and progression. The products of these genes will interact with the internal and external milieu and determine the biology of the tumor. They may also be targeted for therapeutic intervention. Thus, recurring aberrations and the genes that drive their selection should provide excellent prognostic markers for gliomas. Since recent studies have documented that tens of aberrations are present in single malignant gliomas, sensitive and specific assays for several aberrations or several genes may be necessary to describe the tumor's biology and to provide good prognostic information. Several genetic schemes have already been proposed to account for the various histologic grades and even the subsets of grades of gliomas,[53, 217] but these are still likely to be incomplete, because assays for genetic aberrations in gliomas are not sensitive or specific enough and because most genes responsible for initiation and progression of these tumors remain undiscovered.

Several methods have been developed to screen tumors for specific genetic aberrations; these draw attention to particular portions of the genome. The techniques include karyotypic analysis, allelotyping, and molecular cytogenetics. Issues of sensitivity and specificity plague these assays. Until these problems are settled, studies of prognosis will remain suspect.

Further, these techniques cannot in themselves prove whether a particular piece of DNA is an oncogene or a tumor suppressor gene. That process requires cloning a gene, determining its function, and showing that its aberrant expression abets malignant progression. As the phenotype of a biologically significant genetic loss or gain becomes clear, specific protein or RNA may replace or augment the genotype as a convenient assay.

Karyotyping is the process of identifying chromosomes in metaphase based on both their morphologic characteristics and their dye staining ("banding") patterns. It requires cells in metaphase that are appropriately prepared and stained to be visualized under a microscope, and an expert in chromosome identification must examine the cells. Each metaphase allows the experimenter to examine each chromosome for abnormalities. However, since metaphase chromosomes are rarely found in gliomas, primary cultures of tumor cells are often used to identify chromosomal aberrations. Because only a few metaphases may be found, even using primary cultures, and because cell culture is inherently selective, it is impossible to know whether results from karyotyping fairly represent the genetic composition of the primary tumor. In addition, the complex chromosomal aberrations found in gliomas often make it difficult to correctly identify chromosome banding patterns.

Most molecular methods that screen for genetic aberrations in cancer rely on polymorphic sites. If one can distinguish both the paternal and the maternal allele at a polymorphic site in DNA that is isolated from a patient's normal tissue, then one can ask whether both alleles are still present in DNA isolated from that patient's glioma. When tumor tissue has more of one than of the other allele, the conclusion is that a piece of tumor DNA has been altered at that site. However, results from these methods may be difficult to obtain and interpret. First, one must know which polymorphic sites will be informative. Thus, these methods may miss regions of the genome that are lost or gained in a substantial proportion of gliomas. Second, the results of the assay depend on the quality of the DNA that is isolated. If multiple genetic subpopulations are present within the tumor, the DNA isolated from the tumor will be heterogeneous, and molecular methods may not be able to distinguish small but important subpopulations.

Recently developed molecular cytogenetic techniques rely on in situ hybridization of DNA probes labeled with fluorescent molecules (Figs. 21–3 and 21–4). These methods allow direct assay of DNA from the tumor to survey regions of genetic loss and gain.[218] They also permit hybridization of probes of specific regions of the genome against tumor cells in interphase to assay individual cells in a tissue sample for deletions and amplifications.[219–221] The limitations of these techniques are related to the size of aberration: mutations must encompass tens of thousands of base pairs to be visualized.

Studies of genetic aberrations in malignant gliomas using these methods have demonstrated gains of chromosome 7 in more than 75% of patients, losses of chromosome 10 in more than half of cases, and significant numeric losses of chromosomes 6, 13, 14, 15, 18, and Y. Smaller aberrations have been found on 1p, 6q, 7q, 8p, 9p, 10q, 11p/q, 13q, and 19q; small extra chromosomes (*double minute chromosomes*) that represent amplified genetic material have been found in more than 30%; and *marker* or unidentified chromosomes that are often present testify to chromosomal rearrangements that occur in the disease.[217, 222–231]

Amplified genetic material present in glioma DNA has been mapped to more than 20 chromosomal regions.[230, 231] Each region is theoretically linked to an oncogene or to several oncogenes selected to promote the survival of tumor cells. Particular genes proposed as candidates for these oncogenes include avian erythroblastic leukemia viral oncogene homolog 1 (ERBB1/epidermal growth factor receptor [EGFR]).

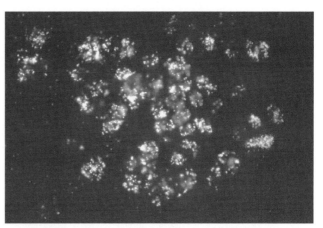

Figure 21–3 (Epidermal growth factor receptor (EGFR) amplification in malignant glioma. Cosmid DNA encoding EGFR was labeled with fluorescein isothiocyanate (FITC) and centromeric sequences from chromosome 7 were labeled with Texas red and hybridized to a touch preparation of glioblastoma multiforme. Each green spot (seen here as white clusters) represents at least one copy of EGFR, and each red spot (seen here as a white dot with a gray penumbra) represents one copy of the centromere for chromosome 7. Hundreds of EGFR copies are sometimes present in a single cell, but some cells register far fewer, which indicates a large degree of heterogeneity for the amplification of EGFR in tumor cells. Normal diploid cells should each contain two copies of the centromere and two copies of the gene (i.e., two red spots and two green spots.)

This gene is located in an amplicon on the short arm of chromosome 7 (7p), close to the centromere,[232] and amplification occurs in more than 30% of malignant astrocytomas.[233–236] ERBB1 encodes a truncated version of EGFR that is constitutively active[237]; interestingly, similar mutated versions of the protein are found in human tumors.[238] Other genes associated with amplicons in gliomas include GLI (a Kruppel zinc finger protein), CDK4 (a cyclin-dependent kinase), SAS (a transmembrane 4 protein), and MDM2 (an inhibitor of p53), all on 12q[239, 240]; the α subunit of platelet-derived growth factor receptor (PDGFRA) on 4q[241–243]; and MET (a cell surface receptor with tyrosine kinase activity) on 7q.[244, 245] Evidence for thepathogenicity of these genes includes the following: (1) each is associated with an amplicon that occurs in gliomas; (2) each has a function and expression pattern compatible with an oncogene; (3) EGFR and PDGFRA have activating rearrangements in gliomas. This evidence does not exclude the possibility that other relevant oncogenes are present in the same region of the genome; the several genes localized to a common region on 12q make this point well. Because more than 20 other amplicons have been described in gliomas, and it is believed that each contains at least one gene that drives the amplification process, it is evident that many oncogenes that have an impact on glioma pathogenesis remain to be discovered.

Multiple chromosomal deletions and other genetic losses have been described in gliomas[229–231] (also see earlier discussion). However, the loss of tumor suppressor activity implies that each copy of the gene in question is inactivated. Genes that are doubly inactivated and that have been proposed as tumor suppressor genes important for glioma pathogenesis include CDK4/MTS1/P16 and MTS2/P15, two inhibitors of cyclin-dependent kinases on 9p[246–248]; TP53, the gene encoding a tumor suppressor gene and stress monitor on 17p[51, 249];

SUMMARY OF DNA COPY NUMBER CHANGES IN PRIMARY GLIOBLASTOMAS

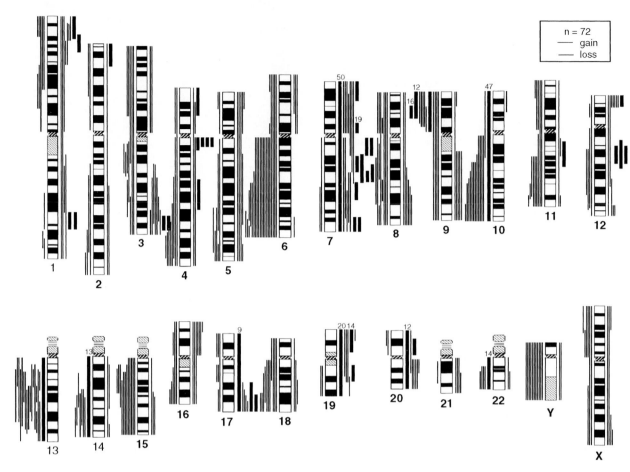

Figure 21–4 Losses and gains of genetic material identified by comparative genomic hybridization in 72 primary glioblastomas multiforme. Ideograms for each chromosome are labeled by chromosome number. Lines represent regions of loss or gain in individual tumors. Some lines represent multiple tumors (note numbers above some lines). Regions of loss are displayed to the left of each ideogram and regions of gain are to the right. The thickest bars to the right of some ideograms represent amplifications. It is evident that a large number of chromosomal regions are recurrently lost or gained in glioblastoma multiforme.

and RB, a negative regulator of proliferation on 13q that normally sequesters a variety of growth-promoting nuclear proteins.[250] The situation for deletions is similar to that in amplicons: there are at least seven regions of the genome in which chromosomal losses occur in over 15% of GBM and in which no tumor suppressor gene has been described.[230, 231] Each of these losses should mark a site or several sites at which tumor suppressor genes drive the loss of chromosomal material.

CONCLUSIONS

A tumor marker measures a variable that predicts disease incidence, progression, recurrence, or survival. The marker must be accurate, reliable, sensitive, and specific. Experiments that confirm and validate its predictive power must be well designed and unbiased.

Because the prevalence of glioma is low in the general population, tumor markers that predict the risk of contracting glioma will require the identification of high-risk groups. Diagnosis of glioma relies heavily on clinical factors and histologic analysis, and prognostic markers that assay proliferation. We expect that future markers will describe cell lineage and differentiation or outline the genetic selections that have led to a malignant phenotype. This interplay of cell lineage and selection will describe the mechanisms that define malignancy and point the way to future therapy.

ACKNOWLEDGMENTS

We thank James Jacobson, Harry Burke, Joe Gray, Dan Pinkel, and Fred Waldman for their comments concerning definitions and characteristics of tumor markers; Lovedeep Grewal, Sehyuck Park, and Atul Patel for valuable data and discussion; Lovedeep Grewal for providing Figure 21–3; Pam Derish for editorial assistance; and Mitchel Berger for extreme patience. This work has been supported in part by the National Brain Tumor Foundation and NIH grants CA13525, CA61147, and CA64898.

REFERENCES

1. Jones HB: On a new substance occurring in the urine of a patient with mollities ossium. Phil Trans R Soc Lond 1848; 138:55–62.
2. MacIntyre W: Case of mollities and fragilitas ossium, accompanied with urine strongly charged with animal matter. Medicochirurg Trans R Soc Lond 1850; 33:211–232.
3. von Rustisky J: Multiple myeloma. Zentralbl Chir 1873; 3:102–111.
4. Kahler O: Zur symptomatologie des multplen myelomas. Wien Med Presse 1889; 30:209–253.
5. Bostwick DG, Burke HB, Wheeler TM, et al: The most promising surrogate endpoint biomarkers for screening candidate chemopreventive compounds for prostatic adenocarcinoma in short-term phase II clinical trials. J Cell Biochem Suppl 1994; 19:283–289.
6. Burke HB, Henson DE: The American Joint Committee on Cancer: Criteria for prognostic factors and for an enhanced prognostic system. Cancer 1993; 72:3131–3135.
7. Baynes RT: An essay toward solving a problem in the doctrine of chance. Phil Trans Soc Lond 1763; 5:370–418.
8. Centor RM: Signal detectability: The use of ROC curves and their analyses. Med Decis Making 1991; 11:102–106.
9. Zweig MH, Campbell G: Receiver-operating characteristic (ROC) plots: A fundamental evaluation tool in clinical medicine. Clin Chem 1993; 39:561–577.
10. Hanley JA: Receiver operating characteristic (ROC) methodology: The state of the art. Crit Rev Diagn Imaging 1989; 29:307–335.
11. Lusted LB: Signal detectability and medical decision-making. Science 1971; 171:1217–1219.
12. Lusted LB: Decision-making studies in patient management. N Engl J Med 1971; 284:416–424.
13. Galen RS, Gambino SR: Beyond Normality: The Predictive Value and Efficiency of Medical Diagnoses. New York, John Wiley, 1975.
14. Kapp JP, Paulson GW, Odom GL: Brain tumors with tuberous sclerosis. J Neurosurg 1967; 26:191–202.
15. Gomez MR: Tuberous Sclerosis, ed 2. New York, Raven, 1988.
16. Shepherd CW, Scheithauer BW, Gomez MR, et al: Subependymal giant cell astrocytoma: A clinical, pathological, and flow cytometric study. Neurosurgery 1991; 28:864–868.
17. Li FP, Fraumeni JJ, Mulvihill JJ, et al: A cancer family syndrome in 24 kindreds. Cancer Res 1988; 48:5358–5362.
18. Malkin D, Li FP, Strong LC, et al: Germ line p53 mutations in a familial syndrome of breast cancer, sarcomas, and other neoplasms. Science 1990; 250:1233–1238.
19. Sorensen SA, Mulvihill JJ, Nielsen A: Long-term follow-up of von Recklinghausen neurofibromatosis: Survival and malignant neoplasms. N Engl J Med 1986; 314:1010–1015.
20. Blatt J, Jaffe R, Deutsch M, et al: Neurofibromatosis and childhood tumors. Cancer 1986; 57:1225–1229.
21. Martuza RL, Eldridge R: Neurofibromatosis 2 (bilateral acoustic neurofibromatosis). N Engl J Med 1988; 318:684–688.
22. Wolff RK, Frazer KA, Jackler RK, et al: Analysis of chromosome 22 deletions in neurofibromatosis type 2-related tumors. Am J Hum Genet 1992; 51:478–485.
23. Bodmer WF, Bailey CJ, Bodmer J, et al: Localization of the gene for familial adenomatous polyposis on chromosome 5. Nature 1987; 328:614–616.
24. Chowdhary UM, Boehme DH, Al JM: Turcot syndrome (glioma polyposis): Case report. J Neurosurg 1985; 63:804–807.
25. Lewis JH, Ginsberg AL, Toomey KE: Turcot's syndrome: Evidence for autosomal dominant inheritance. Cancer 1983; 51:524–528.
26. Tijssen CC, Halprin MR, Endtz LJ: Familial Brain Tumors: A Commented Register. Boston, Martinus Nijhoff, 1982.
27. Farwell J, Flannery JT: Cancer in relatives of children with central nervous system neoplasms. N Engl J Med 1984; 311:749–753.
28. Miller RW: Deaths from childhood leukemia and solid tumors among twins and other sibs in the United States, 1960–67. JNCI 1971; 46:203–209.
29. Draper GJ, Heaf MM, Kinnier WL: Occurrence of childhood cancers among sibs and estimation of familial risks. J Med Genet 1977; 14:81–90.
30. Kuijten RR, Bunin GR, Nass CC, et al: Gestational and familial risk factors for childhood astrocytoma: Results of a case-control study. Cancer Res 1990; 50:2608–2612.
31. Bondy ML, Lustbader ED, Buffler PA, et al: Genetic epidemiology of childhood brain tumors. Genet Epidemiol 1991; 8:253–267.
32. Wrensch MR, Barger GR: Familial factors associated with malignant gliomas. Genet Epidemiol 1990; 7:291–301.
33. Farwell J, Flannery JT: Second primaries in children with central nervous system tumors. J Neurooncol 1984; 2:371–375.
34. Preston MS, Mack W, Henderson BE: Risk factors for gliomas and meningiomas in males in Los Angeles County. Cancer Res 1989; 49:6137–6143.
35. Ryan P, Lee MW, North B, et al: Risk factors for tumors of the brain and meninges: Results from the Adelaide Adult Brain Tumor Study. Int J Cancer 1992; 51:20–27.
36. Peters FM, Preston-Martin S, Yu MC: Brain tumors in children and occupational exposure of parents. Science 1981; 213:235–237.
37. Olshan AF, Breslow NE, Daling JR, et al: Childhood brain tumors and paternal occupation in the aerospace industry. JNCI 1986; 77:17–19.
38. Gold E, Gordis L, Tonascia J, et al: Increased risk of brain tumors in children exposed to barbiturates. JNCI 1978; 61:1031–1034.
39. Zuccarello M, Sawaya R, deCourten MG: Glioblastoma occurring after radiation therapy for meningioma: Case report and review of literature. Neurosurgery 1986; 19:114–119.
40. Marus G, Levin CV, Rutherfoord GS: Malignant glioma following radiotherapy for unrelated primary tumors. Cancer 1986; 58:886–894.
41. Salvati M, Artico M, Caruso R, et al: A report on radiation-induced gliomas. Cancer 1991; 67:392–397.
42. Fontana M, Stanton C, Pompili A, et al: Late multifocal gliomas in adolescents previously treated for lymphoblastic leukemia. Cancer 1987; 60(7):1510–1518.
43. Nowell PC: The clonal evolution of tumor cell populations. Science 1976; 194:23–28.
44. Fishel R, Lescoe MK, Rao MR, et al: The human mutator gene homolog MSH2 and its association with hereditary nonpolyposis colon cancer. Cell 1993; 75:1027–1038.
45. Leach FS, Nicolaides NC, Papadopoulos N, et al: Mutations of a mutS homolog in hereditary nonpolyposis colorectal cancer. Cell 1993; 75:1215–1225.
46. Mikkelsen T, Cairncross JG, Cavenee WK: Genetics of the malignant progression of astrocytoma. J Cell Biochem 1991; 46:3–8.
47. Bishop JM: Molecular themes in oncogenesis. Cell 1991; 64:235–248.
48. Hartwell LH, Kastan MB: Cell cycle control and cancer. Science 1994; 266:1821–1828.
49. Van de Kelft E, De Boulle K, Willems P, et al: Loss of constitutional heterozygosity in human astrocytomas. Acta Neurochir 1992; 117:172–177.
50. Collins VP, James CD: Gene and chromosomal alterations associated with the development of human gliomas. FASEB J 1993; 7:926–930.
51. Fults D, Brockmeyer D, Tullous MW, et al: p53 mutation and loss of heterozygosity on chromosomes 17 and 10 during human astrocytoma progression. Cancer Res 1992; 52:674–679.
52. Watkins D, Rouleau GA: Genetics, prognosis and therapy of central nervous system tumors. Cancer Detect Prev 1994; 18:139–144.
53. Batra SK, Rasheed BK, Bigner SH, et al: Oncogenes and anti-oncogenes in human central nervous system tumors. Lab Invest 1994; 71:621–637.
54. Bailey P, Cushing H: A Classification of the Glioma Group on a Histologic Basis with a Correlated Study of Prognosis. Philadelphia, JB Lippincott, 1926.
55. Daumas DC, Scheithauer BW, Kelly PJ: A histologic and cytologic method for the spatial definition of gliomas. Mayo Clin Proc 1987; 62:435–449.
56. Daumas DC: Histological grading of gliomas. Curr Opin Neurol Neurosurg 1992; 5:924–931.
57. Daumas DC, Scheithauer B, O'Fallon J, et al: Grading of astrocytomas: A simple and reproducible method. Cancer 1988; 62:2152–2165.
58. Kernohan JW, Mabon RF, Suien HS: A simplified classification of gliomas. Proc Staff Meeting Mayo Clin, 1949, pp 2471–2474.
59. Fulling KH, Nelson JS: Cerebral astrocytic neoplasms in the adult: Contribution of histologic examination to the assessment of prognosis. Semin Diagn Pathol 1984; 1:152–163.
60. Berens ME, Rutka JT, Rosenblum ML: Brain tumor epidemiology, growth, and invasion. Neurosurg Clin North Am 1990; 1:1–18.
61. Byar DP, Green SB, Stike TA: Prognostic factors for malignant gliomas. In Walker MD (ed): Oncology of the Nervous System. Boston, Martinus Nijoff, 1983, p 12.

62. Mahaley MS, Mettlin C, Natarajan N, et al: Analysis of patterns of care of brain tumor patients in the United States: A study of the Brain Tumor Section of the AANS and the CNS and the Commission on Cancer of the ACS. Clin Neurosurg 1990; 36:347–352.

63. Prados MD, Gutin PH, Phillips TL, et al: Highly anaplastic astrocytoma: A review of 357 patients treated between 1977 and 1989. Int J Radiat Oncol Biol Phys 1992; 23:3–8.

64. Burger PC, Vogel FS, Green SB, et al: Glioblastoma multiforme and anaplastic astrocytoma: Pathologic criteria and prognostic implications. Cancer 1985; 56:1106–1111.

65. Chandler KL, Prados MD, Malec M, et al: Long-term survival in patients with glioblastoma multiforme. Neurosurgery 1993; 32:716–720.

66. Coons SW, Johnson PC: Regional heterogeneity in the DNA content of human gliomas. Cancer 1993; 72:3052–3060.

67. Perez LA, Dombkowski D, Efird J, et al: Cell proliferation kinetics in human tumor xenografts measured with iododeoxyuridine labeling and flow cytometry: A study of heterogeneity and a comparison between different methods of calculation and other proliferation measurements. Cancer Res 1995; 55:392–398.

68. Onda K, Davis RL, Wilson CB, et al: Regional differences in bromodeoxyuridine uptake, expression of Ki-67 protein, and nucleolar organizer region counts in glioblastoma multiforme. Acta Neuropathol 1994; 87:586–593.

69. Prognostic factors for high-grade malignant glioma: Development of a prognostic index. A Report of the Medical Research Council Brain Tumour Working Party. J Neurooncol 1990; 9:47–55.

70. Eng LF, Vanderhaeghen JJ, Bignami A, et al: An acidic protein isolated from fibrous astrocytes. Brain Res 1971; 28:351–354.

71. Eng LF: Glial fibrillary acidic protein (GFAP): The major protein of glial filaments in differentiated astrocytes. J Neuroimmunol 1985; 8:203–214.

72. Sensenbrenner M, Devilliers G, Bock E, et al: Biochemical and ultrastructural studies of cultured rat astroglial cells: Effect of brain extract and dibutyryl cyclic AMP on glial fibrillary acidic protein and glial filaments. Differentiation 1980; 17:51–61.

73. Herpers MJ, Budka H, McCormick D: Production of glial fibrillary acidic protein (GFAP) by neoplastic cells: Adaptation to the microenvironment. Acta Neuropathol 1984; 64:333–338.

74. Jessen KR, Mirsky R: Nonmyelin-forming Schwann cells coexpress surface proteins and intermediate filaments not found in myelin-forming cells: A study of Ran-2, A5E3 antigen and glial fibrillary acidic protein. J Neurocytol 1984; 13:923–934.

75. Jessen KR, Thorpe R, Mirsky R: Molecular identity, distribution and heterogeneity of glial fibrillary acidic protein: An immunoblotting and immunohistochemical study of Schwann cells, satellite cells, enteric glia and astrocytes. J Neurocytol 1984; 13:187–200.

76. Duffy PE, Graf L, Huang YY, et al: Glial fibrillary acidic protein in ependymomas and other brain tumors: Distribution, diagnostic criteria, and relation to formation of processes. J Neurol Sci 1979; 40:133–146.

77. Deck JH, Eng LF, Bigbee J, et al: The role of glial fibrillary acidic protein in the diagnosis of central nervous system tumors. Acta Neuropathol 1978; 42:183–190.

78. Choi BH, Kim RC: Expression of glial fibrillary acidic protein in immature oligodendroglia. Science 1984; 223:407–409.

79. Herpers MJ, Budka H: Glial fibrillary acidic protein (GFAP) in oligodendroglial tumors: Gliofibrillary oligodendroglioma and transitional oligoastrocytoma as subtypes of oligodendroglioma. Acta Neuropathol 1984; 64:265–272.

80. Rubinstein LJ, Brucher JM: Focal ependymal differentiation in choroid plexus papillomas: An immunoperoxidase study. Acta Neuropathol 1981; 53:29–33.

81. Kepes JJ, Rengachary SS, Lee SH: Astrocytes in hemangioblastomas of the central nervous system and their relationship to stromal cells. Acta Neuropathol 1979; 47:99–104.

82. Haugen OA, Taylor CR: Immunohistochemical studies of ovarian and testicular teratomas with antiserum to glial fibrillary acidic protein. Acta Pathol Microbiol Immunol Scand 1984; 92:9–14.

83. Yen SH, Fields KL: Antibodies to neurofilament, glial filament, and fibroblast intermediate filament proteins bind to different cell types of the nervous system. J Cell Biol 1981; 88:115–126.

84. Hofler H, Walter GF, Denk H: Immunohistochemistry of folliculo-stellate cells in normal human adenohypophyses and in pituitary adenomas. Acta Neuropathol 1984; 65:35–40.

85. Budka H: Non-glial specificities of immunocytochemistry for the glial fibrillary acidic protein (GFAP): Triple expression of GFAP, vimentin and cytokeratins in papillary meningioma and metastasizing renal carcinoma. Acta Neuropathol 1986; 72:43–54.

86. Velasco ME, Roessmann U, Gambetti P: The presence of glial fibrillary acidic protein in the human pituitary gland. J Neuropathol Exp Neurol 1982; 41:150–163.

87. Kepes JJ, Rubinstein LJ, Chiang H: The role of astrocytes in the formation of cartilage in gliomas: An immunohistochemical study of four cases. Am J Pathol 1984; 117:471–483.

88. Martin de las Mulas, J, Espinosa de los Monteros A, Bautista MJ, et al: Immunohistochemical distribution pattern of intermediate filament proteins and muscle actin in feline and human mammary carcinomas. J Comp Pathol 1994; 111:365–381.

89. Achstatter T, Moll R, Anderson A, et al: Expression of glial filament protein (GFP) in nerve sheaths and non-neural cells re-examined using monoclonal antibodies, with special emphasis on the co-expression of GFP and cytokeratins in epithelial cells of human salivary gland and pleomorphic adenomas. Differentiation 1986; 31:206–227.

90. Goldman RD, Steinert PM: Cellular and Molecular Biology of Intermediate Filaments. New York, Plenum, 1990.

91. Lukas Z, Draber P, Bucek J, et al: Expression of vimentin and glial fibrillary acidic protein in human developing spinal cord. Histochem J 1989; 21:693–701.

92. Yang HY, Lieska N, Shao D, et al: Immunotyping of radial glia and their glial derivatives during development of the rat spinal cord. J Neurocytol 1993; 22:558–571.

93. Wilkinson M, Hume R, Strange R, et al: Glial and neuronal differentiation in the human fetal brain 9–23 weeks of gestation. Neuropathol Appl Neurobiol 1990; 16:193–204.

94. Yang HY, Lieska N, Shao D, et al: Proteins of the intermediate filament cytoskeleton as markers for astrocytes and human astrocytomas. Mol Chem Neuropathol 1994; 21:155–176.

95. Dahl D, Bignami A, Weber K, et al: Filament proteins in rat optic nerves undergoing Wallerian degeneration: Localization of vimentin, the fibroblastic 100-Å filament protein, in normal and reactive astrocytes. Exp Neurol 1981; 73:496–506.

96. Dahl D, Rueger DC, Bignami A, et al: Vimentin, the 57 000 molecular weight protein of fibroblast filaments, is the major cytoskeletal component in immature glia. Eur J Cell Biol 1981; 24:191–196.

97. Foisner R, Wiche G: Intermediate filament-associated proteins. Curr Opin Cell Biol 1991; 3:75–81.

98. Eberhard DA, Brown MD, VandenBerg SR: Alterations of annexin expression in pathological neuronal and glial reactions. Immunohistochemical localization of annexins I, II (p36 and p11 subunits), IV, and VI in the human hippocampus. Am J Pathol 1994; 145:640–649.

99. Bianchi R, Garbuglia M, Verzini M, et al: S-100 protein and annexin II2-p11(2) (calpactin I) act in concert to regulate the state of assembly of GFAP intermediate filaments. Biochem Biophys Res Commun 1995; 208:910–918.

100. Jahn R, Schiebler W, Ouimet C, et al: A 38,000-dalton membrane protein (p38) present in synaptic vesicles. Proc Natl Acad Sci USA 1985; 82:4137–4141.

101. Miller DC, Koslow M, Budzilovich GN, et al: Synaptophysin: A sensitive and specific marker for ganglion cells in central nervous system neoplasms. Hum Pathol 1990; 21:271–276.

102. Wiedenmann B, Franke WW: Identification and localization of synaptophysin, an integral membrane glycoprotein of Mr 38,000 characteristic of presynaptic vesicles. Cell 1985; 41:1017–1028.

103. Frankfurter A, Binder LI, Rebhun LI: Limited tissue distribution of a novel beta-tubulin isoform. J Cell Biol 1986; 103:273a.

104. Dale BA, Resing KA, Haydock PV: Filaggrins. In Goldman RD, Seinert P (ed): Cellular and Molecular Biology of Intermediate Filaments. New York, Plenum, 1990, pp 393–412.

105. Matus A: Microtubule-associated proteins: Their potential role in determining neuronal morphology. Annu Rev Neurosci 1988; 11:29–44.

106. Binder LI, Frankfurter A, Rebhun LI: Differential localization of MAP-2 and tau in mammalian neurons in situ. Ann NY Acad Sci 1986; 466:145–166.

107. Binder LI, Frankfurter A, Rebhun LI: The distribution of tau in the mammalian central nervous system. J Cell Biol 1985; 101:1371–1378.

108. Hessler RB, Lopes MB, Frankfurter A, et al: Cytoskeletal immunohistochemistry of central neurocytomas. Am J Surg Pathol 1992; 16:1031–1038.

109. Bansal R, Gard AL, Pfeiffer SE: Stimulation of oligodendrocyte differentiation in culture by growth in the presence of a monoclonal antibody to sulfated glycolipid. J Neurosci Res 1988; 21:260–267.

110. Bansal R, Warrington AE, Gard AL, et al: Multiple and novel specificities of monoclonal antibodies O1, O4, and R-mAb used in the analysis of oligodendrocyte development. J Neurosci Res 1989; 24:548–557.

111. Bansal R, Pfeiffer SE: Reversible inhibition of oligodendrocyte progenitor differentiation by a monoclonal antibody against surface galactolipids. Proc Natl Acad Sci USA 1989; 86:6181–6185.

112. Warrington AE, Pfeiffer SE: Proliferation and differentiation of O4+ oligodendrocytes in postnatal rat cerebellum: Analysis in unfixed tissue slices using anti-glycolipid antibodies. J Neurosci Res 1992; 33:338–353.

113. Svennerholm L, Rynmark BM, Vilbergsson G, et al: Gangliosides in human fetal brain. J Neurochem 1991; 56:1763–1768.

114. Noble M: Points of controversy in the O-2A lineage: Clocks and type-2 astrocytes. Glia 1991; 4:157–164.

115. Raff MC, Abney ER, Cohen J, et al: Two types of astrocytes in cultures of developing rat white matter: Differences in morphology, surface gangliosides, and growth characteristics. J Neurosci 1983; 3:1289–1300.

116. Warrington AE, Barbarese E, Pfeiffer SE: Stage specific, (O4+GalC−) isolated oligodendrocyte progenitors produce MBP+ myelin in vivo. Dev Neurosci 1992; 14:93–97.

117. Gard AL, Pfeiffer SE: Two proliferative stages of the oligodendrocyte lineage (A2B5+O4− and O4+GalC−) under different mitogenic control. Neuron 1990; 5:615–625.

118. Dyer CA, Benjamins JA: Glycolipids and transmembrane signaling: Antibodies to galactocerebroside cause an influx of calcium in oligodendrocytes. J Cell Biol 1990; 111:625–633.

119. Wikstrand CJ, Fredman P, Svennerholm L, et al: Monoclonal antibodies to malignant human gliomas. Mol Chem Neuropathol 1992; 17:137–146.

120. Hakomori S: Bifunctional role of glycosphingolipids: Modulators for transmembrane signaling and mediators for cellular interactions. J Biol Chem 1990; 265:18713–18716.

121. Yates AJ, VanBrocklyn J, Saqr HE, et al: Mechanisms through which gangliosides inhibit PDGF-stimulated mitogenesis in intact Swiss 3T3 cells: Receptor tyrosine phosphorylation, intracellular calcium, and receptor binding. Exp Cell Res 1993; 204:38–45.

122. Van Brocklyn J, Bremer EG, Yates AJ: Gangliosides inhibit platelet-derived growth factor-stimulated receptor dimerization in human glioma U-1242MG and Swiss 3T3 cells. J Neurochem 1993; 61:371–374.

123. Fredman P, Von HH, Collins VP, et al: Sialyllactotetraosylceramide: A ganglioside marker for human malignant gliomas. J Neurochem 1988; 50:912–919.

124. Berra B, Gaini SM, Riboni L: Correlation between ganglioside distribution and histological grading of human astrocytomas. Int J Cancer 1985; 36:363–366.

125. Sung CC, Pearl DK, Coons SW, et al: Gangliosides as diagnostic markers of human astrocytomas and primitive neuroectodermal tumors. Cancer 1994; 74:3010–3022.

126. Sung CC, Pearl DK, Coons SW, et al: Correlation of ganglioside patterns of primary brain tumors with survival. Cancer 1995; 75:851–859.

127. Hakomori S: Role of gangliosides in tumor progression. Prog Brain Res 1994; 101:241–250.

128. Gray JS, Dolbeare F, Pallavicini MG, et al: Quantitative cell-cycle analysis. In Melamed MR, Lindmo T, Mendelsohn ML (eds): Flow Cytometry and Sorting, ed 2. New York, Wiley-Liss, 1990, pp 445–467.

129. Kharbanda K, Karak AK, Sarkar C, et al: Prediction of biologic aggressiveness in human meningiomas: A cell kinetic study using bromodeoxyuridine in cells of primary explant culture. JNCI 1992; 84:194–195.

130. Meyer JS, Marchosky JA, Hickey WF: Cell kinetic classification of tumors of the nervous system by DNA precursor labeling in vitro. Hum Pathol 1993; 24:1357–1364.

131. Dinda AK, Kharbanda K, Kharbanda K, Sarkar C, et al: In-vivo proliferative potential of primary human brain tumors: Its correlation with histological classification and morphological features: I. Gliomas. Pathology 1993; 25:4–9.

132. Labrousse F, Daumas DC, Batorski L, et al: Histological grading and bromodeoxyuridine labeling index of astrocytomas: Comparative study in a series of 60 cases. J Neurosurg 1991; 75:202–205.

133. Fujimaki T, Matsutani M, Nakamura O, et al: Correlation between bromodeoxyuridine-labeling indices and patient prognosis in cerebral astrocytic tumors of adults. Cancer 1991; 67:1629–1634.

134. Ito S, Chandler KL, Prados MD, et al: Proliferative potential and prognostic evaluation of low-grade astrocytomas. J Neurooncol 1994; 19:1–9.

135. Hoshino T, Ahn D, Prados MD, et al: Prognostic significance of the proliferative potential of intracranial gliomas measured by bromodeoxyuridine labeling. Int J Cancer 1993; 53:550–555.

136. Wacker MR, Hoshino T, Ahn DK, et al: The prognostic implications of histologic classification and bromodeoxyuridine labeling index of mixed gliomas. J Neurooncol 1994; 19:113–122.

137. Ritter AM, Sawaya R, Hess KR, et al: Prognostic significance of bromodeoxyuridine labeling in primary and recurrent glioblastoma multiforme. Neurosurgery 1994; 35:192–198.

138. Ito S, Hoshino T, Shibuya M, et al: Proliferative characteristics of juvenile pilocytic astrocytomas determined by bromodeoxyuridine labeling. Neurosurgery 1992; 31:413–418.

139. Prados MD, Krouwer HG, Edwards MS, et al: Proliferative potential and outcome in pediatric astrocytic tumors. J Neurooncol 1992; 13:277–282.

140. Gerdes J, Schwab U, Lemke H, et al: Production of a mouse monoclonal antibody reactive with a human nuclear antigen associated with cell proliferation. Int J Cancer 1983; 31:13–20.

141. Schluter C, Duchrow M, Wohlenberg C, et al: The cell proliferation-associated antigen of antibody Ki-67: A very large, ubiquitous nuclear protein with numerous repeated elements, representing a new kind of cell cycle-maintaining protein. J Cell Biol 1993; 123:513–522.

142. Gerdes J, Lemke H, Baisch H, et al: Cell cycle analysis of a cell proliferation-associated human nuclear antigen defined by the monoclonal antibody Ki-67. J Immunol 1984; 133:1710–1715.

143. Bruno S, Darzynkiewicz Z: Cell cycle dependent expression and stability of the nuclear protein detected by Ki-67 antibody in HL-60 cells. Cell Prolif 1992; 25:31–40.

144. Hall PA, McKee PH, Menage HD, et al: High levels of p53 protein in UV-irradiated normal human skin. Oncogene 1993; 8:203–207.

145. Key G, Becker MH, Baron B, et al: New Ki-67-equivalent murine monoclonal antibodies (MIB 1–3) generated against bacterially expressed parts of the Ki-67 cDNA containing three 62 base pair repetitive elements encoding for the Ki-67 epitope. Lab Invest 1993; 68:629–636.

146. Zhang H, Xiong Y, Beach D: Proliferating cell nuclear antigen and p21 are components of multiple cell cycle kinase complexes. Mol Biol Cell 1993; 4:897–906.

147. Xiong Y, Zhang H, Beach D: Subunit rearrangement of the cyclin-dependent kinases is associated with cellular transformation. Genes Dev 1993; 7:1572–1583.

148. Xiong Y, Zhang H, Beach D: D type cyclins associate with multiple protein kinases and the DNA replication and repair factor PCNA. Cell 1992; 71:505–514.

149. Prelich G, Tan CK, Kostura M, et al: Functional identity of proliferating cell nuclear antigen and a DNA polymerase-delta auxiliary protein. Nature 1987; 326:517–520.

150. Prelich G, Stillman B: Coordinated leading and lagging strand synthesis during SV40 DNA replication in vitro requires PCNA. Cell 1988; 53:117–126.

151. Waga S, Stillman B: Anatomy of a DNA replication fork revealed by reconstitution of SV40 DNA replication in vitro. Nature 1994; 369:207–212.

152. Li R, Waga S, Hannon GJ, et al: Differential effects by the p21 CDK inhibitor on PCNA-dependent DNA replication and repair. Nature 1994; 371:534–537.

153. Waga S, Hannon GJ, Beach D, et al: The p21 inhibitor of cyclin-dependent kinases controls DNA replication by interaction with PCNA. Nature 1994; 369:574–578.

154. Shivji MK, Podust VN, Hubscher U, et al: Nucleotide excision repair DNA synthesis by DNA polymerase epsilon in the presence of PCNA, RFC, and RPA. Biochemistry 1995; 34:5011–5017.

155. Aboussekhra A, Biggerstaff M, Shivji MK, et al: Mammalian DNA nucleotide excision repair reconstituted with purified protein components. Cell 1995; 80:859–868.

156. Wood RD, Aboussekhra A, Biggerstaff M, et al: Nucleotide excision

repair of DNA by mammalian cell extracts and purified proteins. Cold Spring Harb Symp Quant Biol 1993; 58:625–632.

157. Shivji KK, Kenny MK, Wood RD: Proliferating cell nuclear antigen is required for DNA excision repair. Cell 1992; 69:367–374.

158. Busch H, Lischwe MA, Michalik J, et al: Nucleolar Proteins of Special Interest, ed 15. New York, Cambridge University Press, 1982.

159. Hozak P, Roussel P, Hernandez VD: Procedures for specific detection of silver-stained nucleolar proteins on Western blots. J Histochem Cytochem 1992; 40:1089–1096.

160. Lischwe MA, Smetana K, Olson MO, et al: Proteins C23 and B23 are the major nucleolar silver staining proteins. Life Sci 1979; 25:701–708.

161. Buys CH, Osinga J: Selective staining of the same set of nucleolar phosphoproteins by silver and Giemsa: A combined biochemical and cytochemical study on staining of NORs. Chromosoma 1984; 89:387–396.

162. Tsanaclis AM, Robert F, Michaud J, et al: The cycling pool of cells within human brain tumors: In situ cytokinetics using the monoclonal antibody Ki-67. Can J Neurol Sci 1991; 18:12–17.

163. Morimura T, Kitz K, Stein H, et al: Determination of proliferative activities in human brain tumor specimens: A comparison of three methods. J Neurooncol 1991; 10:1–11.

164. Plate KH, Ruschoff J, Behnke J, et al: Proliferative potential of human brain tumours as assessed by nucleolar organizer regions (AgNORs) and Ki67-immunoreactivity. Acta Neurochir (Wien) 1990; 104:103–109.

165. Karamitopoulou E, Perentes E, Diamantis I, et al: Ki-67 immunoreactivity in human central nervous system tumors: A study with MIB 1 monoclonal antibody on archival material. Acta Neuropathol (Berl) 1994; 87:47–54.

166. Karamitopoulou E, Perentes E, Melachrinou M, et al: Proliferating cell nuclear antigen immunoreactivity in human central nervous system neoplasms. Acta Neuropathol (Berl) 1993; 85:316–322.

167. Shibuya M, Ito S, Miwa T, et al: Proliferative potential of brain tumors: Analyses with Ki-67 and anti-DNA polymerase alpha monoclonal antibodies, bromodeoxyuridine labeling, and nuclear organizer region counts. Cancer 1993; 71:199–206.

168. Maier H, Morimura T, Ofner D, et al: Argyrophilic nucleolar organizer region proteins (Ag-NORs) in human brain tumors: Relations with grade of malignancy and proliferation indices. Acta Neuropathol (Berl) 1990; 80:156–162.

169. Hara A, Hirayama H, Sakai N, et al: Correlation between nucleolar organizer region staining and Ki-67 immunostaining in human gliomas. Surg Neurol 1990; 33:320–324.

170. Vigliani MC, Chio A, Pezzulo T, et al: Proliferating cell nuclear antigen (PCNA) in low-grade astrocytomas: Its prognostic significance. Tumori 1994; 80:295–300.

171. Figge C, Reifenberger G, Vogeley KT, et al: Immunohistochemical demonstration of proliferating cell nuclear antigen in glioblastomas: Pronounced heterogeneity and lack of prognostic significance. J Cancer Res Clin Oncol 1992; 118:289–295.

172. Louis DN, Meehan SM, Ferrante RJ, et al: Use of the silver nucleolar organizer region (AgNOR) technique in the differential diagnosis of central nervous system neoplasia. J Neuropathol Exp Neurol 1992; 51:150–157.

173. Frindel E, Malaise E, Tubiana M: Cell proliferation kinetics in five human solid tumors. Cancer 1968; 22:611–620.

174. Wilson GD, McNally NJ, Dunphy E, et al: The labelling index of human and mouse tumours assessed by bromodeoxyuridine staining in vitro and in vivo and flow cytometry. Cytometry 1985; 6:641–647.

175. Steel GG: Growth Kinetics of Tumours. Oxford, Clarendon Press, 1977.

176. Begg AC, McNally NJ, Shrieve DC, et al: A method to measure the duration of DNA synthesis and the potential doubling time from a single sample. Cytometry 1985; 6:620–626.

177. Shibuya M, Ito S, Davis RL, et al: A new method for analyzing the cell kinetics of human brain tumors by double labeling with bromodeoxyuridine in situ and with iododeoxyuridine in vitro. Cancer 1993; 71:3109–3113.

178. Hoshino T, Ito S, Asai A, et al: Cell kinetic analysis of human brain tumors by in situ double labelling with bromodeoxyuridine and iododeoxyuridine. Int J Cancer 1992; 50:1–5.

179. Steel GG: Cell loss from experimental tumours. Cell Tissue Kinet 1968; 1:193–207.

180. Zatterstrom UK, Johansson M, Kallen A, et al: Comparison of BrdUrd and [³H]TdR incorporation to estimate cell proliferation, cell loss, and potential doubling time in tumor xenografts. Cytometry 1992; 13:872–879.

181. Weller M, Malipiero U, Rensing EA, et al: Fas/APO–1 gene transfer for human malignant glioma. Cancer Res 1995; 55:2936–2944.

182. Weller M, Malipiero U, Aguzzi A, et al: Protooncogene bcl–2 gene transfer abrogates Fas/APO–1 antibody-mediated apoptosis of human malignant glioma cells and confers resistance to chemotherapeutic drugs and therapeutic irradiation. J Clin Invest 1995; 95:2633–2643.

183. Alderson LM, Castleberg RL, Harsh GR, et al: Human gliomas with wild-type p53 express bcl–2. Cancer Res 1995; 55:999–1001.

184. Morris SM: The genetic toxicology of 5-bromodeoxyuridine in mammalian cells. Mutat Res 1991; 258:161–188.

185. Pilkington GJ: Tumour cell migration in the central nervous system. Brain Pathol 1994; 4:157–166.

186. Figarella BD, Durbec PL, Rougon GN: Differential spectrum of expression of neural cell adhesion molecule isoforms and L1 adhesion molecules on human neuroectodermal tumors. Cancer Res 1990; 50:6364–6370.

187. Gingras MC, Roussel E, Bruner JM, et al: Comparison of cell adhesion molecule expression between glioblastoma multiforme and autologous normal brain tissue. J Neuroimmunol 1995; 57:143–153.

188. Edvardsen K, Chen W, Rucklidge G, et al: Transmembrane neural cell-adhesion molecule (NCAM), but not glycosyl-phosphatidylinositol–anchored NCAM, down-regulates secretion of matrix metalloproteinases. Proc Natl Acad Sci USA 1993; 90:11463–11467.

189. Couldwell WT, de Tribolet N, Antel JP, et al: Adhesion molecules and malignant gliomas: Implications for tumorigenesis. J Neurosurg 1992; 76:782–791.

190. Paulus W, Baur I, Schuppan D, et al: Characterization of integrin receptors in normal and neoplastic human brain. Am J Pathol 1993; 143:154–163.

191. Gladson CL, Cheresh DA: Glioblastoma expression of vitronectin and the alpha v beta 3 integrin. Adhesion mechanism for transformed glial cells. J Clin Invest 1991; 88:1924–1932.

192. Giese A, Rief MD, Loo MA, et al: Determinants of human astrocytoma migration. Cancer Res 1994; 54:3897–3904.

193. Mikkelsen T, Yan PS, Ho KL, et al: Immunolocalization of cathepsin B in human glioma: Implications for tumor invasion and angiogenesis. J Neurosurg 1995; 83:285–290.

194. Sivaparvathi M, Sawaya R, Wang SW, et al: Overexpression and localization of cathepsin B during the progression of human gliomas. Clin Exp Metastasis 1995; 13:49–56.

195. Rempel SA, Rosenblum ML, Mikkelsen T, et al: Cathepsin B expression and localization in glioma progression and invasion. Cancer Res 1994; 54:6027–6031.

196. Mohanam S, Sawaya RE, Yamamoto M, et al: Proteolysis and invasiveness of brain tumors: Role of urokinase-type plasminogen activator receptor. J Neurooncol 1994; 22:153–160.

197. Yamamoto M, Sawaya R, Mohanam S, et al: Expression and localization of urokinase-type plasminogen activator receptor in human gliomas. Cancer Res 1994; 54:5016–5020.

198. Yamamoto M, Sawaya R, Mohanam S, et al: Expression and localization of urokinase-type plasminogen activator in human astrocytomas in vivo. Cancer Res 1994; 54:3656–3661.

199. Gladson CL, Pijuan TV, Olman MA, et al: Up-regulation of urokinase and urokinase receptor genes in malignant astrocytoma. Am J Pathol 1995; 146:1150–1160.

200. Hsu DW, Efird JT, Hedley WE: Prognostic role of urokinase-type plasminogen activator in human gliomas. Am J Pathol 1995; 147:114–123.

201. Sawaya R, Ramo OJ, Shi ML, et al: Biological significance of tissue plasminogen activator content in brain tumors. J Neurosurg 1991; 74:480–486.

202. Caccamo DV, Keohane ME, McKeever PE: Plasminogen activators and inhibitors in gliomas: An immunohistochemical study. Mod Pathol 1994; 7:99–104.

203. Bindal AK, Hammoud M, Shi WM, et al: Prognostic significance of proteolytic enzymes in human brain tumors. J Neurooncol 1994; 22:101–110.

204. Hoshino T, Nomura K, Wilson CB, et al: The distribution of nuclear DNA from human brain-tumor cells. J Neurosurg 1978; 49:13–21.

205. Frederiksen P, Bichel F: Sequential flow cytometric analysis of single

cell DNA content in recurrent human brain tumours. *In* Laerum OD, Limdino T, Thorud E (eds): Flow Cytometry IV. Bergen, Norway, Universitaetsforlaget, 1980, pp 398–492.

206. Lehmann J, Krug H: Flow-through fluorocytophotometry of different brain tumours. Acta Neuropathol (Berl) 1980; 49:123–132.
207. Barlogie B, Raber MN, Schumann J, et al: Flow cytometry in clinical cancer research. Cancer Res 1983; 43:3982–3997.
208. Danova M, Giaretti W, Merlo F, et al: Prognostic significance of nuclear DNA content in human neuroepithelial tumors. Int J Cancer 1991; 48:663–667.
209. Koss LG, Czerniak B, Herz F, et al: Flow cytometric measurements of DNA and other cell components in human tumors: A critical appraisal. Hum Pathol 1989; 20:528–548.
210. Jimenez O, Timms A, Quirke P, et al: Prognosis in malignant glioma: A retrospective study of biopsy specimens by flow cytometry. Neuropathol Appl Neurobiol 1989; 15:331–338.
211. Salmon I, Kiss R, Dewitte O, et al: Histopathologic grading and DNA ploidy in relation to survival among 206 adult astrocytic tumor patients. Cancer 1992; 70:538–546.
212. Salmon I, Kiss R: Relationship between proliferative activity and ploidy level in a series of 530 human brain tumors, including astrocytomas, meningiomas, schwannomas, and metastases. Hum Pathol 1993; 24:329–335.
213. Salmon I, Kruczynski A, Camby I, et al: DNA histogram typing in a series of 707 tumors of the central and peripheral nervous system. Am J Surg Pathol 1993; 17:1020–1028.
214. Salmon I, Dewitte O, Pasteels JL, et al: Prognostic scoring in adult astrocytic tumors using patient age, histopathological grade, and DNA histogram type. J Neurosurg 1994; 80:877–883.
215. Kros JM, van Eden CG, Vissers CJ, et al: Prognostic relevance of DNA flow cytometry in oligodendroglioma. Cancer 1992; 69:1791–1798.
216. Forsyth PA, Shaw EG, Scheithauer BW, et al: Supratentorial pilocytic astrocytomas: A clinicopathologic, prognostic, and flow cytometric study of 51 patients. Cancer 1993; 72:1335–1342.
217. von Deimling A, von Ammon K, Schoenfeld D, et al: Subsets of glioblastoma multiforme defined by molecular genetic analysis. Brain Pathol 1993; 3:19–26.
218. Kallioniemi A, Kallioniemi OP, Sudar D, et al: Comparative genomic hybridization for molecular cytogenetic analysis of solid tumors. Science 1992; 258:818–821.
219. Gray JW, Kuo WL, Liang J, et al: Analytical approaches to detection and characterization of disease-linked chromosome aberrations. Bone Marrow Transplant 1990; 1:14–19.
220. Gray JW, Pinkel D: Molecular cytogenetics in human cancer diagnosis. Cancer 1992; 69:1536–1542.
221. Feuerstein BG, Mohapatra G: Molecular cytogenetic quantitation of gains and losses of genetic material from human gliomas. J Neurooncol 1995; 24:47–55.
222. Bigner SH, Mark J, Bullard DE, et al: Chromosomal evolution in malignant human gliomas starts with specific and usually numerical deviations. Cancer Genet Cytogenet 1986; 22(2):121–35.
223. Bigner SH, Mark J, Burger PC, et al: Specific chromosomal abnormalities in malignant human gliomas. Cancer Res 1988; 48:405–411.
224. Bigner SH, Mark J, Bigner DD: Cytogenetics of human brain tumors. Cancer Genet Cytogenet 1990; 47:141–154.
225. Bello MJ, de Campos JM, Kusak ME, et al: Molecular analysis of genomic abnormalities in human gliomas. Cancer Genet Cytogenet 1994; 73:122–129.
226. Jenkins RB, Kimmel DW, Moertel CA, et al: A cytogenetic study of 53 human gliomas. Cancer Genet Cytogenet 1989; 39:253–279.
227. Rey JA, Bello MJ, de Campos JM, et al: Chromosomal patterns in human malignant astrocytomas. Cancer Genet Cytogenet 1987; 29:201–221.
228. von Deimling A, Bender B, Jahnke R, et al: Loci associated with malignant progression in astrocytomas: A candidate on chromosome 19q. Cancer Res 1994; 54:1397–1401.
229. Kim DH, Mohapatra G, Bollen A, et al: Chromosomal abnormalities

in glioblastoma multiforme tumors and glioma cell lines detected by comparative genomic hybridization. Int J Cancer 1995; 60:812–819.

230. Schröck E, Thiel G, Lozanova T, et al: Comparative genomic hybridization of human malignant gliomas reveals multiple amplification sites and nonrandom chromosomal gains and losses. Am J Pathol 1994; 144:1203–1218.
231. Mohapatra G, Kim DH, Feuerstein BG: Detection of multiple gains and losses of genetic material in ten glioma cell lines by comparative genomic hybridization. Genes Chromosom Cancer 1995; 13:86–93.
232. Libermann TA, Nusbaum HR, Razon N, et al: Amplification, enhanced expression and possible rearrangement of EGF receptor gene in primary human brain tumours of glial origin. Nature 1985; 313:144–147.
233. Strommer K, Hamou MF, Diggelmann H, et al: Cellular and tumoural heterogeneity of EGFR gene amplification in human malignant gliomas. Acta Neurochir (Wien) 1990; 107:82–87.
234. Torp SH, Helseth E, Ryan L, et al: Amplification of the epidermal growth factor receptor gene in human gliomas. Anticancer Res 1991; 11:2095–2098.
235. Hurtt MR, Moossy J, Donovan PM, et al: Amplification of epidermal growth factor receptor gene in gliomas: Histopathology and prognosis. J Neuropathol Exp Neurol 1992; 51:84–90.
236. Schlegel J, Merdes A, Stumm G, et al: Amplification of the epidermal-growth-factor-receptor gene correlates with different growth behaviour in human glioblastoma. Int J Cancer 1994; 56:72–77.
237. Downward J, Yarden Y, Mayes E, et al: Close similarity of epidermal growth factor receptor and v-erb-B oncogene protein sequences. Nature 1984; 307:521–527.
238. Wells A, Bishop JM: Genetic determinants of neoplastic transformation by the retroviral oncogene v-erbB. Proc Natl Acad Sci USA 1988; 85:7597–7601.
239. Reifenberger G, Reifenberger J, Ichimura K, et al: Amplification at 12q13–14 in human malignant gliomas is frequently accompanied by loss of heterozygosity at loci proximal and distal to the amplification site. Cancer Res 1995; 55:731–734.
240. Reifenberger G, Liu L, Ichimura K, et al: Amplification and overexpression of the MDM2 gene in a subset of human malignant gliomas without p53 mutations. Cancer Res 1993; 53:2736–2739.
241. Fleming TP, Saxena A, Clark WC, et al: Amplification and/or overexpression of platelet-derived growth factor receptors and epidermal growth factor receptor in human glial tumors. Cancer Res 1992; 52:4550–4553.
242. Kumabe T, Sohma Y, Kayama T, et al: Overexpression and amplification of alpha-PDGF receptor gene lacking exons coding for a portion of the extracellular region in a malignant glioma. Tohoku J Exp Med 1992; 168:265–269.
243. Kumabe T, Sohma Y, Kayama T, et al: Amplification of alpha-platelet-derived growth factor receptor gene lacking an exon coding for a portion of the extracellular region in a primary brain tumor of glial origin. Oncogene 1992; 7:627–633.
244. Fischer U, Muller HW, Sattler HP, et al: Amplification of the MET gene in glioma. Genes Chromosom Cancer 1995; 12:63–65.
245. Wullich B, Muller HW, Fischer U, et al: Amplified met gene linked to double minutes in human glioblastoma. Eur J Cancer 1993; 29:1991–1995.
246. Arap W, Nishikawa R, Furnari FB, et al: Replacement of the p16/CDKN2 gene suppresses human glioma cell growth. Cancer Res 1995; 55:1351–1354.
247. Jen J, Harper JW, Bigner SH, et al: Deletion of p16 and p15 genes in brain tumors. Cancer Res 1994; 54:6353–6358.
248. Moulton T, Samara G, Chung WY, et al: MTS1/p16/CDKN2 lesions in primary glioblastoma multiforme. Am J Pathol 1995; 146:613–619.
249. Frankel RH, Bayona W, Koslow M, et al: p53 mutations in human malignant gliomas: Comparison of loss of heterozygosity with mutation frequency. Cancer Res 1992; 52:1427–1433.
250. Henson JW, Schnitker BL, Correa KM, et al: The retinoblastoma gene is involved in malignant progression of astrocytomas. Ann Neurol 1994; 36:714–721.

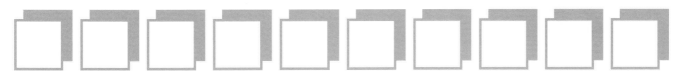

Diagnostic Imaging

LINDSEY C. BLAKE

KENNETH R. MARAVILLA

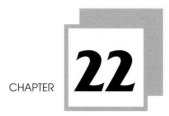

CHAPTER **22**

Computed Tomography

Primary intracerebral gliomas represent 40% to 45% of the approximately 35,000 new brain tumors that develop in adult Americans each year.[1, 2] In adults, the peak incidence of intracranial gliomas occurs in the seventh decade of life; the majority of these are supratentorial, and they tend to be aggressive malignancies. One report suggests an increasing incidence of primary tumors in the elderly.[3] In the pediatric population, intracranial tumors are the second most common site of neoplasm; 70% to 80% are located in the posterior fossa. The majority of pediatric gliomas are low-grade lesions, such as pilocytic astrocytomas, that follow a more benign clinical course.[4] Compared to intracranial gliomas, which are the most common primary intracranial neoplasms, intraspinal gliomas are relatively uncommon, accounting for approximately 18% of all spinal axis tumors.

Neuroradiologic assessment of patients suspected of harboring a central nervous system (CNS) neoplasm has been enhanced with the development of computed tomography (CT) and magnetic resonance imaging (MRI). These imaging modalities have revolutionized the evaluation of patients with intracranial and spinal tumors and have complementary roles in both preoperative diagnosis and treatment planning as well as postoperative assessment and therapy. CT and MRI are used for tumor detection and definition of tumor extent preoperatively, and for demonstrating the degree of tumor resection, identifying postsurgical complications, assessing tumor recurrence, and following tumor response to radiation and chemotherapy postoperatively. This chapter reviews the contemporary use of CT in patients with intracranial and intraspinal gliomas, in both adult and pediatric populations.

CURRENT ROLE OF CT IN EVALUATING INTRACRANIAL GLIOMAS

Prior to MRI, CT was the primary imaging modality for the detection and evaluation of suspected or known intracranial neoplasms. Currently, CT plays a secondary role in this regard, with MRI almost invariably being the study of choice unless specific contraindications to MRI are present. In a study of 80 patients with intrinsic hemispheric tumors, MRI successfully demonstrated all lesions found on CT, as well as additional lesions not detected or seen on CT.[5]

Advantages of MRI include superior soft tissue contrast, which can be generated with a variety of pulse sequences, and which makes MRI more sensitive and specific than CT in detecting primary brain tumors. Multiplanar imaging allows easier discrimination between intra-axial vs. extra-axial lesions and offers better definition than CT of exact tumor location, extent, and relation to adjacent normal structures. Precise tumor location is mandatory, because even a benign tumor that is located in or adjacent to a critical structure, or in a region of eloquent brain tissue such as the Rolandic cortex or Broca's area, may not be entirely resectable surgically. Its higher sensitivity to intravenous contrast agents makes MRI superior to CT for the detection of intratumoral enhancement as well as for identification of leptomeningeal and subependymal tumor involvement.

CT is an acceptable modality for the evaluation of patients with suspected CNS mass lesions and for follow-up of patients with previously confirmed intra-axial tumors. CT routinely reveals the vast majority of intracranial neoplasms. However, in practice, MRI is usually the preferred imaging modality. A very low percentage of tumors may be missed entirely or may be difficult to visualize with routine CT scanning (Fig. 22–1). These are generally small, low-grade neoplasms, which are difficult to detect on CT because they are either isodense with brain parenchyma, produce minimal mass affect, or are located near the calvarium, where the mass may be obscured by bone artifact. Bone artifact is a particular problem in the posterior fossa. The majority of these tumors are clearly demonstrated with MRI.

CT plays an important role in treatment planning, even in patients who have had a prior MRI. Because of its superior definition of cortical bone, CT readily demonstrates the relation of underlying tumor to bony landmarks of the calvarium and sinuses, which are important in planning the craniotomy site or potential radiation ports as well as in marking lesions close to the brain surface for open or stereotactic biopsy.

CT-guided stereotactic biopsy uses three-dimensional coordinates to precisely localize intra-axial brain masses. It is an effective alternative to open biopsy in selected patients, especially if the lesion is diffuse or located deep within the

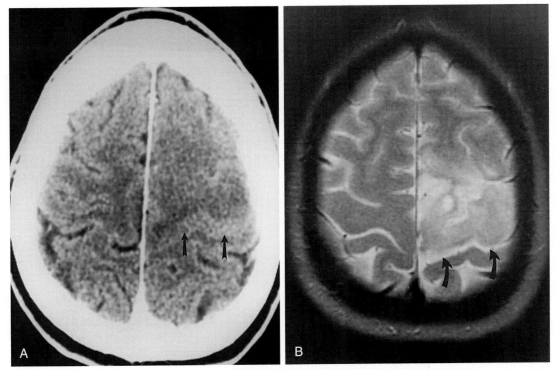

Figure 22-1 Mixed oligoastrocytoma in a 55-year-old woman presenting with new onset seizure. Noncontrast CT (*A*) shows subtle sulcal effacement in the left posterior frontal region with involvement of the precentral gyrus (*arrows*). The high-signal infiltrating mass is more obvious on the T2 (TR/TE, 2000/80) MRI image (*B*), which demonstrates expansion of the motor cortex (*curved arrows* on central sulcus).

brain parenchyma. Even biopsy of intrinsic brainstem lesions can be undertaken successfully. A recent report[6] reviewing complications of 300 consecutive CT-guided stereotactic biopsies demonstrated a low overall complication rate (6.3%) and a 3% incidence of mortality and major morbidity.

CT is more rapid than MRI; consequently it is less prone to motion artifact, and patients generally require little to no sedation. CT can safely image patients with aneurysm clips, pacemakers, and other implantable devices that are contraindicated in MRI. In addition, CT is less expensive and generally more available. Finally, for the patient who is severely claustrophobic, CT requires a far less confining environment that is generally tolerated without problem.

CT TECHNIQUE

CT detects differences in x-ray attenuation based on relative differences in electron density of tissues and uses these data to reconstruct cross-sectional images of the brain and spine. CT is very sensitive to very small amounts of calcium, hemorrhage, and intravenous (IV) iodinated contrast material. Preoperative and postoperative scanning is performed both without and with IV contrast enhancement. In the brain, axial 5-mm thick images are obtained at 5-mm intervals from the foramen magnum to the skull vertex. Direct coronal images are useful for demonstrating the relationship of posterior fossa lesions to the tentorium and to the foramen magnum. Sagittal reformatted images can be performed if midline relationships need to be assessed (Fig. 22–2).

Spiral or helical CT is a relatively recent technique that allows continuous CT data acquisition while simultaneously moving the patient through the CT gantry. This results in a volume data set obtained in a relatively short period of time, usually less than 1 minute. Images can be reconstructed from this data set at desired intervals and viewed in the standard axial projection or in multiplanar or three-dimensional formats. Advantages include less motion artifact, higher resolution, and the ability to perform "dynamic" contrast enhancement during the first passage of the contrast bolus.[7]

Contrast-enhanced scans are obtained after the intravenous injection of approximately 100 to 150 mL of 60% iodinated contrast material. Density changes are produced because of the increased attenuation of x-ray photons by the iodine molecule. The greater the concentration of iodine present in tissue, the higher the degree of enhancement demonstrated with CT. Enhancement is dependent on the loss of integrity of the blood-brain barrier. Contrast agents accumulate in regions of blood-brain barrier disruption within the extracellular spaces of the tumor. Separate portions of the same tumor may have varying degrees of blood-brain barrier compromise. This, together with necrosis, may account for the heterogeneous enhancement pattern present in some neoplasms.

Normal anatomic structures that enhance following IV contrast injection include arteries, veins, dural venous sinuses, choroid plexus, pituitary stalk, and pineal gland. Contrast-enhanced images increase the sensitivity of lesion detection by revealing areas of abnormal contrast enhancement. For instance, enhancement may be seen in one or more masses not visualized on noncontrast images. Additionally, enhancement may provide useful information for treatment

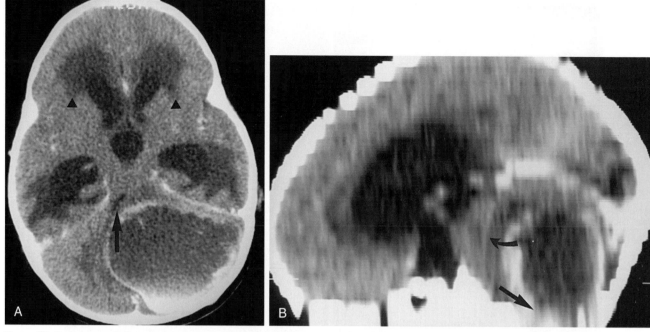

Figure 22–2 Large cerebellar astrocytoma in a 16-month-old child. Axial contrast-enhanced CT (*A*) shows a large hypodense mass in the left cerebellar hemisphere with thin rim enhancement. The fourth ventricle is effaced and displaced to the right (*arrow*). Note hydrocephalus and periventricular transependymal CSF spread (*arrowheads*). Midsagittal (*B*) reformatted image clearly demonstrates the relation of the mass to the foramen magnum (*arrow*) and anterior compression of the brainstem (*curved arrow*).

planning by revealing extension of tumor into a region of the brain that is not surgically resectable or by demonstrating unsuspected involvement of the dura or the ependymal surface.

The presence or absence of enhancement, as well as the degree and pattern of enhancement, generally correlate with tumor grade.[8–10] This is especially true for adult supratentorial gliomas. For example, high-grade gliomas enhance strongly, often with a thick, irregular, ring-like enhancement pattern. Lower-grade gliomas never demonstrate this pattern, and often do not enhance at all (Fig. 22–3). Focal areas of enhancement in regions of tumor may indicate more aggressive tumor grade and cellular proliferation. Such areas of focal enhancement can serve to guide determination of biopsy site. Following radiation or chemotherapy, areas of new contrast enhancement may indicate new growth of recurrent tumor or onset of radiation necrosis. The outer border of tumor enhancement seen on CT or MRI does not correspond to the actual pathologic tumor margin.[11, 12] This is particularly accurate in high-grade gliomas, in which tumor cells may be found in regions of the brain distant from the primary mass and adjacent edema.

Homogeneous enhancement can occur in both low- and high-grade malignancies. Histologically benign lesions that typically have prominent enhancement include pilocytic astrocytoma, pleomorphic xanthoastrocytoma, and ganglioglioma. An enhancing mural nodule within a cyst is suggestive of a low-grade tumor and is most commonly associated with pilocytic astrocytoma.

POSTOPERATIVE EVALUATION

Postoperative CT is done to evaluate for both immediate complications (those occurring shortly after surgery) and delayed changes (those occurring weeks to months following treatment). A noncontrast CT is obtained immediately after surgery, when the patient is still sedated and is difficult to evaluate neurologically, to detect possible early complications such as intracranial hemorrhage, cerebral infarction, swelling, or tension pneumocephalus. CT is the procedure of choice in the immediate postsurgical period because all of the important findings can be demonstrated, and MRI would be difficult to potentially impossible as a result of the condition of the patient and the multiple monitoring devices that are incompatible with the MRI magnet.

A second indication for postoperative CT evaluation is to assess for extent of resection and to estimate residual tumor volume. In patients with a tumor that enhances with contrast, a postoperative CT without and with contrast is obtained 1 to 4 days postsurgery. Areas of enhancement correlate with residual unresected tumor, as it has been shown that postoperative parenchymal enhancement on CT is first seen after the fifth postsurgical day and may last up to 6 months.[13, 14] However, postoperative enhancement has been shown to occur earlier on MRI than on CT, is almost always present at 6 months, and resolves at around 1 year after surgery.[15]

It is important to remember that subtle foci of enhancement on CT may be obscured by high-density blood at the operative site. In addition, nonenhancing tumor cannot be evaluated in this manner. Most nonenhancing gliomas appear as low-density lesions on CT that are inseparable from cerebral edema, which is virtually always present in the postoperative patient.

Further assessment of tumor recurrence or residual tumor growth is best performed with MRI, but it can be accomplished with CT. The frequency of routine follow-up imaging depends on tumor histology, grade, and clinical symp-

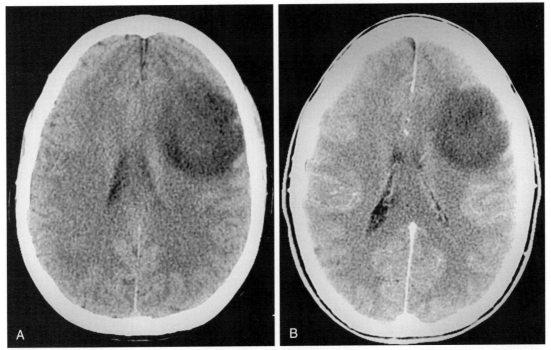

Figure 22–3 Well-demarcated low-attenuation left frontal lobe mass in a 36-year-old woman seen on non–contrast-enhanced (*A*) and contrast-enhanced (*B*) CT. Given large size of the lesions, the lack of mass effect, edema, and enhancement correlate well with this pathologically proved low-grade glioma.

tomatology. For low-grade neoplasms, periodic imaging at 6-month intervals is adequate. More frequent imaging, every 3 to 4 months or less, is necessary for higher-grade lesions or in patients with neurologic deterioration. Imaging should be continued for an indefinite period of time because the likelihood of tumor recurrence increases with increasing time from surgical resection.

PRIMARY INTRACRANIAL GLIAL NEOPLASMS

General

Primary intracranial gliomas are the most common intra-axial CNS tumors. The majority of adult gliomas represent forms of astrocytoma (astroglial neoplasms), ranging histologically from low-grade to anaplastic. Separate portions of the same tumor may contain cells with varying grades of tumor, in which case grading is based on the cells with the most malignant histologic characteristics.

A common classification scheme separates astrocytomas into three groups. Astrocytomas are considered to be benign lesions; their histologic features demonstrate mild hypercellularity with minimal pleomorphism and no vascular proliferation or necrosis. Anaplastic astrocytomas and glioblastomas are considered malignant gliomas. An anaplastic astrocytoma has a moderate degree of pleomorphism and vascular proliferation, but no necrosis. Glioblastoma multiforme, which accounts for as many as 50% of adult astrocytomas, contains similar histologic findings but is accompanied by the hallmark feature of necrosis. Oligodendroglioma and juvenile pilocytic astrocytoma are considered separately

because of a more indolent biologic behavior. This classification scheme was shown to have prognostic value with a 2-year survival of 5% for glioblastoma multiforme and 50% for anaplastic astrocytoma.[16]

CT imaging findings in primary tumors correlate roughly with histologic grade and can guide the differential diagnosis. Findings associated with a higher degree of malignancy include heterogeneity, necrosis, hemorrhage, extensive peritumoral vasogenic edema, marked mass effect, poorly defined margins, irregular contrast enhancement, and involvement of midline structures.[4] Low-grade tumors may occasionally demonstrate some features of high-grade neoplasms.

The differential diagnosis of intracranial gliomas includes infarction, demyelinating disease, metastasis, and abscess. Cerebral infarctions are distinguished by a characteristic clinical history with an abrupt onset of symptoms combined with a wedge-shaped area of low density on CT that follows strict vascular territories. An infarction characteristically involves both gray and white matter. This contrasts with most gliomas, which predominantly infiltrate white matter with only mild involvement of cortex. Infarctions demonstrate progressive evolution of decreased mass effect and decreased density and develop characteristic gyriform enhancement, which can be detected on follow-up scans in 5 to 10 days.[17] Tumors will not show a change in appearance during this short period of time (Fig. 22–4).

A focus of acute demyelination may also present as a focal low-density lesion with mass effect, edema, and enhancement. A solitary lesion may occasionally appear indistinguishable from tumor. MRI is more useful in this instance because it has higher sensitivity to white matter lesions. The MR detection of multiple T2 high-signal white matter foci

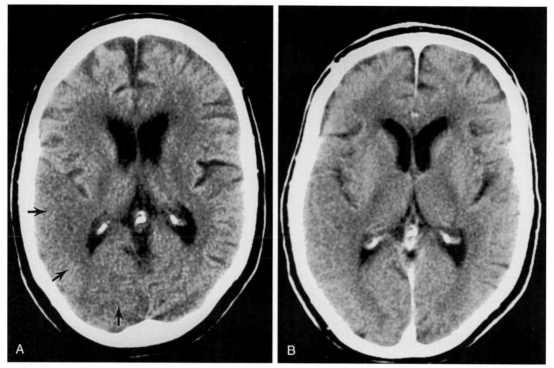

Figure 22–4 Low-grade glioma simulating cerebral infarction. A low-density lesion in the right posterior temporal and occipital lobes (*arrows*) with sulcal effacement on non–contrast-enhanced CT (*A*) resembles an acute cerebrovascular accident. However, both middle and posterior cerebral artery vascular territories are involved. A contrast-enhanced CT (*B*) 4 days later is unchanged, making a low-grade primary neoplasm a more likely diagnosis. Rapid evolution of low density and mass effect would be expected with infarction.

would lead to the correct diagnosis of multiple sclerosis. Over 3 to 6 weeks a tumor will remain stable, whereas a focus of demyelination will demonstrate diminished mass effect, edema, and contrast enhancement.

A solitary metastatic lesion is more commonly round to oval, circumscribed, and centered at the gray-white junction. Like glioblastoma multiforme, a metastasis may have thick nodular ring enhancement and extensive vasogenic edema, although the edema associated with a metastatic lesion is usually greater and out of proportion to the size of the mass. An abscess is commonly hypodense centrally with a peripheral thin, smooth, rim-enhancing border, which is often thinner on the ventricular side of the lesion. A multiloculated abscess or an abscess with daughter lesions may be indistinguishable from a malignant glioma (Fig. 22–5).

Astrocytoma

Low-grade astrocytomas represent approximately 9% of all intracranial tumors and 25% to 30% of intracranial astrocytomas, and they generally occur in children and adolescents. Characteristic CT features reflect the nonaggressive biology of this tumor. The tumor appears either as a subtle isodense mass with imperceptible borders or as a well-delineated slightly low-attenuation lesion with little or no mass effect (Fig. 22–6). Vasogenic edema and enhancement are minimal. Lack of enhancement indicates that there is no significant disruption of the blood-brain barrier. Focal areas of cyst formation or necrosis are distinctly unusual. Approximately 10% to 20% of untreated intracranial gliomas contain calci-

fications; this is especially true in lower-grade malignancies but can also be seen occasionally in high-grade lesions.

Anaplastic Astrocytoma

Anaplastic astrocytomas demonstrate biologic activity between low-grade astrocytoma and glioblastoma multiforme. They represent 25% to 30% of astrocytomas and occur in a relatively older population. Many CT features are similar to those of low-grade glioma, whereas some characteristics reflect its more aggressive behavior, in which case the appearance is indistinguishable from that of glioblastoma multiforme (Fig. 22–7). In general, anaplastic astrocytomas are more poorly defined and demonstrate more vasogenic edema, mass effect, and enhancement than lower-grade gliomas. As many as 89% of anaplastic astrocytomas may demonstrate areas of contrast enhancement by CT.[18] The differential diagnosis includes a solitary demyelinating lesion and metastasis, and biopsy may be required to establish the correct diagnosis.

Glioblastoma Multiforme

Glioblastoma multiforme, the most malignant astrocytoma, is the most common supratentorial primary neoplasm in older adults. Glioblastoma multiforme represents 15% to 20% of all intracranial tumors and 50% of all cerebral gliomas. These aggressive neoplasms are most common in the fifth to seventh decades, are rare in patients younger than

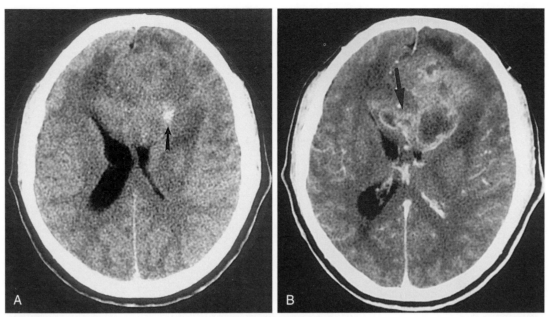

Figure 22–5 Non–contrast-enhanced CT (*A*) of a 37-year-old man who had progressive headaches 1 week after a tooth extraction shows a left frontal mass with a small foci of hemorrhage (*arrow*). Contrast-enhanced CT (*B*) demonstrates a heterogeneous mixed-density mass infiltrating across the genu of the corpus callosum (*large arrow*). Multifocal nodular and irregular ring enhancement patterns with large areas of internal necrosis are characteristic of glioblastoma. A cerebral abscess may have similar imaging characteristics, but typically does not cross the corpus callosum.

30 years, and have a higher frequency in males (3:2).[4] Patients with glioblastoma multiforme have a uniformly poor prognosis with a median survival of 6 to 9 months.

Glioblastomas are frequently large at presentation, and they appear on CT as inhomogeneous mixed-attenuation masses with poorly marginated borders. The epicenter of the

mass is characteristically deep in white matter. The cerebral hemisphere is the most commonly affected site, usually in the frontal or temporal lobes. The corpus callosum and cerebral cortex are frequently invaded, and the overlying leptomeninges and dura are also occasionally involved. A distinct characteristic of supratentorial glioblastoma multi-

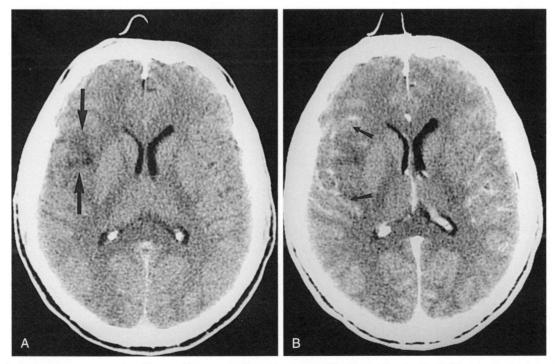

Figure 22–6 Low-grade astrocytoma in a 39-year-old man presenting with seizures. CT without (*A*) and with (*B*) IV contrast enhancement demonstrate subtle low attenuation (*A; arrows*) in the right perisylvian region without mass effect or enhancement. Note distorted sylvian middle cerebral artery branches (*B; arrows*) on contrast-enhanced CT.

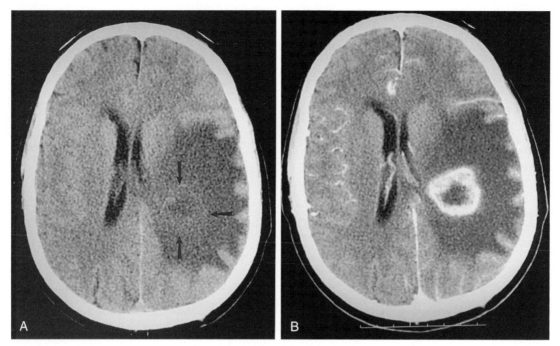

Figure 22–7 Recurrent headaches prompted CT scanning in this 63-year-old man with an anaplastic astrocytoma. Non–contrast-enhanced CT (*A*) shows a subtle mass centered in deep white matter (*arrows*) and contrast-enhanced CT (*B*) demonstrates a rim-enhancing mass with extensive surrounding low-density edema. Imaging features are illustrative of a high-grade glioma. CT cannot reliably differentiate anaplastic astrocytoma from glioblastoma. A typical cerebral abscess has thinner walls.

forme is spread to the subependymal ventricular surface and seeding of the subarachnoid pathways. Distant metastases outside the CNS are rare.

Focal areas of hyperdensity on CT (Fig. 22–8) represent either histologic areas of densely packed malignant cells with high nuclear-to-cytoplasmic ratio or foci of hemorrhage. The presence of hemorrhage secondary to necrosis is a common finding at autopsy with glioblastoma multiforme,

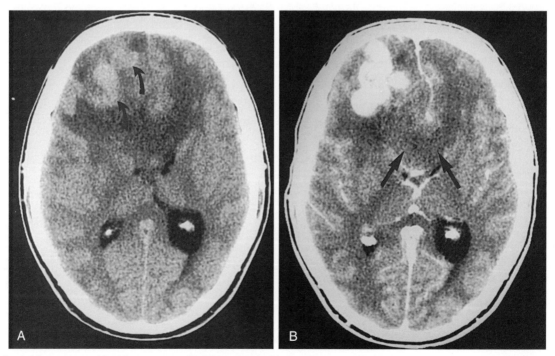

Figure 22–8 Axial pre-contrast (*A*) and post-contrast (*B*) CT images of a 31-year-old man. *A* shows a hyperdense mass (*arrows*) in the right frontal lobe, suggesting dense cellularity and high nuclear-to-cytoplasmic ratio. In *B*, note extensive low attenuation in both frontal lobes and thickening of the corpus callosum (*arrows*) from infiltrating tumor and edema. *B* shows marked enhancement typical of malignant gliomas.

and is a differentiating feature from lower-grade astrocytomas. Calcification is rare, but it may be seen in tumors that start out as lower-grade lesions and undergo malignant degeneration.

High-grade gliomas infrequently present on CT as a spontaneous intracerebral hematoma of unknown etiology that can be difficult to distinguish in some cases from hemorrhages caused by hypertension, infarction, or ruptured vascular malformation (Fig. 22–9). Other tumors that have a propensity to bleed are oligodendrogliomas and ependymomas. Characteristically, tumor-induced hemorrhage has a more heterogeneous appearance, with evidence of hemorrhage in different stages of resolution, compared with that of hemorrhagic infarction or hypertensive hemorrhage.[19–20] Extensive edema, focal areas of enhancement within or adjacent to the hemorrhage, and persistent mass effect are additional findings that indicate underlying neoplasm.

Glioblastoma multiforme demonstrates more frequent and more intense enhancement than other gliomas, which reflects greater compromise of the blood-brain barrier. In a series of 295 glioblastomas, 98% demonstrated some contrast enhancement.[18] The most common pattern is thick, heterogeneous, or nodular ring enhancement surrounding areas of low-density necrosis or cyst formation. Characteristically, glioblastomas have moderate to marked mass effect, secondary to both the underlying mass and the associated vasogenic edema. Edema is of low attenuation, it tracks along white matter pathways, and it may be extensive. An exact tumor-edema border cannot be identified with CT, MRI, or even histologic analysis. All grades of glioma may infiltrate midline structures along commissural fibers, giving rise to bihemispheric extension of tumor. However, glioblastomas are more commonly associated with this bilateral or "butterfly" pattern (Fig. 22–10).

Gliosarcoma

Malignant gliosarcoma is an extremely rare subclassification of glioblastoma multiforme with sarcomatous degeneration, and it carries a very poor prognosis. Imaging findings are identical to those of other high-grade glial neoplasms.[21]

Gliomatosis Cerebri

Gliomatosis cerebri is a rare form of disseminated infiltrating low-grade glial tumor that occurs in both children and adults, with a peak incidence between 20 and 40 years of age. The clinical presentation is often nonspecific and mild with respect to the extent of involvement. The disease process may clinically and radiologically mimic that of a demyelinating or dysmyelinating process,[17, 22] occasionally requiring biopsy for definitive diagnosis. This neoplasm consists of astrocytes that diffusely infiltrate the brain along white matter tracts. The tumor follows perineural, perivascular, and subpial pathways, while leaving the underlying neuroanatomic architecture relatively intact. A large segment of one or both hemispheres (Fig. 22–11) may be involved. Extension into the brainstem, cerebellum, and spinal cord is possible.[22, 23]

The CT diagnosis is often difficult because the scan may appear normal or may demonstrate minimal diffuse mass effect without, or with only equivocal, density change or enhancement. Subtle isodense to low-density foci may be seen that expand involved gyri, resulting in effacement of

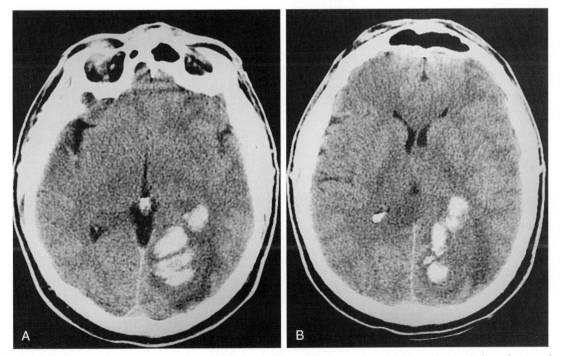

Figure 22–9 Glioblastoma presenting as intracranial hemorrhage. A 52-year-old man presented with sudden headache, seizure, and obtundation. Non–contrast-enhanced CT scans (*A* and *B*) demonstrated a left occipital hemorrhage with minimal mass effect, which initially was felt to represent a hemorrhagic infarction.

Illustration continued on following page

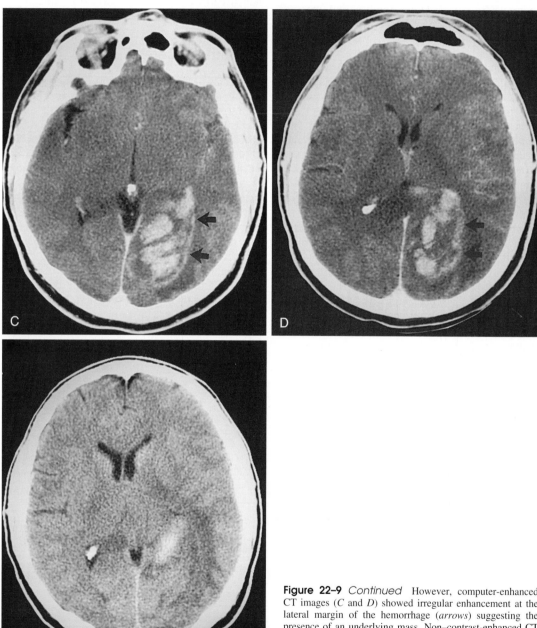

Figure 22–9 *Continued* However, computer-enhanced CT images (*C* and *D*) showed irregular enhancement at the lateral margin of the hemorrhage (*arrows*) suggesting the presence of an underlying mass. Non–contrast-enhanced CT 10 days later (*E*) revealed resolving hemorrhage and increasing mass effect. Glioblastoma multiforme was present at surgery.

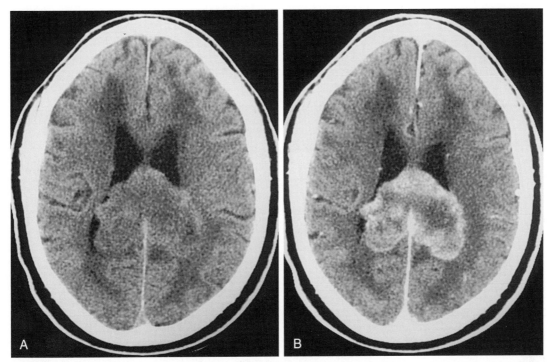

Figure 22–10 A 71-year-old man presented with dementia. CT images without (A) and with (B) contrast enhancement show a lobulated mass straddling the body and splenium of the corpus callosum, spreading laterally to both hemispheres. The appearance is typical of the "butterfly glioma" pattern. Other masses that can have this appearance include lymphoma and metastasis.

adjacent sulci and ventricles without focal mass effect. As tumor cells spread, the gray-white matter interface may become indistinct, and commissural tracts, such as the corpus callosum, may enlarge. Enhancement is uncommon, and when present it is indistinct and has a focal or patchy pattern. A recent study[24] shows that MRI is more sensitive than CT in detecting and defining the extent of the neoplasm, and that it increases the conspicuousness of subtle areas of contrast enhancement.

Multicentric and Multifocal Glioma

The vast majority of gliomas are solitary neoplasms. However, gliomas may rarely present as synchronous multicentric (independent foci without microscopic connection) or multifocal (multiple related foci with parenchymal connection or CSF spread) masses, which may have a striking similarity to metastatic disease (Fig. 22–12). The incidence of true multicentric glioma is estimated at 5% to 7.5%.[1, 25] CT demonstrates two or more separate hypointense masses without apparent connection, generally in the same hemisphere. The majority demonstrate irregular or nodular contrast enhancement, reflecting its occurrence in higher-grade gliomas. Multifocal glioma appears as separate distinct masses because different grades of tumor, with variable regions of blood-brain barrier disruption and enhancement, may exist within the same neoplasm. Two areas of enhancement separated by low-grade tumor may inaccurately display a single lesion as two separate smaller masses.[26] The distinction between multicentric vs. multifocal lesions is usually not possible using CT.

The CT and MRI appearance of multicentric and multifocal glioma may be indistinguishable from metastatic disease without biopsy.[26, 27] Imaging findings favoring synchronous, rather than metastatic lesions include the presence of large irregularly shaped masses with heterogeneous enhancement, lesions centered in deep white matter, and lesions restricted to the same hemisphere. Metastatic lesions are more uniform in size and shape, are located at the gray-white matter junction, and are most often bilateral.

Pleomorphic Xanthoastrocytoma

Pleomorphic xanthoastrocytoma is a rare, slow-growing glial-origin tumor[28] that is considered a more clinically benign subtype of supratentorial astrocytoma. This neoplasm has a peak incidence in the second and third decades and has an equal incidence in males and females. Seizure and headache are the most common presenting symptoms. Pleomorphic xanthoastrocytomas are predominantly found in the superficial temporal lobe near the gray-white matter junction, which reflects their suspected origin from subpial astrocytes. The tumor may involve the superficial cortex, leptomeninges, or dura.[29, 30] On CT, pleomorphic xanthoastrocytomas appear as either a well-circumscribed or a poorly defined mixed-attenuation lesion with mild mass effect and variable amounts of edema. Cystic areas are present in approximately 50% (Fig. 22–13), calcification is uncommon, and hemorrhage is absent. The enhancement pattern of pleomorphic xanthoastrocytoma is different from that of most other low-grade astrocytomas because there is often moderate enhancement of the solid portions of the tumor, which may appear

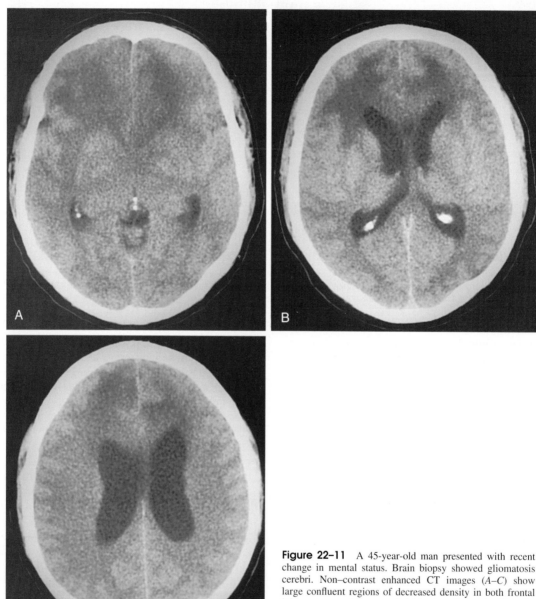

Figure 22–11 A 45-year-old man presented with recent change in mental status. Brain biopsy showed gliomatosis cerebri. Non–contrast enhanced CT images (*A–C*) show large confluent regions of decreased density in both frontal lobes, corpus callosum, and right external capsule. Note the paucity of mass effect given the large areas of involvement. No enhancement was present on CT or MRI, as would be expected with a low-grade glioma.

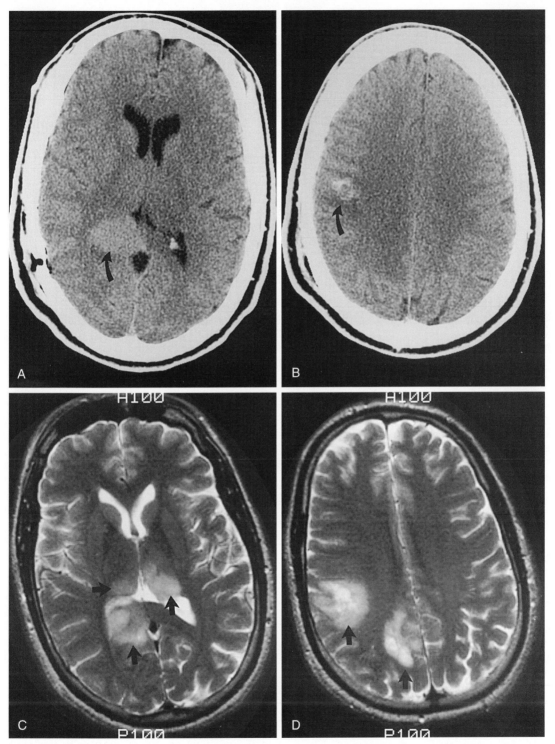

Figure 22–12 A 35-year-old man had multicentric/multifocal mixed-anaplastic glioma, proved with stereotactic biopsy. Non–contrast-enhanced CT (*A* and *B*) demonstrates noncontiguous hyperdense masses in the right posterior frontal lobe and splenium (*arrows*). Additional lesions are seen as high signal foci in the right parietal lobe and bilateral thalami (*arrows*) on T2-weighted (3600/108/8, TR/TE/ETL) MR images (*C* and *D*).

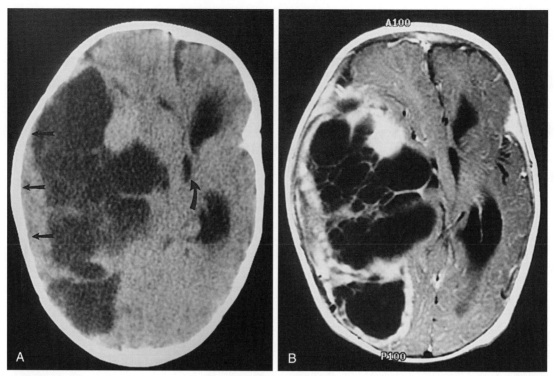

Figure 22–13 Pleomorphic xanthoastrocytoma: non–contrast-enhanced CT (*A*) and T1 post-gadolinium MRI (*B*) in an 8-year-old child demonstrates a very large multicystic right temporal mass with marked midline shift (*curved arrow* on third ventricle). Intense enhancement of peripheral nodules and internal septations is present in this low-grade tumor. Strong enhancement is not unusual in pleomorphic xanthoastrocytoma. Note remodeling of calvarium in *A* (*small arrows*), suggesting a slow-growing process.

gyriform or involve the leptomeninges.[29–32] The prognosis and clinical course are favorable in comparison to those of conventional astrocytomas. However, recurrence may result if the leptomeningeal component is incompletely resected, and the recurring lesion may be of a high histologic grade.

Brainstem Gliomas

Brainstem gliomas are uncommon intracranial tumors that are found most often in the pediatric population, with a peak incidence between the ages of 4 and 13 years. The most common presenting symptoms include multiple cranial nerve palsies and long tract signs, which are steadily progressive. Hydrocephalus is distinctly uncommon, and when present it occurs late in the disease process. The median survival is 4 to 15 months, with a 5-year survival of 30%. Brainstem gliomas account for 10% to 15% of all primary CNS tumors[4] and 20% of all posterior fossa gliomas in children.[33] CT is capable of detecting the majority of brainstem gliomas; in one series,[33] 27 of 28 lesions were identified.

A recent report correlated four distinct growth patterns, as seen on MRI, with tumor grade and prognosis.[34] These growth patterns can be identified with CT scanning, but are less clearly demonstrated with CT than with MRI. Diffuse brainstem gliomas were centered in the pons and demonstrated infiltrating growth rostrally into the midbrain and caudally into the medulla and upper cervical cord (Fig. 22–14). All diffuse tumors were anaplastic astrocytomas and were associated with more rapid clinical deterioration. Focal

medullary, cervicomedullary, and dorsal exophytic morphologic subtypes were associated with a greater incidence of low-grade histologic features and demonstrated a less rapid clinical deterioration. Focal medullary and cervicomedullary tumors are circumscribed lesions without craniocaudal extension. Dorsal exophytic gliomas are limited to the medulla, with exophytic tumor growing posteriorly into the fourth ventricle.

The CT appearance of brainstem gliomas parallels the morphologic categories described previously. On noncontrast CT they appear as isodense to hypodense intra-axial masses that are centered most commonly in the pons and less commonly in the midbrain or medulla. They may be entirely intrinsic, with infiltration into the medulla or midbrain. Early pontine lesions may demonstrate subtle enlargement or distortion with flattening of the ventral pons against the clivus and effacement of the prepontine cistern. Exophytic extension of tumor is not uncommon (Fig. 22–15) and may be seen in the fourth ventricle, cerebellopontine angle, and the prepontine cistern.[35] When the exophytic growth is anterior and the prepontine cistern is involved, the tumor may encase the basilar artery. Tumors originating in the midbrain or tectum are usually low-grade pilocytic astrocytomas.[36] Small tectal masses cause subtle asymmetry of the midbrain. When large, they displace, but do not generally invade, the ipsilateral thalamus and pons. Contrast enhancement is variable; it is usually present in 50% of these masses on MRI. On CT, enhancement is usually minimal and patchy, but ring-enhancing lesions can also be detected. Hydrocephalus is a late finding and occurs with masses that

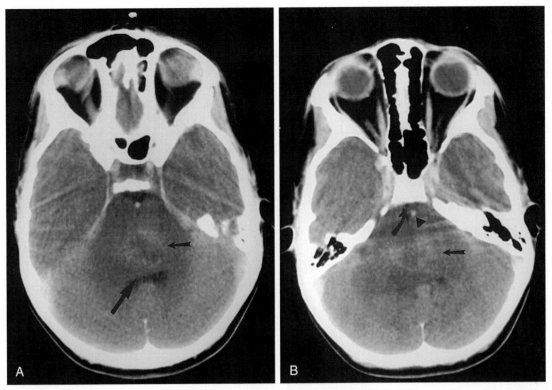

Figure 22–14 Diffuse pontine glioma in a 7-year-old girl with multiple cranial nerve deficits. Computer-enhanced CT (*A* and *B*) shows diffuse expansion and hypodensity within the pons and bilateral brachium ponti. The anterior fourth ventricle is flattened (*large arrow*) and the prepontine cistern (*curved arrow*) is effaced. Note contrast in the basilar artery. The mass has mild central irregular ring enhancement (*small arrows*).

are large enough to obstruct the fourth ventricle. Calcification and hemorrhage are uncommon characteristics.

Oligodendroglioma

Oligodendrogliomas are slow-growing neoplasms arising from oligodendrocytes. These tumors occur more frequently in middle-aged adults, rarely in children, and are slightly more common in males (3:2). Overall, oligodendrogliomas account for fewer than 5% of all intracranial gliomas.[37]

Current immunocytochemical techniques demonstrate that many tumors with a histologic appearance of astrocytoma will partially or completely lack staining for glial fibrillary acidic protein (GFAP), and are therefore diagnosed as mixed oligoastrocytomas or pure oligodendrogliomas, respectively. Using the newer criteria, the incidence of oligodendrogliomas has increased. Most oligodendrogliomas are benign, but anaplastic or malignant grades are occasionally found. Anaplastic transformation to glioblastoma multiforme is rare.

In adults, oligodendrogliomas arise in the white matter of the peripheral cerebral hemisphere with a predilection for the supratentorial compartment, particularly the frontal lobe. Cortical involvement is common. Because of slow growth and peripheral location, calvarial remodeling can be detected in up to 17% of tumors,[38] a finding that is often subtle or nondetectable on MRI. Oligodendrogliomas have the highest incidence of associated calcification (40% to 50%). When present, calcifications usually have a coarse, clumped appearance (Fig. 22–16) and can be seen on plain radiographs

of the skull. Finer intratumoral calcification is seen more often in low-grade astrocytomas. Faint patchy enhancement can be detected in up to 50% of oligodendrogliomas and hemorrhage is frequent (20%) (Fig. 22–17), which is the distinct opposite of what is seen in other low-grade gliomas. Vasogenic edema is not common with lower-grade lesions. Malignant oligodendrogliomas may appear identical to glioblastoma multiforme on both CT and MRI.

A recent series of 39 surgically proved pure oligodendrogliomas in the pediatric population demonstrated a less frequent occurrence of calcification, enhancement, and edema compared with adult oligodendrogliomas.[37] The majority of these lesions, as seen in adult oligodendroglioma, were well-circumscribed low-density neoplasms with little mass effect.

Rarely, oligodendroglioma may occur in the ventricular system. The differential diagnosis in this instance includes a calcified intraventricular astrocytoma, choroid plexus papilloma, meningioma, and central neurocytoma. Intraventricular (central) neurocytoma has been described as a tumor of young adults that is associated with a very favorable prognosis. Almost all of these are located in the lateral or third ventricle, and most have a distinctive attachment to the septum pellucidum. These tumors can be confused radiologically and by light microscopy with oligodendroglioma and ependymoma.[39] Ultrastructural and immunochemical features demonstrate their true neuronal origin.[40]

Ependymoma

Ependymomas arise from ependymal cells lining the ventricular surface or from ependymal rests within the brain paren-

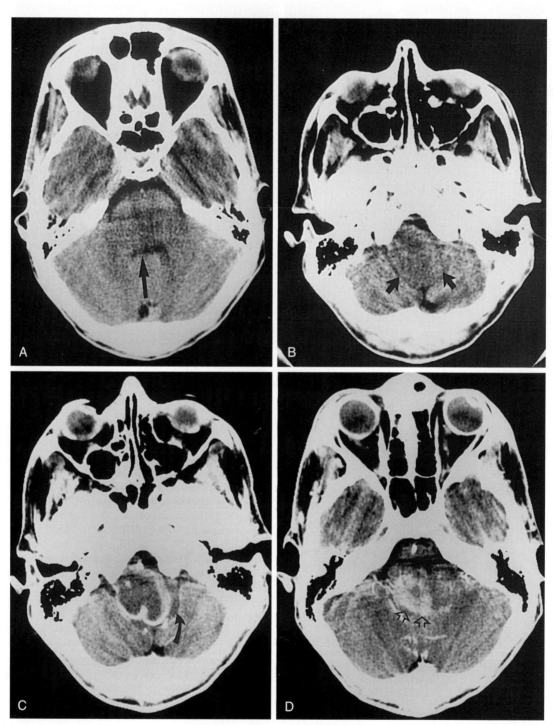

Figure 22–15 Exophytic brainstem glioma. An 18-year-old man underwent CT for head trauma. Non–contrast-enhanced CT at the level of the pons (*A*) demonstrates subtle asymmetry of the pontine tegmentum and effacement of the fourth ventricle (*arrow*) and lobulated enlargement (*B*) of the cervicomedullary junction (*arrows*). The premedullary cistern is effaced. Contrast-enhanced CT images (*C* and *D*) show an exophytic ring-enhancing mass with the epicenter at the cervicomedullary junction. *C*, The mass displaces the medulla posteriorly and to the left (*arrow*). *D*, The mass is growing into the inferior fourth ventricle (*arrows*).

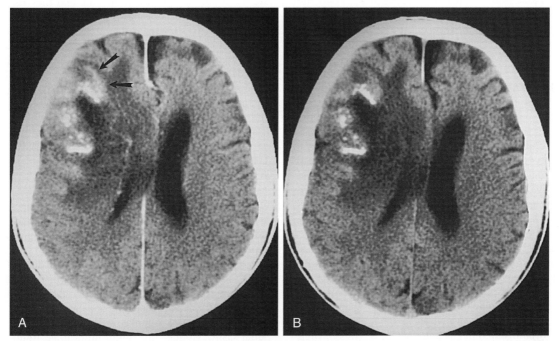

Figure 22–16 Pre–contrast-enhancement (*A*) and post–contrast-enhancement (*B*) CT images of a 74-year-old man. A right frontal mixed-density mass with clumped calcifications (*arrows*) demonstrates mild enhancement along the anterior border after IV contrast (*B*). Oligodendrogliomas are most common in the frontal lobe; they most commonly calcify and often demonstrate mild to moderate contrast enhancement.

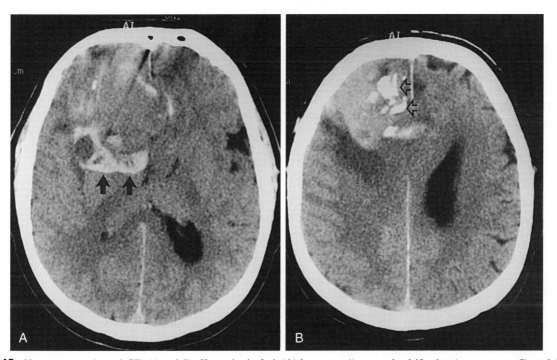

Figure 22–17 Non–contrast-enhanced CTs (*A* and *B*). Hemorrhagic foci (*thick arrows; A*), tumoral calcification (*open arrows; B*), and frontal lobe location led to the correct preoperative diagnosis of oligodendroglioma. Hemorrhage is not uncommon in these tumors.

chyma. These tumors represent 5% of CNS gliomas and 10% of childhood brain tumors. Two-thirds of all ependymomas are infratentorial, and are most commonly located in the fourth ventricle in children. The peak incidence in children is at ages 1 to 5 years, with higher frequency in males. Supratentorial ependymomas are uncommon in the pediatric population (Fig. 22–18); in adults, however, ependymomas are generally supratentorial and intraparenchymal. Histologically, ependymomas range from benign to malignant, with higher-grade tumors being more frequent with increasing age.

Ependymomas on CT are most often well-defined low- to mixed-density lesions that are commonly associated with cyst formation, hemorrhagic foci, and dense punctate calcifications (Fig. 22–19). Ependymoma has the highest frequency of calcification (45%) of all posterior fossa tumors. Moderate to intense heterogeneous contrast enhancement is present in all but rare cases. Fourth ventricular ependymomas expand the ventricle and, with growth, extend the fourth ventricle outlet foramina. When a posterior fossa tumor is present that extends through the foramen of Magendie and the lateral foramen of Luschka and upper cervical canal through the foramen magnum, a diagnosis of ependymoma is likely.[41]

Supratentorial ependymomas can contain regions of high- or mixed-density on CT prior to contrast enhancement, are usually well demarcated, and show moderate to marked enhancement. No correlation has been demonstrated between the degree of enhancement and tumor grade.[42]

Subependymoma, a variant of ependymoma, contains both ependymal cells and astrocytes. These unusual neoplasms are most common in men with a mean age at occurrence of 60 years. They are often found incidentally or at autopsy. Subependymomas are sharply demarcated small or lobulated nodular masses that are most commonly (75%) located in

the fourth ventricle[43] (Fig. 22–20). These noninvasive tumors are not associated with CSF spread, and they have a benign clinical course unless the fourth ventricle becomes obstructed.

Ependymoblastomas constitute a rare embryonal form of ependymoma; they are found most commonly in children and carry an extremely poor prognosis. CT demonstrates a large, mixed-density supratentorial mass with moderate enhancement. This lesion frequently invades the meninges and disseminates into the subarachnoid space.

Cerebellar Astrocytoma/Pilocytic Astrocytoma

Cerebellar astrocytomas are found almost exclusively in children and in adolescents,[2] but they are occasionally found in adults. They are clinically and radiologically distinct from supratentorial astrocytomas. Eighty-five percent[1] are classified as juvenile pilocytic astrocytomas, a distinct subgroup of astrocytoma that is the most common form of posterior fossa tumor in childhood. Juvenile pilocytic astrocytomas are often completely resectable and carry the highest survival rates of all primary gliomas.[44] The remaining 15% of cerebellar astrocytomas are solid infiltrating tumors that are identical to adult supratentorial astrocytomas. Pediatric glioblastoma is exceptionally rare (Fig. 22–21).

Supratentorial juvenile pilocytic astrocytomas commonly involve the optic pathway and hypothalamus, but they may also be intraparenchymal (Fig. 22–22). Although the majority are slow-growing benign lesions, a small percentage have a more aggressive clinical course. It has been shown that the initial CT and MRI features of pilocytic astrocytoma are unreliable for predicting which tumors will act in a more aggressive manner.[45]

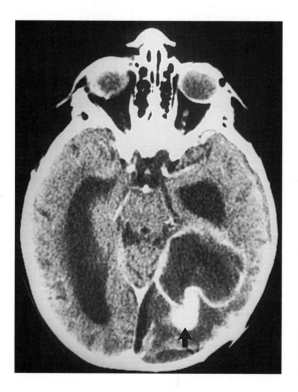

Figure 22–18 A 7-year-old boy with a malignant ependymoma. Contrast-enhanced CT shows a large complex mass in the left occipital horn; note ventricular enlargement. There is dense homogeneous enhancement of the solid nodular component (*arrow*) and enhancement of the thin wall surrounding a large cystic component.

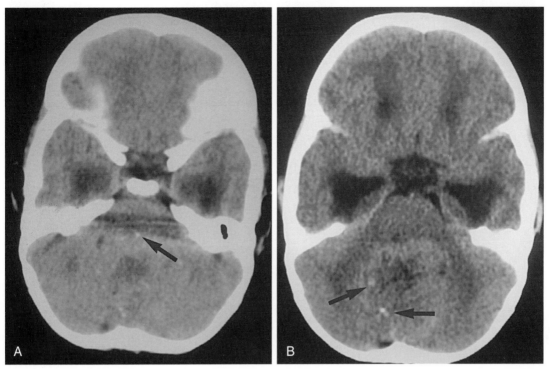

Figure 22–19 A 10-month-old child with a large mixed-density fourth ventricular mass (*A* and *B*) that has multiple punctate calcifications on non–contrast-enhanced CT (*arrows*). Ependymoma was found at surgery. Approximately 50% of ependymomas contain calcifications.

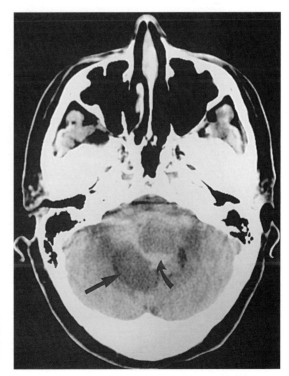

Figure 22–20 Mixed subependymoma/ependymoma. Non–contrast-enhanced CT reveals a complex mass with thick irregular walls along the anterior aspect of a dilated fourth ventricle (*straight arrow*). Cyst contents are of higher density than CSF, and a sediment layer is present (*curved arrow*). Subependymomas are most commonly located in the fourth ventricle.

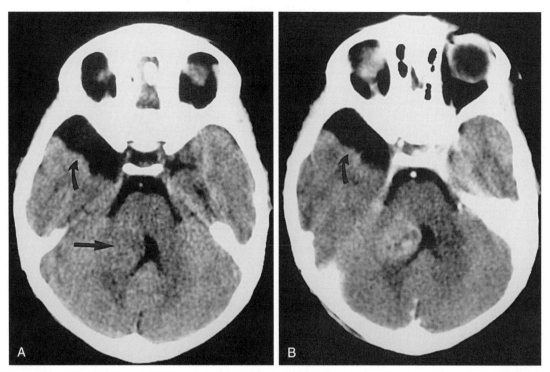

Figure 22–21 Axial non–contrast-enhanced CT (*A*) in a 6-year-old girl shows isodense focal expansion (*straight arrow*) of the right middle cerebellar peduncle, which is deforming the fourth ventricle. Heterogeneous enhancement is present with central foci of low density on contrast-enhanced CT (*B*). Pathology showed glioblastoma multiforme. An incidental temporal tip arachnoid cyst is noted (*curved arrow*).

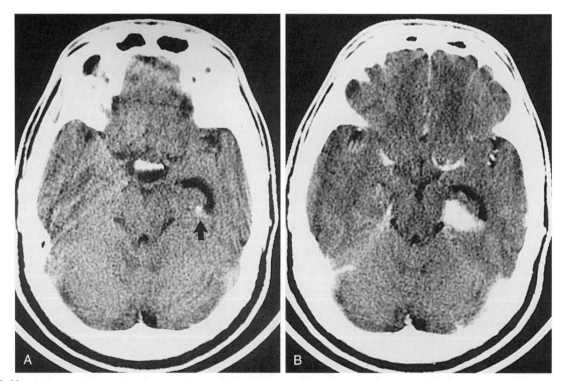

Figure 22–22 A 33-year-old man with seizures and known left mesial temporal mass is seen to have a small isodense temporal lobe mass (*arrow*) with a punctate calcification on non–contrast-enhanced CT (*A*). The lesion demonstrates solid, homogeneous enhancement (*B*). The nonaggressive appearance and paucity of change over 2 years favored a diagnosis of low-grade astrocytoma or ganglioglioma. The pathologic diagnosis was pilocytic astrocytoma.

Cerebellar juvenile pilocytic astrocytomas are usually large tumors, which may be solid (Fig. 22–23), but which more typically appear on CT as round to oval unilocular cystic masses. They are commonly midline masses centered in the cerebellar vermis, and they also occur in the cerebellar hemisphere. An associated sharply circumscribed, solid mural nodule is common. It is isodense on noncontrast CT and enhances intensely[46] (Fig. 22–24). The nodule is nearly always solitary and round or oval, but it may be plaque-like and may extend a variable distance around the cyst.[47] The intense enhancement correlates with hypervascularity seen at pathologic analysis. The cyst wall does not enhance because it is not composed of neoplastic tissue. However, the wall of the cyst may appear slightly hyperdense. This hyperdensity represents displaced, compressed cerebellar tissue. The circumscribed cyst wall makes the lesion more amenable to complete surgical removal. Multiple enhancing nodules and thick, irregular, or septated walls favor the diagnosis of a necrotic infiltrating mass. Calcifications are not characteristic of cerebellar astrocytomas, but they can occur in up to 20%.

Optic Pathway/Hypothalamic Glioma

Astrocytomas of the visual pathway and hypothalamus represent 5% of all primary pediatric CNS neoplasms, and they account for 3% of childhood and 1% of adult gliomas. These are slow-growing masses with low-grade histologic characteristics; they are most often pilocytic astrocytomas.

Because of their slow growth they may be very large at presentation, making the exact structure of origin difficult to define. Surprisingly, vision is preserved even with large tumors.

Optic gliomas are the most common abnormality of brain in neurofibromatosis type 1 (NF1), with an incidence of 30% to 90%. Bilateral lesions are present in 10% to 20%.[48] In NF1, most gliomas arise in the intraorbital optic nerve and extend posteriorly. Gliomas may also originate in the chiasmatic region.

Optic nerve gliomas appear on noncontrast CT as fusiform or lobulated low-density masses that can extend along the optic pathways. Moderate to marked enhancement is common. Optic gliomas may be restricted to the orbital optic nerve, or they may have intracranial extension. Chiasmatic lesions may track anteriorly or posteriorly to involve the optic tracts, radiations, lateral geniculate bodies, and temporal lobes (Fig. 22–25). A series of chiasmatic gliomas in 22 patients demonstrated three patterns based on CT imaging: (1) tubular thickening of the optic nerve and chiasm, (2) a suprasellar mass with contiguous optic nerve expansion, and (3) a suprasellar mass with involvement of the optic tracts.[49]

Axial and direct coronal CT images are excellent for showing the intraorbital extent because of excellent contrast between the tumor along the optic nerve complex and surrounding intraorbital fat as well as with the adjacent bony orbit. Intracanalicular extension of tumor is best demonstrated with MRI; however, this may be inferred in CT if asymmetrical enlargement of the optic canals is present (Fig. 22–26).

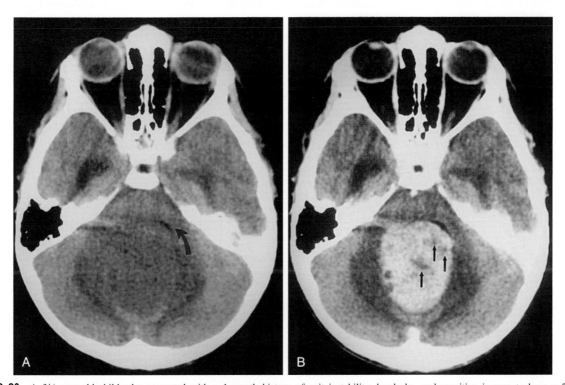

Figure 22–23 A 3½-year-old child who presented with a 1-month history of gait instability, headache, and vomiting is seen to have a 5 × 4 cm-diameter midline cerebellar astrocytoma, causing deviation of the fourth ventricle anteriorly (*arrow*), on non–contrast-enhanced CT. The mass is solid and has low attenuation on non–contrast-enhanced CT (*A*). The lesion demonstrates strong homogeneous enhancement (*B*) and contains small foci of central necrosis (*arrows*). Other tumors to consider include medulloblastoma, ependymoma, and choroid plexus papilloma.

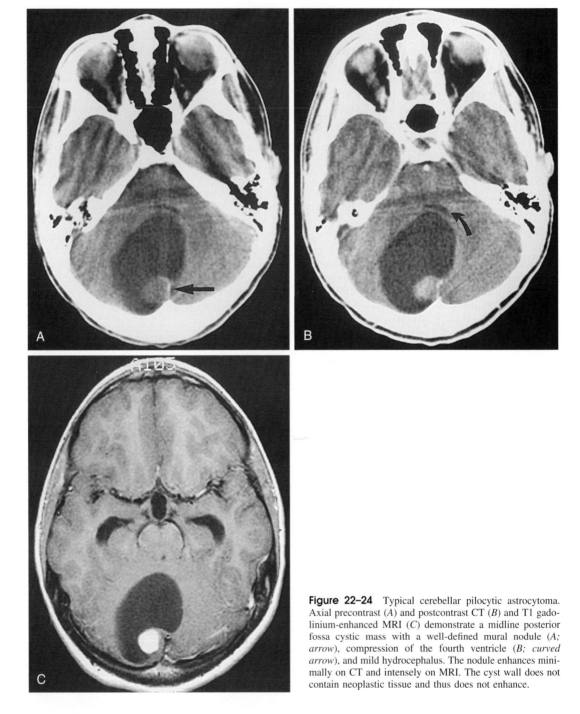

Figure 22–24 Typical cerebellar pilocytic astrocytoma. Axial precontrast (*A*) and postcontrast CT (*B*) and T1 gadolinium-enhanced MRI (*C*) demonstrate a midline posterior fossa cystic mass with a well-defined mural nodule (*A; arrow*), compression of the fourth ventricle (*B; curved arrow*), and mild hydrocephalus. The nodule enhances minimally on CT and intensely on MRI. The cyst wall does not contain neoplastic tissue and thus does not enhance.

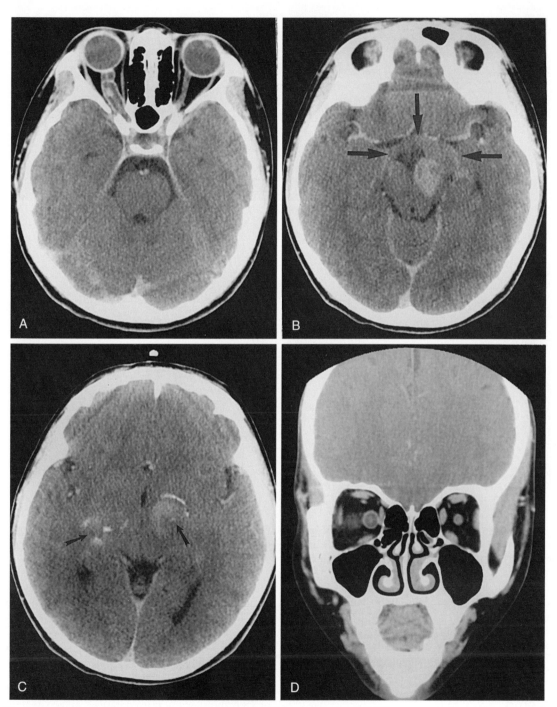

Figure 22–25 Axial (*A–C*) and direct coronal (*D*) contrast-enhanced CT images show typical CT appearance of an optic pathway glioma. There is diffuse, lobulated enlargement of the right optic nerve (*A* and *D*), optic chiasm, optic tracts (*B; large arrows*), and involvement of the optic radiations bilaterally (*C; arrows*).

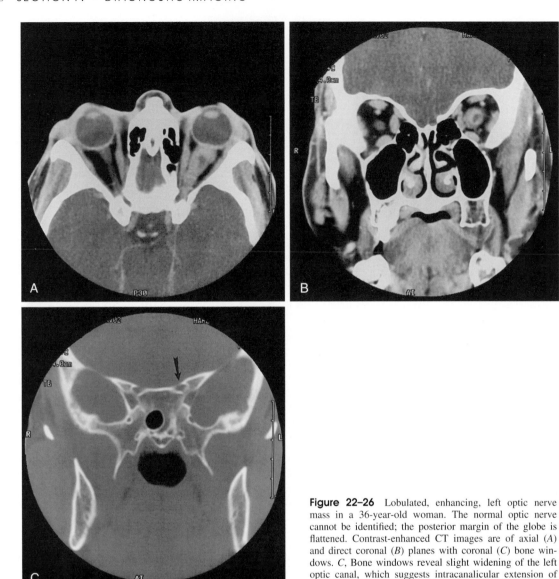

Figure 22–26 Lobulated, enhancing, left optic nerve mass in a 36-year-old woman. The normal optic nerve cannot be identified; the posterior margin of the globe is flattened. Contrast-enhanced CT images are of axial (*A*) and direct coronal (*B*) planes with coronal (*C*) bone windows. *C*, Bone windows reveal slight widening of the left optic canal, which suggests intracanalicular extension of tumor (*arrow*).

Gliomas arising from the hypothalamic region may have a striking resemblance to those that arise within the optic chiasm (Figs. 22–27 and 22–28). The true site of origin may be difficult to discern, especially with large masses. Large hypothalamic and chiasmatic masses can expand into the third ventricle, suprasellar cistern, and interpeduncular fossa and can obstruct the foramen of Monro. Solid portions of the mass enhance homogeneously. Lack of involvement of optic pathway structures in this situation is a clue to the correct site of origin within the hypothalamus.

Ganglioglioma

Gangliogliomas are rare intracranial neoplasms that, although they account for fewer than 1% of all primary CNS tumors and 3% of pediatric brain tumors, are being diagnosed more frequently. Pathologically, gangliogliomas contain a combination of neoplastic glial cells—usually astrocytes—and neuronal cells.[50] *Ganglioglioma* is the term used when the ganglion cell population predominates; when the majority of cells are neurons, the mass is termed a *ganglioneuroma*.

These neoplasms are generally low-grade, slow-growing tumors with a favorable prognosis, and they occur more frequently in children and adolescents, with no sex predilection. The most common location is in the temporal lobe, in which case seizures are a common presentation. They may also be found in the cerebellar hemisphere, less commonly in the brainstem, and rarely in the spinal cord.

The majority are low to isodense well-circumscribed lesions with essentially no mass effect or edema. In a series of 18 pathologically proved cases,[51] approximately half were cystic and, despite their benign nature and slow growth, demonstrated mild to moderate enhancement. Dense or large calcifications are found in 20% to 35%. In one series,[52] calcification was the only CT finding in six patients. Involvement of the leptomeninges and spread into the subarachnoid space rarely occur.[53] Remodeling of the adjacent calvarium may be present in peripherally located tumors (Figs. 22–29

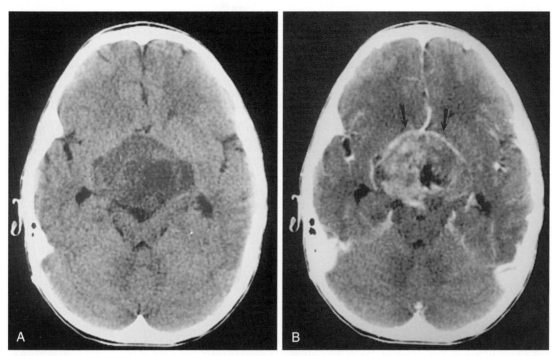

Figure 22–27 A 3-year-old boy who presented with nystagmus was found to have a hypothalamic pilocytic astrocytoma. Precontrast (*A*) and postcontrast (*B*) axial images demonstrate a large suprasellar mixed-attenuation mass, with the epicenter at the hypothalamus. The solid components of the mass enhance; note displacement of the A1 segments of the anterior cerebral arteries (*arrows*).

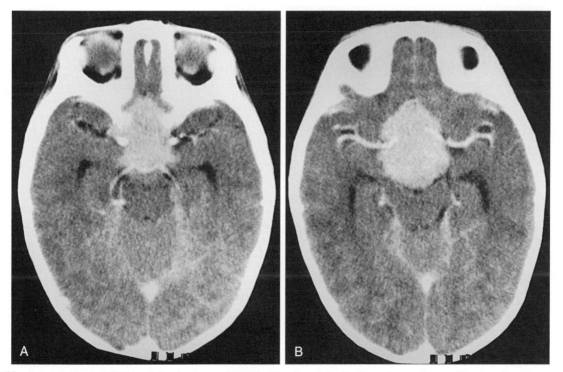

Figure 22–28 Contrast-enhanced CT (*A* and *B*) of a 1-year-old child with a hypothalamic glioma shows a large uniformly enhancing suprasellar mass. The origin of large suprasellar masses is difficult to accurately determine with CT, and sometimes even with MRI. Lack of extension along the optic pathways in a mass this size favors a hypothalamic origin.

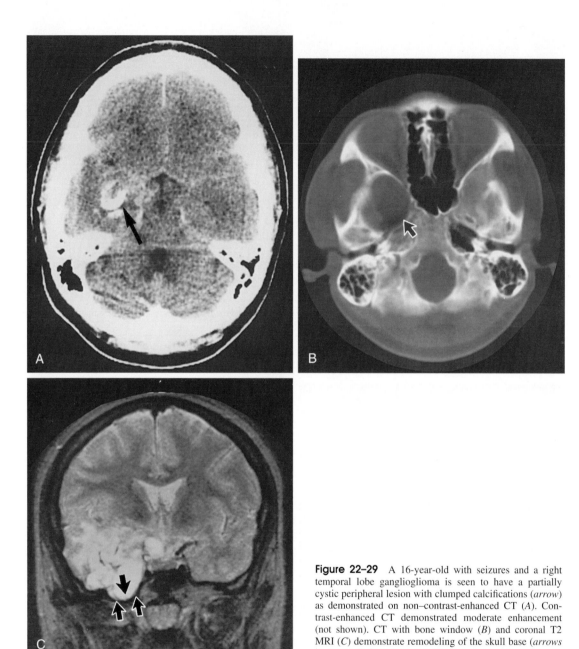

Figure 22–29 A 16-year-old with seizures and a right temporal lobe ganglioglioma is seen to have a partially cystic peripheral lesion with clumped calcifications (*arrow*) as demonstrated on non–contrast-enhanced CT (*A*). Contrast-enhanced CT demonstrated moderate enhancement (not shown). CT with bone window (*B*) and coronal T2 MRI (*C*) demonstrate remodeling of the skull base (*arrows* in *B* and *C*) from long-standing pressure erosion.

and 22–30). The differential diagnosis includes low-grade astrocytoma, oligodendroglioma, and pleomorphic xanthoastrocytoma. Gangliogliomas rarely undergo malignant transformation; any such transformation usually occurs along the glial cell line, resulting in glioblastoma.

Subependymal Giant Cell Astrocytoma

Subependymal giant cell astrocytomas occur in approximately 5% to 15% of patients with tuberous sclerosis. The CT and MRI characteristics of tuberous sclerosis have been well documented.[54] The peak incidence is at ages 5 to 10 years, with tumors occurring as frequently in males as in females. Subependymal giant cell astrocytomas characteristically arise in a subependymal tuber that is present in the wall of the lateral ventricle near the foramen of Monro. Because of this critical location, unilateral hydrocephalus may be a presenting symptom of this neoplasm.

Subependymal giant cell astrocytomas typically appear on CT as circumscribed, low-density, round lesions at the foramen of Monro, often with associated calcifications, cysts, and hydrocephalus. Dense heterogeneous enhancement is typical. Identification of multiple calcified subependymal tubers and cortical hamartomas are clues to the correct diagnosis (Fig. 22–31). CT demonstration of rapid growth or the presence of enhancement within a tuber located at the foramen of Monro is strong evidence of histologic degeneration into a subependymal giant cell astrocytoma. Enhancement of tubers can sometimes be seen with gadolinium-enhanced MRI, and malignant degeneration should not be inferred.

RADIATION EFFECTS

Radiation damage to the brain is variable and can follow either whole-brain radiation, limited-field radiation restricted to the tumor bed, radiosurgery, or brachytherapy. The degree of radiation injury is related to the cumulative dose, the dose rate, and the volume of tumor and normal brain irradiated. Associated CT changes are well recognized and include both focal and diffuse findings. Focal radiation necrosis mimics recurrent tumor both clinically and on CT, especially when it is present at the site of previous tumor resection.[55, 56]

Focal radiation changes occur months to years after therapy. Patients present with focal neurologic deficits or signs of increased intracranial pressure. CT demonstrates a focal hypodense mass with vasogenic edema and variable mass effect. An irregular ring-enhancing lesion may be present, reflecting the disruption of the blood-brain barrier, which gives an appearance similar to recurrent glioma, metastasis, or abscess (Fig. 22–32). Both recurrent tumor and focal radiation necrosis usually occur at the original tumor bed and may be coexistent. Radiation necrosis cannot be differentiated with a high degree of accuracy by conventional CT or MRI. Some reports suggest a definite role for PET as well as for thallium or technetium-HMPAO SPECT imaging in this difficult clinical situation.[57, 58]

The CT and MRI findings of diffuse radiation injury may be found months to years after initial therapy. Typically, bilateral widespread subcortical and deep white matter hypodensities are seen, with sparing of the corpus callosum. A geometric border represents the margin of the radiation port and is a clue to the diagnosis (Fig. 22–33). Focal mass effect and contrast enhancement are not present. The white matter

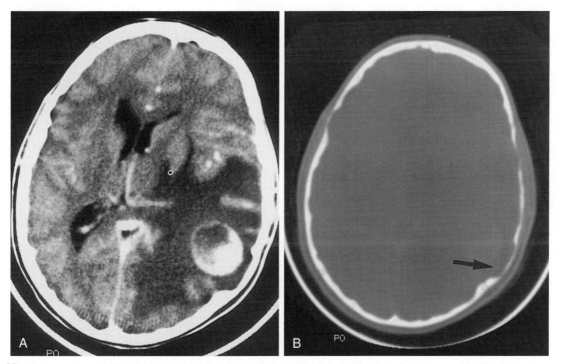

Figure 22–30 Contrast-enhanced CT (*A*) and corresponding bone windows (*B*) of a ganglioglioma in a 12-year-old girl with new onset seizure. A strongly enhancing partially cystic left temporal lobe mass is seen. The enhancement, marked edema, and mass effect suggest an aggressive neoplasm. However, smooth erosion of the adjacent calvarium (*arrow*) is a sign of a slowly growing mass that has been present for some time.

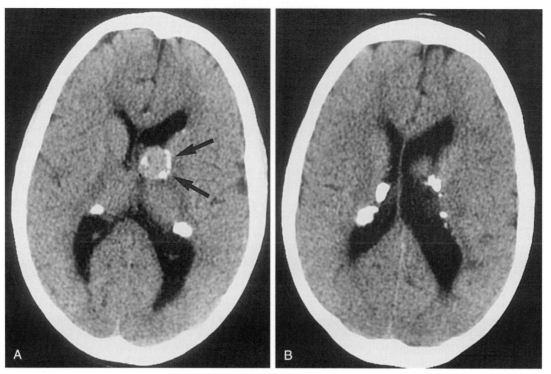

Figure 22–31 Subependymal giant cell astrocytoma in a 10-year-old boy with stigmata of tuberous sclerosis. A sharply circumscribed, round, partially calcified mass (*arrows*) is present at the foramen of Monro on the left (*A*). Note mild enlargement of the left lateral ventricle and multiple calcified subependymal nodules typical of tuberous sclerosis (*B*).

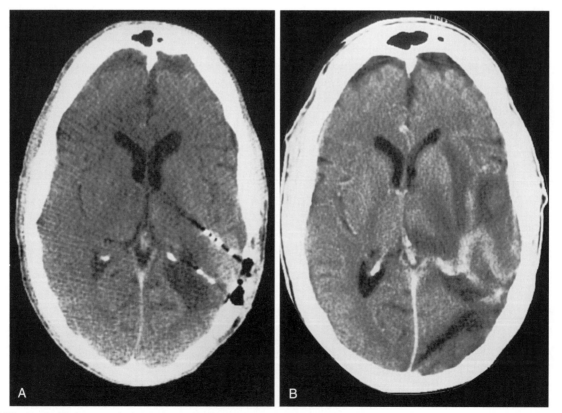

Figure 22–32 Focal radiation necrosis: brachytherapy implants are present at the site of a previously resected tumor on non–contrast-enhanced CT (*A*). Contrast-enhanced CT 5 months later (*B*) shows an area of irregular ring enhancement corresponding to the site of the implants as well as extensive vasogenic edema and mass effect. CT and MRI cannot differentiate recurrent tumor from radiation necrosis.

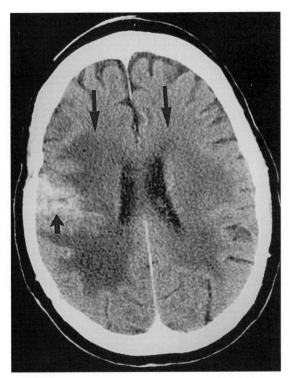

Figure 22–33 Diffuse radiation effects: contrast-enhanced CT shows recurrent right frontal glioblastoma multiforme (*short arrow*). Note diffuse, bilateral, deep white matter regions of low density with sharply defined anterior margins and no mass effect. This is characteristic of diffuse radiation change. The anterior margins (*long arrows*) correspond to radiation ports.

changes are better demonstrated on MRI.[59] Recognition of this common post-radiation change is important and it should not be confused with edema or recurrent tumor.

Additional radiation-induced changes include generalized atrophy and calcification. Atrophy results from deep white matter volume loss, which is seen radiographically as ventriculomegaly with enlarged sulci. Dystrophic calcifications occur in the deep white matter, basal ganglia, or subcortical regions. Radiation-induced tumors are extremely uncommon and usually occur more than 10 years post-radiation; they include gliomas, meningiomas, and malignant mesenchymal tumors.[60]

INTRASPINAL GLIOMAS

Intrinsic spinal cord tumors are approximately 10% as frequent as primary intracranial CNS neoplasms and are more common in adults than in children. It is estimated that 90% to 95% of all intramedullary spinal cord tumors are gliomas. The overwhelming majority (95%) are astrocytomas and ependymomas; glioblastoma multiforme, anaplastic astrocytoma, oligodendroglioma, and ganglioglioma are rare exceptions. Intramedullary tumors represent approximately 5% of CNS tumors and 30% of all spinal tumors in children.[61, 62]

In adults, 60% of intra-axial gliomas are ependymomas, whereas 30% represent astrocytic neoplasms. The frequency ratio of astrocytoma to ependymoma is reversed in children.[41, 63] Spinal cord tumors tend to be more rostrally

located in children, with 50% located in the cervical region compared with 28% at that site in adults. The most common imaging characteristics include focal or fusiform enlargement of the spinal cord, rostral or caudal tumoral cystic components, and contrast enhancement.

Current Role of CT in Intraspinal Neoplasms

MRI is much more sensitive than CT in the detection of intramedullary neoplasms and in the evaluation of these patients, and it is therefore the imaging modality of choice in the overwhelming majority of cases. However, CT may be useful in several specific situations. CT or CT myelography is performed in patients with absolute contraindications to MRI, such as the presence of a pacemaker or an intracranial aneurysm clip. Metal artifacts from prior spinal instrumentation may obscure visualization of the spinal cord. This is becoming a less frequent occurrence since the introduction of non-ferromagnetic hardware. CT is more useful than MRI in demonstrating subtle osseous pathology, such as widening of the spinal canal and thinning of adjacent pedicles. It may also be useful in defining important bony landmarks prior to surgery. MRI is more sensitive than CT in identifying subtle areas of intramedullary contrast enhancement and is more accurate in differentiating between tumor cysts and benign syrinx. Neither CT nor MRI can reliably differentiate astrocytomas from ependymomas.

CT Technique

Axial 1.5-mm slices in the cervical spine and contiguous 3-mm sections in the thoracolumbar region are obtained following intravenous contrast enhancement. Intravenous enhancement is necessary because the majority of cord gliomas do contain focal areas of enhancement regardless of grade, unlike intracranial glial tumors. CT myelography is performed by injecting 10 mL of 60% nonionic iodinated contrast (iohexol and iopamidol are the only currently approved agents for intrathecal use) into the cervical or lumbar subarachnoid space, followed by acquiring CT images at the desired levels. Detection of cyst cavities on CT depends on delayed scanning during CT myelography, because time is needed for intrathecal iodinated contrast agents to permeate the cord and to accumulate in the cyst.

CT and CT myelographic findings suggestive of an intramedullary tumor include fusiform or focal regions of spinal cord enlargement, intra-axial foci of enhancement, and cyst formation. Effacement of the subarachnoid space, obliteration of epidural fat, subtle expansion of the spinal canal, scalloping of the posterior vertebral body, and pedicular erosion are additional important findings (Fig. 22–34). Sagittal and coronal reformatted images are extremely useful for demonstrating the bony relationships of an intrinsic spinal cord lesion (Fig. 22–35).

Drop metastases from intracranial neoplasms occur more frequently in children than in adults, most commonly from medulloblastoma. Astrocytomas, especially glioblastomas multiforme, and ependymomas are the most common glial

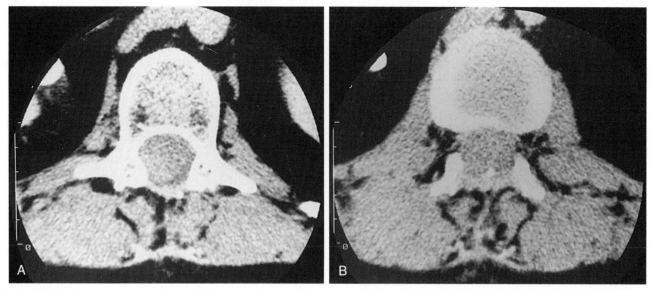

Figure 22–34 Non–contrast-enhanced axial CT images of the spine in a patient with a surgically proved ependymoma (A). The spinal cord is diffusely enlarged, which obliterates the epidural fat. The spinal canal is expanded and the pedicles are remodeled (B). The patient has had a prior laminectomy.

tumors to demonstrate CSF seeding. Multiple nodular filling defects in the subarachnoid space (Fig. 22–36), irregular spinal cord contour, thickened nerve roots, and narrowing of the thecal sac are CT myelographic signs of CSF tumor dissemination.

Intramedullary Ependymoma

Of all CNS ependymomas, one-third are primary intramedullary spinal cord neoplasms.[64] They are the most common spinal cord tumors overall, the most common intramedullary neoplasm in adults (60%), and the second most common tumor in children.[65] The mean age at presentation is 40 years, with a slightly higher incidence in females.

Ependymomas have a predilection for the lower spinal cord, conus, and filum terminale, and they represent the most common (90%) primary cord tumor located in this region.[66] Ependymomas are classified as cellular, which is the most common subtype overall, or myxopapillary, which is the most common subtype in the distal cord and filum.[64] Because the ependymal cells lining the central spinal canal are the site of origin, these masses are usually centrally located within the spinal cord and are associated with a surgical capsule. This results in symmetrical cord expansion with thinning of the residual cord tissue.

CT and CT myelography typically demonstrate a centrally located, focal or fusiform intramedullary mass with sharply defined rostral and caudal margins (Fig. 22–37). All enhance strongly and homogeneously with well-defined borders, a finding that helps differentiate a tumor from a benign syrinx. Because of the capsule, the margin of enhancement has a higher correlation with actual tumor margin than is the case for astrocytomas, which have a more infiltrating growth pattern.[67] Fifty percent are associated with cyst formation. Unlike the findings in intracranial ependymomas, calcifications are rare, and small foci of hemorrhage may be present.

Intramedullary Astrocytoma

Astrocytomas are the most common intramedullary neoplasm in children and the second most frequent spinal cord tumor in adults. The peak incidence is in the third to fourth decades, with a slight male predominance. They are typically slow-growing low-grade fibrillary neoplasms that can be found anywhere in the cord, but which have a predilection for the cervical and upper thoracic spine. Astrocytomas are rare in the filum. In contrast to ependymomas, which are more focal, astrocytomas characteristically infiltrate rostrally and caudally to involve multiple cord segments with no distinct demarcation from normal cord. In addition, astrocytomas are often located eccentrically within the cord, resulting in asymmetrical expansion.

CT imaging shows multisegmental, diffuse, fusiform cord expansion. Rostral or caudal cysts are found in 25% to 35% and tend to be benign. Compared with benign cysts, tumor cysts are smaller, more irregular, and eccentrically located and they have associated enhancement. Despite the low-grade histologic characteristics, nearly all enhance to some degree with IV contrast. The enhancement is best detected with MRI and is less prominent than the strong enhancement typical of ependymoma. Osseous changes are the same as those found with ependymoma.

The differential diagnosis of an intrinsic intramedullary mass includes primary cord neoplasms, the majority of which are gliomas and hemangioblastomas. Generally, astrocytomas are eccentrically located within the cord and are more diffuse than ependymomas. However, ependymomas tend to be centrally located, appear more circumscribed, demonstrate greater enhancement, and are more commonly associated with hemorrhage. Hemangioblastomas are rare in the spinal cord and have a higher incidence in patients with von Hippel–Lindau disease. Hemangioblastomas are hypervascular neoplasms that may appear as a hypodense intra-axial mass with an enhancing nidus on CT myelogra-

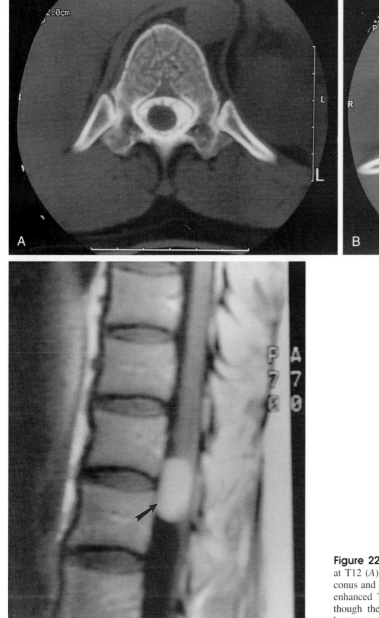

Figure 22–35 Rare exophytic glioblastoma of the conus: CT myelography at T12 (*A*) and L1 (*B*) shows an intramedullary mass diffusely expanding the conus and effacing the subarachnoid space (*open arrows*). Sagittal gadolinium-enhanced T1 MRI demonstrates a strongly enhancing mass (*C; arrow*). Although the mass was easily demonstrated on CT, its overall appearance is better appreciated on MRI. (Case courtesy of R. A. Nugent, M.D., University of British Columbia.)

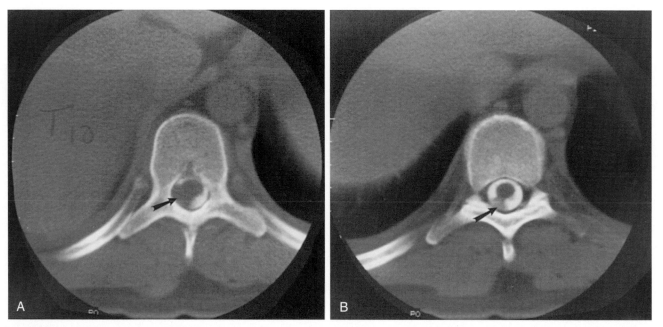

Figure 22–36 CT myelogram in a patient with a brainstem glioma. Axial images (*A* and *B*) demonstrate extramedullary intradural filling defects (*arrows*), which were proved to be drop metastases. MRI is the current modality of choice for detecting subarachnoid tumor dissemination.

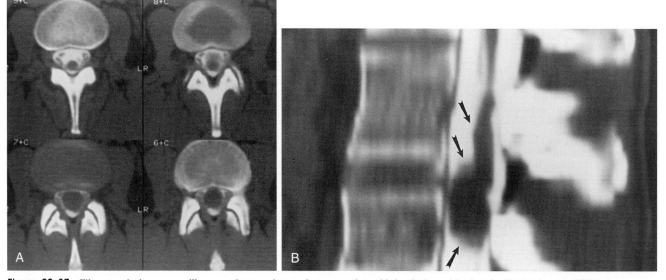

Figure 22–37 Filum terminale myxopapillary ependymoma in a patient presenting with headache and back pain. Xanthochromic CSF was present on lumbar puncture. Axial (*A*) and sagittal reformatted (*B*) images at the L2–3 interspace show an elongated lobulated mass (*arrows*) arising from the filum. At surgery it was noted that the ependymoma had ruptured inside of its capsule and bled, which accounted for the symptoms of subarachnoid hemorrhage. (Case courtesy of R. A. Nugent, M.D., University of British Columbia.)

phy. Serpiginous filling defects in the subarachnoid space represent distended vascular structures. Intramedullary metastases are rare and occur most often with lung and breast carcinoma. Hydrosyringomyelia, demyelinating disease, and an enhancing inflammatory mass are other diagnostic possibilities.

REFERENCES

1. Russell DS, Rubinstein LJ: Incidence, pathogenesis, and other general aspects. *In* Pathology of Tumors of the Nervous System, ed 5. Baltimore, Williams & Wilkins, 1989, p 1–57.
2. Walker AE, Robins M, Weinfeld FD: Epidemiology of brain tumors: The National Survey of Intracranial Neoplasms. Neurology 1985; 35:219–226.
3. Greig NH, Ries LG, Yancic R, et al: Increasing annual incidence of primary malignant brain tumors in the elderly. JNCI 1990; 82:1621–1624.
4. Atlas SW: Intra-axial brain tumors. *In* Atlas SW (ed): Magnetic Resonance Imaging of the Brain and Spine. New York, Raven, 1991, pp 223–326.
5. Lee BCP, Kneeland JB, Cahill PT, et al: MR recognition of supratentorial tumors. AJNR 1985; 6:871–878.
6. Bernstein M, Parrent AG: Complications of CT-guided stereotactic biopsy of intra-axial brain lesions. J Neurosurg 1994; 81:165–168.
7. Heiken JP, Brink JA, Vannier MW: Spiral (helical) CT. Radiology 1993; 189:647–656.
8. Tchang S, Scotti G, Terbrugge K, et al: Computerized tomography as a possible aid to histologic grading of supratentorial gliomas. J Neurosurg 1977; 46:735–739.
9. Butler AR, Horii SC, Kricheff II, et al: Computed tomography in astrocytomas. Radiology 1978; 129:433–439.
10. Thompson JLG: Computerized axial tomography and the diagnosis of glioma: A study of 100 consecutive histologically proven cases. Clin Radiol 1977; 27:431–441.
11. Brant-Zawadski M, Berry I, Osaki L, et al: Gd-DTPA in clinical MR of the brain: I. Intracranial lesions. AJNR 1986; 7:781–788.
12. Earnest F, Kelly PJ, Scheithauer BW, et al: Cerebral astrocytomas: Histopathologic correlation of MR and CT contrast enhancement with stereotactic biopsy. Radiology 1988; 166:823–827.
13. Jeffries BF, Kishore PRS, Singh KS, et al: Contrast enhancement in the postoperative brain. Radiology 1981; 139:409–413.
14. Rao CVGK, Kishore PRS, Bartlett J, et al: Computed tomography in the postoperative patient. Neuroradiol 1980; 19:257–263.
15. Elster AD, DiPersio DA: Cranial postoperative site: Assessment with contrast-enhanced MR imaging. Radiology 1990; 174:93–98.
16. Burger PC, Vogel FS, Green SB, et al: Glioblastoma multiforme and anaplastic astrocytoma: Pathologic criteria and prognostic implications. Cancer 1985; 56:1106–1111.
17. Davis KR, Ackerman RH, Kistler JP, et al: Computed tomography of cerebral infarction: Hemorrhage, contrast enhancement, and time of appearance. Comput Tomogr 1977; 1:71–86.
18. Steinhoff H, Lanksch W, Kazner E, et al: Computed tomography in the diagnosis and differential diagnosis of glioblastomas: A qualitative study of 295 cases. Neuroradiol 1977; 14:193–200.
19. Atlas SW, Grossman RI, Gomori JM, et al: Hemorrhagic intracranial neoplasms: spin-echo MR imaging. Radiology 1978; 164:71–77.
20. Zimmerman RA, Bilaniuk LT: Computed tomography of acute intratumoral hemorrhage. Radiology 1980; 135:355–359.
21. Goldstein SJ, Young B, Markesberry WR: Congenital malignant gliosarcoma. AJNR 1981; 2:475–476.
22. Geremia GK, Wollman R, Foust R: Computed tomography of gliomatosis cerebri. JCAT 1988; 12:698–701.
23. Rippe DJ, Boyko OB, Fuller GN, et al: Gadopentetate dimeglumine-enhanced MR imaging of gliomatosis cerebri: Appearance mimicking leptomeningeal tumor dissemination. AJNR 1990; 11:800–801.
24. Shin YM, Chang KH, Han MH, et al: Gliomatosis cerebri: Comparison of MR and CT features. AJR 1993; 161:859–862.
25. Barnard RO, Geddes JF: The incidence of multifocal cerebral gliomas:

26. Van Tassel P, Lee YY, Bruner JM: Synchronous and metachronous malignant gliomas: CT findings. AJNR 1988; 9:725–732.
27. Kieffer SA, Salibi NA, Kim RC, et al: Multifocal glioblastoma: Diagnostic implications. Radiology 1982; 143:709–710.
28. Kepes JJ, Rubinstein LJ, Ansbacher L, et al: Histopathological features of recurrent pleomorphic xanthoastrocytomas: further corroboration of the glial nature of this neoplasm. Acta Neuropathol 1989; 78:585–593.
29. Lipper MH, Eberhard DA, Phillips CD, et al: Pleomorphic xanthoastrocytoma, a distinctive astroglial tumor: Neuroradiologic and pathologic features. AJNR 1993; 14:1397–1404.
30. Yoshino MT, Lucio R. Pleomorphic xanthoastrocytoma. AJNR 1992; 13:1330–1332.
31. Brown JH, Chew FS: Pleomorphic xanthoastrocytoma. AJR 1993; 160:1272.
32. Blom RJ: Pleomorphic xanthoastrocytoma: CT appearance. JCAT 1988; 12:351–354.
33. Bilaniuk LT, Zimmerman RA, Littman P, et al: Computed tomography of brain stem gliomas in children. Radiology 1980; 134:89–95.
34. Epstein FJ, Farmer JP: Brain stem glioma growth patterns. J Neurosurg 1993; 78:408–412.
35. Stroink AR, Hoffman HJ, Hendrick EB, et al: Diagnosis and management of pediatric brain-stem gliomas. J Neurosurg 1986; 65:745–750.
36. Vandertop WP, Hoffman JH, Drake JM, et al: Focal midbrain tumors in children. Neurosurgery 1992; 31:186–194.
37. Tice H, Barnes PD, Goumnerova L, et al: Pediatric and adolescent oligodendrogliomas. AJNR 1993; 14:1293–1300.
38. Lee YY, Van Tassel P: Intracranial oligodendrogliomas: Imaging findings in 35 untreated cases. AJR 1989; 152:361–369.
39. Goergen SK, Gonzales MF, McLean CA: Intraventricular neurocytoma: Radiologic features and review of the literature. Radiology 1992; 182:787–792.
40. Barbosa MD, Balsitis M, Jaspan TJ, et al: Intraventricular neurocytoma: A clinical and pathological study of three cases and review of the literature. Neurosurgery 1990; 26:1045–1054.
41. Barkovich AJ, Edwards M: Brain tumors of childhood. *In* Barkovich AJ (ed): Pediatric Neuroimaging. New York, Raven Press, 1990, pp 149–204.
42. Centeno RS, Lee AA, Winter J, et al: Supratentorial ependymomas: Neuroimaging and clinicopathologic correlation. J Neurosurg 1986; 64:209–215.
43. Scheithauer BW: Symptomatic subependymoma: Report of 21 cases with review of the literature. J Neurosurg 1978; 49:689–696.
44. Gjerris F, Klinken L: Long term prognosis in children with benign cerebellar astrocytoma. J Neurosurg 1978; 49:179–184.
45. Strong JA, Hatten HP, Brown MT, et al: Pilocytic astrocytoma: Correlation between the initial imaging features and clinical aggressiveness. AJR 1993; 161:369–372.
46. Lee YY, Tassel PV, Bruner JM, et al: Juvenile pilocytic astrocytomas: CT and MR characteristics. AJR 1989; 152:1263–1270.
47. Naidich TP, Zimmerman RA: Primary brain tumors in children. Semin Roentgenol 1984; 19:100–114.
48. Aoki S, Barkovich AJ, Nishimura K, et al: Neurofibromatosis types 1 and 2: Cranial MR findings. Radiology 1989; 172:527–534.
49. Fletcher WA, Imes RH, Hoyt WF: Chiasmal gliomas: Appearance and long term changes demonstrated by computerized tomography. J Neurosurg 1986; 65:154–159.
50. Demierre B, Stichnoth FA, Hori A, et al: Intracerebral ganglioma. J Neurosurg 1986; 65:177–182.
51. Castillo M, Davis PC, Takei Y, et al: Intracranial ganglioglioma: MR, CT, and clinical findings in 18 patients. AJNR 1990; 11:109–114.
52. Tampieri D, Moumdjian R, Melanson D, et al: Intracerebral gangliogliomas in patients with partial complex seizures: CT and MR imaging findings. AJR 1991; 157:843–849.
53. Tien RD, Tuori SL, Pulkingham N, et al: Ganglioglioma with leptomeningeal and subarachnoid spread: Results of CT, MR and PET imaging. AJR 1992; 159:391–393.
54. Altman NR, Purser PK, Post MJD: Tuberous sclerosis: Characteristics at CT and MR imaging. Radiology 1988; 167:527–532.
55. Brismar J, Roberson GH, Davis KR: Radiation necrosis of the brain: Neuroradiological considerations with computed tomography. Neuroradiol 1976; 12:109–113.
56. Tolly TI, Bruckman JE, Czarnecki DJ, et al: Early CT findings after

A histologic study of large hemispheric sections. Cancer 1987; 60:1519–1531.

interstitial radiation therapy for primary malignant brain tumors. AJNR 1987; 9:1177–1180.

57. Schwartz RB, Carvalho PA, Alexander E, et al: Radiation necrosis vs high grade recurrent glioma: Differentiation by using dual-isotope SPECT with 201Tl and 99mTc-HMPAO. AJNR 1991; 12:1187–1192.

58. Doyle WK, Budinger TF, Valk PE, et al: Differentiation of cerebral radiation necrosis from tumor recurrence by [18-F] FDG and 82-Rb positron emission tomography. JCAT 1987; 11:563–570.

59. Valk PE, Dillon WP: Radiation injury of the brain. AJNR 1991; 12:45–62.

60. Kingsley DP, Kendall BE: CT of the adverse effects of therapeutic radiation of the central nervous system. AJNR 1981; 2:453–460.

61. Anderson FM, Carson MJ: Spinal cord tumors in children: A review of the subject and presentation of 21 cases. J Pediatr 1953; 43:190–207.

62. Raffel C, Edwards MSB: Intraspinal tumors in children. *In* Youmans JR (ed): Neurological Surgery, ed 3. Philadelphia, WB Saunders, 1990, pp 3574–3588.

63. Sze G, Twohig M: Neoplastic disease of the spine and spinal cord. *In* Atlas SW (ed): Magnetic Resonance Imaging of the Brain and Spine. New York, Raven, 1991, pp 921–965.

64. Barone BM, Elvidge AR: Ependymomas: A clinical survey. J Neurosurg 1970; 33:428–438.

65. McCormick PC, Torres R, Post K, et al: Intramedullary ependymoma of the spinal cord. J Neurosurg 1990; 72:523–532.

66. Moellekin SMC, Seeger LL, Eckhardt JS, et al: Myxopapillary ependymoma with extensive sacral destruction: CT and MR findings. JCAT 1992; 16:164–166.

67. Epstein FJ, Farmer JP, Freed D: Adult intramedullary spinal cord ependymomas: The result of surgery in 38 patients. J Neurosurg 1993; 79:204–209.

RICHARD L. GOLD

WILLIAM P. DILLON, JR.

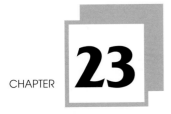

CHAPTER **23**

Magnetic Resonance Imaging

Magnetic resonance imaging (MRI) has become the imaging modality of choice in the evaluation of intracranial and spinal cord tumors. The major advantages of MRI over computed tomography (CT) is its inherent superb tissue contrast and its ability to image directly in multiple planes. MRI has been shown to be more sensitive than CT for both detection and determination of the extent of tumor.[1] In comparing CT and MRI in the evaluation of intracranial neoplasms, Kelly and co-workers[2] found that T2-weighted abnormalities usually extended well beyond the corresponding low-attenuation lesions on CT scan. In addition to increased area of T2 signal abnormalities, Earnest and colleagues[3] found that the region of MRI contrast enhancement was equal to or greater than the region of iodinated contrast present on CT scan. In addition, MRI is less sensitive to bone artifacts than CT, and as a result, it depicts anatomy in the posterior fossa and skull base more clearly.

In CT scanning, the brightness of the image is determined by the ability of the tissue to stop (attenuate) the x-ray beam. Atoms with higher atomic number, having greater electronic density, are able to cause greater attenuation of the x-ray beam than are atoms with lower atomic numbers. However, the differences in attenuation between types of tissue is on the order of only a few percent, which limits contrast resolution in CT scanning. Understanding the nature of the signal from MRI is far less intuitive and requires a basic review of nuclear magnetism.

The nuclei of all atoms contain a varying number of protons and neutrons. Nuclei that have an odd number of neutrons or protons have a net nuclear charge and spin on their axis. Spinning charged particles ("spins") generate a small magnetic field similar to that of a small bar magnet. The hydrogen nucleus, which contains one proton, is well suited for MRI because of its great abundance and its inherently large magnetic field. Although individual hydrogen nuclei possess a magnetic field, these are canceled due to the random orientation of hydrogen nuclei within human tissue. However, when placed in an external magnetic field, such as an MRI scanner, the individual hydrogen nuclei align parallel (in a longitudinal direction) to the magnetic field, creating a net magnetic field within tissue. A 1.5 Tesla MRI scanner has a magnetic field 30,000 times stronger than that of its natural surroundings. Special coils built into the

MRI scanner, which surround anatomic parts during imaging, are used to generate specific radiofrequency (Rf) wave pulses, the energy from which temporarily tips the nuclei away from the longitudinal direction. Immediately after the Rf pulse is turned off, the nuclei slowly realign from the transverse direction to the longitudinal direction, giving off energy that is detected by coils surrounding the body part being imaged (surface or head coils). This sequence of events—Rf pulse on, off, sampling of signal—is repeated hundreds of times to create the images we know as MRI. The time between successful Rf pulses is termed *TR*. The time from Rf to sampling the signal is *TE*. By adjusting the TR and TE, T1- or T2-weighted images are formed. The time required for a spinning nucleus to regain 63% of its original longitudinal direction is referred to as the T1 relaxation time. Due to a different chemical milieu, the T1 relaxation time of a hydrogen nucleus differs between tissues. The T1 relaxation time of a hydrogen nucleus in water is much longer than that of a hydrogen nucleus in fat. This considerable difference in relaxation times is one of the major reasons for the superb tissue contrast of MRI. In addition to losing signal as a proton regains longitudinal magnetization, signal is also lost when adjacent protons interfere with each other's spins. This loss of energy due to spin-spin interaction, is called *T2 relaxation*. T1 and T2 relaxation occur simultaneously and are independent of one another. A tissue may have a short T1 relaxation time and a long T2 relaxation time. Different MR pulse sequences have been designed to emphasize or "weight" the T1 or T2 relaxation times. Contrast between tissues and/or pathology can be achieved by using T1- or T2-weighted sequences that maximize differences in these relaxation times. A long TR and long TE interval result in T2-weighted scans, whereas short T1 and TE intervals emphasize T1 differences.

In summary, a tissue placed in the MRI magnet quickly gains a net magnetic field that is parallel to that of the main magnetic field (longitudinal magnetization). Repetitive short Rf pulses, specific to the nucleus and the strength of the magnet, tip the nuclei to the transverse plane, where signal can be detected. Depending on the inherent T1 and T2 relaxation properties of the tissues, different signal intensities, and, therefore, tremendous contrast differences, will be seen.

Hydrogen nuclei (protons) roaming free within water have low signal intensity on T1-weighted sequences and high signal intensity on T2-weighted sequences. Pathologic processes such as tumor, infection, and infarction all produce an increase in extracellular water. On T1-weighted images, these pathologic regions show decreased signal compared to that of normal brain tissue. Tissue contrast is usually most apparent on T2-weighted images, in which the high signal from edema generated by pathologic processes stands out against the intermediate signal intensity of normal brain parenchyma.

Intracranial neoplasms are usually hypointense on T1-weighted images and hyperintense on T2-weighted images, but they are frequently quite heterogeneous, with regions of high signal on T1 and low signal on T2. Heterogeneity in signal may result from calcification, hemorrhage, necrosis, proteinaceous debris, fibrous stroma, and signal voids from rapidly flowing blood. Table 23–1 lists the most common sources for different signal intensities on T1 and T2.

The introduction of MRI contrast agents in 1988 had a tremendous impact on CNS tumor evaluation. The most commonly used MRI contrast agent is gadopentetate dimeglumine, also known as gadolinium DTPA (Gd-DTPA) (Magnevist, Berlex Laboratories, Wayne, NJ). Gadolinium is a rare earth metal with seven unpaired electrons. These unpaired electrons enable nearby hydrogen protons to realign (relax) more quickly with the main magnetic field and, thus, shorten T1 relaxation time. On T1-weighted images, molecules that realign rapidly with a magnetic field have higher signal intensity than those that realign slowly. Thus, gadolinium, which leaks through the blood-brain barrier, will increase the signal intensity on T1-weighted images. Although gadolinium affects both T1 and T2 relaxation times, the effect on T1 is much greater at the concentration used clinically. Thus, only T1-weighted sequences are obtained routinely after the administration of contrast.

In a normal brain with an intact blood-brain barrier, capillaries are impermeable to gadolinium complexes because of tight endothelial junctions. Regions of the brain normally lacking a blood-brain barrier, such as the pituitary gland, pineal gland, choroid plexus, and dura, normally enhance and should not be mistaken for pathologic lesions.

Neoplasm-induced angiogenesis, especially in more malignant gliomas, results in capillaries with discontinuous basement membranes that lack a blood-brain barrier. These abnormal capillaries permit diffusion of contrast agents such as Gd-DTPA into the extravascular space, which demonstrates enhancement on MRI. The enhancing region within a tumor generally corresponds to the areas of greatest disruption of the blood-brain barrier, reflecting the most solid component of the tumor. The enhancing region provides the greatest diagnostic yield on biopsy.

MRI TECHNIQUE

Multiple MRI sequences have been developed that highlight various soft tissue contrast parameters, such as T1, T2, flow, and magnetization transfer. Unfortunately, a clinician is often faced with a confusing array of acronyms. A basic understanding of the different techniques presently available can be valuable in tailoring an MRI examination.

Spin-Echo Sequence

Spin-echo sequence is by far the most common technique used in intracranial imaging and has become the "gold standard" for evaluating brain and spinal abnormalities. This pulse sequence consists of a 90-degree initial Rf pulse followed by a 180-degree refocusing Rf pulse. This second 180-degree pulse serves to decrease inhomogeneity produced by the imperfect magnetic field. Spin-echo technique offers excellent contrast and spatial resolution, and can be "weighted" to highlight T1 relaxation differences (short TR/TE) or T2 relaxation differences (long TR/TE), although it is somewhat insensitive to areas of calcification and hemorrhage.

Gradient-Echo Technique

The generic term *gradient-echo technique* refers to multiple pulse sequences that differ from spin-echo in two fundamental ways: (1) the initial Rf pulse is usually less than 90 degrees; (2) the 180-degree refocusing Rf pulse is replaced by gradient pulses in order to refocus the signal. Gradient pulses do not completely cancel magnetic field inhomogeneities, caused by hemorrhage, air, calcium, or magnetic field imperfections; therefore, gradient-echo techniques are much more sensitive to foci of calcification and hemorrhage than are spin-echo techniques (Fig. 23–1).

Fast Spin Echo

Fast spin echo is a relatively new scanning technique that employs multiple 180-degree refocusing Rf pulses following an initial 90-degree Rf pulse, producing spin-echo–type contrast in a much shorter time than routine spin echo. One of the main applications of fast spin echo in evaluation of CNS neoplasms is that the faster pulse sequence allows high-resolution imaging in a reasonable scan time. This has been most beneficial in evaluation of temporal lobes and smaller

TABLE 23–1

COMMON CAUSES OF MRI SIGNAL INTENSITY ON T1 AND T2 IMAGES

Decreased Signal	Increased Signal
T1	T1
Edema	Fat
Cyst	Subacute hemorrhage
Calcification	Melanin
Hemosiderin	High protein content
Rapidly flowing blood	Gadolinium enhancement
Tumor	
T2	T2
Calcification	Edema
Acute/early subacute hemorrhage	Cyst
Dense cellularity (lymphoma)	Late/subacute hemorrhage
Rapidly flowing blood	Tumors
High protein content	

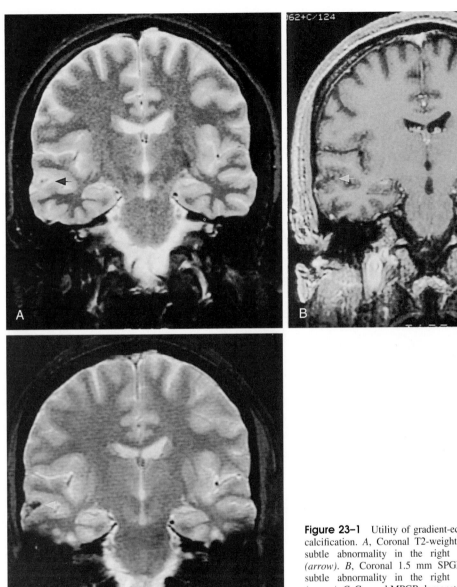

Figure 23–1   Utility of gradient-echo technique in detecting calcification. *A,* Coronal T2-weighted image demonstrates a subtle abnormality in the right superior temporal gyrus *(arrow). B,* Coronal 1.5 mm SPGR sequence confirms the subtle abnormality in the right superior temporal gyrus *(arrow). C,* Coronal MPGR demonstrates increase in the extent of the hypointense signal in the lesion *(arrow).* At surgery, calcification was found in a small oligodendroglioma.

structures, such as the eighth cranial nerve. The major drawback to fast spin echo is that it is less sensitive than spin echo and far less sensitive than gradient echo in detection of hemorrhage or calcification. However, this technique is as accurate as spin echo for detecting edema and is therefore a reasonable pulse sequence for evaluating brain tumors.

Three-Dimensional (Volume) Gradient-Echo Techniques

Three-dimensional gradient-echo sequences image a volume of tissue, which can then be processed as individual thin, contiguous, high-resolution sections (partitions). In addition to providing high resolution similar to that of fast spin echo, three-dimensional (3-D) imaging results in images that can be retrospectively reformatted into any plane. 3-D volume imaging has also been essential in the development of frameless stereotactic surgery. With this technique, 3-D MRI images serve as references for surgical biopsy. One technique utilizes a handheld articulated probe or ''wand'' whose position is continually referenced to a previously acquired MR derived 3-D model of the patient's brain. Thus, the surgeon is able to accurately assess, intraoperatively, the progress of the resection relative to the preoperative MRI study. This technology has found most utility in skull-based lesions and cortical lesions adjacent to eloquent cortex. Newer techniques may utilize intraoperative real-time MR acquisitions for operative manipulations.

LIMITATIONS OF MRI

Despite the improvement of MRI techniques, its limitations and drawbacks must be understood as well.

1. Decreased Sensitivity for Detection of Calcification
Although the gradient-echo sequence is the best MRI technique for detecting calcification, CT remains the most sensitive modality for imaging calcification. Figure 23–2 shows a large oligodendroglioma with extensive regions of calcification best seen on CT.

2. Lack of Specificity
Due to its exquisite sensitivity for detection of increased interstitial water, multiple pathologic processes can demonstrate low signal intensity on T1-weighted images and high signal intensity on T2-weighted images. Three common processes that can simulate intracranial neoplasms are infarctions, abscesses, and demyelination.

Infarction Infarctions, especially in the subacute phase, can occasionally simulate a neoplasm on MR or CT. Fortunately, these lesions are often easy to distinguish based on

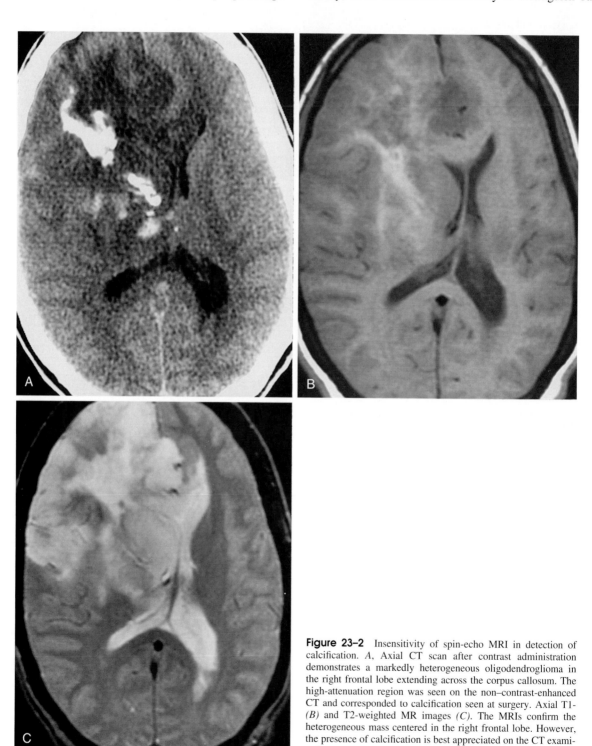

Figure 23–2 Insensitivity of spin-echo MRI in detection of calcification. *A,* Axial CT scan after contrast administration demonstrates a markedly heterogeneous oligodendroglioma in the right frontal lobe extending across the corpus callosum. The high-attenuation region was seen on the non–contrast-enhanced CT and corresponded to calcification seen at surgery. Axial T1-*(B)* and T2-weighted MR images *(C).* The MRIs confirm the heterogeneous mass centered in the right frontal lobe. However, the presence of calcification is best appreciated on the CT examination.

history and clinical findings. Imaging features that favor an infarction include its location within a vascular territory, gyral petechial hemorrhage, and well-defined borders. If this distinction cannot be made, a follow-up study in 2 to 3 weeks can be extremely helpful. Infarction usually changes over this period of time, decreasing in enhancement and mass effect as the infarction evolves from subacute to chronic stages. In general, most tumors remain unchanged or enlarge over the 2- to 3-week period (Fig. 23–3).

Abscesses Cerebral abscesses classically have a thin rim of enhancement compared with the thick rind of enhancement seen in gliomas. However, enough imaging overlap occurs between the two processes that the clinical history is usually vital in making the distinction.

Demyelination Demyelinating disease may occasionally present in a tumefactive fashion, with a large lesion showing enhancement and white matter edema. Additional signal intensity abnormalities in the periventricular white matter and corpus callosum would support a diagnosis of multiple sclerosis. An incomplete ring of enhancement around a demyelinating plaque has also been described (Fig. 23–4).

Radiation Necrosis Necrosis may simulate malignant tumors on MRI or CT. Proton (H^1)-spectroscopy and positron emission tomographic (PET) scanning have shown promise in distinguishing necrosis from tumor.[4]

3. Enhancement Does Not Equate With Histologic Grade
Although it is true that higher-grade gliomas generally enhance more than lower-grade gliomas, benign tumors, such as juvenile pilocytic astrocytoma, can show marked enhancement, which reflects their prominent vascularity. At the other extreme, high-grade malignant tumors may occasionally demonstrate minimal, or no, enhancement. In a study of 20 patients with MRI findings suggestive of a low-grade nonenhancing glioma, Kondziolka and others[5] found that only 50% were proved to be low-grade astrocytoma, whereas 9 of the 20 patients had higher-grade anaplastic astrocytoma, and one patient was diagnosed with encephalitis. The authors concluded that due to the unreliability of predicting histologic grade of tumors, all patients with supratentorial masses should undergo stereotactic biopsies for confirmation. Figure 23–5 illustrates the difficulty of predicting histologic grade on the basis of enhancement.

4. Enhancement Does Not Delineate the Borders of Tumor Cells
Although enhancement on MRI has been shown to be equal to or greater in extent than enhancement seen on CT, stereotactic biopsies have demonstrated viable tumor cells beyond the borders of the abnormal contrast enhancement and T2 abnormalities.[3] The occurrence of viable tumor cells in adjacent tissue that appears normal on MRI corresponds with the infiltrative nature of gliomas at pathologic examination. In a study by Tovi and associates,[6] 14 patients with cerebral gliomas underwent contrast MRI, contrast CT, and PET scanning using C-L-methionine. Areas of tumor with blood-brain barrier disruption seen on MRI and CT were compared with areas with increased accumulation of methionine on PET scan. The authors concluded that

PET scanning correlated best with viable tumor and that contrast MRI can dramatically underestimate the extent of tumor.

GLIOMAS OF THE BRAIN

Astrocytic Tumors

Astrocytic tumors represent the majority of primary brain tumors and are the most common intracranial neoplasm. Multiple histopathologic classification systems of astrocytomas have been developed, including those of Kernohan, the World Health Organization (WHO), Russell and Rubenstein, and Daumas-Duport. The heterogeneous mixture of different cell types within a tumor accounts for the multiplicity of classification systems. Tumor classification is based on the predominant cell type and graded on the basis of pathologic features of malignancy, including cellular pleomorphism, mitosis, vascular endothelial proliferation, and necrosis. Our discussion uses the WHO classification scheme published in the second edition of *Histological Typing of Tumours of the Central Nervous System*[10] (Table 23–2).

ASTROCYTOMA

Astrocytoma is a term applied to diffusely infiltrating tumors composed of well-differentiated neoplastic astrocytes. They account for approximately 25% of hemispheric gliomas in adults and 20% to 30% of pediatric cerebellar tumors. They typically occur in early adult life, with a peak incidence in the fourth and fifth decades. In adults, these tumors tend to involve the regions of the brain with the greatest amount of white matter, with the frontal lobe being the most common location.

Microscopically, astrocytomas are ill defined and show a tendency to diffusely infiltrate the surrounding brain. The diffuse infiltration often results in enlargement and distortion of the invaded structures. Mild pleomorphism and hypercellularity may be present, although necrosis and endothelial proliferation are not seen. Calcification may be present in approximately half of cases. Histologically, astrocytomas can be subdivided into fibrillary (most common), protoplasmic, and gemistocytic.

TABLE 23–2
ASTROCYTIC TUMORS (WHO CLASSIFICATION)

Astrocytoma
Variants
Fibrillary
Protoplasmic
Gemistocytic
Anaplastic (malignant) astrocytoma
Glioblastoma
Variants
Giant cell glioblastoma
Gliosarcoma
Pilocytic astrocytoma
Pleomorphic xanthoastrocytoma
Subependymal giant cell astrocytoma

Data from Kleihues P, Burger PC, Scheithauer BW: Histological Typing of Tumours of the Central Nervous System, ed 2. Berlin, Springer-Verlag, 1993.

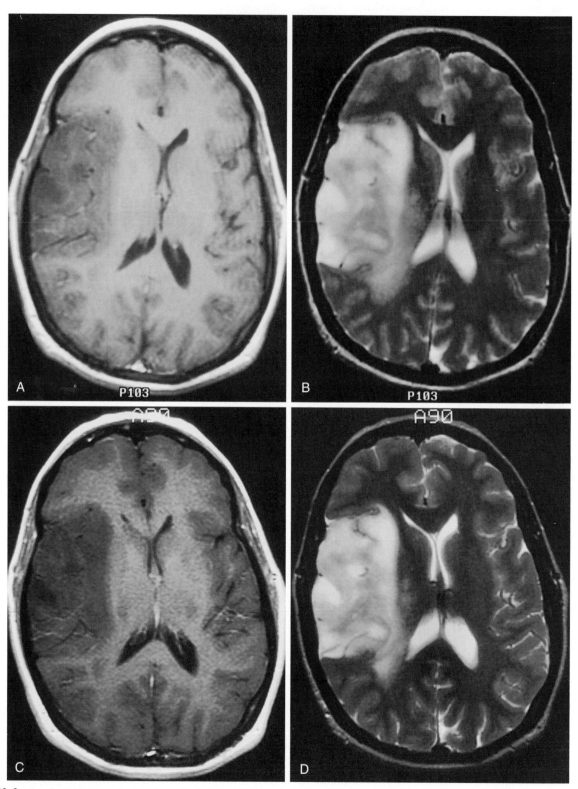

Figure 23–3   Anaplastic (malignant) astrocytoma simulating a middle cerebral artery infarction. Axial T1-weighted postcontrast *(A)* and axial T2-weighted *(B)* images demonstrate a non-enhancing mass infiltrating the right insular cortex that may be mistaken for a right middle cerebral artery infarction. However, follow-up images 2 months later *(C and D)* do not show the expected evolution of an infarction. Biopsy revealed anaplastic (malignant) astrocytoma.

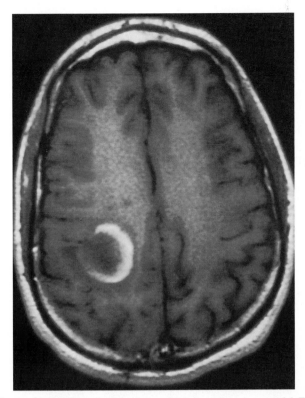

Figure 23–4 Demyelinating plaque simulating a neoplasm. Axial T1-weighted postcontrast image shows an enhancing lesion in the right parietal lobe. No other lesions were detected. This was a focal area of demyelination on biopsy. The incomplete ring of enhancement has been described in demyelinating plaques.

On MRI, astrocytomas are usually well-defined, homogeneous masses that are hypointense on T1 and hyperintense on T2 sequences. Mass effect and associated edema are often minimal. They are often superficial in location, and thickening of the overlying gray matter may be present. Fibrillary astrocytomas usually involve the white matter, whereas protoplasmic astrocytomas are more likely to involve the cortex.[7] Calcification may be present and can be missed on a standard spin-echo MR, but it may be seen on a gradient-echo sequence. Enhancement is variable, although the majority of tumors demonstrate minimal, if any, enhancement.[8] At the present time, the MRI appearance is not specific for the diagnosis of astrocytoma, as appearance of higher-grade glial tumors can be radiographically identical to that of astrocytoma (see Fig. 23–5).

ANAPLASTIC (MALIGNANT) ASTROCYTOMA

Anaplastic (malignant) astrocytomas occur later in life than astrocytomas, although they share a similar regional distribution. Pathologically, compared with an astrocytoma, they can have increased hypercellularity, pleomorphism, and mitosis. However, unlike glioblastoma multiforme, necrosis and endothelial proliferation are not typical features.

Anaplastic (malignant) astrocytomas tend to be more heterogeneous on MRI than astrocytomas. Characteristically, these tumors demonstrate less well-defined borders and a greater degree of mass effect, vasogenic edema, and en-

hancement.[9] Cyst and calcification can also be seen. Hemorrhage may be present, but it is more common in the higher-grade glioblastoma multiforme. On noncontrast T1- and T2-weighted images, heterogeneous signal intensity is usually present. Although enhancement is generally greater than that seen in lower-grade gliomas, it must be stressed that these are general principles; we have seen many cases of well-defined, non-enhancing lesions that, on biopsy, have been identified as anaplastic (malignant) astrocytomas.

GLIOBLASTOMA MULTIFORME

Glioblastoma multiforme is the most common astrocytic tumor, representing 50% of astrocytic tumors and 15% to 20% of all intracranial tumors. The peak incidence occurs at age 45 to 60 years. It is typically located in the cerebral hemispheres. Although most are frontotemporal in location, they can occasionally be seen in the cerebellum, brainstem, and spinal cord.[10] The tumor frequently infiltrates into adjacent lobes and deep structures, such as the corpus callosum. A characteristic feature of a glioblastoma is spread across the corpus callosum to involve the contralateral cerebral hemisphere. When enhancing, this may result in a ''butterfly'' appearance (Fig. 23–6).

Pathologically, the diagnosis of glioblastoma multiforme requires a heterogeneous tumor with areas of necrosis and/or prominent vascular proliferation. MRI reflects this complex histology, often demonstrating a heterogeneous signal intensity on both T1- and T2-weighted images. The heterogeneous signal reflects a combination of cysts, hemorrhage, and necrosis. Linear, serpiginous punctate regions of low signal on T1 and T2 may represent flow voids from tumor vascularity. The tumors are usually poorly defined, with extensive mass effect and vasogenic edema. Hemorrhage is common in glioblastoma multiforme, and some observers feel that hemosiderin deposition is helpful in distinguishing a glioblastoma from an anaplastic (malignant) astrocytoma.[9] Hemosiderin is best appreciated on gradient-echo images, where it appears markedly hypointense.

Enhancement is usually greater in glioblastoma than in other astrocytic tumors, and almost all glioblastomas enhance to some degree. These tumors usually demonstrate heterogeneous enhancement, although an irregular thick rim or nodular enhancement can also be seen.[8]

Glioblastoma multiforme is almost always associated with a large region of high signal seen on T2-weighted images. This consists of both vasogenic edema and microscopic tumor infiltration of the white matter tracts. MRI is insensitive to the exact margin of tumor as vasogenic edema, and tumor infiltration of the white matter tracts have similar signal intensities on MRI. Infiltration of central gray matter is less common. In most cases, the extent of microscopic invasion is limited to a 2- to 3-cm margin surrounding the enhancing tumor.

Glioblastoma is the most common of the glial tumors to spread to the ependyma and leptomeninges. Contrast-enhanced MRI has been shown to be far more sensitive than contrast CT in detecting leptomeningeal spread.[11] An early indication of leptomeningeal spread is enhancement of the pial surfaces of the cranial nerves and brainstem (Fig. 23–7).

Gliosarcoma is a rare variant of glioblastoma. It is presumed to originate from malignant transformation of the

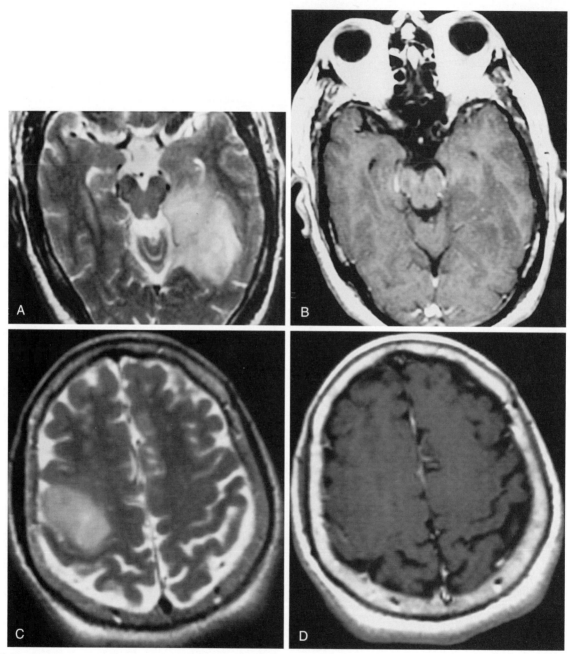

Figure 23–5 Difficulty of determining histologic grade on the basis of enhancement. Axial T2-weighted *(A)* and postcontrast T1-weighted *(B)* images show a region of T2 signal abnormality in the left medial temporal lobe without obvious enhancement. Axial T2-weighted *(C)* and postcontrast T1-weighted *(D)* images show a well-defined region of signal intensity abnormalities in the posterior right frontal lobe.

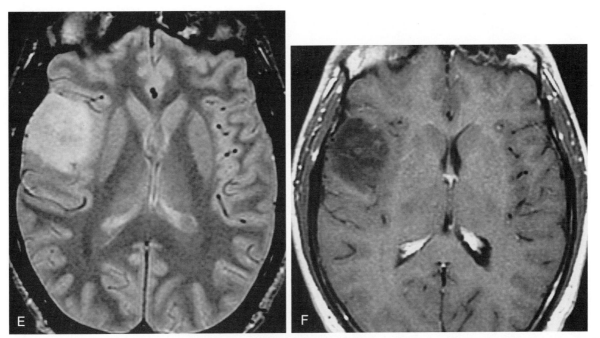

Figure 23–5 *Continued (E and F)* Axial T2-weighted *(E)* and postcontrast axial T1-weighted *(F)* images show a well-defined lesion in the right insular cortex without obvious enhancement. These three lesions are well-defined radiographically without obvious enhancement. However, the three lesions were found to be astrocytoma (A), anaplastic (malignant) astrocytoma (B), and glioblastoma multiforme (C).

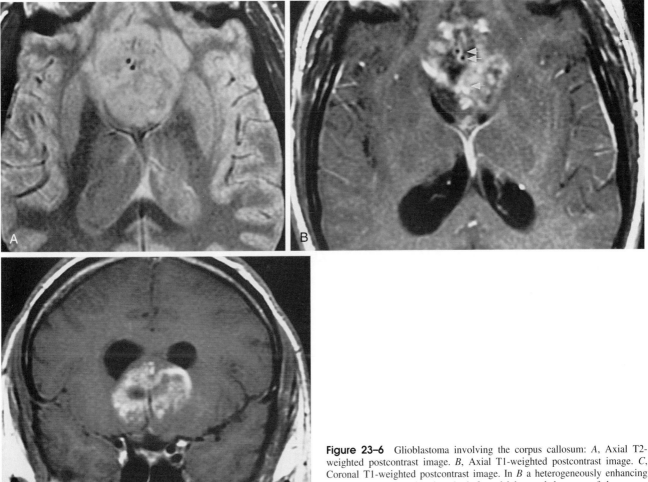

Figure 23–6 Glioblastoma involving the corpus callosum: *A*, Axial T2-weighted postcontrast image. *B*, Axial T1-weighted postcontrast image. *C*, Coronal T1-weighted postcontrast image. In *B* a heterogeneously enhancing mass is present that involves both frontal lobes and the genu of the corpus callosum *(arrow)*. The A₂ segments of both anterior cerebral arteries are encased by the tumor *(double arrows)*.

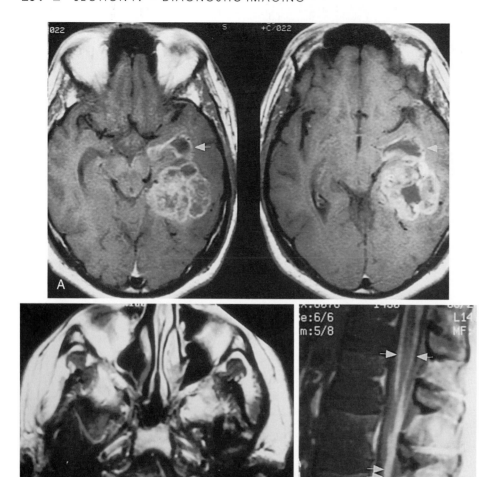

Figure 23–7 Ependymal and subarachnoid spread of glioblastoma. *A,* Axial T1-weighted postcontrast image reveals a large heterogeneously enhancing mass in the medial left temporal lobe. Enhancement is seen in the ependyma of the left temporal horn *(arrows)*. *B,* Axial T1-weighted postcontrast image demonstrates abnormal enhancement surrounding the medulla *(arrow)*. *C,* Sagittal T1-weighted postcontrast image of the lumbar sacral spine reveals marked enhancement coating the conus *(arrow)*, and cauda equina *(double arrows)*.

hypertrophic vascular elements seen in a glioblastoma.[12] About 79 cases have been described in the literature as of 1987.[12] They are most commonly found in the temporal lobes and may demonstrate dural enhancement mimicking a meningioma.

BRAINSTEM GLIOMAS

Brainstem gliomas account for approximately 10% of pediatric CNS neoplasms and 25% of posterior fossa neoplasms in children. The peak incidence is between ages 3 and 10 years, and there is no sex predilection. Presenting symptoms usually result from involvement of cranial nerves (especially the sixth and seventh), corticospinal tracts, and cerebellum.[13] One third of patients have hydrocephalus at the time of diagnosis.

MRI has greatly facilitated the diagnosis of brainstem gliomas. Sagittal images often demonstrate pontine enlargement with an undulating contour of the ventral surface of the pons and mass effect on the fourth ventricle. T2-weighted sagittal images facilitate radiotherapy treatment planning. It is important that patients being evaluated for brainstem tumors be imaged in both the axial and sagittal planes.

The pons is the most common site of origin of brainstem gliomas, accounting for 80% to 90% of cases. The MR appearance of a pontine glioma is typically that of an intra-axial expansile mass that is hypointense on T1 and hyperintense on T2 images. Contrast enhancement is usually irregular and has been reported in up to 50% of cases. Exophytic growth is a common feature of pontine gliomas. In a review of 87 brainstem gliomas, Barkovich and co-workers[13] found that 82% of pontine gliomas were exophytic, with most growing ventrally into the prepontine cistern surrounding the basilar artery and, less commonly, into the cerebellar pontine angle. Longitudinal extension into the midbrain and medulla and axial extension into the middle cerebellar peduncle and cerebellum were common. None of the diffuse pontine gliomas were confined to the pons in their review (Fig. 23–8).[13] Hemorrhage or cysts have been reported in up to 25% of pontine gliomas, although a more recent review showed that these occurred in fewer than 5% of patients.[13]

Diffuse pontine gliomas have a poor prognosis because although they are predominantly low-grade histologically, they frequently contain foci of anaplastic cells. At autopsy, 70% to 80% of pontine gliomas have malignant areas.[13]

It is important to note that not all masses in the pons represent tumor. The differential diagnosis of pontine signal intensity abnormalities includes encephalitis, infection, infarction, and demyelination. However, the identification of diffuse and exophytic growth essentially confirms a neoplastic etiology, which may obviate the need for biopsy.

MRI has facilitated the identification of two subtypes of brainstem gliomas that usually have a much better prognosis than pontine gliomas. The first, accounting for 10% of cases, consists of tumors that originate in the cervicomedullary junction and extend exophytically from the dorsal brainstem. The dorsal exophytic component is frequently a large superodorsal cyst behind the medulla invaginating into the fourth ventricle.[14]

A second subtype primarily involves the tectum. Patients usually present with hydrocephalus due to the compression of the aqueduct. On MRI, these tumors are usually nonenhancing, well-circumscribed masses and are best identified by morphologic changes and increased T2 signal (Fig. 23–9). Treatment is often limited to CSF shunting and to long-term observation.

PILOCYTIC ASTROCYTOMA

Cerebellar astrocytomas are the most common type of posterior fossa tumors in children. Approximately, 75% to 85% of cerebellar astrocytomas are pilocytic astrocytomas, with a peak incidence in the first decade. The remaining 15% to 25% of cerebellar astrocytomas are the diffuse, infiltrating fibrillary type, which most commonly occur in adolescents and young adults.

Pilocytic astrocytomas are typically located in the midline, (e.g., optic nerves, third ventricle, thalamus, median temporal lobes, brainstem), and in the cerebellum. The cerebral hemispheres are affected less frequently.[10] These tumors are distinguished from other astrocytomas by their distinctive pathologic appearance. Grossly, pilocytic astrocytomas are often cystic, with solid tumor confined to a mural nodule in the wall of the cyst. Vascular endothelial proliferation is prominent, which accounts for the intense enhancement of the tumor. However, unlike other astrocytomas, the intense contrast enhancement does not indicate an unfavorable prognosis.

Most cerebellar pilocytic astrocytomas occur in the midline, with approximately 15% limited to the cerebellar hemispheres. They are usually well demarcated and smoothly marginated and are often round or oval in configuration.[15] These tumors can be cystic, solid, or solid with areas of necrosis and/or cysts. Approximately 50% are cystic with a solid, enhancing tumor nodule in the wall of the cyst. The remainder of the cyst wall is composed of nonenhancing, non-neoplastic, compressed cerebellar tissue (Fig. 23–10). The cyst is hypointense on T1-weighted images and hyperintense on T2-weighted images. The cyst fluid may have higher signal on T1 relative to CSF due to increased protein content.

Approximately 40% of pilocytic astrocytomas are predominantly solid with a cystic center. The cyst walls in these tumors are composed of tumor cells that usually enhance. A well-defined mural nodule is not usually present. Fewer than 10% of pilocytic astrocytomas are completely solid tumors. These are usually round to oval, lobulated, well-defined

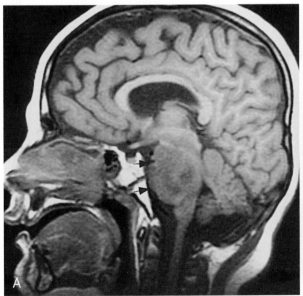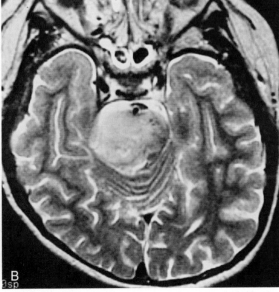

Figure 23–8　Brainstem glioma. *A,* Sagittal T1-weighted image shows expansion and contour abnormality of the pons. The normal, smooth convex ventral border of the normal pons is lost *(arrows)*. *B,* Axial T2-weighted image shows a heterogeneous region of increased T2 signal intensity in the right ventral aspect of the pons.

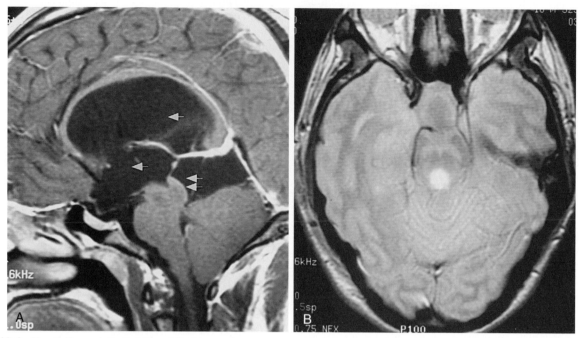

Figure 23–9   Tectal glioma. *A,* Sagittal T1-weighted image demonstrates marked hydrocephalus *(arrows)* with enlargement and deformity of the tectum *(double arrows). B,* Axial proton density images reveal marked hyperintensity in the region of the tectal plate. This lesion was not biopsied and treatment was limited to CSF shunting.

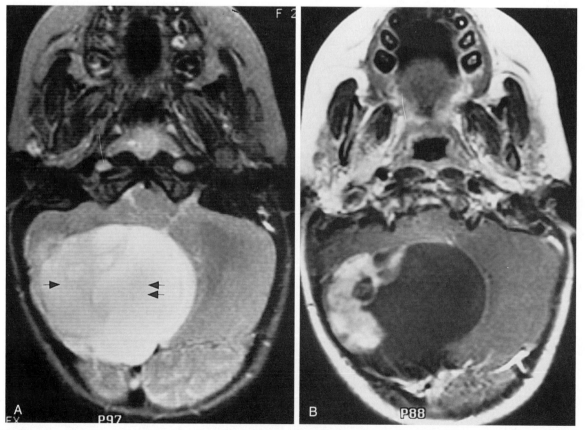

Figure 23–10   Pilocytic astrocytoma. *A,* Axial T2-weighted image shows a large mass centered in the right cerebellar hemisphere. The solid component of the tumor *(arrow)* is slightly lower in signal intensity than the adjacent cyst *(double arrows). B,* Postcontrast axial T1-weighted image shows marked enhancement of the solid portion of the tumor.

masses that show heterogeneous or homogeneous enhancement.

Supratentorial pilocytic astrocyomas also tend to show marked contrast enhancement. Cystic components and calcifications are seen less commonly than with infratentorial pilocytic astrocytoma (Fig. 23–11).[14]

PLEOMORPHIC XANTHOASTROCYTOMA

Pleomorphic xanthoastrocytoma is a rare, usually benign, tumor primarily located in the supratentorial cortex of the temporal lobes. The most common presenting symptoms are seizures and headaches. Males and females are equally affected. Although it can occur at any age, it usually presents in childhood and adolescence. On gross examination, the tumor is often composed of a cystic mass with a mural nodule adjacent to a dural surface. At surgery, leptomeningeal involvement is commonly seen and may account for occasional tumor recurrences.

MRI typically demonstrates a cortically based mass located primarily in the temporal lobes. The tumor mass shows nonspecific low signal intensity on T1 and high signal on T2. There is usually a marked enhancement of a tumor nodule. Cysts are frequently seen and may constitute the bulk of the tumor mass. Clinical utility of an MRI scan includes visualization of the cystic component of the mass in orthogonal planes. This is useful information from a surgical perspective, because it allows decompression of the cyst before excision of the solid portion of the lesion is undertaken.[16]

Leptomeningeal and gyral enhancement have been reported in up to a third of patients in one series. Mass effect

and edema are usually minimal, and extensive peritumoral edema may indicate more aggressive lesions.[17] Calcification is rarely seen.

SUBEPENDYMAL GIANT CELL ASTROCYTOMA

Subependymal giant cell astrocytoma is almost exclusively seen in the setting of tuberous sclerosis. Tuberous sclerosis is a phakomatosis with cutaneous, intracranial, cardiac, and renal manifestations. The four major intracranial abnormalities are cortical tubers, subependymal nodules, white matter lesions, and subependymal giant cell astrocytomas. These lesions all share very similar histopathologic features, with giant cells surrounded by areas of gliosis and demyelination.[18] Cortical tubers, subependymal nodules, and white matter lesions are present in more than 90% of patients, whereas subependymal giant cell astrocytomas occur in only 10% of patients with tuberous sclerosis. The peak age is between 8 and 18 years, with no gender predilection. These benign tumors are slow growing and noninvasive, and they rarely recur after excision.[18]

Subependymal giant cell astrocytoma occurs in a subependymal location, almost always at the foramen of Monro, and projects into the ventricle. Obstructive hydrocephalus is common. On MRI, these masses are predominantly hypointense to white matter on T1 and heterogeneously hyperintense on T2. Heterogeneous signal on T2 most likely reflects calcification and hemorrhage. Braffman and associates[18] found that 3 of their 9 patients with subependymal giant cell astrocytomas showed linear, serpentine flow voids, most likely representing tumor vessels. Marked contrast enhancement is the rule, although peritumoral edema is uncommon.

The most common explanation for the pathogenesis of subependymal giant cell astrocytomas is that they arise from subependymal nodules.[18] Radiologically, the distinction between the two entities may be difficult. However, subependymal nodules tend to be small; most range in size between 1 and 10 mm, whereas subependymal giant cell astrocytomas are usually larger than 2 cm. Enhancement can be seen in both lesions, although it tends to be greater in subependymal giant cell astrocytomas. Finally, linear signal voids, interval growth, and obstructive hydrocephalus all favor a diagnosis of subependymal giant cell astrocytoma.[18] The diagnosis should be suspected when interval growth and enhancement of a subependymal "tuber" is identified on sequential MR or CT examinations.

Oligodendrogliomas

Oligodendrogliomas are uncommon brain tumors, representing approximately 4% to 7% of intracranial gliomas.[19] They are relatively slow-growing tumors and characteristically produce a chronic history of seizures or headaches. Males are affected slightly more than females, and the peak incidence occurs between the fourth and sixth decades. These tumors tend to occur in the peripheral aspects of the frontal and parietal lobes.[19] Intraventricular and cerebellar sites and locations on the spinal cord are rare.[8]

Macroscopically, oligodendrogliomas are solid, infiltrative lesions with well-defined borders. They frequently contain

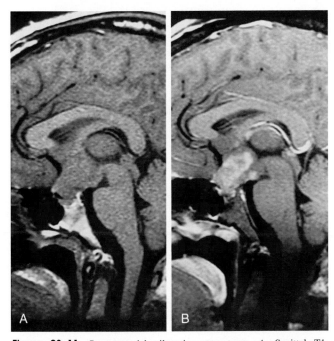

Figure 23–11 Supratentorial pilocytic astrocytoma. *A*, Sagittal T1-weighted image, precontrast. *B*, Sagittal T1-weighted postcontrast image reveals a solidly enhancing mass in the suprasellar and third ventricular region. Unlike infratentorial pilocytic astrocytomas, a large macrocystic component is not as common in supratentorial pilocytic astrocytomas.

other glial tumor cells, usually astrocytes, and are "mixed" in up to half of cases. These tumors are generally round or oval and are rarely multilobulated.[20] Calcification has been reported in up to 30% to 70% of oligodendrogliomas (see Figs. 23–1 and 23–2). Cystic degeneration and hemorrhage occur in up to 20% of lesions. There is no correlation between calcification, hemorrhage, or cyst formation and tumor purity or grading.[20]

On MRI, oligodendrogliomas are predominantly isointense with gray matter on T1-weighted images and hyperintense on T2. Heterogeneous signal is typical and reflects a combination of calcification, hemorrhage, and cystic change. Gradient-echo imaging is far more sensitive to calcification and hemorrhage than are spin-echo sequences (see Fig. 23–1). Approximately half of oligodendrogliomas demonstrate faint, patchy enhancement, whereas the remainder show no evidence of enhancement. Peritumoral edema is usually mild or absent.[8] In 6 of 35 patients in one series, overlying calvarial erosion was associated with the peripherally located oligodendrogliomas.[20]

The MR appearance of oligodendrogliomas is not pathognomonic. However, the presence of tumor calcification, peripheral location, minimal amount of peritumoral edema, and calvarial erosion may suggest the proper diagnosis.[20]

Ependymoma

Ependymomas represent 2% to 6% of all gliomas. They arise from ependymal cells, which are usually related to

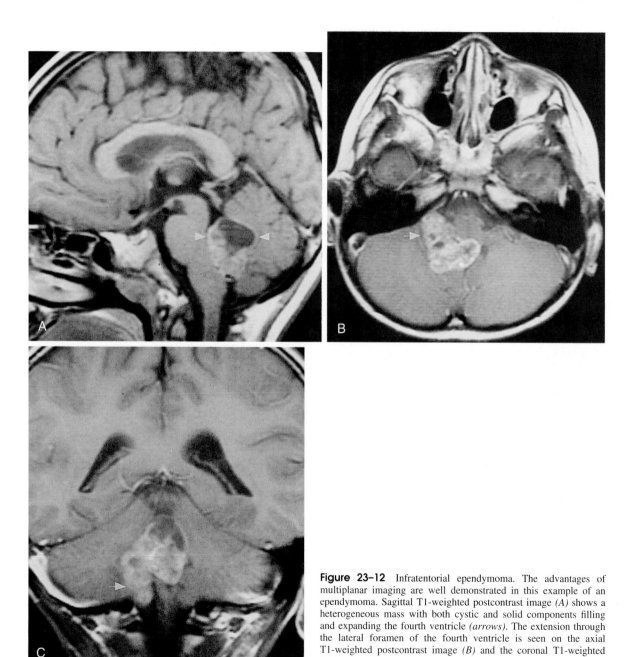

Figure 23–12 Infratentorial ependymoma. The advantages of multiplanar imaging are well demonstrated in this example of an ependymoma. Sagittal T1-weighted postcontrast image *(A)* shows a heterogeneous mass with both cystic and solid components filling and expanding the fourth ventricle *(arrows)*. The extension through the lateral foramen of the fourth ventricle is seen on the axial T1-weighted postcontrast image *(B)* and the coronal T1-weighted postcontrast image *(C) (arrow)*.

the ventricular system or the central canal of the cord. Ependymomas are common tumors in children; they account for 10% of pediatric CNS neoplasms. Intracranial ependymomas are usually found in children, whereas intraspinal ependymomas are most often seen in adults.[19] Seventy percent of intracranial ependymomas are infratentorial in location, arising from the floor of the 4th ventricle. The peak age at occurrence is 1 to 5 years, and males and females are equally affected. These tumors often extend through the foramina of the fourth ventricle into the vallecula, cerebellopontine angle, foramen magnum, and the upper cervical subarachnoid space. This morphology has been termed *plastic ependymoma* by Courville and Broussalian,[21] but it should be noted that other tumors, especially PNET (medulloblastoma), can exhibit similar morphologic features. Sagittal and coronal MRI is particularly suited for evaluation of the extraventricular extension of tumor (Fig. 23–12).

The majority of supratentorial ependymomas are parenchymal in location rather than intraventricular, with the reported frequency of a parenchymal origin ranging from 56% to 85% (Fig. 23–13).[8] These parenchymal tumors are thought to arise from ependymal rests. They are most frequent in the frontal and parietal lobes, although any portion of the cerebral hemispheres can be affected. These lesions tend to be larger than infratentorial ependymomas. In one series, 94% of the tumors were larger than 4 cm.[22] They are usually well defined and homogeneous, although larger tumors may contain cysts.

Anaplastic ependymoma is an ependymal tumor with histologic evidence of anaplasia. MRI signal characteristics cannot accurately differentiate anaplastic ependymoma from the much more common ependymoma. However, a supratentorial location can be suggestive, as anaplasia has been reported in up to 86% of supratentorial ependymomas.[23]

On gross pathologic examination, ependymomas are extremely heterogeneous with areas of calcifications, cysts, and occasional hemorrhage. MRI reflects this complex pathology. The solid portions of the tumor are hypointense on T1-weighted images and hyperintense to white matter on proton-density and T2-weighted images. Foci of signal heterogeneity within solid tumors represent methemoglobin, hemosiderin, necrosis, calcification, and encased native vessels. Calcification is seen in half of the cases and can range in size from punctate foci to large nodules.[24] Ependymoma is the most common of the childhood posterior fossa tumors to calcify. Calcification may be missed on spin-echo sequences but is more apparent on gradient-echo pulses. Cysts are more common in supratentorial ependymomas and usually have slightly higher intensity than CSF on T1-weighted and proton-density images due to increased protein content. Almost all ependymomas enhance with contrast. Enhancement is usually patchy and irregular, unlike the more homogeneous enhancement of a medulloblastoma.

Subependymoma

Subependymomas are rare, benign neoplasms that contain both astrocytes and ependymal cells. They are generally sharply marginated, lobulated tumors that arise beneath the ventricular lining and extend into the ventricle. Even when large, subependymomas are usually asymptomatic and rarely undergo malignant degeneration or subarachnoid spread. These tumors are much more common in men, with a mean age at occurrence of approximately 60 years. The most frequent location for subependymomas is the fourth ventricle (75%), but they can occur at other sites, including the lateral ventricles.[8] Solid tumors tend to be homogeneous, whereas larger lesions can have focal areas of cysts, calcifications, and hemorrhage. Symptomatic subependymomas are related to ventricular outflow obstruction.

On MRI, subependymomas demonstrate nonspecific signal intensity. T2 signal is increased and may be heterogeneous, especially in larger lesions. Enhancement has been reported to range from patchy to homogeneous. In our experience, enhancement has usually been moderate to intense. The key to preoperative diagnosis of a subependymoma depends on identifying its intraventricular location, the most common site being the fourth ventricle (Fig. 23–14). Lesions in the lateral ventricle are usually adjacent to the septum pellucidum.[19] The differential diagnosis includes other intraventricular neoplasms, such as ependymoma, oligodendroglioma, meningioma, choroid plexus papilloma, and astrocytoma.[19]

SPINAL CORD GLIOMAS

MRI is the modality of choice in the assessment of intramedullary lesions of the spinal cord. Conventional myelography

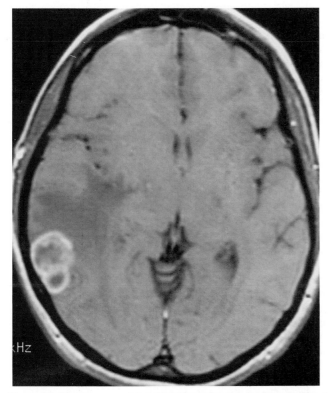

Figure 23–13 Supratentorial anaplastic ependymoma. Axial T1-weighted postcontrast image shows a lobulated enhancing mass in the posterior right temporal lobe with a nonenhancing center and a marked amount of adjacent white matter edema.

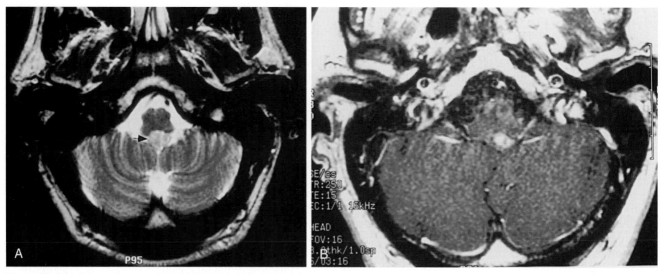

Figure 23-14   Subependymoma. *A*, Axial T2-weighted image reveals a well-defined lesion in the inferior aspect of the fourth ventricle *(arrow)*. *B*, Axial T1-weighted postcontrast image reveals enhancement of the tumor. This is the most common location of a subependymoma.

and postmyelography CT still have an important role in the workup of extradural and intradural extramedullary disease, but MRI has replaced these modalities in the evaluation of intramedullary lesions. New techniques for motion compensation, such as gradient moment nulling, help suppress pulsatile artifact from flowing CSF. These techniques now make it possible to visualize the spinal cord in detail not available previously. At our institution, evaluation for spinal tumors includes a sagittal T1, sagittal fast spin-echo T2, axial gradient echo, and postcontrast T1-weighted images in two planes, usually axial and sagittal.

Intramedullary tumors are often associated with cord expansion and increased signal intensity on T2 images. Although noncontrast MRI is quite sensitive for detection of cord expansion and of signal intensity changes within the cord, the delineation and characterization of the lesions are improved dramatically with the use of paramagnetic contrast material.[25] Unlike gliomas of the brain, of which up to 50% do not enhance, the large majority of spinal cord gliomas enhance after contrast administration, even those of low histologic grade. Of the 55 reported cases of intramedullary gliomas, enhancement was seen in 54 cases.[25] We have seen only one documented case of a nonenhancing spinal cord astrocytoma at our institution out of approximately 300 cases reviewed over the last several years. Enhancement delineates the solid tumor nidus from adjacent edema and proteinaceous reactive cord cysts. T2-weighted images of cord tumors often demonstrate increased signal throughout a large region of cord enlargement, whereas enhancement corresponding to the actual tumor nidus is limited to a much smaller region (Fig. 23–15). Although it is clear that enhancement does not always correlate with exact tumor margins, which is similar to the situation found with intracranial gliomas, separation of tumor nidus from associated edema is of utmost significance in performing precise preoperative tumor localization and operative resection.

Adjacent cysts often accompany intramedullary tumors. The cysts may either be neoplastic cysts or reactive, nonneoplastic cysts. Non-neoplastic cysts lined with reactive

glial cells are seen both rostral and caudal to cord tumors. In a review of 155 spinal cord tumors associated with cystic cavities, Poser found that 75% of the cysts were adjacent to the tumor but were separated from the actual tumor nidus.[26] These reactive cysts are generally drained at surgery and are not excised. Benign reactive cysts need to be distinguished from true intratumoral cysts, which are lined by neoplastic cells and require surgical excision. On noncontrast MRI, both reactive and neoplastic cysts can appear similar. They both can have proteinaceous and xanthrochromic fluid, which will be higher in signal intensity than CSF on T1 images and similar to CSF on T2 images. Contrast-enhanced MRI has proven an extremely useful technique in this situation. Benign reactive rostral and caudal cysts do not demonstrate contrast enhancement, whereas the margin of neoplastic intratumoral cysts often enhances.

MRI with contrast enhancement is also extremely useful in the initial workup of expansile intramedullary processes. A common clinical dilemma is the evaluation of a syrinx cavity. Syringohydromyelia can be the result of a variety of processes including neoplasm, trauma, and Chiari malformation. Lack of enhancement of a syrinx cavity strongly reduces the likelihood of a underlying cord neoplasm. Conversely, a region of a cord expansion, increased T2 signal, and enhancement suggests, but is not pathognomonic, of a cord tumor. Non-neoplastic processes, such as multiple sclerosis, infarction, venous hypertension from vascular malformations, and transverse myelitis, can acutely expand the cord contour and can have a variable degree of enhancement.[27] The clinical history is often most helpful in distinguishing these processes. A repeat MRI after a 6- to 8-week interval may best help to distinguish neoplastic from nonneoplastic cord processes. Myelography is required to confirm the presence of abnormal veins in suspected cases of dural arteriovenous fistula.

Spinal Cord Ependymomas

Ependymomas are the most common intramedullary neoplasm of the spinal cord. They most commonly involve the

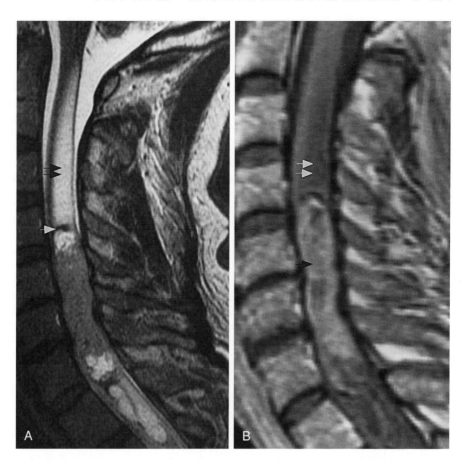

Figure 23–15 Spinal cord ependymoma. *A,* Sagittal T2-weighted fast spin-echo image shows a heterogeneous multilobulated mass in the mid–cervical cord. A hypointense rim is visible in the cephalad aspect of the lesion consistent with old blood products *(white arrow).* An adjacent flame-shaped region of T2 hyperintensity is visible in the upper cervical cord *(double black arrows). B,* Sagittal T1-weighted postcontrast image illustrates that although the tumor nidus enhances *(black arrow),* the region of cord edema does not demonstrate enhancement *(double white arrows).* The hypointense ''cap'' seen in *A* is characteristic of an ependymoma.

lower thoracic cord, conus, and filum. The peak age at incidence of cord ependymomas is the third through the sixth decades, which is much later than that for intracranial ependymomas. There is a 3:2 male predominance.

Ependymomas tend to be central in location and to expand the cord in a centrifugal growth pattern, reflecting the origin of the ependymal cells lining the central canal.[28] On noncontrast MRI, ependymomas are usually isointense on T1-weighted images with respect to the spinal cord, and their boundaries may be difficult to define unless they are capped by syrinx cavities. On T2-weighted images, ependymomas usually have a multilobulated appearance and are hyperintense in comparison with the normal cord. However, this hyperintensity is difficult to distinguish from associated tumor edema. Hemorrhage is frequently associated with ependymomas, especially at the superior and the inferior borders of the tumor. Hemorrhage appears hypointense on both T1- and T2-weighted images at the tumor margins, corresponding to a relatively firm pseudocapsule seen at surgery. Previous hemorrhage is thought to induce the pseudocapsule. In a study by Nemoto and colleagues,[29] 35 intramedullary tumors showed this hypointense rim, and all were identified as ependymomas at pathologic examination.

Ependymomas show intense, homogeneous, sharply marginated enhancement on contrast MRI scans. This appearance differs from astrocytomas of the cord, which tend to enhance in a more patchy, diffuse fashion.[28]

The most common subtype of ependymoma is myxopapillary ependymoma. The myxopapillary subtype is the most common lesion of the conus and filum. On MRI, myxopapillary ependymoma shares imaging features of other ependymomas. Hemorrhage occurs more frequently in the myxopapillary subtype. These tumors can occasionally present with subarachnoid hemorrhage or, more commonly, with chronic pial siderosis from chronic small subarachnoid hemorrhages. This may be seen on T2-weighted sequences as a thin, hypointense signal along the pial surface of the spinal cord and intracranial structures.

Spinal Cord Astrocytoma

Astrocytomas represent between 20% to 30% of gliomas of the spinal cord. These tumors tend to occur more frequently in children and represent approximately 60% of intramedullary tumors in this age group. They occur anywhere within the cord, although they most frequently occur in the cervical and upper thoracic regions.

On noncontrast MRI, astrocytomas appear as nonspecific regions of cord expansion, isointense to normal cord on T1 sequences and increased in signal on T2-weighted images. Focal regions of decreased signal on T1- or T2-weighted images corresponding to prior hemorrhage and hemosiderin are less frequently seen in astrocytomas than in ependymomas. After contrast administration, astrocytomas enhance in a patchy, irregular pattern as compared with the intense, homogeneous, sharply marginated enhancement of ependymomas.[28] In addition, the enhancement tends to be more eccentrically located, usually in the posterior aspect of the spinal cord.[28]

In summary, MRI offers superb delineation of intrinsic tumors of the spinal cord. Paramagnetic contrast material helps delineate the tumor nidus from adjacent edema and associated benign rostral and caudal cysts, which assists in presurgical and radiation therapy planning.

MRI FINDINGS AFTER THERAPY

Surgery and/or radiation therapy are the mainstays in the treatment of intracranial and spinal cord neoplasms. One of the important roles of MRI is to monitor the effectiveness of these therapies and to evaluate for recurrent disease. Several important issues need to be addressed regarding the utility of post-treatment MRI examinations.

Postsurgical Changes on MRI

The extent of the tumor resection is one of the major issues in the postoperative patient. A gross total resection appears to increase significantly both the length and quality of survival when compared with a subtotal resection.[30] Determining the extent of residual tumor is made more difficult by enhancement normally seen at the resection site. The mechanisms underlying this non-neoplastic postoperative enhancement are not fully understood, but they may include blood-brain barrier disruption, luxury perfusion, and neovascularity.[30] In a study of 78 patients who underwent resection of intracranial gliomas, Forsting and co-workers[30] found that enhancement in the resection site began as early as the fourth postoperative day and was difficult to distinguish from residual tumor. Elster and DiPersio[31] have found that

the surgical enhancement usually resolves within 1 year. At the present time, we recommend that postoperative imaging for assessment of residual enhancing tumor be performed within the first 48 to 72 hours after surgery.

In addition to enhancement at the surgical site, the underlying dura frequently enhances after craniotomy.[31] This enhancement is nonspecific and can also be seen after lumbar puncture and CSF shunting procedures. Such dural enhancement can persist for many years.

The Effect of Steroids on Contrast Enhancement

Cairncross and colleagues[32] have shown that corticosteroids may alter the enhancement pattern of tumors. They found that corticosteroids reduce both the extent and the intensity of contrast enhancement as well as the amount of peritumoral edema. Because the systemic effect of steroids evolves over several weeks, it is recommended that patients receive stable or decreasing doses of corticosteroids to accurately assess the degree of therapeutic response in gliomas. Steroids may also increase the sulcal size and, of course, decrease the vasogenic edema produced by neoplasm.

Radiation Necrosis

Radiation injury to the brain is becoming increasingly recognized because of the sensitivity of MRI. It is important to distinguish the injury resulting from radiation and tumor growth. Radiation injury has been classified as acute or late radiation injury.[33] Late radiation injury usually occurs

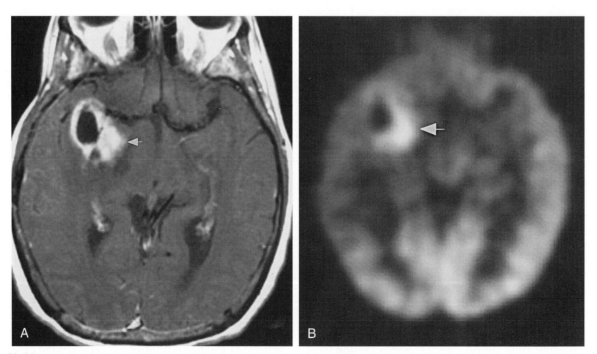

Figure 23–16 The role of PET and MRI spectroscopy in evaluation of radiation necrosis. This 44-year-old woman was diagnosed 4 years earlier with a mixed malignant glioma and underwent surgical resection. Gamma knife radiosurgery for local recurrence was performed 6 months prior to this examination. *A,* Axial T1-weighted postcontrast image demonstrates a nodular region of enhancement medial to the surgical cavity *(arrow). B,* PET examination demonstrates a region of marked FDG uptake in the medial aspect of the mass corresponding to the region of enhancement seen on MRI *(arrow).* MRI spectroscopy in this region (not shown) demonstrated a marked increase in the choline peak consistent with a recurrent tumor. At surgery, viable tumor cells were confirmed in the medial aspect of the mass.

months to years post-therapy and is irreversible. Late radiation injury may be diffuse or focal in location. Diffuse white matter injury is seen on MRI as nonenhancing, confluent areas of high signal within periventricular white matter, sparing the corpus callosum. Focal late radiation injury usually manifests as necrosis on MRI. When necrosis develops after irradiation for cerebral tumors, it occurs most frequently near the site of the original tumor, even after whole-brain irradiation. This may be due to vasogenic edema making the tissue adjacent to the tumor more susceptible to injury. When one encounters a patient with clinical deterioration and a prior history of radiation therapy, the distinction between late radiation necrosis and recurrent tumor is difficult to make on MRI. Unfortunately, late radiation necrosis and recurrent tumor share many MRI features. Both can present as a region of decreased T1 signal and increased T2 signal with significant enhancement and extensive vasogenic edema. Although MRI cannot usually distinguish these two entities, PET, using the glucose metabolite tracer ^{18}F-2-fluoro-2-D-deoxyglucose, has been used in this clinical setting. PET is a functional imaging study that measures cerebral glucose metabolic activity. Glucose activity is usually decreased in a region of necrosis and increased in areas of recurrent tumor (Fig. 23–16). This technique has shown some promise in evaluation of recurrent high-grade gliomas. However, lower-grade gliomas have a baseline lower metabolic activity that is often equal to surrounding gray matter, and these lesions are not as easily distinguished from radiation necrosis.[34]

In addition to PET, MR spectroscopy has been utilized in the evaluation of the metabolism of intracranial tumors. Spectroscopy can measure maps of energy metabolism in a specific region of interest. Several molecules relevant to tumor metabolism on proton-H[1]-spectroscopy include N-acetylaspartate (NAA) and choline. Choline is present in phospholipid membranes and can be used to assess cell membrane synthesis, which is increased in tumor growth.[35] NAA is a marker for normal neuronal cells. Although unable to distinguish between histologic grades of gliomas, a study by Fulham and associates[36] showed that an increase in choline with either minimal or no reduction in NAA was an earlier sign of tumor recurrence than could be established by either MRI or PET imaging. Radiation necrosis, however, is associated with diminished levels of choline and NAA. MR spectroscopy may potentially have the capability of evaluating response to therapy. The role of MR spectroscopy in the management of gliomas awaits larger clinical studies.[35]

REFERENCES

1. Lee BCP, Kneeland JB, Cahill PT, et al: MR recognition of supratentorial tumors. AJNR 1985; 6:871–878.
2. Kelly PJ, Daumas-Duport C, Kispert DB, et al: Imaged-based stereotaxic serial biopsies in untreated intracranial glial neoplasms. J Neurosurg 1987; 66:865–874.
3. Earnest F IV, Kelly PJ, Scheithauer BW, et al: Cerebral astrocytomas: Histopathologic correlation of MR and CT contrast enhancement with stereotaxic biopsy. Radiology 1988; 166:823–827.
4. Valk PE, Laxer KD, Barbaro NM, et al: High-resolution (2.6-mm) PET in partial complex epilepsy associated with mesial temporal sclerosis. Radiology 1993; 186:55–58.
5. Kondziolka D, Lunsford LD, Martinez AJ: Unreliability of contempo-

6. Tovi M, Lilja A, Bergstrom M, et al: Delineation of gliomas with magnetic resonance imaging using Gd-DTPA in comparison with computed tomography and positron emission tomography. Acta Radiol 1990; 31:417–429.
7. Piepmeier JM, Fried I, Makuch R: Low-grade astrocytomas may arise from different astrocytic lineages. Neurosurgery 1993; 33:627–632.
8. Masters LT, Zimmerman RD: Imaging of supratentorial brain tumors in adults. Neuroimaging Clin North Am 1993; 3:649–669.
9. Dean BL, Drayer BP, Bird CR, et al: Gliomas: Classification with MR imaging. Radiology 1990; 174:411–415.
10. Kleihues P, Burger PC, Scheithauer BW: Histological Typing of Tumours of the Central Nervous System, ed 2. Berlin, Springer-Verlag, 1993.
11. Sze G, Abramson A, Krol G, et al: Gadolinium-DTPA in the evaluation of intradural extramedullary spinal disease. AJNR 1988; 9:153–163.
12. Maiuri F, Stella L, Benvenuti D, et al: Cerebral gliosarcomas: Correlation of computed tomographic findings, surgical aspect, pathologic features, and prognosis. Neurosurgery 1990; 26:261–267.
13. Barkovich AJ, Krischer J, Kun LE, et al: Brainstem gliomas: A classification system based on magnetic resonance imaging. Pediatr Neurosurg 1990; 16:73–83.
14. Packer RJ, Vezina G: Pediatric glial neoplasms including brainstem gliomas. Semin Oncol 1994; 21:260–272.
15. Lee Y, Van Tassel P, Bruner JM, et al: Juvenile pilocytic astrocytomas: CT and MR characteristics. AJNR 1989; 10:363–370.
16. Yoshino MT, Lucio R: Pleomorphic xanthoastrocytoma. AJNR 1992; 13:1330–1332.
17. Tien RD, Cardenas CA, Rajagopalan S: Pleomorphic xanthoastrocytoma of the brain: MR findings in six patients. AJR 1992; 159:1287–1290.
18. Braffman BH, Bilaniuk LT, Naidich TP: MR imaging of tuberous sclerosis: Pathogenesis of phakomatosis, use of gadopentetate dimeglumine, and literature review. Radiology 1992; 183:227–238.
19. Atlas SW. Intraaxial brain tumors. In Atlas SW (ed): Magnetic Resonance Imaging of the Brain and Spine. New York, Raven Press, 1991, pp 223–236.
20. Lee Y, Van Tassel P: Intracranial oligodendrogliomas: Imaging findings in 35 untreated cases. AJNR 1989; 10:119–127.
21. Courville CB, Broussalian SL: Plastic ependymomas of the lateral recess: Report of eight verified cases. J Neurosurg 1961; 18:792.
22. Armington WG, Osborn AG, Cubberley DA, et al: Supratentorial ependymoma: CT appearance. Radiology 1985; 157:367–372.
23. Pfleger MJ, Gerson LD: Supratentorial tumors in children. Neuroimaging Clin North Am 1993; 3:671–687.
24. Zee CS, Segall HD, Nelson M: Infratentorial tumors in children. Neuroimaging Clin North Am 1993; 3:705–714.
25. Sze G: MR imaging of the spinal cord: Current status and future advances. AJR 1992; 159:149–159.
26. Poser CM: The relationship between syringomyelia and neoplasm. In American Lecture Series, #262. Springfield, Il, American Lectures in Neurology, 1956, pp 28–32.
27. Dillon WP, Norman D, Newton TH, et al: Intradural spinal cord lesions: Gd-DPTA-enhanced MR imaging. Radiology 1989; 170:229–237.
28. Parizel PM, Baleriaux D, Rodesch G, et al: Gd-DTPA-enhanced MR imaging of spinal tumors. AJNR 1989; 10:249–258.
29. Nemoto Y, Inoue Y, Tashiro T, et al: Intramedullary spinal cord tumors: Significance of associated hemorrhage at MR imaging. Radiology 1992; 182:793–796.
30. Forsting M, Albert FK, Kunze S, et al: Extirpation of glioblastomas: CT and MR follow-up of residual tumor and regrowth patterns. AJNR 1993; 14:77–87.
31. Elster AD, DiPersio DA: Cranial postoperative site: Assessment with contrast-enhanced MR imaging. Radiology 1990; 174:93–98.
32. Cairncross JG, MacDonald DR, Pexman JH, et al: Steroid-induced CT changes in patients with recurrent malignant glioma. Neurology 1988; 38:724–726.
33. Valk PE, Dillon WP: Radiation injury of the brain. AJR 1991; 156:689–706.
34. Di Chiro G, Brooks RA: PET-FDG of untreated and treated cerebral gliomas. J Nucl Med 1988; 29:421–422.
35. Byrne TN: Imaging of gliomas. Semin Oncol 1994; 21:162–171.
36. Fulham M, Bizzi A, Dietz M, et al: Mapping of brain tumor metabolites with proton MR spectroscopic imaging: Clinical relevance. Radiology 1992; 185:675–686.

MICHAEL J. FULHAM

GIOVANNI DI CHIRO

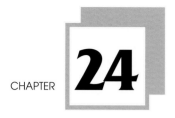

CHAPTER **24**

Positron Emission Tomography and ¹H-Spectroscopic Imaging

In many centers, the accepted neuroradiologic evaluation for a patient with a suspected glioma includes a determination of abnormal anatomy and integrity of the blood-brain barrier with computed tomography (CT) or magnetic resonance imaging (MRI) and an assessment of the degree of tumor vascularity with angiography. Management decisions are then made on the basis of the grade of malignancy of the suspected tumor, the size and location of the tumor, the age of the patient, the clinical symptoms, and the degree of neurologic deficit.[1, 2] Anatomic imaging is also the tool of choice for stereotactic biopsy and volumetric resection.[3–6] Treatment decisions after surgery and the assessment of tumor response are often based on the degree of contrast enhancements seen on anatomic imaging studies.[7] However, the shortcomings of these modalities in evaluating tumor biology and tumoral response to therapeutic regimens are recognized by experienced clinicians.[8–14] The recent introduction of functional imaging modalities, such as positron emission tomography (PET), single photon emission computed tomography (SPECT), and MR spectroscopy (MRS) have provided the opportunity to refine the noninvasive evaluation of brain tumors and to improve management through the measurement of tumor metabolism and metabolites. The emerging role of PET and MRS in the management of patients with brain tumors is presented in this chapter. SPECT radiotracers, which have been used in the evaluation of brain tumors,[15] are not considered; they are included in Chapter 25.

POSITRON EMISSION TOMOGRAPHY

Positron emission tomography was developed in the mid-1970s with the promise of providing quantitative measurements and anatomic localization of biochemical processes in vivo.[16–18] PET began in the research environment, and with the use of a variety of ligands it has provided insights into many aspects of brain tumor biology, from glucose and oxygen metabolism to blood flow, pH, status of the blood-brain barrier, amino acid uptake, presence/concentration of receptors, and the pharmacokinetics of delivery of chemotherapeutic agents. In the last decade, however, PET has been applied to the clinical management of patients with gliomas.[19, 20] The most widely used PET ligand in neuro-oncology is ¹⁸F-2-fluoro-2-deoxyglucose (FDG). FDG PET provides a noninvasive measurement of glucose metabolism.[21, 22] In the following text, the physical and practical aspects of PET and its role in the management of glioma patients are presented.

PET Methodology

PHYSICS OF PET

Positron emitters are unstable radioisotopes that have an excess number of protons and a positive charge. A *positron* is an anti-particle of an electron. It has the same mass as an electron, but it has a positive rather than a negative charge. Positron emission stabilizes the nucleus by removing the positive charge, and one element is therefore converted into another element with an atomic number that is 1 less than the number of the positron emitter. Once ejected from the nucleus, the positron travels a small distance (1 to 2 mm) in tissue before colliding with a surrounding electron to form a *positronium*. The positronium has a very short life and almost instantaneously annihilates, converting its mass into energy in the form of two photons that are emitted 180 degrees apart. The PET scanner detects these γ-rays, or 511 keV photons, rather than the positrons. The simultaneous production of annihilation photons in opposite directions is the fundamental basis for the detection and localization of the positron emitter in tissue. The PET scanner has multiple rings of detectors that are composed of inorganic crystals that scintillate (e.g., bismuth germanate). The detectors are connected to photomultiplier tubes; with sophisticated electronic circuitry and by using the technique of coincidence detection, the PET scanner is able to locate the annihilation

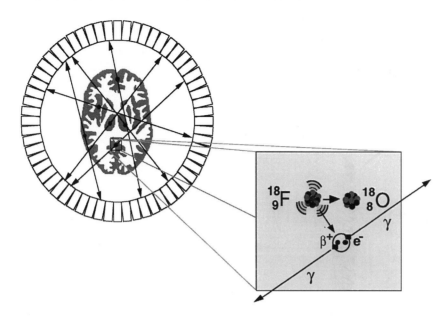

Figure 24–1 Transverse section through PET scanner showing ring of detectors and brain in center of field of view. Schematic illustration shows positron emission (^{18}F to ^{18}O), positron annihilation, and coincidence detection.

events and to provide a three-dimensional distribution of the tracer (Fig. 24–1).

Positron emitters are produced by charged particle accelerators, either linear accelerators or cyclotrons. A cyclotron accelerates charged particles to high velocities and energies, and the particles are then extracted from the beam and aimed at a small target chamber containing a gas. The accelerated ions induce a nuclear reaction within the target to produce the positron-emitting isotope. Various chemical synthetic steps are then performed to incorporate the radioisotope into a particular compound (ligand or tracer). The most common PET positron emitters are ^{18}F (half-life [$t_{1/2}$] = 110 minutes), ^{11}C ($t_{1/2}$ = 20 minutes), ^{13}N($t_{1/2}$ = 10 minutes), and ^{15}O ($t_{1/2}$ = 2 minutes). The short half-lives of these isotopes usually mean that the cyclotron must be in close proximity to the PET scanner.

Since the first PET scan in a human was reported in 1979,[21] major improvements in instrumentation (Fig. 24–2) and radiochemistry have been accomplished.[23] Five-millimeter in-plane and z-axis resolution are standard attributes of current scanners, and many aspects of cellular biology can now be studied with radioligands. Many of the present generation of PET scanners have extended (15 cm) fields of view and wide apertures that allow the entire brain or large regions of the body to be scanned without the need for multiple bed movements.[24] PET resolution is determined by the following: (1) type of detector, (2) distance that a positron travels in tissue before annihilation, (3) random and scatter coincidences, and (4) reconstruction algorithms. However, it is likely that the next generation of PET scanners will approach the theoretical "finite" in-plane spatial resolution in PET of about 2 mm.[25]

FDG PET METHOD

PET achieves functional imaging by combining the principles of the tracer kinetic method and tomographic image reconstruction. In the tracer method, a radiolabeled biologically active compound (tracer) participates in a biochemical process, and a mathematical model is derived to describe the kinetics of the process. The application of FDG to the measurement of cerebral glucose metabolism is based on the [^{14}C]deoxyglucose (DG) autoradiographic method developed by Sokoloff and co-workers in the albino rat.[26] This method was later validated in humans by Phelps and colleagues.[22] The three-compartment FDG model is illustrated in Figure 24–3. FDG is an analog of glucose and is taken up by cells and phosphorylated by hexokinase to become fluorodeoxyglucose-6-phosphate (FDG6P). However, because it is

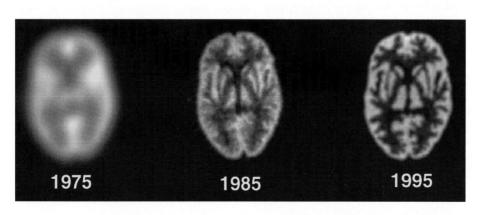

Figure 24–2 Simulations in a Hoffman brain phantom at the level of the deep nuclei and the insula show the improvements in PET resolution over two decades.

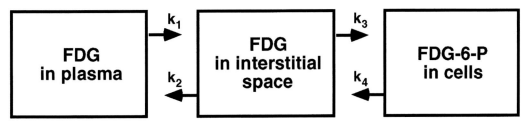

Figure 24–3 The FDG three-compartment model. Rate constants k_1, k_2, and k_3 describe movement of FDG between plasma and tissue, and k_4 describes dephosphorylation of FDG-6-phosphate.

*FDG*6P it cannot participate in other steps of the glycolytic cycle, and so is effectively "trapped" in the cell. Thus, the phosphorylation of FDG to FDG6P reflects cellular glucose utilization. For the clinical evaluation of glucose metabolism, a modification[27] that allows for dephosphorylation of FDG6P (k_4), of the Sokoloff three-compartment model[26] with standard gray matter rate constants ($k_1 = 0.1020$, $k_2 = 0.1300$, $k_3 = 0.0620$, $k_4 = 0.0068$) and a lumped constant value of 0.4180 is used. The input function of the mathematical model is the time-activity of FDG in plasma, which is obtained from counting the radioactivity in timed blood samples taken throughout the study.

Sokoloff's laboratory also demonstrated that in the mammalian nervous tissue DG uptake is mainly localized in synaptic terminals rather than in cell soma.[28, 29] Thus, FDG PET images reflect levels of synaptic activity that are either excitatory or inhibitory, as both require energy utilization. There are two exceptions: (1) high-grade cerebral tumors and (2) seizure foci during the ictus, in which somal glucose utilization predominates. The introduction of the FDG PET method to the evaluation of gliomas was based on the work of Warburg, who demonstrated that "anaerobic glycolysis" increases with increasing grade or with malignancy of tumors.[30, 31]

SCANNING PROTOCOL

Patients are studied after a 6-hour fast. Hyperglycemia results in decreased cerebral FDG uptake and "noisy" images, because the tracer dose of FDG competes with glucose for facilitated uptake. In small children, a 4-hour fast is used. Many centers perform neurologic FDG PET studies without measurement of glucose utilization; however, we routinely perform quantitative studies with blood sampling using the "arterialized venous" method because we believe that it aids in grading gliomas.[22] In patients who have complex partial seizures, video electroencephalographic (EEG) monitoring is carried out throughout the study so that any seizures that occur during the uptake or scanning period are detected. Occasionally a clinically inapparent seizure may produce glucose hypermetabolism, which can be confused with a high-grade tumor. Throughout the study the patient's eyes are patched and the ears are plugged. The typical adult injected dose of FDG is 5.3 MBq (megabecquerels)/kg for neurologic studies using a wide-aperture whole-body PET scanner. An uptake period of 30 minutes is allowed before the patient is positioned on the scanning bed. A thermoplastic mask is used to limit head movement. Motion degrades the quality of the images, and although a number of algorithms are available to correct for motion,[32, 33] we think that

it is better to limit movement than to correct for it after the event.[34] Measured attenuation correction is done with a postinjection method, which together with "off-camera" uptake allows accurate attenuation correction and increased patient throughput.[35] Scan duration is typically 30 to 50 minutes.

IMAGE ANALYSIS

All FDG PET scans are evaluated visually and quantitatively. In published reports, various reference regions have been suggested as the region to which tumoral glucose metabolism should be compared to eliminate systematic errors in the evaluation of tumor grade: (1) the identical region to the tumor but in the contralateral hemisphere, (2) contralateral/ipsilateral cerebral cortex, and (3) white matter. Our practice at the National Institutes of Health (NIH) has been to compare glucose utilization in the tumor to that in normal white matter of the centrum semiovale of the contralateral cerebral hemisphere.[36, 37] This reference region was chosen because white matter contains glial cells and axons of afferent and efferent neurons. From the work of Kadekaro and associates,[28] axons have minimal glucose utilization; thus, white matter glucose utilization reflects glial glucose metabolism. Although the hemisphere contralateral to a brain tumor may exhibit reduced glucose metabolism due to interruption of association fibers between the hemispheres, so-called transcallosal diaschisis,[38, 39] our data and those of others suggest that this effect on contralateral glucose utilization is small.[40–43]

For quantitative analysis, the most metabolically active part of the tumor is sought as the best reflection of tumor grade; the value is then normalized to the maximum value of white matter glucose metabolism. In a large number of patients we reported that average values for the ratio of tumor-to–white matter glucose metabolism are 1.3 for low-grade tumors, 4.2 for anaplastic astrocytomas, and 6.5 for glioblastomas multiforme.[37] Recently, Delbeke and co-workers[44] suggested a cut-off of 1.5 to separate low- from high-grade gliomas. In addition, we register the FDG PET study to anatomic imaging as part of routine clinical practice using commercial (surface contour matching) and in-house software.[34] Finally, it is important to recognize the characteristics (sensitivity, slice thickness) and limitations (resolution) of the PET device when interpreting scans. It is not surprising that a PET device with in-plane and z-axis resolution will have difficulty detecting a 2-mm thin rim of tumor because of partial volume effects; similarly, 10-mm thick transaxial MR sections coupled with a 5-mm interspace gap may miss similar-sized lesions.

Tumor Grading and Malignant Degeneration

Various pathologic classifications[45, 46] have been used for astrocytomas, and newer classifications have been introduced,[47] but this chapter uses the new WHO classification of brain tumors[48]: grade I indicates a pilocytic astrocytoma; grade II, low-grade astrocytoma; grade III, anaplastic astrocytoma; and grade IV, glioblastoma multiforme. The most critical issue in the evaluation of a patient with a glioma is determination of the tumor grade, because patient outcome and therapeutic options are determined largely by histologic grade.[1, 2] Additional management issues include the following:

1. Should the lesion be biopsied stereotactically? If so, what part of the lesion best reflects tumor biology?

2. What is the local extent of the lesion? How far does the tumor extend into surrounding neural tissue?

3. What is the best management plan for a patient with a low-grade glioma? What is the best tool to detect malignant degeneration?

4. When clinical deterioration occurs in a brain tumor patient months after surgery, radiation, and chemotherapy, is it due to recurrent tumor or is it because of the effects of treatment?

5. Which scan best evaluates response or lack of response to treatment?

6. What PET ligand can best answer these questions?

Anatomic imaging is the standard investigative procedure in most institutions for patients with suspected gliomas. It is a general principle that, in the appropriate clinical context, a mass lesion that enhances after intravenous iodinated or paramagnetic contrast agents is considered to be a high-grade tumor, and, similarly, that a lesion without enhancement is regarded as a low-grade tumor,[47, 49–53] with few exceptions (see Special Tumors).[37, 54–56] Treatment planning and longitudinal follow-up are also based on contrast-enhanced anatomic imaging, and MRI is preferred to CT because of its greater sensitivity in detecting and delineating tumor extent.[9, 57] However, a number of reports demonstrate the unreliability of contrast enhancement in determining tumor grade and tumor extent. Chamberlain and colleagues[57a] showed that 31% of highly anaplastic and 54% of moderately anaplastic astrocytomas did not enhance on CT. In smaller series, Kelly and associates noted lack of contrast enhancement in 9 of 10 anaplastic astrocytomas, and Kondziolka and co-workers[14] reported that in 9 of 19 patients with solid lesions that were suspected of being astrocytomas and that did not enhance on MRI, anaplastic astrocytomas were found on stereotactic biopsy specimens.[14, 58]

Since the first report from Di Chiro and co-workers at the NIH in 1982, FDG PET has proven superior to anatomic imaging in grading gliomas.[10] Glucose hypermetabolism relative to white matter is seen in high-grade tumors (anaplastic astrocytoma, glioblastoma multiforme), and in low-grade astrocytomas, glucose metabolism is slightly greater or less than that in white matter. These findings have been duplicated at other centers[59–62] with one exception. Tyler and colleagues[63] found no correlation between glucose metabolism and grade in 16 patients with brain tumors (two with low-grade astrocytomas). They compared average, rather than maximal, tumoral glucose metabolism to contralateral brain with an inferior resolution PET scanner. Partial volume error secondary to instrumentation and regional analysis, which included necrosis in the value for tumoral glucose metabolism, were major factors in the spuriously low metabolic values seen in high-grade tumors.[36]

Prospective comparisons of FDG PET to MRI with gadolinium-DTPA (Gd-DTPA) have also been performed.[64, 65] Davis and associates reported findings in 22 gliomas, whereas Melisi and co-workers analyzed 160 FDG PET studies from 113 patients with gliomas, the majority of whom had been treated. Both studies reported similar findings—that FDG PET and enhanced MRI were generally complementary—but Melisi and colleagues noted that 20%

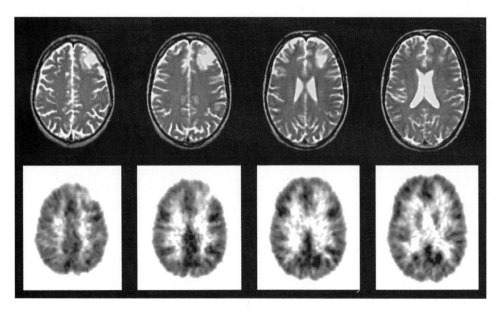

Figure 24–4 Registered transaxial T2-weighted MRI and FDG PET scans in a 35-year-old man with an incidental finding of low-grade astrocytoma. MRI shows signal hyperintensity in left frontal lobe. On FDG PET, the region of hyperintensity is hypometabolic. Note that thin rim of tissue in white matter is relatively hypometabolic when compared with surrounding cortex consistent with tumor infiltration; same cortex on MRI has increased signal intensity. (Note: For this and all subsequent FDG PET scans, regions of high glucose utilization are gray-black and areas of low glucose utilization are white.)

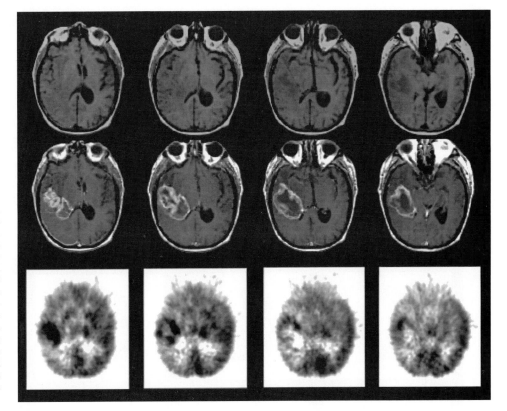

Figure 24–5 Registered transaxial MR imaging and FDG PET scans in a 72-year-old man with a glioblastoma. T1-weighted images *(top row)* show a large mass in the right temporo-occipital lobes with mass effect. Enhanced T1-weighted images *(middle row)* show irregular enhancement in lesion and central hypointensity, which suggests necrosis. On FDG PET *(bottom row)*, lack of complete correspondence between enhanced MRI and PET is seen. Glucose hypermetabolism is most marked in anterolateral temporal lobe, but posterior extent of lesion is hypometabolic and necrotic *(bottom row).*

of cases showed a lack of correspondence between FDG PET and MRI. This group consisted of (1) patients with high-grade tumors that did not enhance on MRI and (2) patients with radiation necrosis that demonstrated avid Gd-DTPA enhancement but reduced glucose utilization on FDG PET. Typical examples of FDG PET and MRI findings in patients with low-grade and high-grade tumors are shown in Figures 24–4 through 24–8. Tumor heterogeneity is characteristic of many gliomas, and pathologic grading may be incorrect if the operative specimen or biopsy sample is not representative of the tumor.[66] In the patient who is the

subject in Figure 24–5, a partial surgical resection of a glioblastoma multiforme was done. The bulk of tissue sent to the pathologist was taken from the posterior margins of the lesion, which, although it enhanced avidly on MRI, was hypometabolic on PET and consistent with necrosis. The neuropathologist could not make a diagnosis of glioma on the basis of the pathologic specimen. The capability of FDG PET to depict tumor heterogeneity has been used to advantage to guide stereotactic biopsy and resection.[67, 68] Levivier and associates reported the diagnostic yield of FDG PET–guided stereotactic biopsy in 43 patients, 38 of whom

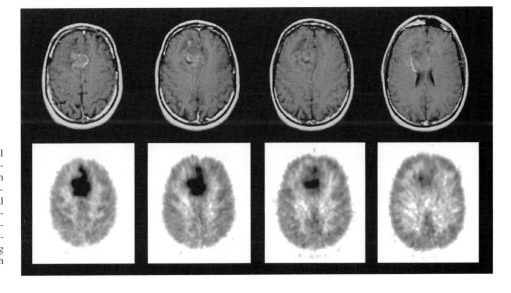

Figure 24–6 Registered transaxial MRI *(top)* and FDG PET scans *(bottom)* in a 44-year-old man with an anaplastic oligodendroglioma. On enhanced T1-weighted images, minimal enhancement is seen in a large bifrontal mass that involves the corpus callosum. FDG PET shows markedly increased glucose utilization involving the white matter and the cortex of both mesial frontal lobes.

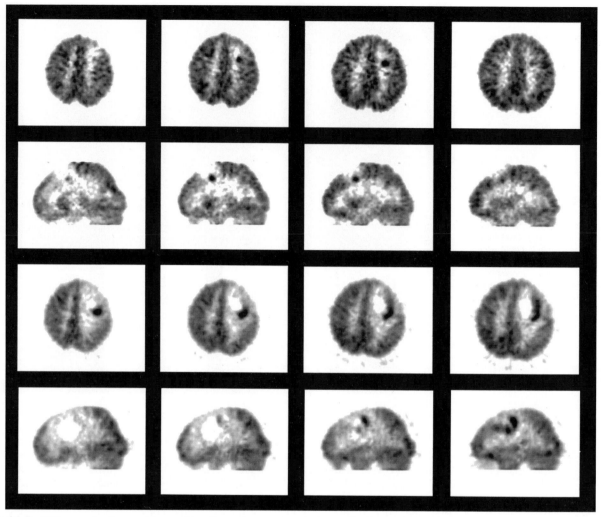

Figure 24–7 PET scans of a 51-year-old man with malignant degeneration of a low-grade glioma. The first PET scan, transaxial (*top*) and sagittal (*second row*) images, shows a large area of hypometabolism in the left sensorimotor cortex with small focus of glucose hypermetabolism consistent with malignant degeneration. The second PET scan (*third and fourth rows*) shows an increase in the size of the hypermetabolic focus curving around a necrotic center.

had brain tumors.[68] They found that FDG PET–guided biopsies were more successful in obtaining diagnostic tissue specimens when compared to CT-guided trajectories, and that the difference was statistically significant.

FDG PET can distinguish between anaplastic astrocytomas and glioblastomas multiforme when areas of marked hypometabolism are present in the lesion, indicating necrosis (see Figs. 24–5 and 24–8). In our experience, the highest tumoral glucose utilization was seen in a glioblastoma multiforme; however, the amount of glucose utilization in these tumors is extremely variable. If the tumor is growing so rapidly that it outgrows its blood supply, only a thin rim of active tumor may be present surrounding a central region of necrosis (see Fig. 24–5). Glucose utilization in this rim is always greater than that in white matter, but it may not be greater than that in normal contralateral cerebral cortex; the PET scanner underestimates the true amount of glucose utilization because of partial volume effects. In addition, FDG PET cannot separate glioma subtypes (e.g., astrocytoma vs. oligodendroglioma), although anaplastic oligodendrogliomas (see Fig. 24–6) show markedly increased glucose

utilization when compared with the usual slow-growing oligodendrogliomas, which are hypometabolic.

Delineating the "true" extent of a glioma, low- or high-grade, is a difficult task with available neuroimaging modalities. The problem is of microscopic invasion beyond the macroscopic abnormality seen at operation and on imaging.[58, 69, 70] Although microscopic resolution is beyond the capability of neuroimaging for the foreseeable future, it is hoped that future PET scanners with finite in-plane resolution and improvements in resolution in MR spectroscopic imaging (see following section) will improve the detection of tumor beyond current limits.

The management of patients with low-grade gliomas is controversial. Some clinicians utilize surgery followed by radiation therapy, others perform a biopsy followed by radiotherapy, and others prefer to manage patients conservatively and to await clinical deterioration before intervention.[1, 2, 13, 71–76] The natural history of low-grade gliomas is uncertain, and many clinicians have patients who have had seizures for 15 to 20 years before an underlying low-grade tumor was found. A large percentage of these tumors (some investiga-

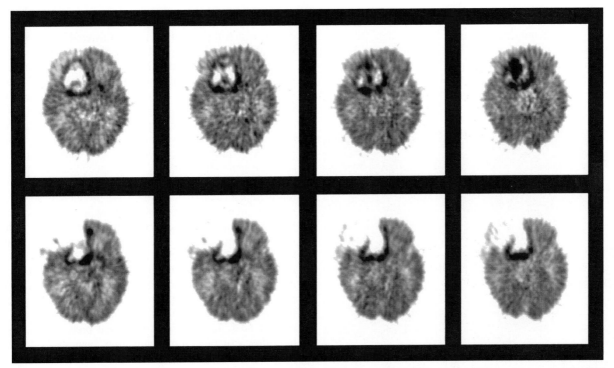

Figure 24–8   Transaxial aligned preoperative (*top row*) and day 7 postoperative (*bottom row*) FDG PET scans in a 45-year-old woman with glioblastoma. *Bottom row* shows extensive residual hypermetabolic tumor at edges of resection.

tors argue that this applies to all of these tumors) will undergo malignant degeneration. Our own practice is to manage patients with low-grade astrocytomas or presumed low-grade astrocytomas conservatively. Anatomic and FDG PET studies are done on a yearly basis, or earlier if there is clinical deterioration, because of PET's ability to detect early malignant change.[12, 77] An example is shown in Fig. 24–7: a 51-year-old man presented with a generalized tonic-clonic seizure 5 years before the FDG PET scan was performed. At the time of the scan, the patient was seizure-free and asymptomatic. The tumor involved eloquent cortex and the focus of malignant change was deep in white matter. When FDG PET detected the focus of hypermetabolism the CT scan was unchanged. Despite the FDG PET findings, observation of the patient was decided as the next step. Right arm weakness developed in the patient 10 months later, and on the second scan the focus of glucose hypermetabolism was much larger; biopsy revealed a glioblastoma. This illustrates an important issue: Once malignant degeneration is detected, when is the best time for intervention? The results for high-grade tumors treated with aggressive local therapies, such as brachytherapy or radiosurgery, are better if the tumor volume is small.[78] But is intervention justified when the patient is asymptomatic? Most neurosurgeons are reluctant to operate on patients who are asymptomatic, but FDG PET data, as first reported by Patronas and co-workers[79] and later by others,[60, 80, 81] demonstrate shortened survival in brain tumor patients with glucose hypermetabolism. The importance of FDG PET in the longitudinal follow-up of patients with low-grade astrocytomas and its ability to detect malignant change is undisputed; trials are now required to arrive at the optimal management for these patients.

Residual Tumor and Treatment Response

Pivotal to the evaluation of new investigational protocols for the treatment of gliomas is an accurate indicator of tumor biology that can be monitored to assess response. In addition to clinical findings, the degree of enhancement on MRI is currently used as the gold standard to measure tumor response in clinical trials.[7] This approach has limitations. Glantz and colleagues have shown that FDG PET performed early in the postoperative period more easily identified residual tumor (see Fig. 24–8) and predicted early recurrence more reliably than CT or the surgeon's estimates of the extent of tumor resection.[82] Cairncross and associates showed that contrast enhancement on anatomic imaging performed 4 days after operation could be due to postsurgical changes rather than residual tumor.[83] Corticosteroids also have a profound effect on the degree of contrast enhancement, peritumoral edema, and, to a lesser extent, the apparent volume of enhancing tumor.[84-88] Up to a 50% reduction in the enhancing volume of anaplastic tumors has been reported following corticosteroid administration.[84, 85, 88] Glantz and co-workers also noted that steroid dose did not affect tumoral FDG uptake in patients studied before and after corticosteroids.

Recurrent Tumor and Radiation Necrosis

Clinical deterioration in a glioma patient months or years after treatment is generally due to tumor recurrence. Structural imaging often reveals a mass lesion with surrounding edema and marked contrast enhancement. Unfortunately, radiation and chemonecrosis have clinical and radiologic pictures identical to those of recurrent tumor (Fig. 24–9A). Radiation necrosis generally appears a year or more after irradiation with doses greater than 50 Gy. The incidence of radiation necrosis is directly proportional to the dose and

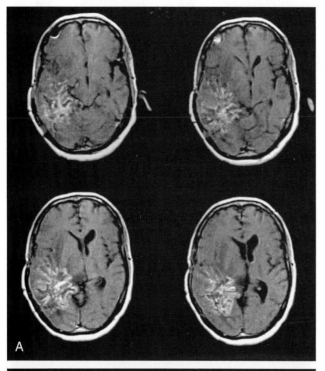

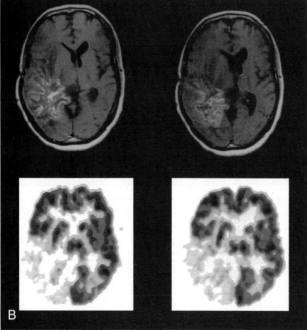

Figure 24–9 Images of a 51-year-old man with anaplastic astrocytoma and radiation necrosis, 2 years after interstitial brachytherapy and external beam irradiation. *A,* Transaxial gadolinium-enhanced MRI shows extensive irregular enhancement in right temporo-occipital lobes. *B,* On FDG PET scan, marked glucose hypometabolism is seen in regions of gadolinium enhancement.

inversely proportional to the number of fractions or the time during which the radiation is administered.[89, 90] However, it is an idiosyncratic phenomenon that cannot be predicted or always explained on the basis of dose, distribution, and fractionation of the radiotherapy. The pathologic injury of radiation necrosis is mainly confined to white matter, whereas with chemonecrosis the gray matter is also affected, and blood vessels undergo fibrinoid necrosis.[91] Furthermore, the pathologic diagnosis of recurrent tumor vs. radiation necrosis is problematic, because both viable and necrotic cells are generally found in tissue specimens removed from radionecrotic areas. Unequivocal evidence of tumor recurrence depends on the presence of pseudopalisading about necrotic areas.[91] Di Chiro and colleagues first reported that FDG PET was able to differentiate hypometabolic radiation necrosis (Fig. 24–9B) and chemonecrosis from recurrent hypermetabolic tumor.[92, 93] Doyle and colleagues and Valk and associates reported similar findings in patients with malignant gliomas who had been treated with interstitial brachytherapy.[62, 94] Valk and co-workers also compared the PET result with clinical outcome and found an overall accuracy of 84%. In aggressive treatment protocols that deliver high doses of radiation locally (e.g., gamma knife therapy and brachytherapy), necrosis is regarded as an expected therapeutic effect rather than as a complication of treatment.[78]

Special Tumors

A number of rarer brain tumors have distinctive neuropathologic features and are now included in the latest classification of brain tumors, but the functional and anatomic characteristics of these tumors are only now being described.[48]

GANGLIOGLIOMA

These tumors are composed of well-differentiated but atypical neuronal elements and neoplastic glia. They are slow growing, although they occasionally undergo anaplastic change.[66] They occur at any age, and although they are commonly found in the temporal lobes—where they can produce refractory epilepsy—they may occur anywhere in the neuraxis. The tumors may be solid or cystic and contain areas of calcification.[54] Castillo and colleagues reported that temporal lobe tumors were generally solid.[54] In a large series reported by Zentner and associates, enhancement on MRI was found in 16 of 36 patients.[55] On FDG PET these tumors are hypometabolic (Fig. 24–10A), which is consistent with their behavior but in contrast to that of pilocytic astrocytomas.

PILOCYTIC ASTROCYTOMA

The pilocytic astrocytoma is regarded as a low-grade astrocytoma with a good prognosis.[66] Pilocytic astrocytomas occur in a younger age group than do astrocytomas, and they are most commonly seen in the midline cerebellum and the hypothalamus, less frequently in the optic nerves and the brainstem; when found in the cerebral hemispheres they usually occur in the temporal lobes.[66] Fulham and co-workers recently reported functional and structural imaging (CT and MRI) results in five patients with pilocytic astrocytomas

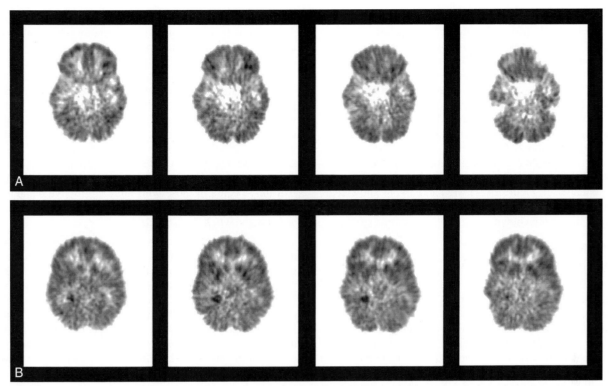

Figure 24–10 *A,* Transaxial FDG PET scans of a 47-year-old man with a 21-year history of epilepsy and a biopsy-proven right anteromesial temporal lobe ganglioglioma, which is markedly hypometabolic. MRI with Gd-DTPA, not shown, showed avid contrast enhancement. *B,* A 27-year-old woman with a 20-year history of complex partial seizures with focus of markedly increased glucose metabolism in right hippocampus (video EEG monitoring showed no seizure during scan). The lesion enhanced avidly after contrast on MRI (not shown).

in which glucose metabolism was significantly higher than that in low-grade astrocytomas (see Fig. 24–10*B*) and was similar to that found in anaplastic astrocytomas.[37] On structural imaging, all tumors enhanced avidly after contrast, but little surrounding edema was noted. Given the usual interpretation of glucose hypermetabolism, these data suggested that the prognosis for pilocytic astrocytomas was not benign.[11, 79] These results provoke important questions:

1. Does a subset of patients with aggressive pilocytic astrocytomas exist?

2. Conversely, do these findings invalidate the FDG PET assessment of brain tumors and violate the general principles used in this evaluation (i.e., that low-grade tumors have reduced glucose metabolism and that high-grade tumors are hypermetabolic)?

3. Do these data reveal an important exception to these principles and reflect a biologic peculiarity in pilocytic tumors?

Fulham and colleagues reported that the condition of all patients was stable and that they showed no evidence of disease progression after a long follow-up period despite evidence of high tumoral glucose metabolism and contrast enhancement on MRI, which indicated that the tumors were behaving in a benign fashion. However, for the following reasons, it is apparent that pilocytic astrocytomas are enigmatic tumors:

1. Although regarded as benign, pilocytic astrocytomas may undergo malignant degeneration and metastasize many years after the original diagnosis.[95–99]

2. High proliferative indices, using Ki-67 labeling, and chromosomal abnormalities that are usually seen in high-grade tumors have been reported in pilocytic astrocytomas.[100–103]

3. Based on morphologic criteria, which correlate well with clinical outcome, pilocytic astrocytomas would be incorrectly classified as aggressive tumors by the Daumas-Duport grading system.[47]

4. The blood vessels of pilocytic astrocytomas have poorly developed tight junctions in their vascular endothelium, which explains the intense enhancement on structural imaging studies; but such vessels are also usually found in malignant tumors.[104, 105]

Although the mechanism for the paradoxical increase in glucose utilization in these tumors was unexplained, the authors speculated that it was related to expression of the glucose transporter.[106–109] It is important to recognize that the occurrence of a combination of intense gadolinium enhancement on MRI in a hypermetabolic tumor with little surrounding edema in the appropriate anatomic location in a younger patient does not always signify a high-grade tumor; pathologic confirmation is needed for accurate prognosis.

DYSEMBRYOPLASTIC NEUROEPITHELIAL TUMOR

Dysembryoplastic neuroepithelial tumors were first identified in tissue resected from patients with refractory epilepsy and reported by Daumas-Duport and associates in 1988.[110] The pathologic, clinical, and radiologic characteristics of the "simple" and "complex" forms of these tumors can be found in a review by Daumas-Duport.[111] The main features are: (1) cortical location; (2) nodular architecture, with nodules that look like astrocytoma, oligodendroglioma, or oligoastrocytoma; (3) foci of dysplastic cortex; and (4) presence of a "glioneuronal" element arranged in columns perpendicular to the cortex. Patients typically have longstanding epilepsy, and MRI shows the involved cortex to be expanded and hyperintense on T2-weighted images. In the complex forms, the large cortical nodules may appear to be located in white matter. In Figure 24–11 MRI and, to our knowledge, the first FDG PET description of a dysembryoplastic neuroepithelial tumor are shown.

PLEOMORPHIC XANTHOASTROCYTOMA

In 1979, Kepes and co-workers described the histologic and clinical features of pleomorphic xanthoastrocytomas.[112] Pleomorphic xanthoastrocytomas are characterized by a superficial location, often involving the meninges, and pleomorphic, lipid-laden, glial fibrillary acid protein–positive neoplastic cells that are associated with an abundant reticulin network. Young adults are affected most often. The tumors are usually found in the temporal lobes and, less commonly, in frontal and parietal lobes.[66] Until recently, all tumors had been found in the supratentorial compartment, but cerebellar pleomorphic xanthoastrocytomas in two patients have been described.[113, 114] Interestingly, in both cases, the cerebellar tumors appeared more than a decade after an earlier pleomorphic xanthoastrocytoma had been removed. Pleomorphic xanthoastrocytomas enhance avidly on CT and MRI.[115–117] A

single report has been published of FDG PET findings in a 19-year-old man with a recurrent pleomorphic xanthoastrocytoma.[115] The tumor recurred 10 and 15 months after the original subtotal resection, and on each occasion recurrence was associated with clinical and radiologic deterioration. The tumor was hypermetabolic relative to white matter, and peak glucose utilization in the lesion was similar to that seen in anaplastic astrocytomas[37, 115]; this is consistent with the clinical behavior of the tumor, although necrosis and mitoses were not seen in the original specimen. Further FDG PET studies are required to determine if all pleomorphic xanthoastrocytomas demonstrate increased glucose utilization or if it only occurs in those with more aggressive behavior.

GLIOMATOSIS CEREBRI

Nevin first used the term *gliomatosis cerebri* to describe a diffuse overgrowth of the nervous system with neoplastic glia in 1938.[118] Russell and Rubinstein regard it as an example of a diffuse astrocytoma.[66] The lesion has been reported in all age groups and has a peak incidence in the fifth decade. It is notoriously difficult to diagnose because the initial symptoms are vague or nonspecific. Seizures, headache, and focal neurologic signs typically appear late in the course of the disease. The white matter is usually extensively infiltrated with bland neoplastic astrocytes, but it can occasionally be confined to gray matter. The neoplastic cells have a proliferative potential similar to that of low-grade gliomas.[119] Both CT and MRI underestimate the extent of the disease.[120, 121] There have been two PET reports of patients with gliomatosis cerebri. Mineura and colleagues used [¹¹C]methionine-PET in a 32-year-old patient with bilateral gray and white matter involvement of the temporo-occipital lobes. Extensive areas of abnormal [¹¹C]methionine uptake

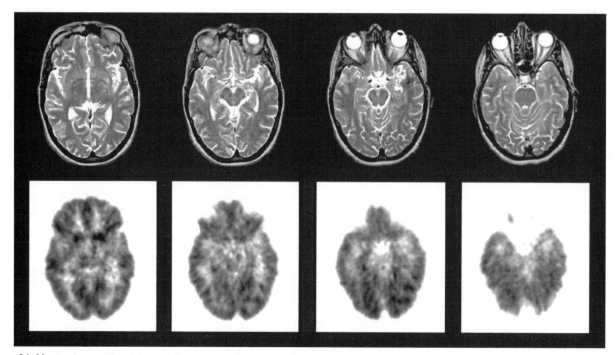

Figure 24–11   Registered T2-weighted MRI *(top)* and FDG PET scans *(bottom)* in a 30-year-old woman with long-standing complex partial seizures and a complex form of dysembryoplastic neuroepithelial tumor. MRIs show thickened left mesial temporal gyrus with nodular regions of hyperintensity. Lesion on FDG PET shows heterogeneous glucose metabolism with areas of normal and reduced glucose metabolism.

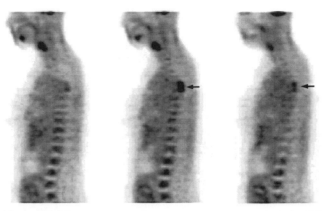

Figure 24–12 Sagittal FDG PET scans done with whole-body PET tomography. Tumor in midthoracic cord *(arrow)* is hypermetabolic to surrounding cord, which is consistent with an aggressive tumor.

corresponded to signal intensity changes on MRI.[122] Dexter and associates reported FDG PET and MRI findings in a 16-year-old girl who presented with an isolated third nerve palsy as the initial manifestation of gliomatosis cerebri, which was largely confined to gray matter.[123] The tumoral involvement was hypometabolic on FDG PET, consistent with a low-grade tumor.

SPINAL CORD TUMORS

The availability of PET tomographs with wide apertures allow functional imaging of the spinal cord. Few data exist on the role of PET in the evaluation of spinal cord tumors.[124, 125] The small studies reported by Di Chiro and co-workers and Alavi and colleagues were performed with early generation PET devices, but the improved PET instrumentation that is now available may allow the noninvasive grading of spinal tumors and also may be used to assess response to therapy and to detect radiation necrosis. An example is shown in Figure 24–12 of a spinal cord tumor in a 25-year-old woman who had development of progressive paraparesis in the last trimester of pregnancy. She had had Lhermitte's sign for many years, but it had become much more frequent during her pregnancy. In the latter half of her pregnancy she noticed increasing difficulty walking and a spastic paraparesis was found on examination at week 36. The FDG PET

scan was done after an elective cesarean section. Pathologic examination revealed an anaplastic ependymoma.

Other PET Ligands

A variety of other PET ligands have been used to evaluate glioma biology (Table 24–1). Glioma oxygen metabolism has been studied with PET. Rhodes and associates showed that gliomas extract a lower fraction of oxygen than normal brain, which suggests that gliomas are adequately oxygenated.[126] Rottenberg and co-workers also demonstrated with [¹¹C]-dimethyl-2,4-oxazolidinedione-PET that, surprisingly, the pH of brain tumors was more alkaline than that of normal brain.[127] This was later confirmed with phosphorus MR spectroscopy.[128] However, after FDG, the greatest effort in neuro-oncologic PET has been focused on the measurement of cerebral protein synthesis in animals and humans.[129, 130] The measurement of tumoral protein synthesis has been attempted with a number of tracers, and the largest experience has been obtained with [¹¹C]methionine.[50, 131–136]

AMINO ACID TRANSPORT

In early work [¹¹C]methionine-PET was compared to CT and MRI without Gd-DTPA and was found to be better at delineating the tumor margin, particularly for low-grade gliomas.[50, 132, 137] But it is apparent from subsequent studies that [¹¹C]methionine-PET is unable to differentiate low- from high-grade tumors on an individual basis.[134, 136] Ogawa and colleagues reported the largest series thus far; in 2 of 15 patients with low-grade astrocytomas, methionine did not accumulate in the tumors, and tumor identified with PET beyond the structural abnormality on CT could only be confirmed pathologically in half of the cases.[136] Furthermore, [¹¹C]methionine-PET is not able to separate recurrent tumor from radiation necrosis,[138] and uptake has been reported in a brain abscess.[139] The mechanism of [¹¹C]methionine uptake seems to be related mainly to a saturable process (capillary transport) rather than to increased amino acid requirements for protein synthesis. Weinhard and associates reported the PET findings with [¹⁸F]fluorotyrosine (F-Tyr) uptake, as compared with that of FDG and ⁶⁸Ga-EDTA, in 13 patients with gliomas.[140] Low-grade astrocytomas were confirmed in

TABLE 24–1
PET LIGANDS IN NEURO-ONCOLOGY

PET Radiotracer/Receptor Ligand	Ligand (Half-Life)	Biologic Parameter
(¹⁸F)fluorodeoxyglucose (¹⁸F)fluoromisonidazole (¹⁸F)fluorotyrosine	¹⁸F (~110 min)	Glucose metabolism Tissue hypoxia Amino acid transport
(¹¹C)methionine (¹¹C)PK 1195 (¹¹C)thymidine (¹¹C)putrescine (¹¹C)tyrosine (¹¹C)dimethyl-2,4-oxazolidinedione	¹¹C (~20 min)	Amino acid transport Peripheral benzodiazepine receptors Cellular proliferation (?) Integrity of blood-brain barrier Amino acid transport pH
¹⁵O-water ⁸²Rb (rubidium) ⁶⁸Ga (gallium)-EDTA	¹⁵O (~2 min) ⁸²Rb (~76 sec) ⁶⁸Ga (~68 min)	Cerebral blood flow Integrity of blood-brain barrier Integrity of blood-brain barrier

3 of 5 patients, anaplastic astrocytomas were found in 2 and glioblastomas multiforme in 5 of 6 patients. They found increased F-Tyr uptake in most tumors irrespective of grade. Kinetic analysis of the data also revealed that the F-Tyr tumoral accumulation was due to increased amino acid transport rather than to irreversible incorporation into proteins. [¹¹C]Putrescine was proposed as a tracer for tumoral DNA synthesis in the late 1980s, since putrescine serves as a precursor to the polyamines spermidine and spermine, and increased polyamine metabolism is associated with malignancy.[141] However, subsequent studies revealed that [¹¹C]putrescine was merely a good tracer to depict blood-brain barrier (BBB) disruption.[142, 143] Preliminary data with 2-[¹¹C]thymidine-PET have recently been published.[144] [¹¹C]Thymidine is attractive because ³H- or ¹⁴C-labeled thymidine incorporation into DNA on autoradiography have been used to evaluate cellular proliferation.[145] Vander Borght and co-workers noted 2-[¹¹C]thymidine uptake in gliomas, regardless of grade, and benign meningiomas.[144] The mechanism of uptake is unclear, and whether uptake reflects disruption of the blood-brain barrier or incorporation into DNA is unresolved. However, based on current data, it appears unlikely to be of clinical value.

TISSUE HYPOXIA

It is a general principle in radiation oncology that tumor cells that are irradiated under normal oxygen tensions are more sensitive to low linear energy transfer (LET) ionizing radiation than hypoxic tumor cells.[146–148] Animal data support hypoxic radioresistance in experimental and animal tumors, but human data are few.[149, 150] Demonstration of tumor hypoxia in vivo in humans is not a simple task, and it requires the invasive placement of oxygen electrodes into the tumor[151]; however, tumor hypoxia has been reported in untreated patients with gliomas.[152] Despite these difficulties, considerable research effort has been directed at altering the tumor milieu with chemical radiosensitizers and with bioreductive agents in hopes of improving cell kill with radiotherapy. Valk and colleagues reported the noninvasive depiction of tissue hypoxia with PET [¹⁸F]fluoromisonidazole (FMISO) in three patients with high-grade gliomas.[153] Yang and associates have also recently reported the development of [¹⁸F]fluoro-erythronitroimidazole, which is cheaper and more hydrophilic than FMISO.[154] Misonidazole and fluoromisonidazole have high electron affinity and are selectively reduced and incorporated into viable hypoxic cells. In the report of Valk and co-workers, marked FMISO uptake was seen in two patients (anaplastic astrocytoma, glioblastoma multiforme), and in the third patient (glioblastoma multiforme) there was no tracer uptake. These data are preliminary and results from a larger number of patients are needed, but they suggest that PET ligands that depict hypoxia might be useful in the selection of patients for treatment with radiosensitizing agents. In addition, the clinical utility of these ligands could then be measured against tumor radiation response.

PERIPHERAL BENZODIAZEPINE RECEPTORS

Experimental evidence suggests that benzodiazepines may regulate glial cell proliferation via the peripheral benzodiaze-pine receptors,[155] and experimental and postmortem human studies have shown a high density of peripheral benzodiazepine receptor binding sites in brain tumors, which suggests their potential use as a marker of cell density in human gliomas.[156–161] Two peripheral benzodiazepine receptor ligands, Ro 5-4864 and PK 11195, have been labeled with ¹¹C and used in human PET studies.[162] Junck and co-workers reported, as had other investigators,[163] that no specific binding to astrocytomas took place with [¹¹C]Ro 5-4864.[162] Evidence was found, however, of [¹¹C]PK 11195 uptake in human gliomas,[162] but definitive evidence of the specificity of its binding to tumoral peripheral benzodiazepine receptor was not provided.[164] Later, Pappata and colleagues found specific tumor binding in a single patient with [¹¹C]PK 11195.[164] In the small series of Junck and associates (nine patients), no meaningful data regarding tumor grading were obtained. Unfortunately, increased peripheral benzodiazepine receptor binding is also found in ischemic and inflammatory lesions,[161, 165] which suggests that [¹¹C]PK 11195 may not be useful in separating recurrent tumor from radiation necrosis. In the final analysis, therefore, few, if any, PET ligands are as valuable as FDG for patient management on an individual basis.[166]

Cerebellar Diaschisis

"Crossed" cerebellar diaschisis is an interesting physiologic phenomenon that is commonly seen in patients with gliomas. It refers to a reduction in blood flow and glucose metabolism in the cerebellar hemisphere contralateral to (or "crossed" from) the supratentorial lesion (Fig. 24–13). The term *diaschisis* was first introduced by Von Monakow in 1910 to describe a "state of reduced or abolished function . . . after a brain injury and acting on a neural region remote from the lesion."[167, 168] Diaschisis was first imaged in 1980 when Baron and co-workers reported "cerebellar diaschisis" to denote a reduction in contralateral cerebellar hemispheric blood flow and oxygen utilization, using ¹⁵O PET, in patients with supratentorial infarction.[169] Their observation was confirmed by others and was extended to patients with cerebral gliomas for blood flow (with ¹⁵O PET) and for glucose metabolism (with FDG PET).[76–79] The mechanism for this phenomenon appears to be an interruption of the corticopontocerebellar (CPC) pathway. The CPC pathway arises from all lobes of the cerebral hemispheres but with major inputs from prefrontal cortex, sensorimotor cortex, and occipital lobes.[169, 170] The CPC pathway has its first synapse in the pons, and second-order neurons then cross to the contralateral cerebellar hemisphere via the middle cerebellar peduncle to terminate in the cerebellar cortex.[171] Fulham and colleagues recently demonstrated with FDG PET in brain tumor patients that there is ipsilateral pontine glucose hypometabolism in cerebellar diaschisis consistent with this hypothesis, and also that there is relative preservation of glucose metabolism in the dentate nucleus of the hypometabolic cerebellar hemisphere.[170] Cerebellar diaschisis does not appear to have a clinical accompaniment and can be seen with any supratentorial injury (e.g., tumor, stroke, or trauma). Its time course is variable,[172] and reversibility has been noted in stroke; but in patients with brain tumors and a fixed deficit

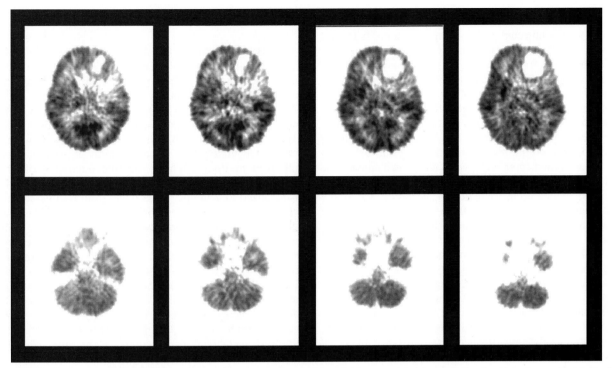

Figure 24–13   Transaxial FDG PET scans in a woman with a left frontal lobe glioblastoma and right cerebellar diaschisis show reduction in glucose metabolism in right cerebellar hemisphere.

induced by a tumor, the cerebellar diaschisis is often persistent.

Corticosteroids and Cerebral Glucose Metabolism

Corticosteroids are commonly administered, often for prolonged periods, for the symptomatic relief of cerebral edema in patients with brain tumors. Common consequences of long-term corticosteroid therapy include centripetal obesity with cushingoid facies, abdominal striae, disordered sleep patterns, and neuropsychiatric disturbances that range from mild behavioral changes to major psychoses.[173, 174] Adrenal glucocorticoids are known to affect cell glucose utilization throughout the body, and experimental studies have shown an effect on brain glucose utilization; but the mechanism for neuropsychiatric abnormalities in patients receiving long-term corticosteroid therapy is unclear.[175, 176] Fulham and associates recently reported a marked reduction in cerebral glucose metabolism in brain tumor patients who had cushingoid features after prolonged exogenous corticosteroid administration, which may provide insights into the neuropsychiatric effects of corticosteroids.[43] They measured cerebral glucose metabolism with FDG PET in 45 patients (56 studies) with unilateral gliomas. Patients were divided into the following groups: (1) Patients with cushingoid features who had been treated with combinations of radiotherapy and chemotherapy. (2) Patients not taking dexamethasone but treated with radiotherapy. (3) Patients not taking dexamethasone who had not been treated with radiotherapy. They found a significant reduction in cerebral glucose metabolism in the cushingoid patients when compared with normal vol-

unteers and the other two patient groups. In addition, serial FDG PET scans were done in eight patients, and a progressive reduction in glucose metabolism was seen over time. In one patient, administration of steroids was stopped, and a concomitant increase in cerebral glucose metabolism was seen. This reduction in glucose metabolism was not a reflection of tumor infiltration or cerebral atrophy, and it was independent of radiotherapy, concurrent anticonvulsant medication, and transhemispheric functional disconnection (transhemispheric diaschisis).[38, 39] The mechanism for dexamethasone-induced cerebral glucose hypometabolism is unclear, but the authors speculate that it may be due to a direct effect on neurons and neuroglia or mediated via glucose transport.

MAGNETIC RESONANCE SPECTROSCOPY

Background

Magnetic resonance spectroscopy is a procedure by which nuclear MR signals are obtained from nuclei that are constituents of molecules other than water. This chapter does not attempt to explain the detailed physics of MR; instead, our aim is to provide sufficient data to appreciate the factors involved in the practical use of MRS. A number of reviews of MRS are available for interested readers.[128, 177–185]

In routine clinical MRI the signal used to create the image arises from water proton nuclei (¹H). In MRS the signals are much weaker and are generated by nonradioactive nuclei that are parts of other solutes or metabolites. Nonwater ¹H, ³¹P, and ¹³C are the most important nuclei for biology. These nuclei can be made to produce electronic signals in a receiving coil when subjected to a strong magnetic field and irradiated with radiofrequency energy. The signals are analyzed to reveal the frequencies present. The analysis involves Fourier transformation, which causes the radiofrequencies emitted by the sample of interest to appear as peaks on a plot of signal intensity against signal frequency, thus producing an NMR spectrum (Fig. 24–14). The horizontal or frequency axes are normalized to the frequency of a strong signal of known origin, and the location of peaks are given as parts per million (ppm) relative to the known signal. The signal strength (the vertical axis) is proportional to a number of factors, including the number of nuclei in the tissue volume being studied. Signals from different isotopes are distinguishable because they occur at different frequencies in any given magnetic field, and nuclear signals from different solutes can also be separated from one another by the property of "chemical shift." Chemical shift refers to the fact that within a molecule containing magnetic nuclei, the electron clouds in the chemical bonds change the local magnetic field strength, so that nuclei of the same species spin at different frequencies. Thus, the three phosphorus nuclei in ATP all spin at different frequencies from one another as well as from phosphorus nuclei in phosphocreatine (PCr) and in inorganic phosphate (P_i) (see Fig. 24–14).

MRS signals are weak because the solutes that produce them occur in low concentrations, in the order of 0.5 mM. The impact of these weak signals is that MRS has poorer sensitivity and resolution when compared with the signal from water ^{1}H in clinical MRI. The low signal strength in MRS therefore means that some solutes cannot be measured with MRS. For instance, virtually all neurotransmitters with the exception of glutamate, glutamine, and γ-aminobutyric acid, are beyond detection with MRS. In addition, molecular motion is required for a solute to be detected with MRS, and most macromolecules (e.g., myelin, proteins, nucleosides, phospholipids) are inaccessible because of their limited mobility. Both ^{31}P and ^{1}H-MRS have been used in the evaluation of brain tumors, but the discussion in this section pertains only to the application of ^{1}H-MRS, which has an inherently stronger signal, better resolution, and greater sensitivity than ^{31}P-MRS.

In ^{1}H-MRS there are four brain metabolites of interest: N-acetyl-aspartate, which occurs at 2.02 ppm; choline-containing compounds (Cho), which occur at 3.20 ppm; creatine-containing compounds (Cre), which occur at 3.93 and 3.04 ppm; and lactate (Lac), which occurs at 1.33 ppm. N-acetyl-aspartate was first discovered in the CNS in 1957 by Tallan.[186] It is found only in the CNS. Its role is uncertain, but it may function as a storage form of aspartate and be involved in lipid synthesis and the regulation of protein synthesis.[187, 188] Simmons and co-workers confirmed that it is localized to neurons.[189] The signal from choline-containing compounds includes contributions from phosphorylcholine, glycerophosphorylcholine, and choline, which are components of phospholipid metabolism and are all well represented in cell membranes. Thus, increased choline signal intensity may reflect increased membrane synthesis and cellularity.[187, 190, 191] The creatine signal intensity includes creatine and phosphocreatine, which provide reserves of high- and low-energy phosphates in the cytosol and are used for cellular, synthetic, and transport functions.[187] Lactate is the terminal metabolite of glycolysis within the cytosol and the initial substrate for the mitochondrial tricarboxylic acid cycle.[192] In Figure 24–15 ^{1}H-MRS spectra from a patient with a low-grade astrocytoma are shown. The top spectrum is from a single voxel (27 cm^3) placed in the hemisphere contralateral to the tumor, and the bottom spectrum shows the reduction in N-acetyl-aspartate signal intensity, presence of lactate, and slight elevation of choline signal in the astrocytoma.

Technical Factors

MRS places more stringent demands on the quality and strength of the magnetic field than does clinical MRI. Clinical MRI can be performed quite satisfactorily at 0.5 Tesla (T), but stronger fields are needed for MRS. Most current MRS work is being performed at 1.5 to 2.0 T, with some experimental studies done at 4.0 T. Signal-to-noise ratios are improved at higher field strengths. Good magnetic field homogeneity is critical for MRS, and poor field homogeneity manifests as difficulty in distinguishing signals from one another and from noise. "Shimming" is used to make small, empirically determined field corrections to optimize field homogeneity. Much research was spent in the early 1980s to refine techniques for localizing the solute signals from a defined volume of interest.[177] In the late 1980s, MRS data were obtained from cubic or rectangular volumes of interest of varying volumes, usually greater than 12 cm^3, using a variety of localization methods.[192–195] These methods have acronyms such as ISIS, PRESS, and STEAM.[177] All of these methods employ some technique to suppress the unwanted signal from water ^{1}H and from mobile lipids in the scalp and the skull.[196] Single-voxel methods have a number of limitations: (1) there is no image, only a spectrum is provided; (2) the measurement of metabolites is influenced by partial volume effects; and (3) the early studies often took up to 2 hours for acquisition of lesion and control volumes.[192] A major improvement was seen with the introduction of

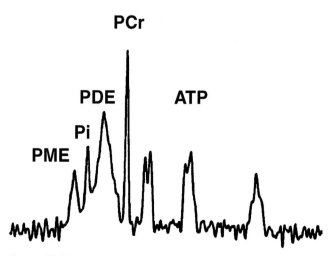

Figure 24-14 ^{31}P MRS spectrum in normal volunteer shows peaks detected.

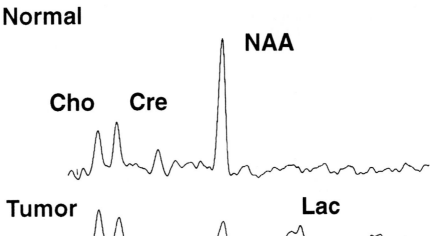

Figure 24–15 ¹H-MRS spectra from uninvolved normal hemisphere (*top*), and tumor (*bottom*) in a 28-year-old woman with a low-grade astrocytoma. Tumor spectrum shows decreased *N*-acetyl-aspartate, increased choline, and elevated lactate signal intensities.

spectroscopic imaging or "chemical shift imaging" methods, which used gradient-based phase-encoding to resolve two of the spatial dimensions. These methods permitted the simultaneous acquisition of spectra from a large number of voxels within a slice of tissue.[197–200] Spectra from multiple voxels from a normal volunteer are shown in Figure 24–16. The metabolite signal intensities can then be displayed in a tomographic format with a volume resolution of about 1 cm³.[201–203]

The first ¹H spectroscopic imaging (¹H-MRSI) studies were limited to a number of voxels, but Fulham and colleagues reported spectroscopic imaging in 50 brain tumor patients using a single-slice technique.[203] The slice had a thickness of 15 mm and comprised a 32 × 32 matrix to provide an array of 1,024 ¹H spectra, in which each spectrum was produced by the nuclei in a voxel, the volume of which was 0.8 cm³. The study duration was about an hour. Single-slice metabolite maps of patients with low- and high-grade gliomas are shown in Figures 24–17 and 24–18. A further improvement has been the introduction of a multi-slice tech-

nique by Duyn and associates.[204] Their method provides four oblique or transaxial slices with a section thickness of 13 mm, and in-plane resolution of 12 mm without time, resolution, or signal-to-noise penalties. Thus, four slices are obtained in under 1 hour, and the technique offers major advantages for the evaluation of tumor heterogeneity and the advancing edge of the tumor.

Clinical Application

Most ¹H-MRS studies, single-voxel and single-slice spectroscopic imaging, have addressed the standard questions of an imaging modality that evaluates patients with brain tumors: tumor grading, assessment of tumor response, and differentiation of radiation necrosis from recurrent tumor.[192, 193, 201–203, 205–209] Thus far, there are few reported studies using multi-slice spectroscopic imaging. The hypotheses that have been tested include the following:

1. Tumor grade correlates with the presence of lactate sig-

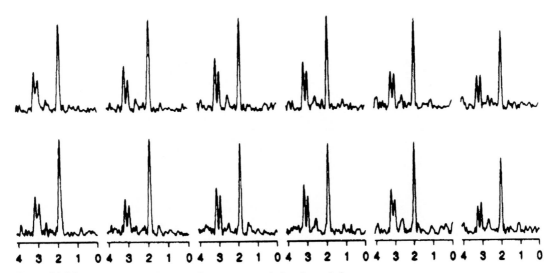

Figure 24–16 Multiple ¹H-MRS spectra from spectroscopic imaging technique.

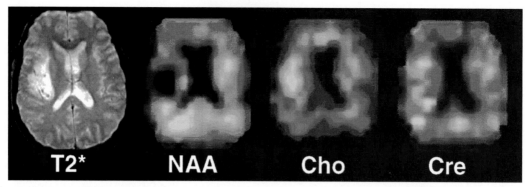

Figure 24–17 Single-slice ¹H-MRSI metabolite maps in a 45-year-old woman with a low-grade astrocytoma. Hyperintense lesion in region of right insula and temporal lobe (T2∗ scan accentuates field inhomogeneities). *N*-acetyl-aspartate is markedly reduced in center of lesion with a gradient to normal tissue; choline is increased and creatine is increased only at margins of lesion. Lactate was not detected (map not shown).

nal. Tumors have a derangement of the respiratory control of glycolysis and an increased dependence on inefficient "anaerobic glycolysis" with net production of lactic acid.

2. Because choline signal intensity reflects constituents of membranes, increased choline is correlated with tumor grade.

3. In radiation necrosis, increased choline signal is not found.

4. MRS is able to detect tumor response to various therapies.

The main findings in relation to the four metabolites are as follows: *N*-acetyl-aspartate signal is decreased in all tumors, high- and low-grade, and also in patients with proven radiation necrosis.[203] At the margins of some low-grade gliomas the loss of *N*-acetyl-aspartate signal intensity is less marked, consistent with tumor infiltration of normal tissue. A reduction in *N*-acetyl-aspartate signal intensity is nonspecific for tumor grade and indicates necrosis or replacement of neuronal tissue with tumor. In Figure 24–19, a scatter plot of normalized (to opposite hemisphere) *N*-acetyl-aspartate signal intensity in 48 patients, adapted from Fulham and colleagues,[203] shows the wide variation in this metabolite across tumor grades. Choline signal intensity is increased in the majority of solid brain tumors. Solid high-grade gliomas have higher normalized (to opposite hemisphere) values for choline intensity than solid low-grade gliomas. However, the

normalized choline signal intensity value is not a discriminator of tumor grade in individual cases. Necrotic high-grade lesions have low values for choline signal intensity as indicated in Figure 24–20, which is a scatter plot of choline signal intensity across tumors, in data from Fulham and associates.[203] It is of interest to note that some patients with low-grade astrocytomas do not have increased choline signal intensity despite a reduction in *N*-acetyl-aspartate signal intensity. An example is shown in Figure 24–21 from a multislice ¹H-MRSI study. The reason for this is uncertain, and work in this area continues, but it may represent a very early stage in a glioma or be related to a particular histologic type. A progressive increase in choline signal as a tumor undergoes malignant degeneration has also been reported.[203] The NIH group also found a reduction in choline signal intensity after radiotherapy and in cases of proven radiation necrosis.[203]

Much emphasis has been placed on the detection of lactate with ¹H-MRS in gliomas.[193, 201, 202, 206, 208] Some investigators[201, 202] have stressed the importance of lactate as a potential predictor of malignancy. However, the NIH group[192, 203] found that the presence of lactate was not helpful because the majority of patients in whom lactate signal was detected had been treated, and lactate was also found after surgery and in subacute radiation necrosis. Hence, when lactate is detected in treated tumors it is impossible to establish whether it arises from the tumor per se or reflects an effect

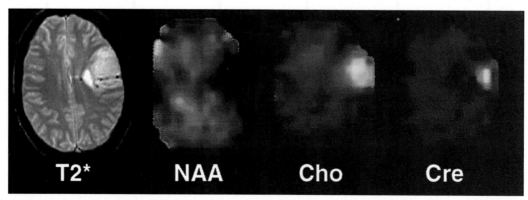

Figure 24–18 Single-slice ¹H-MRSI metabolite maps in a 35-year-old woman with a solid glioblastoma. Hyperintensity is seen in the lesion, with a thin band of hypointensity due to hemosiderin following biopsy. *N*-acetyl-aspartate is reduced and choline is markedly increased compared to surrounding brain. Creatine also increased, but in different distribution to choline.

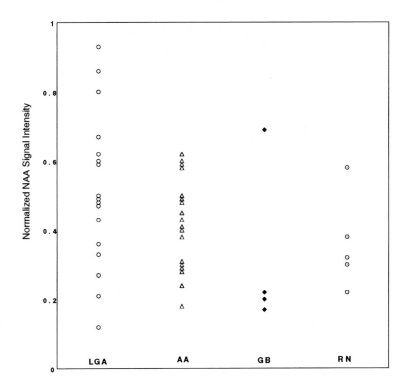

Figure 24–19 Scatter plot of normalized *N*-acetyl-aspartate (NAA) signal intensity values shows considerable variation in NAA levels across the different groups. Abbreviations: LGA = low grade astrocytoma; AA = anaplastic astrocytoma; GB = glioblastoma; RN = radiation necrosis.

of therapy. Similar inconsistencies are found in untreated gliomas. Herholz and co-workers[202] reported lactate signal in 7 of 12 low-grade and only 3 of 6 high-grade untreated gliomas. The findings with creatine signal intensity are also inconsistent. The NIH group found decreased tumoral creatine signal intensities in the majority of patients, but a real increase was seen in about 40% of lesions, mainly at the edge of low-grade tumors.[192, 203] Most studies with ¹H-MRS and

³¹P-MRS have reported normal[205, 210, 211] or decreased[201, 212] creatine/phosphocreatine values. Segebarth and colleagues first suggested the possibility that ¹H-MRSI could detect pathologic tissue before any abnormality was seen with T2-weighted MRI.[205] Their speculation was based on a single unconfirmed case in which a decreased *N*-acetyl-aspartate signal was observed, without changes in choline, in the "contralateral hemisphere" in the region of the sylvian

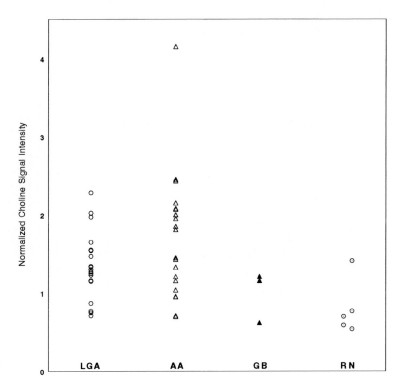

Figure 24–20 Scatter plot of normalized choline signal intensity values shows overlap between low- and high-grade tumors. Lowest value is seen in glioblastoma.

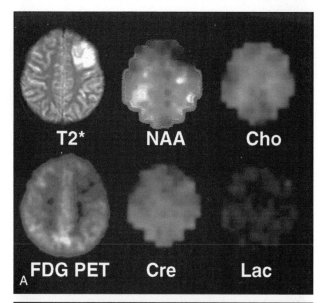

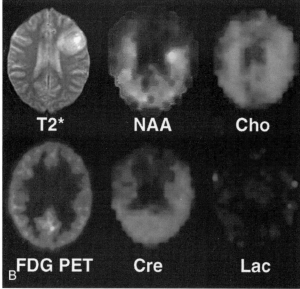

Figure 24–21 Multislice ¹H-MRSI metabolite maps and FDG PET scans in a 28-year-old woman with a low-grade astrocytoma. Two of four slices are shown. *A,* Lesion is clearly seen on MRI and FDG PET scan. *N*-acetyl-aspartate (NAA) is reduced but choline is not markedly elevated; creatine is slightly increased. *B,* NAA is reduced but, again, choline is not markedly increased.

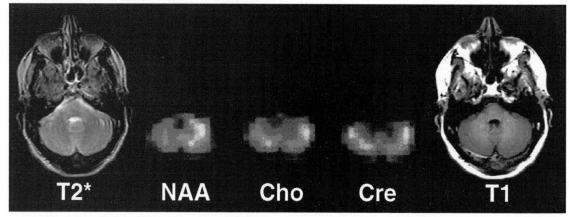

Figure 24–22 Single-slice¹H-MRSI metabolite maps, T2- and T1-weighted MRIs of cerebellum in a 38-year-old man with a 3½-year history of right crossed cerebellar diaschisis. Metabolite maps show a marked reduction in *N*-acetyl-aspartate in right cerebellar hemisphere compared to left. Minimal asymmetry is noted on choline and creatine maps. Atrophy is not seen on MRI.

fissure. The location raises the possibility that the *N*-acetyl-aspartate signal reduction was spurious and due to partial volume effects. Multi-slice ¹H-MRSI coupled with serial stereotactic biopsies should resolve this issue.

Finally, just as with PET, ¹H-MRSI has detected transsynaptic metabolite abnormalities in a single patient with cerebellar diaschisis.[213] Fulham and associates found a marked reduction in *N*-acetyl-aspartate signal intensity and a minimal reduction in choline and creatine signal intensities in the diaschitic cerebellar hemisphere of a patient with a 3.5-year history of cerebellar diaschisis (Fig. 24–22) when compared with normal volunteers. In the seven normal volunteers, choline and creatine were more heavily concentrated in the cortex and *N*-acetyl-aspartate signal was more prominent in white matter of the middle cerebellar peduncles than in the cortex, which suggests a differential distribution and a localization of *N*-acetyl-aspartate in axons rather than in cell bodies.

SUMMARY

Most current MR scanners are sold with spectroscopy capabilities; however, this capability is for single-voxel examinations rather than ¹H-MRSI. Unfortunately, ¹H-MRSI is still limited to a few centers that have the resources and personnel to fine tune the MR hardware and to develop acquisition and analysis software. However, ¹H-MRSI provides functional data that otherwise are limited to PET centers. Although ¹H-MRSI is not the absolute functional surrogate of PET, it is, in our opinion, valuable for the longitudinal evaluation of patients with low-grade gliomas in the detection of malignant degeneration, for the evaluation of treatment response, and for the detection of radiation necrosis. ¹H-MRSI has limitations in evaluating some gliomas in which regional inhomogeneities result from superficial dural clips placed during surgery or from areas of hemorrhage; at present, it provides no more data for tumor grading than does clinical MRI. However, technical developments will shorten data acquisition times and data analysis procedures, which at present are long, cumbersome, and require experienced operators to check validity of spectra. Overall, we think that ¹H-MRSI will provide useful additional information that can be used for clinical management.

ACKNOWLEDGMENT

We wish to thank P.K. Hooper, Chief Technologist, PET Department Royal Prince Alfred Hospital, Sydney, for his expert help with the illustrations for this chapter.

REFERENCES

1. Jaeckle KA: Clinical presentation and therapy of nervous system tumors. *In* Bradley WG, Daroff RB, Fenichel GM, et al (eds): Neurology in Clinical Practice, ed 1, vol 2. Butterworth-Heinemann, Stoneham, Mass, 1991, pp 1008–1030.
2. Shapiro WR, Shapiro JR: Primary brain tumors. *In* Asbury AK, McKhann GM, McDonald WI (eds): Diseases of the Nervous System: Clinical Neurobiology, ed 2, vol 2. Philadelphia, WB Saunders, 1992, pp 1074–1092.
3. Apuzzo MLJ, Chandrasoma PT, Cohen D, et al: Computed imaging stereotaxy: Experience and perspective related to 500 procedures applied to brain masses. Neurosurgery 1987; 20:930–937.
4. Kelly PJ, Daumas-Duport C, Kispert DB, et al: Imaging-based stereotaxic serial biopsies in untreated intracranial glial neoplasms. J Neurosurg 1987; 66:865–874.
5. Kelly PJ: Computer assisted volumetric stereotactic resection of superficial and deep seated intra-axial brain mass lesions. Acta Neurochir 1991; 52:26–29.
6. Kelly PJ: Stereotactic resection and its limitations in glial neoplasms. Stereotact Funct Neurosurg 1992; 59:84–91.
7. Macdonald DR, Cascino TL, Schold SC, et al: Response criteria for phase II studies of supratentorial malignant glioma. J Clin Oncol 1990; 8:1277–1280.
8. Jaeckle KA: Neuroimaging for central nervous system tumors. Semin Oncol 1991; 18:150–157.
9. Byrne TN: Imaging of gliomas. Semin Oncol 1994; 21:162–171.
10. Di Chiro G, DeLaPaz R, Brooks RA, et al: Glucose utilization of cerebral gliomas measured by [18F]fluorodeoxyglucose and positron emission tomography. Neurology 1982; 32:1323–1329.
11. Di Chiro G: Positron emission tomography using [18F]fluorodeoxyglucose in brain tumors: A powerful diagnostic and prognostic tool. Invest Radiol 1987; 22:360–371.
12. Fulham MJ: PET with [18F]fluorodeoxyglucose (PET-FDG): An indispensable tool in the proper management of brain tumors. *In* Hubner KF, Collmann J, Buonocore E, et al (eds): Clinical Positron Emission Tomography. St Louis, Mosby–Year Book, 1992, pp 50–60.
13. Gruber ML, Hochberg FH: Systematic evaluation of primary brain tumors (editorial). J Nucl Med 1990; 31:969–971.
14. Kondziolka D, Lunsford LD, Martinez AJ: Unreliability of contemporary neurodiagnostic imaging in evaluating suspected adult supratentorial (low-grade) astrocytoma. J Neurosurg 1993; 79:533–536.
15. Biersack HJ, Grunwald F, Kropp J: Single photon emission computed tomography imaging of brain tumors. Semin Nucl Med 1991; 21:2–10.
16. Phelps ME, Hoffman EJ, Mullani NA, et al: Application of annihilation coincidence detection to transaxial reconstruction tomography. J Nucl Med 1975; 16:210–223.
17. Ter-Pogossian MM, Phelps ME, Hoffman EJ, et al: A positron emission transaxial tomograph for nuclear medicine imaging (PETT). Radiology 1975; 114:39–93.
18. Phelps ME, Mazziotta JC: Positron emission tomography: Human brain function and biochemistry. Science 1985; 228:799–809.
19. Kuhl DE, Wagner HN, Alavi A, et al: Positron emission tomography: Clinical status in the United States in 1987. J Nucl Med 1988; 29:1136–1143.
20. Report of the Therapeutics and Technology Assessment Subcommittee of the American Academy of Neurology. Assessment: Positron Emission Tomography. Neurology 1991; 41:163–167.
21. Reivich M, Kuhl D, Wolf A, et al: The [18F]fluorodeoxyglucose method for the measurement of local cerebral glucose utilization in man. Circulation Research 1979; 44:127–137.
22. Phelps ME, Huang SC, Hoffman EJ, et al: Tomographic measurement of local cerebral glucose metabolic rate in humans with [18F]2-fluoro-2-deoxy-D-glucose: Validation of method. Ann Neurol 1979; 6:371–388.
23. Frost JJ, Wagner HN (eds): Quantitative Imaging: Neuroreceptors, Neurotransmitters and Enzymes. New York, Raven Press, 1990, p 199.
24. Weinhard K, Dahlbom M, Eriksson L, et al: The ECAT EXACT HR: Performance of a new high resolution positron scanner. J Comput Assist Tomogr 1994; 18:110–118.
25. Phelps ME: Positron Emission Tomography (PET). *In* Mazziotta JC, Gilman S (eds): Clinical Brain Imaging: Principles and Applications. Philadelphia, FA Davis, 1992, pp 71–107.
26. Sokoloff L, Reivich M, Kennedy C, et al: The 14C-deoxyglucose method for the measurement of local cerebral glucose utilization: Theory procedure and normal values in the conscious and anesthetized albino rat. J Neurochem 1977; 28:897–916.
27. Brooks RA: Alternate formula for glucose utilization using labelled deoxyglucose. J Nucl Med 1982; 23:538–539.
28. Kadekaro M, Vance WM, Terrell ML, et al: Effects of antidromic stimulation of the ventral root on glucose utilization in the ventral horn of the spinal cord in the rat. Proc Natl Acad Sci 1987; 84:5492–5495.

29. Schwartz WJ, Smith CB, Davidsen L, et al: Metabolic mapping of functional activity in the hypothalamo-neurohypophysial system of the rat. Science 1979; 205:723–725.

30. Warburg O: Metabolism of Tumors. London, Arnold & Constable, 1930.

31. Warburg O: On the origin of cancer cells. Science 1956; 123:309–314.

32. Green MV, Seidel J, Stein SD, et al: Head movement in normal subjects during simulated PET brain imaging with and without head movement. J Nucl Med 1994; 35:1538–1546.

33. Fulton RR, Hutton BF, Braun M, et al: Use of 3D reconstruction to correct for patient motion in SPECT. Phys Med Biol 1994; 39:563–574.

34. Eberl S, Kanno I, Fulton RR, et al: An automated inter-study image registration technique for SPECT and PET studies. J Nucl Med 1996; 37:137–145.

35. Hooper PK, Meikle SR, Eberl S, et al: Validation of post injection transmission measurements for attenuation correction in neurologic FDG PET studies. J Nucl Med 1996; 37:128–136.

36. Di Chiro G, Brooks RA: PET-FDG of untreated and treated cerebral gliomas. J Nucl Med 1988; 29:421–422.

37. Fulham MJ, Melisi JW, Nishimiya J, et al: Neuroimaging of juvenile pilocytic astrocytomas: An enigma. Radiology 1993; 189:221–225.

38. Andrews RJ, Bringas JR, Alonzo G, et al: Corpus callosotomy effects on cerebral blood flow and evoked potentials (transcallosal diaschisis). Neurosci Lett 1993; 154:9–12.

39. Andrews RJ: Transhemispheric diaschisis: A review and comment. Stroke 1991; 22:943–949.

40. Ginsberg MD, Castella Y, Dietrich WD, et al: Acute thrombotic infarction suppresses metabolic activation of ipsilateral somatosensory cortex: Evidence for functional diaschisis. J Cereb Blood Flow Metab 1989; 9:329–341.

41. Dauth GW, Gilman S, Frey KA, et al: Basal ganglia glucose utilization after recent precentral ablation in the monkey. Ann Neurol 1985; 17:431–438.

42. Katoaka K, Hayakawa T, Yamada K, et al: Neuronal network disturbance after ischemia in rats. Stroke 1989; 20:1226–1235.

43. Fulham MJ, Brunetti A, Aloj L, et al: Decreased cerebral glucose metabolism in patients with brain tumors: An effect of corticosteroids. J Neurosurg 1995; 83:657–664.

44. Delbeke D, Meyerowitz C, Lapidus RL, et al: Optimal cutoff levels of F-18 fluorodeoxyglucose uptake in the differentiation of low grade from high grade brain tumors with PET. Radiology 1995; 195:47–52.

45. Ringertz N: Grading of gliomas. Acta Pathol Microbiol 1950; 27:51–64.

46. Burger PC, Vogel FS, Green SB: Glioblastoma and anaplastic astrocytoma: Pathologic criteria and prognostic considerations. Cancer 1985; 56:1106–1111.

47. Daumas-Duport C, Scheithauer B, O'Fallon J, et al: Grading of astrocytomas: A simple and reproducible method. Cancer 1988; 62:2152–2165.

48. Kleihues P, Burger PC, Scheithauer BW: The new WHO classification of brain tumours. Brain Pathology 1993; 3:255–268.

49. McCormack BM, Miller DC, Budzilovich GN, et al: Treatment and survival of low-grade astrocytoma in adults: 1977–1988. Neurosurgery 1992; 31:636–642.

50. Lilja A, Bergstrom K, Spannare B, et al: Reliability of computed tomography in assessing histopathological features of malignant supratentorial gliomas. J Comput Assist Tomogr 1981; 5:625–636.

51. Joyce P, Bentson J, Takahashi M, et al: The accuracy of predicting histologic grades of supratentorial astrocytomas on the basis of computerized tomography and cerebral angiography. Neuroradiology 1978; 16:346–348.

52. Butler AR, Horii SC, Kricheff II, et al: Computed tomography in astrocytomas. Radiology 1978; 129:433–439.

53. Leeds NE, Elkin CM, Zimmerman RD: Gliomas of the brain. Semin Roentgenol 1984; 19:27–43.

54. Castillo M, Davis PC, Takei Y, et al: Intracranial ganglioglioma: MR, CT, and clinical findings in 18 patients. AJNR 1990; 11:109–114.

55. Zentner J, Wolf HK, Ostertun B, et al: Gangliogliomas: Clinical, radiological, and histopathological findings in 51 patients. J Neurol Neurosurg Psychiatry 1994; 57:1497–1502.

56. Lee Y-Y, van Tassel P, Bruner JM, et al: Juvenile pilocytic astrocytomas: CT and MR characteristics. AJR 1989; 152:1263–1270.

57. Atlas SW: Intraaxial brain tumors. In Atlas SW (ed): Magnetic Resonance Imaging of the Brain and Spine. New York, Raven Press, 1991, pp 223–326.

57a. Chamberlain MC, Murovic JA, Levin VA: Absence of contrast enhancement on CT brain scans of patients with supratentorial malignant gliomas. Neurology 1988; 39:1371–1374.

58. Kelly PJ, Daumas-Duport C, Scheithauer B, et al: Stereotactic histological correlations of computerized tomography and magnetic resonance imaging-defined abnormalities in patients with glial neoplasms. Mayo Clin Proc 1987; 62:450–459.

59. Kim CK, Alavi JB, Alavi A, et al: New grading system of cerebral gliomas using positron emission tomography with F-18 fluorodeoxyglucose. J Neurooncol 1991; 10:85–91.

60. Alavi JB, Alavi A, Chawluk J, et al: Positron emission tomography in patients with glioma: A predictor of prognosis. Cancer 1988; 62:1074–1078.

61. Coleman RE, Hoffman JM, Hanson MW, et al: Clinical application of PET for the evaluation of brain tumors. J Nucl Med 1991; 32:616–622.

62. Valk PE, Budinger TF, Levin VA, et al: PET of malignant cerebral tumors after interstitial brachytherapy: Demonstration of metabolic activity and clinical outcome. J Neurosurg 1988; 69:830–838.

63. Tyler JL, Diksic M, Villemure J-G, et al: Metabolic and hemodynamic evaluation of gliomas using positron emission tomography. J Nucl Med 1987; 28:1123–1133.

64. Davis WK, Boyko OB, Hoffman JM, et al: [18F]2-fluoro-2-deoxyglucose-positron emission tomography correlation of gadolinium-enhanced MR imaging of central nervous system neoplasia. AJNR 1993; 14:515–523.

65. Melisi JW, Fulham MJ, Patronas N, et al: Comparison of Gd-DTPA enhanced MRI with PET-FDG in assessment of gliomas. Proceedings of the Congress of Neurological Surgeons. Orlando, Fla, 1991, pp 264–266.

66. Russell DS, Rubinstein LJ: Tumours of central neuroepithelial origin. In Russell DS, Rubenstein LJ (eds): Pathology of Tumours of the Nervous System, ed 5. Baltimore, Williams & Wilkins, 1989, pp 83–350.

67. Hanson MW, Glantz MJ, Hoffman JM, et al: FDG-PET in the selection of brain lesions for biopsy. J Comput Assist Tomogr 1991; 15:796–801.

68. Levivier M, Goldman S, Pirotte B, et al: Diagnostic yield of stereotactic brain biopsy guided by positron emission tomography with [18F]fluorodeoxyglucose. J Neurosurg 1995; 82:445–452.

69. Burger PC, Dubois PJ, Schold SC: Computerized tomographic and pathologic studies of untreated, quiescent, and recurrent glioblastoma multiforme. J Neurosurg 1983; 58:159–169.

70. Earnest F, Kelly PJ, Scheithauer BW, et al: Cerebral astrocytomas: Histopathologic correlation of MR and CT contrast enhancement with stereotaxic biopsy. Radiology 1988; 166:823–827.

71. Fazekas JT: Treatment of grades I and II brain astrocytomas: The role of radiotherapy. Int J Radiat Oncol Biol Phys 1977; 2:661–666.

72. Sheline GE: Radiation therapy of brain tumors. Cancer 1977; 39:873–881.

73. Peipmeier JM: Observations on the current treatment of low grade astrocytic tumors of the cerebral hemispheres. J Neurosurg 1987; 67:177–181.

74. Laws ERJ, Taylor WF, Clifton MB, et al: Neurosurgical management of low-grade astrocytoma of the cerebral hemisphere. J Neurosurg 1984; 61:665–673.

75. Cairncross JG: The biology of astrocytomas: Lessons learned from chronic myelogenous leukemia—hypothesis. J Neurooncol 1987; 5:11–27.

76. Cairncross JG: Low grade glioma: To treat or not to treat? Arch Neurol 1989; 46:1238–1239.

77. Francavilla TL, Miletich RS, Di Chiro G, et al: Positron emission tomography in the detection of malignant degeneration of low-grade gliomas. Neurosurgery 1989; 24:1–5.

78. Gutin PH, Leibel SA, Wara WW, et al: Recurrent malignant gliomas: Survival following interstitial brachytherapy with high-activity iodine-125 sources. J Neurosurg 1987; 67:864–873.

79. Patronas NJ, Di Chiro G, Kufta C, et al: Prediction of survival in glioma patients by means of positron emission tomography. J Neurosurg 1985; 62:816–822.

80. Holzer T, Herholz K, Jeske J, et al: FDG PET as a prognostic indicator in radiochemotherapy of glioblastoma. J Comput Assist Tomogr 1993; 17:681–687.

81. Schifter T, Hoffman JM, Hanson MW, et al: Serial FDG PET studies in the prediction of survival in patients with primary brain tumors. J Comput Assist Tomogr 1993; 17:509–516.

82. Glantz MJ, Hoffman JM, Coleman RE, et al: The role of F18 FDG PET imaging in predicting early recurrence of primary brain tumors. Ann Neurol 1991; 29:347–355.

83. Cairncross JG, Pexman JHW, Rathbone MP, et al: Postoperative contrast enhancement in patients with brain tumor. Ann Neurol 1985; 17:570–572.

84. Cairncross JG, Macdonald DR, Pexman JH, et al: Steroid-induced CT changes in patients with recurrent malignant glioma. Neurology 1988; 38:724–726.

85. Hatam A, Bergstrom M, Yu Z-Y, et al: Effect of dexamethasone treatment on volume and contrast enhancement of intracranial neoplasms. J Comput Assist Tomogr 1983; 7:295–300.

86. Muller W, Kretzschmar K, Schicketanz K-H: CT analyses of cerebral tumors under steroid therapy. Neuroradiology 1984; 26:293–298.

87. Crocker EF, Zimmerman RA, Phelps ME, et al: The effect of steroid on the extravascular distribution of radiographic contrast material and technetium pertechnetate in brain tumors as determined by computed tomography. Radiology 1976; 119:471–474.

88. Gerber AM, Savolaine ER: Modification of tumor enhancement and brain edema in computerized tomography by corticosteroids: Case report. Neurosurgery 1980; 6:282–284.

89. Sheline GE, Wara WM, Smithe V: Therapeutic irradiation and brain injury. Int J Radiat Oncol Biol Phys 1980; 6:1215–1228.

90. Marks JE, Wong J: The risk of cerebral radionecrosis in relation to dose, time and fractionation. Prog Exp Tumor Res 1985; 29:210–218.

91. Burger PC, Boyko OB: The pathology of central nervous system radiation injury. *In* Gutin PH, Leibel SA, Sheline GE (eds): Radiation Injury to the Nervous System. New York, Raven Press, 1991, p 482.

92. Patronas NJ, Di Chiro G, Brooks RA, et al: Work in progress: [18F]Fluorodeoxyglucose and positron emission tomography in the evaluation of radiation necrosis of the brain. Radiology 1982; 144:885–889.

93. Di Chiro G, Oldfield E, Wright DC, et al: Cerebral necrosis after irradiation and/or intraarterial chemotherapy for brain tumors: PET and neuropathologic studies. AJNR 1987; 8:1083–1089.

94. Doyle W, Budinger TF, Valk PE, et al: Differentiation of cerebral radiation necrosis from tumor recurrence by [¹⁸F]FDG and ⁸²Rb positron emission tomography. J Comput Assist Tomogr 1987; 11:563–570.

95. Bernell WR, Kepes JJ, Seitz EP: Late malignant recurrence of childhood cerebellar astrocytoma: A report of two cases. J Neurosurg 1972; 37:470–474.

96. Kleinman GM, Schoene WC, Walshe TM, et al: Malignant transformation in benign cerebellar astrocytoma. J Neurosurg 1978; 49:111–118.

97. Kocks W, Kalff R, Reinhardt V, et al: Spinal metastasis of pilocytic astrocytoma of the chiasma opticum. Childs Nerv Syst 1989; 5:118–120.

98. Obana WG, Cogen PH, Davis RL, et al: Metastatic juvenile pilocytic astrocytoma: A case report. J Neurosurg 1991; 75:972–975.

99. Mishima K, Nakamura M, Nakamura H, et al: Leptomeningeal dissemination of cerebellar pilocytic astrocytoma. J Neurosurg 1992; 77:788–791.

100. Murovic JA, Nagashima T, Hoshino T, et al: Pediatric central nervous system tumors: A cell kinetic study with bromodeoxyuridine. Neurosurgery 1986; 19:900–904.

101. Tsanaclis AM, Robert F, Michaud J, et al: The cycling pool of cells within human brain tumors: In situ cytokinetics using the monoclonal antibody Ki-67. Can J Neurol Sci 1991; 18:12–17.

102. Germano IM, Ito M, Cho KG, et al: Correlation of histopathological features and proliferative potential of gliomas. J Neurosurg 1989; 70:701–706.

103. Jenkins RB, Kimmel DW, Moertel CA, et al: A cytogenetic study of 53 gliomas. Cancer Genet Cytogenet 1989; 39:253–279.

104. Long DM: Capillary ultrastructure and the blood brain barrier in human malignant brain tumors. J Neurosurg 1970; 32:127–144.

105. Sato K, Rorke LB: Vascular bundles and wickerworks in childhood brain tumors. Pediatr Neurosci 1989; 15:105–110.

106. Mueckler M, Caruso C, Baldwin S, et al: Sequence and structure of human glucose transporter. Science 1985; 29:941–945.

107. Pessin JE, Bell GI: Mammalian facilitative glucose transporter family: Structure and molecular regulation. Annu Rev Physiol 1992; 54:911–930.

108. Guerin C, Laterra J, Hruban RH, et al: The glucose transporter and blood brain barrier of human brain tumors. Ann Neurol 1990; 28:758–765.

109. Guerin C, Laterra J, Drewes LR, et al: Vascular expression of glucose transporter in experimental brain neoplasms. Am J Pathol 1992; 140:417–425.

110. Daumas-Duport C, Scheithauer BW, Chodkiewicz JP, et al: Dysembryoplastic neuroepithelial tumor: A surgically curable tumor of young patients with intractable partial seizures. Neurosurgery 1988; 23:545–556.

111. Daumas-Duport C: Dysembryoplastic neuroepithelial tumors. Brain Pathology 1993; 3:283–295.

112. Kepes JJ, Rubinstein LJ, Eng LF: Pleomorphic xanthoastrocytoma: A distinctive meningocerebral glioma of young subjects with a relatively favorable prognosis: A study of 12 cases. Cancer 1979; 44:1839–1852.

113. Lindboe CF, Cappelen J, Kepes JJ: Pleomorphic xanthoastrocytoma as a component of a cerebellar ganglioglioma: A case report. Neurosurgery 1992; 31:353–355.

114. Glasser RS, Rojiani AM, Mickle JP, et al: Delayed occurrence of cerebellar pleomorphic xanthoastrocytoma after supratentorial pleomorphic xanthoastrocytoma removal. J Neurosurg 1995; 82:116–118.

115. Bicik I, Raman R, Knightly JJ, et al: PET-FDG of pleomorphic xanthoastrocytoma. J Nucl Med 1995; 36:97–99.

116. Blom RJ: Pleomorphic xanthoastrocytoma. CT appearance. J Comput Assist Tomogr 1988; 12:351–354.

117. Rippe DJ, Boyko OB, Radu M: MRI of temporal lobe pleomorphic xanthoastrocytoma. J Comput Assist Tomogr 1992; 16:856–859.

118. Nevin S: Gliomatosis cerebri. Brain 1938; 61:170–191.

119. Hara A, Sakai N, Yamada H, et al: Assessment of proliferative potential of gliomatosis cerebri. J Neurol 1991; 238:80–82.

120. Koslow SA, Classen D, Hirsch WL, et al: Gliomatosis cerebri: A case report with autopsy correlation. Neuroradiology 1992; 34:331–333.

121. Artigas J, Cervos-Navarro J, Iglesias JR, et al: Gliomatosis cerebri: Clinical and histological findings. Clin Neuropathol 1985; 4:135–148.

122. Mineura K, Sasajima T, Kowada M, et al: Innovative approach in the diagnosis of gliomatosis using carbon-11-L-methionine positron emission tomography. J Nucl Med 1991; 32:726–728.

123. Dexter MA, Parker GD, Besser M, et al: MR and positron emission tomography with fludeoxyglucose F18 in gliomatosis cerebri. AJNR 1995; 16:1507–1510.

124. Di Chiro G, Oldfield E, Bairamian D, et al: Metabolic imaging of the brain stem and spinal cord: Studies with positron emission tomography using 18F-2-deoxyglucose in normal and pathological cases. J Comput Assist Tomogr 1983; 7:937–945.

125. Alavi A, Kramer E, Wegener W, et al: Magnetic resonance and fluorine-18 deoxyglucose imaging in the investigation of a spinal cord tumor. J Nucl Med 1990; 31:360–364.

126. Rhodes CG, Wise RJ, Gibbs JM, et al: In vivo disturbance of the oxidative metabolism of glucose in human cerebral gliomas. Ann Neurol 1983; 14:614–624.

127. Rottenberg DA, Ginos JZ, Kearfott KJ, et al: In vivo measurement of brain tumor pH using [11C]DMO and positron emission tomography. Ann Neurol 1985; 17:70–79.

128. Radda G: The use of NMR spectroscopy for the understanding of disease. Science 1986; 233:640–645.

129. Sokoloff L: Cerebral circulation, energy metabolism, and protein synthesis: General characteristics and principles of measurement. *In* Phelps ME, Mazziotta JC, Schelbert H (eds): Positron Emission Tomography and Autoradiography: Principles and Applications. New York, Raven Press, 1986, pp 1–71.

130. Hawkins RA, Huang SC, Barrio JC, et al: Estimation of local cerebral protein synthesis rates with L-(1-11C)Leucine and PET: Methods, model and results in animals and humans. J Cereb Blood Flow Metab 1989; 9:446–460.

131. Lilja A, Bergstrom M, Hartvig P, et al: Dynamic study of supratentorial gliomas with L-methyl-11C-methionine and positron emission tomography. AJNR 1985; 6:505–514.

132. Ericson K, Lilja A, Bergstrom M, et al: Positron emission tomography with ([11C]methyl)-L-methionine, [11C]D-glucose, and [68Ga]EDTA in supratentorial tumors. J Comput Assist Tomogr 1985; 9:683–689.

133. Bergstrom M, Collins VP, Ehrin E, et al: Discrepancies in brain tumor extent as shown by computed tomography and positron emission

tomography using [68Ga]EDTA, [11C]glucose and [11C]methionine. J Comput Assist Tomogr 1983; 11:1062–1066.

134. Derlon JM, Bourdet C, Bustany P, et al: (11C)ʟ-methionine uptake in gliomas. Neurosurgery 1989; 25:720–728.

135. Schober O, Meyer GJ, Gaab MR, et al: Grading of brain tumors by C-11-ʟ-methionine PET. J Nucl Med 1986; 27:890–891.

136. Ogawa T, Shishido F, Kanno I, et al: Cerebral glioma: Evaluation with methionine PET. Radiology 1993; 186:45–53.

137. Mosskin M, Ericson K, Hindmarsh T, et al: Positron emission tomography compared with magnetic resonance imaging and computed tomography in supratentorial gliomas using multiple stereotactic biopsies as reference. Acta Radiol 1989; 30:225–232.

138. Lilja A, Lundqvist H, Olsson Y, et al: Positron emission tomography and computed tomography in differential diagnosis between recurrent or residual glioma and treatment-induced brain lesions. Acta Radiol 1989; 30:121–128.

139. Ishii K, Ogawa T, Hatazawa J, et al: High ʟ-methyl-[11C]methionine uptake in brain abscess: A PET study. J Comput Assist Tomogr 1993; 17:660–661.

140. Weinhard K, Herholz K, Coenen HH, et al: Increased amino acid transport into brain tumors measured by PET of ʟ-(2-18F)fluorotyrosine. J Nucl Med 1991; 32:1338–1346.

141. Hiesiger E, Fowler JS, Wolf AP, et al: Serial PET studies of human cerebral malignancy with [1-11C]putrescine and [1-11C]2-deoxy-ᴅ-glucose. J Nucl Med 1987; 28:1251–1261.

142. Hiesiger EM, Fowler JS, Logan J, et al: Is [1-11C]putrescine useful as a brain tumor marker? J Nucl Med 1992; 33:192–199.

143. Rottenberg DA: Carbon-11-putrescine: Back to the drawing board (editorial). J Nucl Med 1992; 33:200–201.

144. Vander Borght T, Pauwels S, Lambotte L, et al: Brain tumor imaging with PET and 2-[carbon-11]thymidine. J Nucl Med 1994; 35:974–982.

145. Cleaver JE: Frontiers of Biology. Amsterdam, North-Holland Publishing, 1967.

146. Bush RS, Jenkins RDT, Allt WC, et al: Definitive evidence for hypoxic cells influencing cure in cancer therapy. Br J Cancer 1978; 37(suppl III):302–306.

147. Mottram JC: Factors of importance in the radiosensitivity of tumors. Br J Radiol 1936; 9:606–614.

148. Powers WE, Tolmach LJ: A multi-component x-ray survival curve for mouse lymphosarcoma cells irradiated in vivo. Nature 1963; 197:710–711.

149. Moulder JE, Rockwell S: Hypoxic fractions of solid tumors: Experimental techniques, methods of analysis and a survey of existing data. Int J Radiat Oncol Biol Phys 1984; 10:695–712.

150. Cater DB, Silver HB: Quantitative measurements of oxygen tension in normal tissues and in the tumors of patients before and after radiotherapy. Acta Radiol 1960; 53:233–256.

151. Gatenby RA, Kessler HB, Rosenblum SJ, et al: Oxygen distribution in squamous cell carcinoma metastases and its relationship to outcome of radiation therapy. Int J Radiat Oncol Biol Phys 1988; 10:695–712.

152. Kayama T, Yoshimoto T, Fujimoto S, et al: Intratumoral oxygen pressure in malignant brain tumors. J Neurosurg 1991; 74:55–59.

153. Valk PE, Mathis CA, Prados MD, et al: Hypoxia in human gliomas: Demonstration by PET with fluorine-18-fluoromisonidazole. J Nucl Med 1992; 33:2133–2137.

154. Yang DJ, Wallace S, Cherif A, et al: Development of F-18-labeled fluoroerythronitroimidazole as a PET agent for imaging tumor hypoxia. Radiology 1995; 194:795–800.

155. Pawlikowski M, Kunert-Radek J, Radek A, et al: Inhibition of cell proliferation of human gliomas by benzodiazepines in vitro. Acta Neurol Scand 1988; 77:231–233.

156. Olson JMM, Junck L, Young AB, et al: Isoquinolone and peripheral-type benzodiazepine binding in gliomas: Implications for diagnostic imaging. Cancer Res 1988; 48:5837–5841.

157. Starosta-Rubinstein S, Ciliax BJ, Penney JB, et al: Imaging of a glioma using peripheral benzodiazepine receptor ligands. Proc Natl Acad Sci USA 1987; 84:891–895.

158. Richfield EK, Ciliax BJ, Starosta-Rubinstein SR, et al: Comparison of [14C]deoxyglucose metabolism and peripheral benzodiazepine receptor binding in rat C6 glioma. Neurology 1988; 38:1255–1262.

159. Black KL, Ikezaki K, W TA, et al: Imaging peripheral benzodiazepine receptors in brain tumors in rats: In vitro binding characteristics. J Cereb Blood Flow Metab 1990; 10:580–587.

160. Black KL, Ikezaki K, Santori E, et al: Specific high affinity binding

161. Benavides J, Cornu P, Dennis T, et al: Imaging of human brain lesions with an Ω₃ site radioligand. Ann Neurol 1988; 24:708–712.

162. Junck L, Olson JMM, Ciliax BJ, et al: PET imaging of human gliomas with ligands for the peripheral benzodiazepine binding site. Ann Neurol 1989; 26:752–758.

163. Bergstrom M, Mosskin M, Ericson K, et al: Peripheral benzodiazepine binding sites in human gliomas evaluated with positron emission tomography. Acta Radiol 1986; 369:409–411.

164. Pappata S, Cornu P, Samson Y, et al: PET study of carbon-11-PK 1195 binding to peripheral type benzodiazepine sites in glioblastoma: A case report. J Nucl Med 1991; 32:1608–1610.

165. DuBois A, Benavides J, Penney B, et al: Imaging of primary and remote ischemic and excitotoxic brain lesions: An autoradiographic study of peripheral type benzodiazepine binding sites in the rat and cat. Brain Res 1988; 445:77–90.

166. Di Chiro G: Which PET radiopharmaceutical for brain tumors (editorial)? J Nucl Med 1991; 32:1346–1348.

167. Von Monakow C: Neue gesichtspunkte in der Frage nach der Lokalisation im Grosshirn. Wiesbaden, Bergman JF, 1910.

168. West JR: The concept of diaschisis: A reply to Markowitsch and Pritzel. Behav Biol 1978; 22:413–416.

169. Baron JC, Bousser MG, Comar D, et al: Crossed cerebellar diaschisis in human supratentorial infarction (abstract). Ann Neurol 1980; 8:128.

170. Fulham MJ, Brooks RA, Hallett M, et al: Cerebellar diaschisis revisited: Pontine hypometabolism and dentate sparing. Neurology 1992; 42:2267–2273.

171. Brodal A: Neurological Anatomy in Relation to Clinical Medicine. New York, Oxford University Press, 1981, pp 294–391.

172. Feeney DM, Baron JC: Diaschisis. Stroke 1986; 17:817–830.

173. Carlstedt-Duke J, Gustafsson J-A: The molecular mechanism of glucocorticoid action. In Ludecke DK, Chrousos GP, Tolis G (eds): ACTH, Cushing's Syndrome and Other Hypercortisolemic States. New York, Raven Press, 1990, pp 7–14.

174. Carroll BJ: Psychiatric disorders and steroids. In Usdin E, Hamburg DA, Barchas JD, et al (eds): Neuroregulators and psychiatric disorders. New York, 1977, pp 276–283.

175. Muncke A: Glucocorticoid inhibition of glucose uptake by peripheral tissues: Old and new evidence, molecular mechanism and action. Perspect Biol Med 1971; 14:265–289.

176. Kadekaro M, Ito M, Gross PM: Local cerebral glucose utilization is increased in acutely adrenalectomized rats. Neuroendocrinology 1988; 47:329–334.

177. Bottomley PA: Human in vivo NMR spectroscopy in diagnostic medicine: Clinical tool or research probe? Radiology 1989; 170:1–15.

178. Aisen AM, Chenevert T: MR spectroscopy: Clinical perspective. Radiology 1989; 173:593–599.

179. Prichard JW, Brass LM: New anatomical and functional imaging methods. Ann Neurol 1992; 32:395–440.

180. Prichard JW: Magnetic resonance spectroscopy of cerebral metabolism in vivo. In Asbury AK, McKhann GM, McDonald WI (eds): Diseases of the Nervous System: Clinical Neurobiology. Philadelphia, WB Saunders, 1992, pp 1589–1605.

181. Negendank W: Studies of human tumors by MRS: A review. NMR Biomed 1992; 5:303–324.

182. Negendank WG, Brown TR, Evelhoch JL, et al: Proceedings of a National Cancer Institute workshop: MR spectroscopy and tumor cell biology. Radiology 1992; 185:875–883.

183. Weiner MW: The promise of magnetic resonance spectroscopy for medical diagnosis. Invest Radiol 1988; 23:253–261.

184. Ross B, Michaelis T: Clinical applications of magnetic resonance spectroscopy. Magn Reson Q 1994; 10:191–247.

185. Barker PB, Glickson JD, Bryan RN: In vivo magnetic resonance spectroscopy of human brain tumors. Top Magn Reson Imaging 1993; 5(1):32–45.

186. Tallan HH: Studies on the distribution of N-acetyl-ʟ-aspartic acid in brain. J Biol Chem 1957; 224:41–45.

187. Birken DL, Oldendorf WH: N-acetyl-ʟ-aspartic acid: A literature review of a compound prominent in 1H-NMR spectroscopic studies of the brain. Neurosci Biobehav Rev 1989; 13:23–31.

188. Miller BL: A review of chemical issues in 1H NMR spectroscopy: N-acetyl-ʟ-aspartate, creatine and choline. NMR Biomed 1991; 4:47–52.

189. Simmons ML, Frondoza CG, Coyle JT: Immunocytochemical local-

ization of *N*-acetyl-aspartate with monoclonal antibodies. Neuroscience 1991; 45:37–45.

190. Agris PF, Campbell ID: Proton nuclear magnetic resonance of intact Freund leukemia cells: Phosphorylcholine increase during differentiation. Science 1982; 216:1325–1327.

191. Tanaka C, Naruse S, Horikawa K, et al: Proton magnetic resonance spectra of brain tumors. Magn Reson Imaging 1986; 4:503–508.

192. Alger JR, Frank JA, Bizzi A, et al: Metabolism of human gliomas: Assessment with H-1 MR spectroscopy and F-18 fluorodeoxyglucose PET. Radiology 1990; 177:633–641.

193. Bruhn H, Frahm J, Gyngell ML, et al: Noninvasive differentiation of tumors with use of localised H-1 MR Spectroscopy in vivo: Initial experience in patients with cerebral tumors. Radiology 1989; 172:541–548.

194. Ernst T, Hennig J, Ott D, et al: The importance of voxel size in clinical 1H spectroscopy of the human brain. NMR Biomed 1989; 2:216–224.

195. Frahm J, Michaelis T, Merboldt K-D, et al: Localized NMR spectroscopy in vivo: Progress and problems. NMR Biomed 1989; 2:188–195.

196. Moonen CTW, van Zijl PCM: Highly effective water suppression for in vivo proton NMR spectroscopy (dry steam). J Magn Reson 1990; 88:28–41.

197. Kumar A, Welti D, Ernst RR: NMR Fourier zeugmatography. J Magn Reson 1975; 18:69–83.

198. Brown TR, Kincaid BM, Ugurbil K: NMR chemical shift imaging in three dimensions. Proc Natl Acad Sci USA 1982; 79:3523–3526.

199. Maudsley AA, Hilal SK, Perman WH, et al: Spatially resolved high resolution spectroscopy by ''four dimensional'' NMR. J Magn Reson 1983; 51:147–152.

200. Moonen CTW, Sobering G, van Zijl PCM, et al: Proton spectroscopic imaging of human brain. J Magn Reson 1992; 98:556–575.

201. Luyten PR, Marien AJH, Heindel W, et al: Metabolic imaging of patients with intracranial tumors: H-1 MR spectroscopic imaging and PET. Radiology 1990; 176:791–799.

202. Herholz K, Heindel W, Luyten PR, et al: In-vivo imaging of glucose consumption and lactate concentration in human gliomas. Ann Neurol 1992; 31:319–327.

203. Fulham MJ, Bizzi A, Deitz MJ, et al: Metabolite mapping of brain tumors with proton MR spectroscopic imaging: Clinical relevance. Radiology 1992; 185:675–686.

204. Duyn JH, Gillen J, Sobering G, et al: Multisection proton MR spectroscopic imaging of the brain. Radiology 1993; 188:277–282.

205. Segebarth CM, Baleriaux DF, Luyten PR, et al: Detection of metabolic heterogeneity of human intracranial tumors in vivo by 1H NMR spectroscopic imaging. Magn Reson Med 1990; 13:62–76.

206. Arnold DL, Shoubridge EA, Villemure JG, et al: Proton and phosphorus magnetic resonance spectroscopy of human astrocytomas in vivo: Preliminary observations on tumor grading. NMR Biomed 1990; 3:184–189.

207. Demaerel P, Johannik K, Van Hecke P, et al: Localized 1H NMR spectroscopy in 50 cases of newly diagnosed intracranial tumors. J Comput Assist Tomogr 1991; 15:67–76.

208. Gill SS, Thomas DGT, Van Bruggen N, et al: Proton MR spectroscopy of intracranial tumors: In vivo and in vitro studies. J Comput Assist Tomogr 1990; 14:497–504.

209. Ott D, Hennig J, Ernst T: Human brain tumors: Assessment with in vivo proton MR spectroscopy. Radiology 1993; 186:745–752.

210. Segebarth CM, Baleriaux D, De Beer R, et al: 1H Image-guided localized 31P MR spectroscopy of human brain: Quantitative analysis of 31P MR spectra measured on volunteers and on intracranial tumor patients. Magn Reson Med 1989; 11:349–366.

211. Heiss W-D, Heindel W, Herholz K, et al: Positron emission tomography of flourine-18-deoxyglucose and image-guided phosphorus-31 magnetic resonance spectroscopy in brain tumors. J Nucl Med 1990; 31:302–310.

212. Hubesch B, Sappey-Marinier D, Roth K, et al: P-31 MR spectroscopy of normal human brain and brain tumors. Radiology 1990; 174:401–409.

213. Fulham MJ, Dietz MJ, Duyn JH, et al: Transsynaptic reduction in N-acetyl-aspartate in cerebellar diaschisis: A proton MR spectroscopic imaging study. J Comput Assist Tomogr 1994; 18(5):697–704.

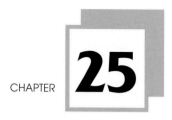

CHAPTER **25**

Single-Photon Emission Computed Tomography

Single-photon emission computed tomography (SPECT) with rotating gamma cameras has become a standard method for acquiring transaxial images of the in vivo distribution of radioactivity. SPECT imaging is used primarily for cardiac perfusion imaging, but it is also widely used for brain and bone imaging. This methodology is quite widespread in that virtually every major nuclear medicine clinic in the United States is equipped with a SPECT system. SPECT imaging has been found to be quite effective in identifying recurrent or residual glioma. In addition, radiopharmaceuticals are being developed that will allow SPECT to detect increased protein synthesis and presence of various receptors using radiolabeled ligands, including antibodies.

SPECT IMAGING SYSTEMS

A SPECT system consists of one or more gamma cameras mounted on a gantry that allows them to rotate around the patient, recording images over 360 degrees (Figs. 25–1 and 25–2). Rotating gamma camera SPECT systems typically have one, two, or three heads. The single-headed systems are most widely available, and almost every large nuclear medicine clinic has at least one. Two-headed systems are primarily designed for whole-body imaging and are not usually used for head imaging. Three-headed systems are optimized for head imaging and produce the highest-quality images. Rotation time is typically 20 to 30 minutes. The images are acquired by a computer and then are used to reconstruct multiple transaxial images of the distribution of activity in the patient. The reconstruction method is usually filtered back-projection, which is the same method used in reconstructing x-ray computed tomographic (CT) images. The image quality is limited by the camera collimators, the proximity of the camera heads to the patient, and the number of counts acquired during the study. Camera collimators are lead plates with many parallel or converging holes, which limit the gamma rays that are detected to those that pass through the holes. Smaller, longer holes yield higher-resolu-

tion but lower counts. Many of the three-headed systems are equipped with fan-beam collimators that converge in only the transaxial plane. This improves resolution but limits the field of view, which is an acceptable trade-off for brain imaging, in which the field of view is substantially larger than the size of the head. The best practical resolution with modern three-headed SPECT systems for brain imaging is about 8 mm, and it is about 12 mm for single-headed systems. Resolution is specified as the apparent width of a point source at half of the peak counts of the image of that point. This is referred to as the *full-width at half-maximum* (FWHM). If two points are imaged 1.0 FWHM apart, then they are just barely distinguishable as two objects. If the count rate is relatively low, such as in thallium 201 images, the images have to be reconstructed with lower resolution (i.e., 12 to 18 mm), or the images would be too noisy to be interpreted.

Another concern in reconstructing SPECT images is loss of counts from deep structures because some of the photons are attenuated before they reach the camera. If attenuation correction is not done, fewer counts will appear to come from deeper regions than from more superficial regions. This is usually corrected by assuming uniform attenuation, using a manually placed ellipse to define the boundary of the head. More sophisticated attenuation correction schemes are being developed that use a low-resolution CT type of image that is obtained using an external source on the side of the head opposite the camera. This more exact attenuation correction is now available and will allow accurate absolute quantitation of activity in the brain.

The other major problem in image quantitation is photon scatter. Some of the gamma rays do not proceed straight from their point of origin to the gamma camera. They may bump into an electron and scatter off at an unpredictable angle. If the angle of scatter is large, then the gamma ray will lose sufficient energy that it can be rejected by the appropriate electronics in the detector. If the angle is small, however, not much energy is lost, and the photon is detected and included in the image. This has the effect of lowering

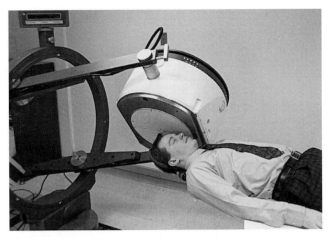

Figure 25-1 Single-camera SPECT system. The patient is suspended on a cantilevered table with his head resting in a specialized head holder. It is often necessary to restrain the patient's head with tape or straps to ensure that the head does not move during the study. The camera is positioned so that it just barely clears the patient as it rotates. Note how the side of the camera nearest the patient is tapered to clear the patient's shoulder.

the contrast in the images and generally adding counts over the entire image that are inappropriate. A number of approximate correction schemes for scatter have been developed, but none is currently in general use. Because of this problem, as well as the problem of inexact attenuation correction, reconstructed SPECT images are not sufficiently quantitative to be used to measure absolute activity in the brain. This also means that ratios of activity from one region to another, such as tumor-to-normal brain, will not be exactly correct and may differ somewhat from one SPECT system to another. Improvements in image processing are likely to lead to adequate corrections in these areas, making quantitative SPECT imaging feasible in the future.

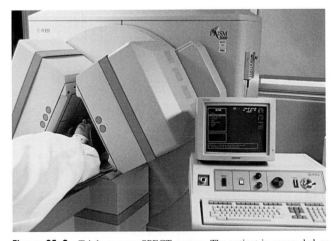

Figure 25-2 Triple-camera SPECT system. The patient is suspended on a cantilevered table in the same way as for the single-camera system. Camera head positioning is partially automatic, in that after one camera head is positioned as close as possible, the other heads automatically align with the first. The main advantages of this system are that data can be acquired approximately three times more rapidly than with a single-headed system and that the collimators that are used result in significantly higher-resolution images.

Practical considerations in doing SPECT imaging include the following:

1. Timing of injection relative to imaging. This depends on the specific radiopharmaceutical being used.

2. Head immobilization. There are various schemes for this. It is important that the head not move during imaging because such movement will blur and/or distort the images. The restraint must be firm but comfortable and should contain no metal parts that would block the gamma rays.

3. Camera positioning. Care must be taken to have the camera pass as close to the patient's head as possible. It must also clear the patient's shoulders. Setting up the acquisition takes a few minutes and must be done carefully to ensure that the images will be of high quality.

Once the imaging data have been acquired they must be reconstructed. Numerous considerations in setting up the reconstruction are not covered in this chapter. (For more details see a modern textbook on SPECT imaging, such as that by Jaszczak.[1]) The most important consideration is the selection of the resolution of the reconstruction filter. This determines the resolution in the final images. If the resolution is too low, the image will appear very smooth with little detail. If the resolution is too high, the image will be excessively noisy and very grainy, making it difficult to interpret. An optimum point is obviously reached somewhere between these two, but there is no widely used objective method to determine this point, and individual preferences vary somewhat. Be aware that if an image looks either too smooth or too noisy, it can be re-reconstructed with a different filter to more closely approximate an optimum resolution.

SPECT imaging is similar to positron emission tomography (PET) imaging in several ways, but significant differences exist between them. Both approaches produce transaxial images of the in vivo distribution of radioactive tracers to define various physiologic parameters. The instruments are quite different: PET scanners are generally configured as a ring of detectors and SPECT scanners usually consist of one, two, or three gamma camera heads that rotate around the patient. Some SPECT systems are now using the ring configuration, and these may become more common. The main differences between PET and SPECT are as follows:

1. Radiotracers used with PET are labeled with positron emitters such as ^{11}C, ^{13}N, ^{15}O, and ^{18}F. This means many interesting organic molecules can be labeled. The most common single photon tracers used with SPECT are ^{99m}Tc, ^{201}Tl, ^{111}In, and ^{123}I. The chemistry of attaching these tracers to molecules with appropriate behaviors is more complex. Little overlap exists between tracers used in SPECT and PET, although tracers with similar behavior are used.

2. The practical resolution of modern PET systems is 6 to 7 mm FWHM, whereas that of SPECT systems is 8 to 12 mm.

3. Scatter and attenuation correction are more accurate with PET than with SPECT. This means the absolute activity

per milliliter of tissue can be accurately determined with PET but not with SPECT.

4. Temporal resolution is better with PET than with SPECT. It is feasible to image at 1-second intervals with PET, although the maximum rate used in most centers is 10-second intervals. With single-headed SPECT systems, 5 minutes is about the most rapid acquisition that is feasible. With three-headed systems it is possible to acquire images at 30-second intervals or less.

5. The sensitivity of PET is about 100 times that of SPECT. This means that less radioactivity has to be injected and that the images have more counts. The newer annular SPECT systems will have higher sensitivity, but it will never approach that of PET because of fundamental differences in how the photons are collimated.

6. The cost of a modern PET system is two to four times that of a modern SPECT system. The most important differences are cost and availability of the systems. Because virtually every nuclear medicine department in the United States has a SPECT system, it is feasible to do these studies almost anywhere. PET will continue to be useful, but it will not be widely available in the near future.

HISTORY

Radionuclide brain scanning began in the early 1960s as the only practical noninvasive method other than angiography for visualizing brain pathology. The early studies were images of breakdown of the blood-brain barrier.[2, 3] Tracers used initially were ^{131}I-albumin, ^{203}Hg-chlormerodrin, and ^{197}Hg-chlormerodrin. Images were first made with rectilinear scanners and later with gamma cameras. In the mid-1960s, ^{99m}Tc-pertechnetate began to be used, with considerable improvement in image quality. It was finally recognized that choroid plexus uptake could be avoided by using either ^{99m}Tc-glucoheptonate or ^{99m}Tc-diethylenetriamine penta-acetic acid (DTPA).[4] The last two agents have become the standard agents for imaging the breakdown of the blood-brain barrier

During the late 1960s and early 1970s, brain scanning was a major part of nuclear medicine practice for the detection and localization of brain tumors and abscesses. However, in the late 1970s, when CT imaging was introduced, nuclear medicine brain imaging virtually ceased, although its diagnostic accuracy for tumor was better than 90%. The only studies that continued were cerebral flow studies to aid in the diagnosis of brain death.

New cerebral blood flow tracers that were retained in the brain in proportion to blood flow became widely available in the 1980s. The first was ^{123}I-isopropyl-*p*-iodoamphetamine (IMP)[5] and the second was ^{99m}Tc-hexamethyl propylene amine oxime (HMPAO).[6] Two brain blood flow radiopharmaceuticals are currently licensed by the FDA: ^{99m}Tc-HMPAO and ^{99m}Tc-ethyl cysteinate dimer (ECD).[7] The behavior of ECD is quite similar to that of HMPAO.

Initial experience[8] with IMP showed it was not taken up by brain tumors, presumably indicating a lack of the appropriate receptors or transporters in the tumors. Although there have been a few case reports of gliomas showing high

uptake of IMP, such uptake is very uncommon and does not seem to correlate with anything else that might be clinically useful. In contrast, ^{99m}Tc-HMPAO seems to be taken up by tumors in proportion to blood flow and can be used to evaluate blood flow.[9] This proportionality has not been validated, but it is based on the observation of definite uptake in the tumors, and the degree of uptake seems to correspond to the expected amount of blood flow for the tumors as a group.

Two other agents have been found to be useful in brain tumor imaging, ^{201}Tl and ^{99m}Tc-methoxyisobutylisonitrile (MIBI).[10–13] These agents have been used for some time as tracers of myocardial perfusion. They are both monovalent cations and are taken up very effectively in the myocardium, such that their distribution in the heart is a map of myocardial perfusion. In the brain, both agents are indicators of breakdown of the blood-brain barrier and concentration by viable tumor. This behavior is particularly useful in trying to determine if viable tumor is present.

Since the early 1960s, enormous strides have taken place in instrumentation development. The earliest brain scans were planar rectilinear images made by physically scanning a focused probe back and forth over the patient's head. These progressed to planar gamma camera images and, finally, to SPECT images. The gamma cameras, collimators, computers, and reconstruction schemes have steadily improved during this period. The improved images have resulted in improved diagnostic accuracy of these studies. This is a trend that is likely to continue for some time. The main areas of improvement will probably be in image reconstruction and in the creation of dedicated brain imaging devices with improved resolution and sensitivity.

Radiopharmaceuticals have also developed over this period, from agents that simply indicated breakdown of the blood-brain barrier to effective tracers of cerebral blood flow and of tumor viability. Newer tracers are beginning to appear on the scene such as L-3[^{123}I]-iodo-α-methyltyrosine (IMT),[14–16] which should be useful in detecting regions of increased protein synthesis, and radiolabeled antibodies, which should allow visualization of a wide variety of specific antigens or receptors on tumors. Radiopharmaceutical development can be expected to continue, and we can therefore expect new tracers to look at tumors in different and more effective ways in the future.

IMAGE REGISTRATION

As SPECT instruments and reconstruction software have improved, it has become increasingly important to be able to accurately align the anatomic CT and magnetic resonance (MR) images with the functional SPECT images. The typical situation in which this is important is in the question of recurrent tumor. Several agents, described in the following paragraphs, show good uptake in tumor and can be used to address this question. Usually, a region of contrast enhancement has been identified with either CT or MRI. If the region of increased uptake in the SPECT images can be shown to coincide with the area of contrast enhancement, then it is highly likely that the abnormality represents recurrent tumor. A positional misalignment of a few millimeters could easily cause a misdiagnosis. Several groups have developed image registration programs using fiducial markers[17] or a method called *principal axes transformation*.[18] These programs are not commercially available currently, but they may become part of the software packages in future SPECT systems.

THALLIUM 201

Thallium 201 is a monovalent cation that behaves much like potassium ion. In well-perfused muscle, such as the heart, it is taken up by the sodium-potassium adenosine triphosphate (ATP) pump and transferred into the myocytes very rapidly. The uptake is fast enough that the extraction fraction is around 70%, and the distribution of activity is essentially the distribution of blood flow. Because of its rapid uptake into tissue throughout the body, the concentration in the blood drops rapidly after injection. Thallium ions do not cross intact blood-brain barrier. Thus, accumulation of thallium in a brain lesion requires breakdown of the blood-brain barrier. Once thallium crosses the blood-brain barrier concentration of thallium will occur in the presence of metabolically active tissue on the other side, creating a region of increased uptake. This is the principle behind the use of ^{201}Tl for imaging of gliomas. The mechanism of transport is not at all specific for tumor, but in nontumor causes of blood-brain barrier breakdown (stroke, radionecrosis, infection) no significant mass of metabolically active tissue is present on the other side of the blood-brain barrier to retain ^{201}Tl significantly. Thus, mild uptake may be seen with these entities, but intense uptake will be seen only with tumors.

The primary use of ^{201}Tl SPECT imaging of gliomas is to discriminate between radionecrosis and recurrent tumor[9, 11, 12] (Fig. 25–3). In addition, more recent studies have shown that quantitative measures of ^{201}Tl uptake may be useful as a prognostic index.[10, 19]

Methodology

As in all brain SPECT studies, the subject must be carefully positioned so the head is fixed in place but the patient is comfortable. There are a wide variety of devices for this purpose. The cameras must be positioned to come as close as possible to the subject's head during the orbits around it. The injected activity of ^{201}Tl reported in the literature varies from 2 to 6 mCi (74 to 222 MBq [megabecquerels]). One group uses 48 μCi/kg. The most common dose used is 4 mCi (148 MBq). Imaging should start 30 to 40 minutes after injection. The optimum timing for start of imaging has not been carefully examined, although one report clearly shows that it is necessary to wait at least 10 minutes after injection.[20] Most studies do not report the type of collimator used. Generally, a high-resolution collimator is most appropriate. Imaging time with a single-head camera is typically 22 minutes (64 stops of 20 seconds each or 128 stops of 10 seconds each over 360 degrees). Multi-headed cameras will need less time. Images should be acquired in a matrix of 128 × 128. Reconstruction should be done with two-dimensional prefiltering, with a ramp filter used for backprojection. Reconstructed resolution has to be chosen to match the expected resolution of the SPECT system. Older single-headed systems will have resolutions of about 18 mm, whereas newer multi-headed cameras with fan-beam collimation will have resolutions of about 10 mm. The thickness of displayed slices should approximately match the transaxial resolution.

These recommendations are meant to be general guidelines. Each nuclear medicine clinic will have its own protocols for brain imaging, which may differ slightly from these recommendations and may be completely appropriate. The main points to watch in evaluating the adequacy of the images is the amount of noise in the images, the degree of smoothing, and the amount of background subtraction. If the images are excessively noisy, either longer acquisition time or more sensitive collimators should be used, a lower resolution filter should be used during reconstruction, or more slices should be added together for display. If images are too smooth then detail will be lost, and a higher-resolution filter should be used during reconstruction. Background subtraction is used to suppress noisy artifacts surrounding the head; if overdone, it will obscure detail in the brain. This is particularly dangerous in ^{201}Tl imaging, in which the lesion

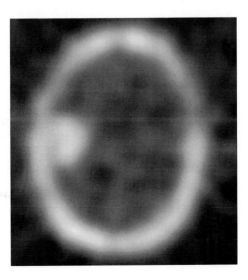
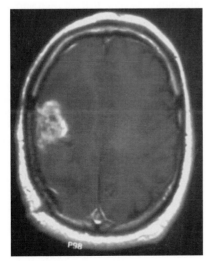

Figure 25–3 Thallium 201 SPECT image *(left)* of a patient with recurrent oligodendroglioma. The tumor had been treated with surgery 6 years before and with gamma knife irradiation 1 year before this study. The MRI image *(right)* showed contrast enhancement in the area of the tumor, which could indicate radiation necrosis or recurrent tumor. The ^{201}Tl SPECT image shows clear uptake activity in the area of concern, indicating recurrent tumor.

uptake may be quite subtle. For this reason, images should be presented with only minimal background subtraction.

The degree of uptake in a lesion can be expressed either as a visual grade (0 to 4 +) or as the result of a semiquantitative method. The most common semiquantitative approach is to place a region of interest over the tumor and over a similar region in the corresponding contralateral portion of the brain. The ratio between tumor counts per pixel and normal brain counts per pixel is then determined. For this approach to be reliable and reproducible, it is essential that the imaging procedure and reconstruction be done in the same manner in all patients. In particular, the time between injection and imaging must be kept constant and the reconstruction parameters must be the same. In addition, the region placement must be done in a consistent manner. Some investigators have used peak count within a tumor as the measure of uptake. Although this is less sensitive to the placement of the region of interest it can vary randomly because of the inherent noise in the images. Whatever method is chosen, make sure it is done consistently.

Recurrence vs. Radionecrosis

Schwartz and co-workers[9] studied 15 glioma patients with ^{201}Tl- and ^{99m}Tc-HMPAO to look for recurrence vs. radionecrosis. They found that four patients with intense ^{201}Tl uptake had recurrent disease, whereas three patients with low uptake had no evidence of recurrence. In the other eight patients with intermediate ^{201}Tl uptake, four showed increased or normal perfusion to the same region, whereas four showed decreased perfusion. All of the subjects with decreased perfusion did not have recurrent tumor. Three of the four subjects with increased or normal perfusion had recurrent tumor. Thus, the overall sensitivity for detecting recurrent disease was 88% (n = 8) with a specificity of 100% (n = 7). ^{99m}Tc-HMPAO was useful in evaluating the group of subjects with intermediate ^{201}Tl uptake. However, no quantitation of ^{201}Tl uptake was attempted.

Most other authors have not used ^{99m}Tc-HMPAO but have used semiquantitative methods to improve accuracy. Table 25–1 shows a summary of recent studies using ^{201}Tl SPECT to detect recurrent glioma. Quantitative analysis was used in all studies except that of Schwartz and colleagues.[9] The quantitative studies generally tried to define a cut-off point to distinguish between tumor and necrosis. The value chosen

in most studies was 1.5, although the optimum value may depend somewhat on the particular SPECT system and how the images are reconstructed. Although the numbers in each study are relatively low, the results are reasonably consistent. Thallium 201 SPECT seems to be very sensitive in the detection of recurrent glioma, but the specificity is not quite as good. It is likely that the average specificity will fall somewhat as larger series with less selection bias are reported in the future.

Comparison of ^{201}Tl SPECT with ^{18}F FDG PET for Diagnosis of Recurrent Glioma

In recent years ^{18}F-fluorodeoxyglucose (FDG) PET imaging has been regarded as the "gold standard" for noninvasive diagnosis of recurrent glioma. This is because gliomas usually show good uptake of FDG, which is taken as an indication of increased glucose metabolic rate, because the spatial resolution of PET is superior to that of SPECT and because FDG PET imaging of glioma has been done for much longer. Several abstracts have directly compared ^{201}Tl SPECT with FDG PET and found that SPECT imaging is at least comparable to PET, and is possibly better.

Maass and colleagues[21] studied 26 patients with high-grade (III to IV) gliomas with both ^{201}Tl SPECT and FDG PET. All SPECT studies were positive. Twenty-three of 26 of the PET studies were positive. SPECT was completely negative in two of five patients with no recurrence. Only two patients without recurrence were studied with PET. Both showed mild hypermetabolism consistent with inflammation. This is the largest study that has been done to date, to our knowledge. Although the numbers are not large, it suggests that ^{201}Tl SPECT is at least as sensitive as FDG PET. Specificity is not well defined because of the very small numbers.

In other studies with somewhat smaller numbers Buchpiquel and others[22] found a sensitivity for ^{201}Tl SPECT of 100% (N = 11) and a specificity of 33% (N = 3). FDG PET had a sensitivity of 82% (N = 11) and specificity of 100% (N = 3). Antar and associates[23] found a sensitivity of 100% (N = 15) for both techniques. Specificity was not reported.

The overall conclusion, based on very limited numbers, is that the two methodologies are at least comparable. As better SPECT systems become available and with careful

TABLE 25–1
ACCURACIES FOR DETECTION OF VIABLE GLIOMA USING SPECT IMAGING WITH THALLIUM 201

Study	Sensitivity		Specificity		Positive Predictive Value		Negative Predictive Value	
	%	No.	%	No.	%	No.	%	No.
Schwartz et al.[9]	100	7	88	8	88	8	100	7
O'Tuama et al.[13]	75	8	90	10	86	7	82	11
Buchpiquel et al.[22]	100	11	33	3	85	13	100	1
Hoh et al.[37]	96	27	0	3	90	29	0	1
Macapinlac et al.[25]	100	11	100	4	100	11	100	4
Maass et al.[21]	91	90	40	5	96	85	20	10
Antar et al.[23]	100	15						

quantitative analysis of the images it is likely that ^{201}Tl SPECT will prove to be a reliable way to noninvasively detect recurrent glioma.

[201]Tl SPECT for Tumor Grading or Prognosis

The rationale for using ^{201}Tl SPECT for determining the prognosis of gliomas is that a more metabolically active, rapidly proliferating tumor should have better vascularity and a more active sodium-potassium ATP pump. This hypothesis has been examined in several studies.

Black and co-workers[10] used an uptake index of tumor activity divided by normal brain activity. They found an index of 1.27 ± 0.40 in 14 patients with low-grade gliomas and an index of 2.40 ± 0.61 in 11 patients with high-grade gliomas. Using a threshold index of 1.5 they could predict tumor grade with 89% accuracy. They also noted that "low-grade" gliomas with relatively high uptake tended to act more like high-grade gliomas. This suggests that ^{201}Tl uptake may provide additional information beyond that provided by histologic grade.

Burkard and colleagues[19] obtained similar results in 22 patients. They found that the threshold index of 1.4 effectively separated the low-grade (I and II) from the high-grade (III and IV) tumors. The grading accuracy with this threshold was 91%.

Oriuchi and others,[24] in a study of 28 patients, examined ^{201}Tl uptake index vs. grade, and also correlated uptake with proliferative activity as measured by bromodeoxyuridine (BUdR). They found that a threshold index of 1.2 effectively separated the grade III to IV tumors from the grade I to II tumors. All of the grade III to IV tumors had indices greater than 1.2, and only one of 14 grade I to II tumors had a higher index (1.77). A significant correlation was observed between the ^{201}Tl uptake index and the BUdR labeling index, with a correlation coefficient of 0.67.

The conclusion to be derived from these studies is that ^{201}Tl SPECT reliably predicts tumor grade. Care must be taken in trying to reproduce these studies because differences in instrumentation and image reconstruction can change the thallium tumor index and can change the appropriate level for the threshold. This may explain why 1.5 seems to be most appropriate in some studies, and 1.2 is appropriate in others.

TECHNETIUM 99m METHOXYISOBUTYLISONITRILE

Technetium 99m MIBI is similar to ^{201}Tl in three respects. It is used as a myocardial perfusion agent, it does not normally cross the blood-brain barrier, and it is taken up by several somatic tumors, including breast cancer and sarcomas. One difference about its behavior in the brain is that it is taken up by the choroid plexus. This uptake cannot be blocked with perchlorate.

O'Tuama and co-workers[13] compared ^{201}Tl uptake with that of ^{99m}Tc-MIBI in a group of 19 children with recurrent brain tumors, mostly gliomas. The quality of the ^{99m}Tc-MIBI images seemed to be better than the ^{201}Tl images. The overall sensitivity was 100% (the same as for ^{201}Tl) and specificity improved to 100% (compared with 91% for ^{201}Tl).

Macapinlac and others[25] studied 23 patients with suspected recurrent brain tumors with ^{201}Tl and ^{99m}Tc-MIBI. Two lesions near the choroid plexus were not seen with ^{99m}Tc-MIBI, and one low-grade astrocytoma was seen with ^{201}Tl, but not with ^{99m}Tc-MIBI.

Darcourt and associates[26] studied nine patients with ^{201}Tl and ^{99m}Tc-MIBI. They found that both agents reliably differentiated between recurrence and radionecrosis. They also found that the tumor-to-nontumor index correlated very highly between the two agents ($r = 0.96$).

Maffioli and colleagues[27] studied 53 patients for suspected tumor recurrence with ^{99m}Tc-MIBI. Most (43) had some type of glioma. The resultant sensitivity was 95%, specificity was 92%, and accuracy was 94%.

Baillet and his group[27a] have shown ^{99m}Tc-MIBI imaging can be used to accurately predict tumor grade in a study of 61 patients. It appears that ^{99m}Tc-MIBI is virtually equivalent to ^{201}Tl in both tumor grading and in detection of recurrent glioma, at least in the portions of the brain relatively distant from the ventricles. ^{99m}Tc-MIBI has the advantage of a higher-energy photon, which means that resultant images are less attenuated. For both economic and radiation dosimetric reasons, it is possible to inject about 10 times the dose of radioactivity with ^{99m}Tc-MIBI than with ^{201}Tl, which means that each image contains more counts and that the quality of the images is much better.

IODINE 123 TYROSINE

Carbon 11 methionine and ^{11}C-leucine have been used to measure amino acid uptake and protein synthesis in gliomas with PET for several years. More recently,[28] a single-photon radiotracer, L-3[^{123}I]-iodo-α-methyltyrosine (IMT), has been synthesized as a reasonable SPECT agent for the same purposes. IMT is apparently transported actively by the carrier system for large neutral amino acids. It is rapidly transported into actively metabolizing tissue, such as tumor, and washes out quite slowly. It is not incorporated into protein and is not significantly metabolized once it is transported into the cell. Metabolism does occur elsewhere in the body, presumably in the liver. This means that a substantial fraction of plasma activity is in the form of metabolites, particularly after 30 to 45 minutes. This must be accounted for if tissue uptake is related to blood activity, as in kinetic modeling analysis.

Typical studies with IMT show glioma-to-normal brain ratios of around 1.5 from 30 to 60 minutes after injection. The uptake ratios are relatively low because significant uptake occurs in normal brain.

Guth-Tougelidis and others[14] studied 13 patients with possible recurrent brain tumor. Their sensitivity was 78% (n = 9) and specificity was 100% (n = 4).

Schober and associates[29] studied 62 patients (54 with glioma) with possibly recurrent tumors. In contrast to ^{201}Tl or ^{99m}Tc-MIBI they found that ^{123}I-IMT uptake did not correlate well with tumor grade. They did find that ^{123}I-IMT was effective in predicting recurrence, but exact sensitivities and specificities were not stated.

Because protein synthesis is likely to be a sensitive measure of tumor well-being, ^{123}I-IMT SPECT imaging is a logical way to evaluate tumor response to therapy. Thus, it may be possible to determine if a tumor is responding to a particular chemotherapeutic agent or to radiation after only 1 or 2 weeks. If a therapy is shown to be ineffective, then a new approach can be tried before the tumor has grown significantly.

RECEPTOR-BASED SPECT IMAGING

Indium 111 octreotide is a somatostatin analog that has recently been approved by the FDA for use in the United States. Most tumors of neuroendocrinologic origin have receptors for somatostatin[30] and can be imaged with ^{111}In octreotide, particularly in instances of a breakdown of the blood-brain barrier. Becker and co-workers[31] found significant uptake in three gliomas studied, and uptake apparently correlated inversely with grade.

Hertel and others[32] also studied several different tumors, including four astrocytomas, and found good uptake of ^{111}In octreotide. Kroiss and associates[33] studied six patients with glioblastoma and found uptake in all tumors, with a tumor-to-normal brain ratio of 1.7 ± 0.5.

Although the number of patients with glioma studied with ^{111}In octreotide is low, the results are encouraging. [111]In octreotide has proved to be very useful in imaging somatic tumors with high densities of somatostatin receptors, such as gastrinomas. It is likely to prove to be a very sensitive way to detect the presence of gliomas. If it can be shown to be highly specific, with no uptake in necrosis or scar, then it may turn out to have a significant role in the diagnosis of recurrent or residual disease.

Another receptor-based agent, ^{99m}Tc-labeled P280, also shows good uptake by gliomas.[34] P280 is a synthetic peptide that binds to the integrin receptor in CNS tumors. Uptake was seen in all eight gliomas imaged, with tumor-to-normal brain ratios of 3.2 to 20. These results are preliminary, but this agent may turn out to be a sensitive detector for presence of glioma.

LABELED MONOCLONAL ANTIBODIES

Use of labeled antibodies would seem to be a highly specific and effective way to image tumors. Numerous investigators have studied hundreds of antibodies over the past decade, with moderate success. A number of considerations, including access to binding sites, circulating antigen, and catabolism of the antibodies, make this approach relatively difficult.

Schold and co-workers[35] have studied monoclonal antibody 81C6, which reacts with the extracellular matrix antigen, tenascin, which is present on gliomas as well as on other tumors and on several normal tissues, such as liver and spleen. Recurrent glioma in 16 patients was imaged with SPECT at 1 and 18 hours following injection of ^{123}I-labeled 81C6. Good uptake was seen in all tumors.

Using a different anti-tenascin antibody, BC-2, Lastoria

and others[36] studied 24 patients with high-grade glioma. The sensitivity was 92%, with tumor-to-normal brain ratios of 2.6 to 11.8. These studies suggest that anti-tenascin antibody imaging may turn out to be a successful approach to imaging gliomas and may also be useful in radioimmunotherapy. These antibodies can be labeled with ^{131}I, which can be used to deliver significant radiation doses to the binding sites. If the localization is highly specific then it becomes possible to deliver a high dose to the tumor without excessively irradiating other tissue. This approach is being explored in other tumors, such as melanoma and lymphoma. It may eventually turn out to be a useful way to boost the radiation dose to the tumor.

One other labeled antibody has been studied with glioma, an anti-epidermal growth factor antibody labeled with [99m]Tc.[32] Three astrocytomas were studied, with good uptake seen in the two high-grade tumors and only weak uptake in the low-grade tumor. This was such a small study that it is impossible to draw any conclusions, although additional studies will certainly be done.

CONCLUSION

Overall, five main agents are being used for SPECT imaging of gliomas. These are ^{201}Tl, ^{99m}Tc-MIBI, ^{123}I-IMT, ^{111}In-octreotide, and labeled antibodies, particularly anti-tenascin antibodies. [201]Tl, ^{99m}Tc-MIBI, and ^{111}In-octreotide are currently approved for administration to humans in the United States, although brain tumor imaging is not regarded as a standard indication for the use of these agents.

The approved agents all seem to be quite sensitive in the detection of recurrent or residual tumor, with sensitivities typically greater than 90%. The specificities of these agents is less well defined because relatively small numbers have been reported. If limited specificity turns out to be a significant problem, appropriate solutions can be brought to bear: semiquantitative analysis should be useful. If the tumor-to-normal brain ratio is very high it is more likely that the lesion is truly a tumor. For equivocal cases it may be appropriate to image with a second tumor imaging tracer or with ^{99m}Tc-HMPAO, a blood flow tracer. Another approach may be to image in a dynamic fashion to determine how rapidly the agent washes out. This seems to be particularly appropriate for [201]Tl. Finally, the SPECT image can be regarded as a map of where tumor recurrence is likely, and, after registration with current CT or MR images, it can be used to guide biopsy to make a definitive diagnosis.

SPECT imaging with ^{123}I-IMT represents the migration of metabolic imaging from PET to the nuclear medicine clinic. When this agent becomes widely available it should be particularly useful in evaluating response to therapy. In doing so, particular care will need to be taken in setting up the SPECT apparatus and in reconstructing the images in a consistent and standardized fashion. Otherwise it will not be possible to directly compare the images taken before and after therapy.

SPECT antibody imaging is another very different approach to visualizing gliomas. The anti-tenascin antibody is the most successful approach thus far, but work with this agent is still in very early stages. Ultimately, this may lead to the development of useful ''boost'' radiotherapy, which may be sufficient to improve the cure rate significantly.

REFERENCES

1. Jaszczak RJ: SPECT: State-of-the-art scanners and reconstruction strategies. *In* Diksic M, Reba RC (eds): Radiopharmaceuticals and Brain Pathology Studied With PET and SPECT. Boca Raton, CRC Press, Fla, 1991, p 93.
2. Goodrich JK, Tutor FT: The isotope encephalogram in brain tumor diagnosis. J Nucl Med 1965; 6:541.
3. Witcofski RL, Maynard CD, Roper TJ: A comparative analysis of the accuracy of the technetium-99m pertechnetate brain scan: Followup of 1000 patients. J Nucl Med 1967; 8:187.
4. Rollo FD, Cavalieri RR, Born M, et al: Comparative evaluation of Tc-99m GH, Tc-99m O4, and Tc-99m DTPA as brain imaging agents. Radiology 1977; 123:379.
5. Winchell HS, Horst WA, Braum L, et al: N-isopropyl (I-123) p-iodoamphetamine: Single pass brain uptake and washout, binding to brain synaptosomes and localization in dog and monkey brain. J Nucl Med 1980; 21:947.
6. Neirinckx RD, Canning LA, Piper JM, et al: Technetium-99m d,l-HM-PAO: A new radiopharmaceutical for SPECT imaging of regional brain perfusion. J Nucl Med 1987; 28:191.
7. Vallabhajosula S, Zimmerman RE, Picard M, et al: Technetium-99m EDC: A new brain imaging agent: In vivo kinetics and biodistribution in normal human subjects. J Nucl Med 1989; 30:599.
8. Hill TC, Holman BL, Lovett R, et al: Initial experience with SPECT (single-photon computerized tomography) of the brain using N-isopropyl I-123 p-iodoamphetamine: Concise communication. J Nucl Med 1982; 23:191.
9. Schwartz RB, Carvalho P, Alexander E, et al: Radiation necrosis vs. high-grade recurrent glioma: Differentiation by using dual-isotope SPECT with 201Tl and 99mTc-HMPAO. Am J Neuroradiol 1991; 12:1187.
10. Black KL, Hawkins RA, Kim KT: Use of thallium-201 SPECT to quantitate malignancy grade of gliomas. J Neurosurg 1989; 71:342.
11. Kim KT, Black KL, Marciano D, et al: Thallium-201 SPECT imaging of brain tumors: Methods and results. J Nucl Med 1990; 31:965.
12. Ancri D, Basset J-Y, Lonchampt MF, et al: Diagnosis of cerebral lesions by thallium 201. Radiology 1978; 128:417.
13. O'Tuama LA, Treves ST, Larar JN, et al: Thallium-201 versus technetium-99m-MIBI SPECT in evaluation of childhood brain tumors: A within-subject comparison. J Nucl Med 1993; 34:1045.
14. Guth-Tougelidis, Müller SP, Mehdorn HM: I-123-α-methyl-tyrosine in brain tumor recurrences. J Nucl Med 1990; 31:766.
15. Langen KJ, Coenen HH, Roosen N: SPECT studies of brain tumors with L-3-[123I] iodo-alpha-methyl tyrosine: Comparison with PET 124IMT and first clinical results. J Nucl Med 1990; 31:281.
16. Biersack HJ, Coenen HH, Stocklin G: Imaging of brain tumors with L-3-[123I]iodo-alpha-methyl tyrosine and SPECT. J Nucl Med 1989; 30:110.
17. Shukla SS, Honeyman JC, Crosson B, et al: Method for registering brain SPECT and MR images. J Comput Assist Tomogr 1992; 16:966.
18. Dhawan AP, Arata L: Knowledge-based multi-modality three-dimensional image analysis of the brain. Am J Physiol Imaging 1992; 7:210.
19. Burkard R, Kaiser KP, Wieler H: Contribution of thallium-201 SPECT
20. to the grading of tumorous alterations of the brain. Neurosurg Rev 1992; 15:265.
21. Ueda T, Kaji Y, Wakisaka S, et al: Time sequential single photon emission computed tomography studies in brain tumour using thallium-201. Eur J Nucl Med 1993; 20:138.
21. Maass AJ, Hoh CK, Khanna S, et al: Evaluation of brain tumors with Tl-201 SPECT studies: Updated correlations with FDG PET and histological results. Clin Nucl Med 1992; 17:760.
22. Buchpiquel CA, Alavi J, Alavi A: Comparison of PET-FDG and SPECT TL-201 in distinguishing radiation necrosis from tumor recurrence in the brain. J Nucl Med 1994; 35:222P.
23. Antar MA, Barnett G, McIntyre WJ: Can brain thallium 201 SPECT substitute for F-18-FDG PET in detecting recurrent brain tumor in the presence of radiation necrosis? Correlation with biopsy/surgery results. J Nucl Med 1994; 35(suppl):223P.
24. Oriuchi N, Tamura M, Shibazaki T, et al: Clinical evaluation of thallium-201 SPECT in supratentorial gliomas: Relationship to histologic grade, prognosis and proliferative activities. J Nucl Med 1993; 34:2085.
25. Macapinlac HA, Scott AM, Zhang JJ: The clinical impact of SPECT/PET co-registration with MRI in patients with brain tumors. J Nucl Med 1994; 35(suppl):7P.
26. Darcourt J, Itti L, Chang L, et al: Tl-201 and Tc-99m-sestamibi SPECT for brain tumor detection: Comparison using MRI coregistration. J Nucl Med 1994; 35(suppl):43P.
27. Maffioli L, Gasparini M, Gramaglia A, et al: Tc-99m sestamibi SPECT in detecting local relapses of intracranial tumors: Preliminary clinical experience. Eur J Nucl Med 1994; 21:S120.
27a. Baillet G, Albuquerque L, Chen Q, et al: Evaluation of single-photon emission tomography imaging of supratentorial brain gliomas with technetium 99m sestamibi. Eur J Nucl Med 1994; 21:1061.
28. Kawai K, Fujibayashi, Saji H: New radioiodinated radiopharmaceuticals for cerebral amino acid transport studies: 3-iodo-alpha-methyl-l-tyrosine. J Nucl Med 1988; 29:778.
29. Schober O, Wagner W, Assman S: Transfer from PET to SPECT: The assessment of ^{123}I-α-methyltyrosine (IMT) in recurrence of primary brain tumors. J Nucl Med 1994; 35(suppl):9P.
30. Scheidhauer K, Hildebrandt G, Luyken C, et al: Somatostatin receptor scintigraphy in brain tumors and pituitary tumors: First experiences. Horm Metab Res Suppl 1993; 27:59.
31. Becker W, Schrell U, Lohner W, et al: In-111-octreotide-SPECT in patients with brain and pituitary tumors. J Nucl Med 1993; 34(suppl):37P.
32. Hertel A, Baum RP, Maul FD: Characterisation of brain tumors using dual-isotope SPECT with thallium, somatostatin-analog, anti-EGF antibody. J Nucl Med 1993; 34(suppl):205P.
33. Kroiss A, Böck F, Auinger C: Localization of brain tumors with indium-111 labeled somatostatin analogue and iodine-123-methyl tyrosine. J Nucl Med 1994; 35(suppl):44P.
34. Muto P, Lastoria S, Varrella P, et al: Brain tumors imaged with Tc-99m labeled synthetic peptide P280. Eur J Nucl Med 1994; 21:S198.
35. Schold SC, Zalutsky MR, Coleman RE: Distribution and dosimetry of I-123-labeled monoclonal antibody 81C6 in patients with anaplastic glioma. Invest Radiol 1993; 28:488.
36. Lastoria S, Varrella P, Castelli L: Brain tumor detection by SPECT using Tl-201 and Tc-99m labeled BC-2 monoclonal antibody. J Nucl Med 1993; 34:115P.
37. Hoh CK, Khanna S, Harris GC, et al: Evaluation of brain tumor recurrence with Tl-201 SPECT studies: Correlation with FDG PET and histologic results. J Nucl Med 1992; 33:867.

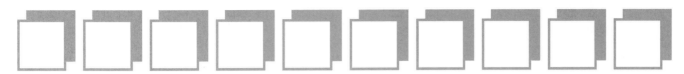

Preoperative Assessment and Management

PATRICK Y. WEN

PETER M. BLACK

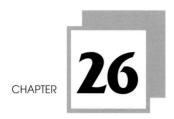

CHAPTER **26**

Clinical Presentation, Evaluation, and Preoperative Preparation of the Patient

In this chapter the clinical features of glioma and the initial evaluation and preoperative management of patients with glioma are discussed.

CLINICAL FEATURES OF GLIOMA

The diagnosis of a probable glioma involves a careful history and examination and the expeditious and cost-efficient use of neuroimaging studies. As a result of the widespread availability of sensitive imaging techniques, such as magnetic resonance imaging (MRI), gliomas are being detected at an earlier stage, at which clinical symptoms and signs are more subtle. Patients with gliomas typically present with headaches, seizures, cognitive or personality changes, and focal neurologic deficits.[1-4] The precise combination of clinical features varies depending on the location, histologic characteristics, and rate of growth of the tumor.

Headache

Headaches are the presenting symptom in approximately 35% of patients with gliomas, and they develop during the course of the disease in 70%.[5] The majority of these headaches are nonspecific and intermittent, and they occur on the same side as the tumor, although they can also be generalized. They are usually dull and nonthrobbing, and are often indistinguishable from tension headaches.[6, 7] Supratentorial gliomas usually produce headaches with a frontal location, as the majority of supratentorial pain-sensitive structures are supplied by the trigeminal nerve. The posterior fossa is innervated by cranial nerves IX and X and upper cervical nerves, and lesions at this site usually produce pain in the occipital region and neck. Posterior fossa tumors occasionally produce headaches focused in the vertex or retro-orbital region.[2]

Certain features of the headache are associated with raised intracranial pressure, which indicates an increased likelihood that an underlying tumor is producing mass effect. These characteristics include headaches that wake the patient at night or that are worse on waking and improve over the course of the day; headaches exacerbated by postural change, coughing, or exercise; and nausea or vomiting.[2, 7]

PAPILLEDEMA

Papilledema is important evidence of increased intracranial pressure being transmitted through the optic nerve sheath. The incidence of papilledema in an older series of patients with brain tumors has been reported to be 50% to 70%.[5] Advances in neuroimaging have resulted in many patients receiving a diagnosis at an earlier stage, and the incidence of papilledema in patients with glioma today is probably much lower. In a review of 100 consecutive patients with malignant gliomas who underwent surgery at Brigham and Women's Hospital, Boston, only 8% had papilledema at the time of diagnosis.[8] Papilledema tends to be more common with slow-growing and posterior fossa tumors and in children. It may be associated with symptoms of transient obscuring of vision, especially with postural change.

Seizure

Seizures are the presenting symptom in approximately one third of patients with gliomas, and they are present at some stage of the illness in 50% to 70% of patients.[5, 9, 10] Approximately half of patients with seizures have focal seizures, and the other half have generalized seizures.

Slow-growing low-grade gliomas are particularly likely to cause seizures,[10, 11] whereas glioblastomas have a lower frequency of seizures, possibly because the decreased lifespan allows less time for development of an epileptic focus.[11] In some early series, seizures occurred in 75% to 95% of patients with oligodendrogliomas, in 65% to 70% of patients with astrocytomas, and in 37% to 50% of patients with glioblastomas.[11-13] Patients with malignant gliomas who present with seizure tend to have a better prognosis,[14] possibly because these tumors are often diagnosed at an earlier stage than tumors in patients presenting with mass effect or focal deficits.

The location of the tumor also affects the frequency of seizures. Supratentorial tumors, especially those located near the rolandic fissure, are particularly likely to cause seizures. Tumors in subcortical areas such as thalamus and the posterior fossa are much less epileptogenic. In one series, seizures occur in 59% of frontal tumors, 42% of parietal tumors, 35% of temporal tumors, and 33% of occipital tumors.[15]

Conversely, 10% of 20% of adult patients with new onset of seizures have brain tumors.[16] Computed tomographic (CT) scanning or MRI should always be part of the evaluation of these patients, especially if they also have focal findings on examination or on electroencephalography (EEG). Among patients who undergo resective surgery to treat intractable seizures, tumors are found in 10% to 20% of adults[9] and in 25% to 46% of children.[17] In children, low-grade astrocytomas are the most common tumor; oligodendroglioma, ganglioglioma, and dysembryoplastic neuroepithelial tumors also occur in children.[11]

Altered Mental Status

Mental status changes are the initial symptom in 15% to 20% of patients with gliomas, and such changes are frequently present in patients by the time of diagnosis.[5] These changes may range from subtle problems with concentration, memory, affect, personality, initiative, and abstract reasoning to severe cognitive problems and confusion. Changes in mentation are especially common in frontal lobe tumors, but they also occur with increased intracranial pressure from the mass effect of a tumor or hydrocephalus or as a result of gliomatosis cerebri. With increasing intracranial pressure, depression of the level of consciousness also occurs, resulting in drowsiness and eventually leading to stupor and coma if treatment is not administered.

Focal Neurologic Symptoms and Signs

Whereas headaches, seizures, and altered mental status may be seen with gliomas in many locations, certain clinical features have specific localizing value.

CORTICAL TUMORS

Frontal lobe gliomas are often clinically silent initially. As the tumor enlarges, personality changes may occur. Symptoms are most prominent when both frontal lobes are involved, but can occur with unilateral lesions. Orbital frontal lesions may cause disinhibition, irritability, impaired judgment, jocularity, and profanity. Dorsal midline lesions may produce lack of initiative (abulia). Lesions over the dorsolateral convexities may produce apathy, reduced drive, and impaired planning.[18] More posterior tumors may produce hemiparesis, seizures, aphasia, urinary frequency, urinary urgency, and gait difficulties. Gaze preference and primitive reflexes, such as forced grasping and snout may be present.

Temporal lobe tumors frequently cause seizures. These include simple partial seizures characterized by olfactory and gustatory hallucinations, déjà vu, and feelings of fear and pleasure, and complex partial seizures characterized by impairment of consciousness, repetitive psychomotor movements, and automatic behavior. Temporal lobe tumors may also cause memory disturbances, visual field defects (superior quadrantopsia), tinnitus, vertigo,[2] and, when the dominant temporal lobe is involved, aphasia. Some patients with temporal lesions have certain behavioral manifestations such as hyperreligiosity, hypergraphia, and hyposexuality.

Gliomas of the parietal lobe can produce contralateral sensory loss involving particularly joint position sense, two-point discrimination, stereognosis, and graphesthesia, although other modalities are also involved. Lesions in the dominant parietal lobe are associated with aphasia, whereas lesions in the nondominant parietal lobe may result in neglect of the contralateral side and the loss of ability to acknowledge deficits (anosognosia). Hemiparesis (arm and face affected more than leg), homonymous visual defects (or neglect), agnosias, apraxias, sensory seizures, and disturbance of visual spatial ability may also be present.

Occipital lobe gliomas may cause homonymous hemianopsia and, less commonly, visual seizures characterized by lights, colors, and formed geometric patterns. Tumors at the parieto-occipital junction may produce visual agnosias such as prosopagnosia (inability to recognize faces), or Balint's syndrome, characterized by a combination of visual disorientation (simultanagnosia), deficit of visual reaching (optic ataxia), and deficit of visual scanning (ocular apraxia).

BRAINSTEM TUMORS

Brainstem gliomas are much more common in children than in adults. They may produce cranial neuropathies, weakness, numbness, ataxia, vertigo, nausea, vomiting, and hiccups. As the tumor increases in size, compression of the aqueduct or the fourth ventricle may occur, producing hydrocephalus.[19]

Thalamic gliomas may produce contralateral sensory loss, hemiparesis, cognitive impairment, and occasionally visual defects and aphasia. Obstructive hydrocephalus occurs commonly and is associated with headache, nausea, vomiting, gait unsteadiness, and urinary incontinence.

PINEAL REGION AND THIRD VENTRICULAR TUMORS

Gliomas in the pineal region are uncommon. They may present either with symptoms of hydrocephalus, resulting from compression of the third ventricle and aqueduct, or with symptoms produced by compression of the tectum of the midbrain. Midbrain compression may result in disturbance of extraocular function, including Parinaud's syndrome, which is characterized by impairment of upgaze and pupillary light-accommodation reflex disturbance. Children occasionally present with precocious puberty.

Gliomas around the third ventricle may produce hydrocephalus. Valsalva maneuvers and positional changes may increase CSF obstruction and lead to severe headaches and occasional leg weakness and syncope. Tumors in this region may also produce memory impairment and symptoms resulting from hypothalamic and autonomic dysfunction. Children with hypothalamic gliomas occasionally have a syndrome characterized by cachexia and anorexia.

CEREBELLAR TUMORS

Headaches and ataxia are the two most common symptoms in patients with cerebellar gliomas. The headaches may be the result of the tumor or hydrocephalus. They are often occipital and are associated with nausea, vomiting, and sometimes neck stiffness. Some patients may experience vertigo. Midline cerebellar lesions may produce truncal ataxia, whereas lesions in the cerebellar hemispheres may cause appendicular ataxia, although frequently the findings are relatively subtle. Examination may also show nystagmus, hypotonia, and cranial nerve and corticospinal tract signs from brainstem compression. Head tilt away from the lesion may occur with incipient tonsillar herniation, which is an important sign of a cerebellar tumor in a child.

Cranial Nerves

Optic gliomas usually present with visual loss and variable visual field defects. Proptosis, nystagmus, and extraocular palsies are much less common presenting features. Other clinical features may also be present that are suggestive of involvement of the hypothalamus. Approximately 35% to 50% of children with optic gliomas have neurofibromatosis, and examination may reveal café au lait spots and other stigmata of this disorder.[20] Lower cranial nerve deficits usually result from brainstem or posterior fossa tumors. Multiple cranial nerve palsies occur with meningeal gliomatosis, in which tumor deposits coat the cranial nerves.

Herniation Syndromes

Occasionally, the progressive mass effect resulting from enlarging gliomas and surrounding edema produces pressure gradients between intracranial compartments, which give rise to herniation syndromes.[21, 22]

CENTRAL TRANSTENTORIAL HERNIATION

Central transtentorial herniation results from progressive involvement of both hemispheres or diencephalon by tumor. The brainstem is displaced downward, leading to a characteristic series of clinical features resulting from rostral-caudal brainstem dysfunction. Impairment of consciousness is the initial manifestation, followed by signs of forebrain dysfunction (Cheyne-Stokes respiration, small reactive pupils, extensor plantar responses, and decorticate posturing), midbrain dysfunction (hyperventilation, decerebrate posturing, pupils fixed in the midposition, and dysconjugate vestibular ocular reflexes), and, finally, medullary dysfunction (ataxic breathing, loss of all brainstem function, and death).

UNCAL HERNIATION

A laterally placed glioma in the frontal or temporal lobe may push the uncus of the temporal lobe medially over the tentorial edge. This often results in entrapment of the oculomotor nerve by the herniating uncus on the free edge of the tentorium. As a result, dilation of the ipsilateral pupil is often the earliest sign of uncal herniation, followed by a complete ipsilateral oculomotor palsy, contralateral hemiparesis, impairment of consciousness, and the progressive brainstem dysfunction seen with central herniation.

TONSILLAR HERNIATION

Gliomas in the posterior fossa can result in herniation of the cerebellar tonsils through the foramen magnum. Tonsillar herniation can cause nuchal rigidity and head tilt and, eventually, respiratory depression and arrest, as a result of compression of the medulla.

UPWARD TRANSTENTORIAL HERNIATION

Posterior fossa gliomas can lead to upward displacement of the brainstem and the anterior cerebellum through the tentorium. Chronic herniation leads to hydrocephalus and spasticity. Acute herniation produces loss of upgaze, impaired consciousness, and death.

SUBFALCINE HERNIATION

Enlarging frontal lobe gliomas can result in displacement of the cingulate gyrus under the falx cerebri. This may lead to compression of the anterior cerebral artery and infarction of the territory it supplies.

False Localizing Signs

Occasionally when tumors produce increased intracranial pressure, shifting of intracranial structures occurs and results in clinical features that suggest involvement of sites distant from the tumor. These are false localizing signs. Examples include abducens nerve (cranial nerve VI) palsy resulting from compression of the nerve as it passes forward over the petrous ligament, and compression of the cerebral peduncle by the free edge of the tentorium cerebelli contralateral to a herniating uncus, which produces hemiparesis on the same side as the lesion.[2]

Differential Diagnosis

The diagnosis of glioma can usually be made on the basis of clinical features and radiologic findings. However, many conditions that produce progressive neurologic deficits or increased intracranial pressure may mimic gliomas. These include the following:

1. Other brain tumors, such as metastatic tumors, primary central nervous system lymphomas, benign brain tumors, and cystic lesions, such as arachnoid and colloid cysts.

2. Non-neoplastic conditions, such as subdural hematomas, brain abscesses, hydrocephalus, benign intracranial hypertension, progressive multifocal leukoencephalopathy, multiple sclerosis, vascular malformations, cerebral infarctions, vasculitis, and Alzheimer's disease.

Although many of these conditions have characteristic

TABLE 26–1
PREOPERATIVE PREPARATION OF THE PATIENT

1. Assessment of the patient's general medical status to exclude complicating medical conditions
   Cardiovascular disorders (e.g., coronary artery disease and hypertension)
   Respiratory disorders (e.g., chronic obstructive airways disease and asthma)
   Renal disorders (e.g., chronic renal failure)
   Hepatic disorders (e.g., hepatitis and cirrhosis)
   Endocrine disorders (e.g., diabetes and hypothyroidism)
   Neurologic disorders (e.g., transient ischemic attacks)
   Hematologic disorders (e.g., coagulopathies)
   Nutritional disorders (e.g., cachexia)
   Genetic/metabolic disorders (e.g., adverse reactions to previous anesthesia, pseudocholinesterase deficiency)
   Tests: Complete blood cell count, bleeding time, prothrombin and partial thromboplastin times, glucose, electrolytes, liver function tests, blood urea nitrogen, creatinine, chest x-ray, electrocardiogram
2. Evaluation of patient's medications
   Exclusion of medications that make surgery unsafe (e.g., aspirin, warfarin)
   Placement of patient on appropriate medications (e.g., anticonvulsants, steroids)
3. Cross-matching blood
4. Obtaining informed consent
5. Psychological and emotional support

From Glick RP, Penny D, Hart A: The preoperative and postoperative management of the brain tumor patient. *In* Morantz RA, Walsh JW (eds): Brain Tumors. New York, Marcel Dekker, 1993, pp 345–366.

radiologic appearances that enable them to be differentiated from gliomas, some require histologic examination for definitive diagnosis. These include other types of brain tumors, brain abscess, inflammatory lesions, demyelinating disease, and hamartomas.

EVALUATION AND PREOPERATIVE MANAGEMENT

Because of the importance of precise histologic diagnosis and grading in the management of patients with glioma, most patients undergo either a stereotactic biopsy or a craniotomy. In addition to the preoperative evaluation and management that is required for all neurosurgical procedures (Table 26–1), several problems occur commonly in glioma patients at the time of diagnosis that may require treatment prior to surgery. These include seizures, increased intracranial pressure from cerebral edema, and hydrocephalus. Despite the frequency and importance of these problems, few formal studies are available to guide optimal management.

Use of Anticonvulsants

The management of patients with gliomas who present with seizures is straightforward and involves the use of standard anticonvulsants, such as phenytoin (Table 26–2). EEG may be useful if the diagnosis of seizures is in doubt, but it is not needed routinely either for patients who give a clear history of seizures or for those who have no symptoms suggestive of seizures. In addition to the usual complications of anticonvulsants (Table 26–3), glioma patients experience an increased incidence of certain side effects, especially drug rashes.

Approximately 15% to 20% of glioma patients who are treated with phenytoin and undergo cranial irradiation develop a morbilliform rash, and a small percentage develop Stevens-Johnson syndrome.[23] The mechanism for this is unknown but it may result from depletion of suppressor T cells by the radiation therapy, which allows the development of a hypersensitivity reaction to phenytoin.[23] Stevens-Johnson syndrome has also been described in glioma patients receiving carbamazepine,[24] whereas patients receiving phenobarbital have an increased incidence of shoulder-hand syndrome.[25]

In addition to producing adverse effects, anticonvulsants also have clinically significant interactions with other drugs commonly administered to brain tumor patients. Phenytoin induces the hepatic metabolism of dexamethasone and significantly reduces the half-life and bioavailability of this corticosteroid.[26, 27] Conversely, dexamethasone may also reduce phenytoin levels.[28] A number of chemotherapeutic agents commonly given to brain tumor patients, such as carmustine, interact with phenytoin, which causes the levels

TABLE 26–2
ANTICONVULSANT THERAPY FOR GLIOMA PATIENTS

Drug	Loading Dose	Maintenance Dose	Therapeutic Levels
Phenytoin (Dilantin)	15 mg/kg	4–7 mg/kg/day	10–20 μg/mL
Phenobarbital	10–20 mg/kg	3–5 mg/kg/day	15–40 μg/mL
Primidone (Mysoline)	Gradual load over 1–2 wk	500–2,000 mg/day	Primidone, 5–12 μg/mL Phenobarbital, 15–40 μg/mL
Carbamazepine (Tegretol)	Gradual load over 1–3 wk	15–25 mg/kg/day in 2–3 divided doses	4–12 μg/mL
Valproic acid (Depakote, Depakene)	Gradual load over 1–3 wk	400–3,000 mg/day in 2–4 divided doses	50–100 μg/mL
Clonazepam (Klonopin)	Gradual load over 1–3 wk	1–15 mg/day in 3 divided doses	Not necessary
Felbamate (Felbatol)	1,200 mg/day, wk 1 2,400 mg/day, wk 2	2,400–3,600 mg/day in 2–3 divided doses	Not necessary
Gabapentin (Neurontin)	300 mg qd, day 1 300 mg bid, day 2 300 mg tid, day 3	900–3,600 mg/day (in 3 divided doses)	Not necessary
Lamotrigine (Lamictal)	Gradual load over several weeks	300–500 mg/day in 2 doses 100–150 mg/day with valproic acid	Not necessary

TABLE 26–3
COMPLICATIONS OF COMMONLY USED ANTICONVULSANTS

Phenytoin (Dilantin) (DPH)
Dose dependent: Drowsiness, ataxia, confusion, nausea, vomiting, constipation, tremor, choreoathetosis
Idiosyncratic: Rashes, blood dyscrasias, hepatitis (often occurs as part of a hypersensitivity syndrome in association with rash, fever, lymphadenopathy, and blood dyscrasias), SLE, pseudolymphoma, possibly lymphoma
Effects of chronic administration: Gingival hyperplasia, coarsening of facial features, hirsutism, cerebellar degeneration, neuropathy, folate deficiency, hypocalcemia, teratogenicity

Carbamazepine (Tegretol) (CBZ)
Dose dependent: Drowsiness, dizziness, diplopia, myoclonus, leukopenia (10%), SIADH
Idiosyncratic: Exfoliative dermatitis, aplastic anemia, thrombocytopenia, pancytopenia, bradyarrhythmias and atrioventricular block (elderly patients), jaundice, lymphatic hyperplasia, lenticular opacities
Drug interactions: DPH, PB, and mysoline decrease CBZ levels; CBZ increases DPH levels and decreases VPA levels

Phenobarbital and Primidone (Mysoline) (PB)
Dose dependent: Drowsiness, ataxia, impaired cognitive function
Idiosyncratic: Hyperactivity and confusion, rash (may be transient), blood dyscrasias, hepatitis, SLE, decreased folate levels (all rare), shoulder-hand syndrome
Drug interactions: Decreases levels of other anticonvulsants

Valproic Acid (Depakote/Depakene) (VPA)
Dose dependent: Sedation, nausea, vomiting, GI discomfort, ataxia, tremor, myoclonus, transaminitis, hyperammonemia
Idiosyncratic: Hepatitis, pancreatitis, alopecia, thrombocytopenia, platelet dysfunction
Drug interactions: VPA increases PB and CBZ levels and decreases total DPH levels; CBZ reduces VPA levels

Clonazepam (Klonopin)
Dose dependent: Sedation, ataxia, dizziness, hypersalivation
Idiosyncratic: Behavioral change, appetite change, thrombocytopenia, increased seizure frequency
Drug interactions: DPH and PB may lower levels of clonazepam; clonazepam does not affect levels of other anticonvulsants

Felbamate (Felbatol)
Dose dependent: Blurred vision, anorexia, nausea and abdominal discomfort, mild tremors, ataxia
Idiosyncratic: Headache, insomnia, rash, fever, hypophosphatemia, aplastic anemia, liver failure
Drug interactions: May increase DPH and VPA levels and decrease carbamazepine levels

Gabapentin (Neurontin)
Dose dependent: Somnolence, ataxia, fatigue, nausea, dizziness, tremors
Idiosyncratic: Rash, leukopenia, dyspepsia, constipation
Drug interactions: Does not interfere with metabolism of other anticonvulsants

Lamotrigine (Lamictil)
Dose dependent: Somnolence, blurred vision, dizziness, headaches, diplopia, ataxia, nausea, vomiting
Idiosyncratic: Rash, Stevens-Johnson syndrome
Drug interactions: Addition of lamotrigine does not affect DPH and CBZ. VPA increases lamotrigine levels and lamotrigine decreases VPA levels

---

Abbreviation: SIADH, syndrome of inappropriate secretion of antidiuretic hormone.
Data from Browne TR, Feldman RG: Epilepsy: Diagnosis and Management. Boston, Brown & Connelly, 1983; and Wyllie E: The Treatment of Epilepsy: Principles and Practice. Philadelphia, Lea & Febiger, 1993.

to fall and can potentially lead to breakthrough seizures,[29] whereas phenobarbital may interfere with certain chemotherapeutic agents.[30]

The role of prophylactic anticonvulsant therapy in glioma patients who have not had a seizure remains controversial. Because the risk of seizures in patients with infratentorial gliomas is very small, anticonvulsant therapy is usually not indicated. The role of anticonvulsant therapy in patients with supratentorial gliomas who have not had a seizure is unknown. Most of these patients are placed on prophylactic anticonvulsant therapy because they are perceived to be at high risk from seizures and because many of them will undergo surgery.

Two small retrospective studies have evaluated the usefulness of anticonvulsant therapy in glioma patients without a history of seizures, and these have produced conflicting results. Boarini and co-workers[31] studied 68 patients, of whom 33 received prophylactic anticonvulsants. Seizures occurred in 39% of untreated patients and in 21% of patients receiving anticonvulsants. Moreover, patients receiving anticonvulsants had fewer generalized seizures. In contrast, Ma-

haley and Dudka[32] studied 59 patients and found that the incidence of seizures was higher in patients who received anticonvulsants (39%) than in patients who did not (28%).

Many glioma patients are treated with anticonvulsants partly because they have had a craniotomy. However, the issue of whether prophylactic anticonvulsant therapy reduces the frequency of seizures after craniotomy is unclear. Early studies, such as that of North and others,[33] found that prophylactic anticonvulsants reduced the frequency of postoperative seizures. However, analysis of their data showed that most of the increased seizure frequency in the patients receiving placebo occurred in the first postoperative week. Foy and associates[34] completed a prospective trial involving 276 consecutive supratentorial craniotomy patients who were randomized postoperatively to receive either carbamazepine or phenytoin or no treatment. No difference was seen in the incidence of seizures (37%) or death between the two groups, suggesting that prophylactic anticonvulsant therapy may not be routinely necessary after craniotomy.

The increased incidence of allergic reactions in patients with brain tumors receiving anticonvulsant therapy and the lack of clear evidence that anticonvulsant therapy reduces the incidence of seizures have led some authors to recommend against the routine prescription of anticonvulsants to brain tumor patients if they have not experienced a seizure.[35] Several prospective randomized studies are currently in progress to evaluate the role of prophylactic anticonvulsants in patients with newly diagnosed gliomas. These studies will provide much-needed guidance on the optimal use of anticonvulsants in such patients.

Treatment of Peritumoral Edema

Peritumoral edema is uncommon with low-grade gliomas, but it occurs frequently with high-grade gliomas and contributes significantly to the mass effect and morbidity associated with these tumors. The edema associated with gliomas is vasogenic in origin.[36] It results from the disruption of the blood-brain barrier, which allows protein-rich fluid to accumulate in the extracellular space.[36] Vasogenic edema tends to spread more readily in the white matter extracellular space in comparison with gray matter, possibly because of lower resistance of white matter to flow.[37]

The breakdown of the blood-brain barrier within gliomas is caused by (1) the production of factors, such as vascular permeability factor (VPF),[38] glutamate,[39] and leukotrienes,[40] which increase the permeability of tumor vessels, and (2) the absence of tight endothelial cell junctions in tumor blood vessels, which develop in response to angiogenic factors such as basic fibroblast growth factor (FGF2)[41] and VPF.[38]

Increased intracranial pressure can be adequately managed with corticosteroids in most glioma patients. Occasionally, when significant intracranial pressure and mass effect are present, other measures may be required.

CORTICOSTEROIDS

The use of corticosteroids for the treatment of peritumoral edema was first described by Galicich and co-workers[42] in 1961, and it has remained the primary treatment since then. It is usually indicated in any glioma patient with more than a minimal amount of peritumoral edema, especially if the edema is contributing to mass effect and symptoms. Corticosteroids produce their anti-edema effect by reducing the permeability of tumor capillaries, which limits the leakage of sodium, protein, and water into the peritumoral extracellular space.[43] Corticosteroids may also increase the clearance of peritumoral edema by facilitating the transport of fluid into the ventricular system, from which it is cleared by CSF bulk flow.[44]

Most patients are usually started on dexamethasone (or an equivalent steroid) at a dose of 16 mg/day. Although this is often given in four divided doses, its biologic half-life is sufficiently long to allow the medication to be administered twice daily.[45, 46] Most patients improve within 48 to 72 hours. In general, headaches tend to respond better than focal deficits. If 16 mg of dexamethasone is insufficient, the dose may be increased, up to 100 mg/day.[37] Steroids improve the patient's symptoms and reduce the morbidity of surgery by reducing cerebral edema and intracranial pressure. Despite the usefulness of corticosteroids, they are associated with a large number of well-known side effects (Table 26–4).

TABLE 26–4
COMPLICATIONS OF CORTICOSTEROID THERAPY

Neurologic	*Common:* Behavioral changes, insomnia, myopathy, hallucinations, hiccups, tremor, reduced taste and smell, cerebral atrophy *Uncommon:* Psychosis, dementia, seizures, dependence, paraparesis (epidural lipomatosis)
Dermatologic	Thin, fragile skin; purpura; ecchymoses; striae; acne; inhibition of wound healing; Kaposi's sarcoma
Rheumatologic	Osteoporosis, avascular necrosis, growth retardation, tendinous rupture
Gastrointestinal	Increased appetite, abdominal bloating, gastrointestinal bleeding and perforation, pancreatitis, liver hypertrophy
Ophthalmologic	Visual blurring, cataract, glaucoma, exophthalmos, uveitis
Cardiovascular	Hypertension, atherosclerosis, arrhythmia (with IV push)
Endocrine/metabolic	Hyperglycemia, hypokalemia, hypophosphatemia, hypernatremia, hyperlipidemia, redistribution of body fat (e.g., centripetal obesity, buffalo hump), amenorrhea
Urogenital	Polyuria, genital burning (with IV push)
Miscellaneous	Opportunistic infections (including candidiasis, *Pneumocystis carinii* pneumonitis), hypersensitivity reactions, neutrophilia, lymphopenia, night sweats
Steroid withdrawal	Pseudorheumatism (very common), headache, lethargy, low-grade fever, adrenal insufficiency, pseudotumor cerebri

Adapted from Delattre JY, Posner JB: Neurologic complications of chemotherapy and radiation therapy. *In* Aminoff MJ (ed): Neurology and General Medicine, ed 2. New York, Churchill Livingstone, 1995, pp 421–446.

Use of H$_2$-Blockers With Steroids Most brain tumor patients receiving corticosteroids are routinely treated with histamine (H$_2$)-blockers to prevent peptic ulceration and upper gastrointestinal (GI) hemorrhage. However, the relationship between corticosteroids, peptic ulceration, and GI bleeding is controversial. The widespread impression that corticosteroids are potentially ulcerogenic originated from observations that stress produced acute ulcers,[47, 48] and from anecdotal studies suggesting that corticosteroids increase and alter the composition of gastric acid secretion.

Theoretically, an association between corticosteroid therapy and peptic ulceration could be established by a prospective randomized clinical trial. However, such a trial is unlikely ever to occur because of the low incidence of peptic ulceration and the difficulty of recruiting a sufficient number of patients. An attempt was made to answer this question in 1976 by Conn and Blitzer,[49] who conducted a retrospective analysis of 42 randomized control trials evaluating the use of corticosteroids in a variety of diseases. This study concluded that there was no statistically significant association between corticosteroid use and upper GI bleeding. Messer and co-workers,[50] in 1983, expanded the analysis to 72 clinical trials. In contrast to the results of the study of Conn and Blitzer, they found that the incidence of peptic ulceration and GI tract bleeding in patients receiving steroids (1.8%

and 2.5%, respectively) was significantly higher than that in controls (0.8% and 1.6%, respectively). However, a reanalysis of the data of Messer and colleagues demonstrated no statistical association between corticosteroids and the occurrence of peptic ulcers.[51] More recently, Carson and colleagues[52] assessed a cohort of ambulatory patients receiving corticosteroids and found a very low incidence of upper GI bleeding (2.8 cases per 10,000 person-months). They concluded that if prophylactic therapy should be used at all, it should be restricted to high-risk patients with a previous history of GI bleeding who are receiving anticoagulation therapy.

In summary, the available data does not definitively support an association between corticosteroids, peptic ulceration, and GI bleeding. Even if an association exists, the overall incidence of peptic ulceration and GI bleeding is very low. There are few data concerning the risk of peptic ulceration and GI bleeding, or the effectiveness of prophylactic therapy with H_2-blockers in glioma patients who often take high doses of steroids. Although these medications are relatively benign, some H_2-blockers (e.g., cimetidine) can produce such CNS side effects as confusion, and most H_2-blockers are expensive. In the absence of data from clinical studies guiding the use of H_2-blockers in brain tumor patients, the use of these medications should probably be restricted to the perioperative period and to patients receiving very high doses of corticosteroids. For most other patients, prophylactic therapy with H_2-blockers is probably unnecessary unless they are at high risk for development of peptic ulcers (i.e., previous history of peptic ulcers, receiving anticoagulation or non-steroidal anti-inflammatory drugs, and old age).

OTHER THERAPIES FOR INCREASED INTRACRANIAL PRESSURE

Corticosteroids may require several days to reduce intracranial pressure from peritumoral edema. Glioma patients occasionally present with significantly increased intracranial pressure from the mass effects of the tumor and edema, and other measures may be required to lower the intracranial pressure until corticosteroids have had a chance to take effect or until the patient has a craniotomy and undergoes a debulking procedure. These measures include the following:

1. Elevation of the head of the bed (30 degrees), which displaces CSF from the intracranial cavity and enhances cerebral venous outflow.

2. Fluid restriction (1 to 1.5 L/day).

3. Use of osmotic agents. Agents such as mannitol, which are relatively impermeable to the blood-brain barrier, are commonly used for the short-term treatment of increased intracranial pressure. These agents decrease intracranial pressure by reducing total brain water, which creates an osmotic gradient toward the intravascular space. Mannitol may also decrease intracranial pressure by increasing erythrocyte deformability and hemodilution with decreased blood viscosity.[53] Mannitol is usually given at an initial dose of 0.75 to 1.0 g/kg followed by 0.25 to 0.5 g/kg every 3 to 5 hours, aiming for a target osmolality of 300 to 310 mOsm/L. The effect of mannitol on intracra-

nial pressure is usually achieved within 10 to 30 minutes after administration, with maximal intracranial pressure reduction occurring within 20 to 60 minutes. Complications of therapy with osmotic agents include hypokalemia, hypochloremic alkalosis, dehydration, hypotension, nonketotic hyperosmolar state, and rebound intracranial hypertension after prolonged use.[53]

4. Use of diuretics. These are effective for the short-term treatment of increased intracranial pressure, especially when used in combination with osmotic therapy. They produce a mild osmotic diuresis (resulting in an osmotic gradient toward the intravascular space), reduce CSF formation, and remove sodium and water from the brain.[53] Loop diuretics, such as furosemide (20 to 40 mg), are used most commonly. Administration of furosemide 15 minutes after administration of mannitol appears to be the most effective in lowering intracranial pressure. The main side effects of loop diuretics are electrolyte disturbance and systemic dehydration.

5. Hyperventilation is an effective short-term measure to reduce intracranial pressure. It produces hypocarbia and lowers intracranial pressure by reducing cerebral blood volume. The reduction in intracranial pressure is rapid, although the maximal effect may follow the change in pCO_2 by 15 to 30 minutes. Usually the pCO_2 is gradually lowered to 25 to 35 mm Hg to achieve the desired intracranial pressure. The intracranial pressure gradually returns to baseline despite hyperventilation, making this an effective treatment for increased intracranial pressure only in the short term.

Hydrocephalus

Gliomas located in the posterior fossa, brainstem, basal ganglia, and diencephalon occasionally obstruct the CSF pathways, resulting in hydrocephalus. Affected patients develop headaches, nausea, vomiting, ataxia, blurred or double vision, urinary incontinence, and obtundation, and a loss of venous pulsation and papilledema may be noted on funduscopic examination. Patients in whom acute obstructive hydrocephalus develops are often very sick and frequently require treatment before definitive surgery for the underlying glioma. Several reviews discuss the management of hydrocephalus in detail.[54, 55, 56] Although medical treatment, especially diuretics, may reduce CSF production for a few days, surgical intervention is usually necessary. Treatment options include insertion of an external ventricular drain to decompress the ventricular system until the obstructing glioma can be resected[56] or placement of a ventriculoperitoneal shunt. In most cases a shunt is preferable, unless it appears that the tumor can be resected completely enough to open up the CSF pathways with certainty.

EMOTIONAL AND PSYCHOLOGICAL SUPPORT

The diagnosis of a glioma inevitably has a devastating and profound effect on the patient and the family. In addition to providing optimal medical care, an important aspect of the preoperative preparation of these patients includes supplying information about the tumor, providing therapeutic options in a compassionate manner, and giving emotional and psychological support. Frequently, the patient and the family will benefit from the help provided by patient support groups, psychiatrists, and societies such as the American Brain Tumor Association (3725 North Talman Ave., Chicago, IL 60618; telephone: 312–286–5571; patient line: 1–800–886–2282), the Brain Tumor Society (84 Seattle St., Boston, MA 02134; telephone: 1–617–243–4229), and the National Brain Tumor Foundation (323 Geary St., Suite 510, San Francisco, CA 94102; telephone: 1–800–934–CURE [2873]).

REFERENCES

1. Thomas DGT, McKeran RO: Clinical manifestations of brain tumors. *In* Thomas DGT (ed): Neuro-oncology: Primary Malignant Brain Tumors. Baltimore, Johns Hopkins University Press, 1990, pp 94–121.
2. Jaeckle KA: Clinical presentation and therapy of nervous system tumors. *In* Bradley WG, Daroff RB, Fenichel GM, et al (eds): Neurology in Clinical Practice. Boston, Butterworth-Heinemann, 1991, pp 1008–1030.
3. Wen PY, Schiff D: Clinical evaluation of patients with astrocytomas. *In* Black PM, Schoene W, Lampson LA (eds): Astrocytomas. Oxford, Blackwell, 1993, pp 26–35.
4. Black PM, Wen PY: Clinical, laboratory, and radiologic diagnosis. *In* Kaye A, Laws E (eds): Encyclopedia of Brain Tumors. Edinburgh, Churchill Livingstone, 1995, pp 191–214.
5. McKeran RO, Thomas DGT: The clinical study of gliomas. *In* Thomas DGT, Graham DL (eds): Brain Tumors: Scientific Basis, Clinical Investigation and Current Therapy. Baltimore, Johns Hopkins University Press, 1980, pp 194–230.
6. Rushton JG, Rooke ED: Brain tumor headache. Headache 1962; 2:139–146.
7. Forsyth P, Posner JB: Headaches in patients with brain tumors: A study of 111 patients. Neurology 1993; 43:678–683.
8. El-Ovahabi M, et al: Unpublished data, 1993.
9. Morris HH, Estes ML: Brain tumors and chronic epilepsy. *In* Wyllie E (ed): The Treatment of Epilepsy: Principles and Practice. Philadelphia, Lea & Febiger, 1993, pp 659–666.
10. Cascino GD: Epilepsy and brain tumors: Implications for treatment. Epilepsia 1990; 3:S37–44.
11. Ettinger AB: Structural causes of epilepsy. Neurol Clin 1994; 12:41–56.
12. Ketz E: Brain tumors and epilepsy. *In* Vinken PJ, Bruyn GW (eds): Handbook of Clinical Neurology. Amsterdam, North Holland Publishing, 1974, pp 254–269.
13. Le Blanc FE, Rasmussen T: Cerebral seizures and brain tumors. *In* Vinken PJ, Bruyn GW (eds): Handbook of Clinical Neurology. Amsterdam, North Holland Publishing, 1974, pp 295–301.
14. Gehan EA, Walker MD: Prognostic factors for patients with brain tumors. Monogr Natl Cancer Inst 1977; 46:189–195.
15. Scott GM, Gibberd FB: Epilepsy and other factors in the prognosis of gliomas. Acta Neurol Scand 1980; 61:227–239.
16. Dam AM, Fuglsang-Frederiksen A, Svarre-Olsen U, et al: Late onset epilepsy: Etiologies, type of seizure, and value of clinical investigation, EEG and computerized tomography scan. Epilepsia 1985; 26:227–231.
17. Drake J, Hoffman HJ, Kobayashi J: Surgical management of children with temporal lobe epilepsy and mass lesions. Neurosurgery 1987; 21:792–797.
18. Kramer KL, Bullard DE: Clinical presentation in the brain tumor patient. *In* Morantz RA, Walsh JW (eds): Brain Tumors. New York, Marcel Dekker, 1993, pp 183–212.
19. Packer RJ, Nicholson S, Vezina G, et al: Brainstem gliomas. Neurosurg Clin 1992; 3:863–880.
20. Cohen ME, Duffner PK: Tumors of the diencephalon and optic pathway. *In* Cohen ME, Duffner PK (ed): Brain Tumors in Children: Principles of Diagnosis and Treatment. New York, Raven Press, 1994, pp 303–328.
21. Plum F, Posner JB: The Diagnosis of Stupor and Coma, ed 3. Philadelphia, FA Davis, 1980.
22. Cohen ME, Duffner PK: Principles of diagnosis. *In* Cohen ME, Duffner PK (ed): Brain Tumors in Children: Principles of Diagnosis and Treatment. New York, Raven Press, 1994, pp 13–26.
23. Delattre JY, Posner JB: Neurologic complications of chemotherapy and radiation therapy. *In* Aminoff MJ (ed): Neurology and General Medicine. New York, Churchill Livingstone, 1989, pp 365–388.
24. Hoang-Xuan K, Delattre J-Y, Poisson M: Stevens-Johnson syndrome in a patient receiving cranial irradiation and carbamazepine. Neurology 1990; 40:1144–1145.
25. Taylor LP, Posner JB: Phenobarbital rheumatism in patients with brain tumor. Ann Neurol 1989; 25:92–94.
26. Werk EE, Choi Y, Sholiton Z, et al: Interference in the effect of dexamethasone by diphenylhydantoin. N Engl J Med 1969; 281:32–34.
27. Chaulk JB, Ridgeway K, Brophy T, et al: Phenytoin impairs the bioavailability of dexamethasone in neurological and neurosurgical patients. J Neurol Neurosurg Psychiatry 1984; 47:1087–1090.
28. Lawson LA, Blouin RA, Smith RB, et al: Phenytoin-dexamethasone interaction: A previously unreported observation. Surg Neurol 1981; 16:23–24.
29. Grossman SA, Sheidler VR, Gilbert MR: Decreased phenytoin levels in patients receiving chemotherapy. Am J Med 1989; 87:505–510.
30. Muller PJ, Tator CM, Bloom M: The effect of phenobarbital on the toxicity and tumoricidal activity of CCNU in a murine brain tumor model. J Neurosurg 1980; 52:359–366.
31. Boarini D, Beck DW, Van Guilder JC: Post-operative prophylactic anticonvulsant therapy in cerebral gliomas. Neurosurgery 1985; 16:290–292.
32. Mahaley M, Dudka L: The role of anticonvulsant medications in the management of patients with anaplastic gliomas. Surg Neurol 1981; 16:399–401.
33. North JB, Penhall RK, Hanieh A, et al: Phenytoin and postoperative epilepsy. J Neurosurg 1983; 58:672–677.
34. Foy PM, Chadwick DW, Rajgopalan N, et al: Do prophylactic anticonvulsant drugs alter the pattern of seizures after craniotomy? J Neurol Neurosurg Psychiatry 1992; 55:753–757.
35. Labar DR: Prophylactic antiepileptic medications after craniotomy. Neurology Alert 1992; 11:27–28.
36. Fishman RA: Cerebrospinal Fluid in Diseases of the Nervous System, ed 2. Philadelphia, WB Saunders, 1992.
37. Bilsky M, Posner JB: Intensive and postoperative care of intracranial tumors. *In* Ropper AH (ed): Neurological and Neurosurgical Intensive Care, ed 3. New York, Raven Press, 1993, pp 309–329.
38. Senger DR, Van De Water L, Brown LF, et al: Vascular permeability factor (VPF, VEGF) in tumor biology. Cancer Metastasis Rev 1993; 12:303–324.
39. Baethmann A, Maier-Hauff K, Schurer L, et al: Release of glutamate and of free fatty acids in vasogenic brain edema. J Neurosurg 1989; 70:578–591.
40. Black KL, Hoff JT, McGillicuddy JE, et al: Increased leukotriene C6 and vasogenic edema surrounding brain tumors. Ann Neurol 1985; 19:592–595.
41. Takahashi J, Fukumoto M, Igorshi K, et al: Correlations of b-FGF expression levels with the degree of malignancy and vascularity in human gliomas. J Neurosurg 1992; 76:792–798.
42. Galicich JH, French LA, Melby JC: Use of dexamethasone in the treatment of cerebral edema associated with brain tumors. Lancet 1961; 81:46–53.
43. Nakagawa H, Groothuis DR, Patlak CS, et al: Dexamethasone reduces brain tumor extracellular space capillary permeability: Implications for diagnosis and therapy. Neurology 1984; 34:184.
44. Eidelberg D: Neurological effects of steroid treatment. *In* Rottenberg DA (ed): Neurological Complications of Cancer Treatment. Boston, Butterworth-Heinemann, 1991, pp 173–184.
45. Vick NA, Wilson CB: Total care of the patient with a brain tumor. Neurol Clin 1985; 3:705–710.
46. Jarden JO, Dhawan V, Moeller A, et al: The time course of steroid action on blood to brain and blood to tumor transport of 82Rb: A positron emission tomographic study. Ann Neurol 1989; 25:239–245.
47. Spiro HM: Is the steroid ulcer a myth? N Engl J Med 1983; 309:45–47.
48. Klompmaker JJ, Slooff MJ, de Bruijn KM, et al: Prophylaxis with ranitidine against peptic ulcer disease after liver transplantation. Transpl Int 1988; 1:209–212.

49. Conn HO, Blitzer BL: Non-association of adrenocorticosteroid therapy and peptic ulcer. N Engl J Med 1976; 294:473–479.

50. Messer J, Reitman D, Sacks HS, et al: Association of adrenocorticosteroid therapy and peptic-ulcer disease. N Engl J Med 1983; 309:21–24.

51. Conn HO, Poynard T: Adrenocorticosteroid administration and peptic ulcer: A critical analysis. J Chron Dis 1985; 38:457–468.

52. Carson JL, Strom BL, Schinnar R, et al: The low risk of upper gastrointestinal bleeding in patients dispensed corticosteroids. Am J Med 1991; 91:223–228.

53. Frank J: Management of intracranial hypertension. Med Clin North Am 1993; 77:61–75.

54. Pudenz RH: The surgical treatment of hydrocephalus: A historical review. Surg Neurol 1980; 15:15–26.

55. Kanev PM, Park TS: The treatment of hydrocephalus. Neurosurg Clin 1993; 4:611–619.

56. Dias MS, Albright AL: The management of hydrocephalus complicating childhood posterior fossa tumors. Pediatr Neurosci 1989; 15:283–290.

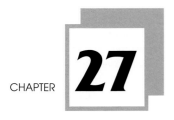

DAVID R. HAYNOR

KEN MARAVILLA

CHAPTER **27**

The Role of Functional Imaging in the Surgical Management of Brain Neoplasms

This chapter discusses the potential for functional imaging in the management of intracranial neoplasms. Although functional imaging is currently limited to research institutions, diffusion into routine clinical use is likely to occur in the next few years. The three main functional imaging techniques are discussed: functional magnetic resonance imaging (fMRI), magnetoencephalography (MEG), and positron emission tomography (PET). The biological and physical basis of each method is briefly sketched and its advantages and limitations, including resource requirements, are discussed. The current state of the art in functional imaging as it relates specifically to the surgical management of brain neoplasms is summarized and the chapter concludes with some speculation about the future.

WHAT IS FUNCTIONAL IMAGING?

The broad term *functional imaging* refers to noninvasive techniques that can be used to localize sites with specific neurologic functions, as distinguished from *metabolic imaging,* which allows the demonstration of areas of metabolic abnormality. In the context of glioma therapy, for example, functional imaging could be used to define the location of eloquent cortex relative to neoplasm for which surgery or radiosurgery is contemplated, whereas metabolic imaging might be used to distinguish recurrent tumor from gliotic scar or radiation necrosis. Functional imaging can also be used to study the localization of brain functions in healthy controls or in patients with non-neoplastic diseases, such as epilepsy.

Functional imaging has several potential roles in the surgical management of cerebral neoplasms. The primary application lies in the possibility of replacing the more invasive and expensive localization methods that are currently used prior to surgery. An example would be the use of the Wada test

(cerebral angiography with intracarotid barbiturate injection) to lateralize language; lateralization of memory is more difficult.[1] Potentially, the use of awake craniotomies could be reduced as language mapping improves. Preoperative mapping of motor cortex, although it may not replace intraoperative stimulation, might allow more precise planning of craniotomies. Functional imaging also offers the opportunity to study how the presence of neoplasm alters the function of nearby normal cortex. Both PET and MEG may be able to more precisely localize tumor-associated epileptic foci, and thereby shorten surgery that is undertaken both to remove a tumor and to reduce seizure frequency. Finally, functional imaging may ultimately be usable to predict the deficits that are likely to occur with a planned operation and to estimate the potential for functional recovery.

Functional imaging techniques operate by detecting physiologic changes that accompany the performance of defined cognitive tasks. These changes are detected either in the form of electrical activity (MEG) or as alterations in blood flow consequent to local neuronal activation (fMRI, PET). The ideal functional imaging technique is easily performed with widely available equipment, requires little in the way of additional personnel training, and can yield reliable information for almost all patients. The relevant physiologic changes can be detected quickly, and *registration* (or precise localization of the metabolic changes on anatomic images such as MRI or CT) is easily accomplished. Although the ideal technique does not exist, fMRI currently comes the closest to meeting the preceding description. The future roles of PET and MEG are likely to be more specialized.

FUNCTIONAL MRI

Within a few seconds of cortical activation by a task, local vasodilation occurs; the increase in local cerebral blood flow

(CBF) can be as much as 30%. The regional change in blood flow is the basis for the signal detected with fMRI. An increase in blood flow is believed to cause a local increase in MR signal by two mechanisms. First, the increase in blood flow generally exceeds the increase in metabolic demand, and local oxygen extraction (measured as a percent of incoming oxygen) actually declines. This results in a local increase in the concentration of oxyhemoglobin (oxyHb) in the capillaries and draining veins and a decrease in the concentration of deoxyhemoglobin (deoxyHb). Unlike oxyHb, deoxyHb is weakly paramagnetic; that is, it causes a local alteration (over a distance of a few tens of microns) in the magnetic field seen by the water protons being imaged. As a result, in the presence of deoxyHb, the magnetic field shows more local inhomogeneity. This results in reduction of the signal arising both from protons within the blood and, because of the range of the paramagnetic effect, within the brain parenchyma. With appropriate MR pulse sequences (T2*-weighted gradient-echo sequences such as GRASS, FFE, or FLASH), the effect of increased local variability in magnetic field is signal loss. As a result, neuronal activation, by causing a local decrease in deoxyHb concentration, causes a slight local *increase* in signal on T2*-weighted images. This increase in signal is known as the BOLD (*blood oxygenation level dependent*) effect. The *inflow effect* is a secondary mechanism of signal increase. With vasodilation, the number of protons entering the slice to be imaged increases. These inflowing spins are less saturated than the stationary spins in the slice being imaged; that is, they have experienced fewer RF pulses and can yield a greater signal on imaging. This effect is the basis of time-of-flight MR angiography, and it also contributes to the signal increase seen with increased local CBF. The combination of the BOLD effect and the inflow effect cause a signal increase of 2% to 10% when appropriate pulse sequences are used. It should be emphasized that fMRI detects a signal *change* with activation, relative to a baseline. Thus, fMRI is not directly suited to measuring resting CBF (in a tumor, for example). However, if a stimulus that causes an overall increase in CBF, such as carbon dioxide inhalation or acetazolamide injection, is applied to the patient, fMRI offers the possibility for detecting areas of abnormal vascular reserve.[2]

The routine application of fMRI must overcome several technical obstacles. As with any functional imaging technique, an appropriate task protocol must be designed and administered reproducibly. Any required equipment must be able to operate in the presence of high magnetic fields; for example, liquid crystal displays must be used for visual stimulation rather than magnetically sensitive CRT displays. Because fMRI seeks to detect small changes between the baseline and activated states, head motion can create significant artifacts. Special equipment for immobilization (e.g., padding, bite bars) must be used, and images must always be checked for the presence of gross motion. Tasks that involve head movement, such as vocalized speech, cannot readily be studied. Other physiologic effects, such as tonic changes in CBF or heart rate, can also create artifacts. To overcome these problems, *correlation* methods have been developed. In these techniques, the stimulus, such as a flashing light used to map visual cortex, is turned on and off repeatedly within a period of a few seconds. If images can

be acquired sufficiently rapidly, it becomes possible to detect only those pixels that change in intensity at the stimulus frequency. Because artifacts are likely to produce signal changes at a frequency different from that of the stimulus, these artifacts are greatly reduced. Moreover, the time delay, or phase offset, between the stimulus change and the change in intensity at a pixel can be studied directly, and it is of independent interest (see following). Compared with other techniques, registration is a minor problem with fMRI, since the images from which the data are derived generally show enough anatomic detail to allow direct correlation with high-resolution anatomic images, and patient motion is limited.

The goal of fMRI is to identify the area of brain parenchyma that is activated by a particular task. The increase in oxyHb and the inflow of unsaturated spins also create significant signal increase in the larger veins draining the activated cortex; this can result in a decrease in the accuracy with which the location of activation can be identified, because these veins drain wide areas of cortex. Several methods, including the use of specialized pulse sequences and discrimination based on time delay,[3] have been proposed for discriminating between parenchymal and venous signals. Most groups currently rely on visual assessment and correlation with conventional MRIs to discriminate venous from parenchymal signal increase. Parenchymal signal is increased relative to venous signal at higher field strengths (3 to 4 tesla [T]), although such magnets are only available at a few sites. A final consideration is the time required for fMRI. With conventional MR scanners and advanced gradient-echo pulse sequences, it is possible to acquire a single, moderate-resolution (128 × 128) slice approximately every 1 to 2 seconds. This allows a single-slice, alternating on/off protocol (sufficient for motor mapping, for example) to be performed in a few minutes. Newer pulse sequences, such as *spiral k-space imaging,* can be used to increase the number of slices acquired per unit of time by a factor of four, using conventional gradients.[4] Multislice protocols, which are required for complex tasks such as language mapping, may require 10 to 15 minutes per task, creating additional problems with patient movement and image registration. With specialized gradient coils, *echo-planar* imaging is possible, in which each slice can be acquired in 30 to 200 msec. This hardware, which is just becoming available for clinical use, adds 10% to 20% to the cost of an MR scanner, but it makes it possible to acquire activation images of the entire brain in a few seconds.

MAGNETOENCEPHALOGRAPHY

MEG[5, 6] is based on detection of the magnetic fields produced by the electrical currents associated with brain activation. The term *magnetic source imaging* (MSI) is often used for the complete functional imaging process, which also requires locating the sources of these fields on anatomic images. When a neuron is activated, small extracellular, intracellular, and transmembrane currents flow. MEG primarily detects the intracellular currents that flow parallel to the scalp and arise from the activation of pyramidal cells in the walls of sulci lying perpendicular to the scalp. This is in contrast to electroencephalography (EEG), which detects the more diffusely generated extracellular currents flowing in the scalp. On the order of 30,000 pyramidal cells (about 1 mm^2 of cortex) must be activated simultaneously to produce a detectable MEG signal. The requirement for simultaneous activation means that the detected signal consists of summated excitatory and inhibitory post-synaptic potentials rather than action potentials, which are much shorter in duration.[7] Compared to fMRI or PET, the MEG signal has a much higher temporal resolution (measured in milliseconds rather than seconds) and is specific for neuronal activity, as opposed to the combined glial-neuronal activity indirectly detected by PET and fMRI via the change in local CBF. Ultimately, combined analysis of both MEG and EEG data may yield still more accurate localization information.[8]

The increase in interest in MEG in the last few years has been a result of major improvements in instrumentation as well as in advances in source modeling. Detectors typically consist of superconducting coil pairs, or gradiometers, attached to devices called SQUIDs (*s*uperconducting *q*uantum *i*nterference *d*evices), which are sensitive to extremely small current fluxes. The weak neuromagnetic fields produced by activation, less than one ten-millionth of the static magnetic field of the earth, induce currents in the coil pairs (much as precessing spins induce signals in the radiofrequency [RF] pickup coils of an MRI scanner), and these currents are detected by the SQUID. By using coil pairs in which the two coils are wound in opposite directions, the effects of stray environmental sources of stray magnetic fields can be reduced. MSI is performed in a magnetically shielded room. In the last few years, MEG systems have evolved from single-channel devices to arrays of as many as 122 gradiometer/SQUID units, allowing simultaneous whole-head magnetic field measurements. The array is contained in a cryostat and is mounted inside a rigid helmet, which is fitted over the patient's head. These systems greatly reduce the time required for a complete set of MEG measurements; a complete examination of somatosensory cortex can be accomplished in approximately an hour. The cost of an MEG setup is comparable to that of a high-end MRI scanner. The total number of active MEG sites worldwide is on the order of 10 to 20.

Once the MEG signals have been detected, they must be localized in space. A new functional image can be formed at each temporal sampling point, and the temporal pattern of activation in the brain is followed. The difficulty is that even the largest currently practicable number of detectors greatly undersample the head. The problem of determining the source distribution that gave rise to the observed current is not well posed, because many possible source distributions can produce the same external magnetic fields. To estimate the true source distribution, therefore, simplifying assumptions must be made. The most common simplification is to model the source distribution at a particular instant in time as being composed of a single dipolar source. A dipolar source generates the same magnetic field as a small bar magnet; estimating the position, orientation, and strength of a single dipolar source from a large number of measurements is relatively feasible. The "effective dipole" produced by a large number of neuronal sources represents something like the centroid of neuronal activation. Accurate calculations also require modeling of the skull anatomy, although MEG

source localization is less sensitive to modeling assumptions than is the case with the EEG. This is primarily due to the fact that the magnetic permittivities of the tissues surrounding the brain differ much less than their electrical conductivities do. Several methods of registration between MEG and anatomic images have been used. Although earlier work was based on the use of fiducial markers, more recently, registration has been performed by digitizing multiple points on the scalp with a hand-held digitizer and then fitting these points to the skin surface derived from MRIs. The transformation between MEG-space and the coordinates of the MR scanner is thereby determined. The locations of the MEG sensors are also digitized; because the locations of the sources are known relative to the sensors, the sources may then be projected onto anatomic images. Although the final accuracy of source location is dependent on several factors (e.g., modeling accuracy, size of the "true" source, noise in the MEG device, registration errors arising from MRI distortion or marker movement), accuracies of 5 to 10 mm are attainable for sources that are well modeled as single dipoles.

With the use of large arrays, interest in more complex models of source distributions (e.g., two or more dipoles) has increased. With more complex models, uncertainty as to the position and strength of the component dipoles increases, and current clinical applications of functional imaging are therefore largely limited to situations in which only a single area, or possibly two widely separated areas, of cortex is activated at one time. Higher-order tasks such as language understanding and generation are therefore difficult to study with MEG, because multiple cortical areas are involved. Clinical MEG studies have been largely limited to primary sensory and motor cortex and to models of interictal spike generation in epilepsy patients. Studies for localization of somatosensory cortex typically take on the order of 30 to 60 minutes.

POSITRON EMISSION TOMOGRAPHY

The use of PET[10] to study normal brain function antedates use of fMRI and MEG; in fact, the uncoupling between metabolism and blood flow that underlies fMRI was first recognized with PET,[11] and the complexity of the paradigms that have been studied with PET to date exceed that of the protocols studied with fMRI.[12] Like fMRI, PET functional imaging rests on the increase in local CBF seen with neuronal activation. Absolute CBF can be measured with PET in the baseline or stimulated condition. During performance of the activated task, a single dose of 10 to 20 mCi of O^{15}-labeled water is given and imaging is performed over the next 40 to 80 seconds. The integrated uptake of the labeled water in a voxel is (nearly) linearly proportional to the absolute local CBF. After a 10-minute period to allow decay of the O^{15} (2-minute half-life), another activation task may be performed. Use of O^{15} requires the presence of an on-site cyclotron (unlike the more common F^{18}-fluorodeoxyglucose PET studies), but otherwise no special additions to a conventional PET scanner are necessary. A variety of techniques have been developed for effective PET-MRI image registration[13]; most require some degree of operator intervention. Because of the short half-life, the radiation dose from O^{15} is small, and 10 to 15 activation sequences can typically be ethically performed in adult volunteers. Current isotopes used for single-photon imaging (SPECT) do not permit multiple activation protocols; therefore, SPECT is considerably less useful for functional imaging than PET.

ACHIEVEMENTS TO DATE IN FUNCTIONAL IMAGING

This section is intended to give the reader an idea of the potential of each of the previously discussed functional imaging methods with respect to surgical management of brain neoplasms.

Review of detailed recent findings with functional imaging with respect to the functional neuroanatomy of vision,[14] motor cortex,[15] auditory cortex,[16] memory,[17, 18] or language[19] are beyond the scope of this chapter. It must be emphasized that, to date, published clinical experience with any of these methods in patients with neoplasms is quite limited. Most studies have consisted of small series of normal volunteers. Experiments have largely focused on determining what parts of the brain are activated during performance of a particular task; this is not the same as identifying regions that are *essential* for performance of the task,[20] or, more generally, as attempting to predict the deficit that would result from a specified resection. It is also important to remember that functional imaging methods identify eloquent cortex but do not directly identify critical white matter pathways.

The early components of the auditory evoked response have been studied with MEG,[9] and auditory cortex has also been mapped with PET[16] and fMRI. All three techniques are capable of reliably locating primary auditory cortex in normal volunteers.

Somatosensory cortex has been studied in patients with lesions near the central sulcus using fMRI,[21] and MEG.[22] MEG correctly localized sensory cortex and, by inference, motor cortex in three patients, two of whom had a normal examination but had tumors near the sensory strip. Similar results were reported by Gallen and co-workers.[23] In the two patients reported on by Jack and associates,[21] intraoperative localization of gliomas relative to sensorimotor cortex was grossly consistent with preoperative mapping of sensory cortex with fMRI. Detailed mapping was not performed in either patient, however, because of protocol limitations or patient cooperation in the case of fMRI, and because of the limited craniotomy size in the case of intraoperative mapping. This work also demonstrates the utility of relating functional images to venous anatomy (as seen on MRI), because the veins are readily identified at surgery. Correlation of intraoperative motor cortex location with localization using fMRI was studied in six patients by Yousry and colleagues.[24] These workers demonstrated good correlation (correct identification of the motor strip) in the patients studied, and also plasticity (manifested by an increase in area of activated cortex) in patients with tumors near the motor strip, compared to controls. PET was used by Frackowiack and co-workers[25] to study the anatomic basis of cortical plasticity in the motor system after stroke. These workers were able to identify areas of cortex that were activated when patients performed motor tasks with the limb that was contralateral to an internal capsule stroke. The homologous areas were not activated when the ipsilateral [unaffected] limb was used, nor were they activated in volunteers. Thus, any of the three functional imaging methods can reliably localize the central sulcus in normal volunteers, and probably in patients with mild weakness as well, and can detect at least gross somatotopic organization. No studies have been performed to see if motor cortex can still be detected in patients rendered hemiplegic by tumor.

fMRI[26] and PET[27] have been used to demonstrate cerebellar activation during cognitive tasks as well as motor learning. Studies of the cerebellum during speech might be of particular interest in view of the well-known occurrence of mutism after operations involving the inferior vermis, particularly in children.[28]

Primary visual cortex is easily detected with any of the three functional imaging modalities. More sophisticated stimulation paradigms have allowed identification of multiple areas of visual association cortex adjacent to primary visual cortex using fMRI[14] or PET.[30]

Most studies of language organization and processing within the brain have been done with PET,[19] although the study of language with fMRI is rapidly accelerating, and it has been shown to accurately predict lateralization of speech in children being worked up for epilepsy surgery.[29] Work has concentrated on single-word (lexical) processing, with few studies of higher linguistic processes. Insight has been gained into the localization of visual and auditory low-level processing that underlies the recognition of written and spoken speech, into speech production, and into semantic processing. Studies of speech generation are limited by the resulting head movement, although covert word generation frequently yields visible changes with either fMRI or PET. Protocols that identify the areas that will produce major language deficits, comparable to the effects of awake stimulation,[31] have not yet been identified, and no validation of methods for detecting lateralization of verbal or object memory has been reported.

THE FUTURE OF FUNCTIONAL IMAGING

The role of functional imaging in neurosurgery is likely to grow. Of the techniques discussed here, fMRI clearly has the greatest potential for widespread use because of its modest incremental cost, the widespread availability of MR scanners, and the possibility of combining preoperative MRI and tailored functional imaging into a single, registered, well-tolerated study. Technical advances, particularly the use of echo-planar imaging and improved coil design, are likely to increase its sensitivity substantially. It has already demonstrated the ability to locate primary and secondary motor, visual, and somatosensory areas in the brain, and language studies are under way. Two major barriers to dissemination remain. First, considerable simplification and streamlining of software and stimulation protocols will be necessary if the technique is to be useful outside of research institutions. Second, additional research is needed to develop and validate clinically usable protocols that can distinguish between cortical areas that are *essential* for important tasks vs. those that are *activated* during the performance of those tasks, if accurate prediction of postoperative deficit is to be achieved.

The roles of MEG and PET in glioma surgery are likely to remain more limited. Although MEG is capable of locating primary sensory cortex, this can also be accomplished with the more widely available techniques of fMRI and PET. The unique strength of MEG is its ability to localize seizure foci by analyzing interictal discharges.[32] It has the potential, therefore, for expediting the workup of patients with seizure disorders, whether related to neoplasm or not, by reducing the need for video-EEG monitoring and subdural grid placement. The principal role for PET in tumor management is likely to rest in its unique ability to study tumor metabolism and biochemistry noninvasively. This will allow chemotherapy and radiation protocols to be tailored more rationally to individual patients.

REFERENCES

1. Dodrill CB: Preoperative criteria for identifying eloquent brain: Intracarotid amytal for language and memory testing. Neurosurg Clin North Am 1993; 4:211–216.
2. Karczmar G, River J, Vijayakumar S, et al: Effects of hyperoxia on T2* and resonance frequency weighted MR images of rodent tumors. NMR Biomed 1994; 7:3–11.
3. Mosely ME, Glover GH: Functional MR imaging: Capabilities and limitations. Neuroimag Clin North Am 1995; 5:161–192.
4. Noll DC, Cohen JD, Meyer CH, et al: Spiral k-space MR imaging of cortical activation. JMRI 1995; 5:49–56.
5. Gallen CC, Hirschkoff EC, Buchanan DS: Magnetoencephalography and magnetic source imaging: Capabilities and limitations. Neuroimaging Clin North Am 1995; 5:227–249.
6. Sato S (ed): Advances in Neurology: Magnetoencephalography, vol 54. New York, Raven, 1990.
7. Barth DS: The neurophysiological basis of epileptiform magnetic fields and localization of neocortical sources. J Clin Neurophys 1993; 10:99–107.
8. Rose DF, Ducla-Soares E: Comparison of electroencephalography and magnetoencephalography, in Sato S (ed): Advances in Neurology: Magnetoencephalography, vol 54. New York: Raven, 1990, pp 33–37.
9. Jacobson GP: Magnetoencephalographic studies of auditory system function. J Clin Neurophys 1994; 11:343–364.
10. Frackowiak RSJ, Friston KJ: Functional neuroanatomy of the human brain: Positron emission tomography—a new neuroanatomical technique. J Anat 1994; 184:211–225.
11. Fox PT, Raichle ME: Focal physiological uncoupling of cerebral blood flow and oxidative metabolism during somatosensory stimulation in human subjects. Proc Natl Acad Sci USA 1986; 83:1140–1144.
12. Wise R, Chollet F, Hadar U: Distribution of cortical neural networks involved in word comprehension and word retrieval. Brain 1991; 114:1803–1817.
13. Van den Elsen PA, Pol EJD, Viergever MA: Medical image matching: A review with classification. IEEE Eng Med Biol 1993; 12:26–39.
14. Tootell RB, Reppas JB, Kwong KK, et al: Functional analysis of human MT and related visual cortical areas using magnetic resonance imaging. J Neurosci 1995; 15:3215–3230.
15. Ashe J, Ugurbil K: Functional imaging of the motor system. Curr Opin Neurobiol 1994; 4:832–839.
16. Elliott LL: Functional brain imaging and hearing. J Acoust Soc Am 1994; 96:1397–1408.
17. Buckner RL, Petersen SE, Ojemann JG, et al: Functional anatomic studies of explicit and implicit memory retrieval tasks. J Neurosci 1995; 15:12–29.
18. Roskies AL: Mapping memory with positron emission tomography. Proc Natl Acad Sci USA 1994; 91:1989–1991.
19. Liotti M, Gay CT, Fox PT: Functional imaging and language: Evidence from positron emission tomography. J Clin Neurophys 1994; 11:175–190.
20. Jackson JH: On the nature of the duality of the brain. *In* Taylor J, Holmes G, Walshe FMR (eds): Selected Writings of John Hughlings Jackson, vol 2. New York, Basic Books, 1958, pp 129–145.
21. Jack CR, Thompson RM, Butts RK: Sensory motor cortex: Correlation of presurgical mapping with functional MR imaging and invasive cortical mapping. Radiology 1994; 190:85–92.
22. Roberts T, Rowley H, Kucharczyk: Applications of magnetic source imaging to presurgical brain mapping. Neuroimag Clin North Am 1995; 5:251–266.
23. Gallen CC, Sobel DF, Waltz T: Noninvasive presurgical neuromagnetic mapping of somatosensory cortex. Neurosurgery 1993; 33:260–268.
24. Yousry TA, Schmid UD, Jassoy AG: Topography of the cortical motor hand area: prospective study with functional MR imaging and direct motor mapping at surgery. Radiology 1995; 195:23–29.
25. Frackowiack RSJ, Weiller C, Chollet F: The functional anatomy of recovery after brain injury. Ciba Found Symp 1991; 163:235–249.
26. Kim SG, Ugurbil K, Strick PL: Activation of a cerebellar output nucleus during cognitive processing. Science 1994; 265:949–951.
27. Roland PE: Partition of the human cerebellum in sensory-motor activities, learning and cognition. Can J Neurol Sci 1993; 20 (suppl 3):S75–S77.
28. Dietze DD, Mickle JP: Cerebellar mutism after posterior fossa surgery. Pediatr Neurosurg 1990–91; 16:25–31.
29. Hertz-Pannier L, Gaillard WD, Motts S, et al: Preoperative assessment of language lateralization by fMRI in children with complex partial seizures: Preliminary study. *In* Abstracts of the 12th Annual Meeting of the Society for Magnetic Resonance in Medicine. Berkeley, Society of Magnetic Resonance in Medicine, 1993, p 1387.
30. Haxby JV, Grady CL, Ungerleider LG, et al: Mapping the functional neuroanatomy of the intact human brain with brain work imaging. Neuropsychologia 1991; 29:539–555.
31. Ojemann G, Ojemann J, Lettich E, et al: Cortical language localization in left, dominant hemisphere: An electrical stimulation mapping investigation in 117 patients. J Neurosurg 1989; 71:316–326.
32. Ebersole JS, Squires KC, Eliashiv SD, et al: Applications of magnetic source imaging in evaluation of candidates for epilepsy surgery. Neuroimag Clin North Am 1995; 5:267–288.

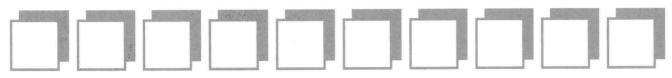

Resection Strategies

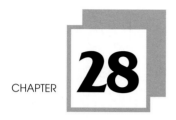

CHAPTER 28

Positioning During Glioma Surgery

Determining optimal positioning of the patient for surgery to remove a glioma is a critical aspect of the planning phase of the procedure. This crucial component of the operative strategy must take into account not only the goals of a radical resection, but also whether physiologic brain mapping will be done, which of necessity requires an increase in the overall exposure obtained by craniotomy.[1] Decisions regarding the positioning and the subsequent opening must take into account potential patterns of tumor regrowth so that the incision will accommodate operations for recurrent tumor.

Positioning must be planned in meticulous detail with regard to careful padding and protection of all the patient's extremities to avoid cutaneous pressure sores or peripheral nerve injury. Moreover, the decision can be made only after giving close consideration to the position that permits the maximum exposure, depending on the anatomic and physiologic aspects of the operative procedure.[1, 2] This chapter concerns positioning of the patient as it relates to four aspects: supine, lateral decubitus, prone or ''Concorde,'' and sitting positions.

SUPINE POSITION

The supine position is sufficient for virtually all gliomas affecting the frontal and anterior parietal lobes. At times, depending on the location of the lesion relative to the temporal lobe or the anterior parietal lobe, it may be necessary to first place a soft roll underneath the patient's shoulder ipsilateral to the operative site to turn the head parallel to the floor. This maneuver is a variation of supine positioning in which a roll is placed under the shoulder and hips to permit the patient's head to be rotated away from the site of the incision to expedite the exposure.

In the standard supine position, the patient's arms are left at the sides, with padding placed beneath the elbows, and each joint should be in flexion; for example, the forearm should be higher than the arm, with the elbow flexed. This positioning can be facilitated by placement of padding beneath the forearms bilaterally. In addition, soft padding should be placed beneath both knees to allow for slight flexion at the hip as well as at the knee. Padding can then

be used to prevent external rotation of the hips bilaterally by slight elevation of the padding beneath the knees in its lateralmost fashion. It is also important to place some soft padding beneath both feet to provide slight dorsiflexion. This is especially important for lengthy operative procedures. Care must be taken not to permit any parts of the extremities to touch each other, out of concern for pressure ulceration of the skin. The head should be slightly flexed to a point at which one to two fingers can be inserted between the chin and the chest.

For lesions involving the anteriormost part of the frontal lobe, the patient's head should be facing forward in a straight-up position. This approach usually requires a bicoronal skin incision to expedite a far-forward craniotomy based on the midline and just above the frontal sinus. In this setting, the craniotomy flap does not need to extend further than the lateral sphenoid wing and sylvian fissure. If the head is flexed too far forward, resection to the very tip of the frontal lobe will be awkward; thus, it is critical not to gain too much of a head-forward position, so as to prevent difficulty in resecting the anterior and inferior frontal lobe. If the lesion is located several centimeters above the gyrus rectus, a curvilinear incision in a reverse ''C'' fashion can be done to facilitate exposure without need for a bicoronal incision. In treating any recurrent tumor that was operated on through a previous incision, all counterincisions must be done perpendicular to the previous incision to prevent ischemic compromise of the scalp flap.

Surgical navigation systems now facilitate positioning of the patient with respect to the location of the lesion during a preplanning stage to determine surgical strategy.[3-5] The lesion can be traced quite nicely underlying the scalp, which helps to determine the overall dimensions of the scalp incision and to verify that the patient is placed in the correct position. It is also important to keep the patient either perpendicular or parallel to the floor to help compensate for the shift that occurs during the course of an operation with loss of cerebrospinal fluid and brain bulk. This aspect of positioning is very important, because the calculated brain shift is different when the patient's head is perpendicular to the floor (e.g., for a posterior frontal lesion) than when it is parallel to the floor (e.g., for a temporal lobe or inferior frontal lobe lesion).

When cortical and physiologic mapping is used during craniotomy to identify motor, sensory, or language pathways, whether the patient is to be awake or asleep, it is critical to plan the exposure to account for the area of the brain to be mapped, because that area often extends beyond the tumor margin, as seen by the navigational device. That is, to accommodate for mapping, it is a general rule of thumb to make the craniotomy bigger than would appear to be necessary[2] (see Chapter 34).

If the lesion involves the temporal lobe or the posterior frontal or anterior parietal lobes, it is necessary, as mentioned earlier, to turn the head far contralateral to the lesion, such that the midline of the head (sagittal suture) is almost parallel to the floor.[2] When this is done, it is important to bring the ipsilateral upper extremity over the chest. Soft padding is placed under the axilla and the wrist, with slight wrist extension effected by the padding. The head should not be positioned low enough to permit the chin to touch the neck, which can allow moisture to accumulate and cause breakdown of the skin over the course of a long operative procedure. Thus it is important, before the final positioning and draping, to feel beneath the contralateral neck and chin to be certain that a space exists of at least a fingerbreadth. It is also important to tape the Foley catheter to the lowermost leg to expedite drainage in a dependent fashion. If the Foley catheter is taped to the topmost leg, it may be difficult for urine to travel uphill until the bladder is overdistended.

LATERAL DECUBITUS POSITION

Tumors involving the parietal lobe, whether inferiorly or superiorly based, and those that occupy the area of the atrium of the lateral ventricle are difficult to approach when the patient is placed in the supine or the modified supine position. For such tumors, the optimal position is the lateral decubitus position, in which the patient's head is actually rotated away from the lesion toward the floor.

To expedite positioning, it is necessary to hang the contralateral arm off of the table by first making a sling or pocket for the arm. This can be done by simply attaching a plywood board to the Mayfield table attachment, which can be inserted away from the table and then taped in place. The board rests on a stool without wheels, which, after it is padded, serves as a pocket for the arm to rest comfortably. The patient should be turned into the decubitus position, and an intravenous (IV) bag padded with thin foam can be inserted under the down-side chest cavity. This fluid-filled bag serves to elevate the chest and to create a pocket in the axilla that is free of any pressure as the arm hangs down on the sling. For small patients or young children, a small (250-mL) IV bag can be used, and a 500- or 1,000-mL IV bag is used for an adult. Fluid can be drained from the IV bag initially to accommodate padding to the overall size of the patient. This ''waterbed'' padding serves to elevate the thorax to create an uncompromised dead space in the axilla, which can prevent any kind of brachial plexus stretch injury. The down-side wrist is elevated to produce slight flexion of the elbow.

The padding is placed on the topmost arm beneath the axilla, and the shoulder is taped in place from side to side and secured beneath the table with cloth tape. This maneuver should allow the shoulders to be perpendicular to the head without any excessive rotation of the shoulders forward or backward, thus preventing stretch on the brachial plexus. On the up-side of the neck, skin and subcutaneous tissue should be loose, which confirms that there is no excessive tension on the brachial plexus. The patient's legs should be slightly flexed forward, and adequate padding should be placed between the legs to ensure that no pressure sores develop. A large roll that is generously padded should be placed behind the back and the hips, and this should be secured in place with sleds or kidney rests, which are secured to the table so that the back and buttocks can rest against the padding. Again, as with the shoulders, the back should be perpendicular to the table. With the patient's head flexed toward the floor, it is then possible for the temporal fossa to be parallel to the floor without the neck being stretched excessively. This positioning of the head is expedited by placing the down-side arm in a padded sling, so that it hangs away from the neck, which allows for further flexion of the head toward the floor. If the lesion is situated very far posteriorly and high in the parietal lobe or in the anterior occipital lobe, this position makes it possible to turn the patient's head toward the floor as much as necessary to facilitate exposure.

Lesions involving the occipital lobe can be approached very effectively with the patient in the decubitus position, especially in the case of a large person, for whom a prone position may actually impede venous drainage and increase intracranial pressure.

PRONE OR ''CONCORDE'' POSITION

The prone position is reserved for lesions involving the occipital lobe or lesions of the posterior fossa or upper spinal cord. The benefit of the prone position is that the patient's head is directly pointed in the midline and perpendicular to the floor. For operations on lesions in the occipital pole, the head should be slightly extended toward the ceiling to make the occipital pole higher than the chest. This positioning reduces obstructive outflow of the venous system and expedites exposure, especially toward the tentorium. Lesions involving the splenium or the posterior body of the corpus callosum can be approached with this position by retracting the parietal and occipital lobes away from the falx. Another way to approach gliomas in this region is to have the patient supine in a semi-slouched position, with the head flexed much more forward than it is in the standard supine position. This position also enables the head to be positioned straight up and perpendicular to the floor to allow for excellent exposure along the falx.

The disadvantage of the prone position is that abdominal pressure is created, which decreases venous outflow. This factor at times gives the illusion of a very tense occipital lobe, and mannitol should be used liberally in this situation in addition to hyperventilation. This is also an ideal position to use in approaching thalamic gliomas by entering the posterior mesial atrium of the lateral ventricle. In this setting, the incision in the cortex can be made approximately 6 cm above the inion and 2 cm lateral to the inion. The ventricle is approached, and the pulvinar is easily identified by the choroid plexus thinned out and stretched over the pulvinar.

The "Concorde" position is ideal for operations on posterior fossa tumors, in that it permits the surgeon to stand behind the patient's head in a 270-degree arc, permitting manipulation with the microscope, which facilitates a view up the fourth ventricle toward the aqueduct. This position is much preferred to a prone position with the surgeon standing at the top of the patient's head, in which it is very difficult for the surgeon to see up the fourth ventricle, especially with the microscope. The "Concorde" position enables the patient's head to be turned down and away from the surgeon, so that an excellent view of the obex and tonsils can be achieved. Again, this positioning allows for superb exposure of the top of the fourth ventricle and aqueduct, which is especially important in operations on tumors that extend superiorly. It is important also to note that with tumors that extend superiorly in the fourth ventricle, the craniectomy must involve the bone overlying the torcular so that the dura can be adequately retracted upward. The "Concorde" position is the ideal position for operations on all tumors involving the fourth ventricle except those that extend inferiorly and do not approach the area of the striae medullaris. For those inferior fourth ventricle lesions and for lesions that extend underneath the arch of C1, it is appropriate to stand at the patient's head and to have the patient in a direct prone position. This positioning is also quite adequate for operating on a cervical cord glioma in which a midline myelotomy is the preferred opening incision. In such a case, a "Concorde" position is not necessary. Also, standing at the top of the patient's head, with the patient prone, expedites making a myelotomy directly on the midline, without extending it to one side or the other, which can be a problem when the surgeon stands on either side of the neck.

When positioning a patient in the prone position or "Concorde" variation it is important that individual shoulder-hip rolls be made to accommodate the size of each patient. Precise length of the roll is determined by measuring the distance between the clavicle and the iliac crest. The thickness of the roll depends on the size of the patient; for example, rolls used for children and small patients should be no thicker than 2 to 3 in. For large patients, however, it is important that the roll be at least 6 to 8 in. or thicker to allow the abdomen to hang down between the rolls, so venous pressure is not created. The rolls should be liberally lined with padding and inserted beneath the patient after the patient is first turned into a prone position. The patient is then logrolled to accommodate each of the shoulder-hip rolls until they are adequately positioned and the head is flexed.

Just before turning the patient to a prone position, the Mayfield tongs should be applied if they are going to be used. It is also important first to create a groove in the padding at the top of the table so that the patient's chin does not hit the padding when the head is flexed. This can be done simply by taping the padding from the surface to the underside of the table to create an indentation. Only cloth tape should be used for this purpose, as it sticks best to the sheet and the table. After this is done, the patient may be turned into the prone position with the shoulder-hip rolls inserted and the head flexed. The arms are kept at the sides

and padded appropriately, with slight flexion of the elbow maintained. The hands are placed in the swimmer's position, with the thumb pointing down toward the floor. Padding is placed under both knees and under both iliac crests to avoid any nerve stretch injuries. The knees are flexed approximately 45 degrees and built up on pillows. The arms are taped in place to the back so that they cannot fall away from the patient's body.

SITTING POSITION

The sitting craniotomy position for glioma surgery is rarely used because of its inherent risks of causing air embolism and cardiac instability. For some indications, however, the sitting position remains well worthwhile. These include tumors involving the superior anterior vermis of the cerebellum (i.e., culmen) and the pineal region. This positioning may be especially helpful in treating patients who have very vascular tumors involving the anterior cerebellum or the pineal region. As mentioned in the previous section, the semislouched position, which is between a supine and a sitting position,[6] can be used for tumors situated along the posterior falx or mesial parietal or occipital lobes. Again, this position can be very helpful when the lesion is expected to be bloody, as it permits blood to fall gently away from the resection cavity. When placing patients in the sitting position, it is important to first build up some padding beneath the buttocks and to secure this in place so that the trunk and the hips do not slide inferiorly. This potential problem can be especially dangerous to a patient who is secured in Mayfield tongs. After padding is placed beneath the buttocks and securely taped to the table, the position is arranged so that the hips are flexed and the legs come to lie just inferior to the chest. Dorsiflexion of both ankles should be achieved to prevent any nerve injury from extensive plantar flexion over the course of a long operative procedure. An overhead bar straddling the patient is then inserted into the table holders, and the Mayfield attachment is inserted into the bar. This maneuver allows forward flexion of the neck. Again, one to two fingerbreadths is the standard rule for determining the degree of flexion forward. The table is then placed in a reverse Trendelenburg position so that the back of the neck is actually forward from a perpendicular position to the floor. This accounts for the dimensions of the tentorium and allows the surgeon to see up and above the top of the cerebellum and up into the pineal region if necessary.

The patient's shoulders and arms should be built up significantly on solid padding to prevent any stretch injury of the brachial plexus. Flexion at the elbows should be adequate, and they can be secured with a sling to the overhead table attachment that is used to secure the Mayfield tongs.

At times, air can come into the venous circulation via the pinholes, and for that reason it is reasonable to wax the pinholes after the patient is in a final position. Attention to detail is critical in operations performed with patients in this position; it is important to wax the bone liberally as well as to place Gelfoam and Surgicel over the dural sinuses to prevent the entry of air. Should there be any sign of venous air embolism, it is important to flood the field with saline irrigation and to lower the head position until the embolism is corrected.

CONCLUSION

The positioning of the patient for surgical treatment of a glioma is as important as the actual resection of the lesion. Improper positioning leads to difficulty during the operative procedure in terms of achieving a radical resectioning of the tumor. Poor positioning may also compromise venous outflow, thus adding to swelling and increased intracranial pressure. Correct positioning is also necessary to allow an extensive craniotomy and to provide flexibility for mapping procedures. Attention to detail in the positioning of the patient will prevent any unnecessary complications related to inadequate exposure.

REFERENCES

1. Berger MS, Ojemann GA, Lettich E: Neurophysiological monitoring during astrocytoma surgery. Neurosurg Clin North Am 1990; 1:65–80.
2. Berger MS, Ojemann GA: Techniques of functional localization during removal of tumors involving the cerebral hemispheres. *In* Loftus C, Traynelis V (eds): Intraoperative Monitoring Techniques in Neurosurgery. New York, McGraw-Hill, 1994, pp 113–127.
3. Maciunas RJ, Berger MS, Copeland B, et al: Interactive image-guided resective surgical techniques for low-grade gliomas. Tech Neurosurg 1996; 2:151–164.
4. Maciunas RJ, Berger MS, Copeland B, et al: A technique for interactive image-guided neurosurgical intervention in primary brain tumors. Neurosurg Clin North Am 1996; 7:245–266.
5. Berger MS, Ojemann GA: Surgical mapping of functional brain. *In* Alexander E III, Maciunas RJ (eds): Advanced Neurosurgical Navigation. New York, Thieme (in press).
6. Bruce JN, Stein BM: Infratentorial approach to pineal tumors. *In* Wilson CB (ed): Neurosurgical Procedures: Personal Approaches to Classic Operations. Baltimore, Williams & Wilkins, 1992, pp 63–76.

FRED G. BARKER II

PHILIP H. GUTIN

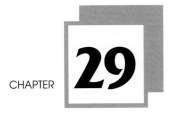

CHAPTER **29**

Surgical Approaches to Gliomas

The principal goal of surgical technique for gliomas is maximal safe resection. Evidence for most glial tumors indicates that extensive surgical resection can prolong survival and, in some cases, offer better quality of life. (See Chapters 56 and 60 for discussions of the rationale for extensive resection.) Some glioma operations are stereotactic biopsies undertaken strictly to provide a pathologic diagnosis. Technique for these procedures is discussed elsewhere in this volume (see Chapter 31), and this chapter focuses on open craniotomy techniques. It is therefore assumed for the purposes of this chapter that one objective of surgery is maximal possible tumor resection. Clearly, this objective must not be achieved at the expense of the patient's quality of life. Surgical technique must be tailored to each individual case to strike the optimal balance between these two sometimes conflicting objectives.

CORTICAL AND SUBCORTICAL TUMORS OF THE CEREBRAL HEMISPHERES

Tumors of the fibrillary astrocytic lineage, such as astrocytomas, anaplastic astrocytomas, and glioblastomas, are often found in the cortical and subcortical portions of the cerebral hemispheres, as are less common gliomas such as oligodendrogliomas, ependymomas, pilocytic astrocytomas, and pleomorphic xanthoastrocytomas. Surgical technique for gliomas varies somewhat for tumors with different histologic characteristics (as predicted on the basis of preoperative imaging and as confirmed by intraoperative pathologic examination), and also depends on tumor location.

Histology

The main influence of histology on operative technique is a consequence of the tendency of various tumor types to have sharp or diffuse borders. Tumors that can be reliably expected to have a sharp, surgically definable border include pilocytic astrocytomas and pleomorphic xanthoastrocytomas. When either of these tumors is found, unless the tumor

intimately involves cerebral structures that must not be sacrificed (e.g., the internal capsule or speech or motor cortex), the goal of surgery should be gross total excision. These tumors do not infiltrate functioning brain, but tend to expand by pushing cerebral structures aside. This makes these tumors excellent candidates for surgical cure. In fact, pilocytic astrocytomas and pleomorphic xanthoastrocytomas of the cerebral or cerebellar hemispheres are almost always completely resectable, and complete resection almost always leads to long-term survival.[1-7] For these tumors, careful attention to definition of the tumor's border is paramount.

Most other histologic types of glioma have diffuse borders, blending imperceptibly into normal brain. It is not uncommon for an astrocytoma or oligodendroglioma to appear to have a distinct border in certain areas, but in deeper regions the border usually becomes less distinct and then disappears entirely. Even a malignant glioma may appear to have sharp margins: in early randomized trials conducted by the Brain Tumor Study Group, about 5% of malignant gliomas were described as "encapsulated."[8, 9] These patients had no better survival than patients with nonencapsulated tumors. Although greater extent of resection predicts longer survival, even in these more malignant tumors, avoiding damage to "eloquent" structures weighs more heavily in surgical planning for higher-grade lesions.

General Technical Considerations

LOBECTOMY VS. LOCAL TUMOR RESECTION

Little agreement exists regarding the proper surgical technique for resection of infiltrating hemispheric gliomas. Two general schools of thought have developed regarding the proper strategy for resection of a diffuse intracerebral mass: (1) internal decompression of the mass and (2) en bloc resection, which sometimes amounts to a lobectomy. These techniques have not been compared prospectively. In a retrospective study of 118 glioblastoma patients who presented during a 12-year period, one group found that there was no survival difference between patients treated with or without lobectomy.[10] With the exception of one study,[11] which used

349

"internal decompression" to mean "less than 25% resection," no large retrospective reports have directly compared these two strategies. The choice between them is thus at present a matter of preference. The surgeon should elect whichever strategy he or she feels will accomplish the greatest extent of tumor resection combined with the lowest risk of morbidity.

We think that in most cases the addition of a lobectomy to a glioma resection poses an unnecessary risk of neurologic deficit. A frequently encountered exception is an astrocytoma or an anaplastic astrocytoma located in the nondominant temporal tip; for these patients, a radical temporal lobectomy is an attractive choice. The frontal pole is another location in which a tumor can often be safely treated with an en bloc resection, sometimes with a surgical margin around the macroscopically abnormal tissue.

OPERATING MICROSCOPE

The routine use of the operating microscope for glioma resection in the cerebral hemispheres has not been shown to convey a survival advantage to patients with glioblastoma, although early postoperative results may be better.[10] Many surgeons feel that the illumination and magnification afforded by the operating microscope constitute an important advantage to the surgeon in distinguishing the subtle differences between glioma tissue and relatively normal surrounding white matter.

VENTRICULAR ENTRY

When attempting a generous resection of a cerebral glioma, the surgeon will often approach or enter the ventricular system. It has been suggested that entry into the ventricles during resection of supratentorial malignant gliomas in children may predispose to dissemination of tumor through the cerebrospinal fluid (CSF).[12] A study of CSF dissemination during surgery for cerebral malignant glioma in adults failed to confirm this finding, although a trend was seen toward earlier CSF dissemination in patients who underwent ventricular entry during surgery.[13] CSF dissemination was more likely in patients with glioblastoma than in patients with lower-grade tumors in this series. Once CSF dissemination became apparent, average survival was only 3 months. It may be prudent to avoid ventricular entry in patients with glioblastoma unless it is absolutely necessary to achieve an adequate resection.

Diffuse Tumors: Surgical Technique

Many diffuse astrocytomas of the cerebral hemisphere present on the cortical surface. For these tumors, after an appropriate craniotomy has been performed, the first step is to inspect the exposed cortex and to attempt to delineate the extent of the tumor as predicted by preoperative imaging studies. Cortical mapping may be performed, if indicated by the location of the tumor. A tentative decision should be reached regarding the extent of the resection to be performed.

If the cortex involved with tumor is determined to be noneloquent, based on imaging or intraoperative mapping,

the cortical surface of the tumor is outlined by cauterizing and cutting the pia and arachnoid surrounding the tumor's borders. Thorough hemostasis of vessels traveling within sulci is necessary before sharp division is performed with microscissors. The incision is deepened through the gray matter and subcortical white matter using bipolar cautery and suction. Self-retaining retractors or rubber dams and cotton pads may be used to maintain definition of the surgical plane while the surgeon works in another area. An attempt is made to stay on the margin of grossly abnormal tissue, as reflected by magnetic resonance imaging (MRI) and the gross appearance of the white matter. Normal white matter is glistening, smooth, white, and relatively avascular. Tumor tissue is slightly darker, often gray or yellow, and is usually more vascular than normal white matter. Bleeding should be controlled as the resection progresses, but the pace of resection should not be allowed to lag or cerebral swelling may supervene. The resection continues around all surfaces of the mass until it can be removed. There is no known advantage to an en bloc resection, and the tumor may be removed primarily with internal suction decompression or morcellation if these techniques will help to minimize retraction of surrounding tissue. Large draining veins on the cortical surface should be preserved to avoid edema and subsequent intraoperative or postoperative swelling. The vein of Labbé must be preserved on the dominant side to avoid postoperative aphasia.

When the tumor does not present on the cortical surface, a corticectomy must be performed to gain access to the mass. A cortical gyrus is chosen that will not cause a postoperative deficit if it is damaged. The crown of the gyrus is electrocoagulated with bipolar cautery and the pia-arachnoid is sharply incised with microscissors. The corticectomy is deepened through gray matter and subcortical white matter in the direction of the tumor until its surface is reached.

Some surgeons prefer to use a cerebral sulcus as a "surgical corridor" to approach the tumor. In this case, a sulcus is split using sharp dissection until its deepest portion is reached, when an incision through cortex becomes necessary. The hypothetical advantages of this approach may be outweighed by the additional time and dissection necessary, but if the tumor is small, focal, and near the depth of a suitable sulcus, this approach can be elegant and attractive.

The surgeon often reaches a distinguishable tumor border as dissection proceeds deeper, but sometimes the tumor blends indistinguishably with surrounding structures, and the "surface" must be defined by measurement of depth of dissection and by comparison with imaging studies. A frame-based or frameless stereotactic system is often helpful when the tumor is not expected to present on the cortical surface. The remaining principles of dissection are as described for cortical tumors. Self-retaining retractors are usually required to maintain exposure as the surgeon works within a cavity.

After the tumor has been removed hemostasis is obtained using standard techniques. Bipolar cautery is preferred, but cotton balls soaked in hot water or dilute solutions of hydrogen peroxide are sometimes required to stop diffuse oozing. Particular care is given to removing all cotton at the end of the procedure, as it can become difficult to distinguish from surrounding brain. A powdered hemostatic agent, such as

Avitene, may be of assistance. Tight packing should not be used in an attempt to stop bleeding within a cavity, as this may simply redirect the hemorrhage into deeper parenchyma or into the ventricular system, causing a hematoma that is not visible to the surgeon. After absolute hemostasis is obtained, the cavity is irrigated and lined with oxidized cellulose mesh. A standard closure of dura, skull, and scalp is performed.

ADVERSE INTRAOPERATIVE EVENTS

Adverse events that can become apparent to the surgeon during a glioma operation include excessive bleeding at the operative site and intraoperative swelling. Bleeding during glioma operations is normally controllable using the techniques outlined earlier. It is best to obtain hemostasis as the operation proceeds, rather than to rely on further tumor removal as a hemostatic aid. Patients with brain tumors may have a variety of coagulation abnormalities, some of which can develop during an operation.[14, 15] If bleeding seems excessive, all hematologic parameters and basic blood chemistries should be rechecked, even though preoperative tests may have been normal. A qualitative platelet disorder may not be apparent on routine screening tests, and should be considered. The most common cause is use of aspirin or nonsteroidal anti-inflammatory agents. Hypothermia severe enough to affect coagulation is rare in glioma surgery, but should be considered.

Cerebral swelling during a glioma operation can be dramatic. Common causes include intraparenchymal hemorrhage, hypercarbia, or occlusion of neck veins due to faulty positioning. Intraoperative ultrasound can be used to exclude hemorrhage. Fluid overload, excess ventilatory pressure, or pneumothorax are less likely causes, but they should be considered. Remedies include drainage of CSF from ventricle or basal cisterns, elevation of the head, administration of mannitol, hyperventilation, and reduction of end-expiratory ventilatory pressure. In extreme cases, pentobarbital may provide a short-lived reduction in intracranial pressure.

Specific Locations Within the Cerebral Hemispheres

The involvement of critical cerebral structures by an infiltrating glioma is usually the major determinant of the possible extent of surgical resection. Other chapters offer detailed descriptions of methods for ensuring that resections of infiltrating tumors remain safe, including intraoperative motor and speech mapping (Chapter 34) and preoperative location of the sensory cortex with magnetic source imaging (Chapter 27). Specialized methods are often employed to ensure completeness of resection, such as intraoperative stereotaxy (Chapter 33) or ultrasound (Chapter 30). When the two goals of resection, (1) safety and (2) completeness, are not mutually compatible, safety should generally take precedence. The principal risks that accompany resections in specific cerebral areas are identified in the following text.

FRONTAL LOBES

When a tumor is located within a single frontal lobe, a gross total or near-total resection can often be safely achieved. The classical frontal lobectomy consists of amputation of the anteriormost 8 cm of the frontal lobe along a flush plane on the nondominant side, opening the frontal horn of the lateral ventricle; on the dominant side, the posterior 2.5 cm of the inferior frontal gyrus (Broca's area) is spared. The anterior cerebral arteries, pericallosal arteries, and contralateral frontopolar artery require careful preservation. With modern imaging and microsurgical techniques, this procedure is rarely indicated except for very large frontal tumors, and a procedure limited to direct resection of the tumor itself using the principles outlined previously will be more suitable.

SUPPLEMENTARY MOTOR AREA

The supplementary motor area is located on the mesial surface of the frontal lobe, immediately anterior to the leg region of the motor strip. It was first described by Penfield and Jasper, who elicited stereotyped behaviors with intraoperative stimulation in this region.[16] Glial tumors such as astrocytomas and anaplastic astrocytomas are sometimes encountered in the supplementary motor area. Resection of supplementary motor area tumors leads to a characteristic syndrome of contralateral weakness and neglect.[17] If the resection is in the dominant hemisphere, mutism may accompany the weakness; speech deficits generally do not result from supplementary motor area resections in the nondominant hemisphere.[17, 18] Both speech and motor deficits resolve over time, with recovery nearly to baseline within weeks.[17, 18] There is a residue of paucity of spontaneous movement or speech, which may reflect the supplementary motor area's role in the planning and initiation of movement.[16, 17] This tends to resolve by a year postoperatively. Studies of patients with infarctions of the supplementary motor area have shown good recovery of contralateral arm and leg function as long as the lesion spares the primary motor cortex in the precentral gyrus.[19] The ipsilateral and contralateral callosomarginal arteries should be preserved when resections are being performed in this area, to avoid possible ischemic damage to the paracentral lobule.

INSULA

Gliomas that are limited to the insular cortex are unusual, but many infiltrating low-grade tumors involve the insula in addition to the frontal and temporal lobes. It is not possible to remove these extensive tumors completely, in either hemisphere, because of expected postoperative motor and/or speech deficits. The safe posterior border on the nondominant side for a partial resection of a frontal mass that extends into the insula is the posterior limb of the internal capsule. This may be identified intraoperatively by subcortical motor mapping.[20] On the dominant side, language deficit is a concern, and resection should not proceed posteriorly past the point at which language sites have been identified in the overlying portion of the frontal lobe.[20]

However, when a small tumor that appears to be limited to a portion of the insular cortex is encountered, safe total resection may be possible. Roper and co-workers[21] reported resection of two low-grade astrocytomas of the nondominant insula that were manifested by complex partial seizures. No new postoperative deficits were seen. Penfield, with Jasper[16] and Faulk,[22] reported resection of the entire insular cortex in four patients undergoing temporal lobectomy for epilepsy without production of any new neurologic deficits. Two of these resections were in the nondominant hemisphere, and the locations of the other two were not specified.

Later reports from the Montreal Neurologic Institute indicated the danger of postoperative hemiparesis after insulectomy.[23, 24] These deficits were attributed to interference with middle cerebral artery circulation, either by direct damage to the arteries or by induction of postoperative vasospasm; direct damage to the underlying internal capsule is another possible mechanism. Evidence from human insular infarctions suggests that damage to the insular region can cause global aphasia on the dominant side[25] and a variety of deficits, including mutism, on the nondominant side[26, 27]; but these reports were based on patients with infarctions that damaged surrounding structures in addition to the insula itself.

FRONTAL OPERCULUM AND PREMOTOR AREA

Broca's and Exner's Areas The dominant frontal operculum includes the region known as Broca's area, which is involved in the direction of complex orofacial movements associated with speech. For this reason, aggressive resections of tumors in this area are rarely performed. However, using speech mapping techniques during awake craniotomies, Obana and co-workers[28] reported successful resections of two small lesions located in the dominant frontal operculum without causing permanent speech deficits. The technique used was repeated removal of small portions of the lesions, with frequent speech testing between removals. Although this technique may be suitable for small, relatively discrete lesions, aggressive resection of a widely infiltrating lesion in this area should be expected to give rise to a significant speech deficit unless the resection stops at the sulcus adjacent to the gyrus that has been identified by speech mapping as the frontal language center.[20] The frontal language site is not consistently located in the most posterior portion of the inferior frontal gyrus: some patients have language sites in the middle frontal gyrus or in the inferior frontal gyrus as far anterior as the pterion.[29]

Another region in the dominant premotor cortex that is potentially important for language function is Exner's area, originally identified as a "writing center." This region is located in the dominant premotor cortex superior to Broca's area. Damage has been reported to cause both agraphia and alexia, sometimes in the absence of spoken language dysfunction or dominant hand weakness.[30, 31]

TEMPORAL LOBES

Many sophisticated techniques for resection of temporal lobe structures have been developed for use in epilepsy surgery. For temporal lobe gliomas, either a lesionectomy or a temporal lobectomy[32–34] is usually performed. For temporal lobectomy, a temporal craniotomy is performed to expose the lateral surface of the temporal lobe to within 2 cm of the pole, affording generous exposure of the planned posterior margin of the resection. This should be anterior to the vein of Labbé. The extent of tissue that can be safely resected varies between the two hemispheres (see following). The posterior margin is incised first, and the resection is deepened until the pia of the sylvian fissure is encountered. The risk to sylvian vessels incurred by splitting the fissure outweighs any theoretical advantage to removing this pia, and a subpial plane is maintained throughout the dissection. The superior margin of the resection is developed inferiorly and medially. The temporal horn of the ventricle is entered, and dissection continues until the floor of the middle fossa is reached. Veins draining the temporal pole are divided and the lobe is removed. Injury to the cerebral peduncle, the anterior choroidal and posterior cerebral arteries, and the structures traversing the tentorial notch must be avoided.

Resections for tumors in the temporal lobes can cause deficits in the visual field and in memory; on the dominant side they can result in speech deficits.

The optic radiations pass laterally from the lateral geniculate body, passing around the tip of the temporal horn of the ventricle, and then backward toward the calcarine cortex. A resection that exposes the tip of the temporal horn may be expected to cause a postoperative visual field deficit (partial or complete contralateral homonymous superior quadrantanopsia) in most patients.[35, 36] Although Penfield stated that resections of less than 6 cm were unlikely to cause visual defects,[37] deficits have been reported after resections as close as 3.0 cm to the temporal pole.[36, 38] These distances are based on experience with temporal lobectomy for epilepsy, and in the presence of a tumor it is possible that the optic radiations may be displaced anteriorly. As resection proceeds posteriorly from the temporal pole, the expected field defect grows larger, until a complete hemianopsia may be seen at approximately 8.0 cm from the temporal pole.[39]

Memory deficit is a known complication of temporal lobectomies that involve the mesial temporal structures on either side.[40] Most authors who have addressed this problem have reported on memory after temporal lobectomies for epilepsy. Deficits are more common after resection of nonsclerosed medial temporal structures, an observation that may be relevant to resections for tumors.[41] Although more extensive resections of medial structures might be expected to result in a higher chance of memory deficit, one study found no significant difference in neurocognitive function after resections of greater than 2.0 cm of medial temporal structures compared with less extensive resections.[42]

Speech deficits can follow tumor resections in the dominant temporal lobe. Some authors have argued that the chance of this complication may be reduced by the use of speech mapping techniques during awake craniotomies (see Chapter 34 for a detailed discussion of these techniques). In one series, permanent speech deficit was significantly more likely when resection was closer than 1 cm to a center identified by mapping as a language site.[43] Sixteen percent of glioma patients in this series had language sites located in the superior temporal gyrus, anterior to the foot of the central sulcus. New postoperative deficits were more likely in high-grade tumors.[43] Another group reported a 7% rate of dysnomia after dominant-sided standard resections (to 4.5 cm from the temporal tip) in epilepsy patients under general anesthesia.[44] The rate of this complication after surgery for temporal lobe tumors has not been specifically reported.

PRIMARY MOTOR AND SENSORY CORTEX

Most surgeons are reluctant to resect astrocytomas located in the primary motor and sensory cortex because of the expected postoperative deficit. However, some tumors that involve only the nondominant face motor cortex can be safely resected, because there is some bilateral cortical representation for facial musculature. The upper face has greater bilateral representation. Resection of tumors involving nondominant face motor cortex has been performed with minimal postoperative deficit.[45–47] To avoid postoperative hand weakness, resection should not be carried beyond a point 2 mm inferior to the lowest elicitable thumb response.[48] Resection of subcortical white matter in this region can also cause motor deficits in the hand, and subcortical mapping should be employed. In the dominant hemisphere, resections in face motor cortex carry a risk of postoperative speech deficit, because some patients have functional language sites in this location.[49] However, resections of inferior motor cortex in the dominant hemisphere have been performed without severe postoperative speech deficit.[50] It is important to preserve the arteries of passage that travel through this gyrus in their path from the sylvian fissure to the inferior frontal gyrus. Some postoperative dysarthria may be expected.[51]

No extensive experience has been reported with intentional glioma resections in the remainder of the primary motor and sensory cortical strips. In the context of surgery for epilepsy, Rasmussen considered that resections of the portions of postcentral gyrus that represent sensation of the face and leg were unlikely to give rise to significant postoperative deficit.[52] Other surgeons have considered the loss of proprioception in the lower limb that follows resection of the leg portion of the postcentral gyrus to be prohibitively disabling.[53]

PARIETAL LOBES

Although the parietal lobes subserve many important cerebral functions, it is possible to remove many intrinsic parietal lesions without causing increased neurologic deficit.[54, 55] Through a parietal craniotomy, the lesion is located either with the aid of triangulation from preoperative imaging or with formal stereotaxis. If the lesion is subcortical, a cortical incision is chosen to minimize deficits. In the dominant hemisphere, an incision on the lateral surface of the parietal lobe will give rise to dysphasia, and an incision in the superior parietal lobule is usually chosen.[56–59] Skin and bone flaps are placed to allow a 6 × 6 cm rectangular exposure centered on the superior parietal lobule. If it is necessary to see the medial surface of the lobe, the edge of the sagittal sinus is exposed. The vein of Trolard is in the surgical field and must be preserved. The entry point is chosen about 9 cm above the inion and 2 cm from the midline.[57] A cortical incision in the coronal plane is preferred by some authors to minimize damage to crossing fibers from the corpus callosum.[58] Exposure through this incision can extend to the atrium of the lateral ventricle. Although the trajectory to the atrium through this incision is usually directly toward the ipsilateral pupil, stereotaxis or intraoperative ultrasound provides a more reliable guide.

Although there is some risk of postoperative occurrence of Gerstmann's syndrome after an incision is made in the dominant superior parietal lobule, Sugita and Hongo[58] did not encounter this complication in 20 dominant parietal operations. Damage to the dominant angular gyrus must be avoided. The medial border of this gyrus is usually about 3.5 to 5.0 cm from the midline.[60] Significant manipulation or retraction through this exposure can cause an inferior homonymous quadrantanopsia or hemianopsia, as well as hemiparesis.

Another approach to tumors in the trigone or its lateral wall is the inferior temporal gyrus approach.[59, 61] With the anteroposterior axis of the head parallel to the floor and the vertex angled slightly down, a craniotomy is made, exposing the lateral temporal lobe and the floor of the middle fossa. A longitudinal corticectomy is made in the inferior temporal gyrus and is deepened until the tumor or trigone is reached. A contralateral superior quadrantanopsia is an expected consequence of this approach, and speech deficit may occur on the dominant side. The vein of Labbé is included in the exposure, and it must not be injured.

Some gliomas are located medial to the trigone. For these tumors, a parasplenial approach may be suitable.[57, 59] Exposure of the edge of the sagittal sinus is necessary, and the surgical corridor passes between the medial portion of the hemisphere and the falx. Another alternative is an approach from the contralateral side of the sagittal sinus, with resection of the falx.[62] It may be advantageous to position the patient with the operative side down, so that gravity retracts the hemisphere away from the falx. Although bridging cortical veins passing into the sagittal sinus can limit the anteroposterior extent of this exposure, these veins may be widely spaced in the parieto-occipital region. Preoperative MRI studies should be reviewed for precise planning of the operative trajectory.

OCCIPITAL LOBES

The classic occipital lobectomy consists of amputation of the occipital lobe 7 cm anterior to its posterior pole (measured along the lateral surface of the lobe, not in the direct anteroposterior plane). On the dominant side, a resection this extensive may injure the angular gyrus, and speech mapping or a less extensive resection is prudent. Occipital lobe operations are performed through an occipital or occipitoparietal craniotomy.[63] The skin flap is usually based inferiorly to preserve the occipital artery, and the bone flap should expose the margins of the sagittal and lateral sinuses so that the medial and inferior surfaces of the lobe can be seen.

With modern imaging, most occipital tumor resections are directed toward a defined target. Extensive tumor resections in the occipital lobe are likely to give rise to contralateral hemianopsia or to a lesser field cut.[64–66] This deficit is well tolerated by most patients unless it occurs in the dominant occipital lobe in conjunction with damage to the splenium of the corpus callosum. Alexia without agraphia may result from this combination of lesions, and alexia or dyslexia after dominant occipital lobectomy alone has also been reported.[60, 67] This deficit is likely to be permanent after resections of the ventrolateral dominant occipital lobe.[67] If a tumor is located in the medial dominant occipital lobe, it is possible that a limited medial resection may be less likely than a lobectomy to cause a permanent reading deficit.

THALAMIC TUMORS

Gliomas located in the thalamus are typically diffuse, infiltrating astrocytomas. Resection of these tumors is not indicated, and stereotactic biopsy may be used to guide further therapy. Some thalamic tumors in young adults and children are pilocytic astrocytomas. Resection of pilocytic thalamic tumors using a stereotactic volumetric technique with low morbidity and mortality has been reported[68] (see Chapter 32). These rare tumors are best treated by surgeons with a professed interest in stereotactic removal of deep-seated lesions.

OPTIC NERVE, CHIASMAL, AND HYPOTHALAMIC TUMORS

Tumors of the anterior visual pathways often represent a dilemma from the standpoint of proper overall management and also constitute a purely technical challenge. The complex decisions regarding timing of surgery are addressed elsewhere in this volume.

Unilateral Optic Glioma

Indications for resection of an optic glioma involving only one optic nerve are limited. In the presence of progressive proptosis and poor visual function, resection may be indicated. When the tumor appears on preoperative MRI studies to be confined to one optic nerve, without involvement of the chiasm, complete resection may be curative and should be the goal. The approach selected should expose the intracranial portion of the opposite optic nerve and the optic chiasm as well as the entire intracranial and intraorbital course of the affected optic nerve.[69] Many surgeons choose a subfrontal approach on the affected side, but some prefer a right-sided approach for an optic nerve tumor on either side.

A frontal or frontotemporal bone flap is elevated on the chosen side. Some surgeons remove the ipsilateral orbital rim and anterior orbital roof as well.[70–73] The flap should cross the midline anteriorly. The intracranial portion of the affected optic nerve is exposed and inspected. CSF may be drained from the suprasellar cisterns to assist in brain retraction during the exposure; a lumbar drain can also be helpful. The proximal extent of the tumor is determined and a site is selected for division of the affected optic nerve. If consistent with a tumor-free surgical margin, the nerve should be divided at least 6 mm from the chiasm, as division of the optic nerve more proximally can damage fibers from the opposite retina, which passes into the proximal contralateral optic nerve through Wilbrand's knee. Injury to these fibers causes a superior temporal field deficit in the opposite eye.[74]

The dura propria is opened over the affected optic nerve, and the dural incision is extended anteriorly along the orbital axis. The roof of the orbital apex and optic canal is removed with high-speed drills and fine punches to expose the periorbita. The periorbita is opened in the axis of the nerve. The annulus of Zinn is defined and divided between the attachments of the superior and medial rectus muscles. Expo-

sure continues through the space between these two muscles. The optic sheath is opened, and the tumor may be centrally debulked with an ultrasonic aspirator. The tumor capsule is then separated from surrounding structures, including the ophthalmic artery and its branches, and the nerve is divided near its insertion into the globe. The proximal division is then made and the nerve is removed. The annulus of Zinn and periorbita are closed with sutures. If the removal of the orbital roof has been extensive, it may now be reconstructed with a thin plate of bone or prosthetic material. A watertight dural closure is performed. If the posterior ethmoid sinuses have been entered during the unroofing of the optic canal, a free fat graft is placed to avoid a postoperative CSF leak. A standard closure of the craniotomy follows, with reconstruction of the orbital rim if it has been removed.

Chiasmal/Hypothalamic Glioma

For large gliomas that involve the chiasm and/or the hypothalamus, the surgical goal is usually debulking of exophytic tumor and fenestration of large cysts, rather than a complete resection. Preservation of visual and endocrine function is of obvious importance. Subtotal resections of hypothalamic gliomas with minimal morbidity have been reported by several groups.[75–78]

Most operations for hypothalamic/chiasmal exophytic tumors are performed through a standard frontal or pterional craniotomy,[75, 77, 79] although some surgeons prefer a transtemporal approach when access to the retrochiasmatic area is important.[80] Resection is limited to the exophytic portions of the tumor, and cysts of significant size are debulked and fenestrated.

When the tumor has grown upward from the chiasm into the third ventricle, a transcallosal approach may be useful.[56, 63, 75, 79, 81, 82] The patient is positioned supine with neck gently flexed and head straight. The craniotomy flap is placed to expose the midline and the area about 6 cm to the right of midline, and it extends about 6 cm anteriorly from just behind the coronal suture. The dura is opened with a U-shaped incision based on the superior sagittal sinus and retracted with sutures, taking care to avoid occlusion of the sinus by torsion. The medial portion of the right hemisphere is gently retracted away from the falx. Dissection proceeds along a line directed from the coronal suture toward the external auditory meatus; this trajectory will be directed toward the foramen of Monro. When the white, glistening corpus callosum is reached, the pericallosal arteries (or artery) are identified and a site for callosotomy is selected. A 2- to 3-cm callosotomy in the anteroposterior axis is made, either between the pericallosal arteries or to one side of them. The ventricle is entered and tumor resection performed with an ultrasonic aspirator. In some patients, tumor removal through the foramen of Monro may be possible; if enlargement of the foramen is necessary, resection of its posteroinferior margin (the anterior nucleus of the thalamus) is preferred to injuring the column of the fornix.[82] Care is required to avoid injuring the internal cerebral vein.

Alternatively, the third ventricle may be entered by the interforniceal or the subchoroidal trans–velum interpositum approach. In the interforniceal approach,[82, 83] an incision is made through the septum pellucidum into the contralateral ventricle. The midline raphe is identified and a split is developed between the two fornices for about 2 cm in a posterior direction from the level of the foramen. Posterior extent is limited by the interhippocampal commissure. Damage to the fornices and internal cerebral veins must be avoided.

The trans–velum interpositum approach[82, 84] may be preferred as a means of entering the third ventricle, because incision of neural structures is minimized. The choroid plexus of the lateral ventricle is elevated medially and superiorly as it enters the foramen of Monro, revealing the velum interpositum beneath. The velum interpositum is incised, affording entry into the midportion of the third ventricle. If necessary, the thalamostriate vein may be divided.

Whichever method of entry into the third ventricle is selected, the goal is tumor debulking, and not a total resection. The tumor is removed with ultrasonic aspiration. Planes are developed between the tumor mass and the walls of the third ventricle. The resection is limited anteriorly as the tumor merges with functioning neural structures. Injury to the anterior cerebral arteries is possible if the resection proceeds too far anteriorly.

TUMORS OF THE CEREBELLUM AND CEREBELLAR PEDUNCLES

Most cerebellar gliomas are cystic juvenile pilocytic astrocytomas. Because complete excision of these tumors is presumably curative (see Chapter 60 on long-term survivors of glioma), and because postoperative cerebellar deficits tend to resolve entirely if the deep nuclei are not injured, an aggressive approach toward these tumors is appropriate. Location of a tumor within the cerebellar hemispheres does not, however, guarantee the surgeon a *carte blanche*, and avoidance of damage to certain structures is crucial to surgical success.

A bilateral suboccipital craniectomy[63, 79] is the appropriate approach for most masses within the cerebellar hemispheres or the vermis, although a unilateral retromastoid craniectomy or craniotomy[85] may suffice for some small, laterally placed tumors. The bilateral suboccipital exposure combines wide access with immediate decompression and is usually preferable. The patient is placed in a prone position with the head flexed. If hydrocephalus is present, an occipital ventriculostomy may be placed at the beginning of the procedure. A midline skin incision is made from the occipital protuberance to the midcervical region. A triangular pericranial graft is taken from the upper portion of the exposed occipital bone for later use in closure. Suboccipital bone is removed as a flap by some authors and is later used for closure; others use a craniectomy. Removal of the neural arch of C1 is performed for masses in the inferior portion of the hemispheres or if a view directed into the fourth ventricle from below is desired. The dura is opened in a Y-shaped manner and retracted with sutures. An incision is made in the cerebellar cortex over the most superficial portion of the tumor or cyst, and dissection proceeds until the pathologic lesion is encountered. If the tumor is a cystic pilocytic astrocytoma, the cyst is evacuated and the cyst cavity is held open with self-retaining retractors. The mural tumor nodule is located and completely resected. If the cyst wall was noted to enhance on preoperative imaging studies, biopsy or resection of the cyst wall should be considered. This will be unnecessary for most cystic pilocytic astrocytomas unless the wall is thick and brightly enhancing. After hemostasis and irrigation, the dura is closed with the pericranial graft in a watertight fashion, and a layered closure of musculature, fascia, and skin is performed.

In the less common malignant gliomas of the cerebellar hemisphere, internal decompression is performed for debulking. A well-defined tumor border may be present in some areas. It is important not to follow the tumor into the cerebellar peduncle and not to damage the deep cerebellar nuclei. Injury of the dentate nucleus causes severe postoperative ipsilateral ataxia. It has been possible to demonstrate atrophy of the contralateral red nucleus after surgical damage to the dentate nucleus.[86]

Cerebellar mutism is another potential complication of cerebellar resection. The anatomic substrate of this phenomenon is still being debated, but evidence points to involvement of the dentate nuclei and the superior vermis in its pathogenesis.[18, 87, 88] Although recovery of speech is typical, the risk of cerebellar mutism is another reason to avoid damage to the dentate nuclei.

Cerebellar Peduncles

A small tumor confined to the cerebellar peduncle may occasionally be encountered. Tomita[89] has reported resection of four cerebellar peduncle tumors in children through a suboccipital craniectomy approach. The peduncle was entered through the lateral fourth ventricular wall, and the tumors were resected with a laser. Postoperative ipsilateral intentional tremor and dysmetria were frequent but transient.

TUMORS OF THE BRAINSTEM AND FOURTH VENTRICLE

Appropriate surgical technique for masses in the brainstem and fourth ventricle is extremely dependent on the location, extent of infiltration, and histologic characteristics of the tumor. With currently available imaging techniques, particularly high-field MRI, it is nearly always possible to distinguish between tumors for which excision is appropriate and those that should be treated with radiation and/or chemotherapy without histologic confirmation.

Diffuse Brainstem Tumors

The diffuse intrinsic brainstem glioma has a characteristic clinical presentation. The peak age at incidence is between 5 and 10 years. The insidious onset of cranial nerve and long tract signs occurs with a median time course of 2 to 3 months between initial symptoms and presentation. Hydrocephalus may be evident. MRI scans typically reveal a diffuse, infiltrating process arising from the pons with hypointense signal on T1-weighted images and hyperintensity on T2-weighted images.

When the clinical presentation and radiographic appearance are typical of diffuse brainstem glioma in a child, stereotactic biopsy, open biopsy, or an attempt at resection are currently believed to be contraindicated.[90] In two studies of biopsy results for brainstem gliomas,[90, 91] including 63 operations, only one patient had an ependymoma; the remainder had astrocytic tumors. Although pathologic results from biopsy of brainstem astrocytomas have prognostic value,[92, 93] this has been supplanted by information available from MRI scans.[94] Biopsies or attempts to resect these lesions carry a significant morbidity (approximately 10%).[90]

When the clinical presentation is markedly atypical or imaging studies suggest a possible brainstem abscess, stereotactic biopsy of the brainstem may be appropriate. In the transfrontal approach, the entry point is parasagittal and precoronal, usually on the nondominant side. A trajectory that remains intraparenchymal from the entry point to the lesion is chosen, with the possible exception of traversing the lateral ventricle. It is important to miss the posterior clinoid process, the free tentorial edge, and the interpeduncular cistern. This trajectory has been used with low morbidity for lesions as caudal as the medulla.[95] An alternative trajectory for targets located in the pons is the transcerebellar transpeduncular route, in which the trajectory passes through the cerebellar peduncle, with a suboccipital entry point over the cerebellar hemisphere.[95–97]

Focal Midbrain Tumors

Focal tumors of the midbrain are usually described as arising from the tectal plate or from the tegmentum of the mesencephalon. Tectal plate tumors are most common in children and in young adults; they present with hydrocephalus, and some also cause eye movement abnormalities or gait ataxia. An indolent clinical course is common, and when the lesion is confined to the tectal plate and does not enhance with gadolinium, progression is unusual.[98–101] Treatment for these lesions consists of a procedure to relieve hydrocephalus. An endoscopic third ventriculostomy or ventriculoperitoneal shunt designed to avoid overdrainage is ideal, because these patients are very sensitive to overshunting.[98, 99] Patients are then followed up with serial MRI scans. Lesions that appear to be enlarging or that develop new enhancement are usually treated with radiotherapy, chemotherapy, or radiosurgery.

If a biopsy of a tectal plate tumor is thought to be necessary, it often can be performed stereotactically.[98, 100] Some authors have reported results of more extensive resections in focal midbrain tectal tumors with enhancement on CT or MRI and radiographically clearly defined borders.[102–104] A supracerebellar infratentorial approach[63, 105] is usually selected. The patient is placed in a semi-sitting or in the Concorde position. A bilateral suboccipital craniectomy is performed, which exposes both lateral sinuses. After dural opening, dissection proceeds in the midline over the top of the vermis until the vein of Galen is seen. The cerebellar precentral vein is divided, and retractors and microscope are repositioned to see the tectum. It frequently is necessary

to split the superior vermis for adequate exposure of the tectal plate.

An alternative approach that may be suitable if the tumor does not extend too far caudally is the posterior interhemispheric approach.[106] The patient is positioned three-quarters prone, right side down. The surgical corridor passes between the falx and the medial right parietal and occipital lobes toward the pineal region and tectal plate. The angulation of the surgical microscope that is necessary to see the tectal plate through the tentorial incisura makes a high parietal craniotomy necessary. Division of the free edges of the falx and tentorium along the side of the straight sinus may afford additional exposure of infratentorial structures. The deep cerebral veins pose an obstacle to surgery of the tectal plate through this exposure, and the surgeon works at a considerable distance from the tumor (10 cm).

Parinaud's syndrome is a common postoperative sequela if the superior colliculi are incised. Auditory hallucinations and the acoustic neglect syndrome have been reported after damage to the inferior colliculi.[104] Although some groups prefer to limit resection to the exophytic portion of tectal tumors, others have attained total resection of tumors extending within the midbrain parenchyma using piecemeal resection with bipolar forceps or an ultrasonic aspirator or laser.[104, 107] Operative mortality of about 10% has been reported for resections of tectal masses.[104, 107]

A focal tumor of the midbrain tegmentum may be encountered rarely. If the tumor appears to have sharp boundaries and extends laterally to the surface of the midbrain, a resection may be attempted through a subtemporal transtentorial approach. Through the point that is exposed on the ependymal surface, the tumor is entered, morcellated, and removed piecemeal.

Focal Pontine Tumors and Dorsally Exophytic Tumors

Focal intrinsic pontine tumors are unusual. An occasional cystic pontine tumor with a brightly enhancing mural nodule may be seen in a child. This appearance is typical of a pilocytic astrocytoma, and some authors recommend an attempt at radical excision.[108] If this is elected, the cyst should be entered through its most superficial point in the floor of the fourth ventricle and the mural nodule removed with a laser.[108] ''Safe entry zones'' in the floor of the fourth ventricle have been described, located 5 mm from the midline both rostral and caudal to the intrapontine portion of the facial nerve.[109] The facial nerve may be located with direct intraoperative stimulation as it courses over the abducens nucleus in the fourth ventricular floor. Alternatively, a midline myelotomy may be used.[110] Difficulty may arise if the tumor cyst collapses when entered, making a handheld narrow-tipped retractor necessary to maintain exposure.[108] It is probably safest to apply gentle lateral retraction rather than to retract medial structures.[109] Many focal pilocytic astrocytomas of the pons are clinically indolent in behavior, resembling tectal plate gliomas.[111] Appropriate management for indolent pontine masses may consist of a biopsy followed by radiation, with resection reserved for clinically aggressive tumors.

The dorsal exophytic tumor of the brainstem is more common. These tumors arise from the floor of the fourth ventricle without a sharp border between tumor and normal pons.[112, 113] They may be resected through a suboccipital craniectomy with splitting of the inferior vermis; alternatively, an incision through the vermis and paravermian lobules directed perpendicular to the vermian axis may be preferable. It is necessary to see the floor of the fourth ventricle above and below the lesion to know the level of the dorsal brainstem, because the tumor blends imperceptibly into the ventricular floor. After separating the mass from its adhesions to the cerebellar tonsils, which are commonly splayed by pressure from the mass, only the exophytic portion of the mass is removed; this is accomplished with an ultrasonic aspirator or a laser. The posterior inferior cerebellar artery may lie between the caudal portion of the exophytic tumor and the cerebellar tonsils. Attempts to remove the portion of the tumor within the pons are likely to cause severe postoperative deficits. Injury to this portion of the pons causes sixth and seventh nerve palsies and potential internuclear ophthalmoplegia.[108] Intraoperative monitoring of somatosensory and brainstem evoked potentials and electromyograms of facial and abducens muscles may help reduce these risks.[114]

Focal Tumors of the Medulla and Cervicomedullary Junction

These tumors may be intrinsic or partially exophytic and can be limited to the medulla or can extend downward into the cervicomedullary junction or the cervical spinal cord. They may be histologically benign or malignant. Many surgeons do not feel that aggressive resection of these tumors offers sufficient benefit to offset the risk of severe postoperative deficits. Others advocate resection.[108, 115, 116]

If resection of a focal cervicomedullary glioma is thought to be indicated, a suboccipital craniectomy is performed, with cervical laminectomies (or, in children, laminotomies) performed as necessary to expose the lower pole of the lesion. Intraoperative ultrasound may be used before or after dural opening to confirm proper exposure. After dural opening, the midline of the rostral cervical spinal cord is determined by identifying the dorsal root entry zones bilaterally. The cord may be distorted by the tumor, and it is important to identify the true midline to avoid the proprioceptive deficit that results when a myelotomy is inadvertently placed over a posterior column. When the midline has been conclusively identified, a midline myelotomy is made over the most superficial portion of the tumor or the associated cyst. Small venules on the surface of the cord may be sacrificed. Some surgeons prefer a laser myelotomy, whereas others use bipolar electrocautery and a sharp blade. Fine pial sutures may be placed for retraction. The border between tumor and cord is identified and carefully followed to define the tumor's margins while it is removed with ultrasonic aspiration or laser. Resection proceeds rostrally and caudally until the limits of safe resection are achieved. Tumors in this location commonly undergo transependymal rupture caudal to the obex. The floor of the fourth ventricle rostral to the tumor is a critical landmark. It is important not to extend a midline myelotomy beyond the obex rostrally and not to injure the posterior inferior cerebellar artery, which often lies between the extension of the tumor into the fourth ventricle and the cerebellar tonsil. Removal of every fragment of tumor is generally an impractical and dangerous goal, particularly at the tumor's rostral pole.[115]

Focal tumors confined to the medulla are more dangerous to remove, and postoperative deficits can be truly devastating. If surgery is elected, the tumor is approached through its most superficial portion, staying at least 1.5 cm rostral to the obex and out of the midline, to avoid injuring lower cranial nerve nuclei. Minimization of retraction and of manipulation of the lower brainstem is essential. Postoperative respiratory embarrassment and swallowing deficit should be anticipated and prepared for with prolonged intubation or a tracheostomy. The dangers of removal of focal tumors in the medulla have been emphasized.[108, 116, 117]

SPINAL CORD TUMORS

Ependymomas and benign and malignant astrocytomas of the spinal cord demand different surgical technique.[118, 119] It is sometimes possible to reach a tentative histologic diagnosis by examining preoperative imaging studies. Ependymomas tend to enhance brightly and homogeneously with gadolinium and to have blunt rostral and caudal poles, sometimes with associated cysts. Astrocytomas are less likely to have sharply defined poles or to be homogeneously enhancing. Intraoperative pathologic results are important, because the degree of aggressiveness in pursuing a gross total resection should be greater in ependymomas. Although recurrence-free survival of low-grade spinal cord astrocytomas in adults has been reported,[120] it is likely that many of these tumors will eventually recur despite "total" resection. Complete excision of an ependymoma is more likely to result in cure and therefore justifies more aggressive (and risky) resection.

The rostral and caudal limits of the tumor on MRI studies guide the extent of the laminectomy, with further assistance from intraoperative ultrasound. The dural opening should expose the entire extent of the tumor and allow further working room at either end. After exposure of the cord, the midline is identified by inspection of the dorsal root entry zones on both sides. A midline myelotomy is the usual choice; care must be taken to remain precisely in the midline to avoid damage to the posterior columns. Bipolar cautery and a sharp knife or a laser are used. If the cord is markedly rotated by the tumor, or if the most superficial portion of the tumor is near the dorsal root entry zone, it may sometimes be preferable to use a myelotomy just posterior to the dorsal root entry zone on one side. Fine pial retraction sutures are placed.

Blunt dissection proceeds in the line of the myelotomy until the tumor is encountered, usually at a depth of about 2 mm. Many surgeons prefer internal decompression of the tumor with an ultrasonic aspirator, followed by excision of the more peripheral portions of the tumor until the border between tumor and cord is reached; some prefer to maintain the tumor intact throughout the dissection. It is not uncommon for astrocytomas of the cord to have a tumor-cord interface in many areas, but usually the rostral and caudal poles of the tumor blend into normal cord structures.[120, 121] In contrast, ependymomas tend to have definable borders throughout, and complete excision is usually feasible.[121, 122] Many intramedullary gliomas grow concentrically with the spinal cord, which is progressively thinned around the circumference of the tumor. The most anterior portion of the tumor is therefore in close proximity to the anterior spinal artery, which must not be injured. After complete removal of the tumor and careful inspection of the tumor bed, attention is paid to meticulous hemostasis and thorough irrigation to remove any blood within the thecal sac. The dura is closed primarily or with a graft of lumbar fascia.

If the tumor is found to be a malignant astrocytoma, the goal of surgery is primarily palliative and every effort should be made to avoid damage to functioning structures. This may be difficult, as the tumor and surrounding cord parenchyma have a tendency to prolapse alarmingly through tiny myelotomies as a result of high pressures within the cord. High-dose steroids, as recommended for spinal cord trauma,[123] may possibly reduce the risk of this undesirable event. When a malignant spinal cord tumor located in the cervical cord is biopsied, sudden postoperative respiratory failure has been known to occur. Patients should be closely monitored in the postoperative period.

Complete resection of the spinal cord in the thoracic or lumbar regions is sometimes discussed as "the only chance for cure" for such patients. Because these tumors commonly spread through the cerebrospinal fluid to other portions of the neural axis, cure is unlikely despite the most radical surgery. No experience with cordectomy has been reported for malignant spinal cord astrocytomas.

REFERENCES

1. Macaulay RJ, Jay V, Hoffman HJ, et al: Increased mitotic activity as a negative prognostic indicator in pleomorphic xanthoastrocytoma: Case report. J Neurosurg 1993; 79:761.
2. Thomas C, Golden B: Pleomorphic xanthoastrocytoma: Report of two cases and brief review of the literature. Clin Neuropathol 1993; 12:97.
3. Hayostek CJ, Shaw EG, Scheithauer B, et al: Astrocytomas of the cerebellum: A comparative clinicopathologic study of pilocytic and diffuse astrocytomas. Cancer 1993; 72:856.
4. Gjerris F, Klinken L: Long-term prognosis in children with benign cerebellar astrocytoma. J Neurosurg 1978; 49:179.
5. Wallner KE, Gonzales MF, Edwards MS, et al: Treatment results of juvenile pilocytic astrocytoma. J Neurosurg 1988; 69:171.
6. Schneider JH Jr, Raffel C, McComb JG: Benign cerebellar astrocytomas of childhood. Neurosurgery 1992; 30:58.
7. Kehler U, Arnold H, Muller H: Long-term follow-up of infratentorial pilocytic astrocytomas. Neurosurg Rev 1990; 13:315.
8. Gehan EA, Walker MD: Prognostic factors for patients with brain tumors. Natl Cancer Inst Monogr 1977; 46:189.
9. Walker MD, Alexander E Jr, Hunt WE, et al: Evaluation of mithramycin in the treatment of anaplastic gliomas. J Neurosurg 1976; 44:655.
10. Höllerhage H-G, Zumkeller M, Becker M, et al: Influence of type and extent of surgery on early results and survival time in glioblastoma multiforme. Acta Neurochir 1991; 113:31.
11. Vecht CJ, Avezaat CJJ, van Putten WLJ, et al: The influence of the extent of surgery on the neurological function and survival in malignant glioma: A retrospective analysis in 243 patients. J Neurol Neurosurg Psychiatry 1990; 53:466.
12. Grabb PA, Albright AL, Pang D: Dissemination of supratentorial malignant gliomas via the cerebrospinal fluid in children. Neurosurgery 1992; 30:64.
13. Elliott JP, Keles GE, Waite M, et al: Ventricular entry during resection of malignant gliomas: Effect on intracranial cerebrospinal fluid tumor dissemination. J Neurosurg 1994; 80:834.
14. Iberti TJ, Miller M, Abalos A, et al: Abnormal coagulation profile in brain tumor patients during surgery. Neurosurgery 1994; 34:389.
15. Sawaya R, Glas-Greenwalt P: Postoperative venous thromboembolism and brain tumors: II. Hemostatic profile. J Neurooncol 1992; 14:127.
16. Penfield W, Jasper H: Epilepsy and the functional anatomy of the human brain. Boston, Little, Brown, 1954.
17. Rostomily RC, Berger MS, Ojemann GA, et al: Postoperative deficits and functional recovery following removal of tumors involving the dominant hemisphere supplementary motor area. J Neurosurg 1991; 75:62.
18. Crutchfield JS, Sawaya R, Meyers CA, et al: Postoperative mutism in neurosurgery: Report of two cases. J Neurosurg 1994; 81:115.
19. Schneider R, Gautier JC: Leg weakness due to stroke: Site of lesions, weakness patterns and causes. Brain 1994; 117:347.
20. Berger MS: Lesions in functional ("eloquent") cortex and subcortical white matter. Clin Neurosurg 1994; 41:444.
21. Roper SN, Levesque MF, Sutherling WW, et al: Surgical treatment of partial epilepsy arising from the insular cortex: Report of two cases. J Neurosurg 1993; 79:266.
22. Penfield W, Faulk ME Jr: The insula: Further observations on its function. Brain 1955; 78:445.
23. Penfield W, Lende RA, Rasmussen T: Manipulation hemiplegia, an untoward complication in the surgery of focal epilepsy. J Neurosurg 1961; 18:769.
24. Silfvenius H, Gloor P, Rasmussen T: Evaluation of insular ablation in surgical treatment of temporal lobe epilepsy. Epilepsia 1964; 5:307.
25. Vignolo LA, Boccardi E, Caverni L: Unexpected CT-scan findings in global aphasia. Cortex 1986; 22:55.
26. Berthier M, Starkstein S, Leiguarda R: Behavioral effects of damage to the right insula and surrounding regions. Cortex 1987; 23:673.
27. Starkstein SE, Berthier M, Leiguarda R: Bilateral opercular syndrome and crossed aphemia due to a right insular lesion: A clinicopathological study. Brain Lang 1988; 34:253.
28. Obana WG, Laxer KD, Cogen PH, et al: Resection of dominant opercular gliosis in refractory partial epilepsy: Report of two cases. J Neurosurg 1992; 77:632.
29. Ojemann G, Ojemann J, Lettich E, et al: Cortical language localization in left, dominant hemisphere: An electrical stimulation mapping investigation in 117 patients. J Neurosurg 1989; 71:316.
30. Anderson SW, Damasio AR, Damasio H: Troubled letters but not numbers: Domain specific cognitive impairments following focal damage in frontal cortex. Brain 1990; 113:749.
31. Penfield W, Roberts L: Speech and brain mechanisms. Princeton, NJ, Princeton University Press, 1959.
32. Maxwell RE: Cerebral lobectomies. In Apuzzo MLJ (ed): Brain Surgery: Complication Avoidance and Management, vol 1. New York, Churchill Livingstone, 1993, p 442.
33. Crandall PH: Cortical resections. In Engel J Jr (ed): Surgical Treatment of the Epilepsies. New York, Raven Press, 1987, p 377.
34. Fried I: Anatomic temporal lobe resections for temporal lobe epilepsy. Neurosurg Clin North Am 1993; 4:233.
35. Cushing H: Distortions of the visual fields in cases of brain tumor (sixth paper): The field defects produced by temporal lobe lesions. Brain 1922; 44:341.
36. Ebeling U, Reulen HJ: Neurosurgical topography of the optic radiation in the temporal lobe. Acta Neurochir 1988; 92:29.
37. Penfield W: Temporal lobe epilepsy. Br J Surg 1954; 41:337.
38. Marino R, Rasmussen T: Visual field changes after temporal lobectomy. Neurology 1968; 18:825.
39. Miller NR: Topical diagnosis of lesions in the visual sensory pathway. In Clinical Neuro-ophthalmology, vol 1. Baltimore, Williams & Wilkins, 1982, p 108.
40. Hermann BP, Wyler AR, Bush AJ, et al: Differential effects of left and right anterior temporal lobectomy on verbal learning and memory performance. Epilepsia 1992; 33:289.
41. Hermann BP, Wyler AR, Somes G, et al: Declarative memory following anterior temporal lobectomy in humans. Behav Neurosci 1994; 108:3.
42. Wolf RL, Ivnik RJ, Hirschorn KA, et al: Neurocognitive efficiency following left temporal lobectomy: Standard versus limited resection. J Neurosurg 1993; 79:76.

43. Haglund MM, Berger MS, Shamseldin M, et al: Cortical localization of temporal lobe language sites in patients with gliomas. Neurosurgery 1994; 34:567.
44. Hermann BP, Wyler AR, Somes G, et al: Dysnomia after left anterior temporal lobectomy without functional mapping: Frequency and correlates. Neurosurgery 1994; 35:52.
45. LeRoux PD, Berger MS, Haglund MM, et al: Resection of intrinsic tumors from nondominant face motor cortex using stimulation mapping: Report of two cases. Surg Neurol 1991; 36:44.
46. Gregorie EM, Goldring S: Localization of function in the excision of lesions from the sensorimotor region. J Neurosurg 1984; 61:1047.
47. Goldring S, Gregorie EM: Experience with lesions that mimic gliomas in patients presenting with a chronic seizure disorder. Clin Neurosurg 1986; 33:43.
48. Pilcher WH, Rusyniak WG: Complications of epilepsy surgery. Neurosurg Clin North Am 1993; 4:311.
49. Ojemann GA, Dodrill CB: Verbal memory deficits after left temporal lobectomy for epilepsy: Mechanisms and intraoperative prediction. J Neurosurg 1985; 62:101.
50. Olivier A: Surgery of epilepsy: Overall procedure. In Apuzzo MLJ (ed): Neurosurgical Aspects of Epilepsy. Park Ridge, Ill, AANS, 1991, p 117.
51. Haglund MM, Ojemann GA: Extratemporal resective surgery for epilepsy. Neurosurg Clin North Am 1993; 4:283.
52. Rasmussen T: Surgery for epilepsy arising in regions other than the temporal and frontal lobes. Adv Neurol 1975; 8:207.
53. Olivier A, Awad IA: Extratemporal resections. In Engel J Jr (ed): Surgical Treatment of the Epilepsies, ed 2. New York, Raven Press, 1993, p 489.
54. Cascino GD, Hulihan JF, Sharbrough FW, et al: Parietal lobe lesional epilepsy: Electroclinical correlation and operative outcome. Epilepsia 1993; 34:522.
55. Williamson PD, Boon PA, Thadani VM, et al: Parietal lobe epilepsy: Diagnostic considerations and results of surgery. Ann Neurol 1992; 31:193.
56. Rhoton AL Jr, Yamamoto I, Peace DA: Microsurgery of the third ventricle: II. Operative approaches. Neurosurgery 1981; 8:357.
57. Heros RC: Brain resection for exposure of deep extracerebral and paraventricular lesions. Surg Neurol 1990; 34:188.
58. Sugita K, Hongo K: Posterior transcortical approach. In Apuzzo MLJ (ed): Surgery of the Third Ventricle. Baltimore, Williams & Wilkins, 1987, p 557.
59. Barrow DL, Dawson RD: Surgical management of arteriovenous malformations in the region of the ventricular trigone. Neurosurgery 1994; 35:1046.
60. Greenblatt SH: Neurosurgery and the anatomy of reading: A practical review. Neurosurgery 1977; 1:6.
61. Nagata S, Rhoton AL Jr, Barry M: Microsurgical anatomy of the choroidal fissure. Surg Neurol 1988; 30:3.
62. Almeida GM, Shibata MK, Nakagawa EJ: Contralateral parafalcine approach for parasagittal and callosal arteriovenous malformations. Neurosurgery 1984; 14:744.
63. Mohsenipour I, Goldhahn W-E, Fischer J, et al: Approaches in Neurosurgery: Central and Peripheral Nervous System. New York, Thieme, 1994.
64. Salanova V, Andermann F, Olivier A, et al: Occipital lobe epilepsy: Electroclinical manifestations, electrocorticography, cortical stimulation and outcome in 42 patients treated between 1930 and 1991: Surgery of occipital lobe epilepsy. Brain 1992; 115:1655.
65. Williamson PD, Thadani VM, Darcey TM, et al: Occipital lobe epilepsy: Clinical characteristics, seizure spread patterns, and results of surgery. Ann Neurol 1992; 31:3.
66. Blume WT, Whiting SE, Girvin JP: Epilepsy surgery in the posterior cortex. Ann Neurol 1991; 29:638.
67. Greenblatt SH: Left occipital lobectomy and the preangular anatomy of reading. Brain Lang 1990; 38:576.
68. Lyons MK, Kelly PJ: Computer-assisted stereotactic biopsy and volumetric resection of thalamic pilocytic astrocytomas: Report of 23 cases. Stereotact Funct Neurosurg 1992; 59:100.
69. Natori Y, Rhoton AL Jr: Transcranial approach to the orbit: Microsurgical anatomy. J Neurosurg 1994; 81:78.
70. Maroon JC, Kennerdell JS: Surgical approaches to the orbit: Indications and techniques. J Neurosurg 1984; 60:1226.
71. Al-Mefty O, Fox JL: Superolateral orbital exposure and reconstruction. Surg Neurol 1985; 23:609.
72. Jane JA, Park TS, Pobereskin LH, et al: The supraorbital approach: Technical note. Neurosurgery 1982; 11:537.
73. McDermott MW, Durity FA, Rootman J, et al: Combined frontotemporal-orbitozygomatic approach for tumors of the sphenoid wing and orbit. Neurosurgery 1990; 26:107.
74. Wilbrand H: Schema des Verlaufs der Sehnervenfasern durch das Chiasma. Z Augenheilk 1926; 59:135.
75. Rodriguez LA, Edwards MSB, Levin VA: Management of hypothalamic gliomas in children: An analysis of 33 cases. Neurosurgery 1990; 26:242.
76. Hoffman HJ, Soloniuk DS, Humphreys RP, et al: Management and outcome of low-grade astrocytomas of the midline in children: A retrospective review. Neurosurgery 1993; 33:964.
77. Wisoff JH, Abbott R, Epstein F: Surgical management of exophytic chiasmatic-hypothalamic tumors of childhood. J Neurosurg 1990; 73:661.
78. Hoffman HJ, Humphreys RP, Drake JM, et al: Optic pathway/hypothalamic gliomas: A dilemma in management. Pediatr Neurosurg 1993; 19:186.
79. Koos WT, Spetzler RF, Lang J: Color Atlas of Microneurosurgery: Intracranial Tumors, vol 1, ed 2. New York, Thieme, 1993.
80. Gillett GR, Symon L: Hypothalamic glioma. Surg Neurol 1987; 28:291.
81. Shucart W: Anterior transcallosal and transcortical approaches. In Apuzzo MLJ (ed): Surgery of the Third Ventricle. Baltimore, Williams & Wilkins, 1987, p 303.
82. Apuzzo MLJ, Litofsky NS: Surgery in and around the anterior third ventricle. In Apuzzo MLJ (ed): Brain Surgery: Complication Avoidance and Management, vol 1. New York, Churchill Livingstone, 1993, p 541.
83. Apuzzo MLJ, Giannotta SL: Transcallosal interforniceal approach. In Apuzzo MLJ (ed): Surgery of the Third Ventricle. Baltimore, Williams & Wilkins, 1987, p 354.
84. Lavyne MH, Patterson RH Jr: Subchoroidal trans-velum interpositum approach. In Apuzzo MLJ (ed): Surgery of the Third Ventricle. Baltimore, Williams & Wilkins, 1987, p 381.
85. Ogilvy CS, Ojemann RG: Posterior fossa craniotomy for lesions of the cerebellopontine angle: Technical note. J Neurosurg 1993; 78:508.
86. Bontozoglou NP, Chakeres DW, Martin GF, et al: Cerebellorubral degeneration after resection of cerebellar dentate nucleus neoplasms: Evaluation with MR imaging. Radiology 1991; 180:223.
87. Cakir Y, Karakisi D, Kocanaogullari O: Cerebellar mutism in an adult: Case report. Surg Neurol 1994; 41:342.
88. Dietze DD Jr, Mickle JP: Cerebellar mutism after posterior fossa surgery. Pediatr Neurosurg 1990; 16:25.
89. Tomita T: Surgical management of cerebellar peduncle lesions in children. Neurosurgery 1986; 18:568.
90. Albright AL, Packer RJ, Zimmerman R, et al: Magnetic resonance scans should replace biopsies for the diagnosis of diffuse brain stem gliomas: A report from the Children's Cancer Group. Neurosurgery 1993; 33:1026.
91. Byrne JV, Kendall BE, Kingsley DP, et al: Lesions of the brain stem: Assessment by magnetic resonance imaging. Neuroradiology 1989; 31:129.
92. Albright AL, Guthkelch AN, Packer RJ, et al: Prognostic factors in pediatric brain-stem gliomas. J Neurosurg 1986; 65:751.
93. Artigas J, Ferszt R, Brock M, et al: The relevance of pathological diagnosis for therapy and outcome of brain stem gliomas. Acta Neurochir Suppl 1988; 42:166.
94. Barkovich AJ, Krischer J, Kun LE, et al: Brain stem gliomas: A classification system based on magnetic resonance imaging. Pediatr Neurosurg 1990; 16:73.
95. Kratimenos GP, Thomas DG: The role of image-directed biopsy in the diagnosis and management of brainstem lesions. Br J Neurosurg 1993; 7:155.
96. Abernathey CD, Camacho A, Kelly PJ: Stereotaxic suboccipital transcerebellar biopsy of pontine mass lesions. J Neurosurg 1989; 70:195.
97. Guthrie BL, Steinberg GK, Adler JR: Posterior fossa stereotaxic biopsy using the Brown-Roberts-Wells stereotaxic system: Technical note. J Neurosurg 1989; 70:649.
98. Pollack IF, Pang D, Albright AL: The long-term outcome in children with late-onset aqueductal stenosis resulting from benign intrinsic tectal tumors. J Neurosurg 1994; 80:681.
99. Chapman PH: Indolent gliomas of the midbrain tectum. Concepts Pediatr Neurosurg 1990; 10:97.

100. Squires LA, Allen JC, Abbott R, et al: Focal tectal tumors: Management and prognosis. Neurology 1994; 44:953.
101. May PL, Blaser SI, Hoffman HJ, et al: Benign intrinsic tectal "tumors" in children. J Neurosurg 1991; 74:867.
102. Hoffman HJ, Vandertop WP: Tumors of the midbrain. Neurosurg Clin North Am 1993; 4:537.
103. Vandertop WP, Hoffman HJ, Drake JM, et al: Focal midbrain tumors in children. Neurosurgery 1992; 31:186.
104. Lapras C, Bognar L, Turjman F, et al: Tectal plate gliomas: I. Microsurgery of the tectal plate gliomas. Acta Neurochir 1994; 126:76.
105. Bruce JN, Stein BM: Supracerebellar approaches in the pineal region. *In* Apuzzo MLJ (ed): Brain surgery: Complication avoidance and management, vol 1. New York, Churchill Livingstone, 1993, p 511.
106. Apuzzo MLJ, Tung H: Supratentorial approaches to the pineal region. *In* Apuzzo MLJ (ed): Brain Surgery: Complication Avoidance and Management, vol 1. New York, Churchill Livingstone, 1993, p 486.
107. Pendl G, Vorkapic P, Koniyama M: Microsurgery of midbrain lesions. Neurosurgery 1990; 26:641.
108. Epstein FJ, Farmer J-P: Intrinsic tumors of the brainstem. *In* Apuzzo MLJ (ed): Brain Surgery: Complication Avoidance and Management, vol 2. New York, Churchill Livingstone, 1993, p 1835.
109. Kyoshima K, Kobayashi S, Gibo H, et al: A study of safe entry zones via the floor of the fourth ventricle for brain-stem lesions. J Neurosurg 1993; 78:987.
110. Wen DY, Heros RC: Surgical approaches to the brain stem. Neurosurg Clin North Am 1993; 4:457.
111. Edwards MS, Wara WM, Ciricillo SF, et al: Focal brain-stem astrocytomas causing symptoms of involvement of the facial nerve nucleus: Long-term survival in six pediatric cases. J Neurosurg 1994; 80:20.
112. Stroink AR, Hoffman HJ, Hendrick EB, et al: Transependymal benign dorsally exophytic brain stem gliomas in childhood: Diagnosis and treatment recommendations. Neurosurgery 1987; 20:439.
113. Pollack IF, Hoffman HJ, Humphreys RP, et al: The long-term outcome after surgical treatment of dorsally exophytic brain-stem gliomas. J Neurosurg 1993; 78:859.
114. Albright AL: Tumors of the pons. Neurosurg Clin North Am 1993; 4:529.
115. Robertson PL, Allen JC, Abbott IR, et al: Cervicomedullary tumors in children: A distinct subset of brainstem gliomas. Neurology 1994; 44:1798.
116. Abbott R: Tumors of the medulla. Neurosurg Clin North Am 1993; 4:519.
117. Abbott R, Shiminski-Maher T, Wisoff JH, et al: Intrinsic tumors of the medulla: Surgical complications. Pediatr Neurosurg 1991; 17:239.
118. McCormick PC, Stein BM: Intramedullary tumors in adults. Neurosurg Clin North Am 1990; 1:609.
119. Epstein FJ, Farmer J-P: Pediatric spinal cord surgery. Neurosurg Clin North Am 1990; 1:569.
120. Epstein FJ, Farmer J-P, Freed D: Adult intramedullary astrocytomas of the spinal cord. J Neurosurg 1992; 77:355.
121. Epstein FJ, Farmer J-P: Removal of spinal intramedullary gliomas. *In* Wilson CB (ed): Neurosurgical Procedures: Personal Approaches to Classic Operations. Baltimore, Williams & Wilkins, 1992, p 200.
122. Epstein FJ, Farmer J-P, Freed D: Adult intramedullary spinal cord ependymomas: The result of surgery in 38 patients. J Neurosurg 1993; 79:204.
123. Bracken MB, Shepard MJ, Collins WF, et al: A randomized, controlled trial of methylprednisolone or naloxone in the treatment of acute spinal-cord injury. Results of the Second National Acute Spinal Cord Injury Study. N Engl J Med 1990; 322:1405.

RAYMOND SAWAYA

MAAROUF A. HAMMOUD

B. LEE LIGON

GREGORY N. FULLER

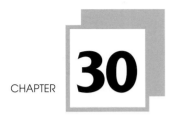

CHAPTER **30**

Intraoperative Localization of Tumor and Margins

Recent studies indicate that optimal management of gliomas is achieved with maximum surgical resection followed by adjuvant radiation therapy and chemotherapy.[1–4] Complicating the surgeon's ability to achieve total excision of a glioma are several of its distinct characteristics. One of these is the presence of neoplastic cells that infiltrate outside the tumor margins as defined by preoperative contrast-enhanced computed tomography (CT) or magnetic resonance imaging (MRI).[5, 6]

Although preoperative imaging studies such as CT and MRI readily identify tumors, they are unable to precisely depict solid tumor margins, infiltrating tumor cells, peritumoral edema, and normal brain tissue adjacent to tumor.[7, 8] CT with contrast enhancement defines the gross bulk of a malignant tumor, but it is less reliable in characterizing the volume of low-grade gliomas that often are non–contrast-enhancing[9, 10]; on CT scans, these tumors appear as hypodense lesions with poorly defined margins,[5] which often cannot be differentiated from edema. Specimens based on CT stereotactic techniques suggest that atypical (tumor) cells may be found beyond regions of low density. MRI studies usually reveal a larger tumor size than does CT, particularly on T2-weighted images.[8] However, MRI, despite being perhaps the most sensitive method for preoperative imaging of a tumor,[11] may not delineate the exact tumor border. Hence, intraoperative detection of tumor margins is paramount for achieving optimal removal of the neoplastic tissue.

Today, the surgeon can utilize any of several adjuvant techniques that provide additional information during surgery and thereby allow for more extensive surgery with maximal accuracy and minimal morbidity. This chapter addresses techniques and developments that offer intraoperative access to the tumors and differentiation of the interface between tumor and normal brain: namely, cortical mapping, ultrasound technology, stereotactic or three-dimensional (3-D) technology, frozen section and smear preparation techniques, laser spectroscopy, and various fluorescence techniques.

CORTICAL MAPPING

Intraoperative brain mapping techniques are especially efficacious when the tumor is located in discrete brain areas. They utilize one of two stimulation procedures, direct cortical stimulation or somatosensory evoked potentials (SSEPs). Their use in neuro-oncology has allowed physicians to maximize the extent of tumor resection and seizure control; they have also been found to minimize operative morbidity. Although both systems are effective, SSEPs are considered by many authors to produce better results.

Direct Cortical Stimulation

The motor cortex was first identified by Fritsch and Hitzig in 1870.[12] Four years later, Bartholow[13] demonstrated the electrical excitability of the human motor cortex; ten years afterward, Sir Victor Horsley identified the motor cortex during standard craniotomies using faradic stimulation and local anesthesia.[14] A landmark study by Penfield and Boldrey[15] showed that electrical stimulation of the cortical surface evoked responses in patients undergoing resection of epileptogenic tissue. Their achievements in 126 patients provided the foundation for practical intraoperative localization of the sensory motor cortex, a necessary procedure for minimizing sensory or motor deficits when the area of intended resection lies in or adjacent to the sensorimotor region. Since that time, improved methods of eliciting movement by applying electrical stimulation to the cortex have been developed. As recently as 1991, a report on 270 patients with intrinsic tumors of the brain and spinal cord noted that direct stimulation methods allowed for greater resection of the tumor and the infiltrated brain adjacent to the tumor nidus, improved seizure control, and less permanent operative morbidity. These authors noted that the advantages of direct stimulation include providing the surgeon with the means to map descending motor pathways during the actual tumor resection.[16]

Somatosensory Evoked Potentials

Mapping of sensory and motor responses elicited by cortical stimulation has two distinct disadvantages: (1) movements may accompany stimulation of the sensory cortex and thereby yield ambiguous identification of the precentral and postcentral gyri, and (2) the necessity of using local rather than general anesthesia is difficult for both the patient and the surgical team, and may be hazardous in the case of certain mass lesions. Because it avoids the problem of ambiguous feedback and is compatible with general anesthesia, the method using SSEPs is considered by some surgeons to be superior to that using cortical stimulation.

In 1987, King and Schell[17] reported their results using cortical sensory potentials under general anesthesia. Both median nerve stimulation and direct cortical stimulation of the motor cortex were performed in 35 consecutive patients who had a mass lesion located in the middle half of the cerebral hemisphere. In five of the 35 patients, the sensory-evoked responses were also monitored during selected portions of the operative procedures. None of the patients who was free of neurologic deficit preoperatively demonstrated neurologic deficits in the immediate postoperative period, and most patients with preoperative neurologic deficits showed improvement in the immediate postoperative period.

In 1988, Wood and co-workers[18] compared results obtained in two groups of patients: the first group consisted of 18 patients who were operated on under local anesthesia, and in whom the sensorimotor cortex was independently localized by electrical stimulation mapping; the second group consisted of 27 patients who were operated on under general anesthesia without electrical stimulation mapping, but in whom SSEPs were recorded. The findings demonstrated that the spatial relationships between SSEPs and the anatomy of the postcentral gyrus, precentral gyrus, and central sulcus provide an accurate and reliable basis for hand area localization that is equally effective, regardless of whether local or general anesthesia is used.

Subsequently, Ebeling and colleagues[19] reported on 50 patients with lesions located in or adjacent to the motor strip; the lesions were microsurgically removed with the use of intraoperative electrophysiologic mapping of the sensorimotor cortex. Using cortical stimulation and/or recording of SSEPs, the authors found that, depending on the patient's preoperative neurologic status, surprisingly good results were obtained. In the 42% who had motor paresis preoperatively, some postoperative recovery (30%) was possible; in patients with no or mild paresis preoperatively, good outcomes with no new deficits or recovery of a preexisting deficit were achieved; for some patients with severe or complete motor paralysis preoperatively, improvement in the motor paresis was also achieved. A few patients with lesions located within the motor area experienced full recovery, a result consistent with those of other reports.[17, 20] They also noted that in addition to achieving low morbidities, the technique enables the surgeon to make intraoperative adjustments in the surgical strategy. By locating the motor strip, which can be achieved only by intraoperative mapping of the precentral and postcentral gyri, the surgeon can identify the sensorimotor region; not only can the motor strip and the pyramidal tract thereby be preserved, but also a more complete resection of the lesion can be achieved.[21–23] Witzmann and associates[24] also noted the latter advantage when continuous monitoring of SSEPs was used during supratentorial tumor removal.

Our own experience has involved the use of intraoperative cortical mapping on 81 patients with primary or metastatic paracentral tumors who underwent craniotomy under general anesthesia. Cortical mapping was used just prior to tumor excision; stimulation of the contralateral median nerve elicited cortical responses that displayed as waveforms $P_{20}N_{30}$ and $N_{20}P_{30}$, which denote motor and sensory cortices, respectively. Mapping showed that 49 lesions (60%) were just anterior to the motor strip, 15 (19%) were just posterior to the sensory strip, and 13 (16%) were in the sensorimotor cortex. Based on postoperative MRI scans, 52 lesions (64%) were totally resected, 21 (26%) were subtotally resected, and 8 (10%) were partially resected. Despite the critical locations of these tumors, the postoperative neurologic outcomes revealed improvement from the preoperative baselines in 23 patients (28%), no change in 50 patients (62%), and deterioration in only 8 patients (10%). Patients with metastatic disease had better results than did those with primary lesions. A positive correlation was found between the extent of parenchymal pathology and the distortion of the cortical tracings.

Cortical mapping does have some drawbacks, however. For instance, it allows localization of only the central area, and even if an impairment to the cortical surface is avoided, motor deficits can occur if the efferent nerve fibers from the motor cortex are injured deep in the white matter during surgical intervention.[25] Nevertheless, as our results indicate, by identifying a safe route as well as allowing maximal resection of the tumor, cortical mapping is a valuable adjunct to surgery on paracentral lesions.

ULTRASOUND TECHNOLOGY

The use of intraoperative ultrasound (IOUS) imaging has been shown to offer significant benefits during neurosurgery[26–28] especially in its ability to provide the surgeon with immediate feedback and to yield images that aid in both the diagnosis and the maximal resection of the tumor.[29–32] For instance, noncystic tumors are readily identified as hyperechoic, and autopsy studies of gliomas using sonographic characterization show a close relationship between neoplastic tissue and echogenic regions.[28]

Procedure

Intracranial ultrasound imaging is usually performed using a real-time sector scanner. This is a self-contained portable unit with a 9 inch television monitor, on which the image that is produced by the transducer is viewed in real time. The transducer can be of different shapes and frequencies (3, 5, 7.5, or 10 MHz). Deep-seated lesions are usually scanned by low-frequency transducers. However, small lesions near the surface are better seen with high-frequency transducers (7.5 MHz). The ultrasound transducer is usually placed in a sterile rubber glove that is kept in place with a sterile rubber band. The cable that connects the transducer to the imaging unit is covered with a sterile plastic drape.

After bone removal, the transducer head may then be placed either on the dura or directly on the exposed brain surface that is moistened with saline solution. Investigation is preferentially performed with the dura closed in order not to exert pressure on the underlying cortex. Moreover, if the bone opening must be extended, the procedure is better and more safely performed while the dura is still closed. However, scanning through the exposed brain surface gives better images in some cases, especially if the dura is thickened or partially calcified.

It has been our custom to scan the entire area of the bone opening in an organized systematic fashion in two perpendicular planes to confirm the presence, size, and location of a lesion. Gentle scanning over the brain surface is then performed in order to locate the shortest and safest route to the tumor. During tumor removal, IOUS is used frequently to evaluate the progress and to detect any residual tumor in cases in which complete excision is the aim. After excision has been completed, the cavity is filled with saline and IOUS is used, preferably with the dura closed, to determine the extent of resection and to detect the presence of any developing hematoma.

Various Uses

LOCALIZATION

The principal use of IOUS imaging is for *localization*. Low-grade, as well as high-grade, gliomas are readily identified by IOUS scanning and are typically echogenic relative to the surrounding brain[28, 33–36] (Fig. 30–1). Autopsy studies of gliomas have shown that this echogenicity is related to both tumor cell density and extracellular constituents.[28] Ultrasound is particularly useful for imaging small subcortical lesions as well as deep-seated ones. The ability of the ultrasound to localize such lesions helps in developing better intraoperative strategies. Tumors located in subcortical areas or in the depth of brain parenchyma can be reached by shorter routes across normal tissue. This is especially helpful in cases in which the lesions are located in or near eloquent areas of the brain. Moreover, after the exact location of a tumor has been defined, opening of the dura can be designed in a better way and restricted to smaller flaps.

DEFINITION OF BORDERS

IOUS is gaining much interest in *defining the borders* of tumors. The appearance of low-grade gliomas may be very similar to that of normal brain during surgery, and they can be extremely difficult to localize and define. The appearance and consistency of high-grade gliomas are usually different from those of normal tissue at the time of surgery, but the actual borders of these tumors cannot be absolutely ascertained. Recent treatment results have shown that both survival and the quality of life for glioma patients depend

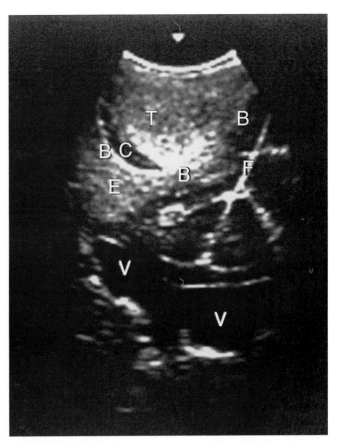

Figure 30–1 Intraoperative ultrasound image of juvenile pilocystic astrocytoma (T) showing the cyst (C), tumor margins (B), falx (F), edema (E), and anterior horns of the lateral ventricles (V).

on the extent of tumor excision, with better prognosis when maximum surgical resection is possible.[1]

IOUS has become an especially valuable adjuvant because it delineates both gliomas and their transition toward normal tissue, regardless of their CT or MRI patterns;[27, 28, 37] it can also differentiate edema from solid tumor and normal brain (which also cannot be achieved with either CT or MRI scans[38, 39]). Sonographically, peritumoral edema either is not visible or, if visible, is less echogenic than the tumor; therefore, it does not interfere with tumor delineation[26, 27, 36] (see Fig. 30–1). LeRoux and co-workers[33] demonstrated in a study that IOUS provided improved intraoperative delineation of solid tumor borders, 73% of which showed sparse atypical cells but no solid tumor on histologic evaluation. Although these studies have shown that IOUS enhances identification of infiltrating tumor cells beyond the tumor margins as indicated by MRI T1 images, and it proffers a means of detecting areas of tumor extension beyond margins of blood-brain barrier breakdown, the user should be cautioned to recognize a potential pitfall: namely, that the nonedematous changes in the peritumoral brain that almost always occur after surgery or irradiation may cause some difficulty in identifying the actual tumor margins.

CHARACTERIZATION

Ultrasound imaging is also used for tumor *characterization*, and studies have indicated that it is more accurate than

CT in differentiating between viable tumor, necrosis, and cysts.[27, 28, 35] Our experience with IOUS reveals the same observation and extends it to apply to MRI as well. Cysts are always imaged as being low in echogenicity on IOUS. In contrast, necrotic areas are imaged as isoechogenic or even hyperechogenic (though less so than the solid tumor).[40] This differentiation by IOUS is especially important if the tumor is located in a deep portion of the brain (and subtotal resection is therefore anticipated) or if the tumor is cystic and can be aspirated with minimal disruption of the overlying brain parenchyma. Enzmann and associates[36] described low-grade gliomas as more homogeneous and less hyperechogenic than high-grade gliomas. However, more recent studies suggest that histopathologic differentiation of gliomas with IOUS seems unlikely.[28, 41]

GUIDANCE

IOUS imaging is also used for *guidance* in tumor biopsy.[28, 41] By determining the location, depth, characteristics, and margins of the tumor, common types of biopsy needles can be passed into the brain within the plane of the ultrasound image toward the tumor. Guidance by real-time IOUS provides reliable knowledge of the position of the needle tip with respect to the tumor and allows multiple biopsies to be taken from different areas of the tumor for more accurate histopathologic diagnoses.

DETECTION OF RESIDUAL TUMOR

Finally, IOUS is helpful in *detecting residual tumor* toward the end of the operation, after complete resection has been attempted (Fig. 30–2). Residual masses that might exist after the course of tumor resection can be evaluated with IOUS, and a decision can be made as to whether or not further resection is appropriate.[29, 31, 32]

Complications

The ultrasound imaging unit requires the assistance of the operating room staff. Although handling the transducer and keeping track of the plane of the image in a three-dimensional orientation is not difficult, it does require some degree of expertise with the technique and an awareness of its potential complications. As with most techniques, certain pitfalls and technical problems accompany the advantages of IOUS. For instance, confluence of cortical sulci may appear as tumors and may be confused with a true mass lesion (Fig. 30–3). This problem can be avoided by intraoperative comparison of the location of this false lesion, called a sulcar pseudomass,[42] with that of the true mass seen on preoperative CT or MRI scans. Scanning the entire area within the bone flap in a systematic fashion helps to ensure that the true lesion is imaged properly.

A pitfall often encountered in patients who have undergone *previous* surgery and have received radiation therapy is that the echogenicity of peritumoral edema may be similar to that of the tumor, with the result that the tumor margin is indistinct (Fig. 30–4); hence, the surgeon may make an excision that is wider than is necessary. Again, the experienced interpreter can usually avoid this problem by carefully inspecting the images in different planes during surgery to distinguish between tumor and edema.

Another pitfall that accompanies using IOUS is mistaking for residual tumor the hyperechogenic rim that appears on IOUS images after complete excision (Fig. 30–5). This is called *acoustic enhancement*[43] and is related to the penetration of the sound through two different media (i.e., tumor tissue before vs. saline-filled cavity after excision). Finally, a small hematoma in the surgical bed cavity may be confused with residual tumor, particularly when hemostatic agents

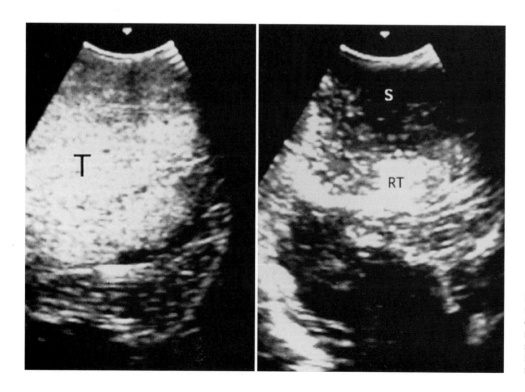

Figure 30–2 *Left,* Intraoperative ultrasound image of purkinjioma (T) of right cerebellar hemisphere before resection. *Right,* Intraoperative ultrasound image of the same tumor during resection, showing residual tumor (RT).

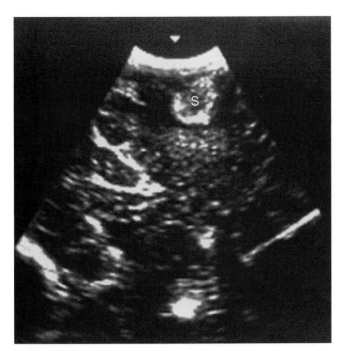

Figure 30–3 Intraoperative ultrasound image demonstrating a sulcar pseudomass (S), which may be confused with a tumor.

such as Oxycel or Surgicel are left in the tumor bed (Fig. 30–6).

In addition to these pitfalls, technical problems can occur during IOUS usage. Thick or calcified dura impedes the degree of sound that penetrates the tissue and interferes with the production of a well-defined tumor image. When this situation occurs, scanning over the brain surface produces much better images. Superficial lesions are better imaged

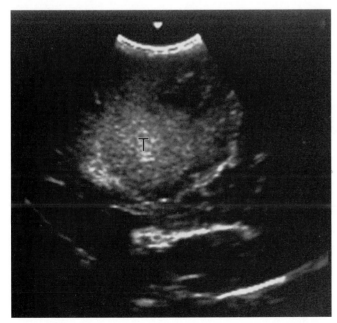

Figure 30–4 Intraoperative ultrasound image of recurrent glioblastoma multiforme (T) showing the ill-defined tumor margins in a patient who had received radiation after the first operation.

with a saline standoff.[44] Bone edges at the site of the craniotomy may interfere with image production, especially in cases in which the craniotomy is inadequately placed and the tumor is superficially located. Finally, air inside the surgical bed cavity produces *dirty shadowing*[45] and precludes the ability of IOUS to detect any residual tumor or to assess the extent of tumor resection. Thus, it is important to continue irrigating the surgical bed with saline during scanning and to position the patient such that the y-axis of the tumor is perpendicular to the floor, so that water will not escape from the surgical bed cavity.

Efficacy

We conducted a prospective study of 30 glioma patients to evaluate the efficacy of IOUS in localizing the tumors, defining the margins, and assessing the extent of resection. Localization was defined as either (1) localized (location of tumor was well-visualized by IOUS) or (2) ill-localized (location of the tumor is not well-visualized by IOUS). Evaluation of the margins was considered to be well defined when the margins of the tumor as seen by IOUS could be clearly visualized and separated from surrounding edema and brain tissue; moderately defined when the margins of the tumor could be visualized by IOUS but could not be clearly separated from surrounding tissue in certain areas; and poorly defined when the margins of the tumor could neither be visualized nor separated from surrounding tissue. In assessing the extent of resection, a comparison was made between the postoperative MRI and the IOUS images taken at the end of the procedure. The extent of tumor resection was considered to be well defined when either no residual tumor was seen because of total excision or residual tumor was clearly seen and further excision was not advisable, or ill defined when the IOUS image did not allow a determination of whether the excision was complete.

Our results showed that in 16 of 30 glioma patients who had no previous therapy, tumors were well localized by IOUS; 13 of these tumors had very well-defined margins, and three had moderately defined margins. In no case was the margin ill defined. The extent of resection was well defined on IOUS in all 16 patients, as confirmed by measurements taken on postoperative MRI (eight patients had total and eight patients had subtotal resections). The remaining 14 glioma patients had previous surgery and radiation therapy; eight of these had recurrent tumors and six had radiation-induced changes. All eight recurrent tumors were well localized by IOUS; two tumors had well-defined margins and six had moderately defined margins. The extent of resection was well defined in the remaining six patients and ill defined by IOUS in two patients. The former was also confirmed by postoperative MRI (three had total and three had subtotal resections). In the six patients whose pathologic findings showed mainly radiation effect, the lesions were well localized in three; however, the margins and the extent of resection were ill defined in all six patients (Table 30–1).

From this study, it is apparent that IOUS not only is helpful in localizing and defining the margins of gliomas, but also is accurate in determining the extent of resection as confirmed by postoperative MRI. This assessment, however,

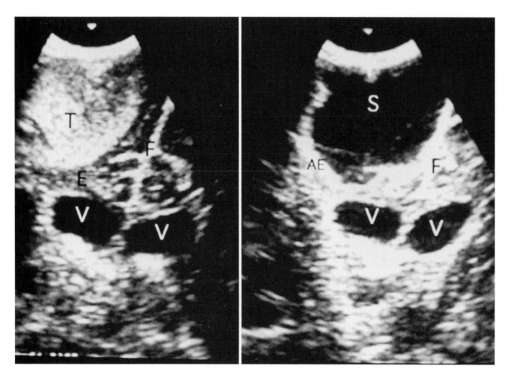

Figure 30–5 *Left*, Pre-resection intraoperative ultrasound image of recurrent anaplastic astrocytoma (T) of the left frontal lobe showing edema (E), falx (F), and anterior horns of the lateral ventricles (V). *Right*, Post-resection intraoperative ultrasound image showing saline (S), falx (F), and anterior horn of the lateral ventricles (V). The hyperechogenic rim (AE) represents "acoustic enhancement" and not tumor.

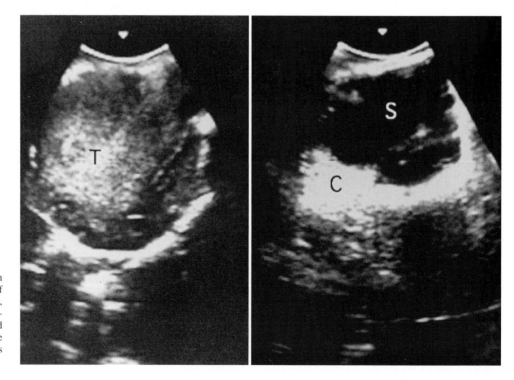

Figure 30–6 *Left*, Pre-resection intraoperative ultrasound image of glioblastoma multiforme (T). *Right*, Post-resection intraoperative ultrasound image showing saline-filled cavity (S) after tumor excision. The hyperechogenic area (C) represents blood clot and not residual tumor.

TABLE 30–1
EFFICACY OF INTRAOPERATIVE ULTRASOUND IN SURGERY

Uses	Patients With No Previous Therapy (N = 16)	Patients With Previous Surgery and/or Radiation (N = 8)	Patients With Radiation-Induced Tumors (N = 6)
Localization			
Well-localized	16	8	3
Ill-localized	—	—	3
Margins			
Well-defined	13	2	—
Moderately defined	3	6	—
Ill-defined	—	—	6
Extent of resection			
Well-defined	16	6	—
Ill-defined	—	2	6
Resection			
Total	8	3	—
Subtotal	8	5	—

does not apply to cases in which the lesion represents radiation effect. IOUS appears to be a promising tool for the achievement of maximal surgical resection of gliomas.

STEREOTACTIC OR THREE-DIMENSIONAL (3-D) TECHNOLOGY

Three-dimensional (3-D) localization of tumors promises to be a highly useful adjunct to surgery. One instrument, a frameless 3-D stereotactic guidance tool, also called a *viewing wand*, is a fully computerized, frameless, CT-stereotactic system that guides the surgeon toward the target by continuously and rapidly locating the operating site. These systems display the patient's preoperative CT or MRI data such that they are correlated with the operating field during surgery.

Procedure

The system has a freely mobile and articulated mechanical arm attached to a computer that contains the patient's preoperative image data. The arm, which can be introduced into the operating field as needed, obtains the 3-D coordinates of the operating point. Specially designed hardware and software enable the computer to interactively display the patient's CT or MRI data as a reconstructed 3-D model or in a tri-planar, reformatted image mode. As the surgeon moves the probe with the arm to the location of interest, the computer displays a model of the probe in correct relation to the 3-D model or tri-planar reformatted display of the patient's anatomy. By first using the mechanical arm to touch a series of landmarks on the patient and then marking the corresponding points on the 3-D model, the surgeon can use the computer to "lock" the patient and model images together. At any time during the operation, the surgeon can place the probe on a structure and, by viewing the screen, determine its location in relation to surrounding structures and the trajectory of the approach (Fig. 30–7).

Efficacy

In one study of 48 patients, the wand was sufficiently accurate in all cases to place a 1.5- or 2-inch trephine over the tumor, and in the 16 cases in which this was correlated with the head-frame system, no significant discrepancies (<3 mm) between the two were found.[46] The viewing wand is especially useful for skull base surgery, which involves an extremely complicated anatomic region in which tumors transcend the normal boundaries of surgical disciplines. When tumors involve the skull base, they result in gross distortion of the anatomic structures.

We have recently assessed the role of 3-D CT/MR imaging in preoperative surgical planning for skull base tumors in several patients. In all patients, the 3-D surgical planning and intraoperative use of the surgical wand facilitated the navigation to and resection of these difficult neoplasms. Furthermore, the viewing wand has been particularly helpful in the resection of multiple brain metastases.

The device promises to shorten the overall time of surgery and anesthesia and to allow for more rapid identification of structures and localization of the tumor.

FROZEN SECTION AND SMEAR PREPARATION TECHNIQUES

Among brain tumors, the gliomas are probably the most susceptible to biopsy sampling bias. In addition to the well-known morphologic variability and attendant implications for tumor grading based on limited tissue samples, current investigation continues to document regional heterogeneity of gliomas with respect to various cellular and molecular features.[47–50] Nonetheless, much useful information can be gained through the intraoperative histologic evaluation of glioma biopsy samples with regard to diagnosis, grading, and relative involvement of surgical margins.

Intraoperative Diagnosis of Gliomas

TISSUE HANDLING

An imperative for maximizing the information that can be obtained from a surgical specimen is its appropriate handling

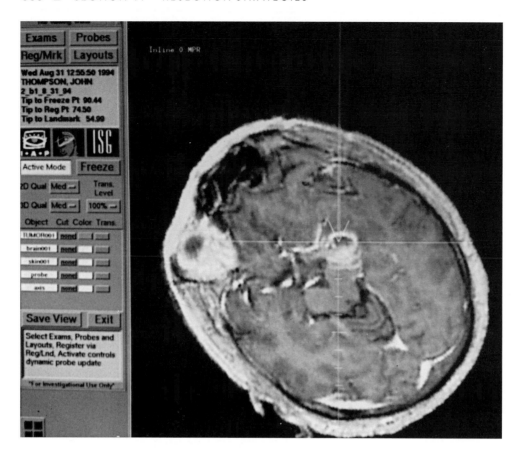

Figure 30–7 Intraoperative MRI guidance using a frameless stereotactic system. The *arrow* points to the location of the tip of the probe during the operative exposure and indicates that the surgeon has already entered the ring-enhancing lesion.

at the time of receipt in the frozen section laboratory. The four principal procedures for which tissue is allocated at the time of frozen section are the following: (1) smear (squash), imprint (touch), or scrape preparations; (2) frozen section; (3) glutaraldehyde fixation for ultrastructural examination (optimal electron microscopy requires prompt fixation of small fragments of tissue in glutaraldehyde as soon as possible after surgical excision; the glutaraldehyde-fixed, plastic-embedded tissue is subsequently placed "on hold" pending examination of permanent sections); and (4) formalin fixation for permanent sections (and subsequent immunostains, if needed). We routinely divide the tissue received at the time of frozen section to provide for all four procedures on every biopsy, including stereotactic needle biopsy specimens. For smear preparations and electron microscopy, only very small (about 1 mm³) fragments of tissue are needed, and, although most surgical cases do not require ultrastructural evaluation for diagnosis, it is prudent to anticipate this possiblity. Although it is technically possible to reprocess tissue for electron microscopy from paraffin blocks, such material is often nondiagnostic and is generally of far inferior quality to tissue that is promptly and appropriately fixed at the time of frozen section. Tissue remaining in blocks cut for frozen section is banked in an ultra–low temperature freezer, where it remains available for special studies that require fresh frozen tissue as needed.

SMEAR (SQUASH) PREPARATIONS

Whereas imprints ("touch") preparations) are useful for neoplasms that tend to shed cells profusely, such as pituitary adenomas, smear preparations are preferable for biopsy specimens of firmer consistency, and they work very well for most gliomas. Scrape preparations, whereby a scalpel blade is drawn across the tissue specimen to collect cellular constituents that are subsequently smeared across a glass slide, is generally required for only the firmest specimens, such as highly desmoplastic tumors.

For smear preparations, a minute fragment (approximately 1 mm³) of tissue is crushed and drawn out into a thin layer between two glass slides in a fashion similar to that used for preparing peripheral blood smears. The slides are then immediately immersed in 95% alcohol (to minimize air-drying artifact) and stained with hematoxylin-eosin. The smear preparation provides a high degree of morphologic detail, particularly with respect to nuclear architecture, that is far superior to that obtained with frozen sections. Although the smear preparation may serve as the sole basis for intraoperative diagnosis,[51–53] we view it as complementary to the frozen section, supplementing rather than supplanting the information provided by cryostat sections.

FROZEN SECTIONS

Cryostat sections complement smear preparations by providing information about tissue architectural features, such as intrinsic tumor cell arrangements (e.g., rosettes, palisading), the relationship of neoplastic cells to the vasculature (e.g., perivascular pseudorosettes), and the interaction between tumor cells and indigenous cellular constituents (e.g., secondary Scherer structures). Particularly helpful in this regard is information gained regarding the nature of the interface between the neoplasm and the surrounding neuropil (specifically, whether the growth is diffusely infiltrative or expansive with discrete "pushing" margins). With very few exceptions, infiltrative neoplasms are either gliomas or lymphomas, whereas discrete boundaries are indicative of metastatic or non-glial (e.g., meningeal) disease.

Features of Specific Gliomas

ASTROCYTOMA

Smear preparations of astrocytomas characteristically show atypical cells with prominent eosinophilic cytoplasm that ranges from the extreme linear fibrillarity of the pilocytic astrocytomas to the large, rounded masses seen in gemistocytic astrocytomas (Fig. 30–8). Clues regarding the grade may be found in the degree of nuclear pleomorphism seen, the presence of necrosis, or the presence of mitotic figures that occasionally are observed in smear preparations of malignant astrocytomas. With respect to nuclear pleomorphism, a strong caveat must be registered regarding juvenile pilocytic astrocytomas (JPAs), which are well known for often showing prominent striking degenerative nuclear atypia (in addition to vascular proliferation and contrast

enhancement on neuroimaging studies) that is otherwise associated with higher-grade neoplasms. In this regard, the Rosenthal fibers characteristic of JPAs frequently may be seen on smear preparations and are often even more striking on frozen sections than on permanent sections.

OLIGODENDROGLIOMA

On smear preparations, oligodendrogliomas exhibit characteristic uniformly rounded nuclei with delicate chromatin surrounded by a very scant to absent rim of cytoplasm that lacks the cytoplasmic processes seen with astrocytomas (Fig. 30–9A). The degree of uniformity is generally striking and is much greater than that observed with most astrocytomas. One caveat in this regard is that central neurocytomas also exhibit exquisitely uniform, rounded nuclei, and until the unmasking of their neuronal nature by electron microscopy and immunohistochemistry, they were routinely misdiagnosed as "intraventricular oligodendrogliomas." An awareness of the distinctive clinicopathologic features of these tumors is essential for avoiding potential misidentification at the time of frozen section.[54]

The nuclear uniformity of oligodendrogliomas is best appreciated on smear preparations; the artifact produced by frozen sectioning usually introduces considerable angularity,

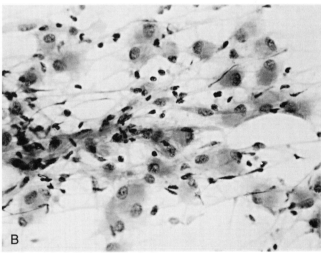

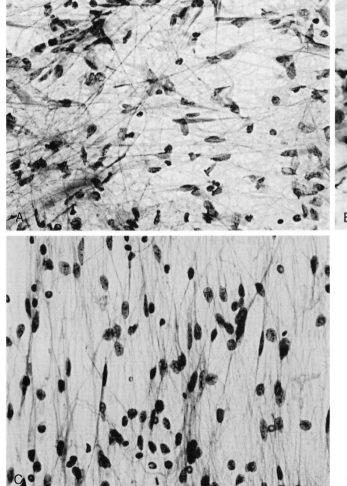

Figure 30–8 Astrocytoma. Smear preparations show the characteristic eosinophilic cytoplasm and fibrillarity common to all astrocytic neoplasms. The spectrum of cytoplasmic morphology is illustrated by typical smear preparations from an anaplastic astrocytoma *(A)*, a gemistocytic astrocytoma *(B)*, and a pilocytic astrocytoma *(C)*. Though varying in amount and architecture, the cytoplasmic fibrillarity seen on smear preparations of astrocytomas contrasts sharply with the nearly "naked nuclei" appearance of oligodendroglioma smear preparations (see Fig. 30–11).

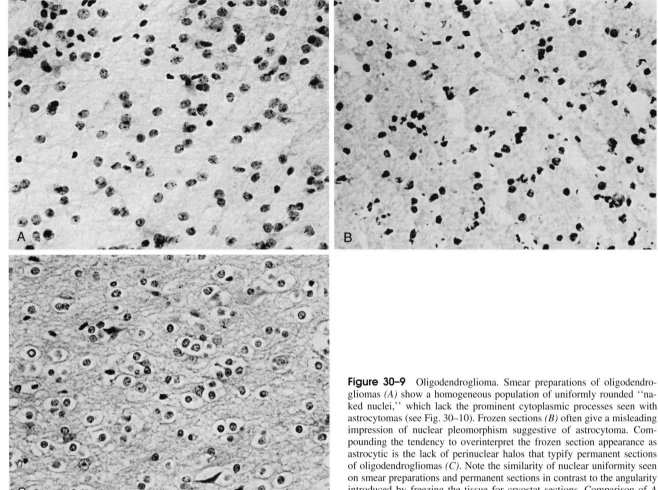

Figure 30–9 Oligodendroglioma. Smear preparations of oligodendrogliomas *(A)* show a homogeneous population of uniformly rounded "naked nuclei," which lack the prominent cytoplasmic processes seen with astrocytomas (see Fig. 30–10). Frozen sections *(B)* often give a misleading impression of nuclear pleomorphism suggestive of astrocytoma. Compounding the tendency to overinterpret the frozen section appearance as astrocytic is the lack of perinuclear halos that typify permanent sections of oligodendrogliomas *(C)*. Note the similarity of nuclear uniformity seen on smear preparations and permanent sections in contrast to the angularity introduced by freezing the tissue for cryostat sections. Comparison of *A* and *B* provides a graphic example of the invaluable additional data.

giving a misleading impression of nuclear pleomorphism that might be interpreted as being astrocytic in appearance (see Fig. 30–9*B*). When these are seen in sections of the cerebral cortex, a common error is to overinterpret such a frozen section artifact as an "infiltrating astrocytoma." The more appropriate diagnosis would be "infiltrating glioma," with a more specific subclassification after analysis of permanent sections. Compounding the tendency to overlook the possibility of an oligodendroglioma in frozen sections is the lack of typical perinuclear halos ("fried egg" appearance) in frozen tissue. Perinuclear halos result from hydropic swelling of oligodendrocyte cytoplasm and are very useful artifacts of delayed fixation that are observed in routinely processed formalin-fixed tissue (see Fig. 30–9*C*) but not in tissue that is rapidly frozen for cryostat sections.

Additional features that may be observed in frozen sections of oligodendrogliomas are cortical invasion with perineuronal and perivascular satellitosis; microcalcifications; and prominent, delicately branching ("chicken wire") blood vessels. Although these features are typical of oligodendrogliomas, they may be absent in many cases. Therefore, any of the typical features described for oligodendrogliomas on squash preparations and frozen sections should serve to alert the surgical pathologist to the possibility of an oligodendro-

glioma or of an oligodendroglial component of a mixed glioma, but they should not be regarded as pathognomonic. In the presence of such features, a frozen section diagnosis of "infiltrating glioma" is appropriate, with a more specific diagnosis deferred to analysis of permanent sections.

MIXED GLIOMA (OLIGOASTROCYTOMA)

These rare neoplasms, which remain the subject of some dispute, exhibit the unequivocal presence of both oligodendroglial and astrocytic components and provide another reason for exercising caution in the interpretation of frozen sections of glial neoplasms.

EPENDYMOMA

Smear preparations of ependymomas often show a tendency of the tumor cells to cluster tightly about vessels (Fig. 30–10*A*). At higher power, nuclei appear round to oval and generally exhibit delicate, uniformly distributed chromatin, with some cells displaying a distinct nucleolus (see Fig. 30–10*B*). The most helpful feature on frozen section is the presence of perivascular eosinophilic anuclear zones (often termed *perivascular pseudorosettes* or *gliovascular rosettes*)

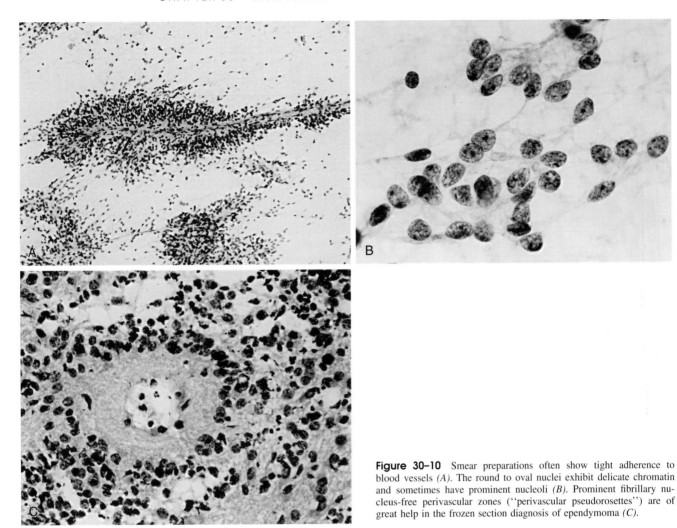

Figure 30–10 Smear preparations often show tight adherence to blood vessels *(A)*. The round to oval nuclei exhibit delicate chromatin and sometimes have prominent nucleoli *(B)*. Prominent fibrillary nucleus-free perivascular zones ("perivascular pseudorosettes") are of great help in the frozen section diagnosis of ependymoma *(C)*.

(see Fig. 30–10*C*). Perivascular pseudorosettes are much more frequently encountered than are "true" ependymal rosettes, which consist of clusters of tumor cells surrounding a central lumen.

PLEOMORPHIC XANTHOASTROCYTOMA VS. GIANT CELL GLIOBLASTOMA

In the large majority of cases, the presence of large, bizarre giant cells and/or multinucleated cells in a squash preparation (Fig. 30–11) is associated with a high-grade glioma. However, one exception warrants comment: the pleomorphic xanthoastrocytoma. As the name implies, the most salient morphologic feature of this low-grade astrocytic neoplasm is striking cellular pleomorphism. The key to avoiding the diagnostic pitfall of overgrading a pleomorphic xanthoastrocytoma as a high-grade glioma at the time of frozen section is an awareness of the entity and its characteristic clinicopathologic features. The clinical setting is especially important in eliciting a high index of suspicion. In particular, a superficial tumor of the cerebral cortex manifesting as a cyst with a mural nodule on neuroimaging studies in conjunction with its occurrence in an adolescent or young adult should immediately suggest to the pathologist

a differential diagnosis that contains, in addition to high-grade cystic glioma, three low-grade neoplasms: pleomorphic xanthoastrocytoma, juvenile pilocytic astrocytoma, and ganglion cell tumor. The importance of communication between pathologist and surgeon with regard to the patient's clinical history, neuroimaging studies, and intraoperative neurosurgical impression cannot be overstressed.

Assessment of Surgical Margins

The difficulty in surgical margin evaluation on gliomas stems from their infiltrative pattern of growth. A gradient of tumor cell density exists from the densest part of the tumor to uninvolved neuropil. Tissue biopsies obtained from brain that is otherwise visually and texturally normal in gross appearance often contains sufficient atypical infiltrating tumor cells to permit a confident microscopic diagnosis of "infiltrating glioma" (Fig. 30–12). Obviously, the more distal the tissue is located from an unequivocal infiltrating tumor edge, the more difficult confident diagnosis becomes. The currently available histologic techniques employing hematoxylin-eosin–stained cryostat sections precludes definitive identification of single infiltrating cells that lack nuclear

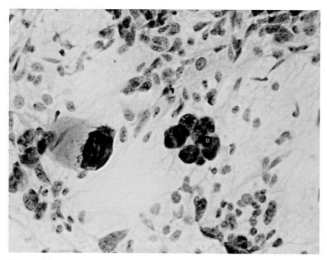

Figure 30–11 Giant cells. The presence of giant cells and marked nuclear pleomorphism is most often associated with high-grade glioma, but may also be seen on smear preparations of the far more rarely encountered pleomorphic xanthoastrocytoma. A high index of suspicion based on a thorough knowledge of the clinicopathologic features of the latter entity mitigates the likelihood misdiagnosis at the time of frozen section. It should also be noted that juvenile pilocytic astrocytomas may also exhibit focal hyperchromatic, pleomorphic nuclei, which, together with vascular proliferation, are a common cause of overgrading of these tumors.

atypia. Nevertheless, frozen section evaluation is useful for determining the presence of microscopic frank disease and, thereby, for facilitating optimal resection. Future development of more specific tumor cell markers combined with rapid detection methods may provide further enhancement of the intraoperative histologic evaluation of gliomas.

DYES AND FLUORESCENCE TECHNIQUES

Dyes

Studies have been instigated to determine the efficacy of dyes, namely indocyanine green (ICG), for intraoperative demarcation of tumor margins. ICG is a water-soluble, dark emerald-green tricarbocyanine dye that contains no more than 5.0% sodium iodide as a contaminant and is reconstituted with sterile water.[57] It has a molecular weight of 744, is almost completely bound to plasma proteins after an intravenous injection, and is excreted unchanged into the bile. Because it undergoes no significant systemic metabolism and does not enter the enterohepatic circulation, it is rapidly cleared after a single pass through the liver following first-order kinetics.[56]

In 1993, Hansen and colleagues,[57] noting some inherent difficulties associated with the aforementioned techniques, reported using an intracerebral rat glioma model to investigate the ability of ICG to stain and demarcate brain tumor margins. ICG injected intravenously into tumor-bearing rats specifically stained the tumor and its margins when administered in doses of 60 to 120 mg/kg; staining was not seen or was variable at doses of 30 mg/kg or less or 30 to 60 mg/kg, respectively. At the higher doses (60 to 120 mg/kg), the

staining intensity, a blue-green color within the tumor mass that was seen with standard ambient lighting conditions, persisted for at least 1 hour. Resection of the blue-green tumor tissue resulted either in margins that were free of tumor or in a very thin rim of neoplastic infiltration (<1 mm). Although the 60- to 120-mg/kg doses required to optimally stain the intracranial tumors in the rat models are well above the median lethal dose (LD_{50}) and are much higher than the 10 mg/kg doses given human patients for liver function or cardiac output determination,[58, 59] the authors noted that (1) the brain tumor model does not adequately simulate the degree and type of vascularity seen in human malignant gliomas, and (2) much lower doses of ICG (<10 mg/kg) would be required in humans with malignant gliomas to achieve a comparable staining effect to that demonstrated in the rat. The dose required to achieve the same efficacy in human brain tumors is currently being determined by a clinical investigation at the University of Washington.[57]

More recently, Haglund and colleagues[60] reported their experience using a new technique, a charge-coupled device camera and enhanced optical imaging, on 22 rat gliomas to determine the efficacy of using ICG to distinguish normal and edematous brain from tumor tissue. In all 22 animals, the peak optical change in the tumor was greater than in the ipsilateral brain around the tumor and the contralateral normal hemisphere. They also reported that the clearance of the dye was significantly delayed in the tumor as compared with the brain around the tumor and the normal brain. Following attempts at complete microscopic resection, the enhanced optical imaging of the tumor margins and the histologic samples demonstrated a specificity of 93% and a sensitivity of 89.5%.

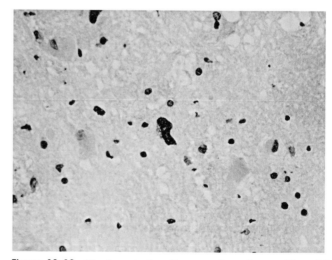

Figure 30–12 Margin evaluation. Frozen sections often provide useful information concerning the degree of involvement of surgical margins because the sensitivity of microscopic examination generally exceeds that of other intraoperative methods of tumor detection. Due to the presence of inconspicuous infiltrating tumor cells that are not detectable by routine hematoxylin-eosin staining of frozen sections, margins can never be proclaimed unequivocally negative. However, the identification of moderate to low densities of infiltrating pleomorphic tumor cells is possible and may facilitate surgical resection.

Fluorescence Techniques

Another attempt to develop a technique for discriminating tumors from normal surrounding tissue involves using laser-induced fluorescence of tissue.[61–63] Tissue fluorescence arises from the superposition of the fluorescence of a number of molecules present in the tissue, with the observed fluorescence spectrum, depending on the following three factors: (1) the absorption and scattering of the excitation light, (2) the emission of fluorescence by the tissue, and (3) the reabsorption and scattering of the emitted light. Studies have shown that fluorescence of human tissue can provide information about the presence of very small amounts of biologic chromophores,[64, 65] and preliminary reports have indicated that the differences in the presence and concentration of biologic chromophores in normal and neoplastic human colon can be measured using fluorescence spectroscopy, which forms the basis of a diagnostic test for colonic neoplasia.[66–68]

Photoradiation Therapy

Photoradiation therapy (PRT), a term for the use of hematoporphyrin and its activation by light, has also been used to delineate malignant tumors in humans. A hematoporphyrin derivative (HpD) prepared by acetylating the parent compound can be given intravenously, is concentrated well in neoplasms, fluoresces red when activated by blue light, and can produce a substantial cytotoxic reaction when activated by light of adequate intensity and proper wavelength.[69] Because HpD clears more rapidly from normal tissue than from tumor, it acts as a tumor-localizing dye.

Used previously to distinguish various tumors, such as those in the lung, bladder, or colon, from normal tissue,[70–72] HpD promises to be an effective means of differentiating neoplasms from normal brain as well. It is excluded by the blood-brain barrier in most animals and in man while being readily absorbed by brain tumor tissue; it reaches peak concentrations within 4 hours and maintains high concentrations for as long as 4 days.[73]

More recently, numerous second-generation photosensitizers, among which are the phthalocyanines, have been studied to determine their efficacy in photoradiation therapy and in tumor margin differentiation. The phthalocyanines have the advantage of having a significantly greater quantum yield than HpD (0.52 vs. <0.1) and a fluorescence peak at 680 nm.[74] Furthermore, they clear the skin rapidly so they avoid the effects of skin phototoxicity associated with HpD, which is the major adverse effect of HpD used for tumor therapy.[69] In 1992, Poon and associates[74] published the first reported use of laser-induced fluorescence to increase the accuracy with which rat brain tumor margins could be defined during resection and to delineate in vivo tumor margins during resection of a tumor model. Using chloro-aluminum phthalocyanine tetrasulfonate ($ClAlPcS_4$) injected intravenously 24 hours before tumor resection, they found contrast ratios of up to 40:1 for glioma-normal brain fluorescence signals. Spatially resolved spectra were acquired in approximately 5 seconds using a fiberoptic probe. The study demonstrates that the efficacy of an intraoperative laser-induced fluorescence system is such that it is capable of detecting tumor margins that could not be identified with the operating microscope.

NAD(P)H, Flavin, and Porphyrin

In preliminary studies at the University of Texas M.D. Anderson Cancer Center, we obtained solid brain tumor and normal brain specimens of different pathologic states from patients undergoing craniotomy for brain tumors. Fluorescence excitation/emission matrix (EEM) is a matrix of fluorescence emission intensities, the columns and rows of which indicate emission wavelengths and excitation wavelengths, respectively. A matrix can be constructed from a series of emission spectra collected for a range of excitation wavelengths (in this case a fluorescence contour map in which the y-axis indicates excitation wavelengths, the x-axis indicates emission wavelengths, and the contour lines connect points of equal fluorescence emission intensity).

Using an autofluorescence measurement system, we recorded fluorescence EEM for samples from four normal brain specimens, six anaplastic astrocytomas, two glioblastomas multiforme (GBM), two meningiomas, three low-grade astrocytomas, five metastatic tumors, one craniopharyngioma, and one olfactory neuroblastoma. The nicotinamide-adenine dinucleotide phosphate (NAD(P)H) fluorescence intensities of normal in vitro brain tissues were greater than those measured in metastatic tumors, low- and high-grade astrocytomas, and medulloblastoma. Flavin fluorescence was greater in normal in vitro brain tissues than in those measured in metastatic tumors and in low- and high-grade astrocytomas, but less than that in medulloblastoma. Porphyrin fluorescence was much greater in normal brain than in metastatic tumors and low-grade astrocytoma, but nearly equal to or slightly less than that of medulloblastomas and high-grade astrocytomas. No remarkable differences in the ratios of NAD(P)H to flavin between in vitro human normal brain and tumors were noted, except for anaplastic astrocytomas and GBM cell aggregates prepared with trypsin, a finding that is similar to those reported elsewhere. These results are subject to considerably more study before definitive conclusions can be drawn, but they suggest that a fluorescence spectroscopic diagnostic system capable of distinguishing brain neoplasms from normal brain tissue is viable, and, if so, portends an immensely practical means of intraoperative identification of infiltrating brain tumors.

CONCLUSION

Preoperative imaging studies such as CT and MRI readily identify tumors, but they are unable to precisely depict the margins of a solid tumor, infiltrating tumor cells, peritumoral edema, and normal brain adjacent to tumor. Specimens based on CT stereotactic techniques suggest that atypical (tumor) cells may be found beyond regions of low density. MRI studies usually reveal a larger tumor size than CT does, particularly on T2-weighted images; but despite being perhaps the most sensitive method for preoperative imaging of a tumor, MRI may not delineate the exact tumor border.

Hence, intraoperative detection of tumor margins is paramount for achieving optimal removal of the neoplastic tissue.

One intraoperative method, brain mapping, is especially efficacious when the tumor is located in discrete brain areas. Two stimulation procedures, direct cortical stimulation and SSEPs, have allowed surgeons to maximize the extent of tumor resection and seizure control; they have also been found to minimize operative morbidity.

IOUS imaging has been shown to offer significant benefits during resection of gliomas, especially in its ability to provide the surgeon with immediate feedback and to yield images that aid in both the diagnosis and the maximal resection of the tumor. From our own experience, IOUS is not only helpful in localizing and defining the margins of gliomas, but it is also accurate in determining the extent of resection as confirmed by postoperative MRI.

Three-dimensional localization of tumors also promises to be a highly useful adjunct to the surgical treatment of gliomas. These fully computerized, frameless, stereotatic systems guide the surgeon toward the target by continuously and rapidly locating the operating site. They display the patient's preoperative CT or MRI data such that they are correlated with the operating field during surgery.

Among brain tumors, gliomas are probably the most susceptible to biopsy sampling bias, and current investigation continues to document regional heterogeneity of gliomas with respect to various cellular and molecular features. Intraoperative histologic evaluation of glioma biopsy samples with regard to diagnosis, grading, and relative involvement of surgical margins provides much useful information. For smear preparations and electron microscopy, only very small (about 1 mm^3) fragments of tissue are needed, and, although most surgical cases do not require ultrastructural evaluation for diagnosis, it is prudent to anticipate this possibility. Smear (squash) preparations are preferred for biopsy specimens of firmer consistency and work very well for most gliomas. Scrape preparation is generally required for only the firmest specimens, such as highly desmoplastic tumors. Cryostat sections complement smear preparations by providing information about tissue architectural features, the relationship of neoplastic cells to the vasculature, and the interaction between tumor cells and indigenous cellular constituents.

Fluorescence of human tissue can provide information about the presence of very small amounts of biologic chromophores. Preliminary reports indicate that the differences in the presence and concentration of biologic chromophores in normal and neoplastic human colon can be measured using fluorescence spectroscopy, which forms the basis of a diagnostic test for colonic neoplasia. Photoradiation therapy, a term for the use of hematoporphyrin and its activation by light, has also been used to delineate malignant tumors in humans. An HpD prepared by acetylating the parent compound can be given intravenously; it clears more rapidly from normal tissue than from tumor, thus acting as a tumor-localizing dye. Studies have been instigated to determine the efficacy of ICG (a water-soluble, dark emerald green tricarbocyanine dye that contains no more than 5.0% sodium iodide as a contaminant and is reconstituted with sterile water) for intraoperative demarcation of tumor margins. It may prove to be beneficial in surgical treatment of gliomas.

Each of these techniques proffers a broader realm of surgical expertise with lower mortality and morbidity rates in the treatment of gliomas. The surgeon must determine the most efficacious method as determined by the specific demands of the individual case; in addition to the preoperative advantages that the advent of imaging studies has provided, advanced means of performing more exact and even more effective treatment of gliomas are now available with these intraoperative techniques.

REFERENCES

1. Ammirati M, Vick N, Liao YL: Effect of the extent of surgical resection on survival and quality of life in patients with supratentorial glioblastomas and anaplastic astrocytomas. Neurosurgery 1987; 21:201.
2. Medical Research Council Brain Tumor Working Party: Prognostic factors for high grade malignant glioma: Development of a prognostic index. J Neurooncol 1990; 9:47.
3. Laws ER Jr, Taylor WF, Bergsrath E, et al: The neurosurgical management of low-grade astrocytoma. Clin Neurosurg 1975; 33:575.
4. Laws ER Jr, Taylor WF, Clifton MB, et al: The neurosurgical management of low-grade astrocytoma of the cerebral hemispheres. J Neurosurg 1984; 61:655.
5. Kelly PJ, Kall BA, Goerss S, et al: Computer-assisted stereotactic laser resection of intra-axial brain neoplasms. J Neurosurg 1986; 64:427.
6. Lunsford LD, Martinez AJ, Lathchaw RE: Magnetic resonance imaging does not define tumor boundaries. Acta Radiol 1986; (suppl 369):254.
7. Johnson P, Hart S, Drayer B: Human cerebral gliomas: Correlation of post mortem MR imaging and neuropathologic findings. Radiology 1989; 170:211.
8. Kelly PJ, Daumas-Duport C, Kispert DB, et al: Imaging-based stereotactic serial biopsies in untreated glial neoplasms. J Neurosurg 1987; 66:865.
9. Lewander R, Bergström M, Bothius J, et al: Stereotactic computer tomography in biopsy of gliomas. Acta Radiol 1978; 19:867.
10. Lilja A, Bergstrom K, Spannare, et al: Reliability of computer tomography in assessing histopathologic features of malignant supratentorial gliomas. J Comput Assist Tomogr 1981; 5:625.
11. Mosskin M, Erickson K, Hindmarsh T, et al: Positron emission tomography compared with magnetic resonance imaging and computed tomography in supratentorial gliomas using multiple stereotactic biopsies as reference. Acta Radiol 1989; 30:225.
12. Fritsch G, Hitzig E: Ueber die elektrische Erregbarkeit des Grosshirns. Arch Anat Physiol Wissensch Med 1870; 37:300.
13. Bartholow R: Experimental investigations into the functions of the human brain. Am J Med Sci 1874; 84:305–313.
14. Northfield DWC: Sir Victor Horsley: His contributions to neurological surgery. Surg Neurol 1973; 1:131.
15. Penfield W, Boldrey E: Somatic motor and sensory representation in the cerebral cortex of man as studied by electrical stimulation. Brain 1937; 60:389.
16. Berger MS, Ojemann GA: Intraoperative brain mapping techniques in neuro-oncology. Stereotact Funct Neurosurg 1992; 58:153.
17. King RB, Schell GR: Cortical localization and monitoring during cerebral operations. J Neurosurg 1987; 67:210.
18. Wood CC, Spencer DD, Allison T, et al: Localization of human sensorimotor cortex during surgery by cortical surface recording of somatosensory evoked potentials. J Neurosurg 1988; 68:99.
19. Ebeling U, Schmid UD, Ying H, et al: Safe surgery of lesions near the motor cortex using intra-operative mapping techniques: A report on 50 patients. Acta Neurochir 1992; 119:23.
20. Gregorie E, Goldring S: Localization of function in the excision of lesions from the sensorimotor region. J Neurosurg 1984; 61:1047.
21. Berger MS, Kincaid J, Ojemann GA, et al: Brain mapping techniques to maximize resection, safety and seizure control in children with brain tumours. Neurosurgery 1989; 25:786.
22. Berger MS, Ojemann GY, Lettich E: Neurophysiological monitoring during astrocytoma surgery. Neurosurg Clin North Am 1990; 1:65.
23. Rostomily RC, Berger MS, Ojemann GA, et al: Postoperative deficits and functional recovery following removals of tumors involving the

dominant hemisphere supplementary motor area. J Neurosurg 1991; 75:62.

24. Witzmann A, Beran H, Böhm-Jurkovic H, et al: The prognostic value of somatosensory evoked potential monitoring and tumor data in supratentorial tumor removal. J Clin Monit 1990; 6:75.

25. Taniguchi M, Cedzich C, Schramm J: Modification of cortical stimulation for motor-evoked potentials under general anesthesia: Technical description. Neurosurgery 1993; 2:219.

26. Gooding GAW, Boggan JE, Weinstein DR: Characterization of intracranial neoplasms by CT and intraoperative sonography. AJNR 1984; 5:517.

27. LeRoux PD, Berger MS, Ojemann GA, et al: Correlation of intraoperative ultrasound tumor volumes and margins with preoperative computerized tomography scans. J Neurosurg 1989; 71:691.

28. McGahan JP, Ellis WG, Budenz RW, et al: Brain gliomas: Sonographic characterization. Radiology 1986; 159:485.

29. Chandler WF, Knake JE: Intraoperative use of ultrasound and neurosurgery. *In* Weiss MH (ed): Clinical Neurosurgical Proceedings of the Congress of Neurological Surgeons. Baltimore, Williams & Wilkins, 1983, p 550.

30. Gooding GAW, Edwards MSB, Rabskin AE, et al: Intraoperative real-time ultrasound in the localization of intracranial neoplasms. Radiology 1989; 146:459.

31. Quencer RM, Montalvo BM: Intraoperative cranial sonography. Neuroradiol 1986; 28:598.

32. Rubin JM, Dohrmann GJ: Efficacy of intraoperative US for evaluating intracranial masses. Radiology 1985; 157:509.

33. LeRoux PD, Winter TC, Berger MS, et al: A comparison between preoperative magnetic resource and intraoperative ultrasound tumor volumes and margins. J Clin Ultrasound 1994; 22:29.

34. LeRoux PD, Berger MS, Wang K, et al: Low grade gliomas: Comparison of intraoperative ultrasound characteristics with preoperative imaging studies. J Neurooncol 1992; 13:189.

35. Chandler WF, Knake JE, McGillicuddy JE, et al: Intraoperative use of real-time ultrasonography in neurosurgery. J Neurosurg 1982; 57:157.

36. Enzmann DR, Wheat R, Marshall WH, et al: Tumors of the central nervous system studied by computed tomography and ultrasound. Radiology 1985; 154:393.

37. Knake JE, Chandler WF, Gabrielson TO, et al: Intraoperative sonographic delineation of low grade brain neoplasms defined poorly by computed tomography. Radiology 1984; 151:735.

38. Brant-Zawadski M, Badami JP, Mills CM, et al: Primary intracranial tumor imaging: A comparison of magnetic resonance and CT. Radiology 1984; 150:435.

39. Hasselink JR, Press GA: MR contrast enhancement of intracranial lesions with Gd-DPTA. Radiol Clin North Am 1988; 26:873.

40. Auer LM, van Velthoven V: Intraoperative ultrasound (US) imaging: Comparison of pathomorphological findings in US and CT. Acta Neurochir (Wien) 1990; 104:84.

41. Sutcliffe JC: The value of intraoperative ultrasound in neurosurgery. Br J Neurosurg 1991; 5:169.

42. Bowerman RA: Tangential sulcal echoes: Potential pitfall in the diagnosis of parenchymal lesions on cranial sonography. J Ultrasound Med 1987; 6:685–689.

43. Rubin JM, Carson PL: Physics and techniques. *In* Rubin JM, Chandler WF (eds): Ultrasound in Neurosurgery. New York, Raven, 1990.

44. Chandler WF: Use of ultrasound imaging during intracranial operations. *In* Rubin JM, Chandler WF (eds): Ultrasound in Neurosurgery. New York, Raven, 1990.

45. Sommer FG, Taylor KJW: Differentiation of acoustic shadowing due to calculi and gas collections. Radiology 1980; 135:399.

46. Barnett GH, Kormos DW, Steiner CP, et al: Use of a frameless, armless stereotactic wand for brain tumor localization with two-dimensional and three-dimensional neuroimaging. Neurosurgery 1993; 33:674.

47. Coons SW, Johnson PC: Regional heterogeneity in the DNA content of human gliomas. Cancer 1993; 72:3052.

48. Coons SW, Johnson PC: Regional heterogeneity in the proliferative activity of human gliomas as measured by the Ki-67 labeling index. J Neuropathol Exp Neurol 1993; 52:609.

49. Figge C, Reifenberger G, Vogeley KT, et al: Immunohistochemical demonstration of proliferating cell nuclear antigen in glioblastomas: pronounced heterogeneity and lack of prognostic significance. J Cancer Res Clin Oncol 1992; 118:289.

50. Onda K, Davis RL, Wilson CB, et al: Regional differences in bromodeoxyuridine uptake, expression of Ki-67 protein, and nucleolar organizer region counts in glioblastoma multiforme. Acta Neuropathol 1994; 87:586.

51. Folkerth RD: Smears and frozen sections in the intraoperative diagnosis of central nervous system lesions. Neurosurg Clin North Am 1994; 5:1.

52. Martinez AJ, Pollack I, Hall WA, et al: Touch preparations in the rapid intraoperative diagnosis of central nervous system lesions: A comparison with frozen sections and paraffin-embedded sections. Mod Pathol 1988; 1:378.

53. Reyes MG, Homsi MF, McDonald LW, et al: Imprints, smears, and frozen sections of brain tumors. Neurosurgery 1991; 29:575.

54. Hassoun J, Soylemezoglu F, Gambarelli D, et al: Central neurocytoma: A synopsis of clinical and histological features. Brain Pathol 1994; 3:297.

55. Deleted in proof.

56. Cherrick GR, Stein SW, Leevy CM: Indocyanine green: Observation of its physical properties, plasma decay, and hepatic extraction. J Clin Invest 1960; 39:592.

57. Hansen DA, Spence AM, Carski T, et al: Indocyanine green (ICG) staining and demarcation of tumor margins in a rat glioma model. Surg Neurol 1993; 40:451.

58. Hillis LD, Firth BG, Winniford MD: Comparison of thermodilution and indocyanine green dye in low cardiac output or left-sided regurgitation. Am J Cardiol 1986; 57:1201.

59. Paumgartner G: The handling of indocyanine green by the liver. Schweiz Med Wochenschr 1975; 105(suppl 17):1.

60. Haglund MM, Hochman DW, Spence AM, et al: Enhanced optical imaging of rat gliomas and tumor margins. Neurosurgery 1994; 35:930.

61. Alfano RR, Tang GC, Pradhan A, et al: Fluorescence spectra from cancerous and normal human breast and lung tissue. IEEE J Quantum Electron QE-23 1987; 23:1806.

62. Anderson PS, Kjellin E, Montan E, et al: Autofluorescence of various rodent tissues and human skin tumor samples. Lasers Med Sci 1987; 2:41.

63. Yuanlong Y, Yanming Y, Fuming L, et al: Characteristic autofluorescence for cancer diagnosis and its origin. Lasers Surg Med 1987; 7:528.

64. Campbell ID, Dwek R: Biological Spectroscopy. Menlo Park, Calif, Benjamin Cummins, 1984.

65. Richards-Kortum RR, Rava RP, Fitzmaurice M, et al: A one-layer model of laser-induced fluorescence for diagnosis of disease in human tissue: Application to atherosclerosis. IEEE Trans Biomed Eng 1989; 36:1222.

66. Cothren RM, Richards-Kortum RR, Sivak MV, et al: Gastrointestinal tissue diagnosis by laser induced fluorescence spectroscopy at endoscopy. Gastrointest Endosc 1990; 36:105.

67. Kapadia CR, Cutruzolla FW, O'Brian KM, et al: Laser-induced fluorescence spectroscopy of human colonic mucosa. Gastroenterology 1990; 99:150.

68. Richards-Kortum RR, Rava RP, Petras RE, et al: Spectroscopic diagnosis of colonic dysplasia. Photochem Photobiol 1991; 53:777.

69. Ransohoff J, Kelly P, Laws E: The role of intracranial surgery for the treatment of malignant gliomas. Semin Oncol 1986; 13:27.

70. Balchum OJ, Profio AE, Razum N: Ratioing fluorometer probe for localizing carcinoma in situ in bronchi of the lung. Photochem Photobiol 1987; 46:887.

71. Profio AE: Laser excited fluorescence of hematoporphyrin derivative for diagnosis of cancer. IEEE J Quantum Electron QE-20 1984; 12:1502.

72. Svanberg K, Kjellén E, Ankerst J, et al: Fluorescence studies of hematoporphyrin derivative in normal and malignant rat tissue. Cancer Res 1986; 46:3803.

73. Wharen RE Jr, Anderson RE, Laws ER Jr: Quantitation of hematoporphyrin derivative in human gliomas, experimental central nervous system tumors, and normal tissue. Neurosurgery 1983; 12:446.

74. Poon WS, Schomacker KT, Deutsch TF, et al: Laser-induced fluorescence: Experimental intraoperative delineation of tumor resection margins. J Neurosurg 1992; 76:679.

ROBERTO SPIEGELMANN

WILLIAM FRIEDMAN

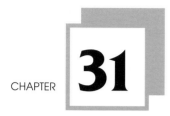

CHAPTER **31**

Closed Biopsy Techniques

With the exception of pilocytic astrocytomas in children, gliomas are, by and large, infiltrative tumors. In addition to the compact tumor mass, isolated tumor cells microscopically infiltrate the surrounding normal brain parenchyma to a variable distance. This characteristic renders gliomas usually incurable by surgery or by any treatment modality aimed at the recognizable tumor mass. Still, surgical intervention is central to the management of these tumors, having three cardinal goals:

1. Tissue diagnosis
2. Treatment of intracranial pressure
3. Cytoreduction to enhance results of other therapies

Tumor debulking to reduce intracranial pressure is certainly a definitive indication for surgery. Whether cytoreductive surgery improves outcome in high-grade gliomas is highly controversial.[1-3]

Tissue diagnosis in gliomas and other intra-axial tumors can be obtained by minimally invasive techniques, often with the advantages of more precise tissue sampling and much less surgical trauma than is possible with open procedures. These techniques can be used as well to reduce increased intracranial pressure produced by tumor cysts or obstructive hydrocephalus.

By shortening operative time, time to recovery, and surgically related complications, closed biopsy techniques can improve the short-term outcome of patients with gliomas.

The various techniques that may be comprised by this denomination are addressed in this chapter. Illustrative case examples from our own series are included.

DEFINITION AND SCOPE

Closed biopsy techniques include every method for tissue diagnosis of intracranial tumors that gains access to the brain through a twist drill or burr hole, uses a needle to harvest the tissue, and produces minimal disruption to intervening brain tissue.

All needle biopsy techniques rely on image guidance to reach the target. These techniques can be classified as follows:

■ Freehand biopsy, which is guided either by ultrasound or by computed tomography (CT). Image guidance is usually contemporaneous with the biopsy procedure. Infrequently, to biopsy superficial, large tumors, freehand biopsy may rely on a preexisting CT.

■ Stereotactic biopsy, which represents the gold standard for image-guided biopsy. Imaging may be provided by CT or magnetic resonance imaging (MRI). More recently, positron-emission tomography (PET) has been explored to increase diagnostic yield in gliomas.

■ Endoscopic biopsy, which is gaining momentum due to miniaturization of endoscopic probes and improved design of ancillary endoscopic instrumentation.

INDICATIONS

Broadly speaking, any intracranial space-occupying lesion that is not deemed appropriate for conventional resection, is amenable to closed biopsy techniques. Management of intracranial tumors without tissue diagnosis is now unacceptable. CT and MRI are clearly unreliable to establish a diagnosis of glioma: a diagnosis different than expected has been obtained by biopsy in 10% to 26% of cases in various series.[4-6] The following case is illustrative.

◻ CASE 1

A 41-year-old man presented with a short history of progressive right spastic hemiparesis. A few days before admission he complained of headaches and gradually became nauseated and confused. On admission, he was partially cooperative and disoriented. He had a marked right hemiparesis. The rest of the clinical examination was unremarkable. CT (Fig. 31–1) showed a hypodense mass lesion in the left thalamocapsular area with irregular, partial peripheral enhancement. Obstructive hydrocephalus was also present. The preoperative diagnosis was glioblastoma.

On stereotactic biopsy, thick, foul-smelling pus was aspirated from each of the hypodense areas. The patient re-

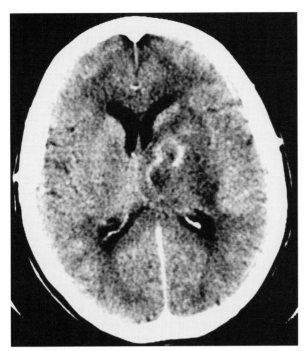

Figure 31-1 This lesion was assumed on clinical examination to be a high-grade glioma. Stereotactic biopsy disclosed an abscess, which was cured by drainage and antibiotics administration.

covered completely and was cured of his cerebral abscess following an antibiotic course of 3 weeks.

regular margins and intense homogeneous enhancement on CT should be further investigated with MRI to rule out the presence of flow void. When necessary, conventional angiography, CT-angiography, or MR-angiography should be performed to rule out this possibility.

Another relative contraindication to closed biopsy techniques are lesions with significant mass effect and midline shift.[7] Although biopsy can be tolerated in patients with these lesions, a small hemorrhage or even slight edema complicating the procedure could result in neurologic decompensation and herniation. The following case is illustrative.

□ CASE 2

A 55-year-old woman presented with gradual onset of hemiparesis. CT and MRI showed a large mass in the left deep centrum, involving the basal ganglia. Some midline shift was present (Fig. 31–2A). Open decompression was judged too risky. It was decided to proceed with stereotactic biopsy. Before surgery, the patient was markedly confused and apathetic, despite steroid treatment. Stereotactic biopsy was completed without operative complications. The tissue was compatible with the diagnosis of glioblastoma. Following the procedure, the patient remained obtunded. Control CT ruled out bleeding in the operative bed or increased midline shift (Fig. 31–2B). Nonetheless, the patient did not recover full consciousness; she died 2 months later.

CONTRAINDICATIONS

Primary vascular lesions are, obviously, an absolute contraindication for closed biopsy techniques. Any lesion with

STEREOTACTIC TECHNIQUES

Stereotaxy was introduced in clinical practice in the late 1940s. For many years the technique was used primarily for

Figure 31-2 *A,* Preoperative CT shows a heterogeneous lesion with substantial midline shift. *B,* Postbiopsy noncontrast CT ruled out bleeding or further edema in the lesion. The amount of midline shift was unchanged. Nonetheless, this patient became obtunded immediately after surgery and did not return to her preoperative status; she died 2 months later.

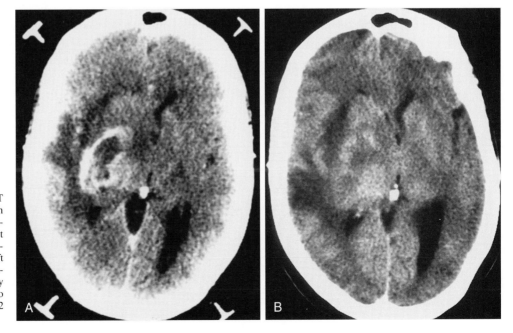

"functional" procedures, such as thalamotomy for control of movement disorders and mesencephalotomy for chronic pain.

With the advent of CT in the late 1970s, pathologic processes within the brain became directly visible in a highly accurate, scaled image format. CT gave impulse to the development of "morphologic" stereotaxy (i.e., the application of stereotaxy to the diagnosis and treatment of pathologic processes within the skull).

Biopsy of intracranial space-occupying lesions is currently the most frequent application of stereotaxy. This is a relatively simple procedure that can be easily mastered by neurosurgeons without specific dedication to the field. Stereotactic technique does not require dexterity. However, more than in any other area of neurosurgery, rigorous planning, careful anatomic evaluation, and attention to detail are mandatory for achievement of proper results.

Limitations of Stereotactic Biopsy

The accuracy of any commercially available stereotactic frame is within the 1-mm range. Therefore, small target size is not a limitation for stereotactic biopsy. Although virtually any intracranial lesion can be reached stereotactically for diagnostic purposes, the technique is best suited for sampling of intra-axial tumors. A stereotactic approach to lesions in the subarachnoid space (suprasellar area, pontocerebellar angle) is highly risky. It may require the blind transgression of a pial-arachnoidal surface that faces away from the skull entry point. In addition, tumor displacements produced by the needle may tear delicate blood vessels attached to the tumor surface. Both events can result in bleeding within the subarachnoid space, a complication that cannot be controlled with stereotactic instrumentation.

Stereotactic Imaging

CT is the standard imaging modality for stereotactic biopsy. Rarely, a tumor is found that cannot be adequately visualized by CT, which necessitates use of an alternative image modality, such as MRI. Even in this event, CT can still be used as the data base for stereotactic coordinates, with MRI used to fine tune the selection of the target (Fig. 31–3).

MRI is certainly more sensitive than CT in detecting some intrinsic brain tumors, and it better reveals their true extent. Nonetheless, the increased acquisition time and the reduced availability of MRI make it a second-line image modality for stereotactic localization. Stereotactic MRI requires the use of specially adapted stereotactic instrumentation constructed with non-ferromagnetic materials (e.g., plastics, carbon fiber, glass fibers, and certain metals). Spatial resolution of MRI is inferior to that of CT due to inhomogeneities in the magnetic field, which tend to increase with field strength and proximity to the magnet. Nonetheless, spatial inaccuracies are not significant enough to compromise targeting in biopsy procedures.

PET has been used as a method of increasing accuracy in biopsy target selection in gliomas.

PET with ^{18}F-labeled fluorodeoxyglucose (PET-FDG) is used to study the brain glucose metabolism. When performed in patients with brain tumors, it has been shown to improve the assessment of tumor heterogeneity and extension. Although PET images have poor anatomic definition, their integration in multimodality stereotactic planning might be helpful to define a biopsy target in the more metabolically active areas of the tumor.

Levivier and co-workers[8] have used the Zamorano-Dujovny (ZD) frame for PET and CT multimodality stereotactic data acquisition. Localization was done using Sturm localizers that were filled with FDG for PET. Stereotactic coordinates of highly metabolic areas seen on PET were measured and transferred to the corresponding CT images.

The technique may eventually become useful to help eliminate undergrading of gliomas by signaling the most highly metabolic area of a lesion. Better spatial resolution will further increase the potential of PET in stereotactic localization for biopsy.

Single-photon emission computed tomography (SPECT) using thallium 210, although it has not yet been used to direct stereotactic biopsy, may complement tumor biopsy in

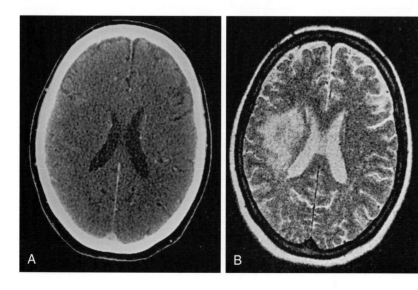

Figure 31–3 A 56-year-old woman presented with focal facial seizures. An abnormal MRI scan was followed up for 6 months; slow enlargement of the abnormal area was noted. An MRI-guided biopsy was eventually performed, which yielded a diagnosis of low-grade glioma. The lesion was barely discernible on stereotactic CT *(A)* but was easily visualized on T2-weighted stereotactic MRI *(B)*.

gliomas by establishing their metabolic activity, which has been shown to correlate well with tumor grade.[9, 10]

Local or General Anesthesia

Except for young children (those younger than 10 to 12 years), we recommend use of local anesthesia for any stereotactic procedure, including biopsy. Local anesthesia has several advantages:

- Continuous monitoring of patient's neurologic status and rapid detection of intraoperative and postoperative complications.

- Immediate recovery and return to activity, even in patients with increased intracranial pressure.

- Simplicity. When biopsy is performed with local anesthesia, the procedure starts at the patient's bedside with application of the stereotactic frame. CT is obtained immediately thereafter, and the patient is transferred to the operating room, where shaving, positioning, etc., are done with the patient's cooperation. When general anesthesia is used, it is usually required before the frame is applied, because the frame represents an impediment to regular intubation. Considerable extra time is then required for stereotactic CT and patient transfer to the operating room. Additional personnel are needed to care for the patient at all stages.

In our experience, even the most apprehensive, emotionally unstable patient can undergo the procedure with local anesthesia. Good preoperative rapport, step-by-step explanations, and continuous reassurance are key to the patient's cooperation. We refrain from use of intraoperative hypnotics or tranquilizers. In patients with increased intracranial pressure, these agents can induce a confusional state that results in loss of cooperation.

Instrumentation

STEREOTACTIC FRAME

Most stereotactic systems consist of two parts: *the coordinate frame* and *the aiming device*. The *frame* is a metallic platform that can be affixed to the skull so that no displacement can take place Fig. 31–4. This attachment is generally achieved with three or four screws that perforate the outer table of the vault. The stereotactic frame serves two purposes: (1) it embodies a cartesian coordinate system to which spatial calculations are referred and, (2) it represents a foundation to which aiming devices can be affixed and directed to the desired intracranial target, with minimal disruption of intervening tissue.[11]

Most currently available frames are mounted to the patient's skull with manually applied screws. This procedure can be completed in less than 5 minutes, and we perform it at bedside. Prepping or shaving is not required. We have not had a single case of screw-related infection in several hundred cases of frame application. Local anesthesia is applied in the scalp points selected for pin penetration in all adult patients. Small children usually require a short period of anesthesia for frame application.

The *aiming device* is a rigid system of precision moving parts that bears a probe holder. The moving parts can perform angular and/or linear translations to direct the probe to any intracranial target.

Several stereotactic frames are commercially available, and virtually all of them are highly accurate and mechanically reliable. Although the instruments of different manufacturers originally employed different geometric approaches to lesion targeting, most vendors currently offer frames that work on the the arc-center (arc-quadrant; arc-radius) principle: The probe is mounted on a semicircular arc. The arc can be moved in three linear dimensions (anteroposterior, lateral, and vertical) so that its center coincides with the intracranial target coordinates. A biopsy needle having a

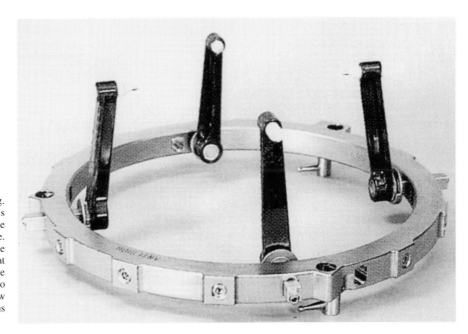

Figure 31–4 The BRW stereotactic base ring. The metallic ring, when attached to the patient's head, becomes a spatial reference frame for the exact localization of any intracranial structure. Manual screws are used for skull fixation. The screws are fastened through threaded holes at the ends of four carbon-fiber posts that produce very little artifact in CT. The posts connect to the metallic ring that usually is positioned below the skull. Most available stereotactic systems use the "base ring" paradigm.

length equal to the radius of the arc will always reach the target, regardless of its position along the arc or of the elevation of the arc above the horizontal plane (Fig. 31–5). This kind of frame allows for infinite trajectories to the target without modifying the arc settings or the probe depth, which provides the surgeon with great freedom to select a approach.

Focal-point frames are equally easy to use. They also work on the arc-radius principle, with one important distinction: The target is brought to the impact point by moving the patient's head toward the center of the fixed arc, instead of by bringing the impact point to the target.

IMAGE LOCALIZER

We have always used a gantry-independent CT localizer, originally designed for the BRW stereotactic system (Fig. 31–6) (Radionics, Burlington, Mass). The Kelly-Goerss localizer is of the same type. Although it requires the use of a small computer to calculate the target, it relieves the surgeon of the need to lock the stereotactic frame to the CT table; and, most important, it allows image acquisition with various CT gantry angulations without loss of accuracy. We have used this feature extensively to simplify both data acquisition and the biopsy procedure itself.

BIOPSY NEEDLE

Cup forceps, corkscrew needles, or side-cutting aspirating needles are available for collection of tissue samples (Fig. 31–7). In our experience with several hundred biopsies, we encountered only one intra-axial tumor that could not be successfully aspirated and sampled with the side-cutting needle (Nashold's or Sedan's needle). That tumor, an unusually firm pineal germinoma, required the use of a corkscrew needle for tissue collection. The side-cutting needle usually

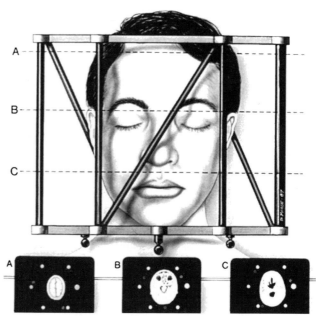

Figure 31–6 The BRW CT localizer is unique in that it allows target localization regardless of the CT gantry angulation in relation to the basal plane of the stereotactic ring. The localizer has three N-shaped arrays of carbon-fiber rods. They produce nine visible fiducial artifacts in any axial CT image. In each N, the distance between the vertical rods is fixed and known. The distance of the diagonal rod from the vertical rods varies in the vertical *[z]* plane (see insets *A–C*). This variability is used to calculate the distance between the base ring and each of the diagonal rods at any axial CT image. The *x* and *y* pixel coordinates of each rod are obtained with the cursor option at the CT screen and fed into a handheld computer. The existence of three N arrangements allows the determination of the height in three different points in space. Consequently, a plane is defined as it passes through the target. This eliminates the need for a fixed relationship between the stereotactic frame and the CT gantry. A tilt in any direction is automatically computed and included in the algorithm for probe trajectory and depth determination. (From Friedman WA, Spiegelmann R: The principles of stereotaxis. *In* Hoff J, Crockard A (eds): Neurosurgery: The Scientific Basis for Clinical Practice, ed 2. London, Blackwell, 1992, pp 956–974.)

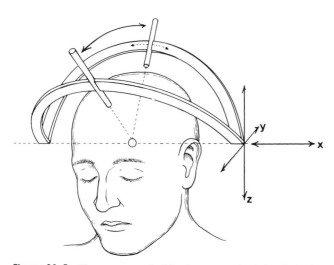

Figure 31–5 The arc-center principle: the stereotactic aiming device is a segment of arc that can be displaced in three orthogonal planes *(x, y,* and *z)* so that its center is brought to coincide with the target. A biopsy needle equal in length to the arc radius will hit the target regardless of its position along the arc or of the position of the arc above the horizontal plane *(arrows)*. (From Friedman WA, Spiegelmann R: The principles of stereotaxis. *In* Hoff J, Crockard A (eds): Neurosurgery: The Scientific Basis for Clinical Practice, ed 2. London, Blackwell, 1992, pp 956–974.)

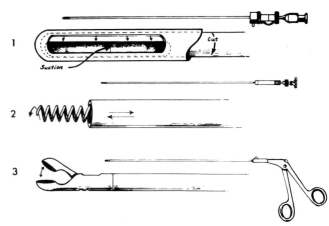

Figure 31–7 The Nashold needle *(1)* is well suited for soft tissue biopsy. Forceful aspiration applied with a syringe drives tissue into the 10-mm side port. A 180-degree rotation of the inner needle cuts the specimen and closes the port. With the spiral needle *(2)*, the spiral is advanced with a rotational movement to trap the target, and then the outer sleeve is advanced to cut and secure the tissue. The pistol grip bronchoscopy forceps *(3)* can be used on tissue of any consistency.

allows quick retrieval of a 1-cm cylinder of tissue with good preservation of histoarchitecture.

Sampling

Gliomas are heterogeneous tumors. Their biologic behavior corresponds well with the histologic characteristics of the tumor; therefore, definition of histologic features has paramount importance not only in diagnosis but also in establishing a prognosis in patients with gliomas. Classification schemes have varied over the years, since Kernohan first divided gliomas into four grades of ascending malignancy. Currently, at least four different classifications are accepted for gliomas.

We have adopted in our work the Ringertz-Burger classification, which corresponds extremely well with clinical behavior and outcome of gliomas. It divides these tumors into categories based on three degrees of malignancy (astrocytoma [grade I], anaplastic astrocytoma [grade II], and glioblastoma [grade III]), with pilocytic astrocytoma constituting a separate group. Grades I and II differ only quantitatively (amount of pleomorphism, mitoses, and vascular proliferation), which leaves some room for subjective incongruity between observers.

The St. Anne-Mayo classification is a four-tiered system that grades the tumor by the presence or absence of four elements (pleomorphism, mitoses, vascular proliferation, and necrosis), which makes it more objective. Grade 1 tumors have none of the elements, and grade 4 tumors have any three of them.[12]

Gliomas frequently have heterogeneous histologic patterns within a single tumor mass. The biologic behavior of the tumor corresponds well with the highest-grade component, regardless of its relative volume at the time of diagnosis. Ideally so, tissue diagnosis in gliomas has to be obtained from the area bearing the highest grade of tumor. One of the frequent arguments against stereotactic biopsy is that the small tissue samples obtained with a needle may lead to undergrading of heterogeneous tumors such as gliomas. In fact, stereotactic biopsy frequently proves to be more accurate than larger tissue samples obtained by conventional surgery (Fig. 31–8). In contrast to biopsy obtained during tumor resection, stereotactic tissue samples are retrieved from *predetermined* areas of the tumor, where imaging studies have indicated that diagnostic tissue is likely to be found.

Biopsy undergrading of glioma can be greatly obviated by obtaining serial biopsy specimens along the needle tract. Obviously, the risk of bleeding increases with the number of samples retrieved in a given case. The surgeon has to decide on the best compromise between adequate sampling and reasonable risk.

High-grade gliomas frequently appear on CT as cystic lesions with a central hypodense area, a bordering irregular ring of enhancement, and a peripheral, ill-defined zone of hypodensity that may contain tumor cells and/or edematous normal tissue (Fig. 31–9). In these lesions, we usually target the central hypodense area first, and then withdraw the needle in 1-cm increments (the length of the side window) along the trajectory, so that the different areas of the tumors can be sampled sequentially. It is well known that the area of contrast enhancement usually contains viable, diagnostic

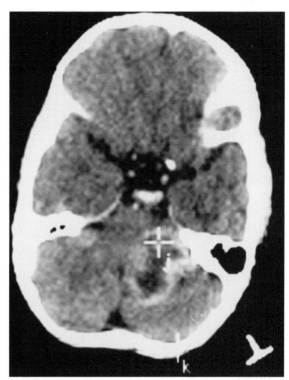

Figure 31–8 The transcerebellar, transpeduncular approach is a very safe technique for lateral brainstem lesions. In this 9-month-old infant, biopsy was compatible with high-grade glioma. Accordingly, resection was not recommended. The tumor was removed subtotally at another institution, where the pathologic diagnosis was pilocytic astrocytoma. The child died as a result of rapid tumor regrowth 2 months after surgery. (From Friedman WA, Spiegelmann R: Reoperative stereotactic neurosurgery and radiosurgery. *In* Little J, Awad I (eds): Reoperative Neurosurgery. Baltimore, Williams & Wilkins, 1992, pp 271–302.)

tissue, whereas the hypodense central areas are generally necrotic and are per se nondiagnostic. Nonetheless, necrotic tissue is also important for tumor grading when other areas are compatible with the diagnosis of glioma. In selected cases, the seemingly necrotic area may contain the greatest amount of diagnostic tissue.

HYPODENSE LESIONS

Low-grade gliomas, with the exception of pilocytic astrocytoma, are characteristically hypodense, ill-defined lesions. They also should be serially biopsied along a trajectory that courses through the center of the lesion. In this manner, not only is diagnostic tissue obtained, but tumor grading is more accurate. The real extent of the tumor can be assessed by careful sampling throughout and beyond the area of hypointensity seen on MRI.[13] This information is instrumental in the design of further therapeutic procedures.

CYSTIC LESIONS

Gliomas may present as primarily cystic lesions, oftentimes with an irregularly enhancing wall. Cysts require special techniques for their sampling. Puncture of the cyst with fluid aspiration immediately modifies the lesion geometry, which may invalidate preselected target coordinates. Edner[14] has recommended cyst puncture with a fine needle. After a few drops of fluid are collected, the needle is withdrawn until no further fluid exits, and a biopsy is taken at that point.

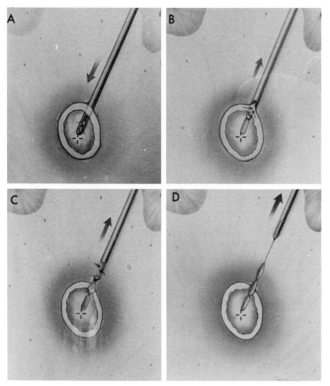

Figure 31–9 The biopsy probe should be aimed at the center of a ring-enhancing lesion (*A*). Although viable tumor is more likely to be retrieved from the ring area (*B*), necrotic tissue, which is usually present in the central hypodense region, helps in tumor grading. Biopsy samples from the peripheral hypodense-isodense areas (*C* and *D*) may define the actual tumor extension better than imaging studies. (From Friedman WA, Spiegelmann R: Reoperative stereotactic neurosurgery and radiosurgery. *In* Little J, Awad I (eds): Reoperative Neurosurgery. Baltimore, Williams & Wilkins, 1992, pp 271–302.)

We prefer to target the center of the cyst. Fluid is then gently aspirated until resistance is felt. This is due to the collapse of the cyst wall around the needle. Further aspiration sucks the cyst wall towards the needle window, allowing the retrieval of diagnostic tissue (Fig. 31–10). The cyst fluid can also be sent for cytologic analysis.

Selection of an Entry Point and Trajectory

If possible, the trajectory to the target should avoid blind crossing of ependymal or pial-arachnoidal surfaces, which substantially increases the risk of brain distortion (due to escape of cerebrospinal fluid [CSF]) and bleeding. Although small vessels tend to be displaced by an advancing blunt needle, the subependymal veins of the lateral ventricles are relatively fixed, which creates a high risk of injury followed by uncontrollable bleeding. As a rule, the surgeon selects the shortest possible track to the target through a non-eloquent brain area, with an entry point away from known vascular avenues (sylvian fissure, venous sinuses).

According to the lesion topography, certain trajectories are standardized.

FRONTAL LOBE AND ANTERIOR BASAL GANGLIA

Because these areas represent the largest volume of brain tissue, they are also the most frequently affected by mass lesions of all etiologies, including gliomas. A precoronal entry point on the side of the lesion, 2 to 3 cm from the midline, is a customary approach to gliomas in these regions. For the pericoronal area, we believe that a standard burr hole is safer than a drill hole, allowing for direct visualization of the cortex and coagulation of the pia before needle advancement. When the target is in the basal ganglia, a more lateralized burr hole avoids penetration of the frontal horn.

An alternative route to targets in these areas is the plane-of-target entry point in the forehead. This technique is advantageous because it allows the sampling of the tumor along a trajectory that can be exactly predetermined in a single axial CT slice (Fig. 31–11), without dedicated computer aids.

Both the target point (usually at the posterior border of the lesion) and the entry point in the forehead are selected in the same CT slice. The entry point is placed so that it creates a trajectory across the entire lesion, away from visible blood vessels. If a gantry-independent CT localizer is used for data acquisition, CT gantry angulation may be modified as needed to obtain the best trajectory. In any case,

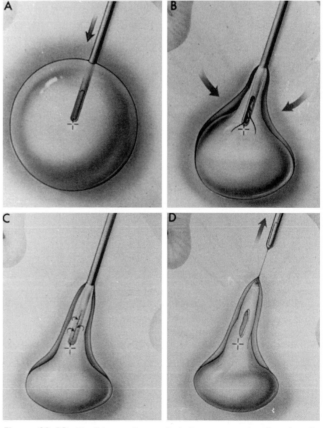

Figure 31–10 For biopsy of a cystic lesion, a target is selected at the center of the cyst (*A*). Fluid is gently aspirated, leading to collapse of the cyst wall onto the needle (*B*); sampling at this point (*C* and *D*) usually yields diagnostic tissue. (From Hood TW, Gebarski SS, McKeever PE, et al: Stereotaxic biopsy of intrinsic lesions of the brain stem. J Neurosurg 1986; 65:172–176.)

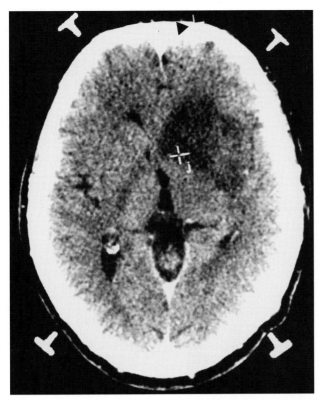

Figure 31–11 In this hypodense lesion, a forehead plane-of-target approach is a simple way of ensuring a needle path through the major diameter of the tumor, with the added safety of an image-determined needle corridor. The small stab wound in the forehead heals without leaving a noticeable scar (the *arrowhead* highlights the entry point).

the entry point is calculated as a second target. In an arc-centered stereotactic apparatus, the coordinates of the entry point serve to fix an arc and collar angulation. The procedure is best planned with a phantom.[15] In the absence of a phantom, the surgeon needs first to set the coordinates of the entry point, and with the arc already mounted on the patient's head, the entry point is marked on the patient's skin. The target coordinates are then dialed in the frame, and arc and collar angulations are fixed when the needle touches the skin mark as it advances toward the target.

A small stab wound is made in the skin and a thin drill (3 mm) is advanced through the bone along the prefixed trajectory. The normally adherent dura is usually pierced with the drill. The needle is then slowly advanced through the opening to the target. Following retrieval of serial samplings by stepped needle withdrawals, the skin wound is closed with a sterile self-adhesive paper strip.

The ability to retrieve serial biopsy specimens along a visible trajectory may result in more precise diagnosis. In addition, this plane-of-target technique, with an image-determined entry point, reduces the likelihood of significant bleeding caused by blind penetration of the cortex. Blind pial penetration of the non-eloquent frontal pole is relatively safe, becuase the pia is devoid of major vessels or bridging veins.

PERI-INSULAR REGION

Stereotactic surgery for lesions in this area is relatively risky because of neighboring middle cerebral branches. Pre-

operative coronal MRI scans and, if necessary, CT or MRI angiograms are sometimes of great help in delineating whether the lesion is mainly lateral or medial to the insula (Fig. 31–12). If it is medial, either a vertical trajectory through a pericoronal entry point or a plane-of-target forehead entry point is suitable.

For lesions lateral to the insula, a horizontal trajectory through a temporal entry point is safest. The use of a prefixed trajectory with a CT-determined entry point is recommended for the temporal approach. A formal burr hole with visualization of the dura and underlying cortex is desirable to avoid bleeding complications from middle meningeal vessels and middle cerebral branches (Fig. 31–13).

PINEAL REGION TUMORS

Pineal tumors represent 0.4% to 1.6% of intracranial tumors in the United States. The diversity of tumors affecting the pineal region is unmatched at any other intracranial location. Stereotactic biopsy is highly recommended, usually following the insertion of a ventriculoperitoneal shunt, because in most pineal region tumors the role of surgery is limited to diagnosis, whereas radiation represents the best treatment modality.[16] *Astrocytomas* comprise 25% of pineal region tumors in some series. As in other locations, they show varying degrees of malignancy.

The pineal area has anatomic characteristics that complicate the stereotactic approach:

1. The gland is completely contained within the quadrigeminal cistern, above the collicular plate.
2. Immediately above the gland is the tela choroidea of the third ventricle, which contains the medial posterior choroidal arteries and the internal cerebral veins, joined here by the veins of Rosenthal and the precerebellar vein that form the great vein of Galen.

Bleeding from these venous channels may be avoided by careful choice of the needle trajectory. MRI is mandatory to identify the relationship of the tumor to the veins. Most intrinsic tumors displace the veins upward and anteriorly. A paramedian, anterior frontal entry point usually successfully reaches the tumor lateral to the internal cerebral vein.

Because the target is usually small and is surrounded by CSF, the standard Nashold needle, with its 10-mm side window, may sometimes be unfit for these lesions: should a portion of the window remain in the subarachnoid space, aspiration of CSF will preclude the production of enough vacuum to suck tissue toward the needle. Instead, tenuous subarachnoid vessels can be aspirated and torn, producing subarachnoid bleeding. Thus, when gentle aspiration results in flow of CSF, the needle should be further introduced a few millimeters. If this does not solve the problem, a corkscrew needle may prove a better option for tissue retrieval.

PERIVENTRICULAR TARGETS

Periventricular lesions may present with partial obstructive hydrocephalus. Biopsy may lead to minimal hemorrhage or edema, which in turn can cause complete obstruction and rapid neurologic deterioration. When preoperative CT suggests impending hydrocephalus, we routinely place a ventriculostomy, stereotactically, through the same entry point used for the biopsy.

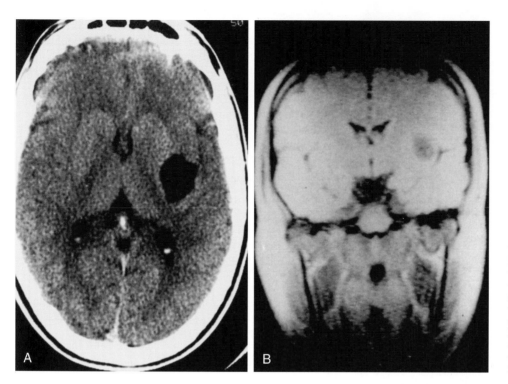

Figure 31–12 Targets in the perisylvian region have an increased risk for bleeding during stereotactic biopsy. Depending on the target position relative to the sylvian fissure, a needle trajectory is selected. Sometimes this may need multimodality imaging. In this case, axial CT *(A)* did not clearly define the location of this cyst. Coronal MRI *(B)* shows that the lesion is medial to the insular cortex. A transfrontal approach was consequently selected for this target.

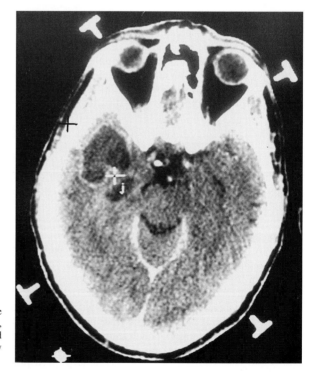

Figure 31–13 For temporal targets, a predetermined trajectory and entry point are particularly important to avoid bleeding complications. In the example shown here, a lateral entry point was selected. This approach requires a formal burr hole to avoid inadvertent piercing of middle meningeal vessels. Alternatively, an occipital entry point may be selected through the major axis of the temporal lobe.

□ **CASE 3**

A 36-year-old woman was admitted to the hospital with a short history of episodic headaches and nausea. CT and MRI disclosed mild hydrocephalus and an isodense/isointense mass in the posterior superior part of the third ventricle (Fig. 31–14*A*). A small calcification was apparent in the center of the lesion. MRI showed upward displacement of the internal cerebral veins. Stereotactic biopsy was carried out under local anesthesia, through a burr hole placed in the right frontal area, just behind the hairline. The center of the lesion was targeted. Likewise, a target was selected in the frontal horn of the right lateral ventricle (Fig. 31–14*B*). Following frozen section confirmation of the presence of tumor (a low-grade glioma) in the tissue samples, a ventriculostomy catheter was introduced stereotactically. The procedure was well tolerated. Ventriculostomy was removed 48 hours later, after ventricular pressure monitoring ruled out increased intracranial pressure. The patient has remained asymptomatic following treatment of the lesion by radiosurgery.

Biopsy should precede ventriculostomy. Failure to do so may result in displacement of intracranial structures following CSF drainage, invalidating preselected target coordinates.

BRAINSTEM

Surgery of intrinsic brainstem tumors has gained momentum in the last few years, due to the identification of a subset of tumors compatible with prolonged survival and amenable to substantial surgical resection.[17–20]

They are almost exclusively confined to the pediatric age group and include focal midbrain gliomas, cervicomedullary junction tumors, and dorsally exophytic transependymal brainstem gliomas.

Still, the majority of brainstem gliomas do not lend themselves to resection. Brainstem tumors in adults are relatively infrequent and are usually more aggressive. For all of these tumors, sound management requires tissue diagnosis, which is obtainable by stereotactic techniques with low morbidity (<5%).[21–23]

The approach to a brainstem target is dictated by its topography. Lesions close to the midline at any level down to the lower medulla can be reached through an entry point placed 2 to 3 cm from the midline, at the coronal suture or slightly posterior to it. The needle usually crosses the lateral ventricle and transits through the ventral brainstem. This trajectory has been used traditionally for many functional procedures (Fig. 31–15).

If the target within the brainstem is relatively lateral, an ipsilateral transfrontal approach may be obstructed by the tentorial edge. A contralateral approach, although feasible, has the potential risk of damaging the normal side of the brainstem. In this situation, the transcerebellar, transpeduncular approach is indicated.[24]

This approach is ideal in that it represents the shortest route to the target, crosses only one parenchymal surface, and transits relatively silent neural tissue. Nonetheless, it is limited to the areas that can be reached through the middle cerebellar peduncle, which represents the intra-axial safety bridge for the needle path. Targets in the upper midbrain or the lower medulla cannot be safely biopsied with this approach, because the needle must cross arachnoid space, which endangers important vessels and nerves.[25]

For the transcerebellar, transpeduncular approach, the patient is place in a prone (which requires general anesthesia), sitting (which has a minimal risk of inducing air emboli), or lateral decubitus position. We prefer the latter, because it does not require special monitoring and can be done with the patient under local anesthesia.[15] A plane-of-target planning

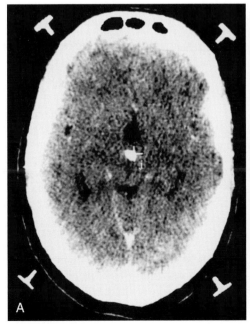

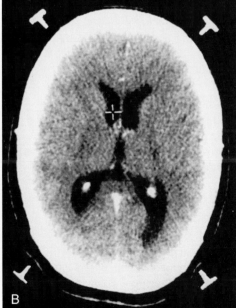

Figure 31–14 This third ventricle lesion has a high risk of producing obstructive hydrocephalus. Targets were selected for biopsy *(A)* and ventriculostomy *(B)*, to be approached through the same entry point.

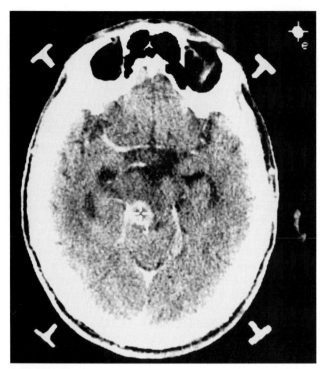

Figure 31–15 A probe introduced through an ipsilateral burr hole just behind the coronal suture easily cleared the tentorial notch in transit to this midbrain target. For a more peripheral target, a contralateral approach is acceptable in the rostral midbrain. In the pons, a transcerebellar, transpeduncular approach may be more suitable.

technique is mandatory to ensure a safe trajectory to the target (see Fig. 31–8).

The transcerebellar transpeduncular approach requires an extremely low mounting position for the stereotactic frame, which may prove difficult or impossible to achieve with a BRW or a Richter-Mundinger frame. Reverse mounting of the ZD or the Kelly-Goerss frame is recommended.

An alternative approach for targets in the brainstem was reported by Apuzzo and Sabshin, who used a parieto-occipital entry point.[26] In this approach, the tentorium is punctured with a trocar, and the posterior fossa target is reached through this transtentorial route. We have not found an indication for this technique.

CEREBELLAR TARGETS

Most cerebellar lesions are best addressed by open resection. In the rare case that may merit a more conservative approach, a suboccipital route with an image-determined (plane-of-target) entry point is indicated.

Postoperative CT

Postoperative CT, although done frequently, is no longer performed routinely in our practice, unless intraoperative bleeding has occurred through the needle. We have learned that clinical status is a good guideline to CT performance and its timing. The following case is illustrative:

❑ CASE 4

A man was admitted with slight progressive right hemiparesis. CT revealed an ill-defined lesion in the left thalamus, with only moderate enhancement. The third ventricle was partially obstructed. Stereotactic biopsy was performed. Tissue was diagnostic for anaplastic astrocytoma. There was no intraoperative bleeding. Nonetheless, immediate postoperative CT (Fig. 31–16A) disclosed a small punctuated hematoma in the operative bed. The patient's neurologic status was unchanged. During the following 4 hours, the right hemiparesis progressed gradually. Repeated CT (Fig. 31–16B) showed some enlargement of the intratumoral hematoma and slight lateral ventricular dilation. Due to slow progression of hemiparesis and the appearance of disorientation, a new CT was obtained 18 hours after the previous one. This showed further enlargement of the hematoma and definite hydrocephalus. A ventriculoperitoneal shunt was implanted. The patient's neurologic status returned to the preoperative condition during the next several weeks.

Pitfalls

Stereotactic biopsy is a relatively simple procedure. Attention to detail avoids situations that can conspire against a successful result.

EXCESSIVE CEREBROSPINAL FLUID LEAK

Because of the need to obtain contemporaneous pathologic examination, the biopsy procedure may be lengthy. Continuous CSF leak through the burr hole can be substantial, particularly in hydrocephalic patients, which can lead to postoperative pneumocephalus (Fig. 31–17) with protracted headaches. This may be minimized by careful intraoperative sealing of the burr hole with bone wax.

INCORRECT PATHOLOGIC INTERPRETATION

Misdiagnosis of pathologic material is particularly frequent in neuroglial tumors. De Divitiis and associates[27] found that these tumors were misdiagnosed in 18% of his cases, whereas the overall error rate for the total series was 8%. High-grade gliomas were implicated in all of the errors: half were misinterpreted as low-grade tumors and in half only "malignant tumor" could be diagnosed. The incidence of this pitfall can be largely reduced by serial sampling along the entire radius of the tumor and beyond, as described previously.

In an early series of biopsies reported by Ostertag and colleagues,[28] excessively small specimens (1 mm³; obtainable with a small biopsy forceps) resulted in 31% of cases in which paraffin sections were not possible to prepare, resulting on reliance on smear preparations alone for diagnosis. In the same series, when results of smear preparations and permanent histologic diagnoses could be compared, a

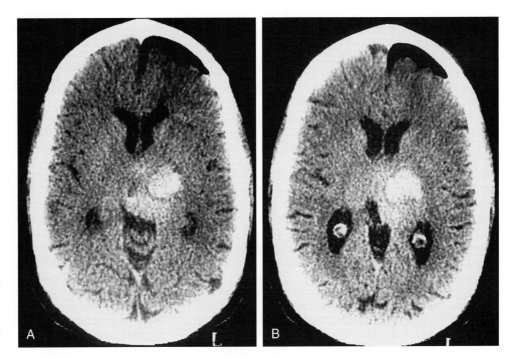

Figure 31-16 This thalamic glioma was biopsied through a frontal approach. Immediately after surgery (A), scattered bleeding points were seen in the operative bed. CT performed 12 hours later following clinical deterioration (B) shows significant enlargement of the hematoma with obstructive hydrocephalus.

12% error was correlated with the former. Smears tended to underestimate tumor malignancy.

The purpose of a biopsy procedure is to obtain a firm histologic diagnosis. Hence, we believe that it should not be terminated until positive confirmation that the collected tissue contains diagnostic material is obtained or, rarely, until reasonable histologic evidence is found to indicate that sampling has been obtained from the entire lesion diameter. In a review of 100 consecutive stereotactic biopsies,[29] it was found that pathologic diagnosis required an average of two frozen sections per case. That is, the first specimen frequently failed to contain diagnostic tissue, but a subsequent biopsy—usually along the same trajectory—was commonly diagnostic.

Close collaboration with an experienced neuropathologist is central to the diagnostic yield of stereotactic biopsy. Different techniques are available for contemporaneous microscopic examination: imprints (touch preparations), smears, and frozen section. All of these are stained by hematoxylin-eosin.

Imprints and smears have the advantages of not requiring special laboratory equipment (such as a cryostat), being faster to prepare than frozen sections, and allowing the preservation of more tissue for paraffin sections.

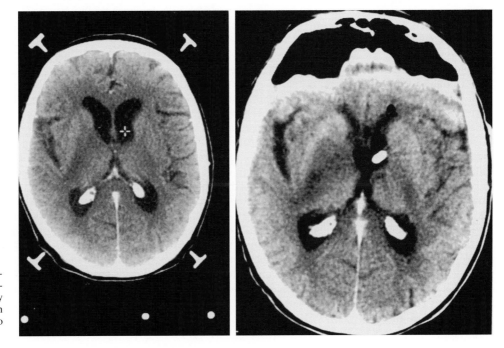

Figure 31-17 Pneumocephalus following ventricular puncture in hydrocephalic patients may be minimized by rapid sealing of the burr hole with bone wax around the biopsy needle, to avoid excessive CSF leak.

Frozen section has proved to be more diagnostically accurate than smears or imprints (99% vs. 92% vs. 82%, respectively) when compared with final diagnosis by paraffin sections. Frozen sections are also more consistently suitable for interpretation (99% of the obtained specimens against 91% of the smears and 86% of the imprints in one series).[30] Imprints and smears are more difficult to obtain in firm, fibrous materials.

Nonetheless, smears or imprints are the procedure of choice for handling tissue in patients with acquired immunodeficiency syndrome (AIDS), to avoid contamination of the cryostat. They are quicker and are as reliable as frozen sections in determining if tissue surrounding tumor margins still contains tumor cells.

Tissue transfer from the operating suite to the pathology laboratory must be fast, and the container used for transport must protect the specimen from desiccation and cell damage. We transfer the tissue in a Petri dish. If possible, CSF or cystic fluid retrieved with the needle is used to moisten the specimen. We avoid the use of "isotonic" solutions, because they may result in cell artifact in these small tissue samples.

In addition, we routinely transfer the tissue personally, and look at the slides along with the pathologist. Often, when diagnostic tissue is not yet obtained, elements in the preparation can help the surgeon to select a new position for the needle.

INCORRECT STEREOTACTIC TECHNIQUE

Because stereotaxy is a blind procedure, errors in the setting of the stereotactic frame can go undetected, leading to sampling from normal brain. The likelihood of these errors can be minimized by simulating the procedure on a phantom device before it is actually performed on the patient.[31] In any case, coordinate verification should be repeated before the needle is introduced.

Rigid structures (brain stimulators, shunt tubing, dural folds) are to be avoided along the planned trajectory, because they may deflect the biopsy needle.

Complications

Morbidity from stereotactic biopsy is in the range of 4% to 5%. Mortality is less than 1%.[23]

In 65 biopsies performed by one of the authors (R.S.) during a 2-year period, three patients (4.6%) experienced transient complications: two (3%) had hemiparesis and one (1.5%) experienced a seizure increase. One patient (1.5%) had permanent deterioration (stupor). There was no operative mortality.

Bleeding in the biopsy bed is usually heralded by blood flowing from the needle. The needle should be kept in place. As long as the blood is allowed to drain, it will likely not accumulate as a hematoma in the tumor bed. Continuous, gentle saline irrigation may avoid blood clotting within the needle. Frequently, the bleeding is self-limited and can be controlled with these maneuvers. Should it continue for more than 15 to 20 minutes, an emergency craniotomy is indicated. The needle is to be left in place to guide dissection toward the bleeding point.

Infective complications are rare with stereotactic biopsy (<1%) and are usually limited to superficial wound infection.[24]

BIOPSY BY FREEHAND TECHNIQUE

Freehand biopsy is usually performed with the patient in the CT scanner, under on-line CT control. The technique is simple and straightforward. When a suitable CT slice is selected that contains both a good target and a safe entry point, depth between both is measured on the CT console.

Savitz[32] has reported his experienced with 227 procedures in 147 patients. All of the procedures were completed under local anesthesia. He reported only one complication (postoperative bleeding).

Freehand biopsy can be used for relatively large and superficial targets. The technique has to its advantage that it does not require specialized equipment, it is simple to perform, and it allows immediate visualization of needle placement and postbiopsy complications. Its disadvantages include the absence of optimal aseptic conditions in the scanner room, the time the scanner has to be dedicated to the procedure, and the reduced space for maneuvering that results from the presence of the CT gantry.

ULTRASOUND-GUIDED BIOPSY

With the advent of small ultrasound probes that fit into burr holes, ultrasound-guided biopsy (USGB) became a practical option for minimally invasive diagnosis in intracranial pathologic lesions.

The technique is suitable for biopsy of lesions 15 mm or larger in the supratentorial compartment. Ultrasound image resolution is currently not good enough to warrant its use in sensitive areas such as the brainstem. Intra-axial tumors are echogenic regardless of their attenuation characteristics on CT (i.e., hypodense or hyperdense). Cysts and ventricles are hypoechoic.[33]

Instrumentation

Currently available USGB sets are burr-hole mounted (Berger[34] and Tsunumi and colleagues[35]). In the biopsy set designed by Berger[34] (Fig. 31–18) the patient's preoperative CT scan is used as a reference guide to place a standard burr hole close to the underlying lesion. The hole is enlarged to 22 mm and the bone edge from the inner table is removed with a rongeur to eliminate false near-field echoes. The set includes a plate that screws into the burr hole and a swivel-socket holder that houses the ultrasound probe and allows its angulation in every direction to place the target at the center of the field of view. Once the target is identified, the holder can be locked. Electronic cursors 1 cm apart superimposed on the ultrasound display measure the distance between the tip of the probe and the target. The probe is then substituted for the biopsy needle, which is rigidly guided to the precalculated depth. Ultrasound visualization is not possible while the needle is in place, but it can be obtained again after withdrawal of the needle. Because the needle

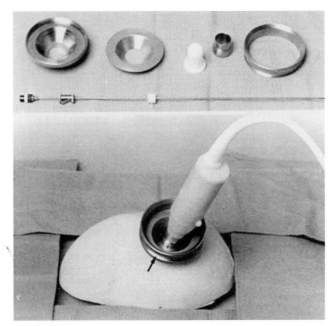

Figure 31–18   Components of Berger's ultrasound-guided biopsy apparatus. *Top,* From left to right: base plate, clamping plate, phantom ultrasound probe, ultrasound probe holder, and locking ring. A biopsy needle is shown below. *Bottom,* The ultrasound transducer inserted into the probe holder. The locking ring *(arrow)* is screwed into the basal plate. (From Berger MS: Ultrasound-guided stereotaxic biopsy using a new apparatus. J Neurosurg 1986; 65:550–554.)

track remains echogenic, immediate postbiopsy ultrasound will show the needle trajectory.

Ultrasound probes 16 mm in diameter are used with the set. A 5-MHz probe is used for near-field lesions (0 to 3 cm from the surface), whereas a 7.5-MHz probe is used for deeper masses (3 to 7 cm from the surface).

Tsutsumi and co-workers[35] have designed an apparatus that allows real-time ultrasound during needle introduction and sampling. Their transducer is 12 mm in diameter with a transmission frequency of 5 MHz. It provides a field of view of 90 degrees, with a dynamic depth focus of 25 to 80 mm. A connector attaches the ultrasound probe to a trocar with engravings at 1-cm intervals. They produce linear echoes that allow depth measurement while the trocar is being introduced. For biopsy, a 12-mm burr hole is trephined. The hole is enlarged in one direction to allow side penetration of the trocar.

Applications

Because of their characteristics, USGB sets are either not suitable or are awkward for mounting where thick muscle or receding bone is present (temporal, posterior fossa). Consequently, cerebellar targets or anterior temporal targets require biopsy with stereotactic techniques, even when they are large enough for ultrasound detection.

The main advantages of USGB are the following:

■ Simplicity. It may be performed without specific training.

■ The whole procedure is performed in the operating room,

obviating the need for preoperative and postoperative CT. Any preoperative CT is suitable to guide burr hole placement.

■ Because hemorrhage becomes echogenic as soon as red blood cells aggregate (within 5 minutes), postbiopsy bleeding can be detected by repeated ultrasound before wound closure.[34]

■ Diagnostic yield of USGB has reportedly ranged between 91%[36] and 95%, with a low complication rate (5% temporary neurologic deterioration and no mortality in one series comprising 38 cases).[37]

Limitations

Ultrasound imaging of intracerebral targets has the following intrinsic limitations, which the clinician should bear in mind:

■ Edema is echogenic, and its presence therefore blurs the real margins of the lesion, making proper targeting difficult.

■ In deep-seated targets, magnification occurs, owing to the fact that the distance between the ultrasonic beam emitted and its reflected echo increases in proportion to the distance covered by the beam itself.

■ Shadowing artifacts may result from the burr hole edge when considerable angulation of the needle becomes necessary.

■ Lateral and depth resolution are dependent on the frequency used as well as on the shape and size of the transducer and the pulse length. Pulse length has an inverse relationship with lateral and deep resolution: the greater the frequency the better the lateral resolution, but the worse the depth resolution. Thus, in using a single wavelength, a compromise between lateral and depth resolution is to be obtained that makes optimal spatial resolution possible.[37]

ENDOSCOPY

Endoscopic neurosurgery has been used for many years with limited indications. The technique has recently gained momentum due to the development of better endoscopic probes and instrumentation designed to allow through-the-scope tissue manipulation and hemostasis. Indications for endoscopic surgery are increasing. In the management of gliomas, the technique can be used to advantage for the diagnosis of intraventricular tumors, allowing concomitant treatment of obstructive hydrocephalus by third ventriculostomy.[38] Endoscopy in fluid-filled spaces has the advantage of providing direct and sharp visualization of anatomy and pathologic lesions. Bleeding can be controlled by monopolar coagulation. Tumor debulking is possible with the concourse of small forceps and laser beams. A detailed description of neuroendoscopy is beyond the scope of this chapter.

REFERENCES

1. Ciric I, Vick NA, Mikhael MA, et al: Aggressive surgery for malignant supratentorial gliomas. Clin Neurosurg 1988; 36:375–386.

2. Coffey RJ, Lunsford LD, Taylor FH: Survival after stereotactic biopsy of malignant gliomas. Neurosurgery 1988; 22:465–473.

3. Scanlon PW, Taylor WF: Radiotherapy of intracranial astrocytomas: Analysis of 417 cases treated from 1960 through 1969. Neurosurgery 1979; 5:301–308.

4. Bosch DA: Stereotactic Techniques in Clinical Neurosurgery. Wien, Springer Verlag, 1986.

5. Frank F, Fabrizi AP, Gaist G, et al: Stereotaxy and thalamic masses. Appl Neurophysiol 1987; 50:243–247.

6. Mundinger F: CT stereotactic biopsy for optimizing the therapy of intracranial processes. Acta Neurochir (Wien) Suppl 1985; 35:70–74.

7. Al-Rodhan NRF, Kelly PR: Stereotactic surgery in the diagnosis and treatment of brain tumors. In Morantz RA, Walsh JW (eds): Brain Tumors: A Comprehensive Text. New York, Marcel Dekker, 1994, pp 493–512.

8. Levivier M, Goldman S, Bidaut L, et al: Positron emission tomography-guided stereotactic brain biopsy. Neurosurgery 1992; 31:792–797.

9. Black KL, Hawkins RA, Kim KT, et al: Use of thallium 210 SPECT to quantitate malignancy grade of gliomas. J Neurosurg 1989; 71:342–346.

10. Burkard R, Kaiser KP, Wieler H, et al: Contribution of thallium 201 SPECT to the grading of tumorous alterations of the brain. Neurosurg Rev 1992; 15:265–273.

11. Spiegelmann R: History, principles and techniques of stereotactic surgery. In Tindall GT, Cooper PR, Barrow DL (eds): The Practice of Neurosurgery. Baltimore, Williams & Wilkins (in press).

12. Coons SW, Johnson PC: Pathology of primary intracranial malignant neoplasms. In Morantz RA, Walsh JW (eds): Brain Tumors: A Comprehensive Text. New York, Marcel Dekker, 1994, pp 45–108.

13. Daumas-Duport C, Monsaingeon V, Szenthe L, et al: Serial stereotactic biopsies: A double histological code of gliomas according to malignancy and 3-D configuration as an aid to therapeutic decision and assessment of results. Appl Neurophysiol 1982; 45:431–437.

14. Edner G: Stereotactic biopsy of intracranial space occupying lesions. Acta Neurochir (Wien) 1981; 57:213–234.

15. Spiegelmann R, Friedman WA: Stereotactic suboccipital transcerebellar biopsy under local anesthesia using the CRW frame. J Neurosurg 1991; 75:486–488.

16. Spiegelmann R, Friedman WA: Pineal region tumors: Diagnosis and management. Contemp Neurosurg 1991; 13:1–7.

17. Boysdton WR, Sanford RA, Muhlbauer MS, et al: Gliomas of the tectum and periaqueductal region of the mesencephalon. Pediatr Neurosurg 1991–2; 17:234–238.

18. Epstein F: Intrinsic brainstem tumors of childhood. In Homburger F (ed): Progress in Experimental Tumor Research. Basel, S. Karger, 1987, pp 160–169.

19. Hoffman HJ, Becker L, Craven MA: A clinically and pathologically distinct group of benign brainstem gliomas. Neurosurgery 1980; 7:243–248.

20. Vandertop WP, Hoffman HJ, Drake JM, et al: Focal midbrain tumors in children Neurosurg 1992; 31:186–194.

21. Abernathey CD, Camacho A, Kelly PJ: Stereotaxic suboccipital transcerebellar biopsy of pontine mass lesions. J Neurosurg 1989; 70:195–200.

22. Coffey RJ, Lunsford LD: Stereotactic surgery for mass lesions of the midbrain and pons. Neurosurgery 1985; 17:12–18.

23. Hood TW, Gebarski SS, McKeever PE, et al: Stereotaxic biopsy of intrinsic lesions of the brain stem. J Neurosurg 1986; 65:172–176.

24. Friedman WA, Spiegelmann R: Reoperative stereotactic neurosurgery and radiosurgery. In Little J, Awad I (eds): Reoperative Neurosurgery. Baltimore, Williams & Wilkins, 1992, pp 271–302.

25. Guthrie B, Steinberg G, Adler J: Posterior fossa stereotaxic biopsy using the Brown-Roberts-Wells stereotaxic system. J Neurosurg 1989; 70:649–652.

26. Apuzzo ML, Sabshin JK: Computed tomographic guidance stereotaxic in the management of intracranial mass lesions. Neurosurgery 1983; 12:277–285.

27. De Divitiis E, Spaziante R, Cappabianca P, et al: Reliability of stereotactic biopsy. Appl Neurophysiol 1983; 46:295–303.

28. Ostertag CB, Mennel HD, Kiessling M: Stereotactic biopsy of brain tumors. Surg Neurol 1980; 14:275–283.

29. Friedman WA, Sceats DJ, Nestok BR, et al: The incidence of unexpected pathological findings in an image-guided biopsy series: A review of 100 consecutive cases. Neurosurgery 1989; 25:180–184.

30. Reyes MG, Fayez Homsi M, McDonald LW, et al: Imprints, smears, and frozen sections of brain tumors. Neurosurgery 1991; 29:575–579.

31. Friedman WA, Spiegelmann R: The principles of stereotaxis. In Hoff J, Crockard A (eds): Neurosurgery: The Scientific Basis for Clinical Practice, ed 2. London, Blackwell, 1992, pp 956–974.

32. Savitz MH: Free hand CT-guided needle for biopsy and drainage of intracerebral lesions: Ten years experience. Int Surg 1992; 77:211–215.

33. Chandler WF, Knake JE, McGillicuddy JE, et al: Intraoperative use of real-time ultrasonography in neurosurgery. J Neurosurg 1982; 57:157–163.

34. Berger MS: Ultrasound-guided stereotaxic biopsy using a new apparatus. J Neurosurg 1986; 65:550–554.

35. Tsutsumi Y, Andoh Y, Sakaguchi J: A new ultrasound-guided brain biopsy technique through a burr hole: Technical note. Acta Neurochir (Wien) 1989; 96:72–75.

36. Di Lorenzo N, Esposito V, Lunardi P, et al: A comparison of computerized tomography-guided stereotactic and ultrasound-guided techniques for brain biopsy. J Neurosurg 1991; 75:763–765.

37. Lunardi P, Acqui M, Maleci A, et al: Ultrasound-guided brain biopsy: A personal experience with emphasis on its indication. Surg Neurol 1993; 39:148–151.

38. Kelly PJ: Stereotactic biopsy and resection of thalamic astrocytomas. Neurosurgery 1989; 25:185–195.

FREDERICK F. LANG, JR.

PATRICK J. KELLY

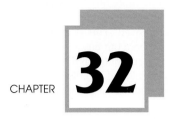

CHAPTER **32**

Computer-Assisted Stereotactic Laser Resection

Glial neoplasms most frequently are ill-defined, irregularly shaped, infiltrating lesions. Despite technical advances in neurosurgery, such as the operating microscope, ultrasonic aspirator, and intraoperative ultrasound, it is often difficult for the operating surgeon (1) to maintain proper orientation in three-dimensional space and (2) to know exactly where resectable tumor ends and where edematous, potentially functional brain tissue begins. For these reasons, general treatment stategies for gliomas (e.g., biopsy vs. resection) are often dictated by the technical aspects of surgery. For example, deep-seated lesions that may benefit oncologically from complete removal are instead biopsied and irradiated. Superficial lesions located near eloquent cortex are often subject to partial removal because of the inability of the surgeon to define the border between tumor and essential cortex.

Since the early 1980s, stereotactic methods based on computed tomography (CT) and magnetic resonance imaging (MRI) have led to the development of computer-assisted stereotactic volumetric surgery.[1-5] This technology, though applicable to any intracranial lesion, is particularly helpful for removal of infiltrating gliomas because it provides the surgeon with precise intraoperative information regarding a tumor's three-dimensional structure and its surgically resectable border.[3, 4, 6]

This chapter provides a comprehensive review of computer-assisted stereotactic surgery in the treatment of glial neoplasms. It aims to convey both the procedural aspects of the technique and the role of the technique as part of a larger management strategy for glial neoplasms.

PRINCIPLES AND PROBLEMS OF GLIOMA SURGERY

Operations are perfomed on patients with gliomas to obtain a tissue diagnosis, reduce intracranial pressure, relieve local compression of surrounding eloquent cortex, and reduce the tumor burden (i.e., cytoreduction).[7] Safe accomplishment of these goals requires a thorough understanding of the macrosurgical and microsurgical anatomy of each glial tumor type.[8-10] Indeed, most of the problems associated with resection of gliomas revolve around their unique surgical anatomy.

Macrosurgical Anatomy of Gliomas

Glial neoplasms can occupy one of three gross anatomic positions: polar, superficial, or deep. Polar lesions are the most surgically accessible, and identifying the lesion during surgery usually presents no difficulty. Consequently, removal of polar lesions does not require special technology. Standard frontal, temporal, or occipital lobectomy can safely and effectively remove these lesions.

Superficial lesions may be near or distant from eloquent cortex. With classic neurosurgical approaches, locating these lesions requires large bone flaps and wide dural openings. This ensures that the center and extensions of the tumor are sufficiently exposed. However, normal surrounding brain is also invariably exposed, which subjects normal eloquent cortex to potential injury, particularly if it protrudes from the dural opening before the tumor has been decompressed.

Classic approaches to deep-seated lesions are accompanied by the same problems as approaches to superficial lesions. In addition, it is often difficult to maintain the correct trajectory between the brain surface and the subcortical target because no landmarks are present to provide orientation. Consequently, shorter rather than safer routes are often undertaken during standard craniotomy for deep-seated gliomas.

Microsurgical Anatomy of Gliomas

Histologic analyses of serial biopsies through specific CT- and MRI-defined areas of glial tumors have demonstrated several regions that correspond to specific imaging features

391

(Table 32–1).[8–12] CT contrast-enhancing areas and MRI T1-weighted gadolinium-enhancing regions correspond to *tumor tissue proper*, characterized by abutting tumor cells that have acquired their own blood supply (neovascularity) and destroyed or displaced intervening normal parenchymal tissue. Because no brain tissue is contained within these areas, they can be removed safely without danger of incurring neurologic deficit. Areas on CT that are hypodense and that are hyperintense on T2-weighted MRI correspond histologically to *isolated tumor cells infiltrating between essentially normal parenchymal structures* without associated neovascularity. These areas cannot be resected, as functional deficit arises with removal of normal intervening brain tissue.

To maximize decompression and cytoreduction and minimize neurologic deficit during glioma surgery, it is essential to remove all tumor tissue proper and to spare infiltrated normal parenchyma. With classic neurosurgical techniques of internal decompression, the surgeon relies primarily on visual inspection and tissue "texture" to locate the surgical border between glial tumor tissue proper and infiltrated normal parenchyma. However, this plane is often not readily apparent at an open surgical procedure. When the tumor lies within "nonessential" brain tissue, the plane of dissection is of little functional consequence, as the surgeon can be quite aggressive in resecting the lesion. However, when the tumor is located near eloquent cortex, neurologic deficit will result if infiltrated parenchyma is resected or damaged. With classic internal decompression procedures, the surgeon often first encounters fragile neoplastic vessels. Bleeding from these vessels further compromises identification of the tumor border, preservation of normal brain, and performance of a complete removal.

Because of the unique gross and microsurgical anatomy of gliomas, the goals of glioma surgery are not often optimized with standard techniques. This may be particularly true for tumor cytoreduction. Cytoreduction should theoretically slow tumor growth rate, because growth rate is determined by the mitotic rate of individual cells, the percentage of mitotically active cells, and the total number of cells.[13, 14] Because most gliomas—with the possible exception of pilocytic astrocytomas—are composed of areas of infiltrating cells within normal parenchyma, complete surgical resection is not possible. Nevertheless, although aggressive surgery may not "cure" most gliomas, it may alter tumor cell biology and kinetics, leading to longer survival and better quality of life.

Complete and safe cytoreduction is best achieved when the entire solid tumor tissue mass (which is usually represented by contrast enhancement on imaging studies) is removed, and infiltrated functional brain tissue is spared. With classic neurosurgical methods, it is impossible to know intraoperatively that all of the imaging-defined contrast-enhancing portion of tumor has been removed. This is particularly difficult when the tumor is not a sphere but has an irregularly shaped volume. The technique of computer-assisted stereotactic volumetric resection was developed to allow surgeons to selectively resect any imaging-defined abnormality.

COMPUTER-ASSISTED VOLUMETRIC STEREOTAXY

Stereotaxy (from Greek *stereos* [solid] + Latin *tactus* [touch]) involves the precise localization of points within three-dimensional space. Stereotactic neurosurgery currently takes two forms: point-in-space and volume-in-space stereotaxy. For the neurosurgeon operating on gliomas, this translates into methods for localizing either points within a tumor for biopsy or volumes of tumor within the brain for resection.

Although the stereotactic method was originally described in 1906 by Horsley and Clarke,[15, 16] use of stereotaxy in the management of intracranial tumors has developed recently, since the advent of CT scanning.[17, 18] Because CT precisely determines the location and configuration of most intracranial tumors, it provides a precise three-dimensional data base that can easily be incorporated into a stereotactic coordinate system. By the early 1980s, methods were established for deriving stereotactic frame coordinates from points selected on CT scan images. These methods led to the development of point-in-space stereotactic procedures, which were used for the biopsy of specific targets within intracranial tumors.[18, 19] More recently, MRI has also become a valuable stereotactic data base. CT- and MRI-based stereotactic biopsy procedures allow for sampling of precise and predetermined areas of a tumor and can safely be used for tumors in deep locations. These methods are generally superior to open biopsy when only a tissue diagnosis is needed, and they have become commonplace in the diagnosis and treatment of gliomas.[18–20]

Development of appropriate computer software has allowed extension of stereotactic methods from point-in-space targets, to volume-in-space targets and interactive volumetric stereotactic surgery.[1–6, 21, 22] In volumetric stereotaxy, planar tumor boundaries defined by stereotactic CT and MRI are reconstructed by the computer into a volume in stereotactic

TABLE 32–1
HISTOLOGIC AND RADIOGRAPHIC CORRELATES OF GLIOMAS AS DEFINED BY SERIAL BIOPSY RESULTS

Histologic Findings	MRI Findings	CT Findings	Resectability
Tumor tissue proper	Gadolinium-enhancing region on T1-weighted image	Contrast-enhancing region	Resectable
Isolated tumor cells within normal parenchyma	Increased intensity on T2-weighted images	Hypodense region	Not resectable
Necrosis	Low signal within enhancing region on T1-weighted image	Hypodensity within enhancing region	Resectable
Edema	Increased intensity on T2-weighted images	Hypodense region	Not resectable

space. This information is reformatted and displayed to the surgeon intraoperatively. With computer-assisted volume stereotaxy, the surgeon is able to precisely localize the tumor in three-dimensional space. Therefore, superficial lesions located near or in eloquent cortex can be approached by a stereotactically positioned craniotomy. This allows for a small trephine opening whose diameter is only slightly larger than the cross-sectional diameter of the CT-enhancing portion of the lesion. Almost no normal brain tissue is exposed by this small craniotomy. Deep-seated tumors located in the thalamus, basal ganglia, or periventricular regions are also easily localized. The trajectory is stereotactically determined. The identification of internal anatomic landmarks used to orient surgeons in nonstereotactic approaches to deep tumors is not required in stereotactic approaches to these lesions. Consequently, stereotactic approaches to deep tumors can employ the safest trajectory through nonessential white matter pathways, even if these are anatomically longer routes.[19]

Computer-assisted stereotactic techniques allow for the intraoperative localization of the CT- and MRI-defined border between tumor tissue proper and surrounding infiltrated parenchyma.[3, 4, 6] In the surgical planning phase of a volumetric stereotactic procedure, the operating surgeon outlines on the computer the region of tumor to be resected. This typically corresponds to the CT contrast-enhancing part of the tumor. This outline is then displayed in the operating room with respect to the position of stereotactically placed trephines or stereotactically directed instruments. In addition, these scaled planar slice images can be projected onto the brain surface by a heads-up display unit attached to the operating microscope, which guides the surgeon during removal of tumor. Because the histologic border of the tumor, which may not be clear on visual inspection, is known to the surgeon using the computer-assisted stereotactic methodology, complete removal of the enhancing glioma tissue proper can be accomplished while the surrounding normal parenchyma is spared. Therefore, volumetric resection maximizes cytoreduction while preventing neurologic deficit.

Technical innovations have increased the facility and accuracy with which stereotactic volumetric operations are performed. In particular, the COMPASS stereotactic system (Stereotactic Medical Systems, New Hartford, NY) was specifically designed for volumetric tumor stereotaxy, and a designated operating room computer system was developed for the transposition of volumetric information derived from axial stereotactic CT scans and MRIs into three-dimensional space and for display in the operating room of the position of stereotactically directed instruments in relation to computer-generated reconstructions of the tumor volume. Digital subtraction angiography has been added to the data base for the stereotactic localization of intracranial vessels that are relevant to the location of the lesion and to the surgical approach. Most recently, functional regions of the brain as defined by magnetoencephalography (MEG) have become an important aspect of the data base. With this technique, functional brain areas can be mapped prior to surgery and their proximity to the tumor mass can be assessed. Functional information can thus be used to further guide tumor resection.

In summary, computer-assisted stereotactic techniques enable the surgeon to accurately locate a tumor within the brain, identify the surgical border between tumor and infiltrated edematous normal brain, and maintain correct three-dimensional orientation during the resection of irregularly shaped neoplasms. The technique can be used in the resection of superficial lesions located near eloquent cortex and in the resection of lesions located deep within the brain. This technology, therefore, overcomes most of the problems associated with the classic internal decompression procedures that have been practiced by neurosurgeons for more than 50 years. Table 32–2 compares classic internal decompression technique and the computer-assisted volumetric stereotactic procedure.

INSTRUMENTATION AND TECHNIQUE

The COMPASS Stereotactic System

The COMPASS stereotactic system evolved from modifications of a standard Todd-Wells stereotactic frame.[21] It utilizes the principles of an arc-quadrant stereotactic frame.[23] Specifically, probes directed perpendicular to the tangent of the arc (which rotates about the vertical axis) and the quadrant, or collar (which rotates about the horizontal axis), and for a depth equal to the radius of the sphere that is defined by the arc-quadrant will always arrive at the center of that sphere. In this system, the patient's head is moved to locate the intracranial target in the arc-quadrant center. The contemporary version of the COMPASS stereotactic frame consists of a removable headholder, a three-dimensional positioning slide apparatus for moving the patient's head, and a fixed arc-quadrant (Fig. 32–1).

HEADHOLDER

The headholder (Fig. 32–2*B*) consists of a round base ring, four vertical supports, and a skull fixation system. The headholder attaches to the patient's skull by means of flanged carbon-fiber pins, which are inserted into four holes drilled in the outer table of the skull, into the diploë.

Detachable micrometers are used to measure the distance between the end of the carbon-fiber pins and the outer face

TABLE 32–2
CONVENTIONAL CRANIOTOMY COMPARED TO COMPUTER-ASSISTED VOLUMETRIC STEREOTACTIC RESECTION

Standard Craniotomy	Stereotactic Resection
Large craniotomy ensures localization of lesion	Trephine craniotomy no larger then lesion, placed stereotactically
Wide dural opening exposes normal and resectable tumor tissue	Small dural opening exposes only resectable tissue
Relies on visual inspection to define tumor-brain border	Tumor border identified by CT/MRI and projected onto surgical field, computer guides resection
Trajectory to deep-seated lesion takes shortest route, not least destructive route; difficult to maintain trajectory	Trajectory defined by stereotaxy, safest route traversed, distance irrelevant, trajectory preplanned

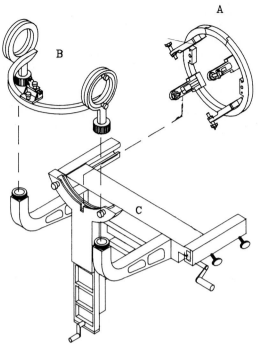

Figure 32–1 Schematic diagram of simplified COMPASS stereotactic frame demonstrates the circular headholder (*A*), 160-mm radius arc-quadrant (*B*), and three-axis slide mechanism (*C*), which attaches to a semipermanent floor stand or to a standard operating table. Hand cranks are shown; these provide mechanical backups to three-axis computer-controlled stepper motors.

of the vertical supports (see Fig. 32–2*A*). These measurements, and the fact that the pins are placed in previously drilled holes in the skull, provide a means for accurate placement of the stereotactic headholder. Thus, data acquisition and surgery need not be performed on the same day, and additional procedures using the same data base can be performed at a later date.

ARC-QUADRANT

The 160-mm radius arc-quadrant attaches to horizontal arms that extend from the base plate of the three-dimensional slide. Probes and retractors are directed by an attachment on the upper face of the arc. The arc-quadrant provides two angular degrees of freedom for approach trajectories: a collar angle (from the horizontal plane) and an arc angle (from the vertical plane).

THREE-DIMENSIONAL POSITIONING SLIDE

The headholder fits into a support yoke of a three-dimensional slide that moves the patient's head within the fixed arc-quadrant. The slide moves the patient's head in *x*, *y*, and *z* directions to place the intracranial target point into the center of the arc-quadrant. Each axis of the three-dimensional slide is moved by gears linked to a computer-controlled stepper motor, which is activated at a remote-control console located outside the surgical field. Hand cranks are provided on each of the three axes for manual backup.

Stereotactic coordinates on the slide are detected by opti-

cal encoders on the *x*, *y*, and *z* axes that transmit the coordinates to digital readout scales and to the computer. In addition, Vernier scales are provided on each axis for direct reading of stereotactic coordinates as a backup to the optical encoders.

The Computer System

Basic software for data acquisition, surgical planning, and interactive surgery evolved over an 8-year period. The computer, although not absolutely necessary, saves a great deal of time in calculating target points; interpolating imaging-defined tumor volumes; cross-registering points and volumes between CT, MRI, and digital angiographic (DA) images; and displaying real-time interactive images during the surgical procedure. The computer makes volumetric stereotactic procedures practical and time-efficient.

HARDWARE

The COMPASS stereotactic frame is supported by a SUN SPARC 10 (SUN Microsystems, Mountainview, Calif) with

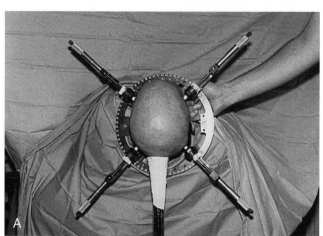

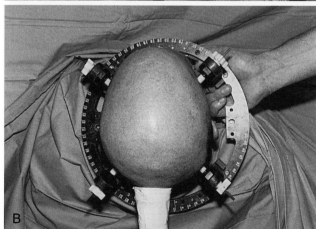

Figure 32–2 The COMPASS stereotactic head frame with (*A*) and without (*B*) attached micrometers. Note indexing marks on base ring of headholder. The headholder fixes to the patient's skull by means of four fixed-length flanged carbon-fiber pins, which insert into twist drill holes made in the outer table of the skull. Micrometers measure the extension of the carbon-fiber pin beyond the plane of the vertical support and provide a mechanism for precise frame reapplication.

three X terminal display monitors mounted in a custom-designed ergonomically efficient workstation-style console (Stereotactic Medical Systems, Rochester, Minn).

SOFTWARE

Data acquisition, surgical planning, and interactive display software run by mouse/cursor and menu interactive devices and by voice recognition systems allow user-friendly interaction with the operating room computer system before and during surgery. Stereotactic tumor resections are possible using manual methods for calculation of stereotactic coordinates and cross-correlation of target points between the different imaging modalities.

Surgical Instruments

LASER

The carbon dioxide (CO_2) laser has been found to have very limited application in the resection of superficial lesions, but it has several advantages in the stereotactic resection of deep tumors. First, the laser is convenient for removing tissue from a deep cavity and is relatively hemostatic. Second, the laser removes tissue by means of a narrow beam of light; thus, one less instrument is neeeded in a narrow surgical field. At present, a Sharplan 1100 CO_2 Laser System (Medical Industries, Tel Aviv, Israel) is used in stereotactic resections.

STEREOTACTIC RETRACTORS

Stereotactic retractors are fixed to the arc-quadrant to provide exposure of deep-seated lesions (i.e., they provide a shaft from the surface of the brain to the surface of deep-seated lesions) (Fig. 32–3). The arc-mounted stereotactic retractor system that is currently employed comprises cylindrical retractors, dilators, and an arc-quadrant adapter. The retractor is a thin-walled hollow cylinder, 140 mm in length and 2 cm in diameter. The retractor cylinder is directed toward the focal point of the stereotactic arc-quadrant. Dilators that fit inside the retractor cylinder are 1 cm longer than the retractor. The distal end of the dilator is wedge-shaped and spreads an incision to the diameter of the retractor so that the retractor cylinder can be advanced. The retractor is used not only to maintain exposure, but also to provide a

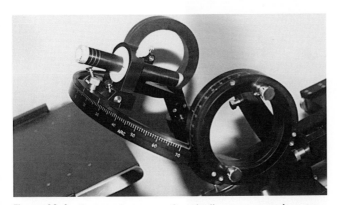

Figure 32–3 Stereotactic retractor, 2 cm in diameter, mounted on stereotactic arc-quadrant of COMPASS stereotactic system.

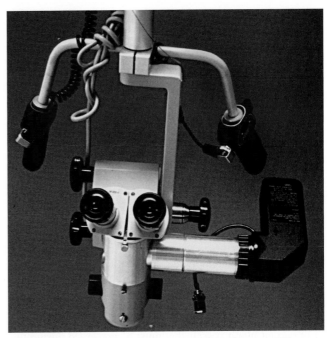

Figure 32–4 Heads-up display unit for operating microscope. This superimposes the computer-generated images on the stereotactically defined surgical field.

fixed stereotactic reference structure within the stereotactic surgical field.

ACCESSORY INSTRUMENTS

Extra-long bipolar forceps with a shaft length of 150 mm are required to control bleeding in the surgical field when working through the stereotactic retractors. In addition, 150- to 160-mm long suction tips, dissectors, and alligator scissors are used.

HEADS-UP DISPLAY FOR THE OPERATING MICROSCOPE

In a specially designed heads-up display unit, the image output of a small video monitor mounted on the operating microscope is optically superimposed on the surgical field viewed through the microscope (Fig. 32–4). The computer-generated image displayed on the video monitor is scaled by a system of lenses to the desired size. Thus, the surgeon sees the actual surgical field with the computer-generated rendition of that field based on CT and MRI superimpositions.

STEREOTACTIC RESECTION PROCEDURES

Computer-assisted volumetric stereotactic resections are performed in three phases: data base acquisition, treatment planning, and interactive procedure.

Data Acquisition The CT- and MRI-compatible stereotactic head frame is placed on the patient's head and secured by means of carbon-fiber pins inserted into ⅛-inch twist drill holes through the outer table of the skull into the diploë. For frame reattachment, detachable micrometers are used to measure the carbon-fiber fixation pins with respect to the fixed vertical support elements of the headholder. This provides a mechanism for accurate repeated placement of the frame for subsequent data acquisition or surgical procedures.

After application of the headframe, the patient undergoes stereotactic CT, MRI, digital angiography, and MEG. The stereotactic head frame is secured to a CT table adaptation plate. A CT localization system, which consists of nine carbon-fiber localiztion rods arranged in the shape of the letter N, and located on either side of the head anteriorly, is used to create nine reference marks on each CT slice (Fig. 32–5). Stereotactic CT scanning is done on a General Electric 8800 or 9800 CT scanning unit that focuses on 5-mm adjacent slices throughout the lesion, with use of a medium body format.

The MRI-compatible stereotactic head frame is similar to that described for CT, except that it is constructed entirely of carbon fiber and molybdenum disulfate, and it has no metal parts. The MRI localization system consists of capillary tubes filled with copper sulfate solution, which also create nine reference marks on each MRI.

Stereotactic digital angiography is used for the localization of important blood vessels that must be preserved during the surgical approach and tumor resection. A digital flouroscopy table adaptation plate receives the stereotactic head frame on the General Electric 3000 or 5000 digital angiographic unit. The digital angiographic localization system consists of lucite plates that contain nine radiopaque reference marks and are located on either side of the head, anteriorly and posteriorly. Thus, 18 reference marks are created on each anteroposterior and lateral digital angiographic image. The mathematical relationships between the fiducial marks and their locations on the digital angiographic images are the basis from which the stereotactic coordinates for intracranial vessels can be calculated, and stereotactic target points derived from CT and MRI can be displayed on angiographic images. Digital angiography is performed with use of a femoral catheterization technique. Orthogonal and 6-degree oblique arterial and venous phases are obtained in orthogonal and 6-degree rotated stereotactic pairs.

MEG is the most recent addition to the data base and is useful in planning resection of infiltrating lesions in or near the sensorimotor areas. When performed in a stereotactic fashion, MEG provides information about the anatomic position of functional motor and sensory cortex and its relationship to the stereotactically localized tumor. A 37-channel neuromagnetic system (Biomagnetic Tehnologies) is used to record magnetic evoked field potentials in response to vibratory stimulation of the fingers. The electromagnetic physiologic data are then overlaid on the stereotactic MRI data. Information about motor cortex is obtained by recording the magnetic fields evoked by repetitive movements of the fingers.

Surgical Planning   After data acquisition, the head frame is typically taken off of the patient. The surgeon then plans the surgical procedure from the computer terminal. Surgical planning involves digitizing the images, contouring the lesion to reconstruct the tumor volume, and determining the optimal surgical approach.

Digitizing the Image for Volume Reconstruction   The archived data tapes from the CT, MRI, and digital angiographic examinations are read into the operating room computer system. The surgeon views each of the CT slices and MRIs that demonstrate the lesion and digitizes them as follows: First, the nine reference marks on each CT slice and MRI are detected automatically by an intensity-detection algorithm. This process suspends the position of each slice in a three-dimensional computer image storage matrix. Second, the outline of the lesion is digitized by the surgeon with the use of an interactive cursor system. The outline of the image is the surgeon's choice. This typically is the contour of the CT contrast-enhancement region, the region of CT hypodensity, or the T1- and T2-weighted signal abnormalities on the MRI slices on serial imaging. Each of these digitized contours is suspended in a separate computer image matrix. A computer program interpolates intermediate slices at 1-mm intervals between each of the digitized contours. By filling in the interpolated and digitized slices with 1-mm cubic voxels, the computer creates separate volumes for CT- and MRI-defined data bases (Fig. 32–6A). Each volume is assigned an identifying gray level for individual or combined display on the monitor.

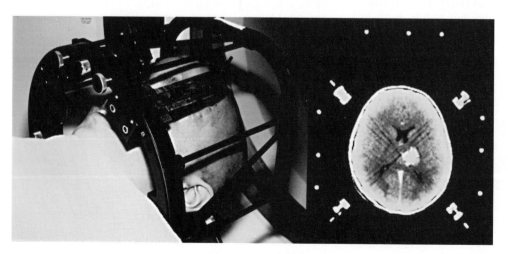

Figure 32–5 Stereotactic localization device for CT (*left*). This consists of nine carbon-fiber rods arranged in the shape of the letter N, which produce nine reference marks on each CT slice from which stereotactic coordinates are calculated (*right*). The MRI localization device is similar and is based on the same principle.

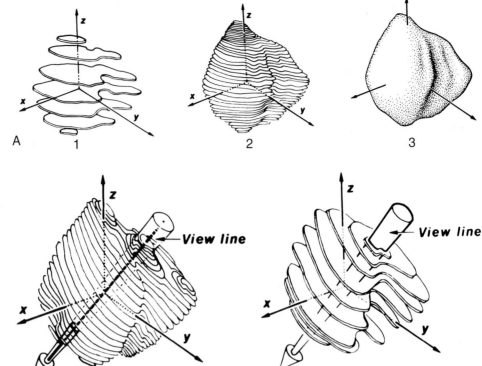

Figure 32–6 *A*, A tumor volume is constructed from digitized contours of the CT- and MRI-defined lesion, which are suspended in a three-dimensional computer matrix (*1*). The computer interpolates intermediate slices at 1-mm intervals (*2*). A tumor volume is created when the computer fills in the intermediate slices with 1-mm cubic voxels (*3*). *B*, The trajectory though the lesion—or surgical viewline—is determined (*left*) and the tumor volume is sliced perpendicular to it (*right*). These slices are presented to the surgeon during the procedure to indicate the CT- and MRI-defined boundaries of the tumor.

Choosing the Surgical Trajectory The object of surgical planning is to select the approach to a tumor that traverses the most expendable brain tissue. Consequently, the surgical approach selected takes into account the three-dimensional shape of the lesion, important overlying cortical regions, subcortical white matter pathways, and vascular structures that must be preserved. In most cases, the stereotactic surgical approach to the lesion is selected on anteroposterior and lateral stereotactic digital angiography images on which the digitized tumor volume has been displayed.

The actual direction of the approach, or the so-called surgical viewline, from the surface of the brain to the target point within the tumor volume is expressed in terms of two angular stereotactic frame settings: an angle from the horizontal plane and an angle from the vertical plane. In the COMPASS system, the viewline is defined by and expressed in terms of patient orientation and by the collar and arc trajectory setting on the stereotactic instrument. The CT- and MRI-defined tumor volumes residing within the computer image storage matrix are then sliced perpendicular to the intended surgical viewline and are displayed on the computer console (see Fig. 32–6*B*). During the surgical procedure, these slice images are displayed on a monitor in the operating room and in the operating microscope via the heads-up display (Fig. 32–7).

The COMPASS stereotactic headholder has indexing marks inscribed around its circumference that align to an indexing mark in the headholder that receives the yoke of the three-dimensional slide system. Thus, the patient's head can be rotated to any position that will provide a comfortable working position for the surgeon. In addition, to avoid possible spatial shifts of the intracranial contents, the surgeon must rotate the patient's head in the stereotactic headholder so that the skull opening is at the least dependent position in the surgical field (i.e., on top). This places the proposed trephine in the most superior position within the surgical field, and the spatial integrity of the brain is maintained by

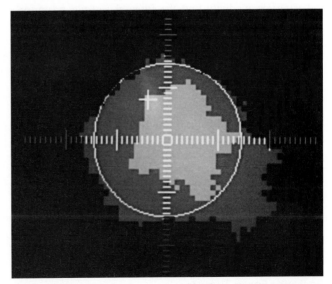

Figure 32–7 Computer display of tumor slice cut perpendicular to the surgical viewline, which indicates the limits of the tumor defined by CT contrast enhancement (*white*) and T2 prolongation of the MRI (*gray*). The circle represents a small trephine that will be used to resect only the CT contrast-enhancing mass. This image will be displayed on a computer monitor in the operating room and into the heads-up display of the operating microscope.

the intact skull's encasing it. This is similar to opening a jar of liquid; the top is directed in the least dependent position and the liquid within the jar does not move.

Surgical Trajectories

A variety of surgical approaches have been developed for various subcortical tumor locations. These include transcortical, transsulcal, transsylvian, and interhemispheric exposures. The actual approach selected depends on the proximity of the tumor to deep sulci that can be split microsurgically and spread wide enough to provide adequate exposure. Experience with lesions in different locations has led to the use of several standard stereotactic approaches.

Thalamic Tumors

The surgical approach employed in the resection of thalamic tumors depends on the relationship of the lesion to normal thalamic structures.[19] The thalamus can be divided into three regions: anterior, posterior ventral, and posterior dorsal. Anterior thalamic lesions are best exposed through an incision in the superior frontal sulcus. The trajectory to the lesions is then directed along the anterior limb of the internal capsule. The patient is supine in the stereotactic headframe. Posterior dorsal lesions are exposed transventricularly by use of a transcortical approach through the superior parietal lobule in the dominant hemisphere or through the posterior corpus callosum interhemispherically in the nondominant hemisphere. The patient is prone in the stereotactic headframe. Posterior ventral lesions are approached by means of a trephine craniotomy at the inferior temporo-occipital junction and an incision through the sublenticular portion of the internal capsule. The patient is rotated into an oblique position in the stereotactic headframe.

Basal Ganglia and Hypothalamic Tumors

Tumors in the basal ganglia and hypothalamus displace the ventricle medially and the internal capsule posteriorly and laterally. These lesions are best approached through an incision in the superior frontal sulcus and the anterior limb of the internal capsule.

Medial Posterior Temporal Lobe Tumors

Medial temporal tumors are particularly challenging lesions because of their proximity to midbrain structures as well as to the choroidal and posterior cerebral arteries. In the nondominant hemisphere, these deep lesions can be exposed via an incision in the superior temporal sulcus. In the dominant hemisphere, injury to speech cortex may result from such an approach. Consequently, these lesions are exposed using a longer, but theoretically safer, trajectory via an inferior occipital trephine craniotomy. The occipital lobe is elevated and an incision through the occipital temporal sulcus at the base of the temporal and occipital lobes exposes the lesion.

Posterior Fossa Tumors

Lesions in the posterior fossa are usually operated on with the stereotactic headframe placed in the inverted position. This provides unlimited access to the posterior fossa. Midline lesions in the cerebellum or brainstem are exposed through the inferior vermis. Lesions of the lateral cerebellar hemisphere are approached with the patient in a prone position (rotation, 180 degrees) in the stereotactic frame. Lateral pontine lesions are approached in a lateral oblique trajectory from posterolateral to anteromedial that traverses the middle cerebellar peduncle.

At the end of the planning session, the computer calculates and displays the stereotactic coordinates of the target as well as the arc and collar angle that are necessary to reach the target along the chosen trajectory. The computer also reformats the tumor volume to account for the desired patient position.

Interactive Stereotactic Surgical Procedures The interactive stereotactic procedure begins with the reapplication of the stereotactic headholder. General endotracheal anesthesia is used. The stereotactic headholder is replaced using the same pinholes in the skull, pin placements, and frame micrometer settings that were used during the data acquisition phase. The patient's head–onto which the headholder has been placed–is then fixed on the stereotactic frame by placing the base ring of the headholder into the receiving yoke of the stereotactic frame. The patient's head in the stereotactic headholder is rotated to the planned position. The head of the operating table is usually raised to place the position of the intended trephine in the least dependent position of the surgical field (usually equivalent to the collar angle) and to provide maximal brain relaxation. Mannitol administration and spinal drainage are never used.

After preparing and draping the head, the stereotactic arc-quadrant is positioned. The selected arc and collar approach angles are set on the instrument. Through a stab incision in the scalp, a pilot hole is drilled in the outer table of the skull by a stereotactically directed ⅛-inch drill. This pilot hole is the entry point along the planned stereotactic viewline and will be the center of the planned trephine. The scalp is then opened by a simple linear incision. A craniotomy is performed using a power trephine centered on the pilot hole. After the bone plug is removed, dural tack-up sutures are secured to drill holes around the edge of the craniotomy defect. The dura is then palpated. If it is tight and nonpulsating, it should not be opened. Maneuvers to reduce intracranial pressure by table position, hyperventilation, and barbiturate anesthesia are undertaken until the brain relaxes. The dura is then opened in a cruciate fashion, and the leaves are tacked back. From this point forward, the technical aspects of the stereotactic surgical procedure depends on whether the lesion is superficial or deep.

Superficial Lesions In the approach to superficial lesions (Fig. 32–8), the size of the trephine selected is equal to or slightly larger than the largest cross-sectional area of the tumor as viewed from the selected surgical approach angles that were determined during the planning phase. Because the pilot hole on which the trephine was turned was placed by means of the stereotactic frame, the location of the circular trephine in space is known. The edges of the cranial defect can be used as a fixed reference structure to which the computer-generated slices of the CT- and MRI-defined tumor volumes are referred. In each computer image display, a circle having the same exact size as the trephine is super-

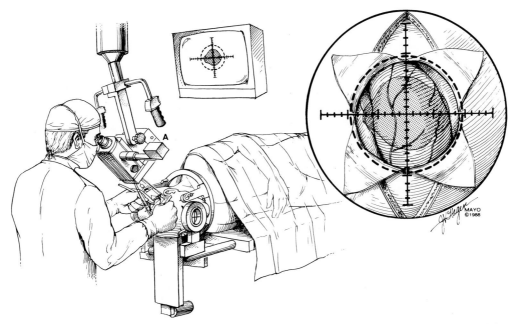

Figure 32–8 Illustration of method employed for the stereotactic resection of a superficial tumor. A trephine opening of the skull is performed, which is centered on a pilot hole drilled by means of the stereotactic frame. The computer displays the position of a tumor slice in proper position with respect to the location of the trephine at a specified distance along the viewline on the display monitor and into the heads-up display unit of the operating microscope (*A*). The image is sealed in the heads-up display and the microscope moved until the configuration of the trephine in the image display is exactly the same size as the actual trephine in the surgical field, and the image aligns to the trephine. The surgeon then uses the tumor slice image as a template that will aid in identification of the surgical plane between CT- and MRI-defined tumor and surrounding brain tissue. This facilitates isolation of the tumor from surrounding brain tissue. (From Kelly PJ: Volumetric stereotactic surgical resection of intra-axial brain mass lesions. Mayo Clin Proc 1988; 63:1186–1198.)

imposed on the surgical field by means of the heads-up display on the operating microscope. The surgeon superimposes the graphic image of the trephine over the actual trephine in the surgical field, using the most superficial computer-generated tumor slice as a template. A section of cortex having the same size and configuration as the superficial computer-generated slice image is removed with bipolar forceps and scissors. This cortex is nonviable when the tumor extends to within 1 cm of the surface. A plane is then developed around the tumor, using suction and bipolar forceps.

During tumor resection, the computer displays 1-mm thick slice configurations of the lesion at successively deeper levels in the correct spatial relationship to a circle that represents, in size and position, the location of the stereotactically placed trephine within the surgical field. It is best to first isolate the lesion from surrounding brain tissue and to keep the specimen intact. Computer displays of deep tumor slices along the viewline provide information on the expected configuration of the tumor as it will appear during the procedure. Measurements may be taken from the edges of the trephine opening and compared with the tumor-generated slice images. Slice depth can be determined by measuring from the level of the cranium at the edge of the trephine to the depth in the brain at which the surgeon is working. This is measured simply on the bipolar forceps with a millimeter ruler. This measurement, added to the distance from the outer surface of the probe carrier assembly on the stereotactic arc-quadrant, is subtracted from 135 mm (the distance from the outer surface of the probe carrier assembly to the focus of the arc-quadrant), which provides the distance in millimeters from the plane of the surgical field to the focal

point plane of the stereotactic arc-quadrant. The computer-generated tumor-slice image corresponding to this plane may then be displayed. If the surgeon notes that hyperventilation, mannitol administration, or loss of subarachnoid fluid has resulted in the brain collapsing away from the dura and inner table of the skull, the amount of collapse can be measured and the depth of the slice images updated accordingly.

In contrast to classic neurosurgical internal tumor decompression, the interior of the lesion should not be entered until late in the procedure, because the walls of the lesion may collapse and render subsequent computer-generated slice images inaccurate. Employing this method, we have found that intermediate and high-grade gliomas can be totally removed as intact specimens with negligible bleeding. In addition, infiltrated areas of brain parenchyma in low-grade gliomas located in nonessential brain tissue can be resected in the same way.

Deep Tumors Volumetric stereotactic resection of deep tumors (e.g., periventricular, basal ganglia, or thalamic tumors) requires stereotactic retractors, extra-long bipolar forceps, dissecting instruments, and the CO_2 laser.

The stereotactic retractors are mounted on the stereotactic arc-quadrant. The position of these retractors also is indicated on the computer display terminal in the operating room and in the heads-up display unit of the operating microscope. The position of the cylindrical retractor is shown as a circle in the computer display in relationship to the tumor slice (Fig. 32–9). During surgery, the computer-generated image of the retractor can be superimposed on the actual view of the retractor in the operating microscope by means of the heads-up display device.

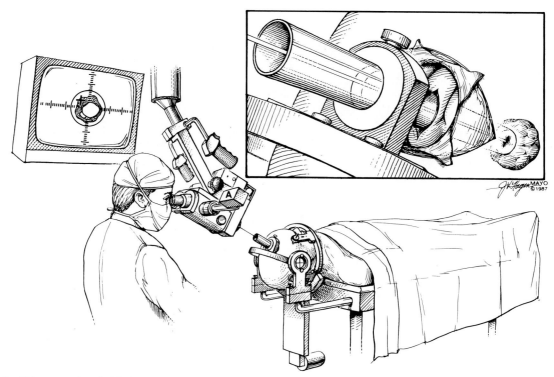

Figure 32–9 The stereotactic cylindrical retractor is employed during the resection of deep-seated lesions. The computer displays the configuration of a cross section of the retractor (*circle*) with respect to a selected slice through the tumor volume cut perpendicular to the surgical viewline. This information is displayed on a computer monitor in the operating room as well as in the heads-up display unit of the operating microscope (*A*). (From Kelly PJ: Volumetric stereotactic surgical resection of intra-axial brain masslesions. Mayo Clin Proc 1988; 63:1186–1198.)

The stereotactic resection of deep tumors is performed under general anesthesia, and the stereotactic headholder is again placed on the patient, who is then positioned in the stereotactic frame. The selected target point within the tumor volume is positioned into the focal point of the stereotactic arc-quadrant.

As previously described, the scalp is opened with a linear or slightly curved incision. A 1.5-inch trephine craniotomy is performed, and a cruciate opening of the dura is accomplished. A linear incision is made in the cortex, and the subcortical white matter incision is progressively deepened with the stereotactically directed CO_2 laser. Alternatively, a convenient sulcus can be split microsurgically and the cortical incision made in the depths of this sulcus.

The direction of the subcortical incision should be through nonessential brain tissue and in a direction parallel to major white matter fibers. As the incision is deepened, the stereotactic retractor is advanced to maintain the developing exposure. The computer has calculated the range of the tumor along the surgical viewline. At the outer border of the tumor, the laser beam is deflected laterally, a dilator is placed through the retractor, and the retractor is advanced. This creates a shaft from the surface to the outer border of the tumor. Using the computer display that demonstrates the relationship of the computer-generated tumor slice images to the edges of the retractor as a guide, the surgeon creates a plane of dissection around the lesion with the laser or with suction and bipolar forceps. The length of the suction and bipolar forceps is 10 to 15 mm longer than the stereotactic retractor; the plane between tumor and brain tissue can

therefore be developed for 10 to 15 mm beyond the end of the retractor, using the computer-generated slice images as a guide, which helps the surgeon to identify and develop that plane. Once the plane has been developed entirely around the tumor to a uniform depth, tumor tissue within the retractor is removed with 65 to 85 W of defocused laser power. In general, tumor is removed slice by slice, extending from the most superficial slices to the deepest. Hemostasis is secured using the extra-long bipolar forceps.

In our experience, shifting of a deep tumor occurs rarely, except in the following circumstances: (1) the tumor is associated with a tumor cyst that is entered early in the procedure, or (2) the tumor is adherent to the walls of the lateral or third ventricle, the opening of which causes loss of ventricular fluid.

Tumors larger than the retractor opening can be removed as follows: First, one side of the tumor is positioned under the retractor, and the surgeon uses the laser to create a plane between this side of the tumor and the brain tissue (Fig. 32–10A). The display image is then translated on the computer display terminal to position the other side of the lesion under the retractor. The computer calculates new stereotactic frame adjustments that are duplicated on the servomotor-driven slide mechanism of the frame by remote control. This side of the tumor is then separated from brain tissue with bipolar forceps or with the laser (see Fig. 32–10B). After isolating the lesion from surrounding brain tissue, it may be vaporized by laser or removed by biopsy forceps and by suction to the level to which the plane between tumor and surrounding brain has been developed (see Fig. 32–10C).

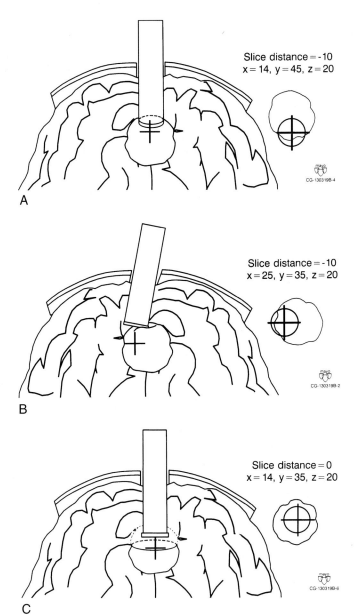

Slice distance = -10
x = 14, y = 45, z = 20

CG-130319B-4

Slice distance = -10
x = 25, y = 35, z = 20

CG-130319B-2

Slice distance = 0
x = 14, y = 35, z = 20

CG-130319B-6

Figure 32–10 Method for resection of large subcortical tumor by translations. *A,* The image of the stereotactic cylindrical retractor is moved on the screen and the computer calculates new stereotactic coordinates that place the edge of the tumor under the retractor. *B,* After developing the plane between the posterior part of the tumor and the brain, the retractor image is translated on the computer screen, and coordinates are executed to place the right side of the tumor under the retractor on the stereotactic frame; plane is developed here as the surgeon is guided by the slice images, which help in the identification of that plane. *C,* After circumscribing the superficial parts of the tumor from the brain, the circumscribed portion is resected and the retractor is advanced to a new level.

Then the plane between residual tumor and brain tissue proceeds using the translations and edge dissection techniques described. Tumors are never "internally decompressed" during stereotactic resection procedures—the walls of the tumor cavity would close inward and render the stereotactic images inaccurate. In stereotactic resection, the edges of the tumor are separated from surrounding brain tissue and tumors are removed in layers, with the surgeon proceeding from the most superficial layers to the deepest.

GLIOMA TREATMENT STRATEGIES

The two most critical features of a glial neoplasm for surgical decision-making using computer-assisted stereotactic technology are the gross anatomic location and the microsurgical anatomy of the tumor. Gross anatomic location is determined from the axial, coronal, and sagittal MRIs. Information about the microsurgical histology can be gleaned from a careful analysis of enhanced and non-enhanced CT and MRIs. An algorithm for the treatment of specific tumor types is given in Figure 32–11.

High-Grade Astrocytomas and Oligodendrogliomas

CT contrast-enhancing neoplasms with surrounding areas of hypodensity are most typically grade III or IV astrocytomas or high-grade oligodendrogliomas. Grade IV astrocytomas are often distinguishable by a central area of hypodensity corresponding to central necrosis. With these tumors, the volume of the enhancing tumor (tumor tissue proper) is determined using computer-assisted volumetric reconstruction, which is compared with the entire T2 prolongation volume (tumor tissue proper plus infiltrating tumor cells in normal parenchyma).

When the contrast-enhancing volume (tumor tissue proper) is *less than one-third* the total volume of the lesion, as indicated by CT hypodensity ("edema") and/or the region of T2 prolongation on the T2-weighted MRI (tumor tissue plus infiltrating tumor cells within normal parenchyma), little value is likely to be gained by surgical removal of the enhancing mass. In patients with such lesions we recommend stereotactic computer-assisted biopsy of the enhancing portion of the mass to obtain a tissue diagnosis. This is followed by radiation and chemotherapy, if appropriate. Accurate biopsy is necessary so that the enhancing portion of the lesion is sampled, as this theoretically represents the highest-grade area of the tumor.

When the contrast-enhancing volume is *greater than one-third* the total volume of the lesion, as indicated by CT hypodensity ("edema") and/or the region of T2 prolongation on the T2-weighted MRI, resection of the contrast-enhancing tumor tissue mass is usually recommended in patients younger than 65 years. Patients older than 65 years should undergo stereotactic biopsy of the contrast-enhancing mass followed by radiation, as we have found that the benefit of surgery in this subset of patients is questionable.[24]

High-grade gliomas located in the poles of a lobe are best removed using standard frontal, temporal, and occipital lobectomy techniques, because removal of the enhancing tumor as well as of the surrounding infiltrating tumor cells may be undertaken with little chance of neurologic deficit. Tumors in these locations do not require specialized stereotactic technology.

For high-grade gliomas located near eloquent cortex or deep wthin the brain, volumetric stereotactic resection is recommended to preserve neurologic function. In these locations, only the enhancing region of the tumor should be removed, as this contains tightly packed tumor cells without intervening functional parenchyma. The surrounding hypo-

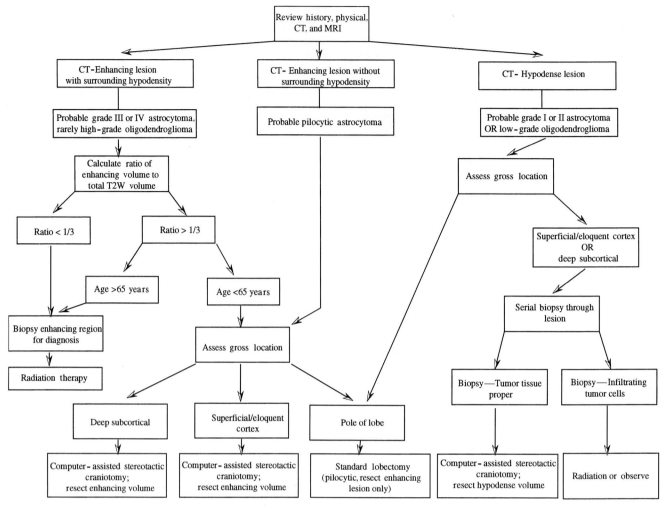

Figure 32–11 Algorithm for surgical decision-making in glial tumors.

dense region contains infiltrating tumor cells within normal parenchyma. In eloquent cortex, removal of this hypodense region may result in undesirable neurologic deficit. For superficial lesions, computer-assisted stereotactic trephine craniotomy is employed. The outer borders of the trephine are just beyond the edge of the enhancing portion of the tumor, as described previously. An en bloc volumetric resection of the entire CT-enhancing part of the tumor is performed by establishing a plane between CT-enhancing tumor and surrounding CT hypodensity, as guided by the computer-generated image projected through the heads-up display. For deep-seated lesions, one of the various trajectories described previously is undertaken. Computer-assisted stereotaxy allows for accurate intraoperative localization of the lesion. The entire CT-enhancing region of the tumor is removed, and surrounding CT hypodense regions are spared.

Pilocytic Astrocytomas

CT-enhancing neoplasms *without* surrounding hypodensity are most typically pilocytic astrocytomas. These lesions are curable by complete surgical resection because no infiltrating

tumor cells occur in the area surrounding the enhancing tumor tissue proper. Therefore, resection of all of the enhancing tumor without removal of the surrounding normal functional brain is the goal of surgery. The algorithm for resection of these lesions is also based on tumor location. Superficial and deep lesions are resected with computer-assisted stereotactic methods, whereas standard methods are employed for polar lesions. Most of these lesions are located in deep structures, such as the thalamus, and are particularly amenable to computer-assisted craniotomy.

Low-Grade Astrocytomas and Oligodendrogliomas

Hypodense lesions on CT most typically represent low-grade astrocytomas or oligodendrogliomas. The typical histologic finding for these lesions is infiltrating tumor cells within normal parenchyma, although tumor tissue proper may rarely be identified. When such lesions are located in nonessential cortex, such as the frontal or temporal poles, complete resection of the hypodense lesion is recommended.

When such lesions are located near eloquent cortex or

deep within the brain, serial stereotactic biopsy is recommended, with specimens taken from the edges as well as through the center of the lesions, because removal of these hypodense tumors could result in major neurologic deficit. In most cases, serial biopsies demonstrate tumor cells amidst intact and presumably functional parenchyma. In these cases, in which the infiltrative lesion involves eloquent cortex, resection by stereotactic or other techniques is ill-advised, because resection of the tumor amounts to resection of functioning brain parenchyma. These patients should be observed or treated with radiation and/or chemotherapy as deemed appropriate for the cell type and grade of the tumor.

On rare occasions, the serial biopsy shows that the majority of the CT hypodense mass comprises closely packed tumor cells that do not enhance. These lesions can be safely resected from most anatomic locations using computer-assisted stereotactic techniques, because no functional parenchyma is found within the lesion. In these instances, the volume resected corresponds to the CT hypodense region as well as to the region defined by T1 and T2 prolongation on the MRI.

CLINICAL EXPERIENCE

Using the algorithm in Figure 32–11, between July 1984 and July 1993, one of us (P.J.K.) operated on 514 patients with gliomas, using computer-assisted volumetric stereotactic resection. Tumor location and histologic characteristics are outlined in Tables 32–3 and 32–4, respectively. The patients ranged in age from 2 to 82 years. The overall morbidity was 6.8% and mortality was 0.9%. These values

TABLE 32–3
LOCATION OF GLIAL TUMORS IN 519 PATIENTS UNDERGOING STEREOTACTIC RESECTION

Location	Total	Right	Left
Supratentorial			
Central	22	8	14
Frontal	127	58	69
Posterior/deep frontal	22	9	13
Frontoparietal	16	8	8
Frontotemporal	5	1	4
Parietal	71	30	41
Parieto-occipital	8	2	6
Temporal	70	32	38
Temporo-occipital	7	2	5
Temporo-parietal	25	8	17
Occipital	9	3	6
Basal ganglia	8	6	2
Thalamus	51	24	27
Cingulate gyrus	5	1	4
Corpus callosum	3	—	—
Septum pellucidum	3	—	—
Third ventricle	3	—	—
Lateral ventricle	19	11	8
Total	474		
Infratentorial			
Deep cerebellar hemisphere	19	12	7
Vermis	2	—	—
Brainstem	16	—	—
Fourth ventricle	3	—	—
Total	40		

TABLE 32–4
HISTOLOGIC SUBTYPES OF 514 GLIAL TUMORS

Astrocytoma	239
Grade IV	175
Grade III	34
Grade II	23
Grade I	7
Pilocytic astrocytoma	87
Oligodendroglioma	85
Grade 4	5
Grade 3	23
Grade 2	46
Grade 1	11
Mixed oligoastrocytoma	61
Ependymoma	15
Subependymoma	14
Ganglioglioma	13

compare favorably with other surgical glioma series. For example, Ciric and co-workers,[25] Ammirati and associates,[26] and Fadul and colleagues[27] reported morbidities of 12.5%, 16%, and 28%, respectively, using conventional techniques.

High-Grade Gliomas

Of the 514 patients who underwent computer-assisted volumetric stereotactic resection, 175 had grade IV astrocytomas (glioblastoma multiforme) and 34 had grade III astrocytomas. Complete removal of all CT-defined contrast-enhancing portions of high-grade glial neoplasms from neurologically important areas was performed with a low morbidity.[6, 4, 22, 28] Postoperative CT studies demonstrate an absence of contrast enhancement around the surgical defect (Fig. 32–12).

One of us (P.J.K.) reported a median postoperative survival of 50.6 weeks in patients with grade IV astrocytomas treated with complete volumetric resection of the contrast-enhancing tumor and postoperative external-beam radiation therapy (50 to 65 Gy).[28] This compares favorably with series of patients undergoing conventional resection and radiation in which median survivals of 36 to 39.5 weeks have been reported.[29, 30] Salcman reviewed the overall experience of patients with grade IV astrocytomas by combining the results of 17 reports on 1,561 patients.[31] The median survival for patients treated with surgery and radiation was 37 weeks. Of course, comparisons between conventional and stereotactic methods are difficult because of biases associated with nonrandomized patient populations. However, aggressive resection of all CT enhancing tumor using volumetric resection may be associated with a prolongation of survival over conventional tumor debulking methods. In addition, Devaux and co-workers[28] demonstrated that volumetric stereotactic resection followed by radiation led to a statistically significant extension of survival when compared with radiation therapy after biopsy alone (median survival, 50.6 weeks vs. 33 weeks, respectively).

Nevertheless, volumetric stereotactic resection does not cure high-grade gliomas. Following resection, new areas of contrast enhancement on CT scanning developed within low-density areas surrounding the surgical defect within 6 to 9 months of the procedure. Preoperative stereotactic T2-

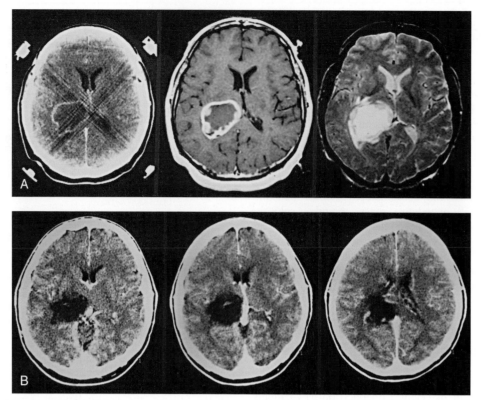

Figure 32–12 *A*, High-grade glial tumor featuring a solid tumor tissue mass defined by CT and MRI contrast enhancement and surrounded by parenchyma infiltrated by isolated tumor cells indicated by increased T2 on MRI. Note that the zone of infiltration (T2 prolongation) in this particular tumor is small in comparison to the volume of the contrast enhancing mass. *B*, The volume of this tumor, defined by contrast enhancement, can be resected with good postoperative results and benefit to the patient in terms of prolongation of survival and quality of life.

weighted MRI in high-grade astrocytomas always demonstrates much larger areas of abnormality than are indicated by contrast enhancement on CT scanning.[11, 12] Examination of stereotactic serial biopsy specimens obtained in patients with high-grade gliomas from the MRI-defined abnormalities outside the contrast-enhancing tumor mass reveals larger areas of intact edematous brain parenchyma infiltrated by aggressive isolated tumor cells.[8–12] In fact, this edematous infiltrated parenchyma usually extends up to, and in some cases beyond, the area of signal prolongation abnormality on the T2-weighted MRI.[11, 12] Although it would be technically possible, using volumetric stereotaxy, to resect the volume defined by the T2-weighted MRI abnormality, and although this, in theory, would substantially prolong postoperative survival,[13,14] unacceptable neurologic deficits would result from removal of the intact, albeit infiltrated, parenchyma. It is this area of infiltrated normal parenchyma in which radiation is most effective. It is toward this histologic area that new innovative treatments must be directed, including biologic response modifiers and genetic therapies. Obviously, as the ratio of infiltrated normal parenchyma to tumor tissue proper increases, the effectiveness of surgery decreases, and the importance of other therapeutic interventions increases.

Low-Grade Gliomas

As defined in the algorithm in Figure 32–11, resectability of low-grade gliomas depends on the histologic composition and the relation to eloquent brain tissue. This strategy holds for non-pilocytic astrocytomas, mixed oligoastrocytomas, and pure oligodendrogliomas. In the majority of cases, stereotactic serial biopsy of the non-enhancing tumors were found to comprise infiltrated intact parenchyma with little tumor tissue proper.[11, 12] Resection of this group of low-grade astrocytomas was *not* performed, because it would have necessitated removal of functionally intact parenchyma infiltrated by tumor cells and would have resulted in an unacceptable neurologic deficit.[6, 22] An example of a nonresectable tumor is shown in Figure 32–13. In this case, serial biopsy confirmed a low-grade astrocytoma composed of infiltrated intact parenchyma deep in the right parietal lobe in a patient whose only symptoms were seizures.

However, some of the infiltrating lesions involve non-eloquent brain tissue and are resectable, as removing the infiltrated parenchyma is not associated with a postoperative neurologic deficit. In our series of 30 patients with grades I and II astrocytomas, 24 patients (80%) had non-enhancing infiltrating lesions located in non-eloquent brain regions. Similarly, of the 57 grades I and II oligodendrogliomas in our surgical series, 42 (74%) were non-enhancing infiltrative lesions located in nonessential brain regions. In each case, the entire hypodense region of the tumor was resected. A resectable non-enhancing low-grade tumor is shown in Figure 32–14. This 37-year-old man presented with motor seizures from a low-grade, non-enhancing, apparently circumscribed lesion in the posterior third of the middle frontal convolution. At stereotactic craniotomy, mapping established

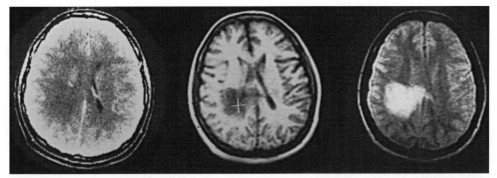

Figure 32–13 CT and MRI of a low-grade astrocytoma, the resection of which is ill advised. Serial biopsy of the lesion revealed isolated astrocytic tumor cells within intact parenchyma. The lesion is located deep within functional parietal lobe. Most low-grade gliomas consist of isolated tumor cells that reside in and infiltrate a volume of intact brain tissue. Resection of these lesions is, in fact, resection of functioning (albeit diseased) brain parenchyma.

that the motor strip was immediately posterior to the tumor. The lesion, found to consist of heavily infiltrated parenchyma without solid tumor tissue, was completely excised, and the patient had no postoperative neurologic deficit.

Occasionally, low-grade gliomas can be composed of solid tumor tissue only and are hypodense and non-enhancing on imaging studies. However, it is impossible to determine on imaging studies whether the lesion is made up of solid tumor tissue that is entirely resectable or if it consists mostly of infiltrated parenchyma that cannot be resected (see Fig. 32–11). In important brain areas, a serial stereotactic biopsy should be performed as a first step. If tumor tissue proper, without any infiltrated parenchyma, is found, the lesion can be resected safely as shown in Figure 32–15. In our experi-

ence, 6 (20%) of 30 low-grade astrocytomas and 15 (26%) of 57 low-grade oligodendrogliomas were composed of tumor tissue proper, which could be resected.

Pilocytic Astrocytomas

Pilocytic astrocytomas are histologically circumscribed and are rarely infiltrative. One of us (P.J.K.) has operated on 87 pilocytic astrocytomas in the 9 years reviewed in this series. These tumors exhibit prominent contrast enhancement on CT and MRI with the histologic borders being defined accurately by the contrast enhancement (i.e., no area of surrounding hypodensity is present on CT, nor is T2-weighted

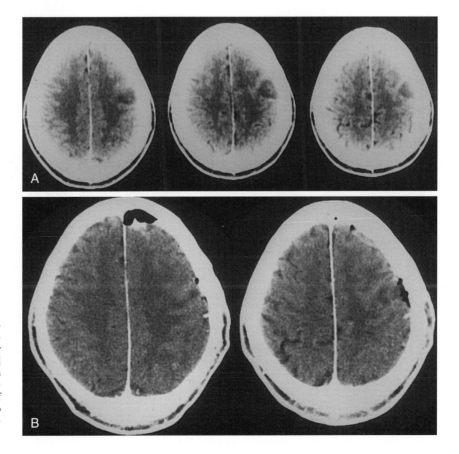

Figure 32–14 *A,* Preoperative CT showing a hypodense non-enhancing tumor located in the posterior frontal area of the left hemisphere. This tumor is resectable because of its location in nonessential brain. *B,* Postoperative CT after gross total resection of volume CT-defined hypodensity. Histologic analysis revealed a low-grade glioma composed of infiltrated brain parenchyma, which contained no tumor tissue. Patient was neurologically intact preoperatively and postoperatively.

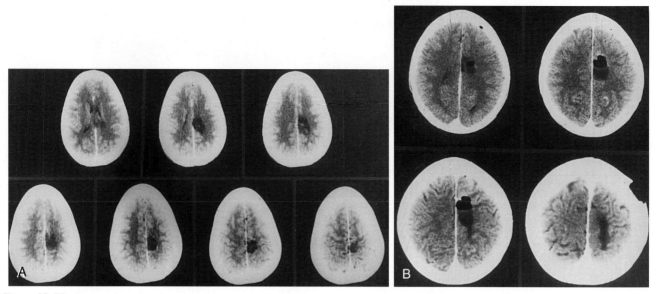

Figure 32–15 Preoperative (*A*) and postoperative (*B*) CT images of a low-grade non-enhancing oligodendroglioma in the deep anterior parietal area. A stereotactic serial biopsy of the lesion prior to resection revealed solid tumor tissue only. This histologic findings made resection possible. The patient was neurologically intact postoperatively.

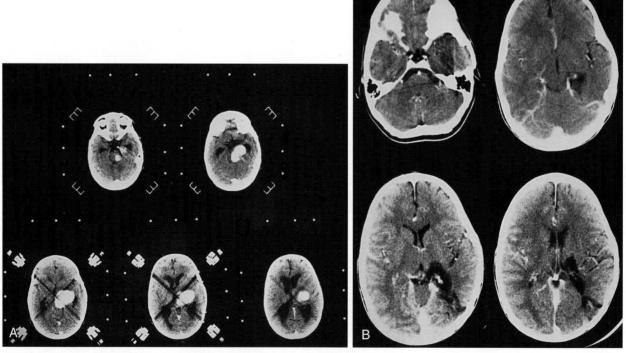

Figure 32–16 Preoperative (*A*) and postoperative (*B*) CT images of large pilocytic astrocytoma that was completely resected from left thalamus and midbrain in a 27-year-old man.

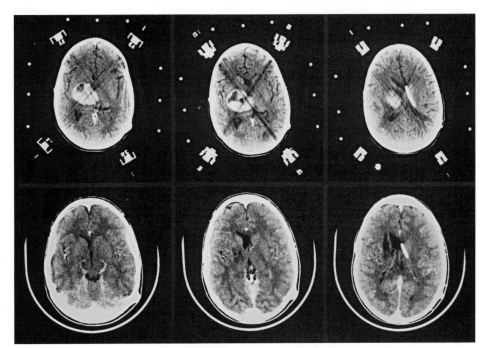

Figure 32–17 Preoperative (*top row*) and postoperative (*bottom row*) CT scans of a 7-year-old girl with a pilocytic astrocytoma involving the right thalamus, internal capsule, and basal ganglia. The patient had a mild hemiparesis preoperatively, which was essentially unchanged postoperatively.

increased signal seen on MRI). Therefore, these lesions are usually resectable and potentially surgically curable (Figs. 32–16 and 32–17). However, many pilocytic astrocytomas are located in deep subcortical locations, such as the thalamus. Resection of lesions in this location using standard craniotomy techniques has been associated with a morbidity of almost 30%.[32] Consequently, many physicians elect to treat these lesions with subtotal resection, radiation, and shunting for hydrocephalus. Computer-assisted stereotactic surgery is ideal for these lesions because it can accurately locate the lesion and define the plane of surgical resection. In a previous series of pilocytic astrocytomas of the thalamus,[19] complete resection (as determined by postoperative CT) was achieved in 73%, and only 5% residual tumor was noted in 26% of cases. At follow-up, 95% of patients were alive and well. None had received postoperative radiation.

CONCLUSION

Computer-assisted volumetric stereotactic craniotomy provides several advantages over conventional freehand neurosurgical techniques in the management of glial neoplasms. The stereotactic method maintains surgical orientation while the procedure extends below the cortical surface, and the approach is preplanned to disrupt as little important brain tissue as possible. Beyond the gross appearance of a tumor at surgery and its apparent margins on visual inspection, the computer display images provide additional information to the surgeon about where tumor boundaries lie in relationship to surrounding brain tissue. The method allows resection of as much of a lesion as desired. This is particularly important in glial neoplasms, in which the infiltrative biologic behavior of the disease process itself renders much of the tumor unresectable and makes the border between resectable and unresectable tumor difficult to identify. With volumetric

stereotactic surgery, the extent of tumor resection in both low- and high-grade glial neoplasms is more controlled, and treatment strategies for each type of glioma can be defined precisely.

REFERENCES

1. Goerss S, Kelly PJ, Kall B, et al: A computed tomographic stereotactic adaptation system. Neurosurgery 1982; 10:375–379.
2. Kelly PJ, Alker GJ: A stereotactic approach to deep seated CNS neoplasms using the carbon dioxide laser. Surg Neurol 1981; 15:331–334.
3. Kelly PJ, Alker GJ, Goerss S: Computer assisted stereotactic laser microsurgery for the treatment of intracranial neoplasms. Neurosurgery 1982; 10:324–331.
4. Kelly PJ, Alker GJ, Kall B, et al: Precision resection of intra-axial CNS lesions by CT-based stereotactic craniotomy and computer monitored CO₂ laser. Acta Neurochir 1983; 68:1–9.
5. Kelly PJ, Kall BA, Goerss SJ: Transposition of volumetric information derived from computed tomography scanning into stereotactic space. Surg Neurol 1984; 21:465–471.
6. Kelly P: Volumetric stereotactic surgical resection of intra-axial brain mass lesions. Mayo Clin Proc 1988; 63:1186–1198.
7. Shapiro WR: Treatment of neuroectodermal brain tumors. Ann Neurol 1982; 12:231–237.
8. Burger PC, Dubois PJ, Schold SC, et al: Computerized tomographic and pathologic studies of the untreated, quiescent, and recurrent glioblastoma multiforme. Neurosurgery 1983; 59:159–168.
9. Daumas-Duport C, Monsaingeon V, Szenthe L, et al: Serial stereotactic biopsies: A double histological code of gliomas according to malignancy and 3-D configuration as an aid to therapeutic decision and assessment of results. Appl Neurophysiol 1982; 45:431–437.
10. Daumas-Duport C, Scheithauer BW, Kelly PJ: A histologic and cytologic method for the spatial definition of gliomas. Mayo Clin Proc 1987; 62:435–449.
11. Kelly PJ, Daumas-Duport C, Kispert DB, et al: Imaging-based stereotactic serial biopsies in untreated intracranial glial neoplasms. J Neurosurg 1987; 66:865–874.
12. Kelly PJ, Daumas-Duport C, Scheithauer BW, et al: Stereotactic histologic correlations of computed tomography and magnetic resonance imaging defined abnormalities in patients with glial neoplasms. Mayo Clin Proc 1987; 62:450–459.

13. Hoshino T: A commentary on the biology and growth kinetics of low grade and high grade gliomas. J Neurosurg 1984; 27:388–400.

14. Hoshino T, Barker M, Wilson CB, et al: Cell kinetics of human gliomas. Neurosurgery 1972; 37:15–26.

15. Clarke RH, Horsley V: On a method of investigating the deep ganglia and tracts of the central nervous system (cerebellum). Br Med J 1906; 2:1799–1800.

16. Horsley V, Clarke RH: The structure and function of the cerebellum examined by a new method. Brain 1908; 31:45–124.

17. Brown RA: A computerized tomography–computer graphics approach to stereotaxic localization. Neurosurgery 1979; 50:715–720.

18. Apuzzo MLJ, Sabshin JK: Computed tomographic guidance stereotaxis in the management of intracranial mass lesions. Neurosurgery 1983; 12:277–285.

19. Kelly PJ: Stereotactic biopsy and resection of thalamic astrocytomas. Neurosurgery 1989; 25:185–195.

20. Coffey RJ, Lundsford LD: Stereotactic surgery for mass lesions of the midbrain and pons. Neurosurgery 1985; 17:12–18.

21. Kelly PJ, Goerss SJ, Kall BA: Evolution of contemporary instrumentation for computer-assisted stereotactic surgery. Surg Neurol 1988; 30:204–215.

22. Kelly PJ, Kall B, Goerss S, et al: Computer-assisted stereotaxic resection of intra-axial brain neoplasms. J Neurosurg 1986; 64:427–439.

23. Leksell L: A stereotaxic apparatus for intracerebral surgery. Acta Chir Scand 1949; 99:229–233.

24. Kelly PJ, Hunt C: The limited value of cytoreductive surgery in elderly patients with malignant gliomas. Neurosurgery 1994; 34:62–67.

25. Ciric I, Rovin R, Cozzens JW, et al: Role of surgery in the treatment of malignant cerebral gliomas. *In* Apuzzo MLJ (ed): Malignant Cerebral Gliomas. Park Ridge, Ill, AANS Publications Committee, 1990, pp 141–153.

26. Ammirati M, Vick N, Liao Y, et al: Effect of the extent of surgical resection on survival and quality of life in patients with supratentorial glioblastomas and anaplastic astrocytomas. Neurosurgery 1987; 21: 201–206.

27. Fadul C, Wood J, Thaler H, et al: Morbidity and mortality of craniotomy for excision of supratentorial gliomas. Neurology 1988; 38:1374–1379.

28. Devaux BC, O'Fallon JR, Kelly PJ: Resection, biopsy and survival in malignant glial neoplasms: A retrospective study of clinical parameters, therapy and outcome. J Neurosurg 1993; 78:767–775.

29. Walker MD, Green SB, Byar DP, et al: Randomized comparison of radiotherapy and nitrosurea for the treatment of malignant glioma after surgery. N Engl J Med 1980; 303:1323–1329.

30. Kreth FW, Warnke PC, Scheremet R, et al: Surgical resection and radiation therapy versus biopsy and radiation therapy in the treatment of glioblastoma multiforme. J Neurosurg 1993; 78:762–766.

31. Salcman M: Survival in glioblastoma: Historical perspective. Neurosurgery 1980; 7:435–439.

32. Greenwood J: Radical surgery of tumors of the thalamus, hypothalamus and third ventricle area. Surg Neurol 1973; 1:29–33.

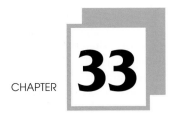

33

Interactive Image-Guided Surgical Technology for Glial Tumor Resection

Malignant primary brain tumors remain a considerable challenge to the expertise of the clinician. Surgery remains the mainstay of glioma therapy. It provides the means of obtaining absolute tissue diagnosis and mapping tumor margins, of performing mechanical cytoreduction, and of guiding focused ionizing radiation with brachytherapy or radiosurgery. Emerging technologies of surgical navigation promise to significantly benefit every neurosurgeon who operates on glial tumors by making precise intraoperative spatial information universally available.

Throughout every operation, a neurosurgeon must maintain a precise sense of complex three-dimensional anatomic relationships. A variety of techniques assist physicians in localizing the relevant pathologic lesion. The advent of digital scanning techniques has resulted in medical images of exquisite detail which revolutionized the planning of certain neurosurgical operations. When the "addresses" of points in one image volume are mapped onto the addresses of points in another image volume or onto physical space itself, these volumes are said to have been *registered* with one another. By registering image spaces with one another and with physical space, medical images become true, point-to-point maps that are capable of precise surgical guidance.

Stereotactic methodology has been employed by neurosurgeons to map image space onto physical space.[33] This is accomplished by application of an external frame of reference to the patient's cranium to register medical images and to provide a mechanical platform (the aiming arc assembly) for a device that precisely accesses a preselected target point. Although most major stereotactic systems have incorporated digital scan imaging information, these apparatus remain structurally very similar to the original plain film devices.

Because stereotactic methodology imposes a restrictive discipline on the surgical process, it cannot be successfully utilized in all cases. These limitations have led some investigators to pursue novel technologies for surgical navigation, referred to as *interactive image-guided neurosurgery*.

INTERACTIVE IMAGE-GUIDED NEUROSURGICAL TECHNOLOGY

The new systems of surgical navigation consist of four fundamental elements:

1. A method for registration of image and physical space.
2. An intraoperative localization device.
3. A computer video display of medical images.
4. Methods of real-time intraoperative feedback.

Registration of Image and Physical Space

Computed tomography (CT), magnetic resonance imaging (MRI), and positron emission tomography (PET) scans are obtained as three-dimensional volumetric data bases, even though they are usually displayed as a series of two-dimensional scan slices along a given axis. The images contain a coordinate system, conferred by the scanner during acquisition, which defines a temporary "address" for each point in that imaging volume. No inherent relationship exists between any of the particular addresses within one image and the addresses assigned to the same points during acquisition of another image. Likewise, no inherent relationship exists outside the scanner between the temporary addresses in any image space for points and the addresses in physical space of corresponding points in the patient's body.

If medical images are to be used as maps for surgical navigation, these sets of medical images must be mapped, or registered, onto one another and onto the physical space of the patient's anatomy. In this way, a quantitative relationship is established on a point-by-point basis between the information in one image and the information in another image or in physical space. This registration can employ information obtained preoperatively, intraoperatively, and postoperatively.

Once registration has been accomplished, then two other techniques may be employed for the processing or manipulating of information in these image volumes. These techniques simply alter the way in which these data are displayed. *Reformatting/reorientation* of an image is the reslicing of that image volume cube along a different axial direction than the one initially chosen for its two-dimensional slice mode of display. *Rendering* is an alternative means of displaying some of the information contained within the original image volume data cube: after defining (or segmenting) a surface (e.g., the skin/air or the skull/skin interface), this surface can be displayed on the two-dimensional video screen in such a way as to prevent the appearance of a photograph of a three-dimensional object in perspective.

Registration techniques may be classified into the following types: (1) point methods, including stereotactic frame systems; (2) curve and surface methods; (3) moment and principal axes methods; (4) correlation methods; (5) interactive methods; and (6) atlas methods.

Point-based registration methods define corresponding points in different images and in physical space, determine their spatial coordinates, and calculate a geometric transformation between the volumes. These points may be intrinsic, and may be based on patient-specific anatomic landmarks. Although this allows registration to be fully retrospective, the selection and definition of anatomic landmarks has proved to be a labor-intensive process that is subject to significant inaccuracies. Extrinsic point-based registration methods, requiring artificially applied markers, do not allow for retrospective registration of images. However, several significant advantages accrue with this technique. Any and all imaging modalities and physical space can be registered as long as a detectable marker can be constructed. The markers may be designed for optimal automatic or semiautomatic detection, allowing for straightforward extraction of their positions from medical images. The advantages of point-based registration methods have led to their widespread use throughout a variety of surgical guidance systems.

Two types of markers have been used: (1) mobile markers, which are taped or otherwise affixed to soft tissue, such as the scalp or skin, and (2) rigidly affixed markers that anchor to the skull or other bone. Mobile markers are easily affixed to soft tissues, but are associated with inconsistent registration accuracy. Rigidly affixed markers require a minor surgical intervention for their application, but this disadvantage is offset by the dramatically increased level of registration accuracy afforded by rigid fixation. Additionally, rigid fixation of markers provides a unique advantage: unlike any other form of registration, this method produces a known geometric relationship between the fiducial markers, thereby precisely defining for each individual patient what the registration accuracy will be for that particular surgical intervention.

Surface-based registration systems fit sets of points extracted from contours in one image set to surface models extracted from contours in other images or physical coordinates of the patient's cranium. This is the only registration technique able to be both fully retrospective and to register image to physical space. The accuracy, however, is less than that of point-based registration methods.

Other registration techniques of limited value to neurosurgeons include those based on principal axes, correlation, and interactive means. None of these techniques can register images to physical space, therefore precluding their surgical use. They are primarily employed by radiologists as retrospective methods for registering sets of medical images.

Anatomic atlases of intracranial landmarks have long been available. Unfortunately, it has proven difficult to adequately define the warping necessary to map such atlas coordinates onto an individual brain distorted by pathologic processes and mass lesions. Nonetheless, to amplify their utility for diagnosis and surgical planning, it is probable that atlas methods will be combined with methods using extrinsic point registration.

Intraoperative Localization Devices

ACTIVE ROBOTIC ARMS

In 1985, Kwoh and colleagues[25] began to use a PUMA Industrial Robot (Westinghouse Electric) for CT-directed stereotactic surgery (Fig. 33–1). The sheer bulk of the PUMA robotic arm proved restrictive when used in a surgical setting. Drake and co-workers[12] reported a clinical series of pediatric brain tumors resected with the aid of the PUMA robotic arm. The Zeiss Corporation has married an active robotic arm mechanism to an optical microscope in the MKM system, which allows access to viewlines that are preoperatively defined as *trajectories*.

PASSIVE LOCALIZATION ARMS

The use of a passive localization arm for neurosurgical guidance was first described by Watanabe and colleagues (Fig. 33–2).[46, 47] This "Neuronavigator" consisted of a personal computer, an image display monitor, and an articulated arm with six joints. The arm endpoint position was determined by digitizing the angles at each of the arm joints. Registration was accomplished with four skin-mounted fiducial markers. This device proved far less intrusive to the surgical procedure than did an active robotic arm. The use

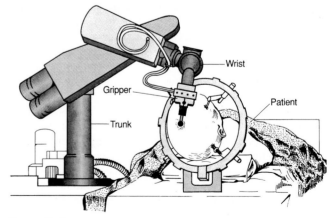

Figure 33–1   Active robotic arm. (From Drake JM, Prudencio J, Holowka S: A comparison of the PUMA robotic system and the ISG Viewing Wand for neurosurgery. *In* Maciunas RJ (ed): Interactive Image-Guided Neurosurgery. Park Ridge, Ill, American Association of Neurological Surgeons, 1993, pp 121–134.)

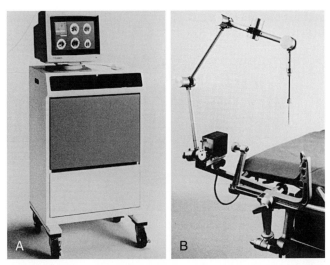

Figure 33–2 Computer video display of intraoperative endpoint position on preoperative images *(A)* and passive articulated localization arm *(B)* of Neuronavigator. (From Watanabe E: The Neuronavigator: A potentiometer-based localization arm system. *In* Maciunas RJ (ed): Interactive Image-Guided Neurosurgery. Park Ridge, Ill, American Association of Neurological Surgeons, 1993, pp 135–148.)

of the arm in "sampling" the surgical space proved to be intuitive in use. Surgery could proceed in a standard fashion, with the localization arm being employed only when necessary. This elegant system had two major practical disadvantages: First, the potentiometers used for angle position detectors in each of the arm joints are not finely incremental and allow for only a coarse measurement of angular displacement. The linearity of potentiometers is also inconstant, introducing fluctuations into the measurement of the angles. The second disadvantage of the system lies in the limited computational abilities supporting the video display of medical images.

The ISG Viewing Wand System (ISG Technologies, Toronto, Canada) has been employed by numerous surgeons during its prolonged preclinical testing.[12] ISG Technologies employs custom-designed and -constructed computer hardware and software for its surgical planning and intraoperative image display programs. The intraoperative localization device (ILD) for the ISG Viewing Wand System is a passive localization arm (FARO Medical Technologies, Miami). The ergonomics of this arm are praiseworthy, although it has a tendency toward backlash and forward drag at times. This six-jointed arm employs electrogoniometers for angular detectors, limiting its accuracy and precision and leaving it vulnerable to environmental electromagnetic interference.

Guthrie and associates[18] have reported on a series of passive localization arms with elegant counterbalancing of the joints (Radionics, Burlington, Mass). The use of high-resolution optical encoders for extreme accuracy in passive localization arms was pioneered by Maciunas and co-workers.[31] Robotics simulation procedures were employed for computer modeling of optimal mechanical and electronic configurations, given the surgical task. Employing 4-mm thick slices for tomograms, intraoperative error was 1.67 ± 0.43 mm. The arm can be sterilized and accepts multiple end-effectors at its terminal link. In this manner, a variety

of surgical tools can be employed in addition to a simple pointer. Rapid movements of the localization arm in physical space are instantly displayed as image changes on the video screen.

SONIC DIGITIZER TRIANGULATION

In 1986, Roberts and colleagues[40] reported on initial investigations into "frameless stereotaxy" (Fig. 33–3). Spark-gap ultrasonic emitters were attached to an operating microscope in a known geometric configuration. Sound detectors for the ultrasonic noises were arrayed throughout the operating room. The combination of the ultrasonic emitters and their detectors created a three-dimensionally registered space through which the microscope moved. The focal length of the optics of the microscope was known, and the microscope's focal point became, accordingly, a virtual end effector for the microscope/spark-gap emitter assembly. In this way, the microscope could be used as an optical ILD for patient landmarks. With the patient in position in the surgical suite, three radiopaque external fiducial markers—which had been attached to the patient's scalp at CT scanning—could be registered to preoperative CT images by aiming the focal point of the microscope at the three markers in sequence. In this manner, the image space of preoperative scan images, the intracranial space of the patient's head, and the extracranial space in which the operating microscope and its ultrasonic emitters and detectors reside were registered. This highly sophisticated technology has proved beneficial during craniotomies by localizing preoperatively defined intracranial targets using the operating microscope.[41]

A fundamental limitation to this system is the use of spark-gap emitters. Because the speed of sound in air is highly temperature dependent, and the distances between ultrasonic emitters and their detectors are long, the temperature fluctuations commonly encountered in surgical suites cause variations in the speed of sound that are sufficient to produce potentially large errors in target position location. The paths between detectors and emitters must be kept clear to prevent signal displacement by intervening structures or

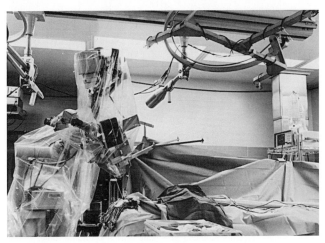

Figure 33–3 Sonic localizing operating microscope fitted with spark-gap emitters. Sound detectors mounted about the operating room. (From Roberts DW, Friets EM, Strohbehn JW, et al: The sonic digitizing microscope. *In* Maciunas RJ (ed): Interactive Image-Guided Neurosurgery. Park Ridge, Ill, American Association of Neurological Surgeons, 1993, pp 105–112.)

materials. Echoes from the multitude of surfaces in the operating suite produce significant interference with surgical localization. Considerable work has been carried out by Roberts and colleagues,[41] as well as others, to correct for temperature fluctuations, echoes, and other sources of error in the system. The error in locating the focal point of the operating microscope in a recent clinical series of 17 patients was 6.33 ± 3.37 mm.

Recently, Barnett and colleagues[4] have incorporated spark-gap ultrasonic emitter technology with a handheld ILD (Picker International, Highland Heights, Ohio) (Fig. 33–4). The spark-gap emitters are carried by this pointing device, rather than being coupled to the operating microscope. The repetitive ultrasonic pulses produced by the ILD are detected by a portable detector/calibration array that is mounted to the side rails of a standard operating table. Software algorithms that compensate for temperature and humidity fluctuation effects are critical to the functionality of the system.

PASSIVE STEREOSCOPIC VIDEO (MACHINE VISION)

Heilbrun and co-workers[18] have proposed a technique of surgical guidance employing *machine vision*, wherein the three-dimensional position of an object in space is determined from its differential position on two-dimensional video images viewed from two different angles (Fig. 33–5). Two video cameras located approximately 1 m apart are aimed at the surgical workspace. A *video localizer*, consisting of a set of eight fiducial objects in a box-like configuration of known dimensions, is placed within the field of view of the two video cameras. A photogrammetric projection algorithm defines the three-dimensional coordinates of the eight fiducial objects. Subsequently, the position and field of view of the video cameras remain unchanged. Thereby, the three-dimensional position of any object in the surgical workspace of the field of view can be determined and tracked. Surgical instruments may be tracked within the

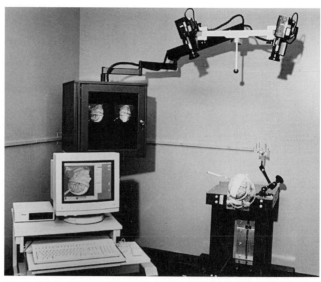

Figure 33–5 Machine vision localization. (From Heilbrun MP, Koehler S, McDonald P, et al: Implementation of a machine vision method for stereotactic localization and guidance. *In* Maciunas RJ (ed): Interactive Image-Guided Neurosurgery. Park Ridge, Ill, American Association of Neurological Surgeons, 1993, pp 179–200.)

surgical space of the video cameras by affixing fiducial markers to the surgical instruments in a known geometric configuration. The registration of image and physical space is accomplished through identifying at least three external fiducial points in each coordinate system for registration.

The advantage of this method is its flexibility, its potential to track standard surgical instruments as stereotactic pointers with minimal modification, and its reliance on readily available video technology. It remains sensitive to line-of-sight considerations, the need for the video cameras to maintain the relationship with the preoperatively defined surgical space, the limitations to the resolution of currently available video technology, and the computation-intensive nature of intraoperative registration.

LIGHT-EMITTING DIODE OPTICAL TRIANGULATION

Several groups have investigated the use of infrared light-emitting diodes (IREDs or LEDs) as an alternative form of optical localization. By having two or more IREDs attached to a surgical instrument, the position in space of that instrument can be tracked over time by a triangulation technique that employs three or more specialized 1,000- to 4,000-element linear charge-coupled devices (LCCDs) with cylindrical lenses. These optical triangulation techniques are highly accurate and precise, are surprisingly robust within the noisy operating theater environment, and are extremely flexible in their use. Line-of-sight considerations apply in this situation, much as they do with sonic digitizer triangulation methods. Unlike sonic digitizers, IRED arrays are insensitive to temperature or humidity fluctuations. Interference from surgical light sources has not proven to be a problem. The infrared wavelength of their emissions is not disruptive to surgery.

Bucholz and Smith[8] have employed an array of two

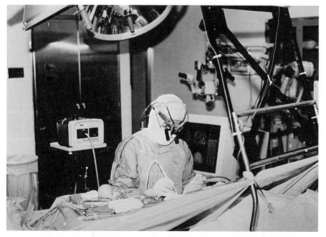

Figure 33–4 Sonic localizing handheld intraoperative localization device (ILD). Sound detectors mounted in a plate on the operating table. (From Barnett GH, Kormos DW, Steiner CP, et al: Frameless stereotaxy using a sonic digitizing wand: Development and adaptation to the Picker Vistar medical imaging system. *In* Maciunas RJ (ed): Interactive Image-Guided Neurosurgery. Park Ridge, Ill, American Association of Neurological Surgeons, 1993, pp 113–120.)

IREDs attached to a surgical bipolar cautery forceps (Codman/JJPI, Raynham, Mass) (Fig. 33–6). Maciunas and colleagues[32] have employed knowledge-based software using center-finding algorithms to better detect the IREDs (Fig. 33–7).[2] To increase the robustness and accuracy of localization, the ILD is studded with an array of multiple IREDs.

MAGNETIC FIELD GUIDANCE

Kato and co-workers[21] and Manwaring[35] have employed magnetic field guidance (Polhemus Navigation Sciences, Colchester, Vermont) of endoscopic dissection (Fig. 33–8). A magnetic field established by a transmitter antenna near the patient's head is measured by a receiving antenna mounted on the surgical instrument. Magnetic field guidance has the attraction of being mechanically simple and inexpensive. Unfortunately, it has proved to be less accurate than other technologies in clinical settings, and it is susceptible to both static and active field distortion in the surgical suite environment due to the presence of common metals as well as to electromagnetic field interference. Goerss and others[17] have used software with algorithms to attempt compensation for static magnetic field inhomogeneities (Regulus Naviga-

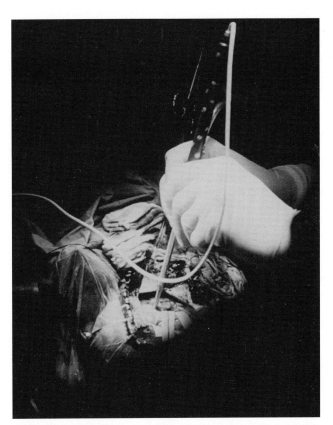

Figure 33–7 Surgical instrument fitted with an array of infrared light-emitting diodes (IREDs). (From Maciunas RJ: The diagnosis and therapy of ganglion cell tumors. *In* Apuzzo MLJ (ed): Benign Cerebral Gliomas. Park Ridge, Ill, American Association of Neurological Surgeons, 1995.)

tional System, Stereotactic Medical Systems, Inc., Rochester, Minn) and to minimize drift and inaccuracies.

Computer Interfaces

The rapid evolution of computer hardware and software has propelled the development of interactive image-guided neurosurgery. Because neurosurgery is a "niche" market for most manufacturers, technical advances have resulted

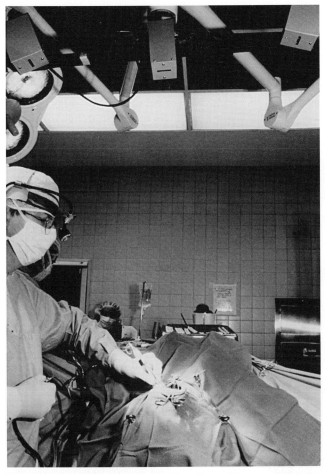

Figure 33–6 Optic triangulation by three linear charge-coupled devices tracking a surgical instrument with infrared light-emitting diodes (IREDs). (From Bucholz RD, Smith KR. A comparison of sonic digitizers versus light-emitting diode-based localization. *In* Maciunas RJ (ed): Interactive Image-Guided Neurosurgery. Park Ridge, Ill, American Association of Neurological Surgeons, 1993, pp 179–200.)

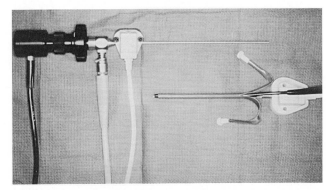

Figure 33–8 An endoscope and shunt catheter stylet fitted for magnetic localization. (From Manwaring KH: Intraoperative microendoscopy. *In* Maciunas RJ (ed): Interactive Image-Guided Neurosurgery. Park Ridge, Ill, American Association of Neurological Surgeons, 1993, pp 217–223.)

either from systematic development of systems at academic institutions by collaborative groups of surgeons, scientists, and engineers, which are translated into distributable product by established medical supply companies, or from ad hoc adaptation of innovations developed for other purposes.

The computer hardware employed tends to be either an image-processing workstation that is fairly generic, commercially available, and interchangeable (and can therefore be upgraded) or a custom high-performance specialized unit that consists of hybrid hardware with machine-specific software and peripherals. Most commonly, the latter characterizes what is typically used in academic research, by small corporations, and by radiologic scanner manufacturers. As systems become commercialized, the considerations of portability of software and upgrading/support of hardware favor the former.

It is interesting to note that most surgical navigation systems have evolved an initial "two-box" solution, wherein an embedded microcomputer serves the ILD by calculating at coordinates in real time and by relaying this information to the image-processing workstation for correlation with spatially registered images.

The surgical ergonomics of treatment-planning software and image-reformatting menus is a field of considerable ongoing research and development. Optimal software will likely allow sufficient flexibility to write menus according to individualized preferences while suppressing extraneous and unselected information. The key to successful development in this sphere is the intimate involvement by a neurosurgeon in directing the clinical interface (Fig. 33–9).

The intraoperative video display of medical images involves a similar interaction by surgeons and engineers (Fig.

33–10). The display of medical images in a surgically meaningful manner is a separate and distinct problem from the display of medical images for diagnostic radiology. Although considerable work on the latter has been carried out, the former is only beginning to come into its own. An ideal standard for intraoperative display appears to be emerging: a high-resolution monitor divided into several 512 × 512 windows for medical images, with color graphic overlays displaying ILD position as a cursor (which is updated at about 20 frames/second). As the expense and complexity of image-processing workstations plummet, the real-time display of ILD position on spatially registered orthogonally reformatted two-dimensional images has become possible. At this writing, the on-line reformatting of medical images is slightly too slow for real-time surgical use. The creation and manipulation of segmented shaded surface and rendered images involves time delays of seconds to hours. Further evolution of computing capabilities over the next decade promises to make this capability a reality for intraoperative use.[16]

Real-Time Intraoperative Feedback

Despite the registration of image to physical space, digital scan information consists of historical data that are subject to becoming outdated during the course of surgical manipulation of tissues. The feedback loop of navigation can be closed by incorporating real-time intraoperative imaging and monitoring: these data are used to refine and modify the patient-specific maps that are being used for surgical guidance. By digitizing the video output from intraoperative

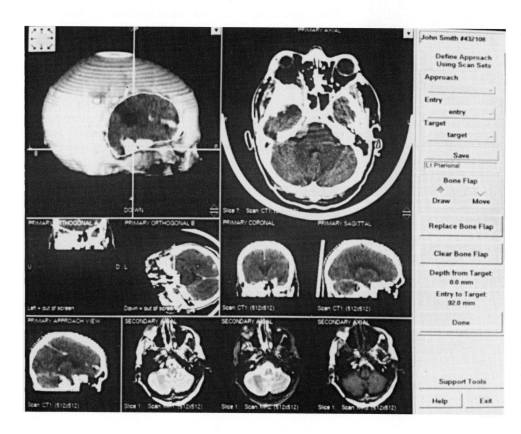

Figure 33–9 A preoperative surgical treatment planning software program. (From Maciunas RJ: The diagnosis and therapy of ganglion cell tumors. *In* Apuzzo MLJ (ed): Benign Cerebral Gliomas. Park Ridge, Ill, American Association of Neurological Surgeons, 1995.)

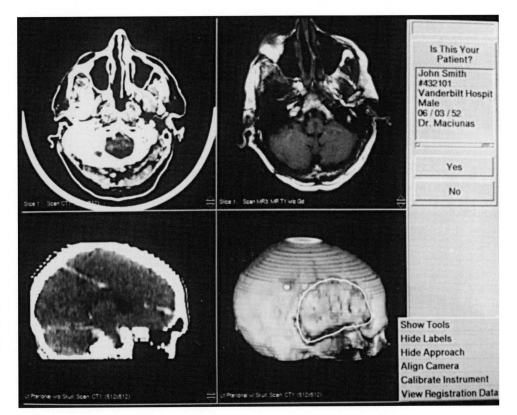

Figure 33-10 An intraoperative multimodality display of image slices and shaded surface renderings. (From Maciunas RJ: The diagnosis and therapy of ganglion cell tumors. *In* Apuzzo MLJ (ed): Benign Cerebral Gliomas. Park Ridge, Ill, American Association of Neurological Surgeons, 1995.)

visualization techniques (ultrasonography, endoscopy, tomography, and electrophysiologic recordings), these images may simply be treated as other sources of spatially registered medical information. Preliminary steps are being taken to incorporate this information into surgical guidance data bases.

Oikarinen and colleagues[38] have spatially registered preoperatively obtained tomographic images with intraoperative ultrasonographic images from a 5-MHz ultrasound sector probe treated as a virtual end effector of the localizing arm; this technique allows direct overlay of text and MRI-derived graphics onto ultrasound images during the operation.

Galloway and co-workers[15] have extended this principle of spatially registered video images to intraoperative ultrasonography, endoscopy, and the registration of intraoperative electrophysiologic data. The additional localization information derived from preoperative medical images provides coarse guidance for initial orientation of the limited field of view that is available through a microneuroendoscope.

Intraoperative tomography offers the promise of high-resolution digital volumetric imaging data for continuous real-time updating of the surgical field. Intraoperative CT has been employed at several centers. Current research and development by scanner manufacturers promises to introduce intraoperative MRI in the near future. The considerable expenditures for such systems have raised concerns about their cost-effectiveness.

CLINICAL APPLICATIONS

Biopsy

In selected cases, patients may undergo stereotactic biopsy as the initial diagnostic/therapeutic intervention. Numerous studies indicate that presumptive diagnoses based on preoperative clinical information and imaging studies alone are incorrect in as many as 25% of cases. With the proliferation of stereotactic techniques, the surgical risk of biopsy has declined significantly. Therefore, empirically prescribed cytotoxic therapy is usually no longer justified. Image-guided fine-needle biopsy, because of its lesser risk, higher yield, and greater cost-effectiveness, has superseded the former practice of performing an open craniotomy for biopsy.

A hallmark of malignant gliomas is heterogeneity. Microscopically, intercellular clonal variability is apparent on histologic preparations. Macroscopically, patterns of topographically distributed cell populations are apparent on imaging studies such as CT, MRI, and PET. Because glial tumors demonstrate considerable heterogeneity, careful preoperative planning is imperative to the achievement of satisfactory biopsy results. This requires precise registration of multiple imaging data sets.

The classic appearance of malignant gliomas is of a mass of solid tumor tissue surrounded by isolated infiltrating tumor cells contained within edematous brain parenchyma. Hochberg[20] noted a correlation, in 29 of 35 cases, between the tumor extent as defined at autopsy and a margin drawn 2 cm beyond the enhancing mass as seen on contrast-enhanced CT. Based on these results, Hochberg advocated a localized approach to gliomas. Far more extensive tumor infiltration and subependymal spread were documented in the meticulous preparations of Burger and colleagues,[9] who stressed the significant involvement of surrounding brain parenchyma by isolated infiltrating tumor cells. Daumas-Duport and others[11] demonstrated that infiltrating tumor cells spread beyond any imaging abnormalities seen during T2-weighted MRI-directed biopsies. It would appear, at the very least, that both the solid tumor tissue and infiltrating tumor cell regions of gliomas are pathologically and clinically significant.

Examining specimens from stereotactic serial biopsies, Daumas-Duport and colleagues[10] classified the parenchymal distribution of gliomas into three spatial types based on their relative components of solid tumor tissue and infiltrating tumor cells. Solid tumor tissue disrupts all underlying parenchyma, whereas infiltrating tumor cells infiltrate intact brain parenchyma. Type I gliomas consist purely of solid tumor tissue. Type II gliomas are composed of a solid tumor tissue mass with a penumbra of infiltrating tumor cells. Type III gliomas consist entirely of infiltrating tumor cells without regions of solid tumor tissue.

Because no single imaging modality can completely elucidate the relevant cytobiology in a given malignant glioma, the correlation of multiple scans is required in clinical practice. The classic imaging appearance of a glioblastoma is that of a solid tumor tissue mass with a rim of enhancement around a variably enhancing central core, having a penumbra of infiltrating tumor cells visualized as a surrounding region of edematous brain. This would correspond to a Daumas-Duport grade 4, spatial type III glial neoplasm. The extent of neovascularization induced by solid tumor tissue is most accurately delimited by reference to contrast-enhanced CT, followed by unenhanced T1-weighted MRI. T1-weighted MRI with gadolinium enhancement, however, is only indirectly and unpredictably correlated with solid tumor tissue margins. Infiltrating tumor cells induce interstitial and intracellular parenchymal edema that appears as nonenhancing hypodensity on CT, as hyperintensity due to prolonged T2 signal on T2-weighted MRI, as hypointensity due to prolonged T1 signal on T1-weighted MRI, and with no enhancement after gadolinium. T2-weighted MRI is more sensitive than non-contrast CT for demonstrating edema and, therefore, extent of involvement by infiltrating tumor cells.[14] The imaging appearances can be altered after adjuvant therapy, and changes in scans do not always correspond to changes in clinical status.

The promising roles for MR spectroscopy, and especially for PET, include intraoperative guidance of stereotactic biopsy to regions of maximal metabolic rate and, presumably, highest tumor grade.

The technique of taking serial biopsy specimens in a stepwise fashion through the bulk of the tumor increases the likelihood of accurate diagnosis. To that end, computer-assisted treatment planning programs are invaluable in selecting a safe and effective trajectory for biopsy. Frozen-section analysis provides reassurance of a diagnostic biopsy prior to removal of the needle, but it should never be considered sufficient to guide further therapy.

Imaging-directed stereotactic serial biopsies of gliomas enable patient-specific mapping of intracranial tumor involvement. This ability to categorize gliomas according to both grade and spatial type may ultimately result in patient-specific regional targeting of multiple tumor therapies, each optimized to target either the solid tumor tissue or the infiltrating tumor cell components of the multicompartmental tumor. Because no viable neural parenchyma exists within solid tumor tissue, this region may be safely ablated by cytoreductive surgery, brachytherapy, or radiosurgery. The infiltrating tumor cells enmeshed in eloquent parenchyma, meanwhile, are better dealt with through techniques that are selective of cell type (e.g., chemotherapy, radiotherapy, or gene therapy).[29, 30]

Craniotomy for Resection

The performance of craniotomy for resection of a glial tumor must proceed in strict accordance with standard neurosurgical principles and technique. Meticulous attention to detail must be maintained during the resection of these frequently extensive tumors, which may be hypervascular and adjacent to eloquent cortex. Surgical resection of intact, functionally eloquent brain parenchyma that is invaded by infiltrating tumor cells is hazardous, as it may result in neurologic deficit. Mechanical cytoreduction is safest within the solid tumor tissue regions of gliomas. Surgical resection of solid tumor tissue is the treatment modality least affected by considerations of cellular heterogeneity, oxygen tension, capillary supply, or cell cycle kinetics.

It has been argued by some that surgery may not be able to regularly achieve a cytokinetically significant reduction of tumor burden, given the degree to which gliomas consist of infiltrating tumor cells. Others contend that surgery cannot serve to reduce any neurologic deficit resulting from cell destruction that is caused by tumor extending into functionally significant areas. However, both the Brain Tumor Study Group (BTSG) and Radiation Therapy Oncology Group (RTOG) controlled trials have demonstrated that survival is related to the degree of surgical resection. Patients who only underwent a biopsy had a shorter median length of survival (6.8 months) and a lower rate of survival at 18 months (15%) than did those who underwent resection (a 12-month median length of survival with a 34% survival rate at 18 months). When feasible, gross total resection of the solid tumor tissue component improves both the length and quality of survival. Reoperation for debulking recurrent solid tumor tissue or focal radionecrosis can also result in prolonged functional survival.[2, 3, 24, 28, 34, 37, 45]

The work of Kelly and others[22, 23] to establish volumetric stereotactic resection techniques has provided a basis for assessing the benefits of surgical resection of deep-seated glial tumors. These techniques have allowed for proper diagnosis and definitive resection of benign and circumscribed gliomas and for radical cytoreduction of the solid tumor tissue component of high-grade gliomas. Volumetric stereotactic resection of centrally located malignant gliomas slightly improves median length of survival for these lesions, up to the level normally associated with radically resected polar lesions.

Although extent of resection of low-grade gliomas has not been analyzed as an influence on outcome in a prospective randomized trial, recent studies suggest improved survival after extensive surgical resection.[26, 27, 36, 39, 44] Berger and co-workers[7] as well as Duong and others[13] have demonstrated that the degree of resection and amount of residual tumor are significantly related to the incidence of recurrence and to the tumor grade at recurrence.

When appropriate, the extent of surgical resection can be benefited by the incorporation of stereotactic methods.

Stereotactically directed craniotomies can provide guidance for the appropriate placement of a bone flap and can direct the transcortical approach to an intraventricular tumor. By selecting several target points along the periphery of a superficially located tumor, a series of ventricular catheters or strings may provide "fenceposts" to better demarcate the extent of the planned resection.

The computer-assisted stereotactic apparatus of Kelly and co-workers[22] offers significant benefit in the sequential image-guided laser resection of deep-seated glial tumors. The restrictive nature of the stereotactic apparatus makes this sort of guidance less applicable in the infant patient population and, depending on surgeon preference, in patients with anterior temporal fossa tumors.

Radiosurgery

Clinically significant recurrence and progression of tumor can result either from local solid tumor tissue regrowth or from diffuse infiltrating tumor cell spread throughout the cerebral hemispheres. Because regrowth of the solid tumor tissue component of glial tumors is essentially a local process, this remains a surgically amenable disease. The principles of radiosurgical management apply to such recurrences of these tumors. Stereotactic radiosurgical treatment of glial tumors is currently under investigation.

Adler[1] has described a method of spatial registration for frameless stereotactic radiosurgery that correlates the extracted surface of the skull from preoperative CT scans with intraoperative projection radiographs. A catalog of rotated and translated projection images is created synthetically from the preoperative CT scan, and it is then compared intraoperatively with orthogonal projection radiographs. The algorithm selects from the catalog the best "fit" between the intraoperative projection images and the synthetic preoperative projection images. This guides the administration of the radiosurgical dosimetry by an active robotic arm coupled to the linear accelerator radiation source.

SURGICAL TECHNIQUE FOR INTERACTIVE IMAGE-GUIDED NEUROSURGERY

The emerging technologies of interactive image-guided neurosurgery offer great promise in the surgical management of glial tumors. The restrictions imposed by stereotactic frame methodology are eliminated, because alternative methods are used to register image space to physical space during surgery. This extends the applicability of image-guided surgery to a wider range of cases. Intraoperative availability of registered image data sets improves the extent of resection. Intracranial shifts encountered during evacuation of cerebrospinal fluid from enlarged ventricles associated with centrally located tumors, however, may limit the role of image guidance to refining the surgical approach to the lesion in these cases.

Of tremendous potential is the fact that intraoperative electrocorticography, motor-evoked potential monitoring, and speech function mapping can all be spatially registered with the preoperatively obtained digital scan images.[6, 15, 42] This capability brings together the two foremost tools in the surgical armamentarium for improving the extent of resection. Once perfected, this may provide the new standard of care for initial management of glial lesions. These technologies represent a broad and rapidly evolving field.

One technique of interactive image-guided neurosurgery is able to achieve extremely accurate registration of image and physical space through the application of implantable fiducial markers acting as external point reference sources. These fiducial markers consist of several subunits that are assembled as indicated. All components of the system may be sterilized and are disposable. A marker base, 13 mm in length and 3 mm in diameter, has a threaded 3-mm portion that anchors firmly in the outer table of the skull. The length of the post of this marker base is designed to provide clearance of other marker components above the scalp (Fig. 33–11).

Four fiducial marker bases are implanted in each patient. A sterile implantation kit allows rapid application of the marker bases. The cranial sites of implantation are selected on an individual basis, depending on clinical circumstances. After local site preparation and sterile draping, 1 mL of 1% lidocaine with epinephrine is instilled at each implantation site. A 3.5-mm scalp incision is made. A sterile guide assembly, preloaded with an obturator, is inserted through the scalp incision until the serrated edges of the metal guide tube are secured on the skull. An anchoring hole is then drilled through the outer table of the skull by inserting a premeasured precision twist drill through the guide cannula. An applicator, preloaded with a marker base, is then advanced down the guide cannula so that the marker base is tightened into the bone of the skull for a positive locking fit. The applicator and guide assembly are then removed; the anchoring post is left in proper position. After application of the marker bases, the patient is transported to the radiology suite for imaging studies.

During scanning, imaging fiducial markers are attached to the anchoring fiducial bases. These imaging fiducial markers

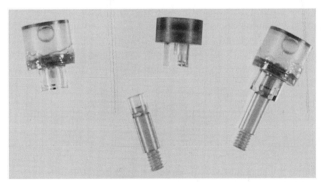

Figure 33–11 Implantable fiducial markers. Pictured are the imaging fiducial marker, the implanted marker base, the intraoperative localization cap, and the assembly of the imaging fiducial marker/implanted marker base. (From Maciunas RJ, Fitzpatrick JM, Galloway RL, et al: Beyond stereotaxy: Extreme levels of application accuracy are provided by implantable fiducial markers for interactive image-guided neurosurgery. *In* Maciunas RJ (ed): Interactive Image-Guided Neurosurgery. Park Ridge, Ill, American Association of Neurological Surgeons, 1993, pp 259–270.)

click into place atop the posts of the fiducial marker bases in a machined keyhole with grooves. Imaging fiducial markers are filled with contrast agents that are visible on CT and on all MRI modalities. Additional fiducial markers have been fabricated with germanium solution for imaging with PET. CT, MRI, and PET scanning proceed routinely. After the imaging studies are completed, the imaging fiducial markers are removed and marker protectors are placed over the fiducial marker bases. Images are transferred to the preoperative treatment-planning computer workstation. The geometric center of these imaging fiducial markers is automatically calculated, and a least-squares fit is used to register one image onto another.

During presurgical treatment planning, the surgeon selects appropriate scan images from the preoperatively obtained data sets as well as from reformatted or rendered displays of the data. The tumor can be digitized as a volume in imaging space and segmented for intraoperative display. A surgically appropriate approach is defined using scan images and a rendered display of the skull and soft tissue images. The surgeon then selects the images deemed most beneficial for intraoperative viewing. These are loaded onto an optical disc and transported to the operative theater.

After the patient is placed in the appropriate surgical position, localization caps are placed over the fiducial marker bases. These caps are fabricated so that their centroid corresponds to the centroid of the imaging fiducial marker. A reference emitter (RE) is attached to the headholder. This RE is an integral component of the optical position sensor mechanism which provides instant interactive visual feedback during surgery. Surgical tools are fitted with IREDs. "Smart" connectors inform the embedded computer system about the geometric configuration of each of a variety of available surgical ILD attachments, allowing multiple probes to be used during a single surgery. All components of the system may be sterilized and are disposable. A precision-milled three-camera LCCD array is placed within the operative theater such that this optical position sensor precisely localizes the RE and all surgical instruments equipped with IREDs. Knowledge-based software with center-finding algorithms is used to detect the IREDs. These spatial coordinates are conveyed to a Hewlett-Packard 712 image-processing workstation with a high-resolution display monitor. Four 512 × 512 images are simultaneously displayed and refreshed at 20 frames/second for real-time display of surgical localization on historically obtained medical images. Graphics capabilities allow the display of rendered, shaded surface displays as appropriate.

Placement of the ILD with a specifically configured tip into the divot of all four of the localization caps ensures precise registration of image and physical space. These are machined with a hemispherical divot such that the centroid of the divot corresponds to the centroid of the imaging marker. The accuracy of target registration for this system is 0.629 ± 0.153 mm.[27]

At this time the system becomes interactive and tracks the position of the ILD with regard to image space at a rate approaching real-time display. This allows the surgeon to progressively define the scalp incision, bone flap, dural opening, and corticotomy size and trajectory to optimally access the neoplasm while minimizing perilesional tissue trauma.

Rendered and shaded surface projection images are most beneficial at this stage of the operation. The rendering of high-resolution thin-cut MRI gradient-echo image sets to portray cortical gyral and sulcal anatomy can be breathtakingly clarifying in planning corticotomies, especially when registered to a cohort of a rendered MR angiogram, a rendered MR venogram, a shaded surface volume projection of the target tumor, and a coregistered preoperative functional MRI or PET map. During resection, periodic positional data sampling with the ILD is carried out as determined to be necessary by the surgeon. Often, an alternating pattern of resection, exposure, and reassessment proves effective in these circumstances. When positional data from the localization probe are not concordant with personal impressions, it is mandatory to carefully assess the significance of the new and critical data. Based on repeated episodes and experience, the surgeon may find that dead reckoning proves to be overcautious or maldirected when applied to debulking of gliomas. It is evident that tissue planes are more distinctive to the naked eye, even under microscopic illumination and magnification, when coupled with exquisite positional information. This is especially true at the margins of highly vascular glioblastomas and of avascular low-grade infiltrative astrocytomas in close approximation to gray matter. Often, the visual correlation of triplanar displays of coronal, sagittal, and axial data is revealing of what lies just beyond the resection margin visible at that time. Preresection passage of "fencepost" catheters can be performed as deemed appropriate. This has proven most practical for accessing deeply subcortical or intraventricular lesions, but it has been cumbersome for removal of a superficial lesion. Shifts of intracranial soft tissue over the duration of the operation have been observed in passing, but this has proved to be remarkably less of a concern than initially feared. Nonetheless, ongoing research at numerous centers is addressing this problem with automated intraoperative nonrigid body reregistration algorithms.

The position of the ILD may be recorded as a data point when needed. In this way, multiple entries of intraoperative electrocorticographic and electrophysiologic data may be recorded on a spatially registered data base (Fig. 33–12). The co-registration of imaging abnormalities and electrophysiologic recordings serves to define the proposed extent of resection. This has repeatedly proved to be beneficial in speeding the progress of resection of tissue from around eloquent regions while affording the surgeon a greater sense of security.

At the conclusion of the resection procedure, the surgical workspace is again sequentially sampled to confirm accomplishment of the preplanned surgical task. On numerous occasions, a humbling reappraisal of subjective intraoperative impressions regarding resectional volumetric estimates is in order. The surgical judgment regarding how to interpret these data is, as always, informed by numerous considerations that are not necessarily demonstrated by imaging studies.

Biopsy of glial tumors proceeds as described, with the exception that the craniotomy is foregone, and a rigid probe holder is employed to advance a side-biting Sedan-type biopsy needle to the requisite target along a predefined

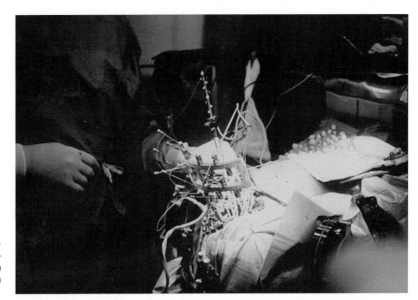

Figure 33-12 Intraoperative spatially registered electrocorticography. (From Maciunas RJ: The diagnosis and therapy of ganglion cell tumors. *In* Apuzzo MLJ (ed): Benign Cerebral Gliomas. Park Ridge, Ill, American Association of Neurological Surgeons, 1995.)

trajectory. This may be deliberated on before the operation takes place or it may be dynamically defined during surgery.

This selfsame probe holder has proven capable of securing a microneuroendoscope for intraventricular exploration and biopsy or membrane fenestration. The video image from the endoscope is handled as simply another digital image to be co-registered with preoperatively obtained tomographic images. The tomograms prove very helpful in providing coarse guidance for endoscopy and for tracking objects just outside the field of view.

Intraoperative ultrasonography promises to make a significant resurgence as the images are correlated to obliquely sliced tomographic images and overlaid on them. The use of ultrasonography to dynamically re-register shifting brain parenchyma during resections has been advocated repeatedly, although the distortions inherent in ultrasonography and the problems of resolution must be addressed first.[5, 15]

Whether these navigational technologies can be demonstrated to benefit cost-effectiveness concerns in a changing medical environment remains to be seen. At present, it can be said that subjective surgical opinions are clear in their appreciation of the utility of this approach to glial tumor surgery.

FUTURE REALITIES

The emerging technologies of interactive image-guided neurosurgery have only begun to be systematically applied to specific clinical situations. As these navigational systems become more robust, flexible, and accurate, their incorporation into much of clinical practice will become irresistible. With precise three-dimensional localization becoming readily available, every practicing neurosurgeon will benefit from greater surgical precision, shorter operating times, and a strengthened appreciation for complex anatomic relationships. Neurosurgical education itself may be further augmented through the integration of preoperative image data bases, intraoperative video recording, and surgical simulation programs. As a result, the learning curve for spatial localiza-

tion by resident trainees will undoubtedly be altered. Finally, the next generation of neurosurgical operations to be developed will undoubtedly be predicated on methods of advanced surgical navigation. The development of technologically intensive solutions to surgical navigation constitutes the lifework of a generation of neurosurgeons and their colleagues in engineering, basic sciences, and industry. Coincident with this evolutionary process in surgical delivery systems is a similarly explosive development of cytobiologically powerful methods for manipulating genomic expression. We can anticipate complementary developments in these two fields, as one provides the vehicle and the other the cargo to effect a new means of surgical healing of disease. It is conceivable that surgical targeting of the fruits of gene therapy may be the first true application of virtual reality to neurosurgery as synthetic images are called on to convey information that can be manipulated intuitively to perform surgical procedures on glial tumors at cellular and molecular levels.

REFERENCES

1. Adler JR Jr: Image-based frameless stereotactic radiosurgery. *In* Maciunas RJ (ed): Interactive Image-Guided Neurosurgery. Park Ridge, Ill, American Association of Neurological Surgeons, 1993, pp 81–89.
2. Afra D, Muller W, Benoist G, et al: Supratentorial recurrences of gliomas, results of reoperations on astrocytomas and oligodendrogliomas. Acta Neurochir 1978; 43:217–227.
3. Ammirati M, Vick N, Liao Y, et al: Effect of the extent of surgical resection on survival and quality of life in patients with supratentorial glioblastomas and anaplastic astrocytomas. Neurosurgery 1987; 21:201.
4. Barnett GH, Kormos DW, Steiner CP, et al: Frameless stereotaxy using a sonic digitizing wand: Development and adaptation to the Picker Vistar medical imaging system. *In* Maciunas RJ (ed): Interactive Image-guided Neurosurgery. Park Ridge, Ill, American Association of Neurological Surgeons, 1993, pp 715–720.
5. Berger MS: Ultrasound-guided stereotaxic biopsy using a new apparatus. J Neurosurg 1986; 65:550.
6. Berger MS, Ojemann GA: Intraoperative brain mapping techniques in neuro-oncology. Stereotact Funct Neurosurg 1992; 58:153–161.
7. Berger MS, Deliganis AV, Dobbins J, et al: The effect of extent of resection on recurrence in patients with low grade cerebral hemisphere gliomas. Cancer 1994; 74:1784–1791.

8. Bucholz RD, Smith KR: A comparison of sonic digitizers versus light emitting diode-based localization. *In* Maciunas RJ (ed): Interactive Image-Guided Neurosurgery. Park Ridge, Ill, American Association of Neurological Surgeons, l993, pp 179–200.

9. Burger PC, Heinz ER, Shibata T, et al: Topographic anatomy and CT correlations in the untreated glioblastoma multiforme. J Neurosurg 1988; 68:698.

10. Daumas-Duport C, Monsaingeon V, Szenthe L, et al: Serial stereotactic biopsies: A double histological code of gliomas according to malignancy and 3-D configuration, as an aid to therapeutic decision and assessment of results. Appl Neurophysiol 1982; 45:431.

11. Daumas-Duport C, Scheithauer B, Kelly PJ: A histologic and cytologic method for the spatial definition of gliomas. Mayo Clin Proc 1987; 62:435.

12. Drake JM, Joy M, Goldenberg A, et al: Computer- and robot-assisted resection of thalamic astrocytomas in children. Neurosurgery 1991; 29:27–33.

13. Duong DH, Rostomily RC, Haynor DR, et al: Measurement of tumor resection volumes from computerized images: Technical note. J Neurosurg 1992; 77:151–154.

14. Galloway RL Jr, Maciunas RJ, Failinger AL, et al: Volumetric measurement of canine gliomas using MRI. Magn Reson Imaging 1990; 8:161.

15. Galloway RL Jr, Berger MS, Bass WA, et al: Registered intraoperative information: Electrophysiology, ultrasound, and endoscopy. *In* Maciunas RJ (ed): Interactive Image-Guided Neurosurgery. Park Ridge, Ill, American Association of Neurological Surgeons, l993, pp 247–258.

16. Galloway RL Jr, Edwards CA II, Lewis JT, et al: Image display and surgical visualization in interactive image-guided neurosurgery. Optical Engineering 1993; 32:1955–1962.

17. Goerss SJ, Kelly PJ, Kall BA, et al: A computed tomographic stereotactic adaptation system. Neurosurgery 1982; 10:375–379.

18. Guthrie BL, Adler JR Jr: Computer-assisted preoperative planning, interactive surgery, and frameless stereotaxy. Clin Neurosurg 1992; 38:112–131.

19. Heilbrun MP, McDonald P, Wiker C, et al: Stereotactic localization and guidance using a machine vision technique. Stereotact Funct Neurosurg 1992; 58:94–98.

20. Hochberg FH, Pruitt A: Assumptions in the radiotherapy of glioblastoma. Neurology 1980; 30:907–911.

21. Kato A, Yoshimine T, Hayakawa T, et al: A frameless, armless navigational system for computer-assisted tomography. J Neurosurg 1991; 74:845–849.

22. Kelly PJ, Kall BA, Goerss DSJ, et al: Computer-assisted stereotaxic laser resection of intra-axial brain neoplasm. J Neurosurg 1986; 64:427.

23. Kelly PJ: Computer-assisted stereotaxis: New approaches for the management of intracranial intra-axial tumors. Neurology 1986; 36:535.

24. Kramer S: The hazards of therapeutic irradiation of the central nervous system. Clin Neurosurg 1968; 15:301.

25. Kwoh YS, Hou J, Jonckheere EA, et al: A robot with improved accuracy for CT-guided stereotactic brain surgery. IEEE Trans Biomed Eng 1988; 35:153–160.

26. Laws ER, Taylor WF, Clifton MB, et al: Neurosurgical management of low-grade astrocytoma of the cerebral hemispheres. J Neurosurg 1984; 61:665–673.

27. Laws ER, Taylor WF, Bergstralh EJ, et al: The neurosurgical management of low-grade astrocytomas. Clin Neurosurg 1985; 33:575–588.

28. Levin VA, Silver P, Hannigan J, et al: Superiority of post-radiotherapy adjuvant chemotherapy with CCNU, procarbazine, and vincristine (PCV) over BCNU for anaplastic gliomas: NCOG 6G61 final report. Int J Radiat Oncol Biol Phys 1990; 18:321.

29. Maciunas RJ, Misulis KE: Comprehensive therapy for malignant gliomas: I. Contemporary Neurosurgery 1991; 18(20):1–6.

30. Maciunas RJ, Misulis KE: Comprehensive therapy for malignant gliomas: II. Contemporary Neurosurgery 1991; 18(21):1–6.

31. Maciunas RJ, Galloway RL, Fitzpatrick JM, et al: A universal system for interactive image-directed neurosurgery. Stereotact Funct Neurosurg 1992; 58:108–113.

32. Maciunas RJ, Fitzpatrick JM, Galloway RL, et al: Beyond stereotaxy: Extreme levels of application accuracy are provided by implantable fiducial markers for interactive image-guided neurosurgery. *In* Maciunas RJ (ed): Interactive Image-Guided Neurosurgery. Park Ridge, Ill, American Association of Neurological Surgeons, l993, pp 259–270.

33. Maciunas RJ, Galloway RL Jr, Latimer J: The application accuracy of stereotactic frame systems. Neurosurgery 1994; 35:682–695.

34. Maciunas RJ: Surgical aspects and general management of ganglion cell tumors. *In* Apuzzo MLJ (ed): Benign Cerebral Gliomas. Park Ridge, Ill, American Association of Neurological Surgeons, 1995, pp 427–444.

35. Manwaring KH: Intraoperative microendoscopy. *In* Maciunas RJ (ed): Interactive Image-Guided Neurosurgery. Park Ridge, Ill, American Association of Neurological Surgeons, l993, pp 217–232.

36. Medbury CA, Straus KL, Steinberg SM, et al: Low-grade astrocytomas: Treatment results and prognostic variables. Int J Radiat Oncol Biol Phys 1988; 15:837–841.

37. Muller W, Afra D, Schroder R: Supratentorial recurrences of gliomas: Morphological studies in relation to time intervals with astrocytomas. Acta Neurochir 1977; 37:75–91.

38. Oikarinen J, Alakuijala J, Louhisalmi Y, et al: The Oulu neuronavigator system: Intraoperative ultrasonography in the verification of neurosurgical localization and visualization. *In* Maciunas RJ (ed): Interactive Image-Guided Neurosurgery. Park Ridge, Ill, American Association of Neurological Surgeons, l993, pp 233–247.

39. Piepmeier JM: Observations on the current treatment of low-grade astrocytic tumors of the cerebral hemisphere. J Neurosurg 1987; 67:177–181.

40. Roberts DW, Strohbehn JW, Hatch JF, et al: A frameless stereotaxic integration of computerized tomographic imaging and the operating microscope. J Neurosurg 1986; 65:545–549.

41. Roberts DW, Friets EM, Strohbehn JW, et al: The sonic digitizing microscope. *In* Maciunas RJ (ed): Interactive Image-Guided Neurosurgery. Park Ridge, Ill, American Association of Neurological Surgeons, 1993, pp 105–112.

42. Rostomily RC, Berger MS, Ojemann GA, et al: Postoperative deficits and functional recovery following removal of tumors involving the dominant hemisphere supplementary motor area. J Neurosurg 1991; 75:62–68.

43. Soffietti R, Chio A, Giordana MT, et al: Prognostic factors in well-differentiated cerebral astrocytomas in the adult. Neurosurgery 1989; 24:686–692.

44. Steiger HJ, Markwalder RV, Seller RW, et al: Early prognosis of supratentorial grade 2 astrocytomas in adult patients after resection or stereotactic biopsy. Acta Neurochir 1990; 106:99–105.

45. Walker MD, Alexander EA Jr, Hunt WE, et al: Evaluation of BCNU and/or radiotherapy in the treatment of anaplastic gliomas. J Neurosurg 1978; 49:333.

46. Watanabe E, Watanabe T, Manaka S, et al: Three-dimensional digitizer (neuronavigator): New equipment for computed tomography-guided stereotaxic surgery. Surg Neurol 1987; 27:543–547.

47. Watanabe E: The neuronavigator: A potentiometer-based localization arm system. *In* Maciunas RJ (ed): Interactive Image-Guided Neurosurgery. Park Ridge, Ill, American Association of Neurological Surgeons, 1993, pp 135–148.

MITCHEL S. BERGER

GEORGE A. OJEMANN

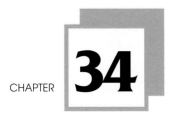

CHAPTER **34**

Techniques for Functional Brain Mapping During Glioma Surgery

Although aggressive surgical resection of both low-grade and high-grade gliomas provides a substantially improved overall survival and quality of life,[1–7] it can risk unacceptable morbidity because glial tumors characteristically infiltrate adjacent normal brain.[8–10] Gliomas occupy the temporal lobe in about 40% of cases.[11, 12] When the temporal lobe that is involved is in the patient's nondominant cerebral hemisphere, radical resection can often be accomplished with no functional deficit except a visual quadrantanopsia, but gliomas occupying the dominant temporal lobe pose significant risk because of the variable location of eloquent sites governing language.[13–15] Tumors of the basal ganglia or thalamus that encroach on the internal capsule present a risk of damage to descending motor pathways.

Although lesions that arise in a rather broad range of areas within the dominant hemisphere can alter language function, it is particularly critical to avoid injury to the sites of language and speech in the perisylvian area because permanent deficits generally occur only with lesions in this area. Although changes in language function frequently arise acutely with the resection of a lesion in the posterior superior frontal cortical areas, recovery soon follows.[16]

There are two approaches to minimize the risk of a language deficit in removal of a tumor that requires resection near the perisylvian cortex in the dominant hemisphere. With the traditional approach, anatomic structures thought to indicate areas not subserving language function provide landmarks for resection. For example, it has been recommended that a temporal resection be restricted to the anterior 4.0 to 4.5 cm or to a point just anterior to the inferior aspect of rolandic cortex, or to a point just anterior to the vein of Labbé. It has also been suggested that the superior temporal gyrus be spared, and the pterion has been proposed as the safe posterior limit for an inferior frontal resection. Such landmarks afford no guidance, however, when resecting a tumor from immediately perisylvian areas—especially those involving the posterior temporal and inferior parietal lobes. Moreover, resection within these safe limits can produce aphasia, particularly when the tumor is in the temporal lobe.[17]

Alternatively, essential functional areas of the brain in each patient can be identified by mapping the functional responses evoked when direct electrical stimulation is applied to cortical and subcortical regions. The mapping procedure can be performed extraoperatively after the implantation of long-term-use electrodes, usually in the subdural space,[18] or intraoperatively during craniotomy. Intraoperative brain mapping is performed by using local anesthesia, with the patient awake and responsive as direct electrical stimulation from a bipolar electrode probe is applied to the cortex at intervals while testing for sites of sensorimotor or language function. Sensorimotor testing is based on sensorimotor responses elicited with stimulation. For the localization of sites governing language function, the patient is asked to respond to questions on a standard repetitive measure of language.

For treating gliomas in either cerebral hemisphere, brain mapping to identify functional regions of the cortex during surgery for gliomas enables the surgeon to preserve eloquent function while safely performing more extensive resection than would otherwise be possible within acceptable limits of morbidity. Brain mapping during the resection of gliomas also permits the surgeon to perform aggressive resection of the tumor nidus and surrounding nonfunctional tissue that may serve to promote tumor regrowth.

Recurrence patterns suggest that gliomas usually recur at the primary resection site or contiguous to it,[19–21] within 2 cm of the contrast-enhancing rim as observed with computed tomography (CT) or magnetic resonance imaging (MRI).[19, 22] The local nature of gliomas is debated,[9, 22] however, as multicentricity has been observed at the time of initial presentation or recurrence in as many as 5% to 7% of cases, and neoplastic infiltration far distant from the disrupted blood-brain barrier has been shown on T2-weighted MRIs in regions that are not contrast-enhanced but have an abnormally high signal intensity.[10, 23] It is argued that more aggressive chemotherapy, irradiation, and new molecular therapeutic modalities can improve survival after surgery. Nonetheless, most patients with glioma die because of a failure to control local tumor recurrence.[20, 24]

421

In a retrospective computerized analysis of tumor volume[25] before and after surgery, we documented that a wide extent of resection of low-grade gliomas improves results in terms of time to tumor progression within the first 5 years,[26] particularly with gross total resection of all tumor seen as signal abnormalities on T2-weighted MRIs. Tumors resected less aggressively often recur with a more malignant phenotype than the original diagnosis. Technical advances make it increasingly feasible to perform radical resection that includes adjacent brain infiltrated by tumor. When considered in combination with more effective adjuvant therapies that are under development, an aggressive surgical approach can afford a definite survival advantage. The only deterrent is the risk of damage to functional parenchyma within and surrounding the tumor.

The often intractable seizures that accompany low-grade gliomas are of related concern. Substantial controversy exists about the origin of seizures in relation to the tumor nidus. The incidence of epilepsy in patients with supratentorial tumors varies among reported series, but it appears generally to occur in association with a slow-growing tumor, such as astrocytoma, ganglioglioma, or oligodendroglioma.[12, 27–32] The slow-growing tumor usually produces structural and chemical changes in the surrounding brain, including neurotransmitter alterations, which contribute to a hyperexcitable cortex.[33, 34] There is also a significant decrease in somatostatin and γ-aminobutyric acid (GABA) immunoreactive neurons in epileptic cortex as compared with adjacent, nonepileptic cortex from the same patient.[35] In treating low-grade gliomas, particularly in children and young adults, these factors must be considered in deciding whether to remove only the tumor or to also resect adjacent epileptogenic cortex that is documented intraoperatively with electrocorticography (ECoG).

To permit resection of neoplastic infiltration in the subcortical white matter, several of the techniques for functional brain mapping during glioma surgery are modified from those used for epilepsy surgery. Direct cortical stimulation was first used in the late 19th century, but it was Cushing,[36] and later Foerster[37] and Penfield and Boldrey,[38] who fostered its neurosurgical use. Penfield and Boldrey,[38] in a large series, showed that the anatomic basis for motor function lay in the precentral gyrus and that that for sensory function lay in the postcentral gyrus, and thereby confirmed earlier observations by Grunbaum and Sherrington[39] and Jackson.[37] Penfield and Roberts[40] developed the first techniques for identifying language function on the cortex with intraoperative stimulation. Table 34–1 summarizes the main sites for localization of functional areas during tumor surgery.

ROLE OF MAGNETIC RESONANCE IMAGING

An accurate preoperative assessment of sensory, motor, and language pathways may one day be achievable with functional MRI based on patterns of change in tissue deoxyhemoglobin concentrations. At present, this technique is most helpful in identifying the rolandic cortex.[41] The individual components of the leg motor cortex are not readily distinguished with functional MRI, however, and cortical sites

TABLE 34–1

PRINCIPAL SITES FOR LOCALIZATION OF FUNCTIONAL AREAS DURING GLIOMA RESECTION

Language and speech	
Dominant hemisphere	Posterior frontal, anterior parietal, temporal, insula
Motor pathways	
Cortical	Rolandic cortex, cerebral peduncle
Subcortical	Corona radiata, internal capsule
Supplementary motor region	Motor cortex and descending motor pathways
Insula	
Dominant hemisphere	Language localization and subcortical motor pathways
Nondominant hemisphere	Subcortical motor pathways
Spinal cord	
Motor pathways	Corticospinal tract or anterior horn cells
Sensory pathways	Primary sensory cortex (only with the patient awake)
Seizures	Electrocorticography (only for epilepsy refractory to medication)

*Adapted from Berger MS, Ojemann GA: Techniques of functional localization during removal of tumors involving the cerebral hemispheres. *In* Loftus C, Traynelis V (eds): Intraoperative Monitoring Techniques in Neurosurgery. New York, McGraw-Hill, 1994, pp 113–127.

governing motor speech, naming, and reading are almost impossible to identify and frequently appear in bilateral representation.[42] Functional MRI is, however, a useful aid in preoperative planning of the surgical resection strategy for lesions within or adjacent to the sensory motor cortex. The relation of a tumor to motor cortex is predicted by identifying consistent landmarks on MRIs. For example, the central sulcus is represented by a pair of mirror-image lines nearly perpendicular to the falx[43–45] that are readily identified near the convexity on T2-weighted axial images. Although this sulcus may be compressed by a large lesion, this landmark is usually identifiable by viewing T1- and T2-weighted images simultaneously. On midline sagittal and lateral parasagittal MRIs (although they are less sensitive), the marginal sulcus and a perpendicular line from the posterior roof of the insular triangle, respectively, localize the combined sensorimotor (rolandic) cortex. By viewing such images collectively, it is possible to gain nearly precise localization of the tumor and motor cortex for lesions of any histologic type or size.

PREOPERATIVE CONSIDERATIONS

In general, only patients with a confirmed history of medically refractory epilepsy are candidates for ECoG during tumor resection. ECoG mapping and removal of seizure foci is usually not done in patients whose seizures are well controlled with antiepileptic drugs.[46, 47] In treating any temporal lobe tumor associated with intractable seizures, it is critical to use strip electrodes to record under the temporal lobe before resection and on the amygdala and the hippocampus after the resection of lateral cortical structures, because patients with such tumors often have seizure foci in those regions. Our experience dictates that intraoperative ECoG is necessary to achieve optimum seizure control in such cases because the seizure activity usually originates in hyperexcitable cortex adjacent to the tumor that is not involved by tumor.[48]

Functional brain mapping is difficult or impossible in certain patients. A thorough neurologic assessment is necessary to determine whether a patient is a good candidate for the procedure. Intraoperative stimulation is unlikely to evoke motor responses in patients who have a dense hemiparesis despite the administration of steroids. Somatosensory evoked potentials (SSEPs) can be used to localize the central sulcus by documenting a phase reversal potential across the sulcus.[49]

Patients who cannot read simple phrases, name common objects, or understand spoken language are not candidates for language mapping. Functional mapping provides no reliable information in patients who have a baseline error rate of more than 25% when tested on object naming. For patients who have a partial expressive dysphasia but no difficulty understanding spoken language, dexamethasone (4 mg every 6 hours for 48 hours) should be given preoperatively in an attempt to improve the possibility of successful performance of mapping before tumor resection. In patients who have a moderate expressive dysphasia, attempts to perform language mapping by repetitively interrupting conversation with stimulation have been proved to be unreliable and should not be attempted.

In children with supratentorial brain tumors whom we have treated, physiologic mapping techniques have proved a safe, reliable, and valuable adjuvant in the resection of tumors within or adjacent to eloquent brain.[50] In children undergoing intraoperative brain mapping to localize language cortex, sensorimotor pathways, and seizure foci, direct cortical and subcortical stimulation, in addition to ECoG, have permitted us to maximize tumor resection, minimize morbidity, and eradicate epileptogenic zones. The epileptogenic zones were always adjacent to, but did not involve, the tumor nidus. Language localization was quite varied in the children tested and was anatomically unpredictable based on preoperative neurologic and radiologic examinations.

Often in children, particularly those younger than 5 to 7 years, the cortex does not respond when direct current is applied with the bipolar electrode probe.[47, 51] As we have elicited stimulation-induced motor responses in a few cases in which an electrode was placed within the central sulcus on the side of the precentral gyrus, it is conceivable that motor cortical neurons are buried deep within the sulcus during early childhood and only migrate to the gyral surface later. Whatever the reason, direct-stimulation mapping can fail in some cases and the surgeon should be prepared to substitute SSEPs as an alternative method for identifying a phase reversal over the central sulcus.[49, 52–54]

Intraoperative brain mapping performed as a one-stage procedure is contraindicated in children younger than early adolescence and in uncooperative adults. However, functional mapping can be accomplished in a two-stage procedure. An initial craniotomy is performed, preceding the operation for tumor resection, to insert a subdural electrode array (plate) *or to place a Silastic electrode grid in contact with the cortical surface* while the patient is under general anes-

thesia. Mapping of the motor, sensory, language, and seizure foci is then performed through the subdural grid when the patient is awake on the hospital ward. This procedure provides critical information, but it can risk infection and may entail faulty contact with the cortical surface owing to blood or cerebrospinal fluid, and it may be contraindicated in patients who have cerebral edema associated with a malignant glioma or metastatic tumor.

It is important to advise patients and their families that swelling during the first 48 hours after surgery often causes a deterioration of speech function, but that speech capabilities will return if they were normal before surgery and if the margin of tumor resection lies more than 1 cm from the nearest essential language site.[55] Motor function will be similarly affected after resection of tumor lying against functional cortical and subcortical descending motor pathways.

SURGICAL PROCEDURE

On the evening before surgery, antiepileptic drug levels are reviewed and, if necessary, are increased to therapeutic levels with extra doses. To enhance the intraoperative recordings, medications are withheld from patients undergoing ECoG in addition to tumor resection, but after the final phase of ECoG, antiepileptic drugs are given in high doses that maintain supratherapeutic levels to avoid postoperative seizures. A week or two after the operation, the dosage can be adjusted to obtain routine therapeutic levels, which are maintained for 6 to 12 months before a trial of dose tapering is attempted.

Surgery is performed with the patient awake. When the patient is brought to the operating room, a Foley catheter is inserted for administering osmotic diuretics. A roll is placed under the patient's left shoulder and the head rests, parallel to the floor, on a soft doughnut (Fig. 34–1). The head is shaved and scrubbed. The scalp is injected with a local anesthetic mixture (e.g., 0.5% lidocaine and 0.25% bupivacaine) to create a wide field block that extends from the zygoma above the orbital rim and posteriorly along the midline to several centimeters behind the pinna of the ear. If the patient is anxious, a small amount of fentanyl may be given, but with care taken not to oversedate the patient. The patient is then given propofol through an intravenous drip to produce a deep hypnotic state. As this drug is not an analgesic, however, the scalp and temporalis muscle must be adequately anesthetized to prevent the patient's experiencing pain. Propofol anesthesia is reestablished after the mapping procedure for those parts of the operation that do not require the patient's cooperation.

Although the site of the scalp incision depends on the tumor location, the incision itself must afford a wide cortical exposure to permit optimum mapping. If the bone flap that is created does not provide adequate exposure of the motor cortex, a strip electrode, with 1-cm intervals between electrodes, can be inserted subdurally to provide stimulation to elicit motor or sensory responses. Sites of language function must always be mapped through a large cortical exposure, however, because, in planning a resection, it is necessary both to isolate the cortical areas governing language and to establish that no language deficit occurs in the areas planned

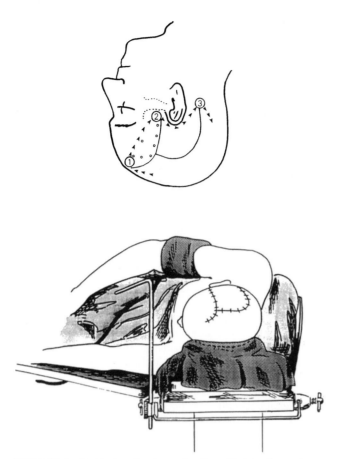

Figure 34–1 Positioning of patient and outline of incision for craniotomy involving a dominant hemisphere tumor, performed with patient awake. The *top* drawing depicts the line of injection of a lidocaine-Marcaine mixture, used to achieve local anesthesia during the awake craniotomy. (From Berger MS, Ojemann GA: Techniques of functional localization during removal of tumors involving the cerebral hemisphere. *In* Traynelis BC, Loftus CM (eds): Intraoperative Monitoring Techniques in Neurosurgery. New York, McGraw-Hill, 1993, pp 113–127.)

for resection. The area to be covered by stimulation mapping must include the area of planned resection as well as the likely sites of language, and the size of the surgical exposure must be planned accordingly. In patients with a temporal lobe tumor, the entire temporal lobe, as well as the inferior parietal and posterior frontal region, must be visible.

The dura is anesthetized by injecting the same local anesthetic mixture along the middle meningeal artery with a 30-gauge needle. Before the dura is opened, the patient is awakened by discontinuing the propofol drip. After about 8 to 15 minutes, when the patient is coherent, the dura may be incised; care must be taken to be certain that patients are awake because coughing while they awaken can cause brain herniation and cerebral edema if the dura is open.

STIMULATION TO LOCALIZE MOTOR FUNCTION

At 15 to 30 minutes before motor mapping is begun, the anesthesiologist is warned to discontinue the paralytic agents and obtain a train of four muscle twitches. For mapping, the

bipolar electrode is placed on the moist cortical surface in parallel to the sulcus.

The motor cortex is localized by using electrical stimulation with a bipolar electrode probe at intervals 5 mm apart. A constant-current generator is used that elicits a train of biphasic square-wave pulses (frequency, 60 Hz) with a 1.25-msec duration per phase; the maximum train duration is 4 seconds. If the patient were asleep, the current necessary to elicit motor responses would vary between 6 and 16 mA. With the patient awake, however, a lower current, in the range of 2 to 6 mA, will be adequate, particularly about the sensorimotor cortex subserving the face and hands. The current is adjusted in 1-mA increments for awake patients, or 2-mA increments for asleep patients, until the desired responses are elicited. Before the cortex is stimulated, the probe may be used briefly to depolarize the temporalis muscle to ensure that the probe is functional and that the paralytic agents are not affecting the patient. As a motor response is evoked from sites on the cortex, each site is marked with a small numbered ticket and is recorded in sequence together with the specific movements evoked.

With the technology available at present, the most practical approach is to identify the primary motor cortex (precentral gyrus) when removing tumors within or adjacent to this region; for example, in supplementary motor areas. With the patient awake, the motor cortex is stimulated with a current as low as 2 mA, especially in the face motor cortex. The primary sensory cortex can be identified by using the same stimulation level. The descending motor pathways in the subcortical white matter and internal capsule are localized with the stimulation as tumor resection proceeds. Because the current spread is minimal,[56, 57] the motor movements induced by the stimulation are evoked from a relatively focal area of cortex, permitting reliable localization of motor function to guide tumor resection and avoid injury to brain subserving the function, particularly in white matter of a grossly normal appearance and consistency.

Tumors that infiltrate the mesial frontal lobe often encroach on the ipsilateral cerebral peduncle. In such a case, it is difficult to dissect the uncus away from the peduncle and its junction with the internal capsule, but repetitive bipolar stimulation can be used during the resection to prevent inadvertent injury to the peduncle. Operations in the subinsular region, basal ganglia, and thalamus can be approached in the same manner. In each case, subcortical stimulation will reveal the internal capsule, which may be infiltrated or displaced by tumor but presents no landmarks to guide the surgeon. Because thalamic tumors usually involve the posterior half of the thalamus, particularly in children, the internal capsule is generally displaced anteriorly. By using a posterior transventricular approach, the initial response to stimulation will be foot and distal leg movement evoked from the posterior limb of the internal capsule. Resection can then proceed from a lateral or mesial aspect. In the case of tumor involving the dominant supplementary motor area that extends beyond 5 cm from the midline, both motor and language mapping are necessary because the high posterior-frontal convexity may harbor essential language sites.[15]

When resecting near the falx, it is usually not possible to see the leg motor cortex because it is hidden by the mass effect of the overlying gyri, but a strip electrode placed between the cortex and the falx will permit mapping of cortical sites associated with leg and foot movements (Fig. 34–2). Resection can then be carried back to within 1 cm of the proximal electrode contact adjacent to the functional sites. This technique is indispensable in the resection of tumors in the supplementary motor region. In some patients, cortical stimulation may evoke a focal motor seizure that is not harmful and usually stops within 10 to 30 seconds. A few minutes after the seizure, stimulation may be continued in the same area.

After functional cortical sites have been identified, the same or a slightly higher current may be used to elicit motor responses from subcortical white matter by using the bipolar electrode to touch and depolarize descending motor axons. As before, each site from which a motor response is evoked is marked with a small numbered ticket and is recorded in sequence together with the specific movements evoked.

After the motor and sensory cortex have been mapped with the patient awake, the ECoG equipment is brought to the operating field. First, the horseshoe-shaped holder is attached to a skull clamp affixed at the edge of the craniotomy, and strip electrodes are placed under the temporal lobe to record epileptic activity from mesial temporal structures. Usually, three strip electrodes are inserted under the lobe, one anteriorly, and one each at a midtemporal and a posterior temporal site. In patients who have an insular or frontal lobe tumor associated with intractable seizures, strip electrodes should be placed inferior to the frontal lobe.

After the placement of strip electrodes, single carbon-tipped electrodes are inserted into the horseshoe holder, one by one, a few centimeters apart, in rows along the lateral cortical surface of the temporal and suprasylvian areas. Each electrode is numbered according to the site where it is inserted into the holder and its placement is recorded. The recording begins and lasts as long as 20 minutes. In consultation, the surgeon and the electroencephalographer identify and record sites of frequent and repetitive spike discharge activity. The distance of this activity from the tumor is documented. Patients who show only a few sites of epileptiform activity may be given an intravenous bolus of methohexital (1 mg/kg) to provoke interictal discharges. For such

patients who show epileptiform activity, it is essential to perform ECoG again after resection to identify additional electrically active sites that, if not discovered, will result in poor postoperative control of seizures. In patients with intractable seizures and temporal lobe tumors, ECoG should always be attempted following resection because their epileptiform activity may be identified only when the exposed hippocampus is recorded.

For localizing sensory and motor pathways, we prefer direct stimulation mapping to the alternative approach involving SSEPs. Direct cortical stimulation is more time-effective and it provides a meticulously detailed map of each gyrus and its contiguous sulci. Moreover, it provides subcortical localization of descending motor or sensory pathways. The only potential difficulty is sometimes encountered when attempting to identify the motor cortex in younger children, which requires that SSEP instrumentation be available in the operating room in case cortical stimulation is not feasible.

An alternate approach for localizing the rolandic cortex is the recording of computer-averaged, short-latency evoked potentials from the cortical surface after the stimulation of large peripheral sensory (e.g., tibial or median) nerves.[58–60] The location of the motor cortex can be inferred by identifying a phase reversal potential across the central sulcus. However, this interpretation can sometimes be difficult to make, especially about the face motor cortex. Although this technique is accurate for mapping the cortex, mass effect can distort the anatomy of the motor strip, which may become particularly confusing as resection progresses. Recording from the cortex is done either with an electrode array, such as is used for language mapping, or with a Silastic electrode grid placed in contact with the cortical surface.[52] Similarly, stimulation can be performed through the grid to elicit motor or sensory responses.[61] It is important to note that general anesthesia can be used with either technique of direct stimulation mapping or SSEPs, but the depth of anesthesia will determine the current level needed to evoke responses. We now use the Silastic electrode grid only when necessary to map motor and language function in children and uncooperative adults.

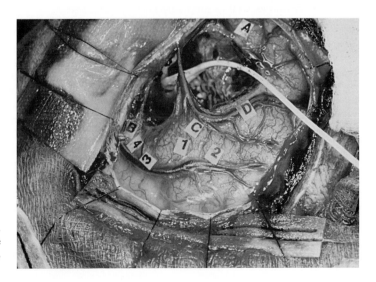

Figure 34–2 Intraoperative photograph demonstrates a strip electrode inserted following resection of the somatosensory cortex. The strip electrode is directed anteriorly to identify the leg motor cortex, which is adjacent to the falx.

STIMULATION TO LOCALIZE LANGUAGE FUNCTION

The localization of language function is usually mapped only in the hemisphere dominant for language, and then usually in the perisylvian area. It is generally assumed that the left hemisphere is dominant for language in right-handed patients, whereas left-handed patients must have dominance established preoperatively by using the intracarotid amobarbital (Amytal) perfusion procedure called Wada testing.[62] Actually, with the exclusion of patients who are left-handed owing to a lesion in the right hemisphere, the difference between left-handed and right-handed patients in regard to laterality of language has no statistical significance.[63] For most patients in both groups, the essential site for language is likely to be confined to the left hemisphere. Nonetheless, a few patients in each group have their essential sites of language function in the right hemisphere or bilaterally, and it may be that slightly more of those patients are left-handed. In about 85% of patients, the site that is essential for language is confined to the left hemisphere, whereas the right hemisphere is language dominant in about 6%, and language is represented bilaterally in about 9% of patients.

We usually establish hemispheric language dominance with Wada testing[62] if any doubt about cerebral dominance remains after the patient is asked about handedness. Indications for this procedure include left-handedness in patients with a tumor in either hemisphere or ambidexterity. Until recently, the usefulness of the Wada procedure in identifying hemispheric language dominance in children was extrapolated from studies in adults. However, its efficacy in children has been confirmed in a retrospective study of 77 consecutive epileptic pediatric patients, 34 of whom underwent intraoperative language mapping.[64] That study showed a strong correlation between left-handedness and an atypical lateralization of speech either bilaterally or to the right hemisphere, and between atypical lateralization of speech and right-sided hemiparesis that indicated early injury to the left hemisphere.

Stimulation mapping that yields a completely negative result affords no assurance that resection of the sites tested will not cause a language deficit. The area covered by stimulation mapping must therefore include the area of planned resection as well as the likely sites of language.

Methodological Issues

The optimal level of stimulation current and the survey measure used for the localization of language are the most important methodological issues in assessing language with stimulation.

ELECTRICAL STIMULATION CURRENT

In selecting current levels for language mapping with stimulation, the current must be strong enough to change cortical function, but not strong enough to elicit seizure activity or afterdischarges (ADs). It is also critical that stimulation effects are not propagated to distant sites, thereby precluding the localizing character of stimulation. At levels higher than 4 to 10 mA, depending on individual differences among patients, stimulation can elicit local ADs, which sometimes propagate to distant structures in a manner similar to that of other epileptic activity. For that reason, the optimal current level is usually set just below the threshold for evoking ADs in the cortical region being mapped, except in special cases. At such current levels, there is little empirical evidence to suggest a propagation of stimulation-induced effects. Were stimulation effects to spread to such deep structures as the thalamus and hippocampus, the behavioral changes evoked would be distinguishing, as they differ from those evoked from cortex.

For the intraoperative mapping of exposed cortex, it is usually possible to select one current that just straddles the AD threshold because intraoperative AD thresholds change little from site to site. ADs are read from the electrocorticogram and are evoked when the cortex is stimulated directly in contact with the recording electrode. Testing of the AD threshold is performed after the first phase of seizure mapping is completed.

When this technique is used to identify motor tracts within spinal cord tumors, the current is reduced to 0.5 mA and then increased gradually in 0.5-mA to 1-mA increments until 4 mA is reached. In our experience, it has not been necessary to exceed that current level.

SURVEY MEASURE

Patients' language capacities are tested before surgery. An extensively used measure of language function is object naming. It appears to be an adequate methodology for mapping before glioma resection because object-naming deficits are a component of all aphasic syndromes caused by glioma. Two respected studies of the relation of stimulation-evoked language changes to changes observed after tumor resection used object naming as the only measure of language, out of a general aphasia battery measuring many language functions, to predict the effects of resection from those of stimulation.[40, 65] However, stimulation of some cortical language sites may not be associated with naming deficits[66]; for example, changes in the ability to read a sentence have been elicited from a rather wider region of cortex than changes in naming, with only partial overlap.[15] Especially for patients undergoing resection in the posterior temporal lobe, we suggest evaluating the effects of stimulation on other language functions, in addition to object naming, before deciding that a cortical site can be resected safely.

Irrespective of the language function measured, the test must consist of many items of approximately equal difficulty, and each item must require only a few seconds for a correct response, as stimulation trains are relatively brief. Because the objective is to identify deficits with stimulation, and because it must be possible to distinguish whether a change during stimulation is a real effect of the current or simply a random event, the test must consist of items that the patient can manage accurately when not under stimulation. To confirm that changes elicited with stimulation are not random events, the patient's performance in the absence of stimulation should also be monitored throughout testing.

After the level of stimulation current has been selected, 10 to 20 sites on the cortical surface—both likely sites of language and sites in the planned area of resection—are marked with a small numbered ticket. Stimulation with the bipolar electrode is applied to one of the numbered cortical sites, and testing begins as the patient responds to repetitive measures of language function. Speech is assessed by first asking patients to count to 10 and to stick out their tongue, and then by using stimulation to block this function. This maneuver verifies that Broca's area and the inferior face motor cortex are intact. Patients are then presented with a series of randomly selected pictures of common objects shown by a slide projector at a rate of one every 4 seconds. Each slide shows a printed "leader phrase" and a drawing of an object. The patient is asked to read the phrase—for example, "this is a . . ."—and then to identify the illustrated object, such as a hat (Fig. 34–3). The electrode contact is maintained until the patient responds either correctly or incorrectly to one slide at a time. Cortical stimulation is then stopped, after which another slide is projected and the patient responds to verify a return to the baseline. Another site is then stimulated as the patient responds to still another slide. For each point of stimulation, the number of the stimulated site, the slides read correctly, and any errors in reading or object identification are recorded. This process continues until each cortical site is stimulated three or more times, and no site is stimulated twice in succession. When a crucial language site is identified, additional stimulation may be done around it to assess how closely surgical resection can approach the site without risking an alteration in function.

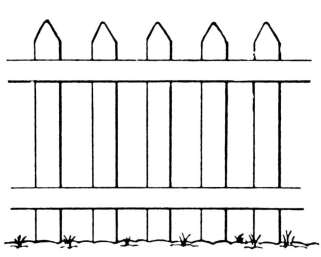

Figure 34–3 One of a slide series of common objects presented to patients during intraoperative mapping of brain regions subserving language function. Patients are asked to read the printed *leader phrase* and then to identify the object illustrated in the drawing. Cortical stimulation of each site is maintained until the patient responds either correctly or incorrectly as one slide is projected. Stimulation is then stopped, another slide is projected, and the patient is asked to respond to confirm a return to baseline. Thereafter, another site is stimulated as the patient responds to still another slide. For each point of stimulation, the site, slides read correctly, and any errors in reading or object identification are recorded. This process continues until each cortical site is stimulated at least three times; no site is stimulated twice in succession. Sites at which the patient makes repeated errors during stimulation appear to be particularly essential to language.

Stimulation mapping of 20 to 30 sites takes about 20 minutes with this technique.

Sites at which the patient makes repeated errors appear to be particularly essential to language (Fig. 34–4). Varied types of errors may be made, but in general only actual disruptions of performance are considered, and minor disruptions such as hesitations are not recorded. With the object-naming technique, such errors usually include anomia, in which the patient has the ability to speak but not to name objects, or the arrest of all speech, for example while counting numbers—which occurs somewhat more often with the stimulation of frontal sites. Reading slowly and with effort is considered a reading error, as is fluent reading during which the patient makes mistakes in verb endings, prepositions, conjunctions, and pronouns, suggesting a relation to syntax.[67]

Regions subserving language and speech must be identified for patients with tumors in the temporal, posterofrontal, or parietal lobes and the insula of the patient's dominant hemisphere. Language mapping is also necessary in the case of tumor involving the dominant supplementary motor area that extends beyond 5 cm from the midline because the high posterofrontal convexity may harbor essential language sites.[15]

In patients with a temporal lobe tumor who have a history of seizures, obtaining a thorough history of any speech dysfunction during or shortly after a seizure can contribute to language localization. Whereas a small mesial temporal tumor generally can be resected through an anterior temporal approach that requires a lateral cortical window no greater than 2 to 3 cm, particularly if the mass is in the superior temporal gyrus, such a procedure can be inadequate if intractable seizures are associated with the mesial temporal mass. In such an instance, resection of lateral cortical seizure foci detected with ECoG may be indicated, in which case prior language mapping is required.

EXTENT OF CORTICAL SURFACE SHOWING FUNCTIONAL ALTERATION WITH STIMULATION

Functional cortical mapping with electrical stimulation is based on the premise that the localized function is represented in the response elicited when current is applied to the surface of the cortex. Only a few studies have investigated the extent of cortical surface showing functional alteration with stimulation. When bipolar stimulation is applied at current levels used for cortical mapping, NADH fluorescence changes removed from the stimulation site take patterns that differ from one application of current to the next at the same site.[68] However, in a study to define the extent of evoked depolarization with similar levels of bipolar stimulation by using the changes in cortical light reflectance that identify neuronal depolarization in visual cortex, those effects were localized between electrode contacts and were relatively uniform between stimulation applications, both in the occipital cortex of monkeys[57] and in human motor and association cortexes.[69] Certainly, the behavioral effects of cortical stimulation are often quite localized, and stimulation at sites only a few millimeters apart differs markedly in its effect.[67]

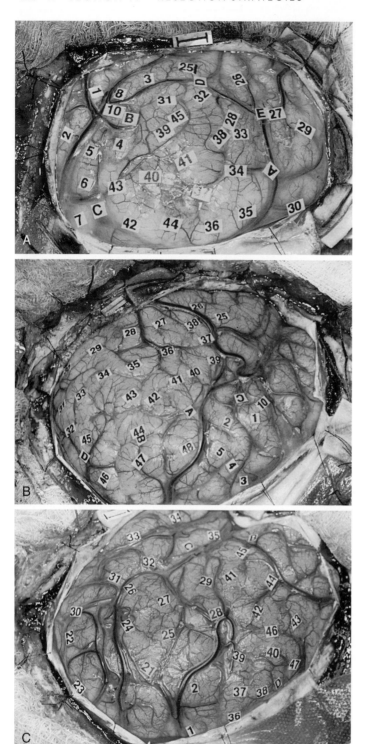

Figure 34–4 *A,* Intraoperative map of brain regions subserving language function in a patient with a large, low-grade glioma in the frontal lobe, as identified by numbers 39, 45, 41, and 40. The motor cortex is designated as 3, 5, 6, 7, involving the face and hand. Speech arrest was found at numbers 8 and 10. Anterior language sites for naming were identified at 25 and 26. *B,* Intraoperative map of the brain showing areas subserving language function in a patient with a diffuse, low-grade glioma involving the dominant hemisphere parietal lobe. The motor cortex involving the face is identified by numbers 1 and 3. The sensory cortex involving paresthesias of the face is identified by numbers 2, 4, and 5. Speech arrest was found at number 10. Areas of stimulation-induced reading deficit are at numbers 33 and 35, with anomia at 42 and 44. *C,* Intraoperative map showing areas subserving language function in a patient with a low-grade glioma involving the face motor area of the dominant hemisphere. The numbers 27, 25, and 24 identify the tumor. Areas at which stimulation induced movements of the face are depicted by numbers 1 and 2. Areas of stimulation-induced anomia are identified by numbers 22 and 32.

Mechanisms of Functional Alteration with Stimulation

The mechanisms through which stimulation affects language functions have not been defined. When electrical current is applied to the surface of the cortex, some neurons and incidentally affected subcortical fibers of both the excitatory and the inhibitory systems are activated, whereas the activity of other neurons and fibers is blocked through depolarization.[70] Although predicting the effects of stimulation based on physiologic changes is therefore impossible, the effects are predictable empirically. Stimulation of the primary motor and sensory cortex usually elicits a positive response. The motor cortex responds with localized movement, somatosensory cortex with localized dysesthetic sensation, primary visual cortex with localized flashes (phosphenes), and, more rarely, the primary auditory cortex with a "buzzing."[71] In some instances, secondary motor and sensory cortex also respond positively, in particular with formed visual responses, such as geometric lines, elicited from secondary visual cortex. Mullan and Penfield[72] and Penfield and Perot[73] reported an "interpretive" and "experiential" response evoked from temporal cortex with cortical stimulation; however, it may be that this response represented evoked local seizures because the experiential response, if not both of the responses evoked, is reported only with ADs that have propagated to medial temporal structures.[74]

Localization of Language Function

Although spontaneous speech usually cannot be elicited with cortical stimulation, Penfield and Roberts[40] showed that at some sites on the association cortex, the application of current elicits no response when the patient is silent but serves to disrupt performance when the patient becomes active in using higher functions such as language—for example, blocking the patient's ability to complete ongoing object naming. It seems likely that when activity is altered, the prevailing effect of stimulation at those sites is either blockade as a result of depolarization or the activation of inhibitory systems. Various types of naming errors were elicited, including the arrest of all speech, anomia, hesitation, and repetitions. Penfield proposed that sites eliciting anomia, which were located in only the left hemisphere, were important to language function because they corresponded approximately to traditional language areas defined in the study of brain lesions. More direct evidence has since supported the relevance to language function of sites at which object naming is disrupted by applied stimulation. One study[7] showed that when the Wepman aphasia battery was given 1 month postoperatively to patients in whom tumor resection in the left anterior temporal lobe had stopped within 2 cm of a site at which repeated anomic errors or arrests were elicited during a naming test, their scores showed subtle increases in errors. However, there were no evident changes on the aphasia battery in patients in whom resection stopped more than 2 cm from those sites at which a change in language function was evoked. No correlation was found in the former group between postoperative aphasic errors and either extent of resection, preoperative language performance, or degree of postoperative seizure control.

Another study of stimulation during object naming investigated the relation between clinically evident aphasia and tumor resections near temporal sites related to language.[75] Cortical mapping with bipolar stimulation was used to localize essential sites of language function in 40 patients undergoing resection of a glioma in the temporal lobe of their dominant hemisphere. The sites of language function were localized to distinct temporal-lobe sectors and compared with those localized in 83 patients without tumors who had undergone language mapping during their treatment for intractable epilepsy. In both groups of patients, the superior temporal gyrus contained significantly more sites of language function than the middle temporal gyrus. In both groups, 12% to 16% of patients also had language sites anterior to the central sulcus in the superior temporal gyrus.

Significantly more language sites were found in the superior temporal gyrus in the group of patients who did not have temporal lobe tumors than in the group of patients with tumors. Variables examined for their effect on preoperative and postoperative language deficits included age, sex, number of language sites, histologic characteristics, tumor size, and the distance of the margin of tumor resection from the nearest language site. The most important variable determining improvement from preoperative language deficits, the duration of language deficits postoperatively, and the permanence of the deficits was the distance of the resection margin from the nearest language site. When the resection margin was within 0.7 cm of a language site, language deficits frequently were permanent, whereas there were no permanent language deficits postoperatively in patients whose resection margin was greater than 1 cm distant from a language site. Patients whose resection margin was within 0.7 to 1.0 cm had deficits, but most recovered within 7 to 30 days after surgery, depending on the distance from the resection margin to a language site. We conclude that cortical sites at which stimulation mapping elicits changes in the ability to perform object-naming tests appear to be essential for language, although the margin of resection can be quite near the site without producing a permanent language deficit.

We would not ordinarily expect that stimulation of the cortical surface would predict the effects of resections that include both the cortical surface and the more extensive deeper cortex. It appears that the cortical language system has a major vertical organization and a preferential location of essential functional areas in crowns of gyri. If critical areas of language function existed deep in the cortex, distant from those on the surface, stimulation of the surface would not reliably predict the effect of resection in the deep cortex. Moreover, in more than 98% of 119 patients in one study,[15] stimulation mapping identified surface sites. This finding indicates that language sites are not randomly distributed throughout the cortex, as substantially more than half of the human cortex is buried. Sulci are not often mapped for language function, but the few studies that are extant have not shown independent sites. In some patients, however, a surface site has extended a short distance into the sulcus.[15, 65] It appears that the connections linking critical language areas must also be organized vertically because surface stimulation also predicts the effect of a resection of white matter back to the essential area. The relation between the effects of surface stimulation and resection appears to also apply to a similar relation between effects of frontal opercular stimulation and results of subinsular resections in the dominant hemisphere.[76]

Stimulation mapping during testing with a measure of language function in adults reveals characteristics of the neurobiology of language that would not be expected from the effect of brain lesions.[77] Such characteristics can be essential to the planning of resections in the dominant cerebral hemisphere. For example, sites that repeatedly evoke errors when tested on one language measure—and are therefore critical to that function—are highly localized in each individual patient, but there are substantial individual differences among individuals in any population of patients in the exact location of these sites.

A study of 117 patients who underwent intraoperative

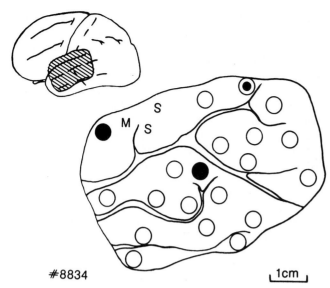

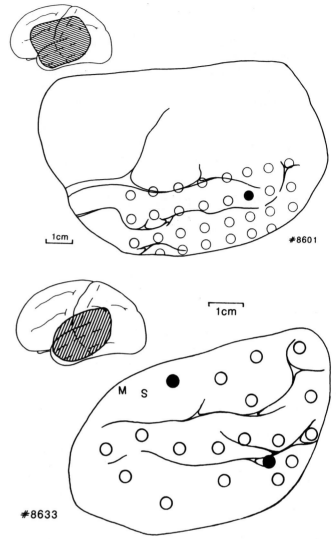

Figure 34–5 Sites essential for naming *(filled circles)* in a 24-year-old woman who had a verbal IQ of 81. Stimulation was at 6 mA, and the control error rate in the absence of stimulation was 3.7%. The *open circles* mark stimulation sites that did not evoke errors; a site of single nonsignificant error is shown by a small dot. M and S identify sites with motor (M) or sensory (S) responses. Note the localized posterior language area with closely spaced surrounding stimulation sites without errors. (From Ojemann GA, Ojemann J, Lettich E, et al: Cortical language localization in the left, dominant hemisphere: An electrical stimulation mapping investigation in 117 patients. J Neurosurg 1989; 71:316–326.)

stimulation mapping of the left dominant perisylvian cortex during object naming[15] showed that the essential sites in most of the patients had a surface area of 2 cm² or less (Figs. 34–5 to 34–7), and only 16% of the patients had a site as large as 6 cm² (Fig. 34–8). There are many examples of highly discrete sites of language function,[15, 65, 78–82] often at both frontal and temporoparietal sites, which have been

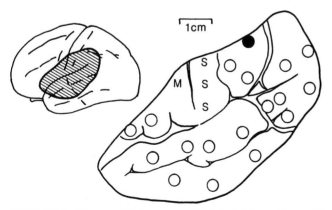

Figure 34–6 Sites essential for naming *(filled circles)* in an 18-year-old woman who had a verbal IQ of 95. Stimulation was at 4 mA, and the control error rate in the absence of stimulation was 0%. The *open circles* mark stimulation sites that did not evoke errors. In this left-handed patient, the intracarotid amobarbital perfusion test showed language in only the left hemisphere. With language residing in this unusual parietal site, no limits are posed on a temporal resection. M and S indicate sites with motor (M) or sensory (S) responses. (From Ojemann GA, Ojemann J, Lettich E, et al: Cortical language localization in the left, dominant hemisphere: An electrical stimulation mapping investigation in 117 patients. J Neurosurg 1989; 71:316–326.)

Figure 34–7 Sites of significant evoked naming errors *(filled circles)* in a 4-year-old boy *(upper)* and a 70-year-old man *(lower)*, both of whom had medial temporal lobe gliomas. The open circles indicate stimulation sites at which no errors were evoked. The boy was stimulated through a chronic subdural grid. Both patients have highly localized temporal language sites. M and S identify sites with motor (M) or sensory (S) responses. (From Ojemann GA, Ojemann J, Lettich E, et al: Cortical language localization in the left, dominant hemisphere: An electrical stimulation mapping investigation in 117 patients. J Neurosurg 1989; 71:316–326.)

identified with language measures such as object naming and word and sentence reading. Some sites have a distinct margin, whereas others are surrounded by an area in which errors are elicited sporadically with stimulation, implying a more graded transition from essential cortex to cortex unrelated to language function.[78, 79] Most patients have several essential perisylvian areas for a language function. Among the 117 patients in the series just mentioned,[15] two thirds had two sites and one quarter had three sites separated by cortex unrelated to language function. Most had one frontal and one or more temporoparietal sites, but some patients had multiple frontal sites.

With all functional mapping methods, there is considerable variation in the exact location of critical language sites (Fig. 34–9).[15, 65, 78, 79] When the left perisylvian cortex was

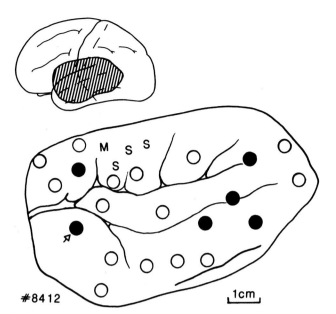

Figure 34-8 Sites essential for naming *(filled circles)* in a 46-year-old woman who had a verbal IQ of 91. Stimulation was at 7 mA, and the control error rate in the absence of stimulation was 6%. The *open circles* mark stimulation sites at which no errors were evoked. Note the relatively large posterior language area, but the very localized anterior language site and a language site in the anterior superior temporal gyrus *(arrow)* in front of rolandic cortex, 4 cm from the temporal tip. M and S identify sites with motor (M) or sensory (S) responses. (From Ojemann GA, Ojemann J, Lettich E, et al: Cortical language localization in the left, dominant hemisphere: An electrical stimulation mapping investigation in 117 patients. J Neurosurg 1989; 71:316–326.)

mapped in the study of 117 patients,[15] language changes in most patients were evoked from only one small area, the posterior inferior frontal lobe, just anterior to the face motor cortex. In some patients, critical sites of language function were localized in "safe" areas, in superior and even middle temporal gyrus in front of rolandic cortex, less than 4.5 cm from the temporal tip. Critical sites of language function have been localized as far forward in the inferior frontal

lobe as the pterion.[15] In contrast, some patients have no temporal language sites, and in those patients an extensive temporal resection poses no risk to language function. In the study of 117 patients,[15] of 90 patients who had frontal and temporoparietal mapping—all of whom were confirmed as left-dominant preoperatively with the Wada testing[62]—16% were found to have language function confined only to frontal sites, with no critical language sites whatever in the temporoparietal region. Conversely, another 15% of those patients had only temporoparietal sites and no frontal sites. Throughout the posterior language area, no specified local area was essential to language function in more than about one third of patients. This variability in the location of language function is far more extensive than the morphologic variability in perisylvian cortex, although that, too, is considerable.[83, 84] Moreover, language function is not related reliably to any particular cytoarchitectonic region. The discrete localization of sites essential to language function in each individual patient, contrasted with the extensive variation in the location of critical language sites across the population, constitutes a strong rationale for stimulation mapping in preference to the use of anatomic landmarks in planning the resection of tumors situated adjacent to such critical areas.

Individual differences in the sites of critical language function seem to be related to the patient's sex and preoperative verbal abilities. In the series of 117 patients[15] who underwent mapping during object naming, evidence suggested that the women were somewhat less likely than the men to have posterior sites of language function. Based on the preoperative use of the verbal intelligence quotient (VIQ) as a measure of verbal ability, patients who had a higher VIQ were somewhat more likely to have essential sites of language function in the middle temporal gyrus, whereas those who had a lower VIQ were somewhat more likely to have their critical language sites in the superior temporal gyrus.[15, 65]

A comparison of effects of electrical stimulation on patients tested with measures of different language functions shows a degree of differential localization. When patients

Figure 34-9 Variability in language localization in 117 patients. Individual maps are aligned, and cortex is divided into zones *(dashed lines)*. The upper number in each zone indicates the number of patients with a site in that zone. The lower number in a circle is the percentage of those patients with sites of significant evoked naming errors in that zone. M and S indicate motor (M) or sensory (S) cortex. (From Ojemann GA, Ojemann J, Lettich E, et al: Cortical language localization in the left, dominant hemisphere: An electrical stimulation mapping investigation in 117 patients. J Neurosurg 1989; 71:316–326.)

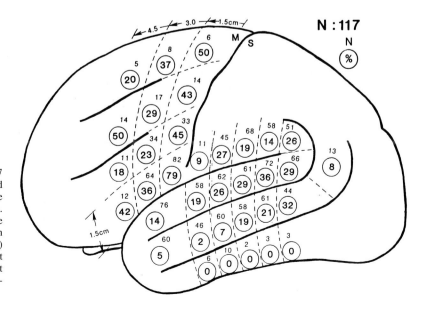

are asked to perform the same language function, object naming, in two different languages, nearly every patient tested has some sites that are essential to object naming in only one of the two languages.[13, 67, 82, 85] Differential sites have been localized in both frontal and temporoparietal lobes. Differential localization was also shown for naming whether patients used an oral or a manual communication system.[86] When the effects of stimulation on object naming and then on reading are tested in the same person, sites often respond with changes elicited for only object naming or for only reading.[65] Patients also may have sites where their tested understanding is defective but their language expression is intact; these are most frequently located in posterior language areas. Some perisylvian sites respond to stimulation with changes on measures of both language expression, including sequential orofacial movement, and perception, which suggests that at those sites resides a mechanism related to both of these two functions,[66, 67] at least in those particular patients.

A study of 14 patients to assess the effects of stimulation on an array of language-related functions, including object naming, reading, recent verbal memory, orofacial mimicry, and speech sound identification, has provided a basis for a model of language organization in lateral cortex. This included a perisylvian area, involving superior temporal and anterior parietal as well as posterior frontal lobes important to speech production and perception, a surrounding zone of specialized sites, some of which were related to syntax, and an even more peripheral area related to recent verbal memory.[67] The stimulation technique for functional brain mapping is a valuable instrument for further defining the extent of separation of language-related functions and the relations among areas important to subserving eloquent function.

Information is relatively sparse regarding the stability of stimulation-derived sites of language localization over time, with or without an intervening brain lesion. In those instances in which repeated mapping was performed after several months without an intervening brain lesion, the comparison of sites with and without language change, as assessed with extraoperative and intraoperative mapping, have generally showed them to be in a similar location.[67] A study in which sites of language function were mapped again several years after static perisylvian brain injuries, such as trauma or stroke, associated with partially recovered aphasias showed language sites located on the edge of the damaged cortex in locations at which language sites are expected in nonaphasic patients (unpublished observations). In patients with recurrent brain tumors and developing aphasias, repeat mapping showed the disappearance of one of the localized areas essential to language after progression of the language deficit, whereas other areas remained stable (unpublished observations).

No findings of functional brain mapping indicate that adults enjoy any degree of plasticity in the localization of essential language function. In our experience with a large series of nonaphasic patients, those who had low-grade intrinsic tumors of the left temporal lobe had fewer sites of language function than did a series of nonaphasic patients with left temporal epileptic foci. This result suggests that the tumor may have slowly destroyed some temporal lan-

guage sites without producing functional deficit. No sign of excessive extratemporal sites was observed, as could be expected with reorganization.

Often, either intraoperative or extraoperative mapping can be used appropriately in planning to treat patients requiring resection (e.g., the many patients, including those with seizure disorders, for whom no intracranial ictal recordings are required, and most adolescents and adults who can cooperate with an awake craniotomy performed with local anesthetic technique). In treating such patients, the main problem with using the intraoperative technique is the limited time available for language mapping. As suggested earlier, however, it is possible to assess many language functions readily at many sites in about 30 minutes, which usually affords all the information necessary to plan the resection. Moreover, the intraoperative technique has several definite advantages, not the least of which is greater flexibility in assessing areas of cortex because effects are not limited by the edges of the electrode arrays. In addition, effects are often better localized, probably because the electrode contact with the cortex can be controlled more finely. The risks of extraoperative mapping and the costs associated with the additional craniotomy, electrode placement, and hospitalization are strong incentives as well. For patients who can be managed equally satisfactorily with either technique, we recommend intraoperative mapping.

FUNCTIONAL SITES WITHIN GLIOMA TISSUE

Some neurosurgeons hold that patients with intra-axial tumors can be treated with a low risk of neurologic deficit if tumor resection is kept within the confines of the grossly abnormal tissue—even when the lesion is located in a presumably functional area—provided that adjacent normal-appearing cortex and subcortical white matter are not disturbed. Our work, in contrast, has shown that functioning motor, sensory, or language tissue can be located in surrounding infiltrated brain as well as within frankly evident tumor.

In our experience with more than 400 patients, intraoperative mapping with bipolar electrode stimulation techniques identified 28 patients who showed evidence of having functional tissue within infiltrative glioma, as was correlated by CT and MRI, intraoperative ultrasound, gross visualization, and histologic confirmation.[56] Direct-stimulation mapping of cortical and subcortical portions of the tumor during resection identified functional sites subserving motor function, sensory function, object naming, reading, or speech arrest. Of 28 patients, 19 had new or worsened neurologic deficits immediately after surgery, but 3 months later only 6 continued to have the new deficit, whereas 18 showed no deficits and 2 improved. Irrespective of the degree of tumor infiltration, edema, evident necrosis, or distortion by tumor mass, functional cortical tissue and subcortical white matter can exist within the tumor or the adjacent infiltrated brain. Intraoperative stimulation mapping can detect functional cortical or subcortical tissue, both within and adjacent to tumor; provide the maximum extent of glioma resection with the least possible injury to eloquent brain in these functional areas; and minimize the incidence of permanent deficit.

SEIZURES ASSOCIATED WITH GLIOMAS

The optimal way to manage patients with intractable epilepsy and an intrinsic neoplasm is a source of controversy, which holds on one hand the view that optimal management need entail only tumor resection, and on the other hand that tumor resection should be preceded by mapping of seizure foci either with ECoG or extraoperative recordings. In our experience, patients who have had tumor resection preceded by ECoG fare far better than have historical controls from series undergoing only tumor resection as reported in the recent literature.[46]

In a series of 45 patients with low-grade gliomas and intractable epilepsy, we retrospectively analyzed preoperative seizure frequency and duration, number of antiepileptic drugs, intraoperative ECoG data from single vs. multiple foci, histologic characteristics of resected seizure foci, and postoperative control of seizures with or without antiepileptic drugs. As compared with patients with single seizure foci, more with multiple seizure foci had a longer preoperative duration of epilepsy. Of the 45 patients, 24 were no longer taking antiepileptic drugs and were seizure-free at the time of this study (mean follow-up interval, 54 months); 17 patients had complete seizure control and were taking antiepileptic drugs at lower doses (mean follow-up interval, 44 months); and 7 of the 17 patients were seizure-free postoperatively, but the referring physician was reluctant to taper the medication. Four patients receiving antiepileptic drugs still had seizures, but they were reduced in frequency and severity. In this series, 41% of the adults vs. 85% of the children were seizure-free while no longer receiving antiepileptic drugs, with mean postoperative follow-up intervals of 50 and 56 months, respectively ($P = 0.016$). On the basis of that experience and many other retrospective studies of similar patients, we recommend ECoG, especially for children and any patients with a persisting seizure disorder, to maximize control of the seizures while minimizing or obviating the need for antiepileptic drugs after surgery.[87]

Many studies emphasize the role of ECoG in tumor resection, but most afford no information about the need for antiepileptic drugs after surgery.[88–90] In one study,[91] about 50% of patients required antiepileptic drugs to reduce seizure frequency by half, despite the intraoperative use of mapping for seizure foci. Reports from the Cleveland Clinic[92, 93] support extraoperative mapping of seizure foci to locate areas adjacent to tumor that require resection to obtain optimal seizure control. The extent of tumor removal was considered as a variable in achieving optimum control of the epilepsy. When the tumor was, for example, an infiltrative low-grade glioma that was not completely resectable, better seizure control was gained by a more radical resection of one or more epileptogenic foci. Nonetheless, all patients required antiepileptic drugs to maintain a reduced seizure frequency. We believe that after resection, ECoG is mandatory to detect hidden seizure foci that are revealed by the initial resection and to obviate any suffering as a consequence of the persistence of epileptogenic regions.

Among other investigators, Spencer and colleagues[94] have advocated tumor resection together with an epilepsy type of operation to remove adjacent mesial temporal or frontal parenchyma without ECoG guidance. As compared with patients undergoing only tumor removal, patients who had this type of surgery for a tumor associated with intractable epilepsy showed a significant reduction in the frequency of seizures. Seizure control was not complete, however, and no information was given about antiepileptic drug usage.

Penfield and others,[29] White and co-workers,[95] Falconer and associates,[96] and Schisano and colleagues[97] advocated tumor removal alone for patients with intractable epilepsy, and the majority of patients continued to have seizures after surgery. Many years later, Goldring and others[98] reported seizure control in 82% of patients after tumor resection without ECoG, although most of their patients had temporal lobe tumors that often required radical removal of mesial structures to maximize tumor resection. They, too, did not mention the use of antiepileptic drugs to maintain this high rate of seizure control. Cascino[99] reported a series of patients undergoing computer-assisted stereotactic tumor resection without removal of adjacent tissue; most of those patients had a reduced seizure frequency and 97% remained on antiepileptic drugs. These investigators considered that for patients with intractable epilepsy associated with an intrinsic tumor, it would not be possible to resect separate seizure foci using their technique, and a second operation might be necessary to control the epilepsy. Hirsch and co-workers[28] believed that tumor resection alone, without ECoG, would control epilepsy refractory to medication in a pediatric series. Only 57% of the children so treated were seizure-free without antiepileptic drugs, whereas 24% continued to have seizures while still taking antiepileptic drugs.

Our data show the efficacy of intraoperative seizure mapping and extraoperative (grid) recordings. The results obtained in pediatric patients have been almost as favorable as those seen in our adult patients, although the adults must rely more greatly on postoperative antiepileptic drugs to maintain a seizure-free status.[46] As this technology becomes more familiar and more widely used, it will provide patients who have tumors associated with intractable epilepsy with a greater opportunity for seizure control.

ACKNOWLEDGMENT

The authors appreciate the editorial collaboration of Susan Eastwood, E.L.S.(D.), in the preparation of this chapter.

REFERENCES

1. Ammirati M, Vick N, Liao Y, et al: Effect of the extent of surgical resection on survival and quality of life in patients with supratentorial glioblastomas and anaplastic astrocytomas. Neurosurgery 1987; 21:201–206.
2. Ciric I, Ammirati M, Vick N, et al: Supratentorial gliomas: Surgical considerations and immediate postoperative results. Neurosurgery 1987; 21:21–26.
3. Wood JR, Green SB, Shapiro WR: The prognostic importance of tumor size in malignant gliomas: A computed tomographic scan study by the Brain Tumor Cooperative Group. J Clin Oncol 1988; 6:338–343.
4. Nelson DF, Nelson JS, Davis DR, et al: Survival and prognosis of

patients with atypical or anaplastic features. J Neurooncol 1985; 3:99–103.

5. Shaw EG, Scheithauer BW, O'Fallon JR, et al: Oligodendrogliomas: The Mayo Clinic experience. J Neurosurg 1992; 76:428–434.
6. Ammirati M, Galicich JH, Arbit E, et al: Reoperation in the treatment of recurrent intracranial malignant gliomas. Neurosurgery 1987; 21:607–614.
7. Ojemann GA, Dodrill CG: Intraoperative techniques for reducing language and memory deficits with left temporal lobectomy. Adv Epileptol 1987; 16:327–330.
8. Burger PC, Heinz ER, Shibata T, et al: Topographic anatomy and CT correlations in the untreated glioblastoma multiforme. J Neurosurg 1988; 68:698–704.
9. Halperin EC, Burger PC, Bullard DE: The fallacy of the localized supratentorial malignant glioma. Int J Radiat Oncol Biol Phys 1988; 15:505–509.
10. Kelly PJ, Daumas-Duport C, Scheithauer BW, et al: Stereotactic histologic correlations of computerized tomography and magnetic resonance imaging defined abnormalities in patients with glial neoplasms. Mayo Clin Proc 1987; 62:450–459.
11. Laws ER Jr, Taylor WF, Bergstrahl EJ, et al: The neurosurgical management of low-grade astrocytoma. Clin Neurosurg 1986; 33:575–588.
12. Piepmeier JM: Observations on the current treatment of low-grade astrocytic tumors of the cerebral hemispheres. J Neurosurg 1987; 67:177–181.
13. Black P, Ronner S: Cortical mapping for defining the limits of tumor resection. Neurosurgery 1987; 20:914–919.
14. Ojemann GA, Creutzfeldt OD: Language in humans and animals: Contribution of brain stimulation and recordings. In Plum F, Geiger S (eds): Handbook of Physiology, Nervous System V, part 2. Bethesda, Md, American Physiological Society Press, 1987, pp 675–700.
15. Ojemann GA, Ojemann J, Lettich E, et al: Cortical language localization in the left, dominant hemisphere: An electrical stimulation mapping investigation in 117 patients. J Neurosurg 1989; 71:316–326.
16. Rostomily R, Berger M, Ojemann G, et al: Postoperative deficits and functional recovery following removal of tumors involving the dominant hemisphere supplementing motor area. J Neurosurg 1991; 75:62–68.
17. Heilman K, Wilder B, Malzone W: Anomic aphasia following anterior temporal lobectomy. Trans Am Neurol Assoc 1972; 97:291–293.
18. Luders H, Lesser R, Hahn J, et al: Basal temporal language area demonstrated by electrical stimulation. Neurology 1986; 36:505–510.
19. Hockberg FH, Pruitt A: Assumptions in the radiation therapy of glioblastoma. Neurology 1980; 30:907–911.
20. Salazar OM, Rubin P, McDonald J: Patterns of failure in intracranial astrocytomas after irradiation: Analysis of dose and field factors. AJR 1976; 126:279–292.
21. Wallner KE, Galicich JH, Krol G, et al: Patterns of failure following treatment for glioblastoma multiforme and anaplastic astrocytoma. Int J Radiat Oncol Biol Phys 1989; 16:1405–1409.
22. Burger P: The anatomy of astrocytomas. Mayo Clin Proc 1987; 62:527–529.
23. Kelly PJ: Image-directed tumor resection. Neurosurgery Clin North Am 1990; 1:81–95.
24. Silbergeld DL, Rostomily RC, Alvord EC Jr: The cause of death in patients with glioblastoma is multifactorial: Clinical factors and autopsy findings in 117 cases of supratentorial glioblastomas in adults. J Neurooncol 1991; 10:179–185.
25. Duong DH, Rostomily RC, Haynor DR, et al: Oligodendrogliomas: The Mayo Clinic Experience. J Neurosurg 1992; 76:428–434.
26. Berger MS, Keles GE, Ojemann GA, et al: Extent of resection affects recurrence patterns in patients with low grade gliomas. Cancer 1994; 74:1784–1791.
27. Arseni C, Petrovici IN: Epilepsy of temporal lobe tumors. Eur Neurol 1971; 5:201–214.
28. Hirsch JF, Rose CS, Pierre-Kahn A, et al: Benign astrocytic and oligodendrocytic tumors of the cerebral hemispheres in children. J Neurosurg 1989; 70:568–572.
29. Penfield W, Erickson TC, Tarlov IM: Relation of intracranial tumors and symptomatic epilepsy. Arch Neurol Psychiatry 1940; 44:300–315.
30. Pilcher WH, Silbergeld DL, Berger MS, et al: Intraoperative electrocorticography during tumor resection: Impact on seizure outcome in patients with gangliomas. J Neurosurg 78:891–902, 1993.
31. Rasmussen TB: Surgery of epilepsy associated with brain tumors. Adv Neurol 1975; 8:227–239.
32. White JC, Liu CT, Mixter WJ: Focal epilepsy: A statistical study of its causes and the results of surgical treatment: Epilepsy secondary to intracranial tumors. N Engl J Med 1948; 238:891–899.
33. Kim JH, Guimaraes PO, Shen MY, et al: Hippocampal neuronal density in temporal lobe epilepsy. Acta Neuropathol 1990; 80:41–45.
34. deLanerole NC, Kim JH, Rommins RH, et al: Hippocampal interneuron loss and plasticity in human temporal lobe epilepsy. Brain Res 1989; 49:387–395.
35. Haglund MM, Berger MS, Kunkel DD, et al: Changes in GABA and somatostatic in epileptic cortex associated with low-grade gliomas. J Neurosurg 1992; 77:109–216.
36. Cushing H: A note upon the faradic stimulation of the postcentral gyrus in conscious patients. Brain 1909; 32:44–53.
37. Foerster O: The motor cortex in man in the light of Hughlings Jackson's doctrines. Brain 1936; 59:135–159.
38. Penfield W, Boldrey E: Somatic motor and sensory representation in the cerebral cortex of man as studied by electrical stimulation. Brain 1937; 60:389–443.
39. Grunbaum ASF, Sherrington GS: Observations on physiology of the cerebral cortex of some of the higher animals. Proc R Soc Lond 1901; 69:206.
40. Penfield W, Roberts L: Speech and Brain Mechanisms. Princeton, NJ, Princeton University Press, 1959.
41. Jack CR Jr, Thompson RM, Butts RK, et al: Sensory motor cortex: Correlation of presurgical mapping with functional MR imaging and invasive cortical mapping. Radiology 1994; 190:85–92.
42. Maldjian J, Atlas S, Howard RS, et al: Functional magnetic resonance imaging of regional brain activity in patients with intracerebral arteriovenous malformation before surgical or endovascular therapy. J Neurosurg 1996; 84:477–483.
43. Berger MS, Cohen W, Ojemann GA, et al: Brain mapping techniques maximize resection, safety, and seizure control in children with brain tumors. Neurosurgery 1989; 25:786–792.
44. Berger MS: Preoperative magnetic resonance imaging localization of the primary motor cortex. Perspect Neurol Surg 1991; 2:23–32.
45. Berger MS: Use of magnetic resonance imaging for intraoperative localization. In Wilkins RH, Rengachary S (eds): Neurosurgery, part V, ed 2. New York, McGraw-Hill, 1995, pp 559–562.
46. Berger MS, Ghatan S, Geyer JR, et al: Seizure outcome in children with hemispheric tumors and associated intractable epilepsy: The role of tumor removal combined with seizure foci resection. Pediatr Neurosurg 1992; 17:185–191.
47. Berger MS, Kincaid J, Ojemann GA, et al: Brain mapping techniques to maximize resection, safety, and seizure control in children with brain tumors. Neurosurgery 1989; 25:786–792.
48. Ghatan S, Berger MS, Ojemann GA, et al: Seizure control in patients with low-grade gliomas: Resection of the tumor and separate seizure foci. Clin Res 1991; 39:105.
49. Woolsey CB, Cividosan TC, Gibson WE: Localization in somatosensory and motor areas of human cerebral cortex as determined by direct recording of epilepsy and electrical stimulation. J Neurosurg 1979; 51:476–506.
50. Berger MS, Kincaid J, Ojemann GA, et al: Brain mapping techniques to maximize resection, safety, and seizure control in children with brain tumors. Neurosurgery 1989; 25:786–792.
51. Goldring S, Gregori EM: Surgical management of epilepsy using epidural recordings to localize the seizure focus. J Neurosurg 1984; 60:457–466.
52. Gregori EM, Goldring S: Localization of function in the excision of lesions from the sensorimotor region. J Neurosurg 1984; 61:1047–1054.
53. Goldring S: Epilepsy surgery. Clin Neurosurg 1983; 31:369–388.
54. Luders H, Leser RP, Morris HH, et al: Chronic intracranial recording and stimulation with subdural electrodes. In Engel JP (ed): Surgical Management of the Epilepsies. New York, Raven Press, 1987, pp 297–321.
55. Skirboll SS, Ojemann GA, Berger MS, et al: Functional cortex and subcortical white matter located within gliomas. Neurosurgery 1996; 38:678–685.
56. Haglund MM, Ojemann GA, Blasdel GG: Video imaging of neuronal activity. In Stamford JA (ed): Monitoring Neuronal Activity: A Practical Approach. New York, Oxford University Press, 1992, pp 85–114.
57. Haglund MM, Ojemann GA, Blasdel GG: Video imaging of bipolar cortical stimulation. Epilepsia 1991; 32(suppl 3):22.
58. Kelly DL, Goldring S, O'Leary JL: Averaged evoked somatosensory responses from the exposed cortex of man. Arch Neurol 1965; 73:1–9.

59. Stohr PE, Goldring S: Origin of somatosensory evoked scalp responses in man. J Neurosurg 1969; 31:117–127.

60. Woolsey CB, Cividosan TC: Study of postcentral gyrus of many by the evoked potential technique. Trans Am Neurol Assoc 1950; 75:50–52.

61. King RB, Schell GR: Cortical localization and monitoring during cerebral operations. J Neurosurg 1987; 27:210–214.

62. Wada J, Rasmussan T: Intracarotid injections of sodium Amytal for the lateralization of cerebral speech dominance. J Neurosurg 1960; 17:266–282.

63. Woods R, Dodrill C, Ojemann G: Brain injury, handedness and speech lateralization in a series of amobarbital studies. Ann Neurol 1988; 23:510–518.

64. Hinz AC, Berger MS, Ojemann GA, et al: The utility of the intracarotid Amytal procedure in determining hemispheric speech lateralization in pediatric epilepsy patients undergoing surgery. Childs Nerv Syst 1994; 10:239–243.

65. Ojemann GA: Some brain mechanisms for reading. In Euler C, Lundberg I, Lennerstrand G (eds): Brain and Reading, vol 1. New York, Macmillan, 1989, pp 47–59.

66. Ojemann GA, Mateer C: Human language cortex: Localization of memory, syntax and sequential motor-phoneme identification systems. Science 1979; 205:1401–1403.

67. Ojemann GA: Brain organization for language from the perspective of electrical stimulation mapping. Behav Brain Sci 1983; 6:189–206.

68. Van Buren J, Lewis D, Schuette W, et al: Fluorometric monitoring of NADH levels in cerebral cortex: Preliminary observations in human epilepsy. Neurosurgery 1978; 2:114–121.

69. Haglund M, Ojemann G, Hochmann D: Optical imaging of epileptiform and functional activity in human cerebral cortex. Nature 1992; 358:668–671.

70. Ranck J: Which elements are excited in electrical stimulation of mammalian central nervous systems: A review. Brain Res 1975; 948:418–440.

71. Penfield W, Jasper H: Epilepsy and the Functional Anatomy of the Human Brain. Boston, Little, Brown, 1954.

72. Mullan S, Penfield W: Illusions of comparative interpretation and emotion produced by epileptic discharge and by electrical stimulation in temporal cortex. Arch Neurol Psychiatry 1959; 81:269–284.

73. Penfield W, Perot P: The brain's record of auditory and visual experience—summary and discussion. Brain 1963; 86:595–696.

74. Gloor P, Olivier A, Quesney L, et al: The role of limbic systems in experiential phenomena of temporal lobe epilepsy. Ann Neurol 1982; 12:129–144.

75. Haglund MM, Berger MS, Shamseldin M, et al: Cortical localization of temporal lobe language sites in patients with gliomas. Neurosurgery 1994; 34:567–576.

76. Berger MS, Ojemann GA: Techniques of functional localization during removal of tumors involving the cerebral hemispheres. In Loftus C, Traynelis V (eds): Intraoperative Monitoring Techniques in Neurosurgery. New York, McGraw-Hill, 1994, pp 113–127.

77. Ojemann G: Cortical organization of language. J Neurosci 1991; 11:2281–2287.

78. Ojemann G, Whitaker H: Language localization and variability. Brain Lang 1978; 6:239–260.

79. Ojemann GA, Whitaker HA: The bilingual brain. Arch Neurol 1978; 35:409–412.

80. Ojemann GA: Effect of cortical and subcortical stimulation on human language and verbal memory. In Plum F (ed): Language, Communication and the Brain. New York, Raven Press, 1988, pp 101–115.

81. Ojemann GA: Cortical organization of language and verbal memory based on intraoperative investigations. Proc Sensory Physiol 1991; 12:192–230.

82. Ojemann GA, Sutherling W: Stimulation. In Engel J (ed): Surgical Treatment of the Epilepsies, ed 2. New York, Raven, 1993.

83. Rubens A, Majowald M, Hutton J: Asymmetry of the lateral (sylvian) fissures in man. Neurology 1976; 26:620–624.

84. Steinmetz H, Ebeling U, Huang Y, et al: Sulcus topography of the parietal opercular region: An anatomic and MR study. Brain Lang 1990; 38:515–533.

85. Rapport RL, Tan CT, Whitaker HA: Language function and dysfunction among Chinese and English-speaking polyglots: Cortical stimulation, Wada testing and clinical studies. Brain Lang 1983; 18:342–366.

86. Mateer CA, Polen SB, Ojemann GA, et al: Cortical localization of finger spelling and oral language: A case study. Brain Lang 1982; 17:46–57.

87. Berger MS, Ghatan S, Haglund MM, et al: Low-grade gliomas associated with intractable epilepsy: Seizure outcome utilizing ECoG during tumor resection. J Neurosurg 1993; 79:62–69.

88. Gonzales D, Elvidge AR: On the occurrence of epilepsy caused by astrocytoma of the cerebral hemispheres. J Neurosurg 1962; 19:470–482.

89. Rasmussen T: Surgical treatment of patients with complex partial seizures. In Penry JK, Daly DD (eds): Complex Partial Seizures and Their Treatment: Advances in Neurology, vol 2. New York, Raven, 1987, pp 415–449.

90. Ribaric IJ: Excision of two and three independent and separate ipsilateral potentially epileptogenic cortical areas. Acta Neurosci 1984; 33(suppl):145–148.

91. Drake J, Hoffman JH, Kobayashi J, et al: Surgical management of children with temporal lobe epilepsy and mass lesions. Neurosurgery 1987; 21:792–797.

92. Wyllie E, Luders H, Morris HH, et al: Clinical outcome after complete or partial cortical resection for intractable epilepsy. Neurology 1987; 37:1634–1641.

93. Awad I: Intractable epilepsy and structural lesions of the brain: Mapping, resection strategies, and seizure outcome. Epilepsia 1991; 32:179–186.

94. Spencer DD, Spencer SS, Mattson RH, et al: Intracerebral masses in patients with intractable partial epilepsy. Neurology 1984; 34:432–436.

95. White JC, Liu CT, Mixter WJ: Focal epilepsy: A statistical study of its causes and the results of surgical treatment: Epilepsy secondary to intracranial tumors. N Engl J Med 1948; 238:891–899.

96. Falconer MA, Driver MV, Serafetinides EA: Temporal lobe epilepsy due to distant lesions: Two cases relieved by operation. Brain 1962; 85:521–534.

97. Schisano G, Tovi D, Nordenstam H: Spongioblastoma polare of the cerebral hemisphere. J Neurosurg 1963; 20:241–251.

98. Goldring S, Rich KM, Picker S: Experience with gliomas in patients presenting with a chronic seizure disorder. In Little JR (ed): Clinical Neurosurgery, vol 33. New York, Raven Press, 1986, pp 15–42.

99. Cascino GD: Epilepsy and brain tumors: Implications for treatment. Epilepsia 1990; 31(suppl 3):37–44.

J. DIAZ DAY

THOMAS C. CHEN

MICHAEL L. J. APUZZO

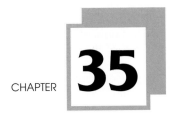

CHAPTER **35**

Tumor Removal Devices

Technological advancements continue to add new ''devices'' to our armamentarium for resecting neoplastic lesions. The goal of this continual evolution of equipment is the reduction of the effects of open surgical manipulation on the surrounding brain. The development of the ultrasonic aspirator and the laser have given us the means to reduce tumor volume in an efficient manner, with reduced disturbance to the surrounding structures. Photodynamic therapy and local hyperthermia are being used as adjuncts for control of tumor growth. Developments in computer technology are contributing to a rapid evolution of stereotactic methods that are less cumbersome and increasingly user-friendly. The current state of development of such complex devices is the focus of this chapter.

TUMOR RESECTION INSTRUMENTATION

The Ultrasonic Aspirator

The ultrasonic aspirator was first developed in 1947 as the CUSA (Cavitron Ultrasonic Surgical Aspirator), by Cooper instruments. It was used initially for removing dental plaque, and its application to neurosurgical procedures began in 1976.[29, 30, 36]

The basic unit consists of an acoustic vibrator, an irrigation system, and a suction system within a self-contained device. The acoustic vibrator converts electrical current into mechanical vibration utilizing an electric coil and a magnetostrictive transducer. As originally produced, alternating current at 23 kHz produces a 100-μm longitudinal vibration that acts to fragment tissue within 1 mm of the tip of the instrument. The irrigation fluid, which emanates from near the tip, suspends the tumor fragments to be removed as an emulsion via the suction apparatus. The Selector unit (Leksell Corp., Atlanta) utilizes a 35-kHz acoustic vibrator (Fig. 35–1). The increase in frequency translates to the delivery of greater power at lower amplitudes. This formula results in decreased tissue disruption to the surrounding area, with more efficient removal of the tumor.

Studies in the laboratory have been carried out to investigate the effects of the instrument on the electrical conduction properties of neural tissue. As an important initial finding, electric current is not passed from the instrument to the tissue. Second, normal electrical conduction has been demonstrated to be preserved within a 1-mm radius of the tip.[38] This work has shown that the instrument may be safely used to dissect tumor adjacent to vital structures without the possibility of disrupting normal function.

The effects on surrounding tissues have also been studied by pathologic analysis. The ideal tissue for fragmentation with the ultrasonic aspirator has a high intracellular fluid content. Brain and fat are examples of two such tissues. The greater collagenous and elastic character of blood vessels makes them more resistant to fragmentation by the instrument, though direct contact can still result in puncture. Cranial nerves in proximity to the working instrument may be spared; however, they are damaged if direct contact is

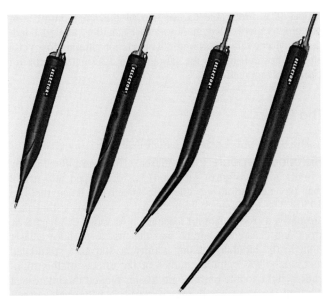

Figure 35–1 The Leksell selector comes in a variety of straight and angled handpieces, allowing for versatility underneath the microscope. The higher-frequency 34 kHz handpiece allows for delivery of greater power at lower amplitudes, decreases tissue disruption, and is good for working in confined spaces.

437

made with the ultrasonic aspirator. Electron microscopy of adjacent tissue shows edema in both myelinated and unmyelinated axons. Large vacuoles are present in both neurons and glial cells. Perivascular spaces demonstrate an increased number of phagocytes; however, the integrity of the small vessels is preserved.[14]

Wide application of the ultrasonic aspirator in neurosurgery has evolved owing to several advantages of the instrument in tumor resection. First, the ultrasonic aspirator requires little manipulation of surrounding tissues to resect tumor. Little heat is generated by the device, and thermal damage to surrounding tissue is therefore minimized. The device simultaneously aspirates as it irrigates and breaks up tumor, minimizing spread of tumor cells. Moreover, it is relatively easy to preserve tissue planes while using the instrument. Despite these advantages, the ultrasonic aspirator does have some limitations. It is not effective in fragmenting very hard tumors. Normal structures coming into direct contact with the vibrating tip are not spared the destructive effects of the instrument. Hemostasis is problematic at times, as the ultrasonic aspirator can only suction blood from the field; it provides no inherent hemostatic action.

From a technical standpoint, several issues are important. The ultrasonic aspirator is a simple instrument to use. However, the instrument works quickly, and its rapid action may cause loss of controlled resection of tumor. Overly rapid and aggressive use may result in extending the fragmentation effects to surrounding tissues that are not intended to be resected. Although the vessels are resistant to the effects of the instrument, direct contact with major vascular structures may result in perforation and a potential disaster. A higher-frequency vibrator helps in this regard, in enabling the use of a lower amplitude. Very hard tumors are resistant to the effects of the instrument and require an alternative strategy. The final point concerns selection of instrument design. Most instruments currently available are somewhat bulky and cumbersome, especially to use under the operating microscope. It is preferable to use one of the small number of designs available that incorporates a smaller, angled handpiece. Moreover, incorporation of suction attenuation via a slotted mechanism that the surgeon can differentially control is also advantageous.[22]

The Laser

HISTORY AND BASIC PRINCIPLES

Historical Aspects. The "laser" (*light amplification by stimulated emission of radiation*) has developed into a tool that has revolutionized scientific endeavors since the late 1950s. The principles on which this device were established are derived from quantum mechanical theories originated by Bohr and Einstein. Maiman was the first to produce a laser light in the laboratory using a ruby crystal as a stimulated medium.[1, 47, 52, 104] Initial studies of the effects of this high-energy light source on biologic tissues piqued the interest of medical researchers with regard to possible "miracle cures" that could result from such application. In the 1960s, the effects of laser energy on central nervous system (CNS) tissues were first investigated. The consequences of high-power laser lesions were devastating to the experimental

animals treated with laser through the intact skull. Such treatment resulted in gross hemorrhage and necrosis, with signs of rapid swelling and herniation. Direct application of laser energy to the cerebral cortex through craniotomy was found to produce local necrosis and hemorrhage.[37, 39, 79] These findings led to the clinical application of the medium as a means of vaporizing tumor tissue.

The first application to the surgery of gliomas was reported in 1966 by Rosomoff and Carroll.[95] These investigators utilized a low-powered ruby laser to directly deliver pulsed sequences of energy to three patients with glioblastomas. Two patients demonstrated necrosis of tumor treated by the laser at postmortem examination. This particular type of laser penetrated tissue deeply and apparently did not instantly vaporize the tissue at surgery. The effects of this type of laser were further characterized by several groups of investigators who showed that irreversible damage occurred to neurons and unmyelinated tissues more than supporting cells. The ruby laser was subsequently abandoned in favor of the less penetrating carbon dioxide (CO_2) laser.[104]

In 1969, Stellar applied the CO_2 laser to surgical resection in three patients with malignant gliomas, taking advantage of its vaporizing effects on tissue.[101] He reported that large blood vessels could not be coagulated using this laser. However, small vessels, 1 mm or less in diameter, were easily controlled. The result was a reduction in surgical blood loss using this tool. This was in accordance with other investigators in varying surgical specialties who found that the CO_2 laser was an efficient tool for incising and vaporizing tissues, but not for coagulation.[104] Despite the early reports of efficacy, widespread use was not seen until the mid-1970s. Designs aimed at reducing the cumbersome nature of the equipment and adapting the laser to the operating microscope took time to develop. The design flaws were largely worked out in Europe and Japan.[104] At the same time, the neodymium:yttrium-aluminum-garnet (Nd:YAG) laser system was developed and applied to neurosurgical procedures in Germany by Beck.[104] Since then, lasers have been used by neurosurgeons as an adjunct to tumor resection operations. Because studies have not clearly demonstrated a difference in outcome, however, this is not a universally employed strategy for tumor resection.[32]

Functional Principles. There are three main properties of laser light that make it unique. The first is monochromaticity, or light of the same wavelength. The second feature is coherence of light, with waves traveling in phase, both spatially and temporally. The great intensity of a laser beam is dependent on this property. The third unique property is collimation. Laser light does not diverge as it travels through space, and the light can travel long distances in a strictly parallel beam.[16, 33]

The apparatus that produces such a beam has several key elements. The first is a medium that can be stimulated by electrical current to produce photons. The medium can exist in any of the three phases of matter: gas, liquid, or solid. The medium is housed in an "optical resonator," in which electrical current is passed through the medium. The energy transfer of the electrical current results in the production of electrons in an excited state. The natural laws governing matter demand that a decay process occur to restore these electrons to their lowest energy state. This process of decay results in the emission of the energy as photons. The photons may then be reflected within the chamber, striking other atoms to elevate other electrons to higher energy states, resulting in amplification of the process. The optical resonator has two mirrors, one at each end of the chamber. One mirror is only partially reflective, allowing emission of the laser beam. Only photons in phase and of the same wavelength are allowed to exit the chamber. This forms the highly intense laser light beam[33, 34] (Fig. 35–2).

Tissue Interactions. The effect of the laser on a particular tissue depends on its intensity and wavelength and on the unique properties of the tissue. Intensity (power/area) is a measure of power density. The area on which the beam strikes the tissue is referred to as the *laser spot*. The size of the laser spot determines what effect the laser will have on the tissue, as a certain power focused on a small area will result in a much higher intensity on the tissue. A small, finely focused laser spot will result in vaporization or incision of the tissue in that confined area. Increasing the laser spot size generally results in coagulation or vaporization over a wider, but more superficial, volume of tissue. The spot size is controlled via a lens system. Tissue that is positioned at the focal point of the lens is subject to the full power of the laser beam via a finely focused, small laser spot. A larger spot is produced by ''defocusing'' the system. Placing tissue beyond the focal length results in coagulation or vaporization. As the beam passes through the tissue in these two modes, the energy is dissipated gradually as the beam becomes increasingly defocused[104] (Fig. 35–3).

Different wavelengths preferentially affect different tissues. The *extinction length* describes the depth at which 90% of the laser light is absorbed. This length changes for various lasers with different wavelengths in relation to certain biologic tissues. Different tissues have varying *absorption coefficients,* which describe the ability of the tissue to absorb a particular wavelength of light. This coefficient is affected by cell type, water content, temperature, and pigmentation. The extinction length values and absorption coefficients are not established for the various available lasers in neural tissues, as it is impossible to control for all of the factors affecting such measurements.[104] The end result is that the laser light may be transmitted, scattered, absorbed, or reflected, depending on the type of laser, the tissue type penetrated, and the varying conditions involved (Fig. 35–4). Light that is reflected has no effect on the tissue itself but may diminish the effect of other light entering the tissue. Transmitted light

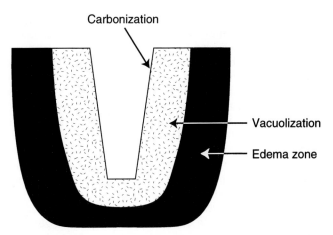

Carbonization

Vacuolization

Edema zone

Figure 35–3 The laser spot may be histologically divided into three layers: (1) carbonization, (2) vacuolization, and (3) edema zone. A small, finely focused laser spot results in vaporization or incision of tissue in that confined area. A more diffuse beam results in coagulation or vaporization.

does not affect the tumor but may cause bystander damage to normal tissue underneath. Scattered light remains within the tissue and permits the laser light to be absorbed over a larger volume. Absorbed light is the most effective, as the energy is directly taken in by the tissue itself.[91] Application of laser light demonstrates its effect on a tissue as a combination of these four reactions. We presently rely on some general observations regarding the interactions of specific laser types to help make choices regarding the appropriate laser to employ, the spot size needed, and how to adjust the focus of the beam.

LASER TYPES UTILIZED IN MICROSURGERY

The CO_2 Laser. The CO_2 laser utilizes a wavelength of 10.6 μm, which is invisible to the human eye. This wavelength resides in the far infrared portion of the light spectrum. Because of its invisibility, this laser must be used with a coaxial pilot beam to guide it during application. This laser has a short extinction length, which results in the absorption of its energy by tissue, mostly at the surface. The vaporization effect on tissues is caused by the rapid heating of intracellular water, which vaporizes the cell instantaneously. Because little energy is transmitted deep into tissues (penetration depth <200 μm), this laser is ideal for tissue surface ablation. The absence of significant transmission in

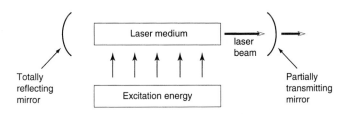

Laser medium

laser beam

Totally reflecting mirror

Excitation energy

Partially transmitting mirror

Figure 35–2 The laser apparatus has several components, including medium that can be stimulated by electrical current to produce photons and two mirrors at each end of the chamber. One mirror is totally reflective and the other mirror is partially reflective, allowing emission of the laser beam.

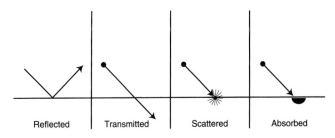

Reflected | Transmitted | Scattered | Absorbed

Figure 35–4 Laser light may be reflected, transmitted, scattered, or absorbed in tissue, depending on the type of laser, the tissue type penetrated, and the conditions involved.

water or in blood, however, are responsible for its poor coagulating properties. Therefore, the CO_2 laser is most advantageous when used to vaporize and remove extra-axial tumors that are fibrous and relatively avascular or lipomatous tumors that involve the skull base or spinal canal.[17, 19, 63, 104]

The CO_2 laser is used either with a handheld apparatus or by attachment to the operating microscope. The microscope-mounted system is preferable. The laser is directed via an articulated arm that is attached to the body of the microscope. This system has different lenses that can be changed by the surgeon to vary the spot size of the laser beam. Precise control over the aim of the laser is through a joystick, controlled either by hand or with a mouthpiece.

This laser finds greatest utility in the debulking of large tumor masses that are in difficult areas of access. In general, this instrument is most applicable in tumors located in the ventricles, brainstem, and spinal cord.[104] The manipulation of adjacent tissues can be decreased in these circumstances by using the laser, which accounts for its value in these sensitive areas.

The two main drawbacks of the CO_2 laser are (1) its wavelength (10.6 μm) reduces its ability to coagulate vessels larger than 1.0 mm, which reduces its efficacy in more vascular tumors; and (2) the beam has to be conducted through an articulated arm, which reduces the flexibility of the laser. Reflection from shiny surfaces is also an avoidable problem with this laser. However, if nonreflective retractor blades and instruments are introduced into the field, this problem should be minimized.

Kelly has developed a computer-assisted stereotatic technique utilizing the CO_2 laser for volumetric resection of deep-seated lesions.[62, 66, 67, 81] This system helps the surgeon to maintain a three-dimensional orientation during resection of such deep lesions. This technique has been reported to be helpful in debulking deep-seated gliomas.[62, 66]

The Nd:YAG Laser.

The Nd:YAG laser possesses a wavelength in the near infrared region of the spectrum at 1.06 μm. This region is also invisible to the human eye, necessitating the use of a co-axial pilot beam for this laser. The surgical application of this laser is enhanced by its ability to be transmitted through a fiberoptic cable. The tissue interaction of the Nd:YAG laser is dominated by minimal tissue absorption, light scattering, and long tissue penetration depth secondary to its poor absorption by water and biologic pigments.[41, 100, 104] As a result, uniform slow heating of a large volume of tissue in an energy dose-dependent manner is possible. Blood vessels measuring 2 to 3 mm in diameter may be easily coagulated.[91] This property has made it useful in the treatment of vascular tumors.[104] The beam is applied to the vascular tumor, coagulating and softening the tumor so that it can be removed by mechanical suction. However, the long tissue penetration depth may result in coagulation of normal tissue or blood vessels underneath a tumor in vital areas of the brain. The use of cottonoids is helpful in protecting the normal brain from laser light reflection, inadvertent irradiation, and damage from hot gases created by tissue vaporization. There has been little experience with the use of this laser in glioma surgery.

Nd:YAG lasers of varying wavelengths have been developed. Long-wavelength Nd:YAG lasers at 1.32 and 1.44 μm have been developed. Roux and colleagues found that the 1.32 μm Nd:YAG laser produced lesions in the rat cortex that were closer to the CO_2 laser than the 1.06 μm Nd:YAG laser.[96, 97] Martiniuk and others[80] found that the 1.44 μm Nd:YAG laser had good photoevaporative effects while maintaining the coagulative properties of the conventional Nd:YAG laser. For a given volume of tissue coagulated, the amount of peripheral edema was less in 1.44 μm lesions, with the aspect ratio (ratio of lesion width to depth) being larger for 1.44 μm lesions. The prototype laser could be switched from 1.06 to 1.32 to 1.44 μm, allowing for endoscopic photovaporization and conventional photocoagulation from a single laser source.[80]

Fasano[31] has developed a combined Nd:YAG and CO_2 laser unit that is attached to an operating microscope. This combination is used to first coagulate and devascularize the tumor with the Nd:YAG laser, then vaporize the tissue with the CO_2 laser. The same authors have reported the successful use of this combination in resecting spinal cord tumors.[31]

The 1.9 μm Wavelength Laser.

The 1.9 μm wavelength laser is an experimental laser with a combined adjunct Nd:YAG (1.06 μm) laser. The advantage of the 1.9 μm wavelength is that it has tissue-ablative capabilities like those of the CO_2 laser. However, because of its shorter wavelength, it has better tissue- and water-penetrating properties, and may be used with irrigation during ablation, which results in decreased thermal injury. Moreover, it may be transmited through conventional fiberoptic delivery systems. The combined Nd:YAG laser may be used in achieving hemostasis.[100]

The Argon Laser.

The argon laser falls into the visible spectrum of light at 0.488 to 0.514 μm, and therefore does not require a co-axial pilot beam for aiming. This laser also may be transmitted through a fiberoptic light cable or aimed via attachment to the microscope. This is a low-energy beam that is most useful for coagulating tissue. The argon laser's action is dominated by its interaction with pigmented tissue components (hemoglobin, melanin, cytochromes). In these areas, it acts like a CO_2 laser secondary to the strong absorption of argon laser energy in these tissues. However, in nonpigmented tissues (minimal absorption and maximal scattering of argon laser energy) the argon laser acts like an Nd:YAG laser, coagulating pial vessels, veins, and small arteries without damage to normal brain. Therefore, the argon laser has the ability to coagulate and vaporize, depending on the tissue involved.[13] Vaporization takes substantially more time with this laser as compared with the CO_2 laser. The argon laser has been reported to be useful in the treatment of small, moderately vascular lesions in critically sensitive areas. It has been used to remove vascular malformations,[27] acoustic neuromas,[43] and hemangioblastomas[27] and to make dorsal root entry zone lesions.[27] This tool has not been reported to be of particular usefulness in the surgery of gliomas.

The Potassium Titanyl Phosphate Laser.

The potassium titanyl phosphate (KTP) laser is a recently introduced

TABLE 35–1
CHARACTERISTICS OF COMMONLY USED LASERS

Laser	Wavelength (μm)	Pigment-Dependent	Maximum Power (W)	Scatter (Tissue)	Absorption (Tissue)	Transmission—Water/Blood	Delivery System	Effect on Tissue
CO₂	10.6	No	100	Low	High	No	Articulated arms	Vaporization
Nd:YAG	1.06	Yes	120	High (precise depth of scatter unpredictable)	Low	Yes	Fiberoptics	Coagulation, poor vaporization
Argon	0.458–0.514	Yes	20	Medium	Medium	Yes	Fiberoptics	Vaporization/coagulation
KTP	0.532	Yes	20	Medium	Medium	Yes	Fiberoptics/small handpieces available	Vaporization/coagulation

instrument that has a wavelength of 0.532 μm. The laser beam is delivered through a fiberoptic cable that may be handheld or attached to the operating microscope. The laser may also be used through the neuroendoscope as it can be transmitted through water. The KTP laser has been found to be effective in coagulating and vaporizing tumor tissue.[41, 42] The extinction length in blood is 0.05 mm, which is near that of the argon laser (0.2 mm), but substantially less than the Nd:YAG laser (7.6 mm).[41] The wavelength of the KTP laser is near that of the argon laser; therefore, the tissue effects would be predicted to be similar. The KTP laser acts on both pigmented and nonpigmented tissues.

Preliminary experience with gliomas has been reported by Gamache and Patterson in the treatment of seven patients.[41] They found this system to be more effective than the CO₂ laser at debulking masses via vaporization because of its greater ability to control blood loss through coagulation of the larger blood vessels. Comparison of the lesions produced by the CO₂ and the KTP laser showed that the KTP laser created a histologically shallower lesion than did the CO₂ laser, and it provided a more hemostatic, less hemorrhagic effect on tissue.[42] As this laser is more widely tested, more data should become available for the treatment of gliomas. The KTP laser is currently being used most often in endoscopic applications.

Operative Technique. For supratentorial tumors, the cortical incision may be made with the focused CO₂ laser at low power over the external surface of the tumor. The ultrasonic aspirator may then be used to progressively remove the glioma. In highly vascularized tumors, a layer-by-layer radiation with defocused Nd:YAG at low power in separate pulses may be used to achieve a devascularization of the tumor. In highly functional areas, defocused CO₂ laser at low power may be used to remove tumor remnants in highly functional areas. Intraventricular glial tumors, such as ependymomas, may be easily coagulated with the Nd:YAG laser. The same principles may be applied to infratentorial tumors. In cystic astrocytomas, the mural nodule may be attached to the brainstem or to important vascular structures. It may be dissected with focused CO₂ laser at low power. Removal of intrinsic brainstem tumors with the laser has been advocated by Fasano.[32] He advocates a vaporization of the tumor, layer by layer, under sonographic control to determine the extent of resection needed. In exophytic brainstem tumors, the exophytic portion is removed

with a CUSA and the intrinsic brainstem portion is removed with the laser.

Advantages and Disadvantages of Lasers for Tumor Resection. The advantages and disadvantages of routinely employing a laser system must be understood before the modality is used. The advantages of a laser system include (1) no-touch surgery, (2) limited effect on restricted areas, (3) shrinkage of mass by drying of tissue, and (4) preservation of normal arterial and venous anatomy. However, lasers must be used by trained personnel who employ safety precautions. Inadvertent damage to the operator's retina or burns may occur if proper precautions are not taken. Removal of a tumor may take hours. No tactile component is available, and resection is dependent on visual differentiation between the tumor and normal brain.[35] Moreover, the benefits of a laser must be weighed from the standpoint of increased hours of surgery, cost, and the cumbersome nature of the instrument. The key issue in the future will be whether the cited surgical advantages of laser surgery warrant the acquisition of new instrumentation.

The characteristics of the commonly used lasers are listed in Table 35–1. Figure 35–5 demonstrates the tissue reaction for the CO₂, argon, and Nd:YAG lasers.

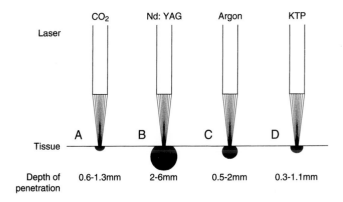

Figure 35–5 Comparative tissue reaction of lasers currently in use in neurosurgery. The CO₂ laser has the least depth of penetration, with most of its energy being absorbed on the tissue surface. The Nd:YAG laser has the highest degree of tissue penetration, making it ideal for coagulation but poor for tissue surface vaporization. The argon and KTP lasers are intermediate in tissue penetration. In nonpigmented tissues, these lasers have high tissue penetration and act like the Nd:YAG laser. In pigmented tissue, with strong absorption, both lasers have good coagulation.

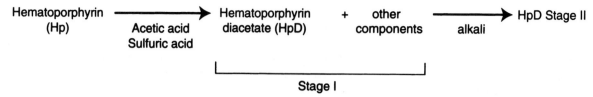

Figure 35–6 Schematic representation demonstrating conversion of hematoporphyrin to hematoporphyrin diacetate and finally to a mixture of hematoporphyrin derivatives, which act as photosensitizers.

PHOTODYNAMIC THERAPY OF MALIGNANT GLIOMAS

The cytotoxic activity of photodynamic therapy depends on the light activation of a photoreactive drug, called a *photosensitizer,* that is selectively bound to tumor. Ideally, the photosensitizer should be selective only for tumor tissue, not exhibit systemic toxicity, absorb light at a wavelength that is readily transmitted through the tissue being treated, and be capable of efficiently destroying malignant tissue when photoactivated. Although a number of photosensitizers have been evaluated in vitro, only hematoporphyrin derivative (HpD) or its purified component (Photofrin II) have been used on a clinical basis (Fig. 35–6). Illumination of HpD by red light initiates a photochemical reaction resulting in a triplet formation of the photosensitizer. The triplet form then forms either a reactive radical or a singlet oxygen reaction that is ultimately lethal to cells[61] (Fig. 35–7). The end result is selective tumor death with an extremely high therapeutic ratio.

HpD has been shown to accumulate in malignant gliomas and does not cross the blood-brain barrier. It is selectively taken up in vitro by higher-grade gliomas, with glioblastoma having the highest cellular uptake.[48, 107] The mechanism for the high uptake by malignant tumors may be related to elevated low-density lipoprotein (LDL) receptors that are present to take up cholesterol for rapidly proliferating cells. The HpD may interact with LDL receptors and be selectively transported into malignant cells, with minimal uptake by normal cells.[61] It is distributed unevenly throughout the tumor and it has been estimated that only 33% to 44% of the tumor cells show fluorescence after systemic administration of the photosensitizer.[11] HpD is especially well localized to endothelial cells. Tumor necrosis after photoradiation may result from injury to the tumor vasculature leading to ischemic damage.[12] Damage to normal brain is minimal. However, endothelial cell injury of normal blood vessels containing HpD has been reported.[23]

To activate the HpD accumulated in the malignant glioma cells, a source of red light must be used. The most commonly used source of light has been the argon laser. However, a gold metal vapor laser has also been used with good effect.

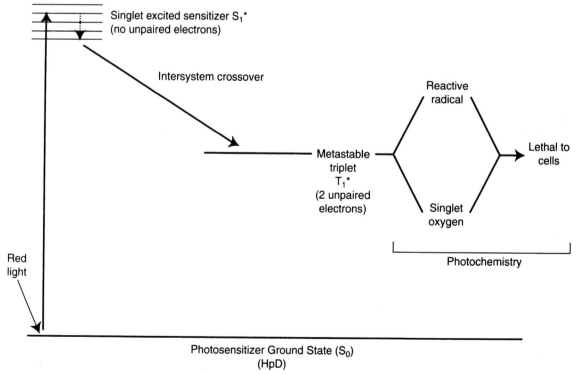

Figure 35–7 Illumination of hematoporphyrin diacetate (HpD) by red light initiates a photochemical reaction resulting in the triplet formation of the photosensitizer. The triplet form then forms either a reactive radical or singlet oxygen reaction, which is ultimately lethal to cells.

Three forms of intratumoral light delivery have been developed. Muller and Wilson have devised an intracavitary photoradiation approach utilizing an inflatable balloon filled with a light-dispersing medium into which an end-emitting, bare-tipped laser fiber is placed. The tumor is decompressed first, then the balloon is placed into the cavity. The amount of energy delivered by the balloon is calculated based on the surface area of the balloon for a given injection volume of dispersion material into the balloon. Light is therefore delivered through the walls of the balloon into the marginal tissues of the tumor resection cavity.[82, 83] The other method uses a standard cut quartz fiber tip from which the laser light is emitted. The fiber tip is attached to a brain retractor arm (Yasargil brain retractor arm) and the fiber tip is moved at regular intervals to completely and evenly cover the surface of the tumor bed.[58] Kaye and others found that the argon laser produced only relatively small doses of light secondary to an ineffective coupling mechanism, and that it had poor mobility. The gold metal vapor laser was portable, produced a much higher-intensity light at 627.8 nm, and produced very high peaks of pulsed light at specific time intervals (10,000 times/second) in contrast with the continuous beam of the argon laser. They found that higher doses of laser light were more effective than lower doses, and that up to 230 J/cm^2 may be administered along with continuous irrigation of the irradiated site, with minimal cerebral edema.[59, 60] Last, stereotactic implantation of acrylic-coated optical fibers, which produce a cylindrical pattern of light emission, may be inserted into the tumor cavity for local control. Although precise insertion is possible, only a certain number of optical fibers may be inserted stereotactically without making too many trajectory passes into the brain. Powers and co-workers[90] found that good local control of the tumor was possible in certain patients. However, the main limitation of this technique remains that the penetration of the argon laser is limited (mean penetration depth 2.9 ± 1.5 mm).

Although photodynamic therapy has yielded good preliminary results, current series are too small in number to conclusively demonstrate whether there is an increase in patient survival. For most series, the effect of photodynamic therapy has been clouded with other variables for patient survival, including extent of tumor resection, past radiation or chemotherapy, and selection of patients with recurrent malignant brain tumors. Moreover, initial series often used much lower doses of energy than would be used systemically for tumor photodynamic therapy. Different ways to improve photodynamic therapy include development of (1) more effective photosensitizers than HpD; (2) better illumination systems capable of delivering light at higher rates (800 to 2000 mW), with increased light penetration of tumor tissue; (3) methods of better localization of HpD into endothelial cells, resulting in more effective tumor necrosis.[88]

USE OF HYPERTHERMIA FOR TUMOR TREATMENT

A wide variety of neoplasms have been shown to be sensitive to damage from temperatures in excess of 40°C over a variable period of time. The site of thermal injury may include the plasma membrane, the nucleus, and inactivation of enzymes within tumor cells. Normal neural tissue, especially neurons, is sensitive to heat damage at temperatures in excess of 43°C. Therefore, it is necessary to restrict high thermal elevation above 44°C to the central tumor nidus and to limit temperature elevations above 42 and 43°C in the adjacent tumor-invaded brain.[44, 91]

A number of techniques have been developed to deliver thermal energy. Laser hyperthermia has been used with the Nd:YAG laser. Cone-shaped, sapphire-tipped optical fibers emitting Nd:YAG laser energy can be positioned at different targets within tumor tissue by stereotactic methods.[102] An exponential falloff of temperature occurs with an increase in the distance from the optical fiber tip in tissue that is similar to that seen with other point-source forms of tissue heating. A number of articles have been published on the integration of laser hyperthermia with magnetic resonance imaging (MRI). Noninvasive rapid-sequence MRI has been used to study the evolution of laser-induced hyperthermic damage of brain tissue. A strong relationship exists between MRI relaxation and tissue temperature. Decreased signal intensity in T1-weighted images is noted in the region of heat injury. The spatial extent of reversible and irreversible thermally induced tissue changes can be demonstrated by MRI.[53, 55] Anzai and colleagues have demonstrated that T2-weighted MRI may be useful for demonstrating three distinct histologic layers caused by thermal injuries, including central ablation, irreversible coagulative necrosis (low signal intensity), and surrounding edema (high signal intensity).[2, 3] Although no difference in survival was apparent in experimental rat models treated with laser hyperthermia, Sugiyama and co-workers reported that in three of five patients (three gliomas, two metastatic lesions) treated with laser hyperthermia (2 to 3 W, 30 to 40 minutes, to maintain peripheral temperature at 42.5 to 43.5°C), tumor recurrence was not detected on CT with up to 31 month follow-up.[102] However, laser interstitial hyperthermia does not provide a curative treatment for spatially disseminated gliomas, in which the "target volume" cannot be adequately defined. As a result, intact tumor cells are likely to be present in the periphery of the irradiated area.[28]

Another method for inducing tumor hyperthermia has been the creation of radiofrequency lesions via stereotactic methods. Although this method is best suited for small metastatic lesions, it is conceivable that it may also be employed for small gliomas. In this technique, a radiofrequency lesion-generator system (480 kHz sine wave signals; Radionics Inc., Burlington, Mass.) may be used to make intratumoral lesions. Anzai and others found that this technique was sufficient for control of metastatic lesions in a number of patients.[4]

Other methods of tumor hyperthermia include the use of ultrasound coupled with MRI. Although this technology is still experimental, it may have some applicability in the future. Focused ultrasound therapy can be applied to both small and large irregularly shaped tumors in any region of the brain where the path to the target is free of bone and air interfaces. High-intensity focused ultrasound may be used to elevate the temperature at the target point to the range of 60 to 70°C until brain tissue is destroyed. Cline and others have performed initial studies using a 5 cm, 10 cm focal length, 1.1 MHz ultrasonic transducer on a 1.5T MRI system on gel phantoms and in vitro bovine muscle specimens. They demonstrated that above a critical thermal dose, the in vitro tissue was irreversibly altered and the focal lesion may be observed on both the MRI and the specimen slice.[20] Darkazanli and co-workers have demonstrated that T2-weighted fast spin-echo images defined the ultrasound-induced lesions clearly within a short period of time.[21]

The advantages of using MRI-guided tumor hyperthermia are its accuracy and ease of applicability. However, the technique is limited by the inherent limitation of having the probe placed into the center of the tumor. In many malignant gliomas and metastatic tumors, the center of the lesion is necrotic. Therefore, the tumor at the periphery or adjacent to the brain is the region that needs to be treated. Unfortunately, it is this region that is treated least with hyperthermia. Long-term applications of this method will need to be evaluated in the future.

Preliminary work has been done on a magnetic stereotaxy system (MSS) at the University of Washington. In this system, a 2 to 3 mm permanently magnetized seed is implanted into the brain and is moved by magnetic force directly through soft tissue. The seed is an alloy made of neodymium, iron, and boron, all of which have a high magnetic content. The prototype model consists of six magnets set up in opposing grids in a cube-like helmet that surrounds the patient's head. The field gradient may be manipulated, resulting in movement of the magnetized seed, which may be detected on x-ray images. These images are then mapped onto preoperative MRI images via a computer-based linkage between real-time biplanar fluoroscopy and the MRI scan. The surgeon is then able to see on the computer screen an MRI with a seed moving through the brain. The advantage of this system is that tumor edges, often visually indistinct in gliomas, may be readily detected on MRI. Therefore, if a heated magnet is moved through a tumor, it may be used for focal thermal radiation, resulting in tumor death even at the tumor periphery. The MSS is still authorized for investigational use only, and checks on its safety are still underway.[45, 50]

INTRAOPERATIVE LOCALIZATION DEVICES

The utility of intraoperative localization lies in sparing critical functional cortex and deep structures while attempting to maximize resection of tumor. This ideally consists of a system that provides real-time information regarding a target volume of tissue. These systems differ from preoperative localization devices and techniques in their ability to provide dynamic output as the procedure progresses. These systems are evolving rapidly, and their increased utilization will undoubtedly lead to constant technological improvements. This discussion focuses on currently available devices that give anatomic localizing information to the surgeon during the procedure.

Frame-Based Stereotaxy

Stereotactic methods are crucial for resecting or debulking gliomas that are in deep areas of the brain. These methods allow tumor exposure with superb accuracy while minimizing the manipulation of adjacent structures. The majority of

stereotactic methods that are currently available do not, however, provide information in real-time. Most techniques rely on preoperative imaging studies as a basis for determining specific coordinates in three-dimensional space. Thus, changes in spatial positioning of structures and lesions that naturally occur as a consequence of shifting fluid and brain matter during craniotomy are not compensated for by most techniques. This fact must be kept in mind when utilizing these methods, allowing for some inaccuracies of localization during the procedure.

Frame-based stereotactic methods are in widespread use for the surgery of deep-seated brain lesions. A number of systems have been well described. All methods rely on preoperative imaging, either computed tomography (CT) or MRI, to generate a set of specific spatial coordinates that describe the intracranial volume. CT and MRI have been demonstrated to be of equal value in preoperative targeting accuracy by Kondziolka and co-workers.[71] Novel methods of adding functional information to the targeting sequence of the procedure include PET, magnetoencephalography, and functional MRI.* These methods are good for tumor localization and operative planning. However, they do not provide real-time feedback during tumor resection. Kelly is credited with the development of a system designed to define a predetermined volume of tumor in stereotactic space and to resect this volume through a limited cranial opening.[62, 64, 65] He has used this system to resect various types of tumors, both intracerebral and intraventricular.[81] The Kelly system, however, is also unable to provide real-time feedback. If used within the ventricular space, this method may offer no advantage over more traditional approaches once CSF is drained from the ventricle or a retractor blade moves adjacent tissues. The system has been used with reportedly good results in the resection of deep-seated gliomas. However, no increase in survival has been reported after radical resection of these tumors.[66]

A system introduced by Reinhardt and others[92] has been developed to free the operative field of cumbersome attachments to the stereotactic frame. It uses sonic stereometry for localization and is composed of a base ring, an ultrasound receiver panel, locatable instruments, and a computer. An ultrasonic transmitter in the instrument handle transmits a signal that is received by the receiver panel. The traveling time of the 24-kHz sonic waves to the receiver panel is measured, and the location of the instrument can be determined with an accuracy of ±1 mm using this information. The location of the instrument is displayed in relation to the preoperative CT scan on the computer screen. As in the previous systems, no compensation for shifts of the intracranial contents can be made.[92]

Frameless Stereotaxy

Frameless stereotactic methods have the advantage of alleviating the steps involved with using an attached head frame for imaging acquisition as an immediate part of the operative procedure. Roberts and colleagues were the first to use such a system based on the sonic stereometric principle.[93, 94] This system utilizes spark-gap generators to produce an ultrasonic frequency signal that is received by a receiver panel mounted

---

*References 40, 51, 56, 68, 73, 75, 86, 87, 98, 103, and 108.

above the microscope. The signals are then converted into spatial information regarding the relationship of the microscope to the patient's head. The three-dimensional information from the preoperative CT or MRI scans is then spatially registered with the operating microscope. Outlines of tumor margin are directed via a beam splitter back through the microscope to be superimposed on the operative field. This provides the surgeon with a comparison between the actual tissue appearance and the boundaries of enhancement, or other imaging characteristic, as seen on preoperative studies. This arrangement, although demonstrated to be reasonably accurate, does not compensate for gross intraoperative shifts of the intracranial contents.

The focus of other frameless stereotactic systems has been on an articulated arm design that acts as a pointer, called a "neuronavigator." Similar systems have been under simultaneous development since the mid-1980s.[25, 26, 46, 57, 70, 105, 106] Watanabe and co-workers first described the use of a six-joint sensing arm that is attached to the Mayfield pin headrest.[105, 106] This system is capable of displaying the location of the tip of the articulated arm in relation to the preoperative CT scan. Fiducial markers are placed at three points on the patient's head. These coordinates serve to synchronize the CT image and the neuronavigator. The pointer can be used to help locate the optimal area for craniotomy and locate intracranial structures (Fig. 35–8). The system is also capable of interacting with other imaging modalities, making it useful in locating blood vessels in conjunction with use of angiograms and MRI scans. Watanabe and associates have reported this instrument's use in the treatment of 35 patients with gliomas.[105] The efficacy with regard to patient outcome has not been analyzed. Real-time localization may be obtained in this system by a combination of ultrasound imaging and transcranial Doppler (TCD). An ultrasound probe may be attached to the tip of the pointer, allowing comparison of the echographic and CT images. This has helped in terms of compensation for shifting of intracranial structures due to craniotomy. The addition of TCD helps to locate intracranial vessels that are not well-demonstrated on the preoperative CT images. Localization of a vessel segment in this way has demonstrated an accuracy to within 2 mm.[105]

The ISG viewing wand system (ISG Technologies, Mississauga, Ontario, Canada) is an available FDA-approved device that also makes use of an articulated arm system.[26] This arrangement includes the articulated arm, acting as a three-dimensional digitizer, and a sophisticated computer graphics workstation. The images in three dimensions may be represented in several different ways to give a comprehensive display of the involved anatomy. This system also relies on preoperative imaging; however, external fiducial markers are not necessary. Rather, the computer uses reproducible anatomic landmarks, such as the eyes and nose, to process targeting information. The average error of the system in testing has fallen to between 1.5 and 2.5 mm.[25] A component of real-time imaging is again provided by combining an ultrasound probe with the tip of the viewing wand. Various instruments, including an endoscope, may be introduced through the modified tips of the articulated arm.[25, 26]

Koivukangas and colleagues have introduced a similar articulated arm system. However, this system makes use of ultrasound in a routine arrangement to make real-time confirmations and comparisons between the open intracranial and the preoperatively digitized intracranial environments.[70, 84] This system provides an improved sense of real-time information. The articulated arm can also be fitted with various types of adaptors at the end of the probe to attach various instruments.

A number of stereotactic pointers are in various stages of development. Few are currently approved by the FDA for general use. This, however, is a rapidly expanding area of interest that should yield many exciting new possibilities for accurate, real-time intraoperative localization of tumor tissue.[5, 6, 57]

Zeiss has produced the MKM model microscope with stereotactic capability, which takes away the need for a robotic pointing arm. The principle of operation is much the same as for the neuronavigators, with the necessary preoperative acquisition of imaging data using fiducial markers placed on the patient's head. The computer sends a signal that translates into a correction in the trajectory of the microscope to stay fixed on any preselected target within the intracranial volume. Thus the microscope acts as its own navigator, always keeping the surgeon directed toward the target volume along a selected trajectory, no matter how the surgeon adjusts the microscope.

Intraoperative Dye for Tumor Localization

A possible adjunctive method for glioma resection may be developed that relies on the properties of selective uptake of particular ligands by glioma cells. The selective uptake of

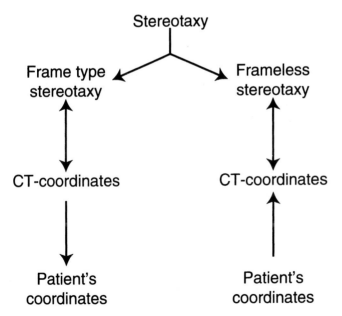

Figure 35–8 Stereotactic surgery may be divided into frame-based and frameless stereotactic procedures. In frame-based systems, the CT-coordinates are translated into the patient's coordinates for accurate localization. Frameless procedures, however, convert the patient's coordinates (via external fiducial markers or patient's skull landmarks) to CT coordinates.

peripheral benzodiazepines by gliomas has been shown by Black and co-workers,[9, 10] Junck and others,[54] and Starosta-Rubinstein and associates.[99] This same idea has been recently applied by Poon and colleagues in a rat glioma model using a laser-induced fluorescence dye.[89] The dye, chloroaluminum phthalocyanine tetrasulfonate ($ClAlPcSO_4$), fluoresces under stimulation from a laser light source. This substance demonstrates selective uptake by glioma cells, thus inferring utility in identifying tumor tissue that is illuminated by the fluorescence-inducing laser light source. This investigation found that animals that had undergone resection guided by this laser-induced fluorescence had a significantly smaller volume of residual tumor as compared with the control animals. Further developments with applications in humans are expected.[89]

Robotics

Robotics have been applied to biopsy situations at the present time, but no reports of a robotic device actually resecting tumor have been presented.[7, 8, 72, 78] The device thus far used consists of a motor-driven articulated arm that is controlled via computer to reach predetermined points in space. The Unimation Puma 200 robot has been suggested by Young[110] and Kwoh and others[72] as a device that could be used for biopsy, resection, drainage of abscesses and hematomas, and implantation of radioactive substances or deep brain electrodes. Drake and colleagues have used the Puma 200 robot for holding the surgical retractor during resection of thalamic astrocytomas in children.[24] The main reservation regarding this type of system is safety. Before a robotic system could be employed in a given procedure, it would need to be specifically designed and tested for neurosurgical application and have an unparalleled safety record. Its main application in the near future will most likely be in the calibration of stereotactic equipment, such as the head frame or the neuronavigator.

Neuroendoscope

A resurgence of interest in the neuroendoscope has occurred since the early 1990s. It has been particularly helpful in fenestrating cysts and loculated ventricles, removing colloid cysts, and visualizing shunt catheter placement.[76, 77] The neuroendoscope has also been used for deep-seated brain tumors. The advantage of the endoscope is its real-time visualization. The guiding tube can be inserted stereotactically into the tumor, then the neuroendoscope can be used as a microscope for viewing the deep and confined operating field. Resection may then be performed using the CO_2 and Nd:YAG laser. The combination of the neuroendoscope with stereotactic methodologies allows for direct intraoperative visualization, hemostasis, assessment of degree of resection, and wide exploration of intracranial cavities or ventricles.[15, 49, 85, 111] Yamasaki and others have combined a Doppler ultrasound and neuroendoscope with stereotactic biopsies of deep-seated vascular tumors. The change in blood velocity may be used to assess nearby blood vessels. The neuroendoscope may be used to directly visualize blood vessels.[109]

Intraoperative Ultrasound

The ultrasound device has been used in the neurosurgical operating theater since the early 1980s. The primary advantage of the use of ultrasound intraoperatively is the ability to gain a picture of the intracranial space in real time. This has led to the widespread use of this tool not only in the surgery of gliomas, but also in other neoplastic, cystic, and infectious processes. Disadvantages of ultrasound include (1) the need for a larger craniotomy to fit the transducer head, (2) its inability to perform preoperative assessment because it can be only be used on an intact dura or exposed brain, and (3) its production of a different image compared with the preoperative CT or MRI.

In the surgical resection of gliomas, some investigators have found particular utility in ultrasound because of its ability to provide added information to preoperative imaging studies.[18, 69] Tumor tends to possess higher echogenicity than surrounding brain. This results in an enhanced view of poorly enhancing tumor or of solid tumor that is adjacent to a cystic or necrotic area that does not show particularly well on CT. LeRoux and colleagues have reported the use of intraoperative ultrasound as a means of enhancing tumor resection in glioma patients. The tumor volume is first estimated via geometric calculations using data from the preoperative CT scans. The calculations were then performed again at surgery using the ultrasound data. Using this method, the boundaries of glioma tissue could be better localized, enabling a more complete resection to be performed. Caution must be exercised in using this method in repeat operations, as hyperechoic signals from significant scarring may lead to ultrasonagraphic overprediction of the size of the lesion.[74]

CONCLUSION

Currently, the ultrasonic aspirator is the most commonly used instrument for the resection of gliomas. New media with more efficient combinations of vaporization and coagulation effects, coupled with streamlined physical designs of the laser itself, may make the laser a more popular tool for glioma resection in the future. Other innovative but still experimental tools for glioma surgery include photodynamic therapy and hyperthermia. Intraoperative localization devices, such as frame-based stereotaxy and the currently available neuronavigators, may aid in intraoperative localization of the tumor. These devices can be used at each stage of planning and performance of the procedure. Technological improvements will come in the form of enhanced capabilities for offering the surgeon updated information in real-time during the procedure, which will eliminate some of the inherent inaccuracies of the current technology.

REFERENCES

1. Absten GT: Physics of light and lasers. Obstet Gynecol Clin North Am 1991; 18:407.
2. Anzai Y, Lufkin RB, Castro DJ, et al: MR imaging-guided interstitial Nd:YAG laser phototherapy: Dosimetry study of acute tissue damage in an in vivo model. J Magn Reson Imaging 1991; 1:553.

3. Anzai Y, Lufkin RB, Hirschowitz S, et al: MR imaging-histopathologic correlation of thermal injuries induced with interstitial Nd:YAG laser irradiation in the chronic model. J Magn Reson Imaging 1992; 2:671.

4. Anzai Y, Lufkin R, DeSalles A, et al: Preliminary experience with MR-guided thermal ablation of brain tumors. AJNR 1995; 16:39.

5. Barnett GH, Kormos DW, Steiner CP, et al: Use of a frameless, armless stereotactic wand for brain tumor localization with two-dimensional and three-dimensional neuroimaging. Neurosurgery 1993; 33:674.

6. Barnett GH, Kormos DW, Steiner CP, et al: Frameless stereotaxy using a sonic digitizing wand: Development and adaptation to the Picker ViStar medical imaging system. In Maciunas RJ (ed): Interactive Image-Guided Neurosurgery. Park Ridge, Ill, American Association of Neurological Surgeons, 1993, p. 113.

7. Benabid AL, Hoffman D, Lavallee S, et al: Is there any future for robots in neurosurgery? Adv Tech Stand Neurosurg 1991; 18:3.

8. Benabid AL, Lavallee S, Hoffmann D, et al: Potential use of robots in endoscopic neurosurgery. Acta Neurochir Suppl 1992; 54:93.

9. Black KL, Ikezaki K, Toga AW: Imaging of brain tumors using peripheral benzodiazepine receptor ligands. J Neurosurg 1989; 71:113.

10. Black KL, Mazziotta JC, Toga AW: Imaging and functional localization for brain tumors. Clin Neurosurg 1992; 39:475.

11. Boggan JE, Walter R, Edwards MSB, et al: Distribution of hematoporphyrin derivative in rat 9L gliosarcoma brain tumor analyzed by digital video fluorescence microscopy. J Neurosurg 1984; 61:1113.

12. Boggan JE, Bolger C, Edwards MSB: Effect of hematoporphyrin derivative photoradiation therapy on survival in the rat 9L gliosarcoma brain tumor model. J Neurosurg 1985; 63:917.

13. Boggan JE, Powers SK: Use of laser in neurological surgery. In Youmans JR (ed): Neurological Surgery, ed 3. Philadelphia, WB Saunders, 1990, p 992.

14. Brock M, Ingwersen I, Roggendorf W: Ultrasonic aspiration in neurosurgery. Neurosurg Rev 1984; 7:173.

15. Bucholz RD, Pittman T: Endoscopic coagulation of the choroid plexus using the Nd:YAG laser: Initial experience and proposal for management. Neurosurgery 1991; 28:421.

16. Cerullo LJ: Application of the laser to neurological surgery. In Wilkins RH, Rengachery SS (eds): Neurosurgery. New York, McGraw Hill, 1985, p 478.

17. Cerullo LJ: Laser in the removal of extraaxial tumors of the brain and spinal cord. In Fasano VA (ed): Advanced Intraoperative Technologies in Neurosurgery. Wien, Springer-Verlag, 1986, p 154.

18. Chandler WF, Knake JE, McGillicuddy JE, et al: Intraoperative use of real-time ultrasonography in neurosurgery. J Neurosurg 1982; 57:157.

19. Chen TC, Rabb C, Apuzzo MLJ: Complex technical methodologies and their applications in the surgery of intracranial meningiomas. Neurosurg Clin North Am 1994; 5:261.

20. Cline HE, Schenck JF, Hynynen K, et al: MR-guided focused ultrasound surgery. J Comput Assist Tomogr 1992; 16:956.

21. Darkazanli A, Hynynen K, Unger EC, et al: On-line monitoring of ultrasonic surgery with MR imaging. J Magn Reson Imaging 1993; 3:509.

22. Day JD, Fukushima T: Suction control of ultrasonic aspirators (letter). J Neurosurg 1993; 78:688.

23. Dereski MO, Chopp M, Chen Q, et al: Normal brain tissue response to photodynamic therapy: Histology, vascular permeability and specific gravity. Photochem Photobiol 1989; 50:653.

24. Drake JM, Joy M, Goldenberg A, et al: Computer- and robot-assisted resection of thalamic astrocytomas in children. Neurosurgery 1991; 29:27.

25. Drake JM, Prudencio J, Holowka S: A comparison of a PUMA robotic system and the ISG viewing wand for neurosurgery. In Maciunas RJ (ed): Interactive Image Guided Neurosurgery. AANS, Park Ridge, Ill, 1993, p 121.

26. Drake JM, Rutka JT, Hoffman HJ: ISG viewing wand system. Neurosurgery 1994; 34:1094.

27. Edwards MSB, Boggan JE, Fuller TA: The laser in neurological surgery. J Neurosurg 1983; 59:555.

28. El-Quahabi A, Guttmann CRG, Hushek SG, et al: MRI guided interstitial laser therapy in a rat malignant glioma model. Lasers Surg Med 1993; 13:503.

29. Epstein F: The cavitron ultrasonic aspirator in tumor surgery. Clin Neurosurg 1984; 31:497.

30. Epstein F: Ultrasonic dissection. In Wilkins RH, Rengachery SS (eds): Neurosurgery. New York, McGraw Hill, 1985, p 476.

31. Fasano VA: Observations on the use of three laser sources in sequence (CO_2-argon-Nd:YAG) in neurosurgery. Lasers Surg Med 1983; 2:199.

32. Fasano VA: Laser neurosurgical techniques. In Fasano VA (ed): Advanced Intraoperative Technologies in Neurosurgery. Wien, Springer-Verlag, 1986, p 107.

33. Fasano VA: Laser physics. In Fasano VA (ed): Advanced Intraoperative Technologies in Neurosurgery. Wien, Springer-Verlag, 1986, p 53.

34. Fasano VA: Principles of laser surgery. In Fasano VA (ed): Advanced Intraoperative Technologies in Neurosurgery. Wien, Springer-Verlag, 1986, p 97.

35. Fasano VA: Laser safety. In Fasano VA (ed): Advanced Intraoperative Technologies in Neurosurgery. Wien, Springer-Verlag, 1986, p 97.

36. Fasano VA: Ultrasonic aspiration in neurosurgery. In Fasano VA (ed): Advanced Intraoperative Technologies in Neurosurgery. Wien, Springer-Verlag, 1986, p 257.

37. Fine S, Klein E, Novak W, et al: Interaction of laser irradiation with biological systems. Fed Proc 1965; 24 (suppl 14):S35–S47.

38. Flamm ES, Ransohoff J, Wuchinich D, et al: Preliminary experience with ultrasonic aspiration in neurosurgery. Neurosurgery 1978; 2:240.

39. Fox JL, Hayes JR, Stein MN, et al: Experimental cranial and vascular studies of the effects of pulsed and continuous wave laser radiation. J Neurosurg 1967; 27:126.

40. Gallen CC, Sobel DF, Waltz T, et al: Noninvasive presurgical neuromagnetic mapping of somatosensory cortex. Neurosurgery 1993; 33:260.

41. Gamache FW, Patterson RH: The use of the potassium titanyl phosphate (KTP) laser in neurosurgery. Neurosurgery 1990; 26:1010.

42. Gamache FW, Morgello S: The histopathologic effects of the CO_2 versus the KTP laser on the brain and spinal cord: A canine model. Neurosurgery 1993; 32:100.

43. Glasscock ME, Jackson CG, Whitaker SR: The argon laser in acoustic tumor surgery. Laryngoscope 1981; 71:1405.

44. Gomer CJ, Ferrario A, Hayashi N, et al: Molecular, cellular, and tissue responses following photodynamic therapy. Lasers Surg Med 1988; 8:450.

45. Grady MS, Howard MA, Molloy JA, et al: Nonlinear magnetic stereotaxis: Three dimensional, in vivo magnetic manipulation of a small object in canine brain. Med Phys 1990; 17:405.

46. Guthrie BL, Adler JR: Computer-assisted preoperative planning, interactive surgery, and frameless stereotaxy. Clin Neurosurg 1992; 38:112.

47. Hecht J, Teresi D: Laser: Super Tool of the 1980s. New York, Ticknor & Fields, 1982.

48. Hill JS, Kaye AH, Sawyer WH, et al: Selective uptake of hematoporphyrin derivative into human cerebral glioma. Neurosurgery 1990; 26:248.

49. Hor F, Desgeorges M, Rosseau GL: Tumor resection by stereotactic laser endoscopy. Acta Neurochirurgica 1992; 54(suppl):77.

50. Howard MA, Grady MS, Ritter RC, et al: Magnetic neurosurgery (abstract). American Society for Stereotactic and Functional Neurosurgery, Marina del Rey, Calif, March 8, 1995.

51. Hu X, Tan KK, Levin DN: Three dimensional magnetic resonance images of the brain: Application to neurosurgical planning. J Neurosurg 1990; 72:433.

52. Jain KK: Lasers in neurosurgery: A review. Lasers Surg Med 1983; 2:217.

53. Jolesz FA, Bleier AR, Jakab P, et al: MR imaging of laser-tissue interactions. Radiology 1988; 168:249.

54. Junck L, Olson JMM, Ciliax BJ, et al: PET imaging of human gliomas with ligands for the peripheral benzodiazepine binding site. Ann Neurol 1989; 26:752.

55. Kahn T, Bettag M, Ulrich F, et al: MRI-guided laser-induced interstitial thermotherapy of cerebral neoplasms. J Comput Assist Tomogr 1994; 18:519.

56. Kamada K, Takeuchi F, Kurichi S, et al: Functional neurosurgical simulation with brain surface magnetic images and magnetoencephalography. Neurosurgery 1993; 33:269.

57. Kato A, Yoshimine T, Hayakawa T, et al: A frameless, armless navigational system for computer-assisted neurosurgery: Technical note. J Neurosurg 1991; 74:845.

58. Kaye AH, Morstyn G: Photoradiation therapy causing selective tumor kill in a rat glioma model. Neurosurgery 1987; 20:408.

59. Kaye AH, Morstyn G, Brownhill D: Adjuvant high-dose photoradiation therapy in the treatment of cerebral glioma: A phase 1–2 study. J Neurosurg 1987; 67:500.

60. Kaye AH, Morstyn G, Apuzzo MLJ: Photoradiation therapy and its potential in the management of neurological tumors. J Neurosurg 1988; 69:1.

61. Kaye AH, Hill JS: Photodynamic therapy of cerebral tumors. Neurosurg Q 1992; 1:233.

62. Kelly PJ, Kall BA, Goerss S, et al: Computer-assisted stereotaxic laser resection of intra-axial brain neoplasms. J Neurosurg 1986; 64:427.

63. Kelly PJ: The stereotactic CO_2 laser: Instrumentation, methodology, and clinical results. In Fasano VA (ed): Advanced Intraoperative Technologies in Neurosurgery. Wien, Springer-Verlag, 1986, p 162.

64. Kelly PJ: Future possibilities in stereotactic surgery: Where are we going? Appl Neurophysiol 1987; 50:1.

65. Kelly PJ, Goerss SJ, Kall BA: Evolution of contemporary instrumentation for computer-assisted stereotactic surgery. Surg Neurol 1988; 30:204.

66. Kelly PJ: Stereotactic imaging, surgical planning and computer-assisted resection of intracranial lesions: Methods and results. Adv Tech Stand Neurosurg 1991; 18:77.

67. Kelly PJ: Prospects for future developments in stereotaxy. In Apuzzo MLJ (ed): Neurosurgery for the Third Millenium. Park Ridge, Ill, AANS, 1992, p 35.

68. Kim SG, Ashe J, Hendrich K, et al: Functional magnetic resonance imaging of motor cortex: Hemispheric asymmetry and handedness. Science 1993; 261:615.

69. Knake JD, Chandler WF, Gabrielsen TO, et al: Intraoperative sonographic delinieation of low-grade brain neoplasms defined poorly by computer-tomography. Radiology 1984; 115:735.

70. Koivukangas J, Louhisalmi Y, Alakuijala J, et al: Ultrasound-controlled neuronavigator-guided brain surgery. J Neurosurg 1993; 79:36.

71. Kondziolka D, Dempsey PK, Lunsford LD, et al: A comparison between magnetic resonance imaging and computed tomography for stereotactic coordinate determination. Neurosurgery 1992; 30:402.

72. Kwoh YS, Hou J, Jonckheere EA, et al: A robot with improved absolute positioning accuracy for CT-guided stereotactic brain surgery. IEEE Trans Biomed Eng 1988; 35:153.

73. Kwong KK, Belliveau JW, Chesler DA, et al: Dynamic magnetic resonance imaging of human brain activity during primary sensory stimulation. Proc Natl Acad Sci 1992; 89:5675.

74. LeRoux PD, Berger MS, Ojemann GA, et al: Correlation of intraoperative ultrasound tumor volumes and margins with preoperative computerized tomography scans: An intraoperative method to enhance tumor resection. J Neurosurg 1989; 71:691.

75. Levivier M, Goldman S, Bidaut LM, et al: Positron emission tomography-guided stereotactic brain biopsy. Neurosurgery 1992; 31:792.

76. Lewis AI, Crone KR, Taha J, et al: Surgical resection of third ventricle colloid cysts. J Neurosurg 1994; 81:174.

77. Lewis AI, Keiper GL, Crone KR: Endoscopic treatment of loculated hydrocephalus. J Neurosurg 1995; 82:780.

78. Lewis MS, Bekey GA: Automation and robotics in neurosurgery: prospects and problems. In Apuzzo MLJ (ed): Neurosurgery for the Third Millenium. Park Ridge, Ill, AANS, 1992, p 65.

79. Liss L, Roppel R: Histopathology of laser produced lesions in cat brains. Neurology 1966; 16:783.

80. Martiniuk R, Bauer JA, McKean JDS, et al: New long-wavelength Nd:YAG laser at 1.44 μm: Effect on the brain. J Neurosurg 1989; 70:249.

81. Morita A, Kelly PJ: Resection of intraventricular tumors via a computer-assisted volumetric steriortactic approach. Neurosurgery 1993; 32:920.

82. Muller PJ, Wilson BC: Photodynamic therapy of malignant brain tumours. Can J Neurol Sci 1990; 17:193.

83. Muller PJ, Wilson PC: Photodynamic therapy: Cavitary photoillumination of malignant cerebral tumours using a laser coupled inflatable balloon. Can J Neurol Sci 1985; 12:371.

84. Oikarinen J, Alakuijala J, Louhisalmi Y, et al: The Oulu neuronavigational system: Intraoperative ultrasonography in the verification of neurosurgical localization and visualization. In Maciunas RJ (ed): Interactive Image-Guided Neurosurgery. Park Ridge, Ill, AANS, 1993, p 233.

85. Otsuki T, Yoshimoto T, Jokura H, et al: Stereotactic laser surgery for deep-seated brain tumors by open-system endoscopy. Stereotact Funct Neurosurg 1990; 54/55:404.

86. Pantev C, Hoke M, Lehnerz K, et al: Identification of sources of brain neruonal activity with high spatiotemporal resolution through combination of neuromagnetic source localization (NMSL) and magnetic resonance imaging (MRI). Electroencephalogr Clin Neurophysiol 1990; 75:173.

87. Pellizzari CA, Chen GTY, Spelbring DR, et al: Accurate three-dimensional registration of CT, PET, and/or MR images of the brain. J Comput Assist Tomogr 1989; 13:20.

88. Perria C, Carai M, Falzoi A, et al: Photodynamic therapy of malignant brain tumors: Clinical results of, difficulties with, questions about, and future prospects for the neurosurgical applications. Neurosurgery 1988; 23:557.

89. Poon WS, Schomacker KT, Deutsch TF, et al: Laser-induced fluorescence: Experimental intraoperative delineation of tumore resection margins. J Neurosurg 1992; 76:679.

90. Powers SK, Cush SS, Walstad DL, et al: Stereotactic intratumoral photodynamic therapy for recurrent malignant brain tumors. Neurosurgery 1991; 29:688.

91. Powers SK: Current status of lasers in neurosurgical oncology. Semin Surg Oncol 1992; 8:226.

92. Reinhardt HF, Horstmann GA, Gratzl O: Sonic stereometry in microsurgical procedures for deep-seated brain tumors and vascular malformations. Neurosurgery 1993; 32:51.

93. Roberts DW, Strohbehn JW, Hatch J, et al: A frameless stereotaxic integration of computerized tomographic imaging and the operating microscope. J Neurosurg 1986; 65:545.

94. Roberts DW, Friets EM, Strohbehn JW, et al: The sonic digitizing microscope. In Maciunas RJ (ed): Interactive Image-Guided Neurosurgery. Park Ridge, Ill, AANS, 1993, p 105.

95. Rosomoff JL, Carroll F: Reaction of neoplasms and brain to laser. Arch Neurol 1966; 14:143.

96. Roux FX, Mordon S, Fallet-Bianco C, et al: Effects of the 1.32 μm Nd-YAG laser on brain thermal and histological experimental data. Surg Neurol 1990; 34:402.

97. Roux FX, Devaux B, Merienne L, et al: 1.32 μm Nd:YAG laser during neurosurgical procedures experience with about 70 patients operated on with the MC 2100 unit. Acta Neurochir 1990; 107:161.

98. Singh M: Neuromagnetic imaging: A new window on brain function. In Apuzzo MLJ (ed): Neurosurgery for the Third Millenium. Park Ridge, Ill, AANS, 1992, p 25.

99. Starosta-Rubinstein S, Ciliax BJ, Penney JB, et al: Imaging of a glioma using peripheral benzodiazepine receptor ligands. Proc Natl Acad Sci 1987; 84:891.

100. Steichen JD, Stewart RB, Louis DN, et al: A new 1.9-μ wavelength laser for neurosurgery. J Neurosurg 1990; 73:611.

101. Stellar S: The carbon dioxide surgical laser in neurological surgery, decubitus ulcers, and burns. Lasers Surg Med 1980; 1:15.

102. Sugiyama K, Sakai T, Fujishima I, et al: Stereotactic interstitial laser-hyperthermia using Nd-YAG laser. Stereotact Funct Neurosurg 1990; 54–55:501.

103. Tan KK, Grzeszczuk R, Levin DN, et al: A frameless stereotactic approach to neurosurgical planning based on retrospective patient-image registration (technical note). J Neurosurg 1993; 79:296.

104. Tew JM, Tobler WD: The laser: History, biophysics, and neurosurgical applications. Clin Neurosurg 1984; 31:506.

105. Watanabe E, Mayamagi Y, Ksougi Y, et al: Open surgery assisted by neuronavigator, a stereotactic, articulated, sensitive arm. Neurosurgery 1991; 28:792.

106. Watanabe ET, Watanabe S, Manaka S, et al: Three-dimensional digitizer (Neuronavigator): New equipment for CT-guided stereotaxic surgery. Surg Neurol 1987; 27:543.

107. Wharen RE, Anderson RE, Laws ER: Quantitation of hematoporphyrin derivative in human gliomas, experimental central nervous system tumors, and normal tissues. Neurosurgery 1993; 12:446.

108. Yamada S, Gallen CC: Biomagnetic technologies: Magnetic source imaging (MSI). Magnes biomagnetometer. Neurosurgery 1993; 33:166.

109. Yamasaki T, Moritake K, Takaya M, et al: Intraoperative use of Doppler ultrasound and endoscopic monitoring in the stereotactic biopsy of malignant brain tumors (technical note). J Neurosurg 1994; 80:570.

110. Young RF: Application of robotics to stereotactic neurosurgery. Neurol Res 1987; 9:123.

111. Zamorano L, Chavantes C, Dujovny M, et al: Stereotactic endoscopic interventions in cystic and intraventricular brain lesions. Acta Neurochir 1992; 54(suppl):69.

MICHAEL TYMIANSKI

MARK BERNSTEIN

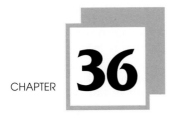

CHAPTER **36**

Closing Procedures and Postoperative Care

Although surgical skills and technical knowledge are essential in neurosurgery, a good outcome is at least as dependent on careful preoperative planning and excellence in postoperative care. A principle of complication avoidance in surgery is meticulous attention to detail in the perioperative period and anticipation of potential pitfalls before their occurrence. This chapter reviews some of the basic principles of craniotomy closure and postoperative care, with particular attention to maneuvers and techniques that serve to minimize later complications. A detailed description of all potential pitfalls is beyond the scope of this chapter. Thus, the goal is to provide a systematic approach to the most common perioperative issues. The reader is directed to the references at the end of the chapter for further details.

HEMOSTASIS: PRINCIPLES AND TECHNIQUES

Due to the rigid confines of the bony cranial vault, expanding intracranial hematomas can produce serious morbidity and loss of life. For this reason, surgical hemostatic control is of utmost importance. A basic understanding of normal biologic hemostasis is essential to the practical application of surgical hemostatic techniques. Biologic hemostasis is the process that terminates blood loss from a disrupted intravascular space, and can be subdivided into four major events: (1) vascular constriction, (2) platelet plug formation, (3) fibrin formation, and (4) fibrinolysis. Normal hemostasis may be seriously altered in patients with cerebral gliomas because of pathologic alterations in neoplastic vessels[175] or as a result of the secretion or aberrant expression of factors that affect hemostasis.[61, 99] Any one or all of the steps involved in hemostasis may be altered by brain neoplasms, producing unexpected hypercoagulable or hypocoagulable states. The most common hemostatic disorder seen in glioma patients is related to a subclinical chronic disseminated intravascular coagulation syndrome.[139]

Tumor-Induced Alterations in Biologic Hemostasis

1. Vascular Constriction. This initial response to vascular injury depends on a local reflex contraction of vascular smooth muscle, which produces luminal constriction. A relative reduction of smooth muscle–containing arterioles in gliomas[32] may impair this process. Furthermore, vascular reactivity to stretch and to vasoactive substances such as thromboxane A_2, serotonins, histamine, and bradykinins (see references 43, 103, 124, and 133) may be impaired in glioma vessels.[113]

2. Platelet Function. Through their interaction with endothelial surfaces, platelets initially form a loose plug to stop bleeding when vascular disruption occurs (primary hemostasis). This is followed by the formation of a compact platelet plug (secondary hemostasis) on activation of the platelet release reaction by factors released from platelets and the injured endothelium (ADP, platelet factor 4, thrombin, Ca^{2+}, and Mg^{2+}).[92, 97, 124, 127] Marked abnormalities in glioma vascular endothelium[112, 151, 175] can result in altered platelet function. For example, adherence to injured endothelium requires von Willebrand Factor (vWF), which is overexpressed in glioma endothelium.[99] Other abnormalities in platelet function have also been reported.[135]

3. Coagulation. Insoluble fibrin clots are produced through a series of stages in which circulating proenzymes (coagulation factors) are converted to activated proteases, resulting ultimately in the cleavage of fibrinogen into fibrin. Several reports attest to the presence of hypercoagulable states in glioma patients.[71, 74, 139, 148]

4. Fibrinolysis. This is the process by which patency of thrombosed blood vessels is restored. It is dependent on the enzyme plasmin, which is derived from the precursor plasma protein plasminogen. Tissue plasminogen levels rise as a consequence of venous occlusion and anoxia, and are actively secreted by glioma cells.[130] However, fibrinolytic activity is frequently reduced in patients with brain neoplasms.[68, 140, 148] A reduction in fibrinolytic activity, coupled with hypercoagulability, is probably the most common hemostatic disorder seen in glioma patients. Thus, this patient population is at an increased risk for spontaneous thrombotic events such as deep vein thrombosis (see following).

Techniques of Surgical Hemostasis

The unpredictability of the glioma patient's hemostatic profile underscores the importance of achieving meticulous intraoperative hemostasis. The control of hemostasis begins preoperatively with a proper history and physical examination, specifically addressing the presence of inherited coagulation and platelet defects, liver disease, vitamin K deficiency, and the use of antiplatelet agents or anticoagulants. The preoperative correction of identified hemostatic defects can transform a potentially fatal operation into a surgical success.

MECHANICAL ISSUES

Intraoperatively, general principles apply. Tumor vessels are generally more difficult to control than normal ones. Therefore, whenever surgery leaves behind a large number of aberrant vessels in the resection bed, hemostasis is more difficult to achieve. Thus, although a gross total macroscopic resection of many gliomas may be impossible, one of the surgical goals should be to excise a sufficient core of abnormal vascularity, preferably leaving behind peritumoral vessels having a greater resemblance to normal brain vessels.[151] An adequate exposure of the surgical field is essential and will greatly facilitate both tumor excision and the task of achieving hemostasis. Any excessive bleeding from exposed surfaces other than the tumor bed should alert the surgeon to the possible presence of a coagulopathy. Otherwise, continuous brisk bleeding sometimes implies a torn blood vessel that has retracted, rather than diffuse bleeding from the tumor bed.

Any bleeding from large feeders, residual tumor vessels, and dural vessels can usually be arrested with the judicious use of bipolar cautery. An irrigating bipolar instrument is especially useful in this instance to prevent sticking of the bipolar tips. Rarely, bleeding may be sufficiently severe to warrant the induction of temporary controlled hypotension.

It is usually pointless to attempt to stop all small tumor bleeders with electrocautery. In many instances, bleeding from small capillaries and arterioles stops spontaneously or when mechanical pressure is applied by temporarily packing the tumor cavity with a moist surgical sponge. The degree of residual bleeding is easily assessed by examining the site after irrigation with clear saline or artificial cerebrospinal fluid (CSF). A Valsalva's maneuver, which creates a transient increase in cerebral venous and capillary pressure, may also be of use in ensuring adequate hemostasis prior to closing a craniotomy.

SURGICAL DRAINS

There are no rigid criteria for the use of drains postcraniotomy, although it is thought that they reduce the incidence of postoperative hematomas.[59] As a principle, it is critical to emphasize that drain placement postcraniotomy can never substitute for meticulous surgical hemostasis. It is commonplace for many neurosurgeons to use extradural drains following routine craniotomy for brain tumor. The drains are frequently omitted when dural closure is incomplete, especially in posterior fossa operations, due to the increased risk of producing a CSF leak. The theoretical risk of increasing postcraniotomy infections with the use of surgical drains has never been demonstrated. However, it is felt that the risk of infection increases with time, and drains should therefore not be left in for more than a few days.[20] An interesting but rarely documented adverse effect of extradural drain insertion is sudden bradycardia and hypotension, as a consequence of the negative intracranial pressure produced by the drain.[84, 100]

CHEMICAL HEMOSTATIC AGENTS

In some cases, the removal of glial tumors produces a friable bed that continues to ooze blood. One option in such a case is to apply a chemical hemostatic agent to the bleeding site. However, chemical hemostatic agents must never be regarded as substitutes for meticulous surgical technique. Commonly used hemostatics include the following:

Oxidized Cellulose.   Oxidized cellulose (Oxycel; Parke-Davis) and oxidized regenerated cellulose (Surgicel; Johnson & Johnson) are absorbable organic acid fabrics having a low pH. In addition to their mechanical hemostatic function, the acidity of these compounds allows them to react with blood to form an artificial clot.[160] They produce a mild tissue reaction[19] and take from several days to a few weeks to be absorbed.[45, 46] Surgicel is thought to have antibacterial action against a variety of microorganisms due to its low pH.[9] One concern regarding the use of Surgicel is the danger of masking a hemorrhagic area with a temporary clot. Also, in excessive quantities, oxidized cellulose can mimic the appearance of tumor, abscess, or hemorrhage on postoperative computed tomographic (CT) scans.[174]

Absorbable Gelatin Sponge.   Gelfoam (The Upjohn Co.) is an absorbable material created from a specially treated gelatin solution. It has no hemostatic action of its own. However, due to its porous structure, it can absorb 45 times its weight in blood.[160] Once in place, the sponge adheres to the wound by the precipitation of fibrin and platelets. The pressure exerted by the blood-saturated sponge aids in mechanical hemostasis. Care should be taken with the use of Gelfoam due to the possibility of creating an expansile mass lesion. Although it is non-antigenic, inflammatory masses due to Gelfoam have been reported.[62]

Microfibrillar Collagen.   Avitene (Avicon Inc.) provides a surface to which platelets can adhere and undergo release reaction. The compound also accelerates the transformation of fibrinogen to fibrin. Because it is a foreign protein, it may increase the risk of infection and abscess formation; hence, only small amounts should be used. Exogenous collagen also has the potential of causing allergic reactions.[9]

Other Hemostatic Agents.   Thrombin (Thrombostat;

Parke-Davis) and fibrin glue (Tisseel; Immuno AG), are compounds intended to directly and indirectly increase fibrin clot formation.[13, 88, 119] Although these compounds are not routinely used as first-line hemostatic agents in glioma surgery, they are frequently used for reconstituting the dura mater (see following).

DURAL CLOSURE

The planning of dural closure begins at the start of the case. In preparing the craniotomy, consideration should be given to preserving pericranial or temporalis fascia flaps or to harvesting a fascia graft in case it is needed at the end of the operation. Care must be taken to avoid tearing the dura during the opening of the craniotomy. This may be difficult, as the dura of older patients is frequently adherent to the overlying bone. If the dura is torn during the drilling of burr holes, further bone can be removed until intact dura is seen, and a separator can be used to disengage the adherent dura from the skull. A Gigli saw guide is sometimes useful in this task. Particular care must be taken when extending a craniotomy over a dural sinus, and any sinus tear should be instantly covered and repaired to avoid the possibility of air embolism. Other dural tears produced during the opening can be left until the end of the operation. When opening the dura, care must be taken not to coagulate the dura excessively. Cautery-induced tissue shrinkage and retraction will hinder subsequent closure.

Important principles of dural closure include meticulous hemostasis of the underlying surgical bed, avoidance of dead spaces, and sealing off any open paranasal sinuses. The latter can be accomplished by overlaying the sinus opening with pericranium or other fascia harvested from the patient. The graft is secured in place with sutures and the seal augmented with fibrin glue.[85, 143] Hemorrhage from the epidural space is almost always venous and can usually be arrested by suturing the dura to the edge of the craniotomy. This is accomplished by passing a suture through the outer layer of the dura and through a small drill hole made obliquely through the outer skull table. Excessive dural traction during tack-up suture must be avoided, as this may cause further bleeding.[8] For large craniotomies, the dead space between the dura and the bone flap can be obliterated with a tack-up suture between the dura and the center of the flap.

Primary dural closure should be sought whenever possible. Many surgeons are proponents of watertight closure. Although this is intuitively and esthetically the most agreeable outcome, the benefits of a watertight closure have never been substantiated for routine craniotomy. The theoretical advantages include a reduction in the incidence of aseptic meningitis, a decrease in the formation of CSF fistulas and subgaleal CSF collections, and facilitation of subsequent reoperation. The use of absorbable suture materials, such as Vicryl (polyglactin 910), provides a theoretical advantage to use of nonabsorbable sutures, as absorbable material decreases the risk of infection, foreign body reaction, and adhesions, which hinder reoperation.[161] Studies show that sutures alone are insufficient for creating a watertight dural barrier, as the defects leak at pressurization within the physiologic range, even if all the dural edges are properly apposed.[30] For this reason, in patients who are at a significant risk of developing a CSF leak, the complementary use of fibrin glue over the suture line is advised.[30, 143, 158]

When the dura is resected due to tumor invasion, and whenever the dural opening cannot be closed primarily, reconstruction is recommended. This is especially applicable when the defect is large, when reoperation is likely, when a paranasal or mastoid sinus is breached, or when a CSF fistula is anticipated. Several reconstructive techniques have been described and are commonly in use. If watertight closure is not deemed crucial, small defects can be covered with a slab of gelatin sponge (Gelfoam). Otherwise, a duraplasty using autologous tissue, such as pericranium or fascia lata,[155] is recommended. This is preferred to numerous prosthetic or lyophilized cadaveric graft materials that have been described.[24, 35, 49, 82, 83, 102, 136, 171] These substances are reported to incite considerable foreign body reactions and occasional hemorrhagic complications.[10, 37, 50, 105, 111, 150, 176] Lyophilized dura substitutes should not be used due to the risk of transmitting Creutzfeldt-Jakob disease.[7, 80, 170] Extensive reconstructions of the dura using autologous tissue flaps[5, 75, 76, 144, 159] may be necessary following resection of skull base neoplasms. These techniques usually involve the use of a combination of autologous tissue flaps, fascial grafts, and the use of fibrin sealant to safeguard against CSF leaks.

CLOSING THE BONE FLAP

The goals in closing the craniotomy are (1) to restore the contour of the cranial vault, (2) to protect underlying structures, (3) to prevent infection and facilitate healing of the skin flap, and (4) to prevent hemispheric collapse, ventricular deformation, and midline displacements (''sinking skull-flap syndrome'').

These goals are easily met in a properly planned craniotomy and by adherence to basic principles. The craniotomy flap should be appropriately placed to prevent the need for additional bone removal, which may result in morcellization of the flap. The cutting instrument should be angled so as to bevel the edge of the craniotomy in a crater-like fashion. This avoids future sinking of the bone flap. In most instances, the use of a Gigli saw produces excellent results, because of the thinness of the saw blade compared with that of most power cutting tools. Bleeding from bone edges should be stopped with the application of bone wax or Gelfoam over the cut surface. Paranasal sinuses and mastoid air cells should be avoided unless otherwise dictated by the need for surgical exposure.

A well-made craniotomy flap is easy to replace. Thus, the routine fixation of bone flaps has received little attention in the neurosurgical literature. The common practice is to pass wire or synthetic suture material through drill holes to approximate the flap. It is preferable to do so at the start of the operation, prior to tacking up the dura. Otherwise, passing the bone suture through a drill hole containing a dural tack-up suture may sever the latter. An alternative is to use separate drill holes for dura and bone sutures. If metallic wire is used, the ends of each stitch should be buried in the drill hole to prevent skin irritation and the possibility of future infection. Recently, the use of titanium craniofacial plates and the principles of rigid fixation have been adapted to cranial flap replacement to achieve superior healing and cosmesis.[149] Two or three x- or y-shaped miniplates are required to provide adequate fixation. The suggestion is that less movement occurs, thereby promoting direct, more rapid bone healing instead of a fibrous union. Although these concepts have been validated in maxillofacial and orthopedic surgery,[41, 126] they remain to be established for routine craniotomy. An epidural Hemovac drain is commonly passed through a separate stab incision and left at the craniotomy site just prior to replacement of the bone flap.

If more than one bony fragment was removed during craniotomy, the pieces should be reconstructed meticulously prior to replacing the flap. Burr holes can be packed with bone dust obtained at the start of the craniotomy, or filled with synthetic bone plugs. In pediatric craniotomies, bone dust may be useful for filling small cranial defects. In frontotemporal craniotomies, the temporalis muscle should be sutured so as to cover the key burr hole.

A cranioplasty is usually indicated when the bone flap cannot be replaced. This includes instances in which bone is invaded by tumor, when the reconstruction of a bony flap from multiple fragments is impossible, or when infection is present. In some craniotomies for glioma, excessive intraoperative brain swelling may impede primary closure. In the case of infection, a cranioplasty should not be considered until the infection is fully treated. Whenever possible, a cranioplasty is preferable to a bony defect, because a functionally important normalization of electroencephalographic (EEG) abnormalities, seizures, and motor and speech function has been reported following cranioplasty, especially in calvarial defects exceeding 100 cm.[21, 42, 153] Other considerations include brain protection and cosmesis. Methyl methacrylate is the cranioplasty material preferred by most neurosurgeons. This attests to the belief that cranioplasty using homologous or cadaveric bone may result in infection and bone resorption, although this may be unfounded.[12, 118] Despite the recommended use in multiple publications of split-thickness cranial grafts, rib, or iliac crest,[41, 125, 164] acrylic remains the preferred material because of tissue tolerance, strength, low cost, ease of application, low infection rate, and compatibility with modern neuroimaging.[12, 17, 95, 125, 131, 132, 157]

REPAIRING THE SKIN FLAP

The goals of skin flap repair are to restore cosmesis and minimize the possibility of subsequent infection. To achieve these, general principles of wound closure apply. These include good skin apposition with eversion of the epidermal edges to maximize skin healing. Also, excellent hemostasis and the elimination of dead spaces are required to prevent the formation of postoperative hematomas and seromas. The skin flap is apposed by suturing together the galea with interrupted, inverted absorbable stitches. It is unnecessary to coagulate scalp vessels, as hemostasis is easily achieved with good approximation of the galeal edges. The skin is usually closed with interrupted nonabsorbable sutures or with surgical staples. Extensive skin flaps, such as those required for a bicoronal craniotomy, may require the insertion of a subgaleal drain for a period of 24 hours to eliminate

the possibility of a seroma. Although the scalp is usually very well vascularized, particular caution must be exercised in patients who have undergone prior surgery, irradiation, or therapeutic embolization of external carotid branches, as the scalp tends to be more friable, less vascular, and more prone to infection. To avoid scalp necrosis, the skin flap should be planned with a consideration of previous skin incisions and scalp vascularity. The use of hemostats may produce less scalp damage than skin clips.

The most common cause of skin flap infection is a stitch abscess, which can be avoided by refraining from strangulating scalp tissue during the closure, and by removing stitches and staples in a timely fashion once the skin flap is sufficiently healed. An erythematous, warm, indurated skin incision can indicate an underlying cellulitis, a postsurgical abscess or empyema, or a bone flap infection. These conditions require immediate investigation, as the treatment is dependent on the location and severity of the infection.

INTRACRANIAL PRESSURE MONITORING

The intracranial space is bounded by the rigid skull and is divided into partial compartments by relatively rigid dural infoldings comprising the falx cerebri and the tentorium cerebelli. As a first approximation, the intracranial contents include brain tissue, CSF, and intracranial blood. Any additional masses must grow at the expense of the above (the Monro-Kellie doctrine). The near incompressibility of the intradural contents accounts for many of the clinically significant aspects of intracranial pressure dynamics. The neurosurgeon is well-acquainted with the classical intracranial volume/pressure relationship that describes an exponential, almost vertical, increase in intracranial pressure (ICP) after a mass lesion reaches a critical volume.[81] Acute diffuse intracranial hypertension compromises the brain by causing (1) brain herniation and (2) a fall in cerebral perfusion pressure (CPP). Local changes in intracranial pressure that shift the intracranial contents[77] can be equally devastating. For this reason, it is common to monitor patients at risk for intracranial hypertension and to intervene when ICP increases or CPP falls.

However, although ICP monitoring is considered by many to be mandatory in head trauma, its role in the perioperative management of gliomas is unclear. Moreover, the relationship between intracranial pressure and brain function is not obvious, to a point at which some have questioned the utility of ICP measurements altogether.[137] For example, many patients with pseudotumor cerebri or obstructive hydrocephalus may appear to function normally with extremely high intracranial pressures. By contrast, a mass lesion in the medial temporal lobe may cause herniation and fatal brainstem compression long before a diffuse rise in ICP is detected. Thus, the cause of intracranial hypertension may be at least as important as the actual level of ICP. This is especially true in patients with brain neoplasms who may present with focal or diffuse intracranial hypertension as a consequence of enlarging localized mass lesions, brain edema, or obstruction of CSF flow or CSF resorption.

Intraoperative Considerations

An awareness of the effect of different operative and anesthetic maneuvers on the patient's ICP is mandatory in all cases, and it begins with proper preoperative planning. Glioma patients with signs, symptoms, or neuroimaging consistent with intracranial hypertension should be premedicated with corticosteroids to reduce brain edema.[3] Patients with large amounts of preoperative brain edema surrounding supratentorial tumors should be considered particularly at risk for developing intraoperative intracranial hypertension.[15] In such instances, consideration should be given to the use of mannitol at the start of the case. In select instances, ventricular drainage may be appropriate. Intraoperative management should be aimed at maintaining the patient's CPP within a normal range (above 60 mm Hg). A sudden intraoperative rise in ICP or the unexpected bulging of brain through the craniotomy should alert the surgeon to the possibility of an unexpected intracranial hemorrhage. If it occurs, then it must be promptly resolved by targeting the cause of the bleed. It should be noted that intracranial pressure is only minimally reduced by the removal of bone, but falls sharply on dural opening. Even the placement of a dural graft does not consistently ensure persistent brain decompression.[165] However, the benefit of a dural opening as an ICP control measure is questionable, as it appears to markedly enhance and accelerate the formation of brain edema.[60] Thus, whenever possible, the preferred management of intraoperative brain bulging should be by pharmacologic and ventilatory therapy rather than by decompressive craniectomy or brain resection.

Postoperative ICP Monitoring

The current literature is insufficient to provide rigid guidelines for the perioperative monitoring of ICP in glioma patients. Constantini and co-workers[39] described, in patients whose ICP was monitored after elective surgery, occurrence of a postoperative sustained ICP elevation that exceeded 20 mm Hg in 18.4% and 12.7% of patients who underwent supratentorial and infratentorial operations, respectively. A similar figure was quoted by Pappadà[120] for infratentorial cases. About half of the patients of Constantini and colleagues had an associated clinical deterioration that correlated with the magnitude of the ICP elevation. More important, about 80% of the patients who had clinical deterioration exhibited an ICP elevation before, or simultaneous with, the deterioration. Risk factors for postoperative ICP elevation were (1) resection of glioblastoma (compared with other gliomas) in 27.2% of cases, (2) repeated surgery in 42.9% of cases, and (3) protracted surgery (greater than 6 hours) in 41.7% of cases. Information gained from ICP monitoring altered the postoperative management of several patients. It was concluded that ICP monitoring was advantageous in immediate postoperative management after elective intracranial surgery and was almost risk free.

Therapy for Increased ICP in Glioma Patients

The goals for ICP management are to prevent ischemic brain injury and brain herniation. The therapy must ideally be directed at the cause of the ICP elevation. Treatment depends on the time-course, magnitude, and etiology of the intracranial hypertension. The initial diagnosis is, thus, crucial to determining the treatment strategy. The stepwise approach depends on the determination of whether the ICP elevation is due to physiologic causes, structural causes, or a combination of both.

Physiologic causes of intracranial hypertension include respiratory abnormalities, such as hypoventilation causing a rise in pCO_2 or endotracheal tube irritation causing a patient to "struggle against" a ventilator. Hypo-osmolar states and hyperthermia may also contribute to intracranial hypertension.[162] Structural causes of elevated ICP include the tumor mass, surrounding edema, hematomas, and hydrocephalus. An initial history, physical examination, and an imaging study (CT or MRI scan) usually suffice to provide the likely diagnosis. Specific treatment can then be planned to reverse the cause of the elevated ICP. For example, if the patient is not intubated and is having respiratory difficulties, intubation may be warranted. Likewise, patients in whom CSF absorption is impaired may benefit from CSF drainage.

When intracranial hypertension persists despite the optimization of the patient's physiologic state and the maximal correction of structural causes, further ICP therapy is warranted. Virtually all glioma patients benefit from perioperative coverage with corticosteroids (see following text). If the ICP elevation persists, mannitol can be used as a 20% solution in doses of 0.25 to 1 g/kg. Patients requiring more than small amounts of mannitol and all patients whose level of consciousness is impaired should be intubated and hyperventilated to create cerebral vasoconstriction and cause a reduction in the blood volume compartment.[26] During osmotherapy, serum osmolality should be kept below 320 mOsm/L, as high serum osmolality will lead to renal damage.[152] Other diuretics, such as furosemide, may help to prevent an untoward rise in serum osmolality.[141, 163] Further reductions in ICP in the ventilated patient may be gained by induction of sedation with opiates or benzodiazepines or by use of paralyzing agents, such as pancuronium.

FLUID AND ELECTROLYTE MANAGEMENT

The goal of perioperative fluid and electrolyte management is to maintain euvolemia by replacing intraoperative and postoperative fluid losses and to avoid osmotic changes that would aggravate postoperative tumor edema. A fluid and electrolyte imbalance is uncommon in uncomplicated craniotomies performed on otherwise healthy individuals. The goal postoperatively is to return the patients to controlling their own oral fluid intake. However, patients who were chronically dehydrated preoperatively may be predisposed to postoperative difficulties.[96] Thus, it is critical during preoperative planning to diagnose and manage chronic dehydration. Likewise, patients with chronic renal insufficiency, those taking diuretics, and those requiring craniotomies because of tumors affecting neuroendocrine function are at particular risk for a postoperative fluid and electrolyte imbalance.[89]

Normal Replacement Therapy

The normal adult fluid requirement is approximately 35 mL/kg/day or 2,500 mL/day. In obese patients, the fluid requirement calculations should be based on ideal, rather than on actual, weight. In the immediate postoperative period, consideration of fluid replacement should include intraoperative fluid losses. The most common electrolyte problem in postcraniotomy patients is overhydration during surgery.[69] This may initially be masked by the intraoperative use of mannitol, producing a normal electrolyte profile with hypovolemia immediately after surgery. However, dilutional hyponatremia can occur following fluid reloading.

Given normal renal function, the adult patient requires about 75 mEq of sodium, 40 mEq of potassium, and 150 g of glucose per day.[147] In the short term, replacement of these constituents is easily achieved by crystalloid therapy. However, it must be borne in mind that these solutions contain little nutritional value, and as such should not be considered for long-term fluid management.[109]

Diabetes Insipidus

This condition is manifest as polyuria with secondary polydipsia. It is most commonly observed after neurohypophyseal injury, but can also occur with hypothalamic tumors.[56] The relative lack of vasopressin causes excess urine water loss and a rise in serum osmolality. The differential diagnosis must include nephrogenic diabetes insipidus and psychogenic polydipsia, though these can be excluded on the basis of simple laboratory investigations. The primary mode of treatment is that of fluid replacement. Patients with neurogenic diabetes insipidus who are awake can be given oral fluids. Treatment with vasopressin will reverse the underlying abnormalities, but should be limited to patients in whom the condition is not expected to resolve spontaneously, who are unable to express thirst, or in whom intravenous fluid replacement is complicated due to other underlying medical conditions. The vasopressin analog desmopressin (DDAVP)[36] is most commonly used either intranasally or intramuscularly.

Hyponatremia and the Syndrome of Inappropriate Secretion of Antidiuretic Hormone (SIADH)

Inappropriate secretion of vasopressin may occur in certain patients with supratentorial neoplasms. The syndrome consists of excessive water retention and hyponatremia in the face of continuing high renal sodium excretion.[14] However, the most common cause of transient water intoxication is overtreatment of diabetes insipidus with either vasopressin or chlorpropamide, associated with continued water ingestion or infusion. Thus, meticulous attention must be paid to water balance to avoid iatrogenic SIADH. Also, gliomas in the region of the hypothalamus may produce disturbances in hunger and thirst.[56] Water intoxication may thus be a complication of neurogenic polydipsia in the absence of elevated ADH.

The most common clinical manifestation of hyponatremia is a change in mentation.[89] This should be treated with fluid restriction (as little as 500 mL/day). Infrequently, this can be supplemented with the antibiotic demeclocycline (300 mg three times a day), which induces a state of partial nephrogenic diabetes insipidus. Severe acute hyponatremia (sodium less than 120 mEq/L) may produce coma and seizures,[89] and constitutes a medical emergency. In the presence of clinical symptoms, fluid restriction should be augmented by the judicious use of hypertonic saline, avoiding a change in serum sodium concentration of more than 20 mEq/L/day, to avoid the complication of central pontine myelinolysis.[11]

Postoperative Transfusion of Blood or Blood Products

The transfusion of postcraniotomy patients solely to correct a laboratory value should be discouraged. Patients with mild, stable postoperative anemia usually do not require therapy and may be treated with oral iron supplements. Only severe anemia that compromises cardiovascular function or oxygen-carrying capacity requires attention. Although anemia following a particular difficult case is frequently due to intraoperative blood loss, special attention should be paid to alternative sources of hemorrhage, particularly the gastrointestinal tract in patients who are taking steroids.

ANTICONVULSANTS

Anticonvulsants are commonly used in the perioperative care of glioma patients. However, specific criteria for their use vary according to different patterns of practice. Although there is little argument about using anticonvulsants once a seizure has occurred, the value of anticonvulsants for seizure prophylaxis is unclear. For example, the role of antiepileptic medication in the patient with a low-grade glioma who has never had a seizure is unproven and must be weighed against the potential morbidity of long-term anticonvulsant therapy. Decisions about anticonvulsant use in glioma patients should be weighed according to current knowledge of seizure risk preoperatively and postoperatively.

Seizure Risk in Unoperated Gliomas (The Preoperative Period)

The value of prophylactic anticonvulsants for glioma patients is unknown. There is certainly a very low incidence of seizures associated with infratentorial neoplasms,[38, 44, 58, 91] which does not mandate the use of prophylaxis in this group of patients.

In the case of supratentorial neoplasms, seizure frequency appears to be inversely related to the degree of malignancy. In a series by Lund,[91] seizure frequency for glial tumors was as follows: oligodendroglioma, 81%; astrocytoma, 66%; ependymoma, 50%; and glioblastoma, 42%. In data compiled by Youmans,[172] seizures were the presenting feature in 50% of oligodendrogliomas, 40% of astrocytomas, 33% of supratentorial ependymomas, and 30% of glioblastomas. The difference in seizure frequency between glioblastomas and other gliomas is borne out in other series as well (29% vs. 68% incidence of seizures in patients harboring glioblastomas vs. other anaplastic gliomas, respectively[94]). However, the increased frequency of seizures in less malignant neoplasms may be a function of lifespan, and data relating the time from symptom onset to time of tumor diagnosis indicate this.[44]

Seizure frequency also correlates with tumor location,[58, 94, 121, 129] with areas around the primary motor cortex being more susceptible than occipital and basicranial locations. Mahaley and Dudka[94] reported preoperative seizures in 40% of patients with frontal, parietal, and temporal lesions as compared with 14% in patients with occipital lesions. With the exception of infratentorial tumors, most surgeons consider the previously quoted incidences of seizures sufficiently excessive to warrant routine seizure prophylaxis and anticonvulsants such as phenytoin or carbamazepine.

Postoperative Seizures

The incidence of seizures after posterior fossa surgery is low, and anticonvulsants may not be warranted.[86] However, a considerable proportion of supratentorial glioma patients who did not suffer seizures preoperatively experience postoperative seizures,[4, 22, 52, 94] although the relationship between seizures and specific factors such as extent of resection is unknown. In a retrospective study, Boarini and co-workers[22] suggested that there tended to be fewer seizures in older patients, females, patients with a higher grade of malignancy, and patients who had a more radical resection of the tumor. Nevertheless, a role for anticonvulsants in further reducing the incidence of those seizures was suggested. However, in a study of postoperative seizures within 48 hours of operation, Fukamachi and associates[54] found a high correlation between the incidence of seizures and CT findings of intracerebral hemorrhage, cerebral edema, and cerebral infarction, suggesting that major operative complications, not the tumor, had a role in triggering postoperative seizures.

Efficacy and Duration of Anticonvulsant Therapy in the Postoperative Period

The current literature provides conflicting evidence regarding the role of the anticonvulsants in the postoperative period, particularly in patients who were seizure-free preoperatively.* Most results suggest the usefulness of a short-term preventive treatment with anticonvulsants after surgery in patients without preoperative seizures. In patients with preoperative epilepsy, medication should be continued after surgery. However, long-term anticonvulsant treatment may not be useful in patients without preoperative epilepsy. In some studies, no significant difference in late seizure occurrence was found between patients receiving preventive treatment and untreated patients.[52] However, properly controlled trials conducted with a standardized therapeutic protocol and an adequate sample size have not been described.

---

*References 1, 22, 44, 52, 54, 78, 86, 94, 98, 114, 115, and 146.

Based on current knowledge, it seems justified to employ routine seizure prophylaxis in all supratentorial glioma cases in the immediate perioperative period. In the long term, the risks of anticonvulsant therapy must be weighed against the probability of a seizure, the consequences of a seizure in a given patient, and the ability of medication to lessen the probability of seizures. About 10% to 15% of patients receiving phenytoin develop a side effect of sufficient severity to warrant intervention,[14] but many toxic responses are preventable or treatable without resorting to discontinuation of therapy. Figure 36–1 shows an algorithm for use of anticonvulsant therapy in glioma patients.

THE USE OF ANTIBIOTICS

Considerable progress has been made in the past decade to rationalize the use of perioperative antibiotics in clean neurosurgical cases. A number of well-controlled, randomized clinical trials have demonstrated that antibiotic prophylaxis is effective in reducing the risk of infection following elective neurosurgical procedures.[21, 57, 64, 104, 123, 145, 167, 173] The relative risk of infection without antibiotic prophylaxis has been estimated to be 5.6 times greater than that with antibiotic prophylaxis.[63, 106] However, no single antibiotic regimen has been demonstrated to be superior to another. The choice of antibiotic must be based on knowledge of the common infecting organisms at a given institution.

A principle of antibiotic usage in neurosurgery is that antibiotics do not effectively cross the blood-brain barrier except when the meninges are inflamed or the blood-brain barrier is disrupted. Thus, it appears that CSF penetration is not the key to the efficacy of perioperative antibiotics. Instead, it appears that most neurosurgical infections begin as soft-tissue infections. Based on this, it is recommended that a dose of antibiotics be given immediately preoperatively to

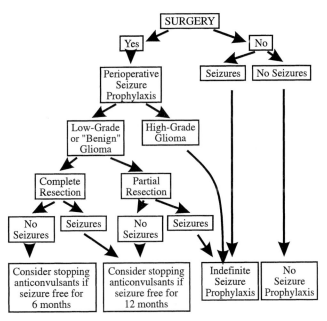

Figure 36–1 Protocol for the use of seizure prophylaxis in glioma patients.

achieve a good tissue levels by the time of the operation. This is the critical antibiotic dose, as no evidence supports the efficacy of postoperative antibiotics. If the preoperative dose has been given, many surgeons choose to continue postoperative antibiotic administration for a period of 24 hours.

There is currently no information to support the benefit of topical antibiotics in neurosurgery. Bacitracin is the most widely used antibiotic, and is generally applied to the operative site near the end of the procedure.

Factors Contributing to Craniotomy Infection

The incidence of infection in clean craniotomies in most hospitals is less than 5%. Thus, it is difficult to determine with certainty which factors contribute significantly to this already low infection rate. Factors such as duration of surgery, patient's age, and whether the procedure is a reoperation remain unproven. Similarly, although studies have addressed the impact on infection risk of ICP monitoring,[166] early diagnosis,[154] and osteoplastic vs. free bone flaps,[128] these retrospective series are insufficient to establish a given risk as significant. In a retrospective study of 9,202 cases, Mollman and Haines[106] found that the presence of a CSF leak and of concurrent non-CNS infection predisposed patients to infection. In another retrospective study, Blomstedt[20] identified CSF leaks as the only significant factor predictive of a higher infection risk. Thus, it is recommended that postoperative CSF leaks be promptly identified and treated.

Also of interest is that the value of removing hair in preparation for neurosurgery is unproven, and that shaving may in fact slightly increase the risk of infection.[6, 168]

CORTICOSTEROIDS IN GLIOMA PATIENTS

Steroid hormones are lipohilic compounds that cross cell membranes to bind to specific cytosolic receptors. The hormone-receptor complex binds to an acceptor site, which in turn alters the transcription rate of certain genes within the cell. Thus, steroids act by altering the rate of protein synthesis from those genes. Glucocorticoid hormones are generally catabolic and anti-inflammatory. However, other effects, such as the stabilization of cell membranes or reduction in brain tumor edema, do not occur at physiologic levels of glucocorticoids, but require considerably higher pharmacologic doses. Thus, some of the pharmacologic effects of steroids may not occur through the classic cytoplasmic receptor–mediated mechanisms.

The primary use of synthetic steroid hormones, such as dexamethasone, in the management of glioma patients is for reduction of peritumoral brain edema,[31, 39, 66, 67, 108] although cytostatic effects on glioma cells in vitro have also been reported.[53, 93] The mechanism by which tumor edema is reduced by steroids is unresolved. One possibility is that dexamethasone inhibits the formation of substances secreted by glioma cells that enhance the permeability of the vascular endothelium.[27] However, the role of vascular permeability

factors has been challenged.[116] Early studies have shown positive correlations between edema extent and the serum protein and sodium content in the edema fluid. The serum protein content is highest in glioblastomas as compared with other brain tumors.[23] However, studies using experimental gliomas in cats have suggested that corticosteroid therapy does not affect increased blood-brain barrier permeability, and has little effect on peritumoral extravasation of serum proteins.[70] In support of this are human MRI studies of brain water content showing that glioma patients receiving dexamethasone improve clinically, but that their brain water content remains unchanged.[16] Steroid effects on edema may be tumor-type specific, because dexamethasone treatment appears to decrease both water and serum protein content in glioblastomas but not in other gliomas and meningiomas.[23] Studies using positron-emission tomographic (PET) scanning show that dexamethasone treatment decreases cerebral blood flow and blood volume and increases the fractional extraction of oxygen thoughout the brain without affecting oxygen utilization.[87] Dexamethasone may thus cause direct vasoconstriction of cerebral blood vessels.

Perioperative Considerations

Most patients with glial tumors receive dexamethasone perioperatively. The presence of tumor edema on the CT or MRI scan is particularly strong indication for preoperative steroid coverage, as these patients are at a high risk for intraoperative intracranial hypertension.[15] Steroid coverage should be continued at least into the immediate postoperative period while the risks of intracranial hypertension and postoperative edema are high. It is recommended to concomitantly administer antacids, blockers of gastric acid production, or H_2 antagonists due to the risks of peptic ulceration.[122]

Consideration should be given to gradually ceasing steroid therapy within a few days of an uncomplicated glioma resection by decreasing the steroid dosage over a period of several days. However, patients with high-grade tumors and patients who continue to suffer from intracranial hypertension due to incomplete tumor resection are maintained on the minimum steroid dosage that palliates symptoms. Patients scheduled to undergo radiotherapy are also maintained on low doses of steroids until this treatment is completed. The palliative benefits of long-term steroid therapy must be weighed against the morbidity of steroid intake. Complications include cutaneous stigmata, immunosuppression,[110] peptic ulceration,[122] steroid myopathy,[47] psychological disturbances,[18] and the development of symptoms and signs of iatrogenic Cushing's syndrome.[101] An important drug interaction to remember is that of steroids with phenytoin: the latter increases the plasma clearance and decreases the bioavailability of dexamethasone.[33, 48, 79]

VENOUS THROMBOEMBOLISM IN GLIOMA PATIENTS

Thromboembolism represents a common and serious problem in patients with brain neoplasms.[90, 107, 134, 138] Most frequently, deep-vein thrombosis (DVT) and pulmonary embolism (PE) remain undetected, such that the estimates of clinically manifest thromboembolic phenomena range from 1% to 7%.[40, 90] However, the incidence of DVT and PE in patients with malignant brain neoplasms is striking when subclinical thromboembolic phenomena are considered. Peripheral venous thrombosis is estimated to occur in up to 40% of glioma patients not receiving antithrombotic prophylaxis,[107, 134] whereas pulmonary embolism may occur in up to 18% of those studied prospectively with ventilation/perfusion scans.[107] Brisman and Mendell detected a PE rate of 8.4% at autopsy.[25] The reasons for such high rates of thromboembolic complications in glioma patients are unknown, although in addition to a markedly altered hemostatic profile,[74, 139] these individuals frequently possess one or more of the specific risk factors for DVT, such as older age, immobility, varicose veins, prior surgery, and the presence of a malignancy. In a large series of patients, Constantini and co-workers[40] identified the following as significant risk factors for thromboembolic complications: (1) operations in the supratentorial area, (2) malignant gliomas, and (3) paraparesis or hemiparesis. Age, sex, and the specific location in the supratentorial area were not found to be statistically significant risk factors.

Thromboembolism Prophylaxis

Thrombosis prophylaxis should be considered in all glioma patients. This includes general measures, such as early postoperative ambulation and the use of graduated stockings or intermittent-pneumatic compression (IPC) garments in the perioperative period.[28, 29, 134] As long as the patient does not already have a documented DVT, use of either graduated stockings or IPC garments should be started preoperatively and maintained until the patient is ambulatory.[65]

Pharmacologic prophylaxis strategies should be considered in high-risk patients as defined in the preceding text. For glioma patients, this consists primarily of low-dose heparin, as other more intense strategies, such as adjusted-dose heparin and adjusted-dose warfarin, are unproven in neurosurgical patients. Typically, low-dose heparin is given at 5,000 IU subcutaneously twice daily, and should be started preoperatively for maximal efficacy.[65] It should be noted that heparin administration does not interfere with primary hemostasis, thus allowing platelet plug formation and hemostasis to occur in heparinized patients.

The risk of hemorrhagic complications in glioma patients treated with prophylactic doses of antithrombotic agents was estimated at 1.9% by Ruff and Posner.[134] It is generally believed that a brain neoplasm is not in itself a contraindication to pharmacologic thromboembolism prophylaxis.[34]

Diagnosis

The classic features of DVT include calf swelling and tenderness and Homans's sign. However, more than 50% of patients with DVT do not have these symptoms and signs. Pulmonary embolism may present with sudden dyspnea, pleuritic chest pain, hemoptysis, or cardiovascular collapse. Because the clinical diagnosis of DVT and PE is unreliable

and nonspecific,[42, 72] a high index of suspicion should be employed, and all patients suspected of harboring a thromboembolic complication should be investigated using laboratory diagnostic techniques. The decision-making algorithm shown in Figure 36–2 is recommended.

Several laboratory techniques have been validated for the diagnosis of DVT and PE. For DVT, these include impedance plethysmography (IPG), Doppler ultrasound, and radioisotope scans with ^{125}I-fibrinogen.[65] IPG and Doppler ultrasound are techniques that detect abnormal egress of blood from the calf by monitoring changes in electrical impedance and by ultrasonography, respectively. ^{125}I-Fibrinogen scans detect the incorporation of the radioisotope into developing thrombus.

The gold standard for the detection of pulmonary embolism is the pulmonary angiogram, which typically shows a filling defect within the pulmonary vasculature. However, due to the invasiveness of angiography,[72] a ventilation/perfusion scan is usually the preferred initial approach.[55] Scans are graded as low, intermediate, and high probability of PE, which corresponds to a probability of 12%, 33%, and 88%, respectively.[156] Patients with high-probability scans should be treated. Those with intermediate or low probability scans should be investigated for DVT as just delineated and treated for PE if DVT is present.[65] If DVT assessment is negative, those patients would have a less than 2% chance of having a recurrent PE. Because the goal of treatment is to prevent PE recurrence, these individuals can be followed by serial IPG or Doppler ultrasound to detect the development of a

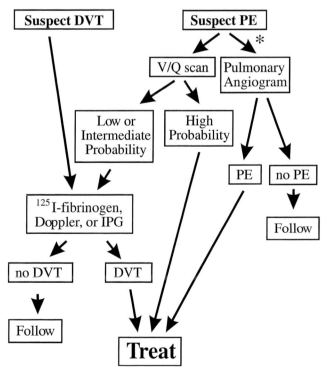

Figure 36–2 A decision tree for the diagnosis and treatment of venous and pulmonary thromboembolism. Pulmonary angiography *(asterisk)* is rarely necessary in the diagnosis of pulmonary embolism (PE) and should be used only when V/Q scanning and/or diagnostic testing for deep venous thrombosis (DVT) cannot be implemented.

new DVT. Pulmonary angiography is thus rarely necessary (see Fig. 36–2).

Thromboembolism Treatment

More than 50% of glioma patients with a documented, untreated, DVT subsequently suffer a PE.[107, 134] Of these, a very high proportion die as a result of this complication. In the series of Constantini and associates,[40] 7 of 19 glioma patients with a PE died within minutes to hours of the onset of symptoms despite the institution of therapy. The diagnosis and treatment of DVT is therefore of paramount importance. After the diagnosis of DVT is confirmed, treatment should follow immediately with the objectives of (1) preventing morbidity and mortality from PE and (2) preventing post-phlebitic syndrome.

Anticoagulant therapy is highly efficacious in preventing death and disability from PE. An intravenous heparin bolus followed by an infusion of heparin should be initiated and maintained with the aim of prolonging the activated pro-thrombin time (APTT) to 1.5 to 2.0 times control level. The oral anticoagulant warfarin can be started simultaneously and adjusted to maintain the international normalized ratio (INR) to between 2.0 and 3.0.[65] Treatment should continue for a minimum of 3 months.[73] Sufficient evidence exists to propose that anticoagulant therapy is safe in patients with glial tumors,[4, 117, 169] especially as compared with the high mortality of not instituting therapy.[40]

Patients with absolute or relative contraindications for anticoagulant therapy (e.g., gastric ulceration, recent intracerebral hemorrhage) benefit temporarily from an inferior vena cava filter.[107, 117] However, some recommend the institution of anticoagulation after the patient has passed the high-risk period for bleeding complications despite the IVC filter.[65] The role of thrombolytic therapy in PE is currently not established and is not recommended.

POSTOPERATIVE CT AND MRI STUDIES

Postoperative neuroimaging in glioma surgery serves three main purposes. First, it rapidly diagnoses structural postoperative complications, such as intracranial hematomas, hydrocephalus, or edema. Second, it assesses the extent of surgical resection. Third, in the follow-up phase, it assesses tumor recurrence, radiation-induced necrosis, and effects of adjuvant therapy or determines the timing of reoperation. The use of neuroimaging as a follow-up tool requires no elaboration.

A postoperative CT scan is useful for differential diagnosis in the patient who fails to awaken from anesthesia following the resection of a brain neoplasm. The immediate differential diagnosis should include incomplete reversal from neuromuscular blocking agents, postoperative hemorrhage, or excessive resection near anatomically critical sites. Similarly, patients who deteriorate neurologically in the early postoperative phase require a CT scan to exclude the presence of a structural lesion. The differential diagnosis in this situation must also include metabolic causes, such as severe hyponatremia, infection, drug reaction, or reaction to excessive use of sedative agents.

Neurodiagnostic imaging is essential in most instances in which the extent of operative resection is felt to have a bearing on future management. This is because the surgeon's subjective intraoperative perception of the extent of tumor removal correlates poorly with the actual amount of tumor tissue remaining.[2] However, the amount of residual tumor in the postoperative contrast CT or MRI scan may be obscured due to postoperative disruption of the blood-brain barrier, formation of neovascularity, or luxury perfusion. Thus, when the aim of imaging is to determine the extent of tumor removal, the study of choice is a gadolinium-enhanced MRI scan, performed within the first 72 hours postoperatively. This early diagnostic time window precedes the appearance of nonspecific enhancement, which impedes the evaluation of residual tumor. Early contrast MRI is superior to contrast-enhanced CT scan in this respect.[2, 51]

REFERENCES

1. Agbi CB, Bernstein M: Seizure prophylaxis for brain tumour patients: Brief review and guide for family physicians. Can Fam Physician 1993; 39:1153–1156, 1159–1160.
2. Albert FK, Forsting M, Sartor K, et al: Early postoperative magnetic resonance imaging after resection of malignant glioma: Objective evaluation of residual tumor and its influence on regrowth and prognosis. Neurosurgery 1994; 34:45–61.
3. Alberti E, Hartmann A, Schutz HJ, et al: The effect of large doses of dexamethasone on the cerebrospinal fluid pressure in patients with supratentorial tumors. J Neurol 1978; 217:173–181.
4. Altschuler E, Moosa H, Selker RG, et al: The risk and efficacy of anticoagulant therapy in the treatment of thromboembolic complications in patients with primary malignant brain tumors. Neurosurgery 1990; 27:74–76.
5. Ammar A: Repair of skull base dural defects: The dura sandwich. Technical note. Acta Neurochir 1992; 119:174–175.
6. Anonymous: Shaving the head: Reason or ritual? Lancet 1992; 340:1198–1199.
7. Anonymous: Creutzfeldt-Jakob disease in patients who received a cadaveric dura mater graft—Spain, 1985–1992. MMWR 1993; 42:560–563.
8. Aoki N: Acute subdural hematoma during tack-up suture of the dura mater: Case report. Neurol Med Chir 1988; 28:994–995.
9. Arand AG, Sawaya R: Intraoperative chemical hemostasis in neurosurgery. Neurosurgery 1986; 18:223–233.
10. Awwad EE, Smith KR Jr, Martin DS, et al: Unusual hemorrhage with use of synthetic dural substitute: MR findings. J Comput Assist Tomogr 1991; 15:618–620.
11. Ayus JC, Krothapolli RK, Arieff AI: Changing concepts in treatment of severe symptomatic hyponatremia: Rapid correction and possible relation to central pontine myelinolysis. Am J Med 1985; 78:897–902.
12. Aziz TZ, Mathew BG, Kirkpatrick PJ: Bone flap replacement vs acrylic cranioplasty: A clinical audit. Br J Neurosurg 1990; 4:417–419.
13. Barton B, Moore EE, Pearce WH: Fibrin glue as a biologic vascular patch: A comparative study. J Surg Res 1986; 40:510–513.
14. Bartter FC, Schwartz WB: The syndrome of inappropriate secretion of anti-diuretic hormone. Am J Med 1967; 42:790–806.
15. Bedford RF, Morris L, Jane JA: Intracranial hypertension during surgery for supratentorial tumor: Correlation with preoperative computed tomography scans. Anesth Analg 1982; 61:430–433.
16. Bell BA, Smith MA, Kean DM, et al: Brain water measured by magnetic resonance imaging: Correlation with direct estimation and changes after mannitol and dexamethasone. Lancet 1987; 1:66–69.
17. Benzel EC, Thammavaram K, Kesterson L: The diagnosis of infections associated with acrylic cranioplasties. Neuroradiology 1990; 32:151–153.
18. Bick PA: Obsessive-compulsive behavior associated with dexamethasone treatment. J Nerv Ment Dis 1983; 171:253–254.
19. Blair SD, Backhouse CM, Harper R, et al: Comparison of absorbable materials for surgical haemostasis. Br J Surg 1988; 75:969–971.

20. Blomstedt GC: Craniotomy infections. Neurosurg Clin North Am 1992; 3:375–385.

21. Blomstedt GC, Kytta J: Results of a randomised trial of vancomycin prophylaxis in craniotomy. J Neurosurg 1988; 69:216–220.

22. Boarini DJ, Beck DW, VanGilder JC: Postoperative prophylactic anticonvulsant therapy in cerebral gliomas. Neurosurgery 1985; 16:290–292.

23. Bodsch W, Rommel T, Ophoff BG, et al: Factors responsible for the retention of fluid in human tumor edema and the effect of dexamethasone. J Neurosurg 1987; 67:250–257.

24. Boop FA, Chadduck WM: Silastic duraplasty in pediatric patients. Neurosurgery 1991; 29:785–787.

25. Brisman R, Mendell J: Thromboembolism and brain tumor. J Neurosurg 1973; 38:337–338.

26. Brodersen P, Gjerris F, Hansen A, et al: Cerebral blood flow and intracranial pressure during hypocapnic halothane anesthesia in brain tumor patients. Acta Neurol Scand 1977; 64:500–501.

27. Bruce JN, Criscuolo GR, Merrill MJ, et al: Vascular permeability induced by protein product of malignant brain tumors: Inhibition by dexamethasone. J Neurosurg 1987; 67:880–884.

28. Bucci MN, Papadopoulos SM, Chen JC, et al: Mechanical prophylaxis of venous thromboembolism in patients undergoing craniotomy: A randomized trial. Surg Neurol 1989; 32:285–288.

29. Bynke O, Hillman J, Lassvik C: Does peroperative external pneumatic leg muscle compression prevent post-operative venous thrombosis in neurosurgery? Acta Neurochir 1987; 88:46–48.

30. Cain JE Jr, Dryer RF, Barton BR: Evaluation of dural closure techniques: Suture methods, fibrin adhesive sealant, and cyanoacrylate polymer. Spine 1988; 13:720–725.

31. Cairncross JG, Macdonald DR, Pexman JH, et al: Steroid-induced CT changes in patients with recurrent malignant glioma. Neurology 1988; 38:724–726.

32. Cervos-Navarro J, Iglesias-Rozas JR: Ultrastructural systematization of vascular changes in gliomas. Zentralb Pathol 1986; 132:49–55.

33. Chalk JB, Ridgeway K, Brophy T, et al: Phenytoin impairs the bioavailability of dexamethasone in neurological and neurosurgical patients. J Neurol Neursurg Psychiatry 1984; 47:1087–1090.

34. Choucair AK, Silver P, Levin VA: Risk of intracranial hemorrhage in glioma patients receiving anticoagulant therapy for venous thromboembolism. J Neurosurg 1987; 66:357–358.

35. Clark RP, Robertson JH, Shea JJ, et al: Closure of dural defects with proplast. Am J Otol 1984; 5:179–182.

36. Cobb WE, Stare S, Reichlin S: Neurogenic diabetis insipidus: Management with DDAVP (1-desamino-8-D-arginine vasopressin). Ann Intern Med 1978; 88:183–188.

37. Cohen AR, Aleksic S, Ransohoff J: Inflammatory reaction to synthetic dural substitute: Case report. J Neurosurg 1989; 70:633–635.

38. Cohen N, Strauss G, Lew R, et al: Should prophylactic anticonvulsants be administered to patients with newly-diagnosed cerebral metastases? A retrospective analysis. J Clin Oncol 1988; 6:1621–1624.

39. Constantini S, Cotev S, Rappaport ZH, et al: Intracranial pressure monitoring after elective intracranial surgery: A retrospective study of 514 consecutive patients. J Neurosurg 1988; 69:540–544.

40. Constantini S, Kornowski R, Pomeranz S, et al: Thromboembolic phenomena in neurosurgical patients operated upon for primary and metastatic brain tumors. Acta Neurochir 1991; 109:93–97.

41. Craft PD, Sargent LA: Membranous bone healing and techniques in calvarial bone grafting. Clin Plast Surg 1989; 16:11–19.

42. Cranley JJ, Canos AJ, Sull WJ: The diagnosis of deep venous thrombosis: Fallibility of clinical symptoms and signs. Arch Surg 1976; 111:34–36.

43. De Clerck F: Effects of serotonin on platelets and blood vessels. J Cardiovasc Pharmacol 1991; 17(suppl 5):S1–S5.

44. Deutschman CS, Haines SJ: Anticonvulsant prophylaxis in neurological surgery. Neurosurgery 1985; 17:510–517.

45. Dimitrijevich SD, Tatarko M, Gracy RW, et al: Biodegradation of oxidized regenerated cellulose. Carbohydr Res 1990; 195: 247–256.

46. Dimitrijevich SD, Tatarko M, Gracy RW, et al: In vivo degradation of oxidized, regenerated cellulose. Carbohydr Res 1990; 198:331–341.

47. Dropcho EJ, Soong SJ: Steroid-induced weakness in patients with primary brain tumors. Neurology 1991; 41:1235–1239.

48. Eadie MJ, Brophy TR, Ohlrich G, et al: Dexamethasone: Pharmacokinetics in neurological patients. Clin Exp Neurol 1984; 20:107–118.

49. Fisher WS, Braun D: Closure of posterior fossa dural defects using a dural substitute: Technical note. Neurosurgery 1992; 31:155–156.

50. Fontana R, Talamonti G, D'Angelo V, et al: Spontaneous haematoma as unusual complication of silastic dural substitute: Report of 2 cases. Acta Neurochir 1992; 115:64–66.

51. Forsting M, Albert FK, Kunze S, et al: Radiologic follow-up after extripation of glioblastoma: Residual tumor and regrowth pattern. AJNR 1993; 14:77–87.

52. Franceschetti S, Binelli S, Casazza M, et al: Influence of surgery and antiepileptic drugs on seizures symptomatic of cerebral tumours. Acta Neurochir 1990; 103:47–51.

53. Freshney RI: Effects of glucocorticoids on glioma cells in culture: Minireview on cancer research. Exp Cell Biol 1984; 52:286–292.

54. Fukamachi A, Koizumi H, Nukui H: Immediate postoperative seizures: Incidence and computed tomographic findings. Surg Neurol 1985; 24:671–676.

55. Fulkerson WJ, Coleman RE, Ravin CE, et al: Diagnosis of pulmonary embolism. Arch Intern Med 1986; 146:961–967.

56. Garnica NAD, Metzloff ML, Rosenbloom AL: Clinical manifestations of hypothalamic tumors. Ann Clin Lab Sci 1980; 10:474–485.

57. Geraghty J, Feely M: Antibiotic prohylaxis in neurological surgery. J Neurosurg 1984; 60:724–726.

58. Gilles FH, Sobel E, Leviton A, et al: Epidemiology of seizures in children with brain tumors: The Childhood Brain Tumor Consortium. J Neurooncol 1992; 12:53–68.

59. Gilsanz FJ, Vaquero J, Lora-Tamayo JI, et al: Circulatory changes caused by a closed, negative pressure drainage system after craniotomy. Neurosurgery 1983; 12:593.

60. Go GK, Hockwalk GM, Kostero-Otte L: The effect of cold-induced brain edema on cerebrospinal fluid formation rate. J Neurosurg 1980; 53:652–655.

61. Goldman CK, Kim J, Wong WL, et al: Epidermal growth factor stimulates vascular endothelial growth factor production by human malignant glioma cells: A model of glioblastoma multiforme pathophysiology. Mol Biol Cell 1993; 4:121–133.

62. Guerin C, Heffez DS: Inflammatory intracranial mass lesion: An unusual complication resulting from the use of Gelfoam. Neurosurgery 1990; 26:856–859.

63. Haines SJ: Antibiotic prophylaxis in neurosurgery: The controlled trials. Neurosurg Clin North Am 1992; 3:355–358.

64. Haines SJ: Ceftizoxime versus vancomycin and gentamicin in neurosurgical prophylaxis: A randomized, prospective, blinded clinical study [letter]. Neurosurgery 1993; 33:949.

65. Hamilton MG, Hull RD, Pineo GF: Venous thromboembolism in neurosurgery and neurology patients: A review. Neurosurgery 1994; 34:280–296.

66. Hatam A, Bergstrom M, Yu ZY, et al: Effect of dexamethasone treatment on volume and contrast enhancement of intracranial neoplasms. J Comput Assist Tomogr 1983; 7:295–300.

67. Hatam A, Yu ZY, Bergstrom M, et al: Effect of dexamethasone treatment on peritumoral brain edema: Evaluation by computed tomography. J Comput Assist Tomogr 1982; 6:586–592.

68. Hindersin P, Koch K, Korting HJ: Changes in blood coagulation and fibrinolysis in brain tumors. Nervenarzt 1989; 60:154–158.

69. Hoff JT, Clarke HB: Adverse postoperative events, in Apuzzo MLJ (ed): Brain Surgery: Complication Avoidance and Management. New York, Churchill Livingstone, 1993, pp 99–126.

70. Hossmann KA, Hurter T, Oschlies U: The effect of dexamethasone on serum protein extravasation and edema development in experimental brain tumors of cat. Acta Neuropathol 1983; 60:223–231.

71. Hsieh V, Molnar I, Ramadan A, et al: Hypercoagulability syndrome associated with cerebral lesions: Prospective study of coagulation during surgery of primary brain tumors (17 cases). Neurochirurgie 1986; 32:404–409.

72. Hull RD, Raskob GE, Hirsh J: The diagnosis of clinically suspected pulmonary embolism: Practical approaches. Chest 1986; 89:417S–425S.

73. Hyers TM, Hull RD, Weg JG: Antithrombotic therapy for venous thromboembolic disease. Chest 1989; 95:37S–51S.

74. Iberti TJ, Miller M, Abalos A, et al: Abnormal coagulation profile in brain tumor patients during surgery. Neurosurgery 1994; 34:389–395.

75. Izquierdo R, Origitano TC, al-Mefty O, et al: Use of vascularized fat from the rectus abdominis myocutaneous free flap territory to seal the dura of basicranial tumor resections. Neurosurgery 1993; 32:192–196.

76. Johnson GD, Jackson CG, Fisher J, et al: Management of large dural defects in skull base surgery: An update. Laryngoscope 1990; 100:200–202.

77. Kuchiwaki H, Misu N, Takada S, et al: Measurement of local directional pressures in the brain with mass. Neurosurgery 1992; 31:731–738.

78. Kvam DA, Loftus CM, Copeland B, et al: Seizures during the immediate post-operative period. Neurosurgery 1983; 12:14–17.

79. Lackner TE: Interaction of dexamethasone with phenytoin. Pharmacotherapy 1991; 11:344–347.

80. Lane KL, Brown P, Howell DN, et al: Creutzfeldt-Jacob disease in a pregnant woman with an implanted dura mater graft. Neurosurgery 1994; 34:737–740.

81. Langfitt TW, Weinstein JD, Kassell NF: Cerebral vasomotor paralysis produced by intracranial hypertension. Neurology 1965; 15:622–641.

82. Laquerriere A, Yun J, Tiollier J, et al: Experimental evaluation of bilayered human collagen as a dural substitute. J Neurosurg 1993; 78:487–491.

83. Laun A, Tonn JC, Jerusalem C: Comparative study of lyophilized human dura mater and lyophilized bovine pericardium as dural substitutes in neurosurgery. Acta Neurochir 1990; 107:16–21.

84. Laurenson VG, MacFarlane M, Davis FM: Negative pressure drainage after craniotomy. Neurosurgery 1985; 17:868.

85. Lee KC, Park SK, Lee KS: Neurosurgical application of fibrin adhesive. Yonsei Med J 1991; 32:53–57.

86. Lee ST, Lui TN, Chang CN, et al: Early postoperative seizures after posterior fossa surgery. J Neurosurg 1990; 73:541–544.

87. Leenders KL, Beaney RP, Brooks DJ, et al: Dexamethasone treatment of brain tumor patients: effects on regional cerebral blood flow, blood volume, and oxygen utilization. Neurology 1985; 35:1610–1616.

88. Lerner R, Binur NS: Current status of surgical adhesives. J Surg Res 1990; 48:165–181.

89. Lester MC, Nelson PB: Neurological aspects of vasopressin release and the syndrome of inappropriate secretion of antidiuretic hormone. Neurosurgery 1981; 8:735.

90. Levi AD, Wallace MC, Bernstein M, et al: Venous thromboembolism after brain tumor surgery: A retrospective review. Neurosurgery 1991; 28:859–863.

91. Lund M: Epilepsy in association with intracranial tumors. Acta Psychiatr Scand 1952; 8:1–149.

92. Luscher TF: Endothelial control of vascular tone and growth. Clin Exp Hypertens 1990; 12:897–902.

93. Maciunas RJ, Mericle RA, Sneed CL, et al: Determination of the lethal dose of dexamethasone for early passage in vitro human glioblastoma cell cultures. Neurosurgery 1993; 33:485–488.

94. Mahaley MS, Jr, Dudka L: The role of anticonvulsant medications in the management of patients with anaplastic gliomas. Surg Neurol 1981; 16:399–401.

95. Malis LI: Titanium mesh and acrylic cranioplasty. Neurosurgery 1989; 25:351–355.

96. Maroon JC, Nelson PB: Hypovolemia in patients with subarachnoid hemorrhage: Therapeutic implications. Neurosurgery 1979; 4:223.

97. Masaki T, Yanagisawa M, Takuwa Y, et al: Cellular mechanism of vasoconstriction induced by endothelin. Adv Second Messenger Phosphoprotein Res 1990; 24:425–428.

98. Mathew E, Sherwin AL, Welner SA, et al: Seizures following intracranial surgery: Incidence in the first post-operative week. Can J Neurol Sci 1980; 7:285–290.

99. McComb RD, Jones TR, Pizzo SV, et al: Immunohistochemical detection of factor VIII/von Willebrand factor in hyperplastic endothelial cells in glioblastoma multiforme and mixed glioma-sarcoma. J Neuropathol Exp Neurol 1982; 41:479–489.

100. McCulloch GAJ, Pattison WJ: Circulatory changes caused by a closed, negative pressure drainage system after craniotomy. Neurosurgery 1981; 9:380–382.

101. McCutcheon IE, Oldfield EH: Cortisol: Regulation, disorders and clinical evaluation, in Barrow DL, Selman W (eds): Concepts in Neurosurgery: Neuroendocrinology. Baltimore, Williams & Wilkins, 1992, pp 117–173.

102. Meddings N, Scott R, Bullock R, et al: Collagen Vicryl: A new dural prosthesis. Acta Neurochir 1992; 117:53–58.

103. Meininger GA, Davis MJ: Cellular mechanisms involved in the vascular myogenic response. Am J Physiol 1992; 263:H647–H659.

104. Mindermann T, Zimmerli W, Gratzl O: Randomized placebo-controlled trial of single-dose antibiotic prophylaxis with fusidic acid in neurosurgery. Acta Neurochir 1993; 121:9–11.

105. Misra BK, Shaw JF: Extracerebral hematoma in association with dural substitute. Neurosurgery 1987; 21:399–400.

106. Mollman HD, Haines SJ: Risk factors for postoperative neurosurgical wound infections: A case control study. J Neurosurg 1986; 64:902–906.

107. Muchmore JH, Dunlap JN, Culicchia F, et al: Deep vein thrombophlebitis and pulmonary embolism in patients with malignant gliomas. South Med J 1989; 82:1352–1356.

108. Muller W, Kretzschmar K, Schicketanz KH: CT-analyses of cerebral tumors under steroid therapy. Neuroradiology 1984; 26:293–298.

109. Nelson PB: Fluid and electrolyte physiology, pathophysiology, and management, in Wirth FP, Ratcheson RA (eds): Concepts in Neurosurgery: Neurosurgical Critical Care. Baltimore, Williams & Wilkins, 1987, pp 69–80.

110. Neuwelt EA, Kikuchi K, Hill S, et al: Immune responses in patients with brain tumors: Factors such as anti-convulsants that may contribute to impaired cell-mediated immunity. Cancer 1983; 51:248–255.

111. Ng TH, Chan KH, Leung SY, et al: An unusual complication of Silastic dural substitute: Case report. Neurosurgery 1990; 27:491–493.

112. Nir I, Levanon D, Iosilevsky G: Permeability of blood vessels in experimental gliomas: Uptake of ^{99m}Tc-glucoheptonate and alteration in blood-brain barrier as determined by cytochemistry and electron microscopy. Neurosurgery 1989; 25:523–531.

113. Nomura T, Ikezaki K, Natori Y, et al: Altered response to histamine in brain tumor vessels: The selective increase of regional cerebral blood flow in transplanted rat brain tumor. J Neurosurg 1993; 79:722–728.

114. North JB, Penhall RK, Hanieh A, et al: Penytoin and postoperative epilepsy: A double blind Study. J Neurosurg 1983; 58:672–677.

115. North JB, Penhall RK, Hanieh A, et al: Postoperative epilepsy: A double-blind trial of phenitoin after craniotomy. Lancet 1980; 1:384–386.

116. Ohnishi T, Sher PB, Posner JB, et al: Capillary permeability factor secreted by malignant brain tumor: Role in peritumoral brain edema and possible mechanism for anti-edema effect of glucocorticoids. J Neurosurg 1990; 72:245–251.

117. Olin JW, Young JR, Graor RA, et al: Treatment of deep vein thrombosis and pulmonary emboli in patients with primary and metastatic brain tumors: Anticoagulants or inferior vena cava filter? Arch Intern Med 1987; 147:2177–2179.

118. Osawa M, Hara H, Ichinose Y, et al: Cranioplasty with a frozen and autoclaved bone flap. Acta Neurochir 1990; 102:38–41.

119. Papatheofanis FJ, Barmada R: The principles and applications of surgical adhesives. Surgery Annu 1993; 25(pt 1):49–81.

120. Pappadà G, Formaggio G, Regalia F, et al: Course of intracranial pressure after extirpation of posterior fossa tumours. Acta Neurochir 1984; 70:11–19.

121. Penfield W, Erickson TC, Tarlov I: Relation of intracranial tumors and symptomatic epilepsy. Arch Neurol Psychiatry 1940; 44:300–315.

122. Pezner RD, Lipsett JA: Peptic ulcer disease and other complications in patients receiving dexamethasone palliation for brain metastasis. West J Med 1982; 137:375–378.

123. Pons VG, Denlinger SL, Guglielmo BJ, et al: Ceftizoxime versus vancomycin and gentamicin in neurosurgical prophylaxis: A randomized, prospective, blinded clinical study. Neurosurgery 1993; 33:416–422.

124. Price JM: Influence of pressure and flow on constriction of blood vessels. J Fla Med Assoc 1991; 78:825–827.

125. Prolo DJ, Oklund SA: The use of bone grafts and alloplastic materials in cranioplasty. Clin Orthop Rel Res 1991; 268:270–278.

126. Rahn BA: Direct and indirect bone healing after operative fracture treatment. Otolaryngol Clin North Am 1987; 20:425–440.

127. Raij L: Mechanisms of vascular injury: The emerging role of the endothelium. J Am Soc Nephrol 1991; 2:S2–S8.

128. Rasmussen S, Ohrstrom JK, Westergaard L, et al: Post-operative infections of osteoplastic compared with free bone flaps. Br J Neurosurg 1990; 4:493–495.

129. Rasmussen T, Blundell J: Epilepsy and brain tumors. Clin Neurosurg 1959; 7:138–158.

130. Reith A, Rucklidge GJ: Invasion of brain tissue by primary glioma: Evidence for the involvement of urokinase-type plasminogen activator as an activator of type IV collagenase. Biochem Biophys Res Commun 1992; 186:348–354.

131. Remsen K, Lawson W, Biller HF: Acrylic frontal cranioplasty. Head Neck J 1986; 9:32–41.

132. Robinson AC, O'Dwyer TP, Gullane PJ, et al: Anterior skull defect reconstruction with methyl methacrylate. J Otolaryngol 1989; 18:241–244.

133. Rubanyi GM, Freay AD, Kauser K, et al: Mechanoreception by the endothelium: Mediators and mechanisms of pressure- and flow-induced vascular responses. Blood Vessels 1990; 27:246–257.

134. Ruff RL, Posner JB: Incidence and treatment of peripheral venous thrombosis in patients with glioma. Ann Neurol 1983; 13:334–336.

135. Sack GH, Jr, Levin J, Bell WR: Trousseau's syndrome and other manifestations of chronic disseminated coagulopathy in patients with neoplasms: Clinical, pathophysiologic, and therapeutic features. Medicine 1977; 56:1–37.

136. San-Galli F, Darrouzet V, Rivel J, et al: Experimental evaluation of a collagen-coated Vicryl mesh as a dural substitute. Neurosurgery 1992; 30:396–401.

137. Saul TG: Is ICP monitoring worthwhile? Clin Neurosurg 1988; 34:560–571.

138. Sawaya R, Cummins CJ, Kornblith PL: Brain tumors and plasmin inhibitors. Neurosurgery 1984; 15:795–800.

139. Sawaya R, Glas-Greenwalt P: Postoperative venous thromboembolism and brain tumors: II. Hemostatic profile. J Neurooncol 1992; 14:127–134.

140. Sawaya R, Ramo OJ, Glas-Greenwalt P, et al: Plasma fibrinolytic profile in patients with brain tumors. Thromb Haemost 1991; 65:15–19.

141. Schettini A, Stahurski B, Young HF: Osmotic and osmotic loop diuretics in brain surgery: Effects on plasma and CSF electrolytes and ion excretion. J Neurosurg 1982; 56:679–684.

142. Segal DH, Oppenheim JS, Murovic JA: Neurological recovery after cranioplasty. Neurosurgery 1994; 34:729–731.

143. Shaffrey CI, Spotnitz WD, Shaffrey ME, et al: Neurosurgical applications of fibrin glue: Augmentation of dural closure in 134 patients. Neurosurgery 1990; 26:207–210.

144. Shaffrey ME, Persing JA, Shaffrey CI, et al: Duraplasty in cranial base resection. J Craniofac Surg 1991; 2:152–155.

145. Shapiro M, Wald U, Simchen E: Randomized clinical trial of intraoperative antimicrobial prophylaxis of infection after neurosurgical procedures. J Hosp Infect 1986; 8:283–295.

146. Shaw MD: Post-operative epilepsy and the efficacy of anticonvulsant therapy. Acta Neurochir 1990; 50:55–57.

147. Shoemaker WC: Fluids and electrolytes in the acutely ill adult, In Shoemaker WC, Thompson WL, Holbrook PR (eds): The Society of Critical Care Medicine Textbook of Critical Care. Philadelphia, WB Saunders, 1984, pp 614–640.

148. Singh VP, Jain D, Mohan R, et al: Haemostatic abnormalities in brain tumours. Acta Neurochir 1990; 102:103–107.

149. Smith SC, Pelofsky S: Adaptation of rigid fixation to cranial flap replacement. Neurosurgery 1991; 29:417–418.

150. Spaziante R, Cappabianca P, Del Basso De Caro ML, et al: Unusual complication with use of lyophylized dural graft. Neurochirurgia 1988; 31:32–34.

151. Stewart PA, Hayakawa K, Hayakawa E, et al: A quantitative study of blood-brain barrier permeability ultrastructure in a new rat glioma model. Acta Neuropathol 1985; 67:96–102.

152. Stuart FP, Torres E, Fletcher D, et al: Effects of repeated and massive mannitol infusion in the dog: Structural and functional changes in kidney and brain. Ann Surg 1970; 172:190–204.

153. Tabaddor K, LaMorgese J: Complication of a large cranial defect: Case report. J Neurosurg 1976; 44:506.

154. Taylor G, McKenzie M, Kirkland T, et al: Effect of surgeon's diagnosis on surgical wound infection rates. Am J Infect Control 1990; 18:295–299.

155. Thammavaram KV, Benzel EC, Kesterson L: Fascia lata graft as a dural substitute in neurosurgery. South Med J 1990; 83:634–636.

156. The PIOPED investigators: Value of the ventilation/perfusion scan in acute pulmonary embolism: Results of the Prospective Investigation of Pulmonary Embolism Diagnosis (PIOPED). JAMA 1994; 263: 2753–2759.

157. Tokoro K, Chiba Y, Tsubone K: Late infection after cranioplasty: Review of 14 cases. Neurol Med Chir 1989; 29:196–201.

158. Toma AG, Fisher EW, Cheesman AD: Autologous fibrin glue in the repair of dural defects in craniofacial resections. J Laryngol Otol 1992; 106:356–357.

159. Ueda K, Inoue T, Harada T, et al: Dura and cranial base reconstruction by external oblique fascia and rectus abdominis muscle flap. J Reconst Microsurg 1992; 8:427–432.

160. Ulin AW, Gollub SS: Surgical Bleeding: A Handbook for Medicine, Surgery and Specialties. New York, McGraw Hill, 1966, pp 404–431.

161. Vallfors B, Hansson HA, Svensson J: Absorbable or nonabsorbable suture materials for closure of the dura mater? Neurosurgery 1981; 9:407–413.

162. Ward JD: Intracranial pressure, head injuries, subarachnoid hemorrhage, non-surgical coma and brain tumors. In Shoemaker WC, Thompson WL (eds): Critical Care, State of the Art, vol II(R)8. New York, Society for Critical Care Medicine, 1981.

163. Ward JD, Moulton RJ, Muizelaar JP, et al: Cerebral hemostasis and protection. In Wirth FP, Ratcheson RA (eds): Concepts in Neurosurgery: Neurosurgical Critical Care. Baltimore, Williams & Wilkins, 1987, pp 187–213.

164. Weber RS, Kearns DB, Smith RJ: Split calvarium cranioplasty. Arch Otol Head Neck Surg 1987; 113:84–89.

165. Wilkinson HA: Intracranial pressure. In Youmans JR (ed): Neurological Surgery. Philadelphia, WB Saunders, 1990, pp 661–695.

166. Winfield JA, Rosenthal P, Kanter RK, et al: Duration of intracranial pressure monitoring does not predict daily risk of infectious complications. Neurosurgery 1993; 33:424–430.

167. Winkler D, Rehn H, Freckmann N: Clinical efficacy of perioperative antimicrobial prophylaxis in neurosurgery: A prospective randomized trial in 159 patients. Chemotherapy 1989; 35:304–312.

168. Winston KR: Hair and neurosurgery. Neurosurgery 1992; 31:320–329.

169. Wolfe MW: Treatment of deep vein thrombosis and pulmonary emboli in patients with primary and metastatic brain tumors. Arch Intern Med 1988; 148:1671.

170. Yamada S, Aiba T, Endo Y, et al: Creutzfeldt-Jacob disease transmitted by a cadaveric dura mater graft. Neurosurgery 1994; 34:740–744.

171. Yamagata S, Goto K, Oda Y, et al: Clinical experience with expanded polytetrafluoroethylene sheet used as an artificial dura mater. Neurol Med Chir 1993; 33:582–585.

172. Youmans JR: Neurological Surgery. Philadelphia, WB Saunders, 1990, p 688.

173. Young RF, Lawner PM: Perioperative antibiotic prophylaxis for the prevention of postoperative neurosurgical infections: A randomized clinical trial. J Neurosurg 1987; 66:701–706.

174. Young ST, Paulson EK, McCann RL, et al: Appearance of oxidized cellulose (Surgicel) on postoperative CT scans: Similarity to postoperative abscess. Am J Roentgenol 1993; 160:275–277.

175. Zama A, Tamura M, Inoue HK: Three-dimensional observations on microvascular growth in rat glioma using a vascular casting method. J Cancer Res Clin Oncol 1991; 117:396–402.

176. Zeman AZ, Maurice-Williams RS, Luxton R, et al: Lymphocytic meningitis following insertion of a porcine dermis dural graft. Surg Neurol 1993; 40:75–80.

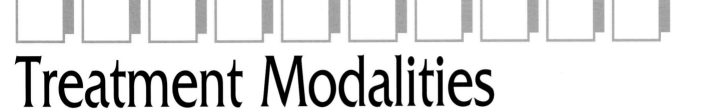

Treatment Modalities

RADIOTHERAPY

DENNIS C. SHRIEVE

DENNIS F. DEEN

DAVID A. LARSON

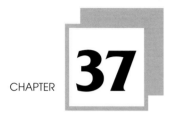

CHAPTER **37**

Basic Principles of Radiobiology and Radiotherapy

For most patients with gliomas, surgery followed by radiotherapy is the mainstay of modern treatment.[1–3] Quite often, when total resection is not feasible, radiotherapy becomes the primary treatment modality. Modern imaging techniques combined with high-energy linear accelerators, computerized treatment planning systems, and better understanding of the biology of the various subtypes of glioma have led to improvements in radiotherapeutic techniques that allow better localization of the volume to be treated and a better ability to spare normal brain and other tissues from unnecessary treatment.[2, 4] However, modern radiotherapy is based on radiobiologic principles. Both the radiation oncologist and the neurosurgeon participating in the care of patients with brain tumors who receive radiotherapy (or radiosurgery) should be aware of these principles and of how they are applied in the treatment of patients. This chapter outlines the radiobiologic principles that provide a basis for this understanding and that serve as background for the following chapters.

RADIATION BIOPHYSICS

Interaction of Radiation With Matter

Radiation energy is absorbed in biologic material mainly through interaction with atomic orbital electrons. Energy imparted may be sufficient to raise the electron to a higher-energy orbit (excitation) or to eject the electron from the atom, creating a charged particle and an energetic free electron (ionization). *Ionizing radiation* transfers energy to the absorbing material in discrete, relatively large amounts in a small volume. The average energy transferred per ionizing event is approximately 33 electron volts (eV), which is

sufficient energy to break chemical bonds and to disrupt molecular structure.[5]

Electromagnetic Radiation

The electromagnetic radiation spectrum includes radio waves, microwaves, infrared light, visible light, ultraviolet light, x-rays, and γ-rays. Although all of these can cause biologic effects under proper conditions, only x-rays and γ-rays have sufficient energy to cause ionization. X-rays and γ-rays do not differ in any way other than in their method of production and site of origin within the atom. γ-rays originate in the nucleus and are the result of radioactive decay. X-rays originate from outside the nucleus, either from energy transition among orbital electrons following radioactive processes or following interaction of accelerated electrons with a heavy metal target in a standard x-ray machine or linear accelerator. Although electromagnetic radiations have the properties of waves (wavelength, frequency, and velocity), this type of radiation may also be considered to have some properties of particles in that energy is contained in discrete packets of energy or photons. Each photon has an energy E related to the wavelength of the electromagnetic radiation,

$$E = h\nu = \frac{hc}{\lambda}$$

or

$$E\ (\text{eV}) = \frac{1.24 \times 10^{-6}}{\lambda\ (\text{m})}$$

where E is expressed in electron volts (eV), h is Planck's

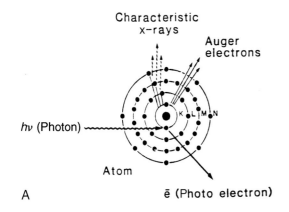

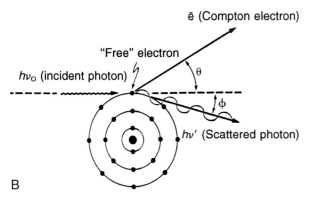

Figure 37–1 Schematic drawing of absorption of photon energy through the photoelectric effect (A) and Compton scattering (B). (From Kahn FM: The Physics of Radiation Therapy. Baltimore; Williams & Wilkins, 1984.)

constant (6.62×10^{-34} J·sec), v is the frequency (cycles/sec), c is the speed of light, and λ is the wavelength in meters.

Thus the characteristic property of ionizing radiation is the size of the packets or *quanta* of energy, which must be sufficient to cause ionizing events. It is also this particulate nature of ionizing radiation that accounts for the random distribution of events throughout the irradiated volume. This in turn explains the nature of cell killing following irradiation that can be described as a certain probability of cell death (or survival) following a particular dose of radiation.

Photons interact with absorbing media through three major processes.[5, 6] The *photoelectric effect* is an important mode of interaction at low energies (<100 keV) and involves the ejection of an orbital electron (Fig. 37–1A). The energy of the incident photon is entirely used up in the process; part of the energy is used to overcome the binding energy of the orbital electron, and the remaining energy is converted into kinetic energy of the ejected electron. The probability of photoelectric interaction is inversely related to the energy of the incident photon and directly related to the cube of the atomic number (Z^3) of the absorbing material. This is the basis of the differential absorption of diagnostic x-rays by bone and soft tissue.

At energies between about 30 and 10 MeV, absorption of photon energy is predominantly through the process of *Compton scattering* (Fig. 37–1B). The incident photon loses a portion of its energy to kinetic energy of the Compton

electron ejected at an angle θ, and a secondary photon of lower energy is deflected at an angle ϕ to conserve momentum. The probability of absorption by Compton scattering is dependent only on electron density and not on Z of the absorbing material.

A third mode of interaction, *pair production*, takes place at energies above 1.02 MeV. An incident photon gives up all of its energy to the nucleus to produce a pair of particles: an electron and a positron. The combined kinetic energy of these particles will be less than the energy of the incident photon by 1.02 MeV (the rest mass of the two particles produced). Pair production becomes an increasingly important mechanism of absorption for photons of energy above 6 MeV (at which energy pair production accounts for 10% of absorption), and is therefore an important mechanism for photons produced by high-energy linear accelerators.

The important similarity of these absorption processes is the production of *energetic electrons*. These fast electrons are responsible for the vast majority of biologic effects. The nuclear DNA is believed to be the most important cellular target for damage produced by ionizing radiation. DNA damage may be produced through a *direct* interaction of the fast electron with the DNA molecule. More often, the fast electron interacts with other molecules in the cell (e.g., H_2O) to produce free radicals that may diffuse to the DNA and cause chemical damage. This *indirect action* of ionizing radiation is responsible for approximately 75% of cellular damage produced by ionizing radiation.[7]

Each of the preceding absorption processes has the end effect of reducing the number of photons as a function of thickness of the absorbing material, a process referred to as *attenuation*. Quantitatively the photon intensity I at a depth of x in an absorbing material may be calculated as

$$I = I_0 e^{-vx}$$

where I_0 is the incident photon intensity and v is the total linear absorption coefficient for the absorbing material and the photon energy (Fig. 37–2).[5]

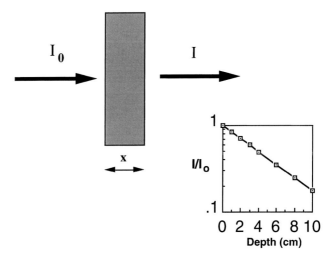

Figure 37–2 Illustration of attenuation of a photon beam with initial intensity I_o. The number of photons I present at any depth x is a characteristic function of the absorbing material and decreases exponentially (*inset*).

Particulate Radiation

Radiotherapy is also delivered using high-energy particles. Electrons are commonly used in general radiotherapy but are of little use in treating brain tumors due to their lack of penetration. However, other particulate radiations are in relatively common use for treatment of intracranial disease. These include protons, neutrons, and heavy charged particles.[8, 9] These particles lose energy through interactions with nuclei in the absorbing material in contrast to photons, which interact with orbital electrons.[7]

Neutrons are absorbed either by *elastic* or *inelastic scattering*. Elastic scattering takes place through interaction of the fast neutron with a hydrogen nucleus (proton). Because the two particles have similar masses, the collision is much like that between two billiard balls, resulting in two energetic particles: a recoil proton and a neutron of lower energy than the original incident neutron. Higher-energy neutrons (>6 MeV) may also interact with larger nuclei (carbon or oxygen) and produce a number of energetic α particles ($^4He_2$) in the process of *inelastic scattering*. These charged particles produced by neutron interactions are much more massive than the fast electrons produced through photon interactions. For this reason, these particles are much less likely to travel through a given thickness of absorbing material without further interactions. The total energy is therefore transferred from the incident neutron to the absorbing material in a relatively small volume. For this reason, neutrons and other particulate radiations are referred to as *densely ionizing*. These energetic particles deposit their total energy while traveling a relatively short distance in the absorbing medium. The average energy lost per unit path length (*linear energy transfer*, or LET) is therefore relatively large. Most biologic damage due to *high LET* radiation is due to the *direct effect* (i.e., effects due to damage in target molecules [DNA] caused by interaction with the energetic particles produced).[7, 10]

The interaction of radiation with matter may be quantified by measurement of the amount of energy absorbed per unit mass. The *gray* (Gy) is now the preferred unit of absorbed dose, defined as the absorption of 1 J/kg. A commonly used unit is the *centigray* (cGy), which is exactly equal to the previously used unit, the *rad*.

CELLULAR RADIOBIOLOGY

Mammalian Cell Survival Curves

The probability of cell survival following x-irradiation is a function of absorbed dose. The shape of the mammalian cell survival curve obtained by irradiating cells in culture (Fig. 37–3) shows little variation between cell lines.[11] The characteristic shape includes a low-dose shoulder region followed by a steeply sloped, or more continuously bending, portion at higher doses. An interpretation of the shoulder region is that an accumulation of damage occurs at low doses such that an additional dose seems to kill cells more efficiently.[7, 12–14] This implies that cells may incur *sublethal damage*, and that lethality may result from the interaction of two or more such sublethal lesions. A simple model for cell

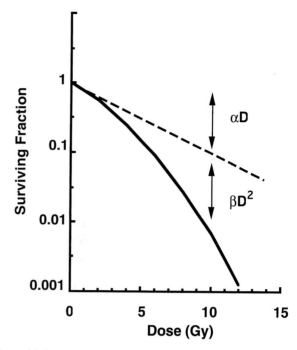

Figure 37–3 Mammalian cell survival curve following x irradiation (*solid line*). The α/β is 10 Gy, a dose at which there is equal contribution to cell killing by single events (αD, *dashed line*) and interaction of sublethal events (βD^2).

killing by ionizing radiation assumes that DNA is the target molecule and that a double-strand break in the DNA is necessary and sufficient to cause cell death (defined as loss of ability to divide). A double-strand break could be produced by a single particle track or by interaction of two single-strand breaks occurring closely in space and time (Fig. 37–4). Single-strand breaks alone may be repaired and therefore represent sublethal damage. Such a model is described by the linear-quadratic formula

$$SF = e^{-(\alpha D + \beta D^2)}$$

where SF is the surviving fraction, D is the dose of radiation

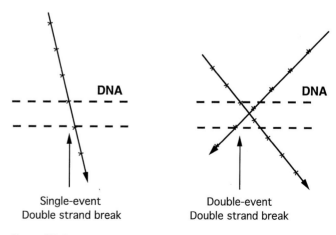

Figure 37–4 Diagrammatic representation of double-strand break production by a single photon or interaction of damage produced by two photon tracks.

in grays, α is the coefficient related to single-event cell killing, and β is the coefficient related to cell killing through the interaction of sublethal events. The ratio α/β is a measure of the relative contributions of these two components to overall cell kill (see Fig. 37–3). α/β is the *dose* at which overall cell killing is equally due to these two components, or

$$\alpha D = \beta D^2$$
$$\text{or}$$
$$D = \alpha/\beta$$

Most mammalian cell survival curves, including those derived from human gliomas, following x-irradiation may be fit well to the linear-quadratic model.[15] Cell survival following a single dose of radiation in vitro reflects the intrinsic *radiosensitivity* of a particular cell type to a particular type of radiation.[16]

Modification of Radiosensitivity

Survival following a particular dose of radiation depends on many factors other than the total absorbed dose. Cellular microenvironment, especially the presence of oxygen, physical parameters, such as the type of radiation (sparsely vs. densely ionizing), the number of doses given, the time interval between doses, and the dose rate all may be altered, resulting in very different survival following a given dose.[7]

THE OXYGEN EFFECT

The most important chemical modifier of radiation damage is molecular oxygen. Cells irradiated in the presence of oxygen are three-fold more sensitive to sparsely ionizing radiation than cells irradiated under anoxic conditions (Fig. 37–5). The *oxygen effect* is quantified by the *oxygen enhancement ratio* (OER), which is defined as the ratio of doses required for a given effect in the presence or absence of oxygen,

$$OER = \frac{D(N_2)}{D(O_2)}$$

where $D(O_2)$ and $D(N_2)$ are the doses in the presence and absence, respectively, of oxygen that are required to achieve a specified level of cell survival. The OER following x-irradiation in vitro is approximately 3.

Free radical species produced in cellular water following irradiation are extremely short-lived.[17] The probability of interaction of these radiation-produced free radicals and DNA depends on diffusion of the free radicals from the point of production to the DNA molecule. The lifetime of free radicals, and the probability of interaction with target molecules, are increased by the presence of oxygen. The mechanism of the oxygen effect is thought to involve the *indirect action* of ionizing radiation only. The competition model for modification of radiosensitivity by oxygen and other electron affinic hypoxic cell sensitizers involves competition between these sensitizing molecules and intrinsic or added reducing species that serve as *radioprotectors* under

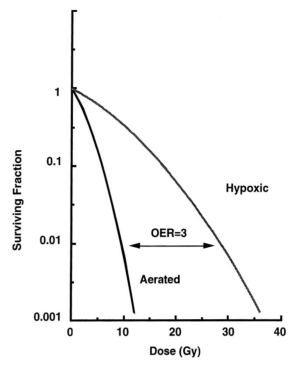

Figure 37–5 Mammalian cell survival curves following irradiation in culture under aerated or hypoxic conditions. Threefold higher doses are required to achieve the same level of cell kill under hypoxic conditions compared with aerated conditions.

certain conditions (Fig. 37–6). Radicals are produced in the target molecule (DNA) through the indirect action. These free radical species are extremely short-lived.[17] Reaction with an electron-affinic compound stabilizes this damage and renders it non-restorable. Reaction with a reducing species (e.g., glutathione) restores the molecule to its native form. These two processes take place in competition with one another at rates determined by the relative concentrations of sensitizer and protector and their respective rate constants. In the presence of oxygen, kinetics greatly favor the production of the peroxy radical and stabilization of DNA damage. Under hypoxic conditions, the reaction with endogenous reducing species takes place, which leads to molecular restoration and is responsible for the relative radioresistance of hypoxic cells. Also under hypoxic conditions, addition of exogenous radiosensitizers that mimic oxygen (but with lower rate constants) may serve to increase cell killing by radiation.[18] The magnitude of the OER depends on the relative contribution to cell killing by the indirect action for a particular type of radiation. Therefore the magnitude of the oxygen effect decreases with increasing LET.[10]

DIFFERENTIAL RADIOSENSITIVITY IN THE CELL CYCLE

Proliferating cells have variable radiosensitivity depending on their position in the *cell cycle*.[19] The cell cycle divides the lifetime of a cell into four phases (Fig. 37–7). The mitotic phase (*M*) is the period of cell division. The *S* phase is the period of DNA synthesis. The time period between mitosis and the beginning of *S* phase is *G1*, and the period

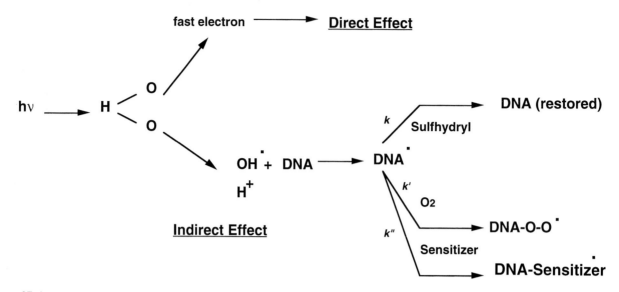

Figure 37–6 The competition model for modification of radiation damage by oxygen. Free radical damage in the DNA, produced via the indirect effect of radiation (hydrolysis of water), reacts with either reducing species (e.g., sulfhydryl compounds such as glutathione), resulting in restoration of a functional molecule, or electron affinic species (such as oxygen), resulting in new radical species (peroxyradicals) that are not restorable to a functional form. The reactions take place in competition, with the reaction constant k' for oxygen being 10 to 100 times higher than that for glutathione (k). Hypoxic cell radiosensitizers may take the place of oxygen under hypoxic conditions.

following *S* phase before mitosis is *G2*. Cells are most radiosensitive during late *G2* and *M*. Cells are most resistant in late *S* phase. *G1* cells are of intermediate sensitivity (Fig. 37–8). The mechanism accounting for the variation in cellular sensitivity through the cell cycle is not clear, but it almost certainly relates to differences in repair capacity in different phases of the cell cycle.

VARIATION OF RADIOSENSITIVITY AND LET

As already mentioned, photons and particulate radiations differ in their mechanisms of absorption, resulting in different LETs. As LET increases, the probability of the occurrence of isolated sublethal events is diminished. The densely

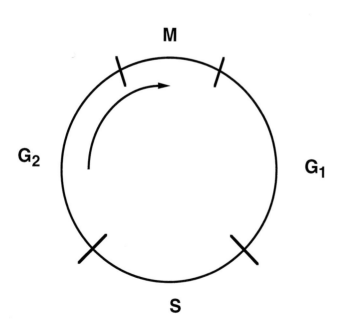

Figure 37–7 The mammalian cell cycle. Following mitosis (M) cells enter the G_1 phase in preparation for DNA synthesis (S phase). The period between completion of DNA synthesis and mitosis is called G_2. Noncycling cells are in a G_1-like phase called G_0.

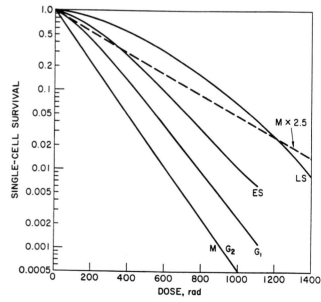

Figure 37–8 Mammalian cell survival curve as a function of position in the cell cycle. M, G_1, and G_2 refer to phases of the cell cycle. ES and LS refer to cells in early and late S phase, respectively. The magnitude of the cell cycle effect is demonstrated by the *dashed line*, which represents a 2.5-fold resistance compared to mitotic cells. (From Sinclair WK: Cyclic x-ray responses in mammalian cells in vitro. Radiat Res 1968; 33:620.)

ionizing nature of high LET particles makes the interaction of damage from different particle tracks an unimportant mechanism of cell killing. This results in cell survival curves with a diminishing shoulder region as LET increases. A comparison of doses required for a specific effect following an exposure to a standard radiation (250 kVp x-rays) and a test radiation results in the *relative biological effectiveness* (RBE). Thus,

$$RBE = \frac{D_{250\ kVp}}{D_{test}}$$

where $D_{250\ kVp}$ is the dose of standard x-rays and D_{test} is the dose of radiation of interest that produces equivalent effects. The specific endpoint and level of effect must be specified (for example, a cell survival of 10%). RBEs range from 0.85 for megavoltage x-rays to more than 5 for heavy particles, depending on the endpoint chosen. A maximum RBE is reached at an LET of approximately 100 keV/μm. Further increase in LET actually results in a lower RBE because the radiation becomes so densely ionizing that dose is wasted, which leads to less efficient cell killing.[10]

DOSE RATE EFFECTS

The rate at which cells are irradiated has profound effects on cell survival as a function of dose.[20] This may be observed by comparing single doses of standard dose rate (2 to 3 Gy/minute) either to multiple smaller doses of radiation or to continuous low-dose radiation. When cells are irradiated with multiple doses (fractionation), the total dose must be increased to achieve the same level of cell kill (or another biologic endpoint). Comparing the survival following a single dose of radiation to that following two doses indicates that survival increases as the interval between radiation doses increases. Maximum survival is achieved when the interval is several hours. This type of split-dose experiment demonstrates the repair of *sublethal damage* between radiation doses (Fig. 37-9).[14, 21]

As mentioned in the preceding text, α/β is a measure of the relative contributions of single lethal (nonreparable) events and interaction of sublethal (reparable) events to overall cell kill. A larger α/β indicates relatively little contribution from interaction of sublethal events. A low α/β indicates a greater contribution from this type of lesion. Therefore, cells with a lower α/β ratio would be expected to be spared to a greater extent by fractionation than would cell types with a larger α/β. This is the basis for fractionated radiotherapy. Tumors and other rapidly proliferating tissues (e.g., skin, mucosa, bone marrow) demonstrate high α/β ratios, whereas many normal tissues, including those of the CNS, have lower α/β ratios.[13, 22]

Repair of sublethal damage also takes place during continuous low-dose rate irradiation, such as occurs during interstitial brachytherapy. As the dose rate is decreased below 100 cGy/min, the total dose required for a given biologic effect must be increased (i.e., there is sparing of irradiated tissues). It is generally accepted that this sparing is due to repair of sublethal radiation damage taking place during the

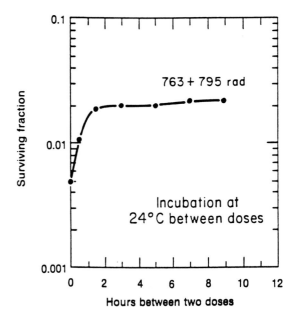

Figure 37-9 Survival of mammalian cells following two doses of x-radiation separated by a variable interval of time. An increase in survival is seen with *split-dose* irradiation compared to *single-dose* (0 time point) irradiation. This reflects repair of *sublethal damage* between radiation doses. This repair is complete within 3 hours. (From Elkind MM, Sutton-Gilbert H, Moses WB, et al: Radiation response of mammalian cells in culture: V. Temperature dependence of repair of x-ray damage in surviving cells (aerobic and hypoxic). Radiat Res 1965; 25: 359.)

period of irradiation.[20, 23] As the dose rate is reduced, the shoulder region of the cell survival curve becomes less pronounced and there is less effect for a given dose. A theoretical limit for the dose rate effect is determined by the initial slope of the survival curve reflecting the "single hit" or α component of cell killing, which does not involve sublethal damage (Fig. 37-10).

A second effect of low–dose rate irradiation is delay of cycling cells in the premitotic phase of the cell cycle (G2 block).[24] It has been clearly shown that radiosensitivity varies with phase of the cell cycle, and that cells in G2 are up to three times as sensitive as the least sensitive population in late S phase (DNA synthesis).[19] Normal glial or neuronal cells are noncycling and remain in a relatively radioresistant state (G0) during low–dose rate irradiation. The choice of dose rate is important, however. Tumor cells being irradiated below a critical minimum dose rate will not be blocked in G2 phase and will continue to divide.[23] If cell proliferation outweighs cell killing, therapy will clearly be ineffective. In addition, this allows for redistribution of cells from a radiosensitive phase of the cell cycle (G2 to M) into more radioresistant phases (G1, S). Marin and co-workers[25] have demonstrated the accumulation of glioblastoma cells in G2 to M phase of the cell cycle during low–dose rate irradiation with[137]Cs. Their data suggest that a minimum dose rate of 25 cGy/hour is necessary to completely inhibit proliferation in the cell lines studied. Cell cycle progression was demonstrated at lower dose rates. It is the practice at most institutions to choose a dose rate of 40 to 60 cGy/hour for interstitial brachytherapy of brain tumors, to take full advantage of

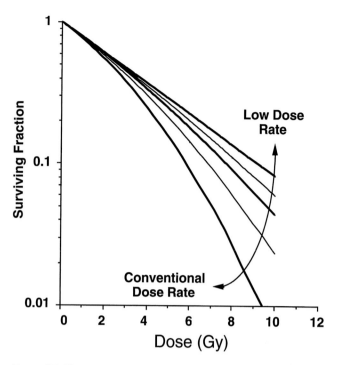

Figure 37–10 Effect of dose rate on mammalian cell survival following irradiation. The lowest curve represents the linear-quadratic model for cell survival at conventional dose rate (2 Gy/min). During low–dose rate irradiation, repair of sublethal lesions occurs at a significant rate before two such lesions may combine to form a lethal event.

dose rate effects and to minimize the chance of tumor progression during treatment.

A third radiobiologic effect of low–dose rate irradiation is the diminished oxygen enhancement ratio (OER) at low dose rates. At conventional dose rate, hypoxic cells, which can constitute a significant fraction of cells present in solid human tumors, including gliomas, require three times the radiation dose for equivalent cell killing when compared with fully aerated cells (i.e., OER = 3). The OER is decreased at low dose rate, likely due to decreased repair of sublethal damage by hypoxic cells.[26] An added effect in in situ tumors is continuous reoxygenation of hypoxic cells during low–dose rate irradiation.[7, 20]

The net effect of low–dose rate irradiation needs to be considered from both a normal tissue and tumor cell point of view. With brachytherapy, the tumor volume receives a higher radiation dose at a higher dose rate than surrounding normal cells. In addition, cycling tumor cells are arrested in the radiosensitive G2 phase of the cell cycle if the dose rate is at least of the order of 25 cGy/hour. Normal glial or neuronal cells remain in a noncycling, radioresistant (G0) state. Hypoxic tumor cells are only marginally less sensitive than their fully aerated counterparts and are continuously undergoing reoxygenation during low–dose rate treatment, conferring full sensitivity. Normal tissues receive a limited dose of radiation at a lower dose rate that enhances repair of sublethal damage. The dose-sparing effects of low–dose rate irradiation have been shown to be greater for normal tissues than for tumors, likely due to a greater increase in repair capacity in normal tissues at low dose rate.[23] These factors together provide the rationale for the treatment or

retreatment of intracranial tumors with interstitial brachytherapy.

TUMOR RADIOBIOLOGY

In Vivo Systems for Experimental Radiotherapy

Until now, the discussion of cellular radiobiology has been in the context of the easily manipulated but artificial in vitro system. More relevant experimental models for studying tumor radiobiology are the transplantable tumor systems. The effects of radiotherapy on experimental tumors transplanted to the flank of mice, for example, may be measured as the probability of tumor cure.[7] Plotting the percentage of tumors cured as a function of radiation dose produces a sigmoidal curve (Fig. 37–11). At low doses, no tumors are cured (i.e., the probability of tumor cure is extremely low). As the tumor dose increases, the probability of tumor cure also increases. The dose that corresponds to a 50% probabil-

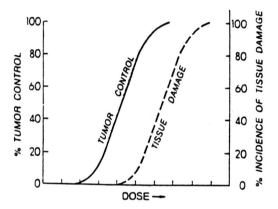

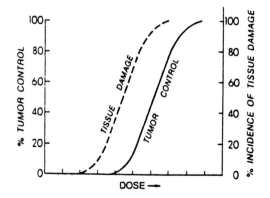

Figure 37–11 Curves schematically comparing doses required for tumor control and those associated with significant damage to normal tissue. *Top,* Depiction of a favorable situation in which a dose regimen resulting in a high rate of tumor control would produce an acceptable rate of significant damage to normal tissue. *Bottom,* An unfavorable situation in which the treatment is unlikely to cure any tumors without substantial risk of injury to normal tissue. Modifications of the treatment regimen that separate the curves in a favorable manner are said to increase the *therapeutic ratio.* (Modified from Rubin P: Clinical Oncology: A Multidisciplinary Approach. New York, American Cancer Society, 1973.)

ity of tumor cure is called the TCD_{50} (tumor cure dose of 50%) and is an expression of the *radiocurability* of the tumor.

If it is assumed that a single surviving cell will repopulate a tumor and cause a failure, then the probability of tumor cure would be

$$P_{cure} = e^{-SF \times N}$$

where SF is the surviving fraction and N is the original number of clonogenic cells in the tumor. $SF \times N$ is therefore the number of surviving cells per tumor, on average. An average of 1 surviving cell per tumor gives rise to a P_{cure} of 37%. The distribution of surviving cells among tumors follows Poisson statistics and illustrates the random nature of cell killing by radiation.[27]

Cell survival may also be measured directly following irradiation of tumors in vivo by removing and dissociating the tumor into single cells and assaying for the clonogenic capacity of individual cells. When this is done following irradiation of tumor in living, air-breathing animals, a biphasic survival curve is produced (Fig. 37–12).[28] The biphasic nature of this curve is due to the presence of a significant number of hypoxic cells in the tumor. The fraction of hypoxic cells may be measured by comparing the survival of tumor cells from air-breathing mice to that of cells from nitrogen-asphyxiated mice. Although experimental tumors have been demonstrated to have a wide range of hypoxic fractions (0% to 90%), most contain between 10% and 20% hypoxic cells.[7]

NORMAL TISSUE RADIOBIOLOGY

The Therapeutic Ratio

The radiation oncologist must be concerned not only with effects of treatment on tumor, but also with normal tissue effects. Normal tissues of particular interest in the treatment of tumors of the central nervous system include brain parenchyma, brainstem and spinal cord, cranial nerves, and the hypothalamic-pituitary axis. Also of interest are effects on the vasculature within both normal and tumor tissue.

The probability of an undesirable normal tissue effect following radiotherapy is, like tumor control probability, a function of dose. This is represented graphically as a sigmoid-shaped curve similar to that obtained for tumor cure (Fig. 37–11). Curves for a wide variety of normal tissue endpoints have been generated. Although each has a similar shape, the relative placement of these curves along the dose axis may be quite different. In clinical radiotherapy the relative position of the curves for tumor cure and relevant normal tissue complication is of primary importance. The relative position of these two curves defines what is known as the *therapeutic ratio*. An optimal therapeutic ratio would be described by curves that allow 100% tumor cure without appreciable probability of normal tissue complication. The opposite extreme would be exemplified by a tumor requiring high-dose radiation for cure located within a critical normal structure with a low tolerance to radiation. The tolerance dose for specific tissues is a function of the volume irradiated, the total dose and dose per fraction used, and the level of acceptable risk.[29–31] For example, the total dose to cause brain necrosis in 5% of patients treated with a single dose of radiosurgery is vastly different than the dose associated with the same risk when conventional fractionation (1.8 to 2 cGy/day) is employed.[29, 30, 32]

Radiation Tolerance of Normal Tissues of the CNS

In general, normal tissue effects are divided into those that occur early (during or within weeks of radiation) and those that occur late (months to years following radiation). Early effects are related to effects on rapidly proliferating tissues, such as skin, bone marrow, and mucosal surfaces. Late effects are related to changes in slowly proliferating or non-proliferating tissues, such as brain, spinal cord, and peripheral nerve.

Acute reactions associated with irradiation of brain tumors are usually not severe. The most common acute side effect of cranial radiation is hair loss, which is associated with the

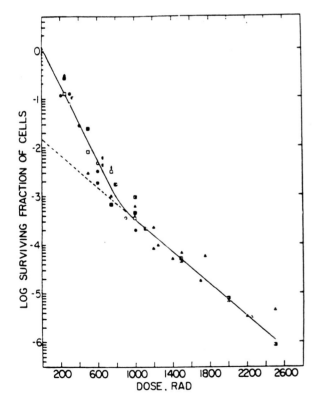

Figure 37–12 Survival curve for mouse tumor cells irradiated as a solid tumor in vivo then removed from the animal, dissociated into single cells, and assayed for clonogenic survival. The biphasic curve indicates the presence of two populations consistent with the presence of radioresistant hypoxic cells in the tumor. (From Powers WE, Tolmach LJ: A multicomponent x-ray survival curve for mouse lymphosarcoma cells irradiated in vivo. Nature 1963; 197:710.)

local dose to the scalp. Other acute effects of cranial irradiation are associated with increased edema or intracranial pressure caused by an acute reaction of the tumor to treatment. These effects are usually minimized by administration of corticosteroids.

Subacute effects of cranial irradiation are related to transient demyelination mediated by radiation injury to oligodendrocytes or through alterations in capillary permeability. The clinical manifestations are transient radiation myelopathy following spinal cord irradiation or a syndrome of somnolence, anorexia, and irritability following cranial irradiation. The *somnolence syndrome* is well described following cranial irradiation in pediatric patients and usually occurs within 10 weeks of the end of treatment.[33, 34] This is a self-limiting process, but patients may benefit from administration of steroids.

Late effects following cranial irradiation occur within several months or up to many years following treatment. Clinical and radiographic changes vary from asymptomatic changes of the white matter and vasculature[35] to changes in cognitive abilities,[36] hypothalamic pituitary dysfunction,[37] cranial neuropathy, and development of frank tissue necrosis and/or second malignancies. With the exception of the development of second malignancies, each of these late effects of cranial irradiation has been shown to be a function of total dose and dose per fraction.

Sheline and others[38] examined 80 cases of cerebral necrosis following cranial irradiation. The interval from completion of radiotherapy to development of necrosis ranged from 4 months to 7.5 years. The total radiation dose, daily dose, and overall treatment time were available for all patients. Plotting the total dose vs. the number of fractions for each case of necrosis described a line representing the threshold for radionecrosis (Fig. 37–13). The authors defined *neuret* as

$$\text{Neuret} = D \times N^{-0.41} \times T^{-0.03}$$

where *D*, *N*, and *T* represent the total dose, number of fractions, and overall time, respectively. From this analysis one finds that the threshold dose for necrosis is 35 Gy in 10 fractions, 60 Gy in 35 fractions, and 76 Gy in 60 fractions when treatments are 5 days/week. This threshold corresponds to approximately 1,700 neuret. This work indicated the relative importance of number of fractions (and, therefore, fraction size) in determining risk of late effects following radiotherapy. Daily dose and total dose have been reconfirmed to be the most important factors determining risk of radionecrosis by Marks and colleagues.[30] They suggested that a dose biologically equivalent to 54 Gy in 30 fractions represented the threshold for radionecrosis. These two clinical studies form the basis of what is considered standard radiotherapy for intracranial tumors. Benign or low-grade tumors receive 54 Gy in 30 fractions, which carries virtually no risk of radionecrosis but is efficacious in a wide range of disease, including meningiomas and low-grade gliomas. This dose corresponds to the more conservative recommendation of Marks and co-workers.[30] Malignant gliomas (anaplastic astrocytomas and glioblastomas multiforme) are less well-controlled by 54 Gy, and the aggressiveness of the disease warrants a higher dose and a small risk of necrosis. Standard doses would be 60 Gy in 30 to 33 fractions, corresponding to a dose just above the threshold found by Sheline and others.[38]

Fraction size has been found to be of primary importance when considering radiation tolerance of optic nerve and other cranial nerves. Harris and Levene[39] showed clearly that daily doses in excess of 250 cGy were associated with an increased risk of visual loss in patients irradiated for pituitary adenoma or craniopharyngioma. Goldsmith and associates[40] recently applied the neuret formula to the analysis of radiation-induced optic neuropathy and found that fraction size was more important than overall time. They proposed a model defining the *optic ret*

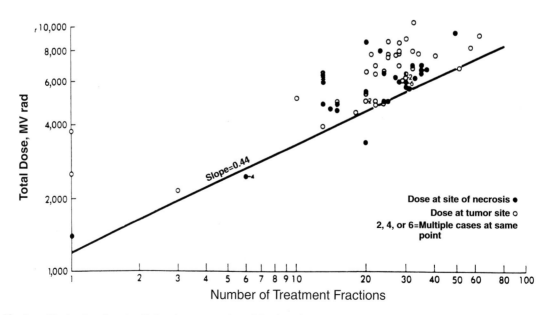

Figure 37–13 Logarithmic plot of total radiation dose vs. number of fractions for cases of radionecrosis following radiotherapy for brain tumors. The line drawn represents an isoeffect line below which the risk of radionecrosis is small. (From Sheline GE, Wara WM, Smith V: Therapeutic irradiation and brain injury. Int J Radiat Oncol Biol Phys 1980; 6:1215.)

$$\text{Optic ret} = D \times N^{-0.53}$$

where the term for overall time has been omitted, emphasizing the relative importance of fraction size. Goldsmith and colleagues[40] have recommended a threshold dose for optic neuropathy of 890 optic ret, which corresponds to 54 Gy in 30 fractions.

Radiation tolerance of the spinal cord is a dose-limiting factor in the treatment of many malignancies: intrinsic spinal cord tumors, spinous metastases, and carcinoma of the head and neck, esophagus, and lung. As with radiation-induced damage to brain parenchyma, the risk of spinal cord injury increases with increasing dose per fraction and total radiation dose. Radiation-associated myelopathy may occur within months of radiotherapy and be transient in nature or may have a delayed time of onset and be permanent in nature. The mechanism of spinal cord injury following radiation involves white matter damage. A dual mechanism of action has been suggested. Extensive demyelination is associated with damage to oligodendrocytes. This process corresponds to a shorter latent period and effects may be transient or progressive, leading to white matter necrosis. A separate mechanism involves damage to the vascular endothelium. Resultant changes in permeability may induce white matter injury and lead to necrosis.[41] Wara and colleagues[42] described the time-dose relationship for radiation-induced spinal cord injury. They used an *effect single dose* (ED)

$$\text{ED} = D(\text{cGy}) \times N^{-0.377} \times T^{-0.058}$$

Based on this formula, the authors suggested that doses of 20 Gy in 5 fractions, 30 Gy in 10 fractions, and 50 Gy in 20 fractions were safe. This corresponds to a single effective dose of about 1,000 Gy and was felt to be associated with a 1% incidence of myelopathy. In practice, the risk is probably much lower. In a review of patients receiving radiotherapy to the cervical spine, Marcus and Million[43] found that 2 of 1,112 patients (0.18%) receiving doses of 30 to 60 Gy had development of myelopathy. It has been estimated that the dose of standard fractionated radiotherapy that would be associated with a 5% incidence of spinal cord injury is 57 to 61 Gy.[44]

EFFECTS OF DOSE FRACTIONATION ON RESPONSE TO RADIATION THERAPY

The radiotherapy of brain tumors utilizes a variety of dose fractionation schemes. These range from large single doses used in radiosurgery to more than 70 total doses given twice daily in hyperfractionation protocols. Another extreme is the continuous low–dose rate irradiation used in brachytherapy with either temporary or permanent implants of radioactive elements. The effective doses associated with normal tissue damage and tumor control are quite disparate in these different modes of radiation therapy.[45]

The effects of dose fractionation have long been known

to influence the outcome of radiotherapy. The effects of fractionated radiotherapy are dependent on the total dose, the size of each fraction, the interval between fractions and the overall time of treatment. The relative contributions of each of these factors varies depending on the endpoint of interest. These effects are explained on the basis of four radiobiologic principles: (1) repair of sublethal damage; (2) reoxygenation of hypoxic cells; (3) reassortment of proliferating cells in the cell cycle; and (4) repopulation.[12] The rationale for fractionated radiotherapy is based on a differential effects between normal tissues and tumors with respect to these processes.

Repair of sublethal damage, as previously discussed, is manifest by the shoulder of the dose-response curve. The α/β ratio is a measure of the relative contributions of reparable and irreparable damage. Tissues with a low α/β ratio have a relatively high proportion of reparable (β-type) damage. These tissues will be significantly spared as the number of fractions is increased, since the number of interfraction intervals and opportunity for repair of SLD increases (Fig. 37–14).[13, 22, 27] In addition, since the term for β-type damage is a function of D^2, lower doses per fraction will be relatively less effective in tissues with a low α/β ratio. Tissues with high α/β ratios have a relatively small contribution from β-type damage and will be spared to a lesser extent by dose fractionation (see Fig. 37–14).[22]

The shapes of dose-effect curves for tissues with low and high α/β ratios indicate the largest differential advantage at low doses per fraction (see Fig. 37–14). The α/β ratio may also be obtained indirectly for tissues and endpoints for which construction of dose-effect curves is not possible. This is accomplished by construction of an isoeffect plot similar to those used to derive the neuret and optic ret. Such curves have been constructed for a variety of endpoints and serve to demonstrate a separation of early- and late-responding tissues in terms of the sparing effects of fractionation (Fig. 37–15).[22]

Reoxygenation of hypoxic cells has been demonstrated in all tumors manifesting a radiobiologically hypoxic population.[46] Following a dose of radiation, relatively sensitive oxygenated cells are preferentially killed and their numbers diminished. Therefore the hypoxic fraction immediately following a dose of radiation is increased and may approach 100%. However, over a period of 12 to 24 hours the tumor will demonstrate reoxygenation and the hypoxic fraction will return to its original value.[7] This principle indicates the important role of fractionation in combating hypoxic cell radioresistance. This is an effect demonstrated in tumors only, as normal tissues contain no radiobiologically hypoxic cells.

Following a single dose of radiation, a cycling population of cells will have lost a larger proportion of cells in radiosensitive phases of the cell cycle. Over a period of 4 to 6 hours the cell population will resume cycling and will *redistribute* cells from relatively resistant phases to more sensitive phases of the cell cycle. This effect has an advantage for tumor cell killing only, and does not apply to noncycling normal tissues.

Although radiotherapy causes a cell cycle delay in late G2, this delay is usually only a maximum of several hours.[7, 24] Therefore, during the interfraction interval, both tumor and

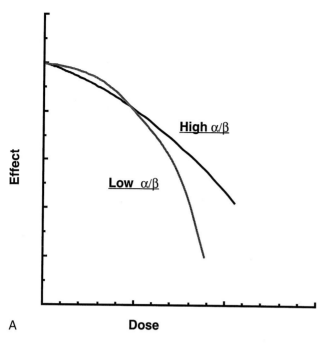

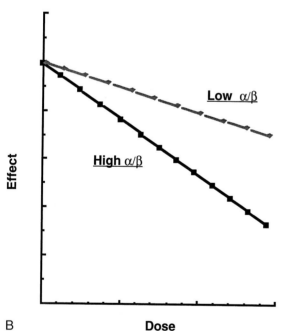

Figure 37–14 *A*, Schematic dose-effect curve for tissue types with high α/β ratio (early-responding tissues and tumors) and low α/β ratio (late-responding tissues, including CNS). The largest differential favoring sparing of late-responding tissues, is in the low dose region of the curves. *B*, When low daily doses are used, as in standard fractionation, the small differential effect is amplified.

normal tissues may proliferate and repopulate, which provides partial compensation for killing by the previous radiation dose. For normal tissues, this is a favorable compensatory mechanism; for tumors, it is counterproductive to the goal of eradication of the tumor. In rapidly proliferating tumors, it may be necessary to increase the dose per fraction or to decrease the interfraction interval to overcome the effects of *tumor repopulation*.

BASIC PRINCIPLES OF RADIOTHERAPY

External Beam Radiotherapy (Teletherapy)

The vast majority of radiotherapy treatments delivered in the United States employ the linear accelerator. Historically, these units have replaced the orthovoltage x-ray units and the ^{60}Co units. The major advantages of the more modern units relate to the higher energies that are available and to the interface with computer verification systems that allow the daily delivery of precise treatments through multiple complex field arrangements. Coupled with modern imaging and CT- or MRI-based treatment planning, present radiotherapy for intracranial disease more reliably delivers therapeutic doses to the tumor volume while excluding normal tissues from the high-dose region. Together these are the most effective means of increasing the therapeutic ratio.[4]

Beam Energy

Modern linear accelerators commonly deliver x-ray beams of nominal energies ranging from 4 to 18 MeV. These nominal energies represent the maximum energy produced by the accelerator, and the beam actually contains a spectrum of energies. The average energy emitted is approximately a third the nominal maximum. Qualitatively, as photon energy increases, dose at the surface *decreases* and the depth at

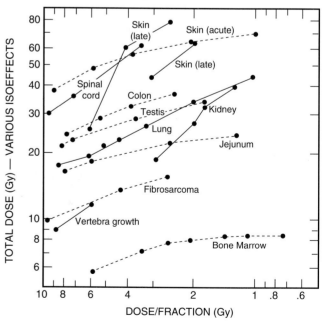

Figure 37–15 Isoeffect plots for various late tissue effects as a function of total dose and dose per fraction. Each point is the combination of dose and fraction size required to cause a particular effect in the various tissues. Early-responding tissues (*dashed lines*) have a shallow slope, demonstrating a modest increase in total dose required as dose per fraction is decreased. Late-responding tissues (e.g., spinal cord, *solid lines*) demonstrate a more rapid rise in total dose required for a given effect as fraction size is lowered, indicating a greater sparing of late-responding tissues by dose fractionation. (From Withers HR: Biological basis for altered fractionation schemes. Cancer 1985; 55:2086.)

which the maximum dose is reached *increases*. The overall effect of higher-energy beams is to have sparing of tissues at the beam entrance and delivery of a more homogeneous dose to deep-seated tumor volumes.

Treatment Planning

Careful treatment planning is an essential component of optimum delivery of modern radiotherapy. For intracranial tumors, CT-based treatment planning offers the most precise information regarding location of tumor and critical normal structures. Definition of the volume to treat is a critical step in the planning process. Postoperative radiotherapy for low-grade and malignant gliomas has been limited to partial brain fields, because adequate imaging with CT and MRI has become available. The contrast-enhancing volume seen with these imaging modalities corresponds to the hypercellular tumor tissue with a compromised blood-brain barrier and perivascular leakage of the iodinated or paramagnetic contrast agent (Fig. 37–16). This tumor tissue does not contain neural parenchyma. This contrast-enhancing region is usually surrounded by a hypodense zone of low-attenuation or ring enhancement that has been shown to correspond to edematous neural parenchyma and is usually infiltrated with individual tumor cells. T2-weighted MRI images reveal larger volumes of edematous tissue than do CT or T1-weighted MRI images (see Fig. 37–16). Infiltration of individual tumor cells has been found to extend at least to the boundary of T2 prolongation.[47]

Comparison of preterminal CT scans with autopsy findings showed that all gross and microscopic tumors occurred within 2 cm of the contrast-enhancing volume in 83% of patients.[48] Studies of patterns of failure following external-beam radiation therapy for glioblastoma multiforme or anaplastic astrocytoma indicated that 78% of recurrences were within 2 cm of the original contrast-enhancing tumor volume defined on CT scan. Fifty-six percent of recurrences were within 1 cm of that margin. Neither extensive edema nor large tumor size was associated with higher probability of more distant recurrence. No unifocal tumor recurred multifocally.[49] Lack of control of tumor growth within the central tumor remains the major cause of failure following external-beam radiotherapy alone.[50]

CT-based treatment planning is recommended in all patients with intracranial tumors. It is most helpful if the patient is imaged in the treatment position. Computer-based treatment planning is rapidly becoming available in more centers.[4, 51] Patients are imaged in the treatment position and the contrast-enhancing tumor volumes are digitized into a treatment planning computer (Fig. 37–17). The treatment volume is based on this contrast-enhancing tumor volume with a 2- to 3-cm margin in three dimensions (see Fig. 37–17). When peritumoral edema is extensive it is not always included in the treatment volume. For smaller tumors, it is usually possible to include the tumor volume and surrounding edema with an adequate margin. Isodose distributions graphically demonstrate the shape of the dose distribution for the particular radiotherapy unit and treatment plan.

Dose Fractionation

The risk of complications following cranial irradiation is clearly a function of total dose and dose per fraction. The risk of cranial nerve damage, pituitary dysfunction, and cerebral necrosis are all diminished when smaller doses per fraction are used. Standard fractionation is considered to be 1.8 to 2.0 Gy/day. A generally accepted total dose used in treating malignant gliomas with these fraction sizes would

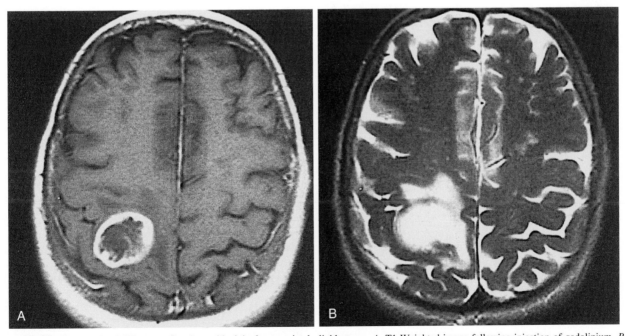

Figure 37–16 Preoperative MRI scans of patient with right frontoparietal glioblastoma. *A*, T1-Weighted image following injection of gadolinium. *B*, T2-Weighted image.

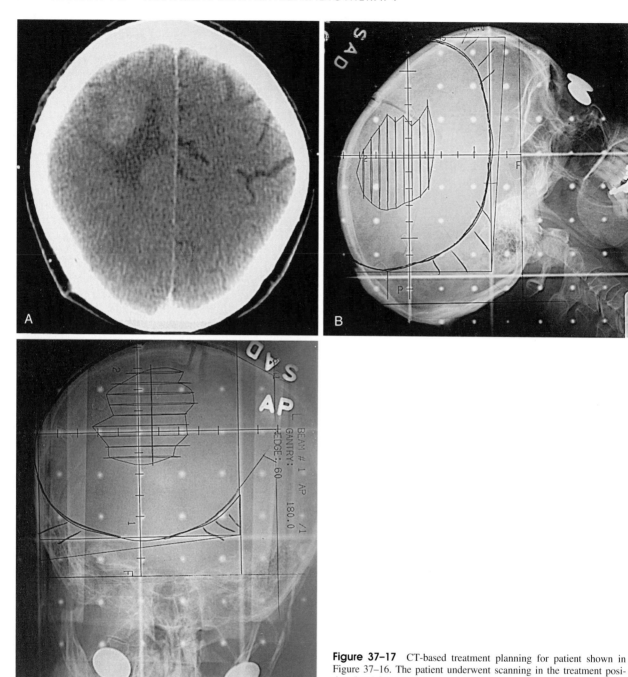

Figure 37–17 CT-based treatment planning for patient shown in Figure 37–16. The patient underwent scanning in the treatment position (head flexed). *A*, Postcontrast CT scan showing tumor and edema. *B*, Lateral simulation film showing tumor volume and treatment portals. *C*, Anteroposterior simulation film.

be 60 Gy in 30 to 33 fractions over 6 to 6.5 weeks.[1] Less agreement exists regarding the proper dose to employ in treating low-grade astrocytomas and oligodendrogliomas.[3] Based on the demonstrated safety of a regimen of 1.8 Gy/day to a total dose of 54 Gy,[30, 40] many centers employ this regimen for the treatment of low-grade gliomas.

Hyperfractionation is defined as the delivery of multiple daily fractions to increase the total dose given over the same period of time.[52] This treatment strategy takes advantage of the difference in sparing of early and late-responding tissues by fractionation. Hyperfractionated regimens have been used in the treatment of pediatric and adult supratentorial and brainstem gliomas.[53] Many regimens have been used. An example might be the delivery of 1.2 Gy twice daily to a total dose of 72 Gy over 6 weeks. This should be compared with a standard fractionation scheme of 2 Gy daily fractions to a total dose of 60 Gy in 6 weeks. These two regimens are currently being compared in a prospective randomized trial by the Radiation Therapy Oncology Group (protocol 9006).

Both the normal tissue and tumor effects must be examined. Using an α/β ratio of 10 for tumor, it can be demonstrated that the hyperfractionated regimen represents a 12% increase in biologically effective dose. The same comparison for normal tissue (using an α/β value of 2 for CNS[54]) indicates a 5% *reduction* in effective dose. Thus, hyperfractionation (and fractionation in general) allows higher biologic doses to be delivered to tumor while maintaining normal tissue doses at or below tolerance levels.

SPECIAL MODALITIES

Interstitial Brachytherapy

The treatment of malignancy by placement of radioactive sources into or next to tumors (brachytherapy) dates to the turn of the century, shortly after the discovery of radium in 1898. Interstitial implantation of focal brain tumors is designed to deliver a high radiation dose to a specified tumor volume while minimizing the dose to surrounding normal brain or other critical structures.[55] This is accomplished by implantation of radioactive ''seeds'' directly into the tumor using stereotactic neurosurgical methods. The result is delivery of continuous low–dose rate radiation to the tumor with rapid fall of dose outside the tumor volume. The biologic rationale for using low–dose rate irradiation is discussed in preceding text. When applied following conventional surgery and external beam radiation therapy, this ''boost'' therapy allows at least twice the total tumor dose to be delivered than with external beam therapy alone.[56, 57] Results to date indicate a substantial benefit of such treatment in highly selected patients with glioblastoma multiforme.[55, 56, 58] The technique has also been demonstrated to be effective in the treatment of recurrent gliomas.[55, 56, 59]

Hyperthermia

Temperatures above 41°C kill cells exponentially as a function of time at temperature.[60] In addition, heat inhibits cellular mechanisms of repair following irradiation. Heat preferentially kills relatively radioresistant S-phase cells and those in acidic environments, such as nutrient-deprived radioresistant hypoxic cells. Thus, heat and radiation are complementary in their mechanisms of cell killing. The combination of external beam radiation and heat has been shown in several nonrandomized trials to result in improved tumor control compared with radiation alone for extracranial squamous cell carcinoma, adenocarcinoma, and melanoma.[61] Hyperthermia has been combined with interstitial implantation of brain tumors in the hope of obtaining improvement in local control.[62]

Stereotactic Radiosurgery

Radiosurgery refers to the delivery of a single high dose of ionizing radiation to a focal intracranial target. An increasing number of centers in the United States are performing this type of treatment. The most common radiosurgery delivery systems are the gamma knife and linear accelerator-based systems. (The details of each are discussed in Chapter 41.) Radiobiologically, radiosurgery is at the opposite end of the spectrum from low–dose rate irradiation. The advantages of

fractionation outlined previously are forfeited by the delivery of a single dose. However, the focal nature of radiosurgery provides a safe and effective treatment for small-volume localized disease.[32] Complication rates following radiosurgery are clearly related to treatment volume, dose, and anatomic site.[29, 63] The single high-dose treatment tends to selectively enhance late effects based on the linear quadratic formulation.[22, 32] This may be advantageous in some situations, such as in the treatment of arteriovenous malformations, but the potential for normal tissue damage and the tolerances of cranial nerves, optic apparatus, and brain parenchyma must always be kept in mind.

Particle Therapy

The use of heavy particles, such as protons or helium and neon ions, in radiotherapy is based on the physical properties of these particles, the characteristics of dose deposition in irradiated tissues, and, in some cases, a biologic advantage related to the LET. Dose deposition is characterized by the Bragg peak (Fig. 37–18).[9] Qualitatively, the entrance dose for particle beams is relatively low. An unaltered beam will deposit more than 50% of its energy over a 2- to 3-cm path at a depth in water that depends on the beam characteristics. The beam may be altered to *spread* the Bragg peak to conform to the thickness of the volume to be treated.[8, 9] Protons and helium ions are used to take advantage of the possible dose distributions. Fast neutrons have been used due to an RBE advantage, and heavy ions, such as neon, have both an increased RBE and dose deposition advantages. (Details are discussed more fully in Chapter 39.)

Radiosensitization

Because of the failure of high-dose radiation therapy to cure a majority of gliomas, an interest has been generated in the

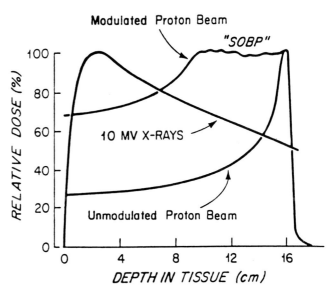

Figure 37–18 Depth dose curves for a 160 MeV proton beam: unmodulated and with spread out Bragg peak (''SOBP''). A curve for 10 MV photons is also shown for comparison. (From Munzenrider JE, Crowell C: Charged particles. *In* Mauch PM, Loeffler JS (eds): Radiation Oncology: Biology and Technology. Philadelphia, WB Saunders, 1994, p 34.)

application of adjuvant therapies that may serve as *radiosensitizers*. By strict definition, a pure radiosensitizer is an agent that enhances the effects of radiation without having any cytotoxic effects of its own. In practice, some agents are used that have some antitumor activity apart from their radiosensitizing effects. A key requirement of a clinically useful sensitizer is a selective radiosensitization of tumor cells relative to normal tissues.

One group of radiosensitizers is targeted at hypoxic tumor cells. The hypoxic cell radiosensitizers are electron-affinic compounds that, in the absence of oxygen, compete with reducing agents for reaction with radiation-induced free radicals (see Fig. 37–6). Such reaction with a free radical in the target DNA molecule prevents restoration of the molecule through hydrogen or electron donation from sulfhydryl compounds. When oxygen is present, these sensitizers have no effect due to the overwhelming reactivity of oxygen, which results in maximum sensitization. The compounds having been studied most extensively in clinical trials have been the 2-nitroimidazole compounds, misonidazole (Ro 07–0582), pimonidazole (Ro 03–8799), and etanidazole (SR 2508). Development of these compounds followed the demonstration of the radiosensitizing properties of metronidazole, a 5-nitroimidazole.[64] Metronidazole and other 5-nitroimidazole compounds, such as nimorazole, are less potent radiosensitizers but have fewer side effects.[65] The dose-limiting toxic effect of the nitroimidazole family of compounds is neurotoxicity.

A second major class of radiosensitizers are the *halogenated pyrimidines*. 5-Bromodeoxyuridine (BUdR) and 5-iododeoxyuridine (IUdR) are analogs of thymidine and are incorporated into the DNA of cells undergoing DNA synthesis. The radiosensitizing properties of these compounds has been known since 1960.[66] The precise mechanism of radiosensitization remains unclear.[67] However, evidence suggests that the presence of these halogenated pyrimidines in the cellular DNA serves to increase radiation-induced damage at the sites of incorporation through a local increase in absorbed energy and migration of DNA-absorbed energy to these sites.[68, 69] The basis for selectivity is the incorporation of these compounds into proliferating cells. In clinical practice, sensitization requires infusion of the radiosensitizer over a period of several days prior to irradiation and during the period of therapy. Clinical trials in this country and in Japan have indicated efficacy of theses sensitizers in the treatment of malignant gliomas.[70, 71]

CONCLUSION

The following chapters discuss in detail the clinical experience with conventional radiotherapy, altered fractionation schemes, radiosensitizers, particle therapy, brachytherapy, hyperthermia, and radiosurgery. This chapter is intended to serve as an introduction and background to these topics and as an outline of the basic principles of radiobiology and radiotherapy, the knowledge of which is necessary for a more advanced discussion.

REFERENCES

1. Leibel S, Scott C, Pajak T: The management of malignant gliomas with radiation therapy: Therapeutic results and research strategies. Semin Radiat Oncol 1991; 1:32.
2. Leibel SA, Scott CB, Loeffler JS: Contemporary approaches to the treatment of malignant gliomas with radiation therapy. Semin Oncol 1994; 21:198.
3. Shaw EG, Scheithauer BW, O'Fallon JR: Management of supratentorial low-grade gliomas. Semin Radiat Oncol 1991; 1:23.
4. Kijewski P: Three dimensional treatment planning. *In* Mauch PM, Loeffler JS, (eds): Radiation Oncology: Biology and Technology. Philadelphia, WB Saunders, 1994, p 10.
5. Johns HE, Cunningham JR: The Physics of Radiology. Springfield, Ill, Charles C Thomas, 1980.
6. Kahn FM: The Physics of Radiation Therapy. Baltimore, Williams & Wilkins, 1984.
7. Hall E: Radiobiology for the Radiologist. Philadelphia, JB Lippincott, 1988.
8. Griffin TW: Particle-beam radiation therapy. *In* Perez CA, Brady LW (eds): Principles and Practice of Radiation Oncology. Philadelphia, JB Lippincott, 1992, p 368.
9. Munzenrider JE, Crowell C: Charged particles. *In* Mauch PM, Loeffler JS (eds): Radiation Oncology: Biology and Technology. Philadelphia, WB Saunders, 1994, p 34.
10. Withers HR: Biological basis for high LET radiotherapy. Radiology 1973; 108:131.
11. Weichselbaum RR, Nove J, Little JB: X-ray sensitivity of human tumor cells in vitro. Int J Radiat Oncol Biol Phys 1980; 6:437.
12. Withers HR: The 4 R's of radiotherapy. *In* Lett JT, Adler H (eds): Advances in Radiation Biology. New York, Academic Press, 1975, p 241.
13. Withers HR: Biological basis for altered fractionation schemes. Cancer 1985; 55:2086.
14. Elkind MM, Sutton H: X-ray damage and recovery in mammalian cells in culture. Nature 1959; 184:1293.
15. Taghian A, Suit H, Pardo F, et al: In vitro intrinsic radiation sensitivity of glioblastoma multiforme. Int J Radiat Oncol Biol Phys 1992; 23:55.
16. Fertil B, Malaise EP: Intrinsic radiosensitivity of human cell lines correlated with radioresponsiveness of human tumors. Int J Radiat Oncol Biol Phys 1985; 11:1699.
17. Boag JW: The time scale in radiobiology. *In* Nygarrd OF, Adler HI, Sinclair WK (eds): Fifth International Congress on Radiation Research. New York, Academic Press, 1975, p 9.
18. Coleman CN, Beard CJ, Hlatky L, et al: Biochemical modifiers: Hypoxic cell sensitizers. *In* Mauch PM, Loeffler JS (eds): Radiation Oncology, Technology and Biology. Philadelphia, WB Saunders, 1994, p 56.
19. Terasima T, Tolmach LJ: Variation in several responses of HeLa cells to x-irradiation during the division cycle. Biophys J 1963; 3:11.
20. Hall E: The biological basis of endocurietherapy: The Henschke Memorial Lecture, 1984. Endocurietherapy/Hyperthermia Oncol 1985; 1:141.
21. Elkind MM, Sutton-Gilbert H, Moses WB, et al: Radiation response of mammalian cells in culture: V. Temperature dependence of repair of x-ray damage in surviving cells (aerobic and hypoxic). Radiat Res 1965; 25:359.
22. Thames HD, Withers HR, Peters LJ, et al: Changes in early and late radiation responses with altered dose fractionation: Implications for dose-survival relationships. Int J Radiat Oncol Biol Phys 1982; 8:219.
23. Fu KK, Ling CC, Nath R, et al: Radiobiology of brachytherapy. *In* Interstitial Collaborative Working Group (eds): Interstitial Brachytherapy. New York, Raven Press, 1990, p 47.
24. Leeper DB, Schneiderman HS, Dewey WC: Radiation-induced cycle delay in synchronized Chinese hamster cells in monolayer culture. Radiat Res 1972; 50:401.
25. Marin LA, Smith CE, Langston MY, et al: Response of glioblastoma cell lines to low dose rate irradiation. Int J Radiat Oncol Biol Phys 1991; 21:397.
26. Ling C, Spiro I, Mitchell J, et al: The variation in OER with dose rate. Int J Radiat Oncol Biol Phys 1985; 11:1367.
27. Withers HR: Biologic basis of radiation therapy. *In* Perez CA, Brady LW, (eds): Principles and Practice of Radiation Oncology. Philadelphia, JB Lippincott, 1992, p 64.
28. Powers WE, Tolmach LJ: A multicomponent x-ray survival curve for mouse lymphosarcoma cells irradiated in vivo. Nature 1963; 197:710.
29. Marks LB, Spencer DP: The influence of volume on the tolerance of the brain to radiosurgery. J Neurosurg 1991; 75:177.
30. Marks JE, Baglan RJ, Prassad SC, et al: Cerebral radionecrosis: Incidence and risk in relation to dose, time, fractionation and volume. Int J Radiat Oncol Biol Phys 1981; 7:243.

31. Emami B, Lyman J, Brown A, et al: Tolerance of normal tissue to therapeutic irradiation. Int J Radiat Oncol Biol Phys 1991; 21:109.

32. Larson DA, Flickinger JC, Loeffler JS: The radiobiology of radiosurgery. Int J Radiat Oncol Biol Phys 1993; 25:557.

33. Littman P, Rosenstock J, Gale G, et al: The somnolence syndrome in leukemic children following reduced daily dose fractions of cranial irradiation. Int J Radiat Oncol Biol Phys 1984; 10:1851.

34. Freeman JE, Johnston PGB, Voke JM: Somnolence after prophylactic cranial irradiation in children with acute lymphoblastic leukemia. Br Med J 1973; 4:523.

35. Leibel SA, Sheline GE: Tolerance of the brain and spinal cord to conventional irradiation. *In* Gutin PH, Leibel SA, Sheline GE (eds): Radiation Injury to the Nervous System. New York, Raven Press, 1991, p 239.

36. Mulhern RK, Ochs J, Kun LE: Changes in intellect associated with cranial radiation therapy. *In* Gutin PH, Leibel SA, Sheline GE (eds): Radiation Injury to the Nervous System. New York, Raven Press, 1991, pp 325.

37. Constine LC, Woolf PD, Cann D, et al: Hypothalamic-pituitary dysfunction after radiation for brain tumors. N Engl J Med 1993; 328:87.

38. Sheline GE, Wara WM, Smith V: Therapeutic irradiation and brain injury. Int J Radiat Oncol Biol Phys 1980; 6:1215.

39. Harris JR, Levene MB: Visual complications following irradiation for pituitary adenomas and craniopharyngiomas. Radiology 1976; 120:167.

40. Goldsmith BJ, Rosenthal SA, Wara WM, et al: Optic neuropathy after irradiation of meningioma. Radiology 1992; 185:71.

41. Delattre JY, Rosenblum MK, Thaler HT, et al: A model of radiation myelopathy in the rat: Pathology, regional capillary permeability changes and treatment with dexamethasone. Brain 1988; 111:1319.

42. Wara WM, Phillips TL, Sheline GE, et al: Radiation tolerance of the spinal cord. Cancer 1975; 35:1558.

43. Marcus RB, Million RR: The incidence of myelitis after irradiation of the cervical spinal cord. Int J Radiat Oncol Biol Phys 1990; 19:3.

44. Schultheiss TE: Spinal cord radiation "tolerance": Doctrine versus data. Int J Radiat Oncol Biol Phys 1990; 19:219.

45. Barendsen GW: Influence of fractionation on normal tissue tolerance. *In* Gutin PH, Leibel SA, Sheline GE (eds): Radiation Injury to the Nervous System. New York, Raven Press, 1991, p 57.

46. Kallman RF: The phenomenon of reoxygenation and its implication for fractionated radiotherapy. Radiology 1972; 105:135.

47. Kelly PJ, Daumas-Duport C, Kispert DB, et al: Imaging-based stereotaxic serial biopsies in untreated intracranial glial neoplasms. J Neurosurg 1987; 66:865.

48. Hochberg FH, Pruitt A: Assumptions in the radiotherapy of malignant glioblastoma. Neurology 1980; 30:907.

49. Wallner KE, Galicich JH, Krol G, et al: Patterns of failure following treatment for glioblastoma multiforme and anaplastic astrocytoma. Int J Radiat Oncol Biol Phys 1989; 16:1405.

50. Sneed PK, Gutin PH, Larson DA: Patterns of failure of glioblastoma multiformae after external beam irradiation followed by implant boost. Int J Radiat Oncol Biol Phys 1994; 29:719.

51. Leibel SA, Scott CB, Loeffler JS: Contemporary approaches to the treatment of malignant gliomas with radiation therapy. Semin Oncol 1994; 121:198.

52. Peters LJ, Ang KK, Thames HD: Altered fractionation schedules. *In* Perez CA, Brady LW (eds): Principles and Practice of Radiation Oncology. Philadelphia, JB Lippincott, 1992, p 97.

53. Shrieve DC, Wara WM, Edwards MSB, et al: Hyperfractionated radiation therapy for brainstem gliomas in children and adults. Int J Radiat Oncol Biol Phys 1992; 24:599.

54. Ang KK, van der Kogel AJ, van der Schueren E: Lack of evidence for increased tolerance of rat spinal cord with decreasing fraction doses below 2 Gy. Int J Radiat Oncol Biol Phys 1985; 11:105.

55. Shrieve DC, Gutin PH, Larson DA: Brachytherapy. *In* Mauch PM, Loeffler JS (eds): Radiation Oncology, Technology and Biology. Philadelphia, WB Saunders, 1994, p 216.

56. Scharfen CO, Sneed PK, Wara WM, et al: High activity iodine-125 implant for gliomas. Int J Radiat Oncol Biol Phys 1992; 24:583.

57. Gutin PH, Prados MD, Phillips TL, et al: External irradiation followed by an interstitial high activity iodine-125 implant "boost" in the initial treatment of malignant gliomas: NCOG study 6G-82-2. Int J Radiat Oncol Biol Phys 1991; 21:601.

58. Loeffler JS, Alexander EA III, Wen PY, et al: Results of stereotactic brachytherapy used in the initial management of patients with glioblastoma. J Natl Cancer Inst 1990; 82:1918.

59. Gutin PH, Leibel SA, Wara WM, et al: Recurrent malignant gliomas: Survival following interstitial brachytherapy with high-activity iodine-125 sources. J Neurosurg 1987; 67:864.

60. Dewey WC, Freeman ML, Raaphorst GP: Cell biology of hyperthermia and radiation. *In* Meyn ER, Whithers RH (eds): Radiation Biology in Cancer Research. New York, Raven Press, 1980, p 589.

61. Overgaard J: The current and potential role of hyperthermia in radiotherapy. Int J Radiat Oncol Biol Phys 1990; 16:535.

62. Sneed PK, Gutin PH, Stauffer PR, et al: Thermoradiotherapy of recurrent malignant brain tumors. Int J Radiat Oncol Biol Phys 1992; 23:853.

63. Nedzi LA, Kooy HM, Alexander E III, et al: Variables associated with the development of complications from radiosurgery of intracranial tumors. Int J Radiat Oncol Biol Phys 1991; 21:591.

64. Urtasun R, Band P, Chapman JD, et al: Radiation and high-dose metronidazole in supratentorial glioblastomas. N Engl J Med 1976; 294:1364.

65. Overgaard J, Overgaard M, Nielsen OS, et al: A comparative investigation of nimorazole and misonidazole as hypoxic radiosensitizers in a C3H mammary carcinoma. Br J Cancer 1982; 46:904.

66. Djordjevic B, Szybalski W: Genetics of human cell lines: III. Incorporation of 5-bromo and 5-iodo-deoxyuridine into the ribonucleic acid of human cells and its effect on radiation sensitivity. J Exp Med 1960; 112:509.

67. McGinn CJ, Kinsella TJ: Bichemical modifiers: Nonhypoxic cell sensitizers. *In* Mauch PM, Loeffler JS, (eds): Radiation Oncology: Technology and Biology. Philadelphia, WB Saunders, 1994, p 90.

68. Zimbrick JD, Ward JF, Myers LS Jr: Studies on the chemical basis of cellular substitution in DNA: I. Pulse and steady-state radiolysis of 5-bromouracil and thymidine. Int J Radiat Biol 1969; 16:505.

69. Fielden EM, Lillicrap SC, Robins AB: The effect of 5-bromouracil on energy transfer in DNA and related model systems: DNA with incorporated 5-BUdR. Radiat Res 1971; 48:421.

70. Phillips TL, Bodell W, Levin VA, et al: Promise and problems in the use of halogenated pyrimidines in the treatment of malignant gliomas. Proceedings of the International Congress on Radiation Research, Toronto, 1991, p 62.

71. Hoshino T, Sano K: Radiosensitization of malignant brain tumors with bromo uridine (thymidine analog). Acta Radiol Ther Phys Biol 1969; 8:15.

72. Sinclair WK: Cyclic x-ray responses in mammalian cells in vitro. Radiat Res 1968; 33:620.

73. Rubin P: Clinical oncology: A multidisciplinary approach. New York, American Cancer Society, 1983.

WALTER J. CURRAN, JR.

CHARLES B. SCOTT

STEVEN A. LEIBEL

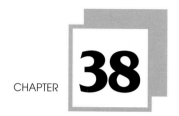

CHAPTER **38**

Issues in the Use of Conventional and Altered Fractionation Radiation Therapy for Pediatric and Adult Gliomas

This chapter summarizes many of the issues related to the application of external beam radiation therapy (RT) to the management of pediatric and adult gliomas. Conventional external beam RT for glial tumors usually involves the administration of once-daily treatments of 1.8 to 2.0 Gy, five times weekly, to total doses of 40 to 70 Gy. The lower dose range has generally been used for low-grade tumors of childhood, such as optic tract gliomas, whereas higher doses are delivered to adult patients with malignant glioma. Sufficient experience has been gained with these treatment regimens to understand both the efficacy and the limitations of such therapy. For tumors with a poor prognosis, such as brainstem or malignant gliomas, there is reason to believe that a substantial increase in the total RT dose could overcome the radioresistance of glial tumor clonogens, which has been observed at traditional RT dose levels, and thus enhance tumor control. However, the tolerance of normal adjacent glial and vascular tissues considerably limits the total RT dose that can be delivered to such tumors. Two strategies designed to circumvent this limitation are three-dimensionally planned conformal radiation therapy (3D-CRT) and altered fractionation regimens.

3D-CRT translates advances in tumor imaging and computer software into the ability to focus the high RT dose region to the tumor target in its entire 3D configuration and to exclude the surrounding normal tissue to the maximum extent possible. Such a treatment approach may involve multiple shaped fields directed at the tumor arranged in coplanar, nonaxial, and non–co-planar orientation, and delivered in either static or dynamic modes.[46] In one comparison of conventional RT and 3D-CRT, 30% less normal brain tissue received high-dose RT when 3D techniques were applied.[76] This reduction in normal tissue exposed to high-dose RT may allow for an escalation in total RT dose delivered to the tumor.[65] Additionally, the integration of magnetic resonance imaging (MRI) into computed tomography (CT)-based 3D-CRT improves tumor volume definition and reduces the likelihood of omitting portions of the tumor from the conformal high-dose volume.[65, 76]

The altered RT fractionation approaches that are most commonly implemented for glial tumor treatment are called *hyperfractionation* and *accelerated hyperfractionation*. Hyperfractionated RT (HRT) is delivered in two or more daily treatments in smaller-than-standard fractions, often in 1.0- to 1.2-Gy fractions. This allows a higher-than-standard total RT dose to be delivered in the usual 6- to 7-week treatment period. The most notable theoretical benefits of HRT are (1) the ability to increase the total RT dose without increasing late normal tissue complications; (2) an increased tumor cell kill for equivalent late normal tissue effects; (3) a reduction in the contribution of hypoxia to radioresistance; and (4) a reduction in late tissue complications, although acute tissue morbidity is similar to that in conventional fractionation schemes.[23, 74, 86]

Accelerated hyperfractionated RT (AHRT) involves multiple daily RT fractions in standard RT dose increments (1.6 to 2.0 Gy), with the total RT dose delivered over a shortened time period. The total RT dose with this technique may be less than or equivalent to that delivered with conventional fractionation. A theoretical advantage of the shortened overall treatment time is a decrease in the opportunity of tumor cell repopulation during treatment.[75, 78, 87] A strong relationship appears to exist between RT fraction size and the risk of late central nervous system injury, particularly radiation necrosis.[69] It has been convincingly demonstrated that fraction size and, conversely, the number of RT fractions influences the risk of late RT injury for neural tissue more strongly than for other organ systems.[24] For these reasons, central nervous system (CNS) tumors, especially relatively radioresistant lesions such as malignant or brainstem gliomas, are especially well suited to an experimental approach using either HRT or AHRT.

PEDIATRIC GLIAL TUMORS

Approximately half of all brain tumors that occur in children are of glial origin. These tumors include, but are not limited to, low-grade gliomas (astrocytomas) and malignant gliomas of the cerebellum, gliomas of the brainstem and the diencephalic region, and low- and high-grade gliomas of the cerebral hemispheres.

Although the successful management of most pediatric brain tumors involves the judicious administration of intermediate- to high-dose cranial radiation, the presence of a glioma in a very young child presents a particularly difficult challenge. The late sequelae of cranial RT for children are inversely related to patient age, and for children younger than 3 years, the developmental and intellectual deficits resulting from multimodality management of brain tumors can be substantial.[40, 57] Several research groups, including the Pediatric Oncology Group (POG), have developed clinical research programs in which children younger than 3 years with a variety of brain tumors received postoperative multiagent chemotherapy as a means of delaying definitive cranial RT for up to 2 years. A phase II POG trial enrolled children younger than 3 years with a variety of brain tumors, including brainstem gliomas and malignant gliomas, to receive up to 1 year of chemotherapy prior to cranial RT. Despite the inclusion of children with tumors not considered to be particularly chemosensitive, definitive RT was successfully delayed in a majority of patients, and overall survival rates appeared superior to those of young brain tumor patients who received postoperative RT only.[17] No evidence exists to suggest that treatment sequelae are reduced in older children or adolescents by using chemotherapy to delay irradiation.

Posterior Fossa Glial Tumors

CEREBELLAR ASTROCYTOMAS

Cerebellar astrocytomas are the most common childhood brain tumors in North America. More than 80% of these are the classic juvenile pilocytic type, or Gilles type A tumor; the diffuse fibrillary type, or Gilles type B tumor, accounts for the remaining 20%. Pilocytic astrocytomas typically arise in a lateralized cerebellar location and appear on imaging studies as well-defined cystic lesions with an enhancing wall. Gross total resection of these lesions can usually be accomplished, with resultant long-term survival of more than 90% of patients without further therapy.[29, 31] The role of postoperative irradiation for incompletely resected pilocytic tumors is not clearly established. Although patient numbers are small, retrospective evidence suggests that the risk of progression following incomplete resection is reduced by posterior fossa irradiation.[1, 29] Among subtotally resected cerebellar astrocytomas reviewed by workers at Washington University in St. Louis, Garcia and co-workers[29] reported that 7 of the 15 patients (47%) not receiving RT suffered relapse, whereas 6 of 25 (24%) who received postoperative RT experienced tumor recurrences. It is important to note that tumor bed recurrences can often be successfully salvaged by a second resection.

Gilles type B astrocytomas tend to arise near the midline of the cerebellum and are less well-demarcated on imaging studies than are pilocytic tumors. Their more infiltrative nature makes complete resection less frequently possible. As with the pilocytic tumors, close observation without adjuvant therapy is recommended following a gross total resection. It is uncertain whether indications for adjuvant RT should differ between type A and B tumors.

HIGH-GRADE CEREBELLAR GLIOMAS

High-grade cerebellar gliomas of childhood are rare, and their prognosis is poor.[7, 42] The largest reported experience was that of 18 from the University of California at San Francisco (UCSF), and in that series, extracerebellar recurrences were noted in both parenchymal and leptomeningeal intracranial locations.[7] Based on this failure pattern, whole-brain RT followed by a posterior fossa "boost" field to 60 Gy appears warranted.

BRAINSTEM GLIOMAS

Brainstem gliomas constitute 20% of childhood brain tumors and are commonly diffuse, infiltrative lesions. The majority arise within the pons; however, a small number of exophytic tumors arise at the cervicomedullary junction and extend in a cranial direction to infiltrate the lower brainstem.[64] A subset of patients has tumors that arise in the superior aspect of the midbrain, specifically the tectum.[80] Both cervicomedullary and high midbrain lesions tend to be histologically benign as compared with the more common pontine tumors. Although focal biopsies of the diffuse pontine tumors are often interpreted as being low grade, autopsy studies reveal malignant or anaplastic foci in 70% to 80% of patients.[2]

Aggressive total or subtotal resection of brainstem tumors is usually possible only for the rare exophytic cervicomedullary tumors. In the past, many children with cranial nerve palsies, long tract signs, and imaging findings consistent with the diagnosis of pontine glioma received definitive irradiation without benefit of tissue confirmation. Although numerous reports have confirmed that surgical intervention for biopsy and, occasionally, subtotal resection can be performed safely, little evidence is present to suggest that such procedures have resulted in either altered management or improved survival.[20] The presence of benign or low-grade histologic findings from a biopsy of a diffuse pontine tumor alters neither management nor the high likelihood that unsampled anaplastic foci are present within the tumor. Patients with either biopsied or unbiopsied tumors are currently eligible for enrollment in brainstem glioma trials conducted by POG and the Children's Cancer Group (CCG).

Standard RT for children with brainstem gliomas involves once-daily treatments to the brainstem using opposing lateral fields in 1.8-Gy fractions to 54.0 to 60.0 Gy. Gadolinium-enhanced MRI, particularly in sagittal imaging, has increased the ability of radiation oncologists to accurately distinguish the extent of infiltration of the brainstem by tumor and to confine the high-dose RT volume to this region. Unfortunately, even with such approaches, the median survival time of children with brainstem gliomas is about 1 year, and the 3-year survival rate is under 20%.[19, 36] The results are less dismal for cervicomedullary junction or tectal tumors, and most long-term brainstem glioma survivors have one of these tumor types.

Hyperfractionated RT has been evaluated for brainstem glioma by POG and CCG and by investigators at UCSF and Children's Hospital of Philadelphia. Total doses ranging from 64.0 to 78.0 Gy in twice-daily 1.0- to 1.2-Gy fractions have been studied in phase I and II trials. No treatment-related fatalities have been reported, and treatment has generally been well tolerated. Several patients have experienced cystic changes within the brainstem that have required either long-term steroid use or surgical intervention (Freedman).[26] Although no clear survival advantage has been identified, tumor response rates to HRT are high.[18, 25, 26, 61] When response is defined as a 50% or greater reduction in the product of perpendicular tumor diameters, response rates of 14% and 17% are reported.[61] When stable disease and minor responses are included among the "responders" group, response rates of up to 77% have been observed.[25, 61] Although no evidence indicates that adjuvant chemotherapy is of benefit to brainstem glioma patients, both CCG and POG are evaluating concurrent chemotherapy-HRT regimens. POG activated a phase III trial in 1992 that compares conventional to hyperfractionated RT, with both treatment arms employing concurrent cisplatin chemotherapy (POG 9239).

POSTERIOR FOSSA EPENDYMOMAS

Ependymomas constitute 5% to 10% of childhood posterior fossa tumors; they arise most commonly from the cells lining the fourth ventricle and less frequently from the lining of the third ventricle or lateral ventricles. Fourth ventricular ependymomas extend through the fourth ventricle in up to 30% of cases and superiorly toward the third ventricle in fewer than 10% of patients.[32] Complete craniospinal imaging and CSF examination must be performed to rule out wider dissemination.

The diagnosis of ependymoma is usually established at the time of resection of a midline posterior fossa mass. Complete surgical resection is associated with a more favorable prognosis in most but not all institutional reviews,[32, 53, 77] and a recently completed phase II trial conducted by POG (trial 8532) and the Radiation Therapy Oncology Group (RTOG) observed no local recurrences among the 10 patients who underwent a gross total resection and posterior fossa RT.[44] The current standard of care for such patients includes maximum tumor resection consistent with preservation of neurologic function followed by postoperative RT.

Institutional reviews have suggested that posterior fossa ependymomas without evidence of neuraxis dissemination at diagnosis can be effectively treated with RT fields limited to the posterior fossa and upper cervical region.[32, 84] Local tumor control rates appear superior among patients receiving at least 45 Gy,[41] and total doses of 54 to 55 Gy with a "shrinking field technique" are generally recommended. In POG trial 8532, 32 patients with either classic or anaplastic fourth ventricular ependymoma without neuraxis dissemination received 54.0 Gy in 1.8-Gy fractions to the posterior fossa and upper cervical region. No isolated recurrences were observed outside the posterior fossa, and the 2-year failure-free survival rate was 68%. Because the predominant site of tumor failure was in the treatment volume that received 54.0 Gy, POG elected to conduct a phase II trial of

hyperfractionated posterior fossa/upper cervical spine RT to 69.6 Gy in 1.2-Gy twice-daily fractionation. The cervical spine dose was limited to 46.8 Gy unless tumor extended through the foramen magnum. Patient accrual was completed in late 1994, and results of this trial are as yet unavailable.[78]

For patients with ependymomas with neuraxis dissemination or ependymoblastoma, intermediate-dose craniospinal RT (36 Gy) is necessary followed by reduced RT field treatment to the primary tumor site to a total dose of 54 to 55 Gy. Patients with supratentorial ependymomas are generally managed with maximal tumor resection followed by whole-brain RT with reduced field treatment to the tumor region to a similar total dose. Goldwein and colleagues[32] concluded from a review of the University of Pennsylvania experience that partial brain RT is adequate for supratentorial lesions.

Supratentorial Brain Tumors

DIENCEPHALIC GLIOMAS

Tumors of the diencephalon, specifically the hypothalamus, thalamus, and optic pathway, are typically low-grade gliomas. The initial approach to a child without neurofibromatosis with a mass lesion in this region is surgical intervention to define the histologic subtype. Patients with bulky, symptomatic tumors may also benefit from surgical debulking. Because 10% to 20% of children with neurofibromatosis who are younger than 10 years may have an asymptomatic low-grade glioma of the optic pathway, biopsy of such lesions is not considered mandatory.[50]

Conventional management of low-grade hypothalamic or thalamic tumors not involving the optic tracts is local field RT to 54.0 to 60.0 Gy. Tumor response or stabilization is observed in the majority of patients, although patients occasionally experience a transient increase in lesion size immediately after treatment. Interest has grown in offering chemotherapy prior to cranial RT as a means of delaying the use of RT in children younger than 5 years.[62] Because the late sequelae of cranial RT for children are inversely related to age, a delay in the delivery of RT of 1 to 2 years may reduce the severity and/or risk of developmental complications.

Many optic pathway tumors found on surveillance scanning of asymptomatic children with neurofibromatosis are slow-growing lesions. Close observation with intervention planned at the time of visual signs or symptoms or tumor enlargement is reasonable. POG recently completed accrual to a study of the biologic behavior of optic pathway tumors (POG trial 8935/8936). On progression of tumors among children younger than 5 years, single-agent carboplatin chemotherapy was employed, followed by local field RT when indicated. For children older than 5 years, local field RT was used at the time of first progression. Historical series detailing results with local field RT describe excellent long-term tumor control and survival. Such tumors are well suited to the potential advantages of 3D-CRT.

LOW-GRADE HEMISPHERIC GLIOMAS

In contrast to adult brain tumors, the majority of pediatric tumors involving the cerebral cortex are of low histologic grade. A variety of low-grade glial neoplasms have been identified in cortical locations; these include juvenile cerebral astrocytoma, pure oligodendroglioma, oligoastrocytoma, supratentorial pilocytic astrocytoma, pleomorphic xanthoastrocytoma, ganglioglioma, and subependymal giant cell astrocytoma. Although enumeration of the distinguishing biologic and histologic details of each of these tumor types appears elsewhere in this book, it is of note that subependymal giant cell astrocytomas occur only among patients with tuberous sclerosis.

Several unifying features regarding hemispheric low-grade gliomas have important therapeutic implications. Recent reports have suggested that gross total resection may be possible in up to 90% of cases in which the lesion is localized and confined to one lobe.[38, 66] Long-term event-free survival rates following such surgery have been reported as ranging from 50% to 95%.[66, 68] Following a gross total resection, close observation with serial imaging and examinations is considered optimal management. Should tumor recurrence be detected, re-operation, prior to initiation of radiation or chemotherapy, should be considered whenever possible.

Optimal management of children who undergo subtotal resection of a cerebral hemisphere low-grade glioma remains controversial. Intermediate-dose irradiation (45 to 55 Gy) to the tumor bed with a small margin has been considered standard therapy, and progression-free survival rates appear to be improved by this therapy.[68, 71, 84] The region of gadolinium enhancement on T1-weighted MRI, with a 1.5 to 2.0 cm margin to the block or field edge, is an adequate RT treatment volume for a well-delineated lesion. A more generous margin may be necessary for more diffuse, less well-marginated tumors. POG and CCG jointly conducted a trial (intergroup trial 0128) in which children aged 5 to 21 years who underwent incomplete resection of low-grade glioma were randomized to immediate partial brain RT to 54.0 Gy vs. close observation. This study was unable to randomize sufficient numbers of patients to answer this question, probably due to the inherent physician biases either in favor of or against postoperative RT. The activity of chemotherapy against low-grade diencephalic tumors has prompted interest in this approach to hemispheric low-grade gliomas, but few current data are available regarding either response rates or progression-free survival.

SUPRATENTORIAL MALIGNANT GLIOMAS

Approximately 30% of childhood cortical gliomas are malignant, and the majority of these meet the World Health Organization (WHO) criteria of anaplastic astrocytoma or glioblastoma multiforme. As with histologically similar gliomas among adults, complete surgical resection is usually not possible, and postoperative partial brain RT results in a prolongation of survival over surgery alone. Children and adolescents with supratentorial malignant gliomas have a superior survival profile to that of adults with histologically similar tumors when treated in a comparable manner.[15, 16] Although the underlying basis for this inverse relationship between age and prognosis in malignant glioma remains elusive, it appears that both response to therapy and prognosis for adult and pediatric hemispheric anaplastic astrocytoma and glioblastoma multiforme patients are sufficiently

different that clinical trials should continue to partition patients by age.

The role of adjuvant chemotherapy appears to have been settled by a recent phase III CCG trial in which 72 children and adolescents with high-grade hemispheric gliomas were randomized between cranial RT alone and cranial RT with a chemotherapeutic regimen that consisted of lomustine, vincristine, and prednisone. Despite a small number of patients, the 5-year progression-free survival rates were significantly superior, and they favored the chemoradiation group over the group with RT alone (46% vs. 18%, respectively; $P = 0.026$).[72] A follow-up randomized CCG trial of 185 patients failed to identify any additional advantage of an aggressive eight-drug chemotherapy regimen with RT over the three-drug/RT regimen.[21] Among the same patients, more aggressive chemotherapy regimens in conjunction with cranial RT are being investigated by CCG, as are altered fractionation radiation schemes by POG. Standard management should consist of maximal surgical resection followed by lomustine, vincristine, and prednisone chemotherapy with cranial RT.

For malignant gliomas, the RT target volume can usually be defined by the gadolinium enhancement on T1-weighted MRI and the bright signal abnormality on T2-weighted images, or by the contrast-enhancing lesion and low-density region surrounding the tumor on CT scan. A 2.0- to 3.0-cm margin on this target is sufficient in most cases for the first 45 to 50 Gy, and a smaller target volume consisting of the enhancing tumor with a 1.5- to 2.0-cm margin should be used to bring the cumulative dose to 55 to 60 Gy. Multifocal or diffuse malignant gliomas may require whole-brain RT to 45 to 50 Gy, followed by a partial-brain RT boost to 55 to 60 Gy.

ADULT GLIAL TUMORS

Supratentorial Low-Grade Gliomas

Supratentorial low-grade gliomas are both a clinically and a histologically diverse group of tumors, which most commonly afflict adolescents and young adults. These patients frequently present with headache or seizure activity, and a non-enhancing mass without edema is seen on imaging. Such a finding elicits clinical management that varies from observation without biopsy to aggressive resection with postoperative intermediate to high-dose partial brain RT. The optimal management for such patients remains controversial, resulting in diverse therapeutic approaches.

The historic institutional series of low-grade glioma patients have suggested an advantage to the use of postoperative RT. Most series have reported on patient data collected over decades, while diagnostic and therapeutic techniques evolved. Retrospective series by Garcia and co-workers[28] and Laws and associates[45] found that only patients older that 30 or 40 years, respectively, appeared to benefit from postoperative RT. However, both series failed to distinguish between results for patients with pilocytic tumors vs. those with non-pilocytic tumors. Because the incidence of pilocytic tumors is much higher among younger patients, a younger cohort of patients will have better survival independent of postoperative management. Sheline and others[69] concluded that only patients with subtotal resection of low-grade gliomas appeared to benefit from postoperative RT. Yet that series also included many young patients with totally resected cerebellar pilocytic astrocytomas, and conclusions from such a group should not be applied to patients with total or near-total resection of ordinary astrocytomas or mixed oligoastrocytomas. A more contemporary report by Berger and co-workers[4] demonstrated the strong relationship of extent of resection to recurrence among 231 patients with non-pilocytic astrocytomas and mixed low-grade tumors managed at the University of Washington Medical Center. The significant correlation existed between residual tumor volume and recurrence rate independent of RT dose. Shaw and colleagues[68] observed a significant advantage to "high-dose" postoperative RT ($\geq$54.0 Gy) among 126 patients with non-pilocytic supratentorial low-grade astrocytomas.

The BTCG attempted to definitively study the question of the role of immediate postoperative RT in BTCG study 8730, in which patients with subtotally resected low-grade gliomas were to be randomized to 50.0-Gy RT vs. no RT. Unfortunately, this trial accrued poorly and was closed in 1991. The EORTC is currently conducting a similar trial. Another management question for low-grade gliomas has been the appropriate RT dose for such patients. An intergroup trial conducted by the North Central Cancer Treatment Group, RTOG, and ECOG from 1986 to 1994 randomized more than 200 low-grade glioma patients to between 50.4 and 64.8 Gy in 1.8-Gy fractions. Preliminary results are expected in 1997. The EORTC randomized 379 patients between 45.0 and 59.4 Gy, and preliminary results demonstrated no improvement in 5-year survival rate (58% vs. 59%) or disease-free survival rate (47% vs. 50%) between those patients assigned to the 45.0- and 59.4-Gy arms, respectively.

Supratentorial Malignant Gliomas

Approximately 33% to 45% of all primary adult brain tumors are malignant gliomas, and 85% of these are glioblastomas multiforme. Using the WHO tumor classification system, the other 15% of patients with malignant gliomas include those with anaplastic astrocytoma, aggressive oligodendroglioma, gliosarcoma, and mixed aggressive oligoastrocytoma. The histopathologic distinction between anaplastic astrocytoma and glioblastoma multiforme is a useful discriminant of patient outcome, with the 5-year survival rate of anaplastic astrocytoma patients being reported at 18% vs. 5% for glioblastoma multiforme patients in a 1980 patterns-of-care study conducted by several American surgical groups.[54] Patient age and performance status have been identified by several groups as the other pretreatment prognostic factors that are strongly predictive of survival outcome in malignant glioma patients.[10]

RANDOMIZED TRIALS OF POSTOPERATIVE RT

Bouchard and Pierce[5] reported in 1960 that glioblastoma multiforme patients who received postoperative cranial RT

had longer survival times than glioblastoma multiforme patients who did not receive RT. This observation was confirmed by the Brain Tumor Study Group (BTSG) in the randomized trial 69–01.[81] A total of 303 adults (222 analyzable) with malignant glioma (90% glioblastoma multiforme and 9% anaplastic astrocytoma) were randomized between (1) supportive management; (2) BCNU (carmustine) chemotherapy; (3) whole-brain RT to 50 to 60 Gy; and (4) both BCNU and whole-brain RT. Significantly superior survival outcomes were seen among the patients receiving cranial RT over those assigned to supportive management, with median survival times of 36 vs. 14 weeks ($P = 0.001$), respectively.[81] A confirmatory trial was reported by the Scandinavian Glioblastoma Study Group (SGSG) in 1981, in which, after aggressive surgical resection, 118 adult malignant glioma patients were randomized between supportive care, whole brain RT to 45.0 Gy in 1.8-Gy fractions, or the same RT regimen with concurrent bleomycin chemotherapy. The median survival time of patients receiving RT with or without bleomycin was 10.8 months as compared with 5.2 months for patients given supportive care. Over a quarter of the irradiated patients maintained an active functional status, whereas none of the untreated patients remained functionally intact.[43]

The subsequent BTSG trial (7201) again demonstrated the survival advantage of regimens containing cranial RT over those without RT. A total of 467 patients (358 analyzable) were randomized between methyl-CCNU chemotherapy alone, whole-brain RT alone, RT plus BCNU chemotherapy, and RT plus methyl-CCNU therapy. All RT-containing regimens had a significantly superior survival compared with the group receiving methyl-CCNU alone.[82] Thus, these three trials clearly established the beneficial role of cranial RT in the primary management of malignant gliomas, and the design of all major trials since that time has included high-dose RT as a primary component of therapy (Table 38–1).

TABLE 38–1
RESULTS OF BRAIN TUMOR STUDY GROUP (BTSG) AND SCANDINAVIAN GLIOBLASTOMA STUDY GROUP (SGSG) PHASE III TRIALS OF POSTOPERATIVE THERAPIES FOR ADULTS WITH SUPRATENTORIAL MALIGNANT GLIOMA

Assigned Treatment	No. of Patients	Median Survival (wk)
BTSG 6901	222	
Supportive care		14
BCNU		19
Standard RT		36*
Standard RT and BCNU		35*
BTSG 7201	358	
Methyl-CCNU		24
Standard RT		36*
Standard RT and methyl-CCNU		42*
Standard RT and BCNU		51*
SGSG	118	
Supportive care		23
Standard RT, with or without bleomycin		47*

*Significantly superior survival compared with that of other arms in each study.

RT DOSE-RESPONSE DATA FOR CONVENTIONAL RT

The first analysis seeking to establish an RT dose response for survival of malignant glioma was published by Walker and colleagues in 1979.[83] The authors analyzed the survival results of three BTSG trials (66-01, 69-01, and 72-01) and concluded that a clear dose response to survival existed between total doses of 50 and 60 Gy.[83] Although issues have been raised regarding the methodology used in this report,[46] its conclusions have helped establish 60.0 Gy given in amounts of 1.8 to 2.0 Gy/fraction over 6 weeks as the standard RT treatment regimen for malignant glioma. Further support was provided by the Medical Research Council trial BR2, in which 443 malignant glioma patients were randomized between a course of 60 Gy in 2.0-Gy fractions vs. 45 Gy in 2.25-Gy fractions without chemotherapy. The median survival times were 12 vs. 9 months, favoring the 60-Gy arm ($P = 0.007$), and overall survival was also improved ($P = 0.04$) (MRC). An intergroup trial conducted by the RTOG and the Eastern Cooperative Oncology Group (ECOG) failed to detect any further improvement in survival among the 281 patients (244 analyzable) randomized between total doses of 60 and 70 Gy.[8]

Very limited information is available regarding the imaging response rate of malignant gliomas to cranial RT. Using standard response criteria, the response rate to RT among evaluable malignant glioma patients entered into several BTCG trials and a Canadian trial were 18% and 16%, respectively.[79, 88] Gaspar and co-workers[30] observed a 35% objective response rate to cranial rate among 71 patients, with a higher rate among anaplastic astrocytoma patients than among those with glioblastoma multiforme (52% vs. 26%, respectively).

RT TARGET VOLUME

Improvements in neuroimaging since the mid-1970s, particularly the development of CT and MRI, have redefined RT treatment planning and target definition for malignant glioma patients. Although the randomized trials in the 1960s and 1970s generally required whole-brain RT to 60 Gy, such treatment is now generally reserved for the small number of patients with multifocal gliomas or gliomatosis cerebri. For the patients with unifocal gliomas, the initial target volume encompasses the primary tumor with or without peritumoral edema with a 2- to 3-cm margin as defined by MRI or CT imaging. This is then followed by a reduction in target volume to include the tumor itself with a 1- to 2-cm margin. Although the specific details of target definition vary among institutions and cooperative groups, partial brain RT is agreed on as the standard approach to most adult malignant glioma patients. Although stereotactic biopsies and autopsy studies have confirmed the presence of tumor cells distant from the primary lesion, the majority of tumor recurrences are manifested at or adjacent to the initial tumor site. Until control of the primary lesion is more successful, it is unlikely that tumor recurrences outside of the tumor bed will have significant clinical consequences. The presence of tumor infiltration of peritumoral regions that are abnormal on T2-weighted MRI and isodense on CT scanning has influenced several groups to use the T2-weighted MRI abnormality as the basis of RT treatment planning. A recent report from Johns Hopkins University drew attention to a high rate of white matter dissemination among 74% of the 30 patients with tumors arising near white matter tracts in the frontal or occipital lobes.[85] Confirmatory observations of this failure pattern are necessary before any change in the standard RT field definition is considered.

This partial brain RT approach has the advantage of decreasing the volume of neural tissue irradiated, and thereby decreasing treatment toxic effects without compromising tumor control. Based on these studies, current standard radiotherapeutic management of malignant gliomas involves delivery of 60 Gy in 1.8- to 2.0-Gy daily fractions using a shrinking field technique as described earlier.

ALTERED FRACTIONATION TRIALS

Both hyperfractionated and accelerated hyperfractionated RT regimens have been investigated for adult malignant glioma patients. The delivery of the smaller than standard RT fractions several times per day is only likely to improve tumor control if the total RT dose is at least 20% higher than the standard total dose. Unfortunately, many of the prior experiences with HRT delivered total doses equivalent to those of standard regimens with no apparent benefit. Both the BTCG and the European Organization for the Research and Treatment of Cancer (EORTC) have reported a lack of advantage to HRT with a dose of 60 or 66 Gy when compared with a once-daily RT regimen in the same total dose range.[14, 39] A randomized trial of 69 patients reported by Fulton and associates[27] indicated a survival advantage of a regimen of 61.4 Gy given in three fractions of 0.89 Gy/day over 58 Gy in once-daily treatments, with 2-year survival rates of 21% and 10%, respectively ($P = 0.05$). However, the same investigators were unable to confirm this difference in a larger phase I and II trial, in which the total HRT dose was escalated to 71.2 and 80 Gy.[27]

From 1983 to 1987 the RTOG conducted a two-step phase I and II trial of HRT with total doses of 64.8, 72.0, 76.8, and 81.4 Gy in twice-daily 1.2-Gy fractionation with BCNU chemotherapy (RTOG 83–02). The intermediate dose of 72.0 Gy was identified as the total dose worthy of phase III testing for several reasons. Patients assigned to this dose had the longest median survival time among all dose levels, and a significantly longer median survival time and 18-month survival rate were observed for this arm over the 81.4-Gy arm in the second randomization (14.0 vs. 11.7 months and 44% vs. 28%, respectively).[59] A subsequent analysis of the quality of life of patients enrolled in this trial also identified 72.0 Gy as the dose with the most favorable "quality-adjusted survival" results.[58] Based on these observations, the RTOG randomized 712 patients on a phase III trial comparing 72.0 Gy HRT with once-daily 60.0 Gy treatments, with all patients receiving BCNU chemotherapy (RTOG 90-06). Enrollment to this trial was completed in March 1994, and a preliminary analysis has identified no survival advantage for any malignant glioma patient subset of HRT over standard therapy (submitted to ASCO, 1996, personal communication, W. Curran).

Accelerated hyperfractionated RT (AHRT) involves the delivery of standard RT dose increments (1.6 to 2.0 Gy) in multiple daily treatments and results in the completion of an

RT course over a shortened time period. The final randomization of RTOG 83–02 involved the delivery of twice-daily fractions of 1.6 Gy to total doses of 48.0 and 54.4 Gy with BCNU. Results of this trial demonstrated that the maximum tolerated dose was not reached and that further dose escalation is possible.[13] A phase II trial of higher total doses of AHFT (64.0 and 70.4 Gy), in which postoperative tumor dimensions are being used to determine the total dose delivered, is currently being conducted by the RTOG for glioblastoma multiforme patients (RTOG 94–11). The Brain Tumor Research Center at UCSF will complete accrual in 1995 to a phase III trial for brachytherapy-ineligible glioblastoma multiforme patients; in this trial the 70.4 Gy in 1.6-Gy twice-daily fractions regimen is being compared with standard fractionation. Results of this trial and subsequent efforts within the RTOG will help determine the future role of altered fractionation RT for malignant glioma patients.

Another altered fractionation approach to malignant glioma patients is that of *hypofractionation*. This term refers to the delivery of larger-than-standard fractions ranging from 2.5 to 6.0 Gy, with a lower total RT dose and a shorter elapsed time. Because of the larger RT fraction sizes, such an approach has a higher risk of RT-related injury to normal brain in long-term survivors. Because of this, hypofractionated regimens should normally be reserved for patients whose prognosis with standard therapy is very unfavorable. Using data extrapolated from the recursive partitioning analysis of prognostic factors in the RTOG malignant glioma data base, such patients include older glioblastoma multiforme patients with significant neurologic impairment, low performance status, and/or a tumor that cannot be surgically debulked.[11] The advantage of a hypofractionated regimen is mainly its cost effectiveness in terms of patient and facility time and the lesser financial burden of this therapy over standard therapy. If quality-adjusted survival is equivalent between such an approach and standard therapy, then the former would be preferable. In a comparison of results of a hypofractionated regimen of 30.0 Gy given in ten 3.0-Gy fractions with historic outcome of a standard 60-Gy course for patients older than 60 years, investigators at the University of Western Ontario and Duke University observed no survival difference among poor performance status patients.[3] However, an apparent survival advantage in favor of the 60-Gy regimen was seen among those patients over age 60 years with a Karnofsky performance status of 70 or greater.

CONFORMAL RADIATION

Both laboratory and clinical experiences support the premise that 60 Gy is an inadequate RT dose to achieve long-term tumor control for most malignant glioma patients. Clinical experiences with a combination of external beam RT and brachytherapy suggest that durable tumor control rates improve only at cumulative doses of 100 Gy or higher.[33, 52] Unfortunately, only a minority of newly diagnosed malignant glioma patients are eligible for brachytherapy or for a stereotactic radiosurgery boost. A review of potential eligibility for either brachytherapy or stereotactic radiosurgery among over 700 patients treated with HRT or AHRT and chemotherapy on RTOG 83–02 found that only 12% and 20%, respectively, might have been eligible for these modalities.[10, 12] Most patients do not qualify for such approaches because of tumor size. Although aggressive surgical debulking may result in a higher eligibility rate, the only radiotherapeutic alternative for the majority of patients is that of partial brain irradiation.

3D planned conformal RT may allow meaningful RT dose escalation for patients unable to receive either brachytherapy or radiosurgery. When successfully applied, 3D-CRT creates a high-dose RT volume that conforms to the tumor volume in its entire three-dimensional configuration. With the development of high-speed computational software and high-performance workstations, 3D-CRT can be implemented in an increasing number of radiation oncology departments. Multiple co-planar and non–co-planar shaped fields resulting from this approach usually result in a decreased dose to the adjacent normal brain. Currently several institutions are conducting RT dose escalation trials of 3D-CRT, and preliminary results from the University of Michigan suggest that dose escalation of conventionally fractionated RT to at least 90 Gy is possible for selected patients.[65]

ANAPLASTIC ASTROCYTOMA AND AGGRESSIVE OLIGODENDROGLIOMA

Approximately 80% of adult malignant gliomas meet the histopathologic criteria of glioblastoma multiforme, and patients with this lesion constitute the majority of patients entered into clinical trials. Most of the non-glioblastoma multiforme malignant glioma patients have anaplastic astrocytoma, and a much smaller number are diagnosed with aggressive oligodendroglioma. Median survival times of these two groups with postoperative RT, with or without chemotherapy, are reported as 3 to 4 years and 4 to 5 years, respectively. Although patterns of tumor recurrence and RT treatment guidelines are essentially similar to those for glioblastoma multiforme patients, the higher likelihood for long-term survival places these patients at higher risk for long-term sequelae of therapy. Several phase II trials have suggested that new systemic approaches currently show greater promise for these patients than for glioblastoma multiforme patients. Multi-agent chemotherapy such as procarbazine, CCNU, and vincristine (PCV) have been demonstrated to induce high response rates among patients with aggressive oligodendroglioma,[6] and this regimen is under study in a phase III trial (RTOG 94–02). The halogenated pyrimidine bromodeoxyuridine (BUdR) has demonstrated promising activity as a radiosensitizer for anaplastic astrocytoma patients[49] and is under study in another phase III trial (RTOG 94–04). In both studies, the RT delivered in both the control and investigational arms is 59.4 Gy in 1.8-Gy fractionation. The possible advantage observed by NCOG of using brachytherapy in the initial treatment of eligible glioblastoma multiforme patients was not observed for anaplastic astrocytoma patients; therefore, subsequent trials for anaplastic astrocytoma patients have not included brachytherapy. The value of stereotactic radiosurgery for such patients remains uncertain.[33]

REFERENCES

1. Akyol FH, Atahan IL, Zorlu F, et al: Results of postoperative or exclusive radiotherapy in grade I and grade II cerebellar astrocytoma patients. Radiother Oncol 1992; 23:245–248.

2. Barkovich AJ, Krishner J, Kun L, et al: Brainstem gliomas: A classification system based on magnetic resonance imaging. Pediatr Neurosci 1991; 16:73–83.

3. Bauman GS, Gaspar LE, Fisher BJ, et al: A prospective study of short-course radiotherapy in poor prognosis glioblastoma multiforme. Int J Radiat Oncol Biol Phys 1994; 29:835–839.

4. Berger MS, Deliganis AV, Dobbins J, et al: The effect of extent of resection on recurrence in patients with low grade cerebral hemisphere gliomas. Cancer 1994; 74:1784–1791.

5. Bouchard J, Pierce CB: Radiation therapy in the management of neoplasms of the central nervous system, with a special note in regard to children: Twenty years' experience, 1939–1948. Am J Roentgenol 1960; 84:610–628.

6. Cairncross G, Macdonald D, Ludwin S, et al: The National Cancer Institute of Canada Clinical Trials Group: Chemotherapy for anaplastic oligidendroglioma. J Clin Oncol 1994; 12:2013–2017.

7. Chamberlain MC, Silver P, Levin VA: Poorly differentiated gliomas of the cerebellum: A study of 18 patients. Cancer 1990; 65:337–340.

8. Chang CH, Horton J, Schoenfeld D, et al: Comparison of postoperative radiotherapy and combined postoperative radiotherapy and chemotherapy in the multidisciplinary management of malignant gliomas. Cancer 1983; 52:997–1007.

9. Corn BW, Yousem D, Scott CB, et al: White matter changes are significantly correlated with RT dose: Observations from a randomized dose escalation trial for malignant glioma (RTOG 83-02). Cancer 1994; 74:2828–2835.

10. Curran WJ, Scott CB, Horton J, et al: Recursive partitioning analysis of 1,578 patients on three Radiation Therapy Oncology Trials malignant glioma trials. J Natl Cancer Inst 1993; 85:704–710.

11. Curran WJ, Scott CB, Nelson JS, et al: Survival comparison of radiosurgery eligible and ineligible malignant glioma patients treated with hyperfractionated radiation therapy and BCNU: A report of RTOG 83-02. J Clin Oncol 1993; 11:857–862.

12. Curran WJ, Scott CB, Weinstein AS, et al: Survival comparison of brachytherapy eligible and ineligible malignant glioma patients treated with twice-daily radiotherapy and BCNU: A report of RTOG 83-02 (abstract). Radiother Oncol 1992; 24:S11.

13. Curran WJ, Scott CB, Nelson JS, et al: A randomized trial of accelerated hyperfractionated radiation therapy and BCNU for malignant glioma: A preliminary report of Radiation Therapy Oncology Group 83-02. Cancer 1992; 70:2909–2917.

14. Deutsch M, Green SB, Strike T, et al: Results of a randomized trial comparing BCNU plus radiotherapy, streptozotocin plus radiotherapy, BCNU plus hyperfractionated radiotherapy, and BCNU following misonidazole plus radiotherapy in the postoperative treatment of malignant glioma. Int J Radiat Oncol Biol Phys 1989; 16:1389–1396.

15. Dropcho EJ, Wisoff JH, Walker RW, et al: Supratentorial malignant gliomas in childhood: A review of 50 cases. Ann Neurol 1987; 22:355–364.

16. Duffner PK, Cohen ME, Myers MH, et al: Survival of children with brain tumors: SEER program, 1973–1980. Neurology 1986; 36:597–601.

17. Duffner PK, Horowitz ME, Krishner JP, et al: Postoperative chemotherapy and delayed radiation in children less than 3 years of age with malignant brain tumors. N Engl J Med 1993; 328:1725–1731.

18. Edwards MSB, Levin V, Wara W: Hyperfractionation radiation therapy for brain stem glioma in children. J Neurooncol 1990; 5:170–175.

19. Eifel PJ, Cassidy JR, Belli JA: Radiation therapy of tumors of the brain stem and midbrain in children: Experience of the Joint Center for Radiation Therapy and Children's Hospital Medical Center (1971–1981). Int J Radiat Oncol Biol Phys 1987; 13:847–852.

20. Epstein FJ, McCleary EL: Intrinsic brain-stem tumors of childhood: Surgical indications. J Neurosurg 1986; 64:11–15.

21. Finlay JL, Boyett JM, Yates AJ, et al: Randomized phase III trial in childhood high-grade astrocytoma comparing vincristine, lomustine, and prednisone with the eight-drugs-in-1-day regimen. J Clin Oncol 1995; 13:112–123.

22. Fowler JF: Total dose in fractionated radiotherapy: Implications of new radiobiologic data. Int J Radiat Biol 1984; 46:103–120.

23. Fowler JF: The linear-quadratic formula and progress in fractionated radiotherapy. Br J Radiol 1989; 62:679–694.

24. Fowler J: Potential for increasing the differential response between tumors and normal tissue: Can proliferation rate be used? Int J Radiat Oncol Biol Phys 1986; 12:641–645.

25. Freeman CR, Kirscher JP, Sanford RA, et al: Hyerfractionated radiation therapy in brain stem tumors: Results of treatment at the 7020 cGy dose level of Pediatric Oncology Group #8495. Cancer 1991; 68:474–481.

26. Freeman CR, Kirscher JP, Sanford RA, et al: Final results of a study of escalating doses of hyperfractionated radiotherapy in brain stem tumors in children: A Pedriatric Oncology Group study. Int J Radiat Oncol Biol Phys 1993; 27:197–206.

27. Fulton DS, Urtasun RC, Shin KH, et al: Misonizadole combined with hyperfractionation in the management of malignant glioma. Int J Radiat Oncol Biol Phys 1994; 10:1709–1712.

28. Garcia DM, Fulling KH, Marks JE: The value of radiation therapy in addition to surgery for astrocytomas of the adult cerebrum. Cancer 1985; 55:919–927.

29. Garcia DM, Marks JE, Latifi HR, et al: Childhood cerebellar astrocytoma: Is there a role for postoperative irradiation? Int J Radiat Oncol Biol Phys 1990; 18:815–818.

30. Gaspar LE, Fisher BJ, Macdonald DR, et al: Malignant glioma-timing of response to radiation therapy. Int J Radiat Oncol Biol Phys 1993; 25:877–879.

31. Glabbeke MV, Karim ABMF, Hamars H, et al: No improvement in survival by an increased radiation dose given postoperatively to patients with low grade brain tumors: An EORTC randomized phase III study (abstract). Proc Am Soc Clin Oncol 1995; 14:145.

32. Goldwein JW, Leahy JM, Packer RJ, et al: Intracranial ependymomas in children. Int J Radiat Oncol Biol Phys 1990; 19:1497–1502.

33. Gutin PH, Prados MD, Phillips TL, et al: External irradiation followed by interstitial high activity iodine-125 implant "boost" in the initial treatment of malignant glioma: NCOG study 6G-82-2. Int J Radiat Oncol Biol Phys 1991; 21:601–606.

34. Gjerris F, Klinken L: Long-term prognosis in children with benign cerebellar astrocytoma. J Neurosurg 1978; 49:179–184.

35. Halperin EC: Multiple-fraction-per-day external beam radiotherapy for adults with supratentorial malignant gliomas. J Neurooncol 1992; 14:255–262.

36. Halperin EC, Wehn SM, Scott JW, et al: Selection of a management strategy for pediatric brain stem tumors. Med Pediatr Oncol 1989; 17:116–125.

37. Healey EA, Braners PD, Kupsky WJ, et al: The prognostic significance of postoperative residual tumor in ependymoma. Neurosurgery 1991; 28:666–672.

38. Hirsch J-F, Rose CS, Pierre-Kahn A, et al: Benign astrocytic and oligodendrocytic tumors of the cerebral hemispheres in children. J Neurosurg 1989; 70:568–572.

39. Horiot JC, Van den Togaert, W Ang KK, et al: European Organization for Research on Treatment of Cancer trials using radiotherapy with multiple fractions per day: A 1978–1987 survey. Front Radiat Ther Oncol 1988; 22:149–161.

40. Jannoun L, Bloom HJG: Long-term psychological effects in children treated for intracranial tumors. Int J Radiat Oncol Biol Phys 1990; 18:747–753.

41. Kim YM, Fayos JV: Intracranial ependymomas. Radiology 1977; 124:805–808.

42. Kopelson G, Linggood RM: Infratentorial glioblastoma: The role of neuroaxis irradiation. Int J Radiat Oncol Biol Phys 1982; 8:999–1003.

43. Kristiansen K, Hagen S, Kollevold T, et al: Combined modality therapy of operated astrocytomas grade III and IV: Confirmation of the value of postoperative irradiation and lack of potentiation of bleomycin on survival time. A prospective multicenter trial of the Scandinavian Glioblastoma Study Group. Cancer 1981; 47:649–652.

44. Kun L: Personal communication, 1995.

45. Laws ER, Taylor WF, Clifton MB, et al: Neurosurgical management of low-grade astrocytoma of the cerebral hemispheres. J Neurosurg 1984; 61:665–673.

46. Leibel SA, Scott CB, Pajak TF: The management of malignant gliomas with radiation therapy: Therapeutic results and research strategies. Semin Radiat Oncol 1991; 1:32–49.

47. Leibel SA, Kutcher GJ, Mohan R, et al: Three-dimensional conformal radiation therapy at the Memorial Sloan-Kettering Cancer Center. Semin Radiat Oncol 1992; 2:274–289.

48. Leibel SA, Sheline GE, Wara WM, et al: The role of radiation therapy in the treatment of astrocytomas. Cancer 1975; 35:1551–1557.

49. Levin VA, Prados MR, Wara WM, et al: Radiation therapy and bromodeoxyuridine chemotherapy followed by procarbazine, lomustine and vincristine for treatment of anaplastic gliomas. Int J Radiat Oncol Biol Phys 1995; 32:75–83.

50. Lewis RA, Gerson LP, Axelson KA, et al: Von Recklinghausen neurofibromatosis: II. Incidence of optic gliomata. Ophthalmology 1984; 91:929.

51. Loeffler JS, Alexander E, Shea WM, et al: Radiosurgery as part of the initial management of patients with malignant gliomas. J Clin Oncol 1992; 10:1379–1385.

52. Loeffler JS, Alexander E, Wen P, et al: Results of stereotactic brachytherapy used in the initial management of patients with glioblastoma. J Natl Cancer Inst 1990; 82:1918–1921.

53. Lyons MK, Kelly PJ: Posterior fossa ependymoma: Report of 30 cases and review of the literature. Neurosurgery 1991; 9:659–665.

54. Mahaley SM, Mettlin C, Natarajan N, et al: National survey of patterns of care for brain tumor patients. J Neurosurg 1989; 71:826–836.

55. Medical Research Council Brain Tumor Working Party: A Medical Research Council trial of two radiotherapy doses in the treatment of grade 3 and 4 astrocytoma. Br J Cancer 1991; 64:769–774.

56. Meis JM, Martz KL, Nelson JS: Mixed glioblastoma and sarcoma: A clinicopathologic study of 26 Radiation Therapy Oncology Group cases. Cancer 1991; 67:2342–2349.

57. Mulhern RK, Hancock J, Fairclough D, et al: Neuropsychological status of children treated for brain tumors: A critical review and integrative analysis. Med Pediatr Oncol 1992; 20:181–191.

58. Murray KJ, Nelson DF, Isaacson S, et al: Quality-Adjusted Survival Analysis of Malignant Glioma Patients Treated With Twice-Daily Radiation and Carmustine: A Report of RTOG 83-02. ASTRO Scientific Program, New Orleans, 1993.

59. Nelson DF, Curran WJ, Scott CB, et al: Hyperfractionated radiation therapy and *bis*-chlorethyl nitrosourea in the treatment of malignant glioma: Possible advantage observed at 72.0 Gy in 1.2 Gy b.i.d. fractions: Report of RTOG protocol 8302. Int J Radiat Oncol Biol Phys 1993; 25:193–207.

60. Packer RJ, Allen JC, Goldwein JL, et al: Hyperfractionated radiotherapy for children with brainstem gliomas: A pilot study using 7,200 cGy. Ann Neurol 1990; 27:167–173.

61. Packer RJ, Allen JC, Goldwein JL, et al: Outcome of children with brain stem gliomas after treatment with 7800 cGy of hyperfractionated radiotherapy. Cancer 1994; 74:1827–1834.

62. Packer RJ, Siegal KR, Bilaniuk LT, et al: Treatment of chiasmatic/hypothalamic gliomas of childhood with chemotherapy: An update. Ann Neurol 1988; 23:79–85.

63. Recht LK, Lew R, Smith TW: Suspected low grade glioma: Is deferring treatment safe? Ann Neurol 1992; 31:431–436.

64. Robertson PL, Allen JC, Abbott R, et al: Pediatric cervicomedullary tumors: A distinct subset of brainstem tumors (abstract). Neurology 1993; 43:248.

65. Sandler HM, Radany EH, Greenberg HS, et al: Dose escalation using 3D conformal radiotherapy for high grade astrocytomas (abstract). Int J Radiat Oncol Biol Phys 30 1994; S1:214.

66. Sanford RA, Kun LE, Langston JW, et al: Pitfalls in the management of low grade gliomas. Concepts Pediatr Neurosurg 1991; 11:133–149.

67. Shapiro WR, Green SB, Burger PC, et al: Randomized trial of three chemotherapy regimens and two radiotherapy regimens in postoperative treatment of malignant glioma. J Neurosurg 1989; 71:1–9.

68. Shaw EG, Daumas-Duport C, Scheithauer BW, et al: Radiation therapy in the management of low-grade supratentorial astrocytomas. J Neurosurg 1989; 70:853–861.

69. Sheline GE: Radiation therapy of brain tumors. Cancer 1977; 39:873–881.

70. Sheline GE, Wara WM, Smith V: Therapeutic irradiation and brain injury. Int J Radiat Oncol Biol Phys 1980; 6:1215–1228.

71. Shibamoto Y, Kitakubu Y, Takahashi M, et al: Supratentorial low-grade astrocytoma: Correlation of computed tomography findings with effect of radiation therapy and prognostic variables. Cancer 1993; 72:190–195.

72. Sposto R, Ertel IJ, Jenkin RDT, et al: The effectiveness of chemotherapy for treatment of high grade astrocytoma in children: Results of a randomized trial. J Neurooncol 1989; 7:165–177.

73. Taghian A, Suit H, Pardo F, et al: In vitro intrinsic radiation sensitivity of glioblastoma multiforme. Int J Radiat Oncol Biol Phys 1992; 23:55–62.

74. Thames HD, Hendry JH, Moore JV: The high steepness of dose-response curves for late-responding normal tissues. Radiat Oncol 1989; 15:49–53.

75. Thames HD, Peters LJ, Withers HR, et al: Accelerated fractionation vs. hyperfractionation: Rationales for several treatments per day. Int J Radiat Oncol Biol Phys 1983; 9:127–138.

76. Thornton AF, Hegarty TJ, Archer P, et al: Three-dimensional treatment planning of astrocytomas: A dosimetric study of cerebral radiation (abstract). Int J Radiat Oncol Biol Phys 1989; 17:125.

77. Tomita T, Mclone DG, Das L, et al: Benign ependymomas of the posterior fossa in childhood. Pediatr Neurosci 1988; 14:277–285.

78. Trott K-R, Kummermehr K: What is known about tumor proliferation rates to choose between accelerated fractionation or hyperfractionation? Radiother Oncol 1984; 3:1–10.

79. Urtasun R, Feldstein ML, Partington J, et al: Radiation and nitroimidazoles in supratentorial high-grade gliomas: A second clinical trial. Br J Cancer 1982; 46:101–108.

80. Vandertop WP, Hoffman JH, Drake JM, et al: Focal midbrain tumors in children. Neurosurgery 1992; 31:186–194.

81. Walker MD, Alexander E, Hunt WE, et al: Evaluation of BCNU and/or radiotherapy in the treatment of anaplastic gliomas. J Neurosurg 1978; 49:333–343.

82. Walker MD, Breen SB, Byar DP, et al: Randomized comparisons of radiotherapy and nitrosoureas for the treatment of malignant glioma after surgery. N Engl J Med 1980; 303:1323–1329.

83. Walker MD, Strike TA, Sheline GE: An analysis of dose-effect relationship in the radiotherapy of malignant gliomas. Int J Radiat Oncol Biol Phys 1979; 5:1725–1731.

84. Wallner K, Gonzales M, Sheline GE: Treatment of oligodendrogliomas with or without postoperative radiation. J Neurosurg 1988; 69:171–176.

85. Wie BA, Grossman SA, Wharam M, et al: Dissemination of high-grade astrocytomas along white matter tracts: Observations and therapeutic implications (abstract). Proc Am Soc Clin Oncol 1993; 12:177.

86. Withers HR: Biologic basis for altered fractionation schemes. Cancer 1985; 55:2086–2095.

87. Withers HR, Taylor JMG, Masciejewski B: The hazard of accelerated tumor clonogen repopulation during radiotherapy. Acta Oncol 1988; 27(fasc 2):131–146.

88. Wood JR, Green SB, Shapiro WR: The prognostic importance of tumor size in malignant gliomas: A computed tomographic scan study by the Brain Tumor Cooperative Group. J Clin Oncol 1988; 6:338–343.

KEITH J. STELZER

GEORGE E. LARAMORE

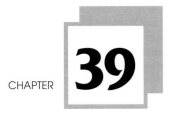

CHAPTER **39**

Particle Beam Therapy

The search for more effective forms of radiation therapy for gliomas and other tumors has led to the development of various types of particle beams. Some of these beams, particularly neutrons, enhance tumor cell kill by providing a high relative biologic effectiveness (RBE). Other beams, such as protons and helium nuclei (α-particles), exhibit dose distribution features that may be utilized to escalate radiation dose to tumor volumes while maintaining normal tissue doses to acceptable levels of risk. Still other particle beams, such as negative π-mesons (pions) and neon ions, provide partial advantages with respect to both RBE and dose distribution. Finally, boron neutron capture therapy represents an attempt to selectively sensitize tumor cells to neutron beam radiation by localizing boronated compounds within tumor cells. This chapter discusses the physical and biologic principles of particle beam radiation as well as the clinical results that have been observed in the treatment of gliomas with these beams.

FAST NEUTRON BEAM

Physical and Biologic Principles

Neutrons are uncharged particles of 1.0 atomic mass unit. Most modern treatment facilities use a cyclotron to provide high-energy protons that impact on a beryllium target, resulting in a high-energy, or fast, neutron beam. These fast neutron beams typically have a broad energy spectrum distributed around average energies of 10 to 30 MeV. Dose penetration profiles are similar to those of typical 4 to 6 MeV x-ray beams used in radiotherapy. An isocentric treatment gantry equipped with a variable multileaf collimator to shape fields integrated with a computerized treatment planning system allows the delivery of conformal neutron radiotherapy that meets the standards achievable with linear accelerator–generated x-ray systems.[1]

Fast neutrons collide with intracellular nuclei and hydrogen nuclei to generate recoil protons and α-particles. These charged recoil particles interact with intracellular targets, such as deoxyribonucleic acids (DNA), to cause ionizations that lead to cell injury and death. The density of the ionizations along a neutron path is greater than that along a photon

(e.g., x-ray) path. Linear energy transfer, or LET, describes the average energy transferred from a beam of radiation to the surrounding medium per distance of medium traversed, and so it directly depends on the density of ionizations.

The biologic importance of LET is reflected in its relationship to RBE. Relative biologic effectiveness for a beam of radiation is calculated from the ratio of biologically isoeffective doses for a reference beam of radiation, such as 250 keV x-rays, and the radiation beam of interest. For example, if the doses to achieve a certain biologic endpoint are 0.5 and 2 Gy for neutrons and 250 keV x-rays, respectively, then the RBE is 4. The RBE varies with the endpoint that is chosen and with experimental conditions. However, a general relationship exists between RBE and LET (Fig. 39–1). The relationship is such that RBE increases to a maximum as LET increases to approximately 100 keV/μm, then decreases at higher LET. The pattern of this relationship is due

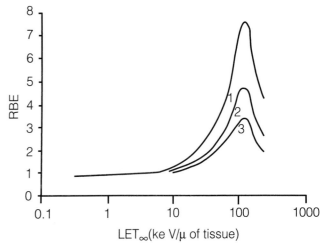

Figure 39–1 Relationship of relative biologic effectiveness (RBE) to linear energy transfer (LET) in mammalian cell culture. The curves 1, 2, and 3 correspond to the biologic endpoint of cell survivals of 0.8, 0.1, and 0.01. The RBE increases to a maximum at an LET of approximately 100 keV/μm, then decreases at higher LET. Also note that the actual value for RBE depends on the endpoint measured. (From Barendsen GW: Responses of cultured cells, tumours and normal tissues to radiations of different linear energy transfer. Curr Top Radiat Res Q 1968; 4:293.)

to the increased probability of cell death at a given dose of more densely ionizing (high LET) radiation. Very high LET radiation provides an excess of ionizations within individual cells, resulting in a portion of radiation dose that is ''wasted'' in causing more ionizations than are necessary for cell death.

The killing of tumor cells with neutrons offers several theoretical advantages that relate to high LET. One advantage is higher RBE, as just described. Another is the lack of dependence on oxygen for tumor cell death as compared with use of photon beams, which require oxygen free radical generation to indirectly ionize DNA. This oxygen effect is most likely to be important in hypoxic regions of tumors, which should be more sensitive to neutron than to photon radiation. Finally, with neutrons as compared to photons, cell death is less dependent on the phase of the cell cycle.

Although neutron radiation has theoretical advantages, as just described, the clinical utility of high LET beams depends on a differential effect between tumor and normal tissues. For example, if the RBE for neutrons is 9 for tumor cells, but only 3 for normal dose-limiting tissues, then the therapeutic gain will be a factor of 3. Conversely, if the RBE for both tumor and normal tissues is 3, the therapeutic gain is nonexistent. The apparent similarity of neutron RBE between gliomas and neuronal tissues is reflected in the narrow therapeutic window described in clinical studies.[2]

Clinical Results

In 1973, a pilot study of fast neutron beam radiotherapy for patients with high-grade astrocytomas was initiated at the University of Washington, Seattle.[3, 4] The neutron beam was generated with a physics laboratory–based cyclotron that was modified for therapy. The first 26 patients received only neutron radiation. Most patients received whole-brain neutron radiation to a dose of 18 Gy at 1.5-Gy per fraction, two fractions per week. Autopsy data from these early patients showed good tumor control but poor survival as a result of CNS deterioration.[3] Subsequently, the regimen was changed to deliver two fractions per week of neutrons (0.6 Gy per fraction) and three fractions per week of photons (1.8 Gy per fraction). Most of the latter patients received approximate doses of 6.5 Gy of neutrons and 30 Gy of photons to the whole brain, plus ''boost'' doses of 1.5 Gy of neutrons and 7.5 Gy of photons to the region of highest tumor burden. The average survivals were 9.4 and 7.6 months for the neutron and mixed photon/neutron groups, respectively. By comparison, a group of 68 patients treated with photons alone at the same institution had an average survival of 13.3 months. Fifteen patients underwent autopsy. In all 15 cases the tumor was replaced by a mass of coagulation necrosis with a surrounding zone of demyelinization. Only one patient had evidence of tumor recurrence. Diffuse white matter degeneration and demyelinization was found in areas far from the tumor volume. The results suggested that neutron radiation caused greater tumor cell kill than photons, but this higher control did not translate to improved survival due to injury of normal brain tissue.

The Royal Marsden Hospital, London, conducted a pilot trial from 1973 to 1976 in which patients with high-grade astrocytomas were sequentially allocated to treatment with photons or neutrons from the Medical Research Council Cyclotron at Hammersmith Hospital, London.[5] Both types of radiation were delivered using a three-field technique with generous margins around the tumor, such that most of the brain received some radiation. Neutron doses were 15.6 Gy in 12 fractions to the first 18 patients and 13 Gy in 12 fractions to the next 11 patients (one additional patient received 14 Gy). The neutron dose reduction was instituted after it was found that some patients were dying without tumor but with fatal brain damage. Conversely, the initial photon dose of 50 Gy was subsequently increased to 55 Gy because patients were dying of recurrent tumor. The median survival, regardless of treatment, was approximately 10 months. In patients treated with neutrons, a trend toward longer survival was observed in patients treated to 15.6 Gy compared with those treated to 13 Gy; however, the number of patients in each subgroup was too small to determine statistical significance. Moderate to gross residual tumor was present in 86% of the photon group but in only 31% of the neutron group, on analysis of autopsy or second craniotomy specimens. In brain regions distant from the tumor bed, only edema was noted in the photon group, whereas white matter degeneration and focal vascular necrosis was observed in the neutron group.

The results of the University of Washington and Royal Marsden Hospital series were remarkably similar with respect to patient survival and post-treatment histologic findings. The neutron doses were selected based on an estimated RBE of 3.[4] Subsequent experiments in mammals demonstrated that the neutron RBE in central nervous system tissue with fractionated radiation was higher, in the range of 4.2 to 5.2.[6, 7] It was suggested that too high a neutron dose was delivered to a large volume of normal brain.[6]

Results from the Middle Atlantic Neutron Therapy Association (MANTA) appear to contradict those from the University of Washington and the Royal Marsden Hospital.[8] Thirty-one patients with high-grade astrocytomas were treated with neutron or combined neutron/photon radiotherapy. In patients treated with neutrons alone, the dose ranged from 16.4 Gy in 12 fractions to 22.4 Gy in 28 fractions, with a median dose of about 21 Gy. Most of the patients receiving the combined neutron/photon radiotherapy were treated with 50 Gy of photons to the whole brain and 4.7 to 6.2 Gy of neutrons with a reduced field. The median survival for these patients was similar to that reported from the other two institutions.[4, 5] However, the MANTA study found histologic confirmation of persistent disease in seven of eight specimens that were examined by autopsy or repeated biopsy. The reason for the discrepancy of histologic findings between these two series is unclear, but the difficulty in differentiating reactive astrocytes from tumor cells has been acknowledged.[4]

Sixty-two patients with high-grade astrocytomas were treated with fast neutron radiation at the Midwest Institute for Neutron Therapy at Fermilab, Batavia, Ill.[9] Patients were treated with one of three regimens to a total dose of 16 to 18 Gy in six fractions over 2 to 6 weeks. The different regimens were not randomized, and differences existed in treatment volume. Nevertheless, this analysis was carried out to look for large differences in survival as a function of overall treatment time. The median survival for the three regimens ranged from 9.3 to 11.4 months, with no difference between treatment time intervals.

Only one group has suggested a survival benefit with neutrons in patients with high-grade astrocytomas.[10, 11] This series from the neutron facility in Orleans, France, had 98 patients suitable for evaluation who were treated for glioblastoma multiforme with a "concentrated" schedule. These patients received large-volume photon radiation to 18 Gy in three fractions over 3 days, followed 2 to 3 weeks later by a primary site boost with neutrons for an additional 6 or 7 Gy in three fractions. Median survival was 8 months both for patients who had undergone surgery and for those who had not. Compared to historical controls treated with photons alone, the survival of the non-operated cohort appeared to be superior for the patients treated with a neutron boost. Among patients undergoing subtotal resection, survival appeared better for patients receiving the higher-dose (7 Gy) neutron boost compared with the historical controls treated with photons alone. This was not a randomized study, and comparability of performance status between the photon and neutron boost groups was not mentioned. The authors did state that these groups were equivalent with respect to age, sex ratio, and tumor location.

To enhance the effectiveness of neutrons on tumor cell kill within hypoxic regions, the hypoxic cell radiation sensitizer misonidazole was used in combination with neutron radiotherapy at the Fermilab facility.[12] Twenty-four patients were suitable for evaluation on this Radiation Therapy Oncology Group (RTOG) study (79–03) for high-grade astrocytomas. Of the 23 pathology specimens submitted for review, 18 were identified as glioblastoma multiforme and five as anaplastic astrocytoma. Patients received whole-brain neutron radiation to a dose of 12 Gy followed by a boost to the tumor bed to a total of 18 Gy, delivered in six weekly fractions of 3 Gy each. Overall median survival was 12 months, with subgroup median survivals of 10 months for glioblastoma multiforme and 20 months for anaplastic astrocytoma. Ten of 22 patients with follow-up computed tomographic (CT) scans demonstrated radiographic evidence of tumor response. There was histologic evidence of tumor response in seven of 13 examined specimens, and all 13 of these specimens had white matter vascular changes with radiation-induced necrosis. No survival advantage was apparent to use of neutron radiation plus misonidazole on comparison with results of other studies that used photons or neutrons.

The first randomized trial of radiation with a neutron boost vs. photon radiation alone for high-grade astrocytomas was conducted by the RTOG (trial 76–11).[13] This trial consisted of 158 eligible patients. Patients on the neutron boost arm received whole-brain photon radiation to a dose of 50 Gy, followed by a neutron boost to the tumor bed in 6 to 8 fractions to a total dose estimated to be equivalent to 15 Gy of photons, based on the RBE for each facility's beam. The median survivals were 9.8 and 8.6 months for the neutron boost and photon arms, respectively, and the difference was not statistically significant. Consistent with most of the phase II studies, persistent tumor was observed in all 12 autopsied patients on the photon arm and in only three of 12 autopsied patients on the neutron boost arm.

Two smaller randomized trials of neutrons for gliomas were reported by Duncan and co-workers from the Edinburgh neutron facility.[14, 15] In the first study, 34 patients received whole-brain radiation, which was randomized to 47.5 Gy of photons or 13.8 Gy of neutrons in 20 fractions. Twenty-seven of the 34 patients had high-grade astrocytomas, with the remaining patients having mixed gliomas, low-grade astrocytomas, or other glial tumors. The median survival was 11 months after photon radiation and 7 months after neutron radiation. The trial was discontinued early because four of nine neutron-treated patients examined at autopsy had radiation-induced brain injury.[14] In the second trial, 61 patients with high-grade astrocytomas were randomized to receive photons alone to 45 Gy, or photons to 28.5 Gy plus a neutron boost of 5.1 Gy. The median survival was 4 months in the photon/neutron group compared with 8 months in the photon group (difference not statistically significant). There was evidence of residual tumor in all patients in both arms of the study who died.[15]

Concomitant integration of photon and neutron radiation in the treatment of high-grade astrocytomas has also been attempted.[16–19] The rationale for this concomitant scheme is based on experiments in which a dose of neutrons decreased the shoulder on the cell survival curve in response to a subsequent dose of photons. These data were interpreted to show that the priming dose of neutrons decreased sublethal damage repair after photons, particularly when the time interval between neutrons and photons was less than 2 hours.[20] The Edinburgh group reported the results of a phase I trial using a "mixed schedule" of two radiation fractions per day, one each of photons and neutrons, in patients with high-grade astrocytomas.[16] Twelve fractions were delivered over 4 weeks with the photon and neutron fractions given each day separated by 2 to 3 hours. The total doses were 6.36 and 20.4 Gy for the neutron and photon beams, respectively. No clinical signs of radiation-induced toxic effects were evident, and the median survival of 6.9 months was similar to that observed historically with conventional photon radiation.

The National Institute of Radiological Sciences, Chiba, Japan, reported the results of combined photon plus neutron radiotherapy for high-grade astrocytomas.[17] The neutron radiation was delivered through localized fields either sequential to the photon radiation as *boost therapy* or concomitant with the photon radiation as *mixed-beam therapy*. The average neutron and photon doses were 5.7 and 36.9 Gy, respectively. The median survival was 15.5 months, with no difference between either form of combined therapy.

The RTOG (trial 80–07) conducted a randomized dose-searching trial in 190 patients of a concomitant neutron boost with whole-brain photon radiation.[18] Whole-brain photon radiation was delivered at 1.5 Gy per fraction, 5 days per week, to a total dose of 45 Gy. Two days per week, neutron radiation was given within 3 hours prior to the photon radiation, directed at the tumor volume determined by CT scan. The neutron doses were randomized among six levels from 3.6 to 6 Gy. Overall, the median survival was 11.5 months, with no difference between neutron dose levels. Autopsies in 35 patients revealed both brain injury and viable tumor at all doses, with no evidence of a therapeutic window. Although patients with anaplastic astrocytoma had a higher median survival than those with glioblastoma multiforme (22 months vs. 9.9 months), anaplastic astrocytoma patients appeared to have a lower survival with higher neutron boost doses. This inverse relationship between neutron dose and survival in anaplastic astrocytoma patients was not statistically significant. The high-dose group included 24 anaplastic astrocytoma patients, and the low-dose group included only 6 anaplastic astrocytoma patients. Laramore and colleagues[21] later included these results in an analysis of RTOG data that suggested a correlation between more aggressive therapy (neutrons or chemotherapy plus photons) and decreased survival in patients with anaplastic astrocytoma.

The University of Chicago reported 44 patients with high-grade astrocytomas treated with whole-brain photon radiation and a concomitant neutron boost.[19] This institution participated in RTOG 80–07, but had a better outcome than that reported for the overall study. The protocol was continued at the University of Chicago using the 5.2-Gy boost dose of neutrons in addition to the 45-Gy whole-brain radiation photon dose. Neutrons were delivered 5 to 20 minutes prior to photons on 2 days/week. This short time interval was in contrast to the 2 to 3 hours used at other institutions on RTOG 80–07. Overall, the median survival was 10 months. However, the median survival for the 10 patients with anaplastic astrocytoma was 40.3 months, almost double that seen on the RTOG study. Possible reasons for the conflicting results are that in the University of Chicago series only 10 patients had anaplastic astrocytoma, the median age was only 45.5 years, the median Karnofsky score was 95, and the interval between neutrons and photons was short.[88]

A pilot study of neutron interstitial brachytherapy using californium-252 in 56 patients with high-grade astrocytomas has been reported from the University of Kentucky, Lexington.[22] After tumors were surgically debulked, ^{252}Cf sources were afterloaded into catheters placed under CT guidance. The radioactive sources were removed after delivery of 3 Gy over 4 to 6 hours to the residual tumor target. Patients then received external beam photon radiation to doses of 60 to 70 Gy. Median survival was 10 months, with recurrent tumor found in all autopsy specimens. The rationale for this interstitial treatment was the common finding of tumor eradication in association with normal brain injury in previous studies that used external beam neutrons. Interstitial ^{252}Cf therapy represents an attractive technique to better localize a neutron boost to the tumor volume. However, the results of this pilot study were not better than those expected with conventional photon radiation.

A summary of the fast neutron trials that included at least 10 patients with high-grade astrocytomas is presented in Table 39–1. The average of the reported median survivals weighted by the number of patients with follow-up in each trial is 10 months. No difference is apparent between the results using neutrons alone or those using neutrons in combination with photon radiation. The fast neutron trials to date have failed to demonstrate a therapeutic window that would allow improvement beyond the survival achieved with conventional photon radiotherapy. More precise neutron dose localization using ^{252}Cf implantation also resulted in a median survival of 10 months. Although dose escalation studies with this technique of brachytherapy have been pro-

TABLE 39–1

SURVIVAL AFTER FAST NEUTRON RADIATION FOR HIGH-GRADE ASTROCYTOMAS

Study	No. of Patients*	Median Survival (mo)
Neutrons		
Laramore et al.[4]	26	9.4
Herskovic et al.[8]	17	11
Catterall et al.[5]	30	10
Kurup et al.[12]	24	12
Duncan et al.[14]	18	7
Saroja et al.[9]	62	11
Total	177	10.3†
Neutrons and Photons		
Laramore et al.[4]	10	7.6
Herskovic et al.[8]	13	8
Mizoe et al.[17]	39	15.5
Breteau et al.[11]	98	7
Griffin et al.[13]	80	9.8
Duncan et al.[15]	31	4
Duncan et al.[16]	50	6.9
Laramore et al.[18]	190	11.5
Kolker et al.[19]	44	12
Batterman[58]	22	9
Total	557	9.8†

*Number of patients with follow-up.
†Average of median survivals weighted by the number of patients from each individual study.

posed,[22] it remains to be determined if the degree of increased brain toxic effects will negate improvement in tumor eradication.

BORON NEUTRON CAPTURE THERAPY

Physical and Biologic Principles

Boron neutron capture therapy is a form of binary therapy. Two agents, which individually are non-lethal, are combined to effect tumor cell death. Barth and others have reviewed the physical and biologic principles of boron neutron capture therapy.[23] One component of boron neutron capture therapy is the target, consisting of boron-10, a stable isotope of boron. Low-energy neutrons, referred to as *thermal neutrons* (.025 eV) or *epithermal neutrons* (1 to 10,000 eV), are the other component of this binary system. Either of these components alone would not cause cell death except at very high doses. However, ^{10}B represents a large target for collision with thermal neutrons. This collision results in recoil particles, which consist of α particles and lithium-7 nuclei. These recoil particles are of high LET and have a short path length, approximately the diameter of a cell, which results in a high RBE.

The therapeutic utility of boron neutron capture therapy faces two major challenges. The first challenge is the development of boronated compounds that may be selectively incorporated into tumor cells. The initial experiments to develop these compounds were undertaken at the Massachusetts General Hospital, Boston, with emphasis on localization within gliomas.[24, 25] After studying 140 boronated compounds in animals, the six most favorable compounds were tested in humans. Sweet and colleagues administered these compounds intravenously, and measured their levels in tumor and in normal brain tissue that had been removed at surgery. The tumor-to-normal brain ratios of boronated compounds increased over 15 to 45 minutes in the range of 3:1 to 5:1.[25] Clinical trials of the most favorable of these initial compounds were not encouraging, and further animal experimentation led to the development of sulfhydryl-containing boronated compounds.[26] One of these compounds, ^{10}B-sodium-mercaptoundecahydrododecaborate (^{10}B-Na$_2$B$_{12}$H$_{11}$SH, or BSH), has been used by Hatanaka and others in the largest clinical experience with boron neutron capture therapy for brain tumors.[27, 28] The levels of BSH within brain tumors and normal tissues vary with dose, dose rate, route of administration, time of measurement after administration, tumor histologic characteristics, extent of tumor necrosis, and individual differences in clearance. Because of the variables and the limited availability of human data, it is not possible to characterize the clinical pharmacokinetics of BSH with a high degree of certainty. It does appear that after intravenous administration of BSH the concentration of boron reaches a maximum in brain tumors after 3 hours and declines thereafter.[29] Blood concentrations decline at a faster rate, such that tumor-to-blood ratios rise from less than 1 at 3 hours to 1.5 or 2 at 24 hours postinjection. The ratio of boron in tumor to "normal" peritumoral brain was found to be greater than 3 at all times. However, large variations in boron concentration within a tumor corresponding to histologic heterogeneity have been documented.[30] The Brookhaven National Laboratory, Upton, NY, reported the distribution of BSH after a 25-hour continuous infusion in a terminally ill patient with malignant astrocytoma.[31] Tissues were examined post-mortem for ^{10}B content 19 hours after discontinuation of the infusion. A 5- to 15-fold preference was found for distribution of ^{10}B within tumor in the brain and spinal cord compared with normal central nervous system parenchyma.

The second important challenge to the clinical application of effective boron neutron capture therapy is the delivery of an adequate dose of low-energy neutrons to tumors located deep within the brain. Most of the clinical experience with boron neutron capture therapy has utilized thermal neutrons. These thermal neutrons are derived from nuclear reactors after slowing through a scattering material, such as heavy or light water or graphite. Epithermal neutrons may be obtained by filtering fast neutron beams with aluminum, sulfur, cadmium, lithium, and bismuth. The dose distribution as a function of depth has been detailed for thermal and epithermal neutron beams that are available at the Massachusetts Institute of Technology Research Reactor in Cambridge, Mass.[32] It was determined that the thermal neutron beams would be useful for tumors at relatively shallow depths in the brain (5 cm or less). Conversely, epithermal beams would be advantageous at depths of greater than 6 cm through bilateral fields.

Several studies that have been carried out in animals suggest selective and efficacious tumor cell killing with boron neutron capture therapy. Results from a rat glioma model have been reported.[33, 34] The therapeutically refractory F-98 anaplastic glioma cells were implanted into the brains

of rats, and boron neutron capture therapy was conducted 12 or 13 days after implantation using BSH and a thermal neutron beam.[33] For experiments in which adequate body shielding and head stabilization were employed, boron neutron capture therapy with a thermal neutron fluence of 4×10^{12}/cm^2 resulted in a median survival of 39 days, compared with 28 days for untreated controls ($P = .005$), and 36.5 days for the same radiation without BSH ($P < .03$). The microvascular response to boron neutron capture therapy in this model was studied in detail. In rats without transplanted tumors, no changes were evident immediately after boron neutron capture therapy or 10 months later. Eighteen months after boron neutron capture therapy, minimal changes were evident on electron microscopy; these consisted of clusters of vesicles bound to the cell membrane of pericytes, but no endothelial cell damage was observed. In contrast, the rats with implanted gliomas demonstrated increased peritumoral edema 3 days after boron neutron capture therapy along with peritumoral necrosis 7 days after therapy. These changes were attributed to a pathologic endothelial response as supported by histologic evidence of vascular proliferation with breakdown of the blood-brain barrier.[34]

Additional experiments have investigated the issue of normal brain tolerance using a model consisting of 9L rat gliosarcoma tumors implanted into rat brains.[35] Animals were treated with either boron neutron capture therapy using p-boronophenylalanine (BPA) and thermal neutrons (7.5 MW-minute) or with 250 kV x-rays (22.5 Gy). Rats that survived at least 6 months after treatment were studied for histopathologic changes attributable to treatment. Long-term survivors after boron neutron capture therapy were found to have relatively normal brains, whereas those treated with x-rays had significant damage to neurons and loss of blood-brain barrier integrity. No viable tumor was found in the long-term survivors regardless of treatment. This study supports the hypothesis that a therapeutic gain can be achieved with boron neutron capture therapy relative to x-ray therapy.

It has been suggested that the increased survival after boron neutron capture therapy in rats with implanted glial tumors was due to a "tumor bed" effect involving endothelial cells and normal tissue components. To investigate this hypothesis, rats were implanted with F98 anaplastic glioma tumors and injected intravenously with BSH 14 to 17 hours prior to thermal neutron radiation.[36] Controls were implanted with tumors but did not receive boron neutron capture therapy. A "pretreatment" group received boron neutron capture therapy 4 hours prior to tumor implantation. The mean survival for the group treated with boron neutron capture therapy after tumor implantation was 33 days. The control and "pretreatment" groups had significantly shorter mean survival times of 26 days after implantation. Furthermore, the size of tumors measured at the time of death was equivalent between all groups. It was concluded from these data that the increased survival after boron neutron capture therapy was attributable to direct effects on tumor cells or peritumoral neovascularity and not to a "tumor bed" effect.

Animal studies have also provided information on optimal timing for neutron radiation after BSH administration.[37] In the F98 rat glioma model, delivery of thermal neutron radiation 13.5 hours after intravenous administration of BSH resulted in longer survival compared with survival after delivery of radiation 3, 6, 18.5, or 23.5 hours subsequent to administration of BSH. Pharmacokinetic studies indicated a concentration in tumor of only 1.1 μg of ^{10}B per gram of tissue at 12 hours after injection with BSH, which was below the level required for tumor eradication.

Thermal neutron dose-response data and comparison of outcome with x-irradiation have been evaluated.[38] Rats with intracerebrally implanted GS-9L gliosarcomas received a sulfhydryl boron dimer by continuous intravenous infusion from 11 through 14 days after tumor implantation. The boron concentrations were approximately 30 μg/g in tumor and only 1.4 μg/g in brain parenchyma. On day 14, animals were exposed to thermal neutrons at doses of 5.0 or 7.5 MW-minute. These doses gave estimated thermal neutron fluences within the tumors of 2×10^{12} or 3×10^{12} neutrons/cm^2. With boron neutron capture therapy using the lower neutron radiation dose, the median survival after implantation was 60 days. At the higher neutron radiation dose the median survival had not been reached after more than 10 months. Median survival after tumor implantation with boron neutron capture therapy was superior to that in untreated animals (21 days), animals treated with equivalent doses of thermal neutrons without the boronated compound (26 or 28 days), and animals receiving x-rays at doses of the same gray-equivalents (Gy-equivalents) (26 or 31 days). Similar improvement in survival with boron neutron capture therapy has been observed in rat and mouse glioma models with BPA given orally[39, 40] or intraperitoneally.[41] Although BPA has been considered primarily as an agent for treatment of melanoma with boron neutron capture therapy, it also appears to have favorable pharmacokinetic and tumor cytotoxic response characteristics in this glioma model.

Hawthorne[42] has reviewed a wide variety of boronated compounds with potential for use in boron neutron capture therapy. The clinical usefulness of boron neutron capture therapy will depend on development of innovative boronated compounds and/or delivery systems to provide favorable tumor concentrations and selectivity.

Another consideration in boron neutron capture therapy is the possible use of fast neutron beams. Hospital-based fast neutron facilities with treatment capabilities comparable to linear accelerators are currently in use. Laramore and co-workers[43] have investigated the thermal neutron "contamination" of the fast neutron beam at the University of Washington Medical Center cyclotron. A mathematical model predicted a 10- to 100-fold enhancement of tumor cell kill by boron neutron capture therapy with a fast neutron beam and 3×10^9 to 6×10^9 ^{10}B per cell. To test this model, V-79 cell cultures were radiated with fast neutrons through a water phantom at a depth of 5 to 6 cm with or without ^{10}B-containing medium. The in vitro data were consistent with the predictions of the mathematical model within a factor of two. It was suggested that boron neutron capture therapy using fast neutron beams to achieve a "concomitant boost" was worthy of further study and could provide a means of treating deeper tumors, such as lung and prostate lesions, that are problematic for thermal or epithermal neutron beams.

Clinical Results

Early human trials of boron neutron capture therapy were undertaken at the Massachusetts General Hospital using *para*-carboxybenzeneboronic acid made with ^{10}B, after preclinical evaluation of 140 compounds.[25] Sixteen patients with glioblastoma multiforme were treated with boron neutron capture therapy 2 to 3 weeks after craniotomy from 1960 to 1961. Patients received the drug intravenously, and the patients were then exposed to thermal neutrons from the core of the nuclear reactor at the Massachusetts Institute of Technology. Patients were exposed for 30 to 105 minutes with scalp, muscle, and bone reflected out of the field. The median survival was only 6 months, and it was concluded by the investigators that the neutron dose was too low. Neuropathologic evaluation in 14 of these cases revealed significant endothelial damage, which was attributed to poor selectivity in ^{10}B distribution and suboptimal beam factors.[44]

In 1975, Hatanaka[45] reported two previously untreated patients with glioblastoma multiforme who were alive without neurologic deficit 3 years after treatment with boron neutron capture therapy using BSH. Other patients who were treated with boron neutron capture therapy after failing initial conventional radiotherapy with ^{60}Co exhibited significant toxic response. An updated summary of 38 patients treated with boron neutron capture therapy for grade 3 and 4 gliomas before July 1985 revealed a median survival of 41 weeks and a 5-year actuarial survival of 19%.[46] Sixteen of these patients had tumors no deeper than 6 cm. Among these 16 patients with shallow tumors, the median survival was 110 weeks and the 5-year actuarial survival was 58%. These results were compared with those in 46 patients with grade 3 and 4 gliomas who were treated with surgery, conventional radiation, and chemotherapy, due to unavailability of the reactor or shortage of ^{10}B. The conventionally treated patients had a median survival of 50 weeks and a 5-year actuarial survival of only 5%.

More recently, Hatanaka and Nakagawa[46] have presented the results of long-term survivors who were treated with boron neutron capture therapy for brain tumors.[46] Of 87 patients treated for intracranial tumors before May 1987, 18 patients (21%) lived longer than 5 years. Of 53 patients treated before May 1982, nine (17%) lived at least 10 years. Among these nine long-term survivors, the three patients for whom prior conventional radiotherapy had failed were incapacitated from toxic effects of retreatment. The six long-term survivors who underwent boron neutron capture therapy without prior radiation had no functional deficit. It should be noted that only four of these nine long-term survivors had a diagnosis of glioblastoma multiforme. Although it appears that boron neutron capture therapy has the capability to cure some cases of glioblastoma multiforme, determination of the frequency of these cures and comparison to conventional radiotherapy cannot be achieved until controlled clinical trials are undertaken.

Human clinical trials of boron neutron capture therapy for malignant gliomas have recently resumed at the Brookhaven National Laboratory reactor. Unlike the case of the Japanese trial, BPA is being used as the ^{10}B-carrier. Trials will also soon start in Europe using BSH as the ^{10}B-carrier.

CHARGED PARTICLE BEAMS
Physical and Biologic Principles

The primary advantage of charged particle beams is improved dose distribution. Unlike neutrons, charged particles such as protons, α particles, pions, and heavier ions (e.g., neon and carbon) exhibit a Bragg peak type of dose deposition. The Bragg peak is illustrated in Figure 39–2 and represents a large deposition of dose near the end of the path of a charged particle beam. The Bragg peak may be broadened by passing the beam through filters of varying thickness. The result is a composite dose distribution that conforms to the target. This improved dose distribution has been the basis for attempting escalation of radiation doses to tumor without increasing toxic effects in normal tissue. Dose-volume analyses comparing three-dimensional treatment plans for high dose x-ray or proton beam radiation in patients with astrocytomas have illustrated the potential sparing of normal brain tissue volume with protons.[47, 48] Some charged particle beams, such as pions, neon ions, and carbon ions, also exhibit increased LET in addition to a Bragg peak dose distribution. However, the gain in LET for these charged particles is small in comparison to that of neutrons, and its clinical significance is unclear.

The unique interactions of pions with tissues deserve special consideration. A therapeutic role for pions was first proposed in 1961 by Fowler and Perkins.[49] These particles have a mass between that of an electron and a proton. Pions exhibit a Bragg peak dose distribution, and at the end of their path, they interact with tissue atoms with the release of characteristic x-rays and eventual capture by the nucleus. The result of this capture is fragmentation of the nucleus into various combinations of protons, neutrons, and α particles, producing the so-called ''star'' of ionizing fragments.

Clinical Results

Neuropathologic effects of proton beam radiation for intracranial neoplasms in humans were reported from the Massa-chusetts General Hospital.[50] Ten patients were treated for various intracranial tumors. Histologic grading of radiation injury was found to correlate with radiation dose. The relationship between injury and proton dose was similar to that observed for x-rays.

Early clinical results for the treatment of malignant gliomas were reported by Graffman and colleagues in 1975,[51] in which seven patients were treated with fractionated high-energy protons. Subsequent histologic evaluation was available in four cases, all of which showed tumor necrosis combined with viable tumor cells. No evidence of injury to normal brain tissue was observed. The authors concluded that the RBE of high-energy protons was similar to that of ^{60}Co γ-radiation, and that dose escalation with protons was feasible.

Austin-Seymour and others[52] reported on seven patients treated with protons to an average dose of 73.1 cobalt Gy-equivalents for intermediate- to high-grade gliomas. One patient was alive 68 months after radiation and the others died 2 to 62 months after treatment.[52]

The Japanese experience with proton beam radiation has been reported to include five patients with glioblastoma multiforme. All five patients have had local failure, and two patients have died. Median follow-up was not specified.[53]

The results of a phase I and II clinical trial of heavy charged particle radiation were reported from the Lawrence Berkeley Laboratory, Berkeley, Calif, in 1985.[54] Thirty-three previously untreated patients with primary or recurrent gliomas were treated with helium, neon, or carbon ion beams. A broad range of doses was used in this study due to uncertainty about RBE factors. The estimated total tumor doses ranged from 48 to 72 photon Gy-equivalents. Among the 17 patients with glioblastoma multiforme, the median survival was 13.9 months, with no patients surviving to 3 years. However, findings seemed to confirm a dose-response relationship for survival. For patients with anaplastic astrocytoma, the median survival was only 7.6 months, with no evidence of a dose-response relationship. It was emphasized that these patients were treated with gradually escalating doses and evolving treatment planning and beam delivery techniques.

Limited data exist on the use of pions for the treatment of high-grade gliomas. Among 230 patients treated at the Los Alamos Meson Physics Facility, Los Alamos, NM, 42 had glioblastoma multiforme or anaplastic astrocytoma.[55] Median survival was 10 months in patients with glioblastoma multiforme and 22 months in patients with anaplastic astrocytoma. A pilot study was performed at the University of British Columbia, Vancouver, in which 53 patients with high-grade astrocytomas were treated with escalating doses of pions.[56] Initially, patients received whole-brain photon radiation followed by a focal pion boost. Later, patients received only pion radiation to a field consisting of the gross tumor volume plus 2 cm. The pion dose was escalated from 17.5 to 36 Gy. A significant improvement in survival was observed for patients receiving localized pions at doses of 30 to 33 Gy compared with treatments of combined whole-brain x-irradiation plus a lower boost dose of pions. The longest median survival in any of the treatment groups was 14.3 months for the 33 Gy pion group. However, the survival decreased on further escalation to a pion dose of 36 Gy. It

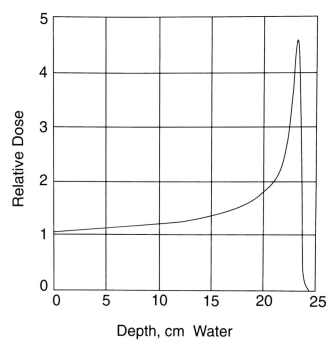

Figure 39–2 Depth-dose distribution showing the Bragg peak for protons from the Uppsala synchrocyclotron. (From Larsson B: Pre-therapeutic physical experiments with high energy protons. Br J Radiol 1961; 34:143.)

should be noted that a large portion (43%) of the patients in this study had anaplastic astrocytoma. Among patients with glioblastoma multiforme, the median survival was only 7.8 months.

Another small study from Switzerland included 20 patients with high-grade astrocytomas who were treated with pions.[57] The proportion of patients with glioblastoma multiforme is unclear in this report. Fifteen patients were alive 9 months after therapy, but only one of these patients had local tumor control.

CONCLUSIONS

Particle beam radiation offers theoretical advantages over conventional photon radiation with respect to relative biologic effectiveness, oxygen enhancement ratio, and/or dose distribution. However, no clinical evidence of a therapeutic gain has been established. Efforts continue with charged particle radiation to allow safe localized dose escalation in an attempt to improve control of high-grade astrocytomas. With recent advances in epithermal neutron beams and tumor-selective agents for delivery of boronated compounds, boron neutron capture therapy may offer the greatest opportunity to enhance survival of patients with high-grade astrocytomas.

REFERENCES

1. Stelzer KJ, Laramore GE, Griffin TW, et al: Fast neutron radiotherapy: The University of Washington experience. Acta Oncol 1994; 33:275.
2. Laramore GE: Neutron radiotherapy for high grade gliomas: The search for the elusive therapeutic window. Int J Radiat Oncol Biol Phys 1990; 19:493.
3. Parker RG, Berry HC, Gerdes AJ, et al: Fast neutron beam radiotherapy of glioblastoma multiforme. AJR 1976; 127:331.
4. Laramore GE, Griffin TW, Gerdes AJ, et al: Fast neutron and mixed (neutron/photon) beam teletherapy for grades III and IV astrocytomas. Cancer 1978; 42:96.
5. Catterall M, Bloom JG, Ash DV, et al: Fast neutrons compared with megavoltage x-rays in the treatment of patients with supratentorial glioblastoma: A controlled pilot study. Int J Radiat Oncol Biol Phys 1980; 6:261.
6. Hornsey S, Morris CC, Myers R, et al: Relative biological effectiveness for damage to the central nervous system by neutrons. Int J Radiat Oncol Biol Phys 1981; 7:185.
7. Stephens LC, Hussey DH, Raulston GL, et al: Late effects of 50 MeVd→Be neutron and cobalt-60 irradiation of rhesus monkey cervical spinal cord. Int J Radiat Oncol Biol Phys 1983; 9:859.
8. Herskovic A, Ornitz RD, Shell M, et al: Treatment experience: Glioblastoma multiforme treated with 15 MeV fast neutrons. Cancer 1982; 49:2463.
9. Saroja KR, Mansell J, Hendrickson FR, et al: Failure of accelerated neutron therapy to control high grade astrocytomas. Int J Radiat Oncol Biol Phys 1989; 17:1295.
10. Breteau N, Destembert B, Sabattier R: An interim assessment of the experience of fast neutron boost in glioblastomas, rectal and bronchus carcinomas in Orleans. Strahlenther Onkol 1985; 161:787.
11. Breteau N, Destembert B, Favre A, et al: Fast neutron boost for the treatment of grade IV astrocytomas. Strahlenther Onkol 1989; 165:320.
12. Kurup PD, Pajak TF, Hendrickson FR, et al: Fast neutrons and misonidazole for malignant astrocytomas. Int J Radiat Oncol Biol Phys 1985; 11:679.
13. Griffin TW, Davis R, Laramore G, et al: Fast neutron radiation therapy for glioblastoma multiforme. Results of an RTOG study. Am J Clin Oncol 1983; 6:661.
14. Duncan W, McLelland J, Jack WJ, et al: Report of a randomised pilot study of the treatment of patients with supratentorial gliomas using neutron irradiation. Br J Radiol 1986; 59:373.
15. Duncan W, McLelland J, Jack WJ, et al: The results of a randomised trial of mixed-schedule (neutron/photon) irradiation in the treatment of supratentorial grade III and grade IV astrocytoma. Br J Radiol 1986; 59:379.
16. Duncan W, McLelland J, Davey P, et al: A phase I study of mixed (neutron and photon) irradiation using two fractions per day in the treatment of high-grade astrocytomas. Br J Radiol 1986; 59:441.
17. Mizoe JE, Aoki Y, Morita S, et al: Fast neutron therapy for malignant gliomas: Results from NIRS study. Strahlenther Onkol 1993; 169:222.
18. Laramore GE, Diener-West M, Griffin TW, et al: Randomized neutron dose searching study for malignant gliomas of the brain: Results of an RTOG study. Int J Radiat Oncol Biol Phys 1988; 14:1093.
19. Kolker JD, Hapern HJ, Krishnasamy S, et al: "Instant-mix" whole brain photon with neutron boost radiotherapy for malignant gliomas. Int J Radiat Oncol Biol Phys 1990; 19:493.
20. Ngo FQH, Han A, Elkind MM: On the repair of sublethal damage in V79 Chinese hamster cells resulting from irradiation with fast neutrons combined with X-rays. Int J Radiat Biol 1977; 32:507.
21. Laramore GE, Martz KL, Nelson JS, et al: Radiation Therapy Oncology Group (RTOG) survival data on anaplastic astrocytomas of the brain: Does a more aggressive form of treatment adversely impact survival? Int J Radiat Oncol Biol Phys 1989; 17:1351.
22. Patchell RA, Maruyama Y, Tibbs PA, et al: Neutron interstitial brachytherapy for malignant gliomas: A pilot study. J Neurosurg 1988; 68:67.
23. Barth RF, Soloway AH, Fairchild RG, et al: Boron neutron capture therapy for cancer. Cancer 1992; 70:2995.
24. Soloway AH, Wright RL, Messer JR: Evaluation of boron compounds for use in neutron capture therapy of brain tumors: I. Animal investigations. J Pharmacol Exp Ther 1961; 134:117.
25. Sweet WH, Soloway AH, Brownell GL: Boron-slow neutron capture therapy of gliomas. Acta Radiol Ther Phys Biol 1963; 1:114.
26. Soloway AH, Hatanaka H, Davis MA: Penetration of brain and brain tumor: VII. Tumor-binding sulfhydryl boron compounds. J Med Chem 1967; 10:714.
27. Hatanaka H, Kamano S, Amano K, et al: Clinical experience of boron-neutron capture therapy for gliomas: A comparison with conventional chemo-immuno-radiotherapy. In Hatanaka H (ed): Boron Neutron Capture Therapy for Tumors. Nigata, Japan, Nishimura, 1986, p 349.
28. Hatanaka H, Nakagawa Y: Clinical results of long-surviving brain tumor patients who underwent boron neutron capture therapy. Int J Radiat Oncol Biol Phys 1994; 28:1061.
29. Stragliotto G, Schupbach D, Gavin PR, et al: Update on biodistribution of borocaptate sodium (BSH) in patients with intracranial tumors. In Soloway AH, Barth RF, Carpenter DE (eds): Advances in Neutron Capture Therapy. New York, Plenum, 1993, p 719.
30. Haritz D, Gabel D, Klein H, et al: Results of continued clinical investigations of BSH in patients with malignant glioma. In Soloway AH, Barth RF, Carpenter DE (eds): Advances in Neutron Capture therapy. New York, Plenum, 1993, p 727.
31. Finkel GC, Poletti CE, Fairchild RG, et al: Distribution of ^{10}B after infusion of $Na_2{}^{10}B_{12}H_{11}SH$ into a patient with malignant astrocytoma: Implications for boron neutron capture therapy. Neurosurgery 1989; 24:6.
32. Choi JR, Clement SD, Harling OK, et al: Neutron capture therapy beams at the MIT Research Reactor. Basic Life Sci 1990; 54:201.
33. Clendenon NR, Barth RF, Goodman JH, et al: Enhanced survival in a rat glioma model following BNCT. Strahlenther Onkol 1989; 165:222.
34. Goodman JH, McGregor JM, Clendenon NR, et al: Ultrastructural microvascular response to boron neutron capture therapy in an experimental model. Neurosurgery 1989; 24:701.
35. Coderre J, Rubin P, Freedman, et al: Selective ablation of rat brain tumors by boron neutron capture therapy. Int J Radiat Oncol Biol Phys 1994; 28:1067.
36. Goodman JH, McGregor JM, Clendenon NR, et al: Inhibition of tumor growth in a glioma model treated with boron neutron capture therapy. Neurosurgery 1990; 27:383.
37. Clendenon NR, Barth RF, Gordon WA, et al: Boron neutron capture tharapy of a rat glioma. Neurosurgery 1990; 26:47.
38. Joel DD, Fairchild RG, Laissue, et al: Boron neutron capture therapy of intracerebral rat gliosarcomas. Proc Natl Acad Sci USA 1990; 87:9808.
39. Coderre JA, Joel DD, Micca PL, et al: Control of intracerebral gliosar-

comas in rats by boron neutron capture therapy with *p*-boronophenyla-lanine. Radiat Res 1992; 129:290.

40. Saris SC, Solares GR, Wazer DE, et al: Boron neutron capture therapy for murine malignant gliomas. Cancer Res 1992; 52:4672.

41. Matalka KZ, Barth RF, Staubus AE, et al: Neutron capture therapy of a rat glioma using boronophenylalanine as a capture agent. Radiat Res 1994; 137:44.

42. Hawthorne MF: The role of chemistry in the development of boron neutron capture therapy of cancer. Angewandte Chemie 1993; 32:950.

43. Laramore GE, Wootton P, Livesey JC, et al: Boron neutron capture therapy: A mechanism for achieving a concomitant tumor boost in fast neutron radiotherapy. Int J Radiat Oncol Biol Phys 1994; 28:1135.

44. Asbury AK, Ojemann R, Nielsen SL, et al: Neuropathologic study of 14 cases of malignant brain tumors treated by boron-10 slow neutron capture therapy. J Neuropathol Exp Neurol 1972; 31:278.

45. Hatanaka H: A revised boron-neutron capture therapy for malignant brain tumors: II. Interim clinical result with the patients excluding previous treatments. J Neurol 1975; 209:81.

46. Hatanaka H, Nakagawa Y: Clinical results of long-surviving brain tumor patients who underwent boron neutron capture therapy. Int J Radiat Oncol Biol Phys 1994; 28:1061.

47. Tatsuzaki H, Urie MM, Linggood R: Comparative treatment planning: Proton vs x-ray beams against glioblastoma multiforme. Int J Radiat Oncol Biol Phys 1991; 22:265.

48. Archambeau JO, Slater JD, Slater JM, et al: Role for proton beam irradiation in treatment of pediatric CNS malignancies. Int J Radiat Oncol Biol Phys 1991; 22:287.

49. Fowler PH, Perkins DH: The possibility of therapeutic applications of beams of negative π-mesons. Nature 1961; 189:524.

50. Nielsen SL, Kjellberg RN, Asbury AK, et al: Neuropathologic effects of proton-beam irradiation in man: I. Dose-response relationships after treatment of intracranial neoplasms. Acta Neuropathol 1972; 20:348.

51. Graffman S, Haymaker W, Hugosson R, et al: High-energy protons in the postoperative treatment of malignant glioma. Acta Radiol Ther Phys Biol 1975; 14:443.

52. Austin-Seymour M, Munzenrider JE, Goitein M, et al: Progress in low-LET heavy particle therapy: Intracranial and paracranial tumors and uveal melanomas. Radiat Res 1985; 8:S219.

53. Tsunemoto H, Morita S, Ishikawa T, et al: Proton therapy in Japan. Radiat Res 1985; 8:S235.

54. Castro JR, Saunders WM, Austin-Seymour MM, et al: A phase I-II trial of heavy charged particle irradiation of malignant glioma of the brain: A Northern California Oncology Group study. Int J Radiat Oncol Biol Phys 1985; 11:1795.

55. Bush SE, Smith AR, Zink S: Pion radiotherapy at LAMPF. Int J Radiat Oncol Biol Phys 1982; 8:2181.

56. Goodman GB, Skarsgard LD, Thompson GB, et al: Pion therapy at TRIUMF: Treatment results for astrocytoma grades 3 and 4: A pilot study. Radiother Oncol 1990; 17:21.

57. Greiner R, von Essen CF, Blattman H, et al: Results of curative pion therapy at SIN. Strahlenther Onkol 1985; 161:797.

58. Batterman JJ: Fast neutron therapy for advanced brain tumors. Int J Radiat Oncol Biol Phys 1980; 6:333.

PENNY K. SNEED

PHILIP H. GUTIN

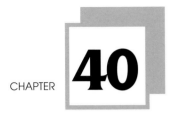

CHAPTER **40**

Interstitial Radiation and Hyperthermia

Brachytherapy means treatment at short range and refers to placement of radiation sources directly inside a tumor, as in interstitial irradiation, or in close proximity to a tumor. The rationale for interstitial radiation of malignant gliomas lies in the fact that radiation has proven efficacy, but the dose is limited by the tolerance of normal brain tissue. Interstitially implanted radiation sources allow delivery of a high tumor dose while limiting dose to surrounding brain tissue. Continuous low-dose-rate radiation has radiobiologic advantages. Hyperthermia is being investigated in combination with brachytherapy in an attempt to improve local control through direct tumor cell kill, tumor reoxygenation, and radiosensitization. This chapter reviews the pertinent physics and radiobiology of interstitial radiation and hyperthermia, patient selection, treatment techniques, and results.

RATIONALE

Analyses of successive Brain Tumor Study Group (BTSG) trials and one prospective randomized trial have demonstrated increased survival of patients with malignant gliomas treated with increasing doses of postoperative external beam radiation therapy over a range from 45 to 62 Gy.[1, 2] However, the risk of brain necrosis increases with doses above 60 to 70 Gy[3, 4] and external beam radiotherapy doses greater than 60 Gy have not generally been associated with increased survival.[5, 6] Although tumor cells may infiltrate well beyond the edge of contrast enhancement visualized on computed tomography (CT) or magnetic resonance imaging (MRI),[7, 8] most recurrences manifest locally after conventional radiotherapy.[9–14]

Radiation Physics Considerations

The use of interstitial brachytherapy allows escalation of the local tumor dose while limiting dose to surrounding tissues because of the very rapid falloff in dose rate outside of an array of radiation sources. The dose from a point source of radiation decreases with the square of the distance away from the source and also decreases due to attenuation in

tissue. Computerized treatment planning makes it possible to design an array of radiation sources that produces an isodose contour that conforms well to a three-dimensional tumor volume.

The most commonly used isotopes include iodine 125 and iridium 192. Iodine 125 emits x-rays with an average energy of 28.5 keV and has a half-life of 59.6 days.[15] Temporary implants designed to deliver 0.4 to 0.6 Gy/hour typically utilize high-activity 5 to 20-mCi ^{125}I sources loaded individually into catheters. Iridium 192 has a half-life of 74.2 days and emits both 0.67-MeV β-particles and γ-rays with an average energy of 0.37 MeV. Due to much lower energy, ^{125}I can be easily shielded with a 0.5-mm layer of lead, whereas ^{192}Ir requires shielding with a considerable thickness of lead.

Remote afterloaders are available for low-dose-rate, pulse-simulated low-dose-rate, or high-dose-rate brachytherapy. Low-dose-rate afterloaders withdraw sources into a shielded safe whenever the patient's room is entered, eliminating radiation exposure of hospital personnel. Pulse-simulated low-dose-rate and high-dose-rate remote afterloaders step a single high-activity ^{192}Ir source through a sequence of treatment positions using varying dwell times to create optimized isodose contours. Treatments using low-dose-rate and pulse-simulated low-dose-rate afterloaders generally take place over many hours or several days, whereas high-dose-rate treatments take minutes to deliver and are often given in multiple fractions of 5 to 8 Gy, weekly or twice weekly.

Radiobiologic Considerations

Interstitial radiation using temporary implants is typically given at a dose rate of about 0.3 to 1.0 Gy/hour, in contrast to a dose rate of about 2 to 4 Gy/minute for external beam radiotherapy. Continuous low-dose-rate radiation tends to make proliferating tumor cells accumulate during G_2, a radiosensitive phase of the cell cycle, whereas noncycling neuronal cells tend to remain in G_1, a more radioresistant phase.[16] Another well-known radiobiologic effect has to do with the fact that hypoxic cells, which are commonly found within malignant gliomas, are three times more resistant to radiation than are normally oxygenated cells. This "oxygen

499

effect'' is less for low-dose-rate radiation, probably due to impaired repair of sublethal radiation damage under hypoxic conditions.[17, 18] In addition, hypoxic tumor cells tend to become reoxygenated during the course of low-dose-rate radiation.[19] Finally, repopulation of tumor cells is less of a concern than with standard external beam radiotherapy, because interstitial radiation given continuously at 0.4 to 0.6 Gy/hour inhibits mitosis.[19]

Hyperthermia Background

At temperatures higher than about 41°C, heat kills cells directly as a function of time and temperature, and heat inhibits the repair of sublethal and potentially lethal radiation damage. Cells that tend to be resistant to radiation are the most sensitive to heat, including low-pH and nutrient-deprived hypoxic cells and those in the S phase of the cell cycle.[20] Hyperthermia may also lead to reoxygenation of hypoxic regions of tumors, thereby increasing sensitivity to radiation.[21]

A large number of uncontrolled trials in which comparable superficial, extracranial malignant tumors were treated with external beam radiation alone or radiation combined with superficial hyperthermia have demonstrated improved tumor response and local control with hyperthermia,[22, 23] and three prospective, randomized trials have shown that adjuvant hyperthermia yields significantly better results than radiation alone in the treatment of melanoma and advanced head and neck cancers.[24–26] One randomized trial comparing interstitial radiotherapy and interstitial thermoradiotherapy for extracranial tumors failed to show a benefit of hyperthermia, but quality assurance was poor during most of the trial.[27]

Interstitial hyperthermia techniques have been reviewed extensively elsewhere.[28, 29] The major available applicators include implanted microwave antennas, needle electrode pairs (between which radiofrequency current passes), or hot sources (such as hot water tubes, resistively heated wires, or inductively heated ferromagnetic seeds or wires).

Recently, interest has increased in simultaneous, continuous, long-duration interstitial thermoradiotherapy, heating tumors to 41°C for many hours in conjunction with low-dose-rate or high-dose-rate brachytherapy. This strategy may maximize thermal radiosensitization and allow for accumulation of a much larger thermal dose than has been possible previously.[30–32]

PATIENT SELECTION

Patient selection for interstitial brachytherapy of brain tumors varies among institutions. In Europe, experience with permanent and temporary implants for low-grade gliomas is extensive.[33, 34] Most of the experience in North America is with malignant gliomas, using interstitial irradiation to treat recurrent disease or using it as a ''boost'' in conjunction with external beam radiotherapy for primary malignant gliomas.

In general, patients should have a Karnofsky performance status of at least 70, and tumors suitable for brachytherapy are unifocal, well-circumscribed, and less than 5 to 6 cm in diameter. Most centers do not use brachytherapy for malignant gliomas in the brainstem or cerebellum because of poor biologic reserve in the event of necrosis. Interstitial radiation is not indicated in patients with very large diffuse tumors, corpus callosal involvement, or subependymal spread.

At the University of California, San Francisco (UCSF), interstitial brachytherapy is offered to patients with technically implantable primary glioblastoma multiforme (to be used in conjunction with external beam radiotherapy) and patients with recurrent glioblastoma multiforme or recurrent anaplastic astrocytoma. Brachytherapy has been used occasionally for recurrent or persistent solitary brain metastases in the setting of controlled systemic disease,[35] and intraoperative permanent implantation of low-activity sources in suture is sometimes performed when skull base or dural-based tumors have been subtotally resected or totally resected with positive microscopic margins.[36] This chapter focuses on the use of temporary interstitial implants for malignant gliomas.

TECHNIQUE

Initial Treatment

All patients undergo surgery initially to obtain a histopathologic diagnosis and, in most cases, to reduce tumor burden. At UCSF, this is followed by external beam radiotherapy, generally encompassing the contrast-enhancing tumor with a 2- to 3-cm margin and treating with daily fractions of 1.8 Gy to a total dose of 59.4 Gy over 6 to 7 weeks. Oral hydroxyurea is administered as a radiosensitizer during the course of external beam radiotherapy, at 300 mg/m^2 every 6 hours, given every other day. The recently completed Brain Tumor Cooperative Group (BTCG) brain brachytherapy trial called for interstitial implantation prior to external beam radiotherapy to obviate the potential for tumor progression to an unsuitable size during external beam radiotherapy.

For patients with technically implantable primary glioblastomas multiforme at UCSF, the interstitial brachytherapy boost is usually performed within 3 weeks after external beam radiotherapy. For patients with recurrent malignant gliomas, no further external beam radiotherapy is administered, but tumor debulking several weeks prior to brachytherapy is performed as needed to help reduce mass effect in patients who are symptomatic and require high-dose steroid therapy.

Most patients implanted at UCSF prior to October 1990 also received adjuvant PCV chemotherapy beginning two weeks postimplantation; this consisted of procarbazine (60 mg/m^2 orally on days 8 to 21), lomustine (CCNU) (110 mg/m^2 orally on day 1), and vincristine (1.4 mg/m^2 intravenously on days 8 and 29). Chemotherapy cycles were repeated every 6 to 8 weeks for 1 year or until documentation of disease progression. A retrospective analysis done in 1990 failed to show a significant benefit of PCV chemotherapy in patients with glioblastoma multiforme, so very few patients with glioblastoma multiforme were given adjuvant PCV chemotherapy after October 1990. More recent retrospective analyses show that a survival advantage may be associated with adjuvant PCV chemotherapy. This issue requires further study.

Brachytherapy Treatment Preplanning

Modern series have employed CT- or MRI-guided stereotactic placement of implant catheters to house radiation sources. A stereotactic base ring (such as the Leksell, Brown-Roberts-Wells, or Cosman-Roberts-Wells frame) is applied to the patient's skull; local anesthesia is used in adults and general anesthesia is used in children. The patient then undergoes CT or MRI with a localizing system mounted on the base ring. A contrast scan is obtained with contiguous 3-mm axial images. Digital imaging information is transferred to the computer treatment planning station via magnetic tape or an information network. Imaging slices are called up on the treatment planning station and the target volume is outlined on each image. At UCSF, the target is outlined immediately outside the edge of contrast enhancement seen on CT images, with no additional margin.

The treatment planner then empirically "places" catheters and radiation sources within the target volume in the preplanning program and makes adjustments until a suitable isodose contour is achieved that conforms well to the target volume; the number of catheters is kept to a minimum. At UCSF this process requires approximately 1 hour of time using software developed in-house.[37] We do not attempt to have a uniform dose distribution within the target volume, and catheters do not need to be parallel or to conform to any particular spacing. We typically orient catheters perpendicular to the skull surface and use 2 to 6 catheters, depending on the tumor size and irregularity, with 2 to 3 ^{125}I sources per catheter, often spaced apart from each other with 3- to 4-mm long spacers, though any length spacer may be used (Fig. 40–1). We aim for a 0.4- to 0.6-Gy/hour isodose contour, which covers 95% to 98% of the target volume as evaluated by a dose-volume histogram.

Brain brachytherapy treatment planning software has been developed at Memorial Sloan-Kettering Cancer Center, New York, with computer optimization of catheter and ^{125}I source locations.[38] Remote afterloaders can be programmed to optimize dose distribution by varying the dwell times of the source along the length of the implant catheters.[39]

At some centers, catheters are implanted through a rigid template and are planned to be parallel to each other and to conform to the template spacing, often 1.0 cm apart.[40, 41] This method can also produce an isodose contour that conforms well to the target volume. More catheters tend to be used and the dose distribution within the target volume tends to be more uniform than in the previously discussed method.[42] Also, the dose to normal surrounding tissue tends to be higher for ^{192}Ir than for ^{125}I sources due to energy-dependent differences in radiation attenuation by tissue.[42]

Brain Implant Procedure

After the treatment plan has been approved by the radiation oncologist and the neurosurgeon, the list of stereotactic coordinates for target points and stereotactic frame angles is taken to the operating room. At UCSF, where ^{125}I sources are used, the physicist makes up inner catheters containing the appropriate sources and spacers in the radiation source room while the neurosurgeon is implanting afterloading outer catheters in the operating room.

The implant procedure is performed using local anesthesia in adults and general anesthesia in children; the patient is placed in a semi-sitting position and the stereotactic frame is attached to the operating room table. Prophylactic antibiotics are administered. For each catheter to be implanted, target point coordinates are set on the stereotactic phantom base, frame angles are set on the arc or arc-ring assembly, and the catheter trajectory is confirmed as accurate. The arc or arc-ring system is then transferred to the base frame on the patient, the skin is anesthetized and incised, and a small hole is drilled through the skull with a 3.4-mm twist drill. The dura is perforated with successively larger K-wires and then the hole in the dura is enlarged with a blunt dilator, and a trial pass is made with the implant catheter. At UCSF, closed-end Silastic catheters are used with an outside diameter of 2.16 mm and an inside diameter of 1.57 mm. The arc-ring assembly is then removed and a 2-0 nylon purse-string suture is placed in the scalp around the twist drill hole to later secure the skin around the brain catheter and to prevent leakage of cerebrospinal fluid. The target depth is checked with the arc-ring assembly on the phantom base. The tip of the Silastic brain implant catheter, stiffened by an inner stylet, is dipped in mineral oil and passed through the guide on the arc-ring assembly mounted on the patient base ring, through a numbered plastic collar on the scalp surface, and through the twist drill hole to the planned depth. Then the catheter is glued to the collar with a small amount of cyanoacrylate glue, the catheter is trimmed off about 6 mm from the collar, and the purse-string suture is tied. The numbered inner catheters containing ^{125}I radiation sources and spacers are sterilized in a lead-lined pan. After all brain implant catheters have been placed individually as just described, the tip of each inner catheter is dipped in mineral oil and afterloaded into the correspondingly numbered brain implant catheter. The inner catheters are trimmed off about 1 cm from the collar and are secured in place with a surgical clip (see Fig. 40–1).

Burr holes may be used as an alternative to twist drill holes, especially in areas in which concern about bleeding

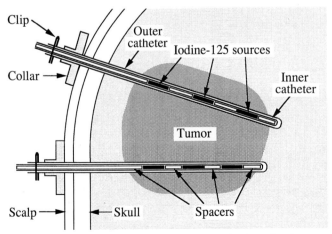

Figure 40–1 Schematic diagram of a brain implant showing two afterloaded catheters within a tumor volume. Each nylon inner catheter containing the ^{125}I sources is fixed to the Silastic outer catheter with a surgical clip, and the outer catheter is glued to a Silastic collar, which is sutured to the scalp.

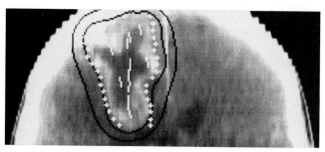

Figure 40–2 Actual ^{125}I source positions and resulting 0.45 and 0.25 Gy/hour isodose contours displayed on a coronal reconstruction of the preimplant CT scan by the treatment planning software after source position verification. Isodose contours can be viewed in any plane.

is increased, such as near the sylvian fissure or sagittal or transverse sinuses.

Orthogonal radiographs are taken in the operating room through a fiducial marker box that is mounted on the patient base ring immediately after source loading before removal of the base ring. This allows source positions to be entered back into the preplanning program and allows actual source positions and radiation isodose contours to be displayed on the preimplant CT images[43] (Fig. 40–2). An actual dose-volume histogram is calculated and reviewed to help determine the adequacy of the implant. At UCSF, the brachytherapy dose is generally prescribed at the isodose contour that encompasses 95% to 98% of the target volume, usually in the range of 0.4 to 0.6 Gy/hour. If planned and actual source positions differ enough to adversely affect the tumor coverage, adjustments may be made later that evening or the next morning at the patient's bedside; this is accomplished by removing the surgical clip, withdrawing the inner catheter, and replacing it with a sterilized corrected inner catheter (with altered spacer lengths and/or source activity).

Implant techniques differ for template-guided stereotactic brain implants.[40, 44] Centers using remote afterloaders may verify source positions in the operating room with dummy sources. Brain implant catheters are later connected to a low-dose-rate or pulse-simulated low-dose-rate afterloading device in a special patient room or to a high-dose-rate afterloader in a shielded room.[39]

Radiation Protection

Radiation protection depends on the type of source used. Iodine 125 is shielded adequately by a 0.5-mm thickness of lead. Operating room personnel wear lead aprons and the surgeon has additional protection from leaded glasses, a thyroid lead shield, and leaded vinyl rubber surgical gloves. Once the inner catheters are in place and the base ring has been removed at the end of the operative procedure, the patient is given a cloth hat containing a thin, malleable layer of lead within two or more of the hat's four compartments, which provides shielding to a dose rate below 1 milliroentgen (mR)/hour at 1 m. The patient is then hospitalized in a private room, only wearing the hat when visitors or hospital personnel (who also wear lead aprons) enter the room.

Shielding of afterloaded ^{192}Ir wires or ribbons is more cumbersome, requiring hospitalization of the patient in a

special private room with thick lead shields. Lead aprons and lead-lined hats are not used, as they do not afford protection against the more energetic γ-rays of [192]Ir.

In the case of remote afterloaders, radiation protection is not a concern. Sources are automatically withdrawn into the low-dose-rate afterloader safe whenever visitors or hospital personnel are in the room with the patient, and high-dose-rate treatments are delivered over minutes in a special shielded room.

Implant Removal

After the desired radiation dose has been delivered, usually in 4 to 7 days, implant catheters are removed, either at the bedside (in the case of catheters placed via twist drill holes) or in the operating room (in the case of catheters placed via burr holes). A suture is placed to close each catheter site. Patients are then observed in the hospital overnight and discharged to home the following morning.

Hyperthermia Technique

At UCSF, hyperthermia treatments are administered within 15 to 30 minutes before and after brachytherapy using 915-MHz helical coil microwave antennas[45] and multisensor fiberoptic thermometry probes inserted into the same catheters that are used for ^{125}I sources. Instead of a small number of more centrally placed catheters (Fig. 40–3A), hyperthermia implants typically consist of catheters placed within 5 mm inside the perimeter of contrast enhancement, evenly spaced 1.2 to 1.7 cm apart for heating antennas, and of one to three additional catheters placed through the tumor center and/or the tumor periphery for thermometry (see Fig. 40–3B). Dummy sources are loaded into the brain implant catheters in the operating room for source position verification prior to hyperthermia. The morning after the implant procedure, the patient is transported to the hyperthermia suite, where dummy sources are removed and microwave antennas and thermometry probes are inserted using sterile technique. The treatment goal is to attain steady-state tumor temperatures after 5 to 10 minutes of heating and then to maintain steady-

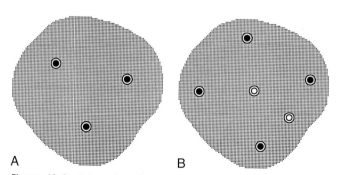

Figure 40–3 Schematic end-on views of a typical catheter arrangement for brachytherapy alone (A) and for combined hyperthermia and brachytherapy (B). For hyperthermia, the catheters tend to be placed more peripherally than for brachytherapy alone, and additional catheters are required for thermometry. Antenna catheters are fairly evenly spaced 1.2 to 1.5 cm apart about 3 to 5 mm inside the perimeter of the target volume.

state temperatures for 30 minutes, with a minimum tumor temperature of 42.5 °C. A maximum tumor temperature of up to 50 °C is allowed in a necrotic center or resection cavity as long as normal tissue temperatures remain below 43.5 °C. Patients are monitored clinically during hyperthermia for any adverse effects.

PATIENT EVALUATION AND MANAGEMENT

Patients are evaluated with contrast CT or MRI brain imaging studies, neurologic examination, and assessment of Karnofsky performance status every 2 months for 1 year, every 3 months the following year, and then every 4 to 6 months. Positron emission tomography (PET) and/or MR spectroscopy scans are sometimes obtained to help distinguish between radiation necrosis and tumor progression.[46] In a review of 34 patients who underwent 40 PET scans at UCSF to help distinguish between tumor recurrence and radiation necrosis, and in whom further follow-up yielded a clinical diagnosis, the overall accuracy of PET for differentiating between active tumor and necrosis was 84%.[46]

Patients are given anticonvulsant medications and corticosteroids as needed. Steroids are tapered and then discontinued whenever possible in patients who are stable or improving.

Reoperation is generally recommended for patients with clinical deterioration and/or steroid dependency and in whom imaging studies show an enlarging contrast-enhancing lesion with associated mass effect or edema. A variety of salvage chemotherapy regimens are used in the event of tumor progression.

RESULTS

Implant Boost for Primary Glioblastoma Multiforme

Nonrandomized series reporting results of brachytherapy boost for primary glioblastoma multiforme are listed in Table 40–1, with survival ranging from 7 to 19 months.[33, 47–52] Prospective, randomized trials are in progress in Toronto[53] and in Iowa City,[54] and a multi-institutional protocol was recently completed by the BTCG (trial 8701) in which pa-

tients with newly diagnosed malignant gliomas either were or were not given a brachytherapy boost preceding external beam radiotherapy.[55] Brachytherapy was associated with significantly improved survival ($P < 0.05$).

At UCSF, the first temporary ^{125}I brain implant boost after external beam radiotherapy for a primary glioblastoma multiforme was performed in February 1981. From then through December 1992, 159 consecutive adults with primary glioblastoma multiforme underwent implant boost without hyperthermia, including 98 males and 61 females with Karnofsky performance status that ranged from 70 to 100 (median, 90) and ages that ranged from 18 to 73 years (median, 52 years). Initial surgery consisted of biopsy in 7% of patients, subtotal resection in 66%, and gross total resection in 27%. Overall, 91% of patients received 59.4 to 61.2 Gy using daily 1.8 to 2.0-Gy fractions. Eighty-one percent of patients had focal radiotherapy alone, and 19% had whole-brain radiotherapy with or without a focal boost. The prescribed brachytherapy dose ranged from 35.7 to 66.5 Gy (median, 55.0 Gy) at 0.30 to 0.70 Gy/hour (median, 0.43 Gy/hour) using one to 16 sources (median, seven) in one to six catheters (median, three). The Kaplan-Meier estimated median survival was 84 weeks (19.3 months), with 1-, 2-, and 3-year actuarial survival rates of 85%, 36%, and 20%, respectively (Table 40–2; Fig. 40–4).[51]

The Joint Center for Radiation Therapy (JCRT) in Boston has also reported long-term results of brachytherapy boost (37.7 to 63.2 Gy; median, 50.0 Gy) after external beam radiotherapy to 59.4 Gy at 1.8 Gy per daily fraction. The 56 patients with glioblastoma multiforme treated from February 1987 through July 1993 had a median age of 50 years and a mean Karnofsky performance status of 85 (range, 70 to 100). Brachytherapy patients had a median survival of 18 months with 1- and 3-year survival rates of 83% and 27%, respectively, compared with a median survival of 11 months for a group of matched controls with 1- and 3-year survival rates of 40% and 9%, respectively.[52]

Results have not been favorable for brachytherapy using low-activity ^{125}I sources with a dose rate of about 0.10 Gy/hour. Ostertag and Kreth[34] reported a median survival of only 6 months for 34 patients with glioblastoma multiforme treated with low-activity ^{125}I brachytherapy.

Implant Boost for Primary Anaplastic Astrocytoma

In 1980, Mundinger and co-workers[33] reported on 34 patients with grade III astrocytoma who underwent brachytherapy

TABLE 40–1
BRACHYTHERAPY RESULTS FOR PRIMARY GLIOBLASTOMA MULTIFORME

Study	Isotope	No. of Patients	Karnofsky Performance Status Range (Median)	Median Survival
Chun et al.[47]	[192]Ir	20	>70	14.5 mo
Kumar et al.[48]	[60]Co	30	Not stated	7 mo
Mundinger et al.[33]	[192]Ir/[125]I	17	Not stated	(19% 2-yr survival)
Patchell et al.[49]	[252]Cf	48, GM; 8, grade III AA	>50	10 mo
Selker et al.[50]	[192]Ir	47, GM; 8, AA	(80)	68 wk (15.6 mo)
Sneed et al.[51]	[125]I	159	70–100 (90)	19 mo
Wen et al.[52]	[125]I	56	70–100 (90)	18 mo

Abbreviations: GM, glioblastoma multiforme; AA, anaplastic astrocytoma.

TABLE 40–2
BRACHYTHERAPY RESULTS AT THE UNIVERSITY OF CALIFORNIA, SAN FRANCISCO

Histology Classification	Reference	Study Period	n	Median Survival (wk)	1-yr Survival (%)	3-yr Survival (%)
Primary GM	51	1981–1992	159	84	85	20
Primary high-grade NGM	57	1979–1990	52	158	84	51
Primary low-grade NGM	57	1979–1990	16	226	94	74
Recurrent GM	57	1979–1990	66	51	48	14
Recurrent high-grade NGM	57	1979–1990	45	53	54	23
Recurrent low-grade NGM	57	1979–1990	22	81	64	32

Abbreviations: GM, glioblastoma multiforme; NGM, non-glioblastoma multiforme malignant glioma.

using ¹⁹²Ir or ¹²⁵I from 1970 to 1979. Survival rates were 66% at 3 years and 45% at 5 years.

Scharfen and associates[56] reported on the entire UCSF experience in adults with malignant gliomas undergoing high-activity ¹²⁵I interstitial brachytherapy through June 1990, including 52 patients with high-grade non-glioblastoma gliomas (NGM). These results were updated in a subsequent article.[57] The median survival was 158 weeks (36.4 months) and the 1- and 3-year survival probabilities were 84% and 51% (see Table 40–2). These results were markedly better than those obtained in primary glioblastomas multiforme treated with brachytherapy boost, but they were not superior to overall results for 357 patients with highly anaplastic astrocytoma treated from 1977 to 1989 on a variety of UCSF and Northern California Oncology Group protocols, for whom the median survival was 171 weeks (39.4 months).[58] Thus, we no longer recommend brachytherapy boost as part of the initial therapy of patients with primary anaplastic astrocytoma.

Again, results have not been favorable for brachytherapy using low-activity ¹²⁵I sources. Ostertag and Kreth[34] reported a median survival of only 8 months for 75 patients with

World Health Organization (WHO) classification grade III anaplastic astrocytomas treated with low-activity ¹²⁵I brachytherapy.

Implant for Recurrent Malignant Gliomas

Series reporting results of brachytherapy for recurrent malignant gliomas are listed in Table 40–3, with survival ranging from 7 to 18 months.[48, 50, 53, 57, 59–64]

The review by Scharfen and co-workers[56] of the UCSF brachytherapy experience included 66 adults with recurrent glioblastoma multiforme and 45 with recurrent high-grade NGMs.[56] Updated results found a median survival of 51 weeks for glioblastoma multiforme and 53 weeks for high-grade NGMs, and 1- and 3-year survival probabilities of 48% and 14% for glioblastoma multiforme and 54% and 23% for high-grade NGMs, respectively (see Table 40–2; Fig. 40–5).[57]

Complications

Acute toxic response to high-activity ¹²⁵I brain implants is uncommon. Of 307 consecutive adults with gliomas who underwent brain brachytherapy at UCSF from December 1979 through June 1990, 19 (6%) had grade 3 (severe but not life-threatening) complications, including persistent increased seizure activity, new neurologic deficit, infection, intracerebral hemorrhage, and non–life-threatening pulmonary embolus. Three patients (1%) had grade 4 (life-threatening) complications, including temporary brainstem dysfunction with full recovery, sepsis, and life-threatening pulmonary embolus. Two patients (<1%) had grade 5 (fatal) complications, including fatal sepsis in one patient and fatal pulmonary embolus in the other patient.[56]

Late brain necrosis as a cause of serious disability or death in the absence of tumor is also uncommon. In a review of dose-response relationships for 97 adults with primary glioblastoma multiforme who underwent brachytherapy boost after external beam radiotherapy at UCSF from June 1987 through December 1992, three patients died or were placed in a hospice because of brain necrosis. All three patients received a brachytherapy dose exceeding 60 Gy to 95% of the tumor volume (and a combined external beam

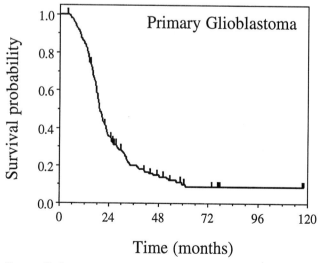

Figure 40–4 Kaplan-Meier survival curve showing the probability of survival from the date of diagnosis for 159 consecutive adults with primary glioblastomas treated with external beam radiotherapy followed by brachytherapy boost, from 1981 through 1993. The median survival was 84 weeks with 1-, 2-, and 3-year survival probabilities of 85%, 36%, and 20%, respectively.

TABLE 40–3
BRACHYTHERAPY RESULTS FOR RECURRENT MALIGNANT GLIOMAS

Study	Isotope	No. of Patients	Karnofsky Performance Status Range (Median)	Median Survival
Bernstein et al.[53]	125I	18 MG	50–100 (80)	44 wk (10 mo)
Fass et al.[59]	125I	20 GM/9 AA	50–100	14.5 mo
Kumar et al.[48]	60Co	19 GM	Not stated	7 mo
Larson et al.[60]	198Au	13 GM	``Good''	9 mo
		20 AA	``Good''	17 mo
Lucas et al.[61]	192Ir	7 GM	Not stated	10 mo
		13 AA	Not stated	11 mo
Matsumoto et al.[62]	192Ir	9 GM	30–100 (80)	18 mo
		14 grade III AA		18 mo
Sneed et al.[57]	125I	66 GM	70–100 (90)	12 mo
		45 NGM (high-grade)	70–100 (90)	12 mo
Selker et al.[50]	192Ir	61 GM	(70)	58 wk (13 mo)
Willis et al.[63]	125I	4 GM/8 AA	≥80	18 mo
Zamorano et al.[64]	125I	23 MG†	Not stated	42 wk (10 mo)

Abbreviations: MG, malignant glioma; GM, glioblastoma multiforme; AA, anaplastic astrocytoma.
*Survival measured from the date of brachytherapy.
†Only patients treated with temporary high-activity 125I implants included.

and brachytherapy dose greater than 120 Gy).[65] Thus, we recommend limiting the brachytherapy dose to 50 to 60 Gy.

Reoperation After Brachytherapy

Reoperation is common after brachytherapy, either for recurrent tumor, radiation necrosis or, in most cases, for a combination of tumor and necrosis. Of 307 adults treated with brachytherapy at UCSF for primary or recurrent malignant gliomas through June 1990, 56% underwent subsequent reoperation at a median of 36 weeks after brachytherapy (range, 4 to 415 weeks). Reoperation rates were similar for primary and recurrent tumors and for glioblastomas multiforme and NGMs. Histologic findings included necrosis only in 5%, tumor only in 29%, and both tumor and necrosis in

66% of specimens. Survival did not depend on histologic findings, but patients with glioblastoma multiforme who underwent reoperation survived significantly longer than those who did not undergo reoperation (median survival, 110 vs. 77 weeks for primary glioblastoma multiforme [*P* = 0.005] and median survival of 84 vs. 35 weeks for recurrent glioblastoma multiforme [*P* = 0.002]).[56] The significance of this finding is unclear, as many selection factors are involved in determining which patients undergo reoperation.

Similar findings were reported by Wen and co-workers[52] based on the JCRT series of 56 glioblastomas multiforme treated with brachytherapy boost after external beam radiotherapy. Sixty-four percent of patients required reoperation. The median survival was 22 months for reoperated patients and 13 months for those who did not undergo reoperation (*P* < 0.02). In comparison, only 15% of patients in the matched control non-brachytherapy group underwent reoperation.[52]

Prognostic Factors

In a review of the entire UCSF experience with high-activity 125I interstitial brachytherapy in 307 adults with primary and recurrent malignant gliomas through June 1990, Scharfen and others[56] found that both histologic diagnosis (*P* = 0.0003 and *P* = 0.032, respectively) and age (*P* = 0.00006 and *P* = 0.00008) were highly significant predictive factors for survival of patients with primary or recurrent tumors.[56] Of note, extent of initial surgery, external beam radiotherapy dose, brachytherapy dose, brachytherapy volume, and Karnofsky performance status were not significant. It is likely that Karnofsky performance status is an important parameter, but in this series Karnofsky performance status only ranged from 70 to 100 and the majority of patients had a Karnofsky performance status of 90.

Sneed and co-workers[51] evaluated prognostic factors in 159 patients with glioblastoma multiforme undergoing brachytherapy boost at UCSF after external beam radiother-

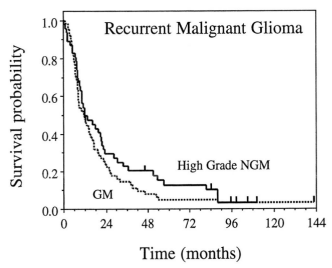

Figure 40–5 Kaplan-Meier survival curves showing the probability of survival from the date of brachytherapy for patients with recurrent glioblastoma multiforme (GM) or recurrent high-grade non-glioblastoma glioma (NGM). The median survival was 51 weeks for GM (n = 66) and 53 weeks for high-grade NGM (n = 45).

apy.[51] Univariate analyses showed that improved survival was associated with younger age ($P < 0.0005$), higher Karnofsky performance status ($P = 0.04$), and the use of adjuvant PCV chemotherapy ($P = 0.018$). A multivariate analysis including age, Karnofsky performance status, and whether or not adjuvant PCV chemotherapy was given showed that age was the only significant variable ($P < 0.0005$) in this population with uniform histologic diagnosis and nearly uniform Karnofsky performance status. For the nine patients aged 18 to 29.9 years, median survival had not been reached (with a median follow-up of 322 weeks in living patients) and the three-year survival rate was 78% ± 14%. In comparison, the 64 patients aged 30 to 49.9 years had a median survival of 102 weeks (23.5 months) and a 3-year survival probability of 29% ± 6%, and the 86 patients aged 50 years or older had a median survival of 76 weeks (17.5 months) and a 3-year survival probability of 6% ± 3%.

Quality of Life

Leibel and colleagues[66] evaluated steroid dependency and Karnofsky performance status in 95 patients treated with brachytherapy for recurrent malignant gliomas at UCSF from January 1980 to January 1988. For the 33 patients who survived at least 18 months, 97% of patients were steroid-dependent prior to brachytherapy and the mean baseline Karnofsky performance status was 87 (range, 80 to 90). At 18 months, 67% of the 33 survivors were steroid dependent and the mean Karnofsky performance status was 79 (range, 50 to 90). At 36 months, 53% of the 17 survivors were steroid dependent and the mean Karnofsky performance status was 76 (range, 40 to 90). It was concluded that quality of life was acceptable in most long-term survivors of brachytherapy.

The JCRT series of 56 glioblastoma multiforme patients given brachytherapy boost yielded similar results. The mean pretreatment Karnofsky performance status of 85.6 (range, 70 to 100) decreased to 77 at 12 months (range, 50 to 90), 71 at 24 months (range, 50 to 90), and 71 at 36 months (range, 40 to 90).[52]

Patterns of Recurrence

In the review by Scharfen and colleagues[56] of 307 adults who underwent brachytherapy at UCSF, with or without external beam radiotherapy for primary or recurrent malignant glioma, noncontiguous sites of failure were noted in only 7% of patients with glioblastoma multiforme or high-grade NGMs.[56] A more in-depth review of a subset of these patients, who received a brachytherapy boost for glioblastoma multiforme on Northern California Oncology Group protocol 6G–82–2, revealed that 77% of failures were local (contiguous with the implant site and within 2 cm of the edge of the implant site), 14% at separate sites in the brain, 5% were subependymal, and 5% were systemic. Another series evaluating patterns of brachytherapy failure reported 88% local failures.[67] Yet another group reported 35% local failures within the brachytherapy target volume,

37% at the tumor margin, and 28% recurrences at distant sites.[52]

Thus, local failure is still a major problem despite very aggressive local therapy. This forms part of the rationale for combining adjuvant interstitial hyperthermia with brachytherapy.

Combined Hyperthermia and Brachytherapy

The UCSF experience with thermoradiotherapy for recurrent malignant gliomas included 25 patients with glioblastoma multiforme and 16 patients with NGM treated from June 1987 through September 1990 on Brain Tumor Research Center (BTRC) protocol 8721.[57, 68, 69] The median patient age was 43 years (range, 18 to 71 years) and the median Karnofsky performance status was 90 (range, 40 to 90). A median dose of 59 Gy was given (range, 32.4 to 63.3 Gy) at a median dose rate of 0.44 Gy/hour (range, 0.37 to 0.70 Gy/hour). Seventy-eight hyperthermia treatments were administered using 1 to 8 microwave antennas and the manual temperature mapping of single and multisensor fiberoptic thermometry probes within one to three dedicated thermometry catheters. Steady-state minimum tumor temperatures ranged from 37.5 to 45.8 °C (median, 40.1 °C) and maximum tumor temperatures ranged from 39.5 to 51.7 °C (median, 45.7 °C). The T90 parameter (the temperature exceeded by 90% of the intratumoral loci monitored) was estimated by interpolation for each patient treatment by fitting a smooth curve through points on a graph of percentage of tumor loci greater than or equal to the index temperature vs. index temperature. The median T90 for this series of 78 treatments was 41.1 °C and a T90 of 41.2 °C or greater was associated with significantly better survival for patients with recurrent glioblastoma multiforme ($P = 0.008$) (Fig. 40–6). The me-

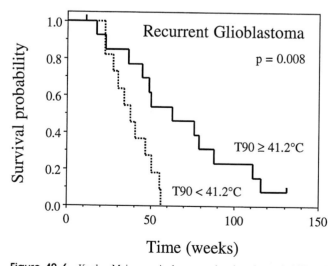

Figure 40–6 Kaplan-Meier survival curves showing the probability of survival from the date of implant with hyperthermia for patients with recurrent glioblastoma multiforme according to the T90 temperature achieved. T90 ≥ 41.2 °C was associated with significantly improved survival ($P = 0.008$; median survival, 38 weeks for T90 < 41.2 °C and 63 weeks for T90 ≥ 41.2 °C).

dian survival for patients with recurrent glioblastoma multiforme and NGM was 49 weeks and 140 weeks, respectively. A multivariate analysis stratified by histologic diagnosis identified both age ($P = 0.04$) and T90 ($P = 0.04$) as significant parameters influencing survival. Acute toxic responses included 13 grade 1 complications (seven transient neurologic changes and six brief seizures), five grade 2 complications (four reversible neurologic changes and one 20-minute seizure), and five grade 3 complications (two reversible neurologic changes, one case of meningitis, one scalp/bone flap infection, and one case of deep venous thrombosis with non-life-threatening pulmonary embolism). No permanent neurologic changes and no deaths were recorded. The reoperation rate after thermoradiotherapy was 46%, similar to that for brachytherapy alone.

This thermoradiotherapy trial showing improved survival for T90 of 41.2 °C or greater in recurrent glioblastomas multiforme laid the groundwork for the ongoing prospective, randomized phase II trial at UCSF, BTRC protocol 6G–90–2, for patients with primary glioblastoma multiforme. Patients are entered into the study after surgery and undergo external beam radiotherapy to 59.4 Gy, 1.8 Gy per daily radiation fraction, with oral hydroxyurea administered on Mondays, Wednesdays, and Fridays. Eligibility for brachytherapy is reassessed with an MRI scan at the conclusion of external beam radiotherapy, and patients are then randomized between arm A (brachytherapy boost alone), or arm B (interstitial microwave hyperthermia for 30 minutes immediately before and after brachytherapy). As of August 1995, 33 patients had received brachytherapy in arm A and 32 had undergone thermoradiotherapy in arm B, with a median T90 of 42.1 °C and 69% of T90s of 41.2 °C or greater. We expect that this protocol will help answer the question of whether or not short-duration, sequential, adjuvant hyperthermia will benefit patients with primary glioblastoma multiforme.

Similar brain thermoradiotherapy techniques have been investigated at Dartmouth, using microwave antennas,[70–72] and at the University of Arizona in Tucson, using inductively heated ferromagnetic seeds.[73, 74] Stea and co-workers[75] reported a retrospective comparison between 25 patients with primary malignant gliomas who were treated with external beam radiotherapy and thermoradiotherapy interstitial boost, and 37 patients who were treated identically but without adjuvant hyperthermia. The median survival was 23.5 months for the thermoradiotherapy group vs. 13.3 months for the nonhyperthermia group. Multivariate analysis showed that hyperthermia ($P = 0.027$), younger patient age ($P < 0.00001$), and histologic diagnosis (anaplastic astrocytoma vs. glioblastoma multiforme, $P = 0.0017$) were all significantly associated with improved survival.

DISCUSSION

We conclude that brachytherapy boost is of value in patients with primary glioblastoma multiforme. In the series from both UCSF and the JCRT, the median survival was 18 to 19 months for patients with primary glioblastoma multiforme who underwent conventional external beam radiotherapy followed by brachytherapy boost, and some long-term survivors

have apparently been cured.[51, 52, 57] These results compare favorably with the usual median survival of about 9 to 11 months for primary glioblastoma multiforme.

At least some of the apparent improvement in survival is due to patient selection factors, but we also believe that the brachytherapy boost has a real impact on survival. Florell and colleagues[76] reviewed an unselected population of conventionally treated patients with malignant gliomas. Forty percent of patients with glioblastoma multiforme were found to have been implant-eligible based on retrospectively reviewed imaging studies and patient performance status. The median survival for implant-eligible patients was 13.9 months, compared with 5.8 months for ineligible patients.[76] However, this still falls short of the 18- to 19-month median survival for patients with primary glioblastoma multiforme treated with brachytherapy boost at UCSF and the JCRT. Findings from matched controls also suggest that there is a survival advantage associated with brachytherapy boost.[52] Two randomized trials are under way[53, 54] and the BTCG trial of conventional external beam radiotherapy with or without a preceding brachytherapy boost showed that brachytherapy was associated with significantly improved survival ($P < 0.05$).[55]

We also think that a role exists for brachytherapy in the treatment of focal recurrent glioblastoma multiforme and NGM. At UCSF, the median survival after brachytherapy was 51 weeks for recurrent glioblastoma multiforme and 53 weeks for recurrent NGM.[57] In comparison, the median survival after reoperation for recurrence has been reported to be 36 weeks for glioblastoma multiforme and 88 weeks for anaplastic astrocytoma,[77] or 29 weeks for glioblastoma multiforme and 66 weeks for anaplastic astrocytoma.[78] No randomized trial has been conducted comparing brachytherapy to other treatment modalities for recurrent malignant gliomas, but we consider the 3-year survival rates of 14% and 23% after brachytherapy for recurrent glioblastoma multiforme and NGM to be encouraging.[57]

In contrast to our experience with primary glioblastoma multiforme and recurrent glioblastoma multiforme and NGM, we do not think that a benefit has been demonstrated for brachytherapy boost in patients with primary NGM. At UCSF, the median survival for these patients was 158 weeks (36 months),[57] but results were not superior to those obtained with non-brachytherapy protocols at UCSF.[58]

The acute toxicity of brachytherapy is acceptable, with only 6% grade 3, 1% grade 4, and fewer than 1% grade 5 complications. The major long-term toxic effects of concern are necrosis and chronic vasogenic edema. Given that about 50% of 3-year survivors are steroid-dependent[66] and that 56% of all patients undergo reoperation (usually showing a combination of tumor cells and necrosis),[56] we appear to have approached the limits of patient tolerance with our brachytherapy techniques and doses. Nevertheless, necrosis rarely leads to death, and quality of life in survivors is good, with an average Karnofsky performance status decrement of about 10 in patients surviving 36 months.[52, 66] It is important to continue to monitor Karnofsky performance status and other measures of quality of life in future protocols, to understand and address the impact of therapy on quality of life.

Appropriate concern has been voiced about the potential

efficacy of brachytherapy, given the infiltrative nature of malignant gliomas.[7, 8] However, the most frequent pattern of disease progression is that of local failure, both in patients undergoing conventional therapy[9–14] and in those treated with an additional brachytherapy boost.[52, 67, 79] This high rate of local failure argues for continued work on strategies to improve local control in addition to better definition of the optimal target volume for brachytherapy and for continued exploration of ways to reduce radiation injury. Research activity has been directed toward finding drugs that are capable of controlling radiation-induced edema and white matter injury without causing the serious side effects of chronic corticosteroid administration.[80]

It is hoped that local control can be improved with the addition of adjuvant hyperthermia. Other research directions include the use of radiation sensitizers with brachytherapy, such as bromodeoxyuridine, or iododeoxyuridine, or etanidazole,[81, 82] and the replacement of brachytherapy with stereotactic radiosurgery or fractionated radiosurgery. Preliminary results with radiosurgery appear to be similar to results obtained with brachytherapy.[83] An aggressive approach has been described using ^{125}I brachytherapy to 60 Gy with concomitant cisplatin administration via infusion as a radiosensitizer, followed by hyperfractionated external beam radiotherapy to an additional 66 Gy with 1.1-Gy fractions given twice daily. It is encouraging to note that the local control rate was reported to be 77% with a median follow-up of 18 months in living patients, although the median survival for 26 patients completing therapy (including 17 with glioblastomas multiforme and nine with anaplastic astrocytomas) was just 16 months.[84] Another interesting approach involves the use of permanently implanted low-activity ^{125}I sources to deliver brachytherapy at an initial dose rate of 0.04 to 0.07 Gy/hour concurrent with external beam radiotherapy.[64] It is likely that a variety of novel approaches will need to be considered if we are to find a way to markedly affect the prognosis for patients with malignant gliomas.

In conclusion, we believe that brachytherapy is applicable to a subset of patients with malignant gliomas who have good Karnofsky performance status and well-circumscribed, supratentorial, solitary lesions less than 5 to 6 cm in diameter, which represents about 30% of patients with malignant glioma.[76] We recommend brachytherapy boost after conventional radiotherapy for primary glioblastoma multiforme and brachytherapy alone for recurrent glioblastoma multiforme and NGMs. Further research is needed both to improve efficacy and to reduce late toxic responses associated with necrosis, chronic cerebral edema, and steroid dependency.

REFERENCES

1. Bleehen NM, Stenning SP: A Medical Research Council trial of two radiotherapy doses in the treatment of grades 3 and 4 astrocytoma. Br J Cancer 1991; 64:769–774.
2. Walker MD, Strike TA, Sheline GE: An analysis of dose-effect relationship in the radiotherapy of malignant gliomas. Int J Radiat Oncol Biol Phys 1979; 5:1725–1731.
3. Marks JE, Baglan RJ, Prassad SC, et al: Cerebral radionecrosis: Incidence and risk in relation to dose, time, fractionation and volume. Int J Radiat Oncol Biol Phys 1981; 7:243–252.
4. Sheline GE, Wara WW, Smith V: Therapeutic irradiation and brain injury. Int J Radiat Oncol Biol Phys 1980; 6:1215–1228.
5. Chang CH, Horton J, Schoenfeld D, et al: Comparison of postoperative radiotherapy and combined postoperative radiotherapy and chemotherapy in the multidisciplinary management of malignant gliomas. Cancer 1983; 57:997–1007.
6. Miller PJ, Hassanein RS, Shankar Giri PG, et al: Univariate and multivariate statistical analysis of high-grade gliomas: The relationship of radiation dose and other prognostic factors. Int J Radiat Oncol Biol Phys 1990; 19:275–280.
7. Burger PC: Pathologic anatomy and CT correlations in the glioblastoma multiforme. Appl Neurophysiol 1983; 46:180–187.
8. Kelly PJ, Daumas-Duport C, Kispert DB, et al: Imaging-based stereotaxic serial biopsies in untreated intracranial glial neoplasms. J Neurosurg 1987; 66:865–874.
9. Bashir R, Hochberg F, Oot R: Regrowth patterns of glioblastoma multiforme related to planning of interstitial brachytherapy radiation fields. Neurosurgery 1988; 23:27–30.
10. Choucair AK, Levin VA, Gutin PH, et al: Development of multiple lesions during radiation therapy and chemotherapy in patients with gliomas. J Neurosurg 1986; 65:654–658.
11. Garden AS, Maor MH, Yung WKA, et al: Outcome and patterns of failure following limited-volume irradiation for malignant astrocytomas. Radiother Oncol 1991; 20:99–110.
12. Gaspar LE, Fisher BJ, Macdonald DR, et al: Supratentorial malignant glioma: Patterns of recurrence and implications for external beam local treatment. Int J Radiat Oncol Biol Phys 1992; 24:55–57.
13. Hochberg FH, Pruitt A: Assumptions in the radiotherapy of glioblastoma. Neurology 1980; 30:907–911.
14. Wallner KE, Galicich JH, Krol G, et al: Patterns of failure following treatment for glioblastoma multiforme and anaplastic astrocytoma. Int J Radiat Oncol Biol Phys 1989; 16:1405–1409.
15. Weaver KA, Anderson LL, Meli JA: Source characteristics. In Anderson LL, Nath R, Weaver KA, et al (eds): Interstitial Brachytherapy: Physical, Biological, and Clinical Considerations. New York, Raven, 1990, pp 3–19.
16. Hall EJ: The biological basis of endocurietherapy: The Henschke Memorial Lecture 1984. Endocurie Hypertherm Oncol 1985; 1:141–152.
17. Hall EJ, Bedford JS, Oliver R: Extreme hypoxia: Its effect on the survival of mammalian cells irradiated at high and low dose-rates. Br J Radiol 1966; 39:302–307.
18. Ling CC, Spiro IJ, Mitchell J, et al: The variation of OER with dose rate. Int J Radiat Oncol Biol Phys 1985; 11:1367–1373.
19. Hall EJ: Radiobiology for the Radiologist. Philadelphia, JB Lippincott, 1994.
20. Dewey WC, Freeman ML, Raaphorst GP, et al: Cell biology of hyperthermia and radiation. In Meyn RE, Withers HR (eds): Radiation Biology in Cancer Research. New York, Raven, 1980, pp 589–621.
21. Oleson JR: Hyperthermia from the clinic to the laboratory: An hypothesis. Int J Hyperthermia 1995; 11:315–322.
22. Overgaard J: The current and potential role of hyperthermia in radiotherapy. Int J Radiat Oncol Biol Phys 1990; 16:535–549.
23. Sneed PK, Phillips TL: Combining hyperthermia and radiation: How beneficial? Oncology 1991; 5:99–108.
24. Datta NR, Bose AK, Kapoor HK, et al: Head and neck cancers: Results of thermoradiotherapy versus radiotherapy. Int J Hyperthermia 1990; 6:479–486.
25. Overgaard J: Thermoradiotherapy of malignant melanoma: The ESHO experience (abstract S11-1). Proceedings of the 14th Annual Meeting of the North American Hyperthermia Society, Nashville, April 29–May 4, 1994, p 87.
26. Valdagni R, Amichetti M: Report of long-term follow-up in a randomized trial comparing radiation therapy and radiation therapy plus hyperthermia to metastatic lymph nodes in stage IV head and neck patients. Int J Radiat Oncol Biol Phys 1993; 28:163–169.
27. Emami B, Scott C, Perez C, et al: Phase III study of interstitial thermoradiotherapy compared with interstitial radiotherapy alone in the treatment of recurrent or persistent human tumors: A prospectively controlled randomized study by the Radiation Therapy Oncology Group (abstract.). Int J Radiat Oncol Biol Phys 1993; 27 (suppl):155.
28. Seegenschmiedt MH, Brady LW, Sauer R: Interstitial thermoradiotherapy: Review on technical and clinical aspects. Am J Clin Oncol 1990; 13:352–363.
29. Stauffer PR: Techniques for interstitial hyperthermia. In Field SB, Hand JW (eds): An Introduction to the Practical Aspects of Clinical Hyperthermia. London, Taylor & Francis, 1990, pp 344–370.

30. Armour EP, Wang ZH, Corry PM, et al: Sensitization of rat 9L gliosarcoma cells to low dose rate irradiation by long duration 41 degrees C hyperthermia. Cancer Res 1991; 51:3088–3095.

31. Armour E, Wang ZH, Corry P, et al: Equivalence of continuous and pulse simulated low dose rate irradiation in 9L gliosarcoma cells at 37° and 41°C. Int J Radiat Oncol Biol Phys 1992; 22:109–114.

32. Armour EP, McEachern D, Wang Z, et al: Sensitivity of human cells to mild hyperthermia. Cancer Res 1993; 53:2740–2744.

33. Mundinger F, Ostertag CB, Birg W, et al: Stereotactic treatment of brain lesions. Appl Neurophysiol 1980; 43:198–204.

34. Ostertag CB, Kreth FW: Iodine–125 interstitial irradiation for cerebral gliomas. Acta Neurochir 1992; 119:53–61.

35. Prados M, Leibel S, Barnett CM, et al: Interstitial brachytherapy for metastatic brain tumors. Cancer 1989; 63:657–660.

36. Gutin PH, Leibel SA, Hosobuchi Y, et al: Brachytherapy of recurrent tumors of the skull base and spine with iodine-125 sources. Neurosurgery 1987; 20:938–945.

37. Weaver K, Smith V, Lewis JD, et al: A CT-based computerized treatment planning system for I-125 stereotactic brain implants. Int J Radiat Oncol BiolPhys 1990; 18:445–454.

38. Anderson LL, Harrington PJ, Osian AD, et al: A versatile method for planning stereotactic brain implants. Med Phys 1993; 20:1457–1464.

39. Woo S, Butler EB, Grant WI, et al: Fractionated high-dose rate brachytherapy for intracranial gliomas. Int J Radiat Oncol Biol Phys 1993; 28:247–249.

40. Beach L, Young AB, Patchell RA: A template for rigid stereotaxic afterloading brachytherapy of the brain. Int J Radiat Oncol Biol Phys 1993; 26:347–351.

41. Lulu BA, Lutz W, Stea B, et al: Treatment planning of template-guided stereotaxic brain implants. Int J Radiat Oncol Biol Phys 1990; 18:951–955.

42. Saw CB, Suntharalingam N, Ayyangar KM, et al: Dosimetric considerations of stereotactic brain implants. Int J Radiat Oncol Biol Phys 1989; 17:887–891.

43. Siddon RL, Barth NH: Stereotaxic localization of intracranial targets. Int J Radiat Oncol Biol Phys 1987; 13:1241–1246.

44. Hamilton AJ, Lulu BA, Stea B, et al: A technique employing Silastic anchoring sheets for securing multiple, percutaneous catheters for stereotactic interstitial brachytherapy for intracranial tumors. Endocurie Hypertherm Oncol 1994; 10:157–160.

45. Satoh T, Stauffer PR, Fike JR: Thermal distribution studies of helical coil microwave antennas for interstitial hyperthermia. Int J Radiat Oncol Biol Phys 1988; 15:1209–1218.

46. Valk PE, Budinger TF, Levin VA, et al: PET of malignant cerebral tumors after interstitial brachytherapy. J Neurosurg 1988; 69:830–838.

47. Chun M, McKeough P, Wu A, et al: Interstitial iridium-192 implantation for malignant brain tumors. Br J Radiol 1989; 62:158–162.

48. Kumar PP, Good RR, Jones EO, et al: Survival of patients with glioblastoma multiforme treated by intraoperative high-activity cobalt 60 endocurietherapy. Cancer 1989; 64:1409–1413.

49. Patchell RA, Maruyama Y, Tibbs PA, et al: Neutron interstitial brachytherapy for malignant gliomas: A pilot study. J Neurosurg 1988; 68:67–72.

50. Selker RG, Eddy MS, Arena V: Pittsburgh brachytherapy experience. Proceedings of the Second Symposium on Stereotactic Treatment of Brain Tumors, New York, Feb 28–March 1, 1991, p 23–24.

51. Sneed PK, Prados MD, McDermott MW, et al: Large effect of age on survival of patients with glioblastoma treated with radiotherapy and brachytherapy boost. Neurosurgery 1995; 36:898–904.

52. Wen PY, Alexander E III, Black PM, et al: Long term results of stereotactic brachytherapy used in the initial treatment of patients with glioblastomas. Cancer 1994; 73:3029–3036.

53. Bernstein M, Laperriere N, Leung P, et al: Interstitial brachytherapy for malignant brain tumors: Preliminary results. Neurosurgery 1990; 26:371–380.

54. Hitchon PW, VanGilder JC, Wen BC, et al: Brachytherapy for malignant recurrent and untreated gliomas. Stereotact Funct Neurosurg 1992; 59:174–178.

55. Selker RG, Shapiro WR, Green S, et al: A randomized trial of interstitial radiotherapy (IRT) boost for the treatment of newly diagnosed malignant glioma (glioblastoma multiforme, anaplastic astrocytoma, anaplastic oligodendroglioma, malignant mixed glioma): BTCG Study 87–01 (abstract). Program of the Congress of Neurological Surgeons, 45th Annual Meeting. San Francisco, Oct 14–19, 1995, pp 94–95.

56. Scharfen CO, Sneed PK, Wara WM, et al: High activity iodine-125 interstitial implant for gliomas. Int J Radiat Oncol Biol Phys 1992; 24:583–591.

57. Sneed PK, Larson DA, Gutin PH: Brachytherapy and hyperthermia for malignant astrocytoma. Semin Oncol 1994; 21:186–197.

58. Prados MD, Gutin PH, Phillips TL, et al: Highly anaplastic astrocytoma: A review of 357 patients treated between 1977 and 1989. Int J Radiat Oncol Biol Phys 1992; 23:3–8.

59. Fass DE, Malkin MG, Arbit E, et al: MSKCC brachytherapy results. Proceedings of the Second Symposium on Stereotactic Treatment of Brain Tumors, New York, Feb 28–March 1, 1991, p 29.

60. Larson GL, Wilbanks JH, Dennis WS, et al: Interstitial radiogold implantation for the treatment of recurrent high-grade gliomas. Cancer 1990; 66:27–29.

61. Lucas GL, Luxton G, Cohen D, et al: Treatment results of stereotactic interstitial brachytherapy for primary and metastatic brain tumors. Int J Radiat Oncol Biol Phys 1991; 21:715–721.

62. Matsumoto K, Nakagawa M, Higashi H, et al: Preliminary results of interstitial ¹⁹²Ir brachytherapy for malignant gliomas. Neurol Med Chir 1992; 32:739–746.

63. Willis BK, Heilbrun MP, Sapozink MD, et al: Stereotactic interstitial brachytherapy of malignant astrocytomas with remarks on postimplantation computed tomographic appearance. Neurosurgery 1988; 23:348–354.

64. Zamorano L, Yakar D, Dujovny M, et al: Permanent iodine-125 implant and external beam radiation therapy for the treatment of malignant brain tumors. Stereotact Funct Neurosurg 1992; 59:183–192.

65. Sneed PK, Lamborn KR, Larson DA, et al: Demonstration of brachytherapy boost dose-response relationships in glioblastoma multiforme. Int J Radiat Oncol Biol Phys (in press).

66. Leibel SA, Gutin PH, Wara WM, et al: Survival and quality of life after interstitial implantation of removable high-activity iodine-125 sources for the treatment of patients with recurrent malignant gliomas. Int J Radiat Oncol Biol Phys 1989; 17:1129–1139.

67. Agbi CB, Bernstein M, Laperriere N, et al: Patterns of recurrence of malignant astrocytoma following stereotactic interstitial brachytherapy with iodine-125 implants. Int J Radiat Oncol Biol Phys 1992; 23:321–326.

68. Sneed PK, Stauffer PR, Gutin PH, et al: Interstitial irradiation and hyperthermia for the treatment of recurrent malignant brain tumors. Neurosurgery 1991; 28:206–215.

69. Sneed PK, Gutin PH, Stauffer PR, et al: Thermoradiotherapy of recurrent malignant brain tumors. Int J Radiat Oncol Biol Phys 1992; 23:853–861.

70. Coughlin CT, Strohbehn JW: Interstitial thermoradiotherapy. Radiol Clin North Am 1989; 27:577–588.

71. Roberts DW, Strohbehn JW, Coughlin CT, et al: Iridium-192 brachytherapy in combination with interstitial microwave-induced hyperthermia for malignant glioma. Appl Neurophysiol 1987; 50:287–291.

72. Ryan TP, Trembly BS, Roberts DW, et al: Brain hyperthermia: I. Interstitial microwave antenna array techniques—the Dartmouth experience. Int J Radiat Oncol Biol Phys 1994; 29:1065–1078.

73. Stea B, Kittelson J, Cassady JR, et al: Treatment of malignant gliomas with interstitial irradiation and hyperthermia. Int J Radiat Oncol Biol Phys 1992; 24:657–667.

74. Stea B, Cetas TC, Cassady JR, et al: Interstitial thermoradiotherapy of brain tumors: Preliminary results of a phase I clinical trial. Int J Radiat Oncol Biol Phys 1990; 19:1463–1471.

75. Stea B, Rossman K, Kittelson J, et al: Interstitial irradiation versus interstitial thermoradiotherapy for supratentorial malignant gliomas: A comparative survival analysis. Int J Radiat Oncol Biol Phys 1994; 30:591–600.

76. Florell RC, Macdonald DR, Irish WD, et al: Selection bias, survival and brachytherapy for glioma. J Neurosurg 1992; 76:179–183.

77. Harsh GR IV, Levin VA, Gutin PH, et al: Reoperation for recurrent glioblastoma and anaplastic astrocytoma. Neurosurgery 1987; 21:615–621.

78. Ammirati M, Galicich JH, Arbit E, et al: Reoperation in the treatment of recurrent intracranial malignant gliomas. Neurosurgery 1987; 21:607–614.

79. Sneed PK, Gutin PH, Larson DA, et al: Patterns of recurrence of glioblastoma multiforme after external irradiation followed by implant boost. Int J Radiat Oncol Biol Phys 1994; 29:719–727.

80. Gobbel GT, Marton LJ, Lamborn K, et al: Modification of radiation-induced brain injury by α-difluoromethylornithine. Radiat Res 1991; 128:306–315.

81. Coleman CN, Noll L, Riese N, et al: Final report of the phase I trial of continuous infusion etanidazole (SR 2508): A Radiation Therapy Oncology Group study. Int J Radiat Oncol Biol Phys 1992; 22:577–580.

82. Djordjevic B, Szbalski W: Genetics of human cell lines: III. Incorporation of 5-bromo and 5-iododeoxyuridine into the deoxyribonucleic acid

of human cells and its effect on radiation sensitivity. J Exp Med 1960; 112:509–531.

83. Shrieve DC, Alexander E III, Wen PY, et al: Comparison of stereotactic radiosurgery and brachytherapy in the treatment of recurrent glioblastoma multiforme. J Neurosurg 1995; 36:275–284.

84. Fontanesi J, Clark WC, Weir A, et al: Interstitial iodine-125 and concomitant cisplatin followed by hyperfractionated external beam irradiation for malignant supratentorial glioma. Am J Clin Oncol 1993; 16:412–417.

DAVID A. LARSON

DENNIS C. SHRIEVE

PHILIP H. GUTIN

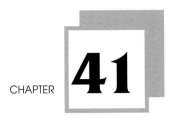

CHAPTER **41**

Radiosurgery

Radiosurgery has evolved considerably since its introduction by Leksell[1] in 1951. It is an external radiation technique in which numerous narrow collimated beams of radiation are stereotactically directed to converge at a radiographically discrete intracranial treatment site. A reference system associated with a stereotactic frame affixed to the patient's skull is used to provide coordinates of the target, and these coordinates are used to direct the radiation beams to the target site. The resultant radiosurgery dose is characteristically high within the target, but beyond the target's perimeter, it drops steeply. Within the target volume, the radiobiologic effects of radiosurgery cause either thrombosis of small blood vessels or reproductive cell death, and they may cause frank necrosis, though such necrosis is usually not required.

Patients who undergo radiosurgery are often selected, treated, and followed up by a team of experts composed of radiation oncologists, neurosurgeons, physicists, nurses, and technologists. This team approach is supported by radiosurgery task forces of societies representing both neurosurgery and radiation oncology.[2, 3]

RATIONALE FOR RADIOSURGERY

Despite advances in surgery, radiotherapy, and chemotherapy in recent years, the outlook for patients with malignant gliomas remains poor. Although most investigators agree that longer survival is associated with higher Karnofsky Performance Score (KPS), younger age, and lower pathologic tumor grade, local failure eventually occurs in the majority of cases, finally resulting in death. Radiosurgery is often used to attempt to improve local control and survival in patients with malignant glioma. The rationale for radiosurgery boost is straightfoward: (1) survival duration increases as the dose of fractionated external beam radiation is increased, at least over the range of 45 to 60 Gy[4, 5]; (2) further escalation of external beam dose given in standard fractions may be associated with increased risk for radiation necrosis; (3) interstitial brachytherapy provides a highly conformal boost and has been shown to increase survival, both in phase I and II[6, 7] and randomized[8] trials; (4) technically, a highly conformal boost can also be delivered with radiosurgery; (5) radiosurgery is noninvasive and often can be delivered as an outpatient procedure. Radiosurgery is therefore attractive from the standpoint of the patient as well as from that of health economics. Although the radiobiologic foundations of radiosurgery are less firm than those of brachytherapy,[9] many physicians now offer radiosurgery as a boost, either as a less-invasive alternative to brachytherapy or as a boost for patients who do not qualify for brachytherapy protocols.

RADIOSURGERY APPARATUS

Radiosurgery is carried out using one of three types of high-energy radiation beams. The most commonly available technology makes use of high-energy x-rays generated by a linear accelerator ("linac"). Fewer facilities use the gamma knife (AB ELEKTA, Stockholm), though it has actually been used to treat more patients than other technologies. A relatively small number of centers use charged particles produced by a cyclotron or a synchrotron to perform radiosurgery, and this technology may be more suited than the others to large target volumes.

Current outcome data for malignant gliomas are similar for linac and gamma knife technologies. Little information exists on the use of charged particle radiosurgery for malignant gliomas, although it has been used successfully for many other indications. For targets with a single isocenter, dose distributions produced by a linac or a gamma knife are similar. For large targets, charged particle techniques are capable of producing more homogeneous dose distributions.[10] Because most radiosurgery targets are small, conclusions about whether a given technology is preferable are usually based on variables such as cost of the apparatus, reliability of the apparatus, ease of operation, staffing requirements, and safety. The results of treatment are probably more closely related to the level of experience of the radiosurgery team than to the type of apparatus used.

For each of the three technologies, the radiosurgery treatment planning system should provide rapid, three-dimensional visualization of the target and the planned isodose distributions.

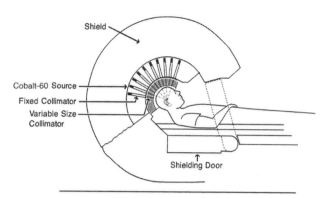

Figure 41–1 Cross-sectional schematic of a gamma knife showing the location of the cobalt 60 sources, their collimators, and the isocenter (point of intersection, within the brain, of all the beams). (From Alexander EI, Coffey R, Loeffler JS: Radiosurgery for gliomas. *In* Alexander EI, Loeffler JS, Lunsford LD (eds): Stereotactic Radiosurgery. New York, McGraw-Hill, 1993.)

Gamma Knife Radiosurgery

In the gamma knife, a central body containing 201 ^{60}Co sources is surrounded by two hemispherical cast-iron shields and a steel entrance door. The sources are located in separate beam channels within the central body, and they are directed radially inward toward a single target point at the hollow center of the radiation unit (Fig. 41–1). Gamma rays are collimated by an iron collimator helmet attached to the treatment table, which contains 201 collimators of 4-, 8-, 14-, or 18-mm diameter.

On the day of radiosurgery, a stereotactic frame is attached to the patient's skull, after which the patient undergoes contrast-enhanced computed tomography (CT) or gadolinium-enhanced magnetic resonance imaging (MRI). Treatment planning is performed, and once isodose curves are judged to be acceptable, which is accomplished by superimposing them on the images to ensure adequate tumor dose and acceptable normal tissue dose, the patient is placed on the treatment table. Next, the table is positioned in such a manner that the patient's head, within the stereotactic frame, is moved into the collimator helmet. The helmet and patient are then moved together into the central body, at which time treatment commences; the patient and apparatus are withdrawn after several minutes. In general the patient will have several additional treatments within the following 1 or 2 hours, each differing from the others by head position within the helmet, size of collimators, plugging pattern of the collimators, and length of treatment, to make the overall isodose surface conform closely to the irregular three-dimensional target contour. It takes about 10 to 20 minutes to place the patient in position and treat each isocenter. The number of isocenters may range from one to more than a dozen.

Linear Accelerator Radiosurgery

Linac radiosurgery is widely available, and the sequence of events on the day of radiosurgery is similar to that for patients treated with the gamma knife: the stereotactic frame is applied, CT or MRI is performed, treatment is planned, and treatment is carried out for a series of isocenters. Most linac facilities use circular collimators attached to the linac gantry to provide narrow radiation beams with little penum-

bra, although some use elliptical, dynamic, or multileaf collimators. Patients are usually treated while they lie supine (Fig. 41–2), although some systems require a patient to be in a sitting position. In most cases, beam-entrance patterns trace a series of non–co-planar arcs on the scalp, each arc corresponding to one of several different couch angles.[11, 12] Circular or helical patterns are produced with the patient-rotator method, in which the sitting patient is rotated about a stationary or moving linac beam.[13] With dynamic radiosurgery, in which both the couch and gantry move simultaneously, the pattern is diamond-shaped.[14] Despite differences in the beam-entrance pattern, the radiation-dose distributions within the target are similar for the various linac techniques. The main differences in dose distribution are chiefly at distances far from the target, but they are probably of little clinical significance. Isodose surfaces can be conformed to the three-dimensional target volume by adjusting the number of isocenters, the shape and size of the collimator opening, the degrees of gantry rotation, and the couch angle. It takes about 20 to 30 minutes to place the patient in position and to treat each linac isocenter, which is slightly longer than the gamma knife procedure.

Charged Particle Radiosurgery

Charged particle radiosurgery, in contrast to linac or gamma knife radiosurgery, requires only a few beams because of the Bragg ionization peak associated with each individual beam (Fig. 41–3). The extent of the Bragg peak along the beam direction and its depth in the brain with respect to the scalp can be adjusted to match the target depth and extent along the beam direction. Each beam has its own irregularly shaped aperture that conforms to the contour of the target, and patients are typically treated with two to six static intersecting beams. The three-dimensional dose distribution produced by a small number of charged particle beams falls

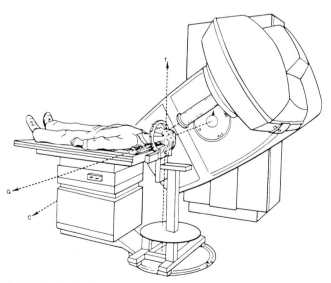

Figure 41–2 Position of patient undergoing linac radiosurgery. *Dotted lines* indicate axes of rotation of the gantry (G), the turntable (T), and the collimator (C). The isocenter is at the point of intersection of the three axes. (From Winston KR, Lutz W: Linear accelerator as a neurosurgical tool for stereotactic radiosurgery. Neurosurgery 1998; 22:455.)

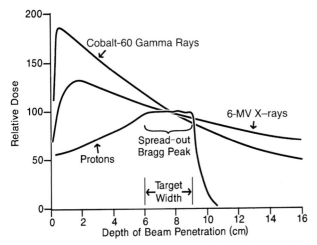

Figure 41–3 Comparison of dose distributions for single radiation beams, with relative dose measured as a function of depth from the scalp to the target and beyond. In this example the target is 3 cm in diameter and is located at a depth of 7.5 cm from the scalp. Single beams of gamma rays or x-rays would be unsatisfactory, because they provide more dose outside the target region than within it. By contrast, a single proton beam deposits more dose to the target than to tissue along the beam entry path. (From Alexander EI, Coffey R, Loeffler JS: Radiosurgery for gliomas. *In* Alexander EI, Loeffler JS, Lunsford LD (eds): Stereotactic Radiosurgery. New York, McGraw-Hill, 1993.)

off rapidly with distance from the target margin, but it is usually quite homogeneous within the target. Figure 41–4 shows treatment dose measured along the beam path for a typical charged particle treatment as well as for typical linac and gamma knife treatments. With charged particles, dose homogeneity within the target is nearly independent of target

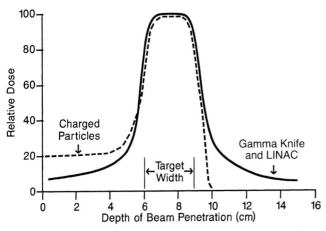

Figure 41–4 Comparison of dose distributions for multiple radiation beams, with relative dose measured as a function of depth along one beam from the scalp to the target and beyond. The dose values were generated by using a complete set of representative beams for each of the three treatment approaches. Each technique is capable of concentrating the dose within the target region. Entry doses appear to the left of the target and exit doses to the right. Charged particles produce almost no exit dose. Entry and exit doses for linac and gamma knife treatments are essentially the same. A charged particle treatment deposits more dose along each of a small number of entry paths than that deposited along each of a large number of entry paths for linac or gamma knife beams. (From Alexander EI, Coffey R, Loeffler JS: Radiosurgery for gliomas. *In* Alexander EI, Loeffler JS, Lunsford LD (eds): Stereotactic Radiosurgery. New York, McGraw-Hill, 1993.)

size. Most treatments are carried out with a single isocenter. Although the total time for treatment is typically a few hours, fabrication of individualized apertures and range-modifying absorbers increases the overall treatment planning time. A typical charged particle beam delivery system is shown in Figure 41–5.

RADIOBIOLOGIC EFFECT AND DOSE

Isodose Prescription

Most of the radiobiologic effect with radiosurgery occurs within the target volume, both because of the steep dose gradient provided by radiosurgery and because the prescription isodose contour (typically 50% to 80%) conforms closely to the three-dimensional configuration of the target volume. As a result, radiosurgery doses are inhomogeneous. This inhomogeneity has important consequences, because radiobiologic effects, measured by biologically effective dose (BED), are not linear with dose: a doubling of dose causes more than a doubling in radiobiologic effect (Fig. 41–6). Therefore, dose inhomogeneities within the radiosurgery target volume may substantially elevate the potential for cure or complication. (Gamma knife and linac techniques are usually associated with greater dose inhomogeneity than are charged particle techniques.) Beyond the target's periphery, the radiobiologic effect decreases rapidly; this allows sparing of normal tissue, but it may also allow sparing of infiltrating tumor cells. Thus, the radiosurgeon treating malignant glioma is faced with a dilemma: should the prescription isodose surface conform tightly or loosely to the enhancing tumor volume? If the prescription isodose surface conforms tightly, the risk of normal tissue complications may be diminished, but the risk of tumor growth just beyond the enhancing volume may be increased. Some practitioners conform the isodose curves very tightly to the three-dimensional treatment volume, whereas others conform them to the three-dimensional target volume plus margin (up to 5 mm or so). Still others simply "cover" the target volume with a few isocenters (minimal attempt made to closely conform isodose surfaces to target volume), so that the margin from enhancing volume to prescription isodose surface for a given patient varies. Current response and complication data are insufficient to demonstrate which of these strategies is best.

Target Categories and Fractionation

Radiosurgery target volumes may be placed in one of four categories (A through D) based on two criteria: (1) whether the radiobiologic response within the target volume is early or late, and (2) whether the target volume does or does not contain normal tissue. Normal intracranial tissue is always late responding; abnormal tissue may be early or late responding.

Category A target volumes have a late response to both normal and abnormal tissue within the target volume (e.g., arteriovenous malformation [AVM]). Category B targets are late responding, but only in tumor tissue, because they contain no normal tissue (e.g., meningioma, pituitary adenoma). Category C targets contain normal tissue as well as early-

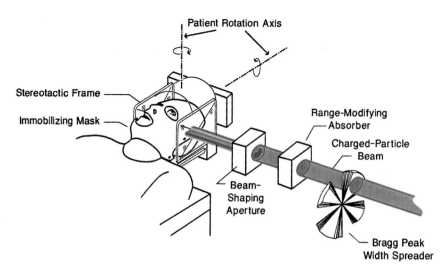

Figure 41–5 Charged particle beam delivery system, including the beam-shaping aperture, the range-modifying absorber, and the Bragg peak width modulator. (From Alexander EI, Coffey R, Loeffler JS: Radiosurgery for gliomas. *In* Alexander EI, Loeffler JS, Lunsford LD (eds): Stereotactic Radiosurgery. New York, McGraw-Hill, 1993.)

responding abnormal tissue (e.g., low-grade glial tumor). Category D target volumes contain predominantly early-responding abnormal tissue (e.g., metastases). Glioblastomas have some radiobiologic properties of both early- and late-responding tissues, and may in fact contain some normal tissue; nevertheless they are usually considered examples of category D.

Theoretical radiobiologic arguments, in some cases supported by much clinical data, indicate that fractionation, in comparison to radiosurgery, may not improve the ratio of cures to complications (therapeutic ratio) for patients with category A or B target volumes, but that it should provide a great improvement for patients with category C or D target volumes.[15] Clinical data on fractionated treatments to a dose sufficient to test this prediction are not available for patients with AVM, nor does there appear to be any motivation to test it. Clinical data for radiosurgery and for fractionated radiotherapy for meningioma are available and show not dissimilar therapeutic ratios.[16, 17] Data for radiosurgery for

low-grade glial tumors (category C) are very limited,[18] and most radiosurgery teams have not recommended radiosurgery as part of the initial treatment of these lesions. For metastases (category D), the therapeutic ratio with radiosurgery appears to be better than that obtained with fractionated treatment, although no studies have used high enough fractionated doses to produce a comparable radiobiologic effect.

For glioblastoma (category D), the therapeutic ratio with brachytherapy would be expected to be substantially more favorable than that obtained with radiosurgery, because the two boost techniques are at opposite ends of the fractionation spectrum. However, current clinical data fail to show a large difference, if any, as discussed in the following section. It is not entirely apparent why fractionation is not more important for glioblastoma, although the explanation may have to do with treatment volume. In most cases, at least for small targets, radiosurgery does not produce damage to a large enough volume of normal tissue to have serious clinical consequences. In any case, most patients with glioblastoma undergo fractionated irradiation as part of their therapy, which may dilute the deleterious effect of that portion of the treatment, which might be "suboptimal."

Dose

As physicians have more thoroughly documented complications of radiosurgery, a trend has developed to reduce radiosurgery dose levels. This is consistent with four principles of radiosurgery: (1) slowly proliferating tissues may require months or even years to demonstrate response; (2) slow response does not necessarily imply radioresistance; (3) the latent interval can be decreased by increasing the radiosurgery dose; and (4) response often reflects proliferative activity rather than intrinsic radiation sensitivity. AVMs, meningiomas, pituitary adenomas, and acoustic neuromas are slowly proliferative radiosurgery targets. In most cases, these or other slowly growing lesions do not require a radiation dose that risks damage to normal tissue to produce a rapid response or to produce tumor necrosis.

Glioblastomas, however, are often rapidly growing, and high dose levels may therefore be warranted, even if risks for necrosis are increased. However, Larson and co-workers[19]

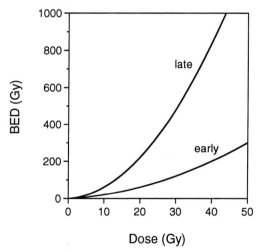

Figure 41–6 The relative biologic effects of different radiosurgery doses can be compared with the biologically effective dose (BED) formalism. The figure shows BED for late- ($\alpha/\beta = 2$) and for early-responding ($\alpha/\beta = 10$) tissue. In either case, radiobiologic effects are not linear with dose: a doubling of dose causes more than a doubling in radiobiologic effect. Within any radiosurgery target volume, dose inhomogeneities may substantially elevate the potential for cure or complication.

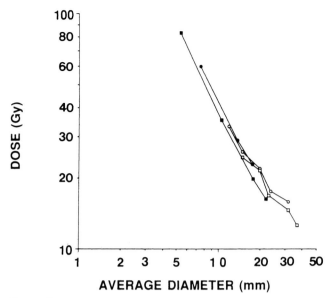

Figure 41–7 Dose-volume isoeffect curves for a 3% risk of radiation necrosis for gamma knife and 6 MV linac radiosurgery, with dose prescribed to either the 80% or the 50% isodose surface (*open circles*, linac 80%; *closed circles*, gamma knife 80%; *open squares*, linac 50%; *closed squares*, gamma knife 50%). Most practitioners use smaller doses for larger tumors to maintain a constant low risk of complications. (From Flickinger JC, Schell MC, Larson DA: Estimation of complications for linear accelerator radiosurgery with the integrated logistic formula. Int J Radiat Oncol Biol Phys 1990; 19:146.)

performed a multivariate analysis of 189 patients with malignant glioma treated with radiosurgery and failed to show that radiosurgery dose level was significantly associated with survival or complications. Lack of a clearcut dose-response relationship has also been noted in patients with glioblastoma undergoing brachytherapy boost.[20] Most practitioners prescribe a smaller dose for larger tumors to maintain a relatively constant risk of complications, based on the integrated logistic model of Flickinger and colleagues (Fig. 41–7).[21]

SURVIVAL

Summary survival data for patients treated with radiosurgery are presented in Table 41–1 (primary tumors) and Table 41–2 (recurrent tumors). Survival for primary glioma patients is measured from the date of pathologic diagnosis, and survival for recurrent glioma patients is measured from the

date of radiosurgery. In both tables, survival results vary considerably, but this can be largely accounted for by differences in selection factors, as discussed later.

The selection of patients who may benefit from radiosurgery has often been difficult, because attempts to identify prognostic factors have often been limited by small numbers of patients, by a narrow spectrum of values of possible prognostic variables, or by failure to analyze several candidate prognostic variables, and published data are in conflict.[22–25]

Larson and associates[19] attempted to overcome these limitations by performing a retrospective analysis of 189 patients with malignant glioma treated with gamma knife radiosurgery at eight different institutions by 23 different physicians. This study was able to explore a broad range of standards for patient selection and treatment. Patients had either unifocal or bifocal tumor, a KPS in the range 40 to 100, tumor volumes in the range 0.3 to 96.0 mL, and minimum tumor doses in the range 5 to 37.5 Gy. With multivariate analysis, the only variables significantly associated with decreased survival from the date of radiosurgery were the following: higher pathologic grade, older patient age, lower KPS, larger tumor volume, and bifocal vs. unifocal tumor.

Larson and co-workers[19] derived an equation to calculate the hazard ratio for individual patients, with larger hazard ratios being associated with shorter survival; they applied the equation to various reported series to obtain an estimated hazard ratio for each series. Table 41–3 presents a summary of surviving fractions following radiosurgery for malignant glioma, and it also shows the estimated hazard ratio calculated according to the model of Larson and others. A statistically significant inverse relationship was found between estimated hazard ratio and survival (Kendall's rank correlation, $P < 0.001$). Larson and co-workers concluded that the wide variations in published survival rates following radiosurgery for malignant glioma could be accounted for mainly by differences in patient populations with respect to pathology, age, KPS, tumor volume, and number of tumors. It was also concluded that subcategories of patients with unfavorable constellations of these variables are unlikely to benefit from radiosurgery.

Because the estimated hazard ratio depends only on the five significant clinical variables mentioned earlier, and not on the technical details of radiosurgery (e.g., dose, isodose percentage, or number of isocenters), the model may apply to brachytherapy data as well, and brachytherapy data have been included in Table 41–3 for comparison. The role of radiosurgery compared to that of brachytherapy is of great

TABLE 41–1
SUMMARY OF REPORTED STUDY GROUP CHARACTERISTICS AND SURVIVAL RATES IN PATIENTS WITH PRIMARY MALIGNANT GLIOMA TREATED WITH RADIOSURGERY

Study	No. of Patients	Glioblastoma (%)	Median Age (yr)	Median KPS*	Median Volume (cc)	Bifocal Tumor (%)	Median Minimum Dose (Gy)	Survival* 1 yr (%)	Survival* Median (wk)
Mehta et al[23]	31	100	57	70	17.4	0	12.0	38	42
Alexander et al[27]	37	62	50	85	4.8	0	12.0	—	104†
Larson et al[19]	57	54	47	90	5.9	7	16.0	67	86

*Survival from date of pathologic diagnosis.
†Glioblastoma only; not reached for anaplastic astrocytoma.

TABLE 41–2
SUMMARY OF REPORTED STUDY GROUP CHARACTERISTICS AND SURVIVAL RATES IN PATIENTS WITH RECURRENT MALIGNANT GLIOMA
TREATED WITH RADIOSURGERY

Study	No. of Patients	Glioblastoma (%)	Median Age (yr)	Median KPS*	Median Volume (cc)	Bifocal Tumor (%)	Median Minimum Dose (Gy)	Survival* 1 yr (%)	Survival* Median (wk)
Shrieve et al[22]	86	84	46	80	10.1	0	13.0	45	41
Hall et al[25]	36	72	47	70	27.0	0	20.0	30	28
Buatti et al[24]	11	55	42	≥90	14.0	0	12.5	—	41
Alexander et al[27]	58	70	45	80	12.0	0	14.0	—	40‡
Dempsey et al[28]	21§	48	40¶	>70	3.7¶	0	≥15.0	—	44‡
Chamberlain et al[29]	20	25	34	80	17.0	15	13.5	—	32
Larson et al[19]	132	50	45	90	6.5	7	16.0	60	67

*Initial pathologic grade.
†Survival from date of radiosurgery.
‡Glioblastoma only; not reached for anaplastic astrocytoma.
§Recurrent and primary tumor patients.
¶Mean.

interest, and the hazard ratio model may account for much of the variation in reported surviving fraction for patients treated with either radiosurgery or brachytherapy. Because this model is independent of the technical details of radiosurgery, it is possible to speculate that brachytherapy and radiosurgery provide similar improvements in survival. However, this must be tested in a clinical trial. Larson and colleagues[19] found that in patients receiving radiosurgery, no relationship was seen between survival and whether or not the patient might have satisfied reasonable brachytherapy criteria. Therefore, any benefits that are conferred on patients undergoing radiosurgery do not appear to be limited to patients with brachytherapy-accessible tumors. It must be reiterated, however, that the true impact of radiosurgery compared to brachytherapy on survival remains unknown, in the absence of a randomized clinical trial.

Although the survival and hazard ratio data in Table 41–3 are highly correlated, with decreasing surviving fractions at 1 or 2 years for increasing hazard ratio, two data points appear to lie several standard errors apart from the general trend. The 1-year surviving fraction for patients with primary glioblastoma treated with brachytherapy by Sneed and colleagues[20, 26] and with radiosurgery by Loeffler (oral communication, 1995) are higher than expected, and they may reflect unidentified prognostic factors, inadequacy of the hazard ratio model, or statistical fluctuations.

COMPLICATIONS

Larson and associates[19] analyzed complications and side effects. Acute complications were seen in 9% of evaluated patients and included acute edema, mass effect, confusion, memory loss, seizures, weakness, and dysphasia. Acute complications have been reported in 0% of patients in some series (Mehta and co-workers,[23] Buatti and colleagues,[24] and Hall and associates[25]) and in 12% of patients reported by Shrieve and co-workers[22] (Table 41–4). It is not obvious how to account for the lack of acute complications in some series and the significant numbers of acute complications in others. The explanation may have to do with differences in

selection and treatment factors or with differences in criteria for scoring acute complications.

Larson and colleagues[19] found chronic complications in 17% of patients followed up for at least 1 year, which included constellations of the following neurologic problems: headaches, numbness, weakness, hemiparesis, ataxia, radionecrosis, cranial nerve damage, Parinaud's syndrome, hemianopsia, apraxia, obtundation, dysarthria, aphasia, tremor, and decreased gait. Other authors have also reported complications: 22% of patients reported by Shrieve and associates[22] (reoperation for necrotic tumor), 13% of patients reported by Mehta and co-workers[23] (clinically significant necrosis), 27% of patients reported by Buatti and colleagues[24] (significant edema leading to reoperation), 19% of primary glioma patients and 21% of recurrent glioma patients reported by Alexander and associates[27] (reoperation for neurologic deterioration), and 19% of patients reported by Hall and co-workers[25] (reoperation). Shrieve and colleagues[22] who recognized that some patients may not survive long enough to experience chronic complications, performed an actuarial calculation that demonstrated a 2-year 50% actuarial risk for reoperation for possible necrotic tumor. Thus, the actuarial risk of chronic complications is substantially higher than that given by a crude calculation.

Larson and associates[19] investigated corticosteroid requirements following radiosurgery and found a 36% rate of chronic corticosteroid use among patients followed up for at least 1 year. Alexander and co-workers[27] reported 46% of 1-year survivors of primary malignant glioma required continuing corticosteroid therapy.

Data on long-term KPS are sparse. However, Larson and colleagues[19] found that approximately half of patients evaluated in any interval ranging from months to years after radiosurgery had stable or improved KPS compared to initial KPS, and approximately half had decreased KPS. Approximately 10% to 25% of patients had a KPS decrease of more than 20 points.

CONCLUSIONS

The use of radiosurgery for malignant glioma has become widespread, either as an alternative to brachytherapy or for

TABLE 41–3
HAZARD RATIOS AND SURVIVING FRACTIONS WITH GREENWOOD STANDARD ERRORS (WHEN AVAILABLE), LISTED IN ORDER OF
INCREASING HAZARD RATIO WITHIN EACH PATHOLOGIC GRADE CATEGORY*

Study	Pathologic Grade†	Tumor Status‡	Treatment§	Hazard Ratio	Surviving Fraction¶		No. of Patients
					1-yr	2-yr	
Larson et al[19]	II	P	RS	1.0	1.00 ± .00	1.00 ± .00	8
Larson et al[19]	II	R	RS	2.5	.80 ± .08	.73 ± .09	35
Sneed et al[20, 26]	II	P	B	2.6	.88 ± .08	.81 ± .10	37
Sneed et al[20, 26]	II	R	B	3.4	.64 ± .10	.46 ± .11	22
Larson et al[19]	III	P	RS**	3.1	1.00 ± .00	.38 ± .29	8
Larson et al[19]	III	P	RS	3.9	.86 ± .09	.48 ± .18	16
Larson et al[19]	III	R	RS**	4.5	.68 ± .12	.61 ± .13	17
Larson et al[19]	III	R	RS	4.6	.65 ± .10	.49 ± .11	27
Sneed et al[20, 26]	III	P	B	5.5	.78 ± .06	.59 ± .07	40
Sneed et al[20, 26]	III	R	B	6.0	.54 ± .07	.29 ± .07	45
Larson et al[19]	IV	R	RS**	9.7	.56 ± .08	.34 ± .08	46
Shrieve et al[22]	II–IV††	R	RS	9.8	.45 ± .11	.19 ± .10	86
Larson et al[19]	IV	P	RS**	10.0	.66 ± .13	.19 ± .15	16
Larson et al[19]	IV	R	RS	11.4	.49 ± .07	.30 ± .06	66
Larson et al[19]	IV	P	RS	11.8	.43 ± .10	.11 ± .09	31
Loeffler et al[7]	IV	P	B	12.8	.74	.24	69
Sneed et al[20, 26]	IV	R	B	14.7	.48 ± .06	.24 ± .05	66
Sneed et al[20, 26]	IV	P	B	13.5	.73 ± .04	.30 ± .04	52
Hall et al[25]	III–IV‡‡	R	RS	16.7	.30	NR	36
Larson et al[19]	II–IV§§	P, R	RS¶¶	18.9	.20 ± .17	.20 ± .17	13
Larson et al[19]	IV	P, R	RS***	27.9	.15 ± .17	.00	14

*In this table survival is measured from the date of radiosurgery, both for primary tumors and for recurrent tumors. The hazard ratio was calculated according to the model of Larson and co-workers[19] using median or mean values of pathologic grade, age, KPS, tumor volume, and number of tumors for each series, and it is independent of technical details of treatment. A hazard ratio value of 1.0 corresponds to a patient with a solitary pilocytic astrocytoma, age = 40, KPS = 100, and tumor volume = 0 cc. The data from Loeffler and colleagues and some data from Sneed and others and Shrieve and associates were based on personal communications. Hazard ratios are highly correlated with 1-year and 2-year survival (Kendall's rank correlation, $P<0.001$).
†Initial pathologic grade: I = pilocytic astrocytoma, II = astrocytoma, III = anaplastic astrocytoma or mixed tumor, IV = glioblastoma.
‡P = primary, R = recurrent.
§RS = radiosurgery, B = brachytherapy.
¶Survival from date of radiosurgery (NR = not reached).
**Brachytherapy criteria satisfied.
††84% IV, 5% III, 11% II.
‡‡72% IV, 28% III.
§§69% IV, 23% III, 8% II.
¶¶Bifocal tumor patients.
***Poor prognosis patients: pathologic grade = IV, KPS<80, and age>45.

patients who do not qualify for brachytherapy trials. Outcome following radiosurgery for glioma is strongly dependent on a relatively small number of selection factors, including pathologic grade, age, KPS, tumor volume, and number of tumor foci. Much of the variation in survival obtained by different groups can be attributed to differences in distributions of significant variables in study populations, and probably to a lesser degree—if at all—on the type of radiosurgery apparatus used. Future trials may be improved by incorporating these variables into their design. Although radiosurgery is attractive from the standpoints of patient comfort and health economics, in the absence of a randomized trial, it is not known how radiosurgery compares to brachytherapy.

TABLE 41–4
SUMMARY OF ACUTE AND CHRONIC COMPLICATIONS IN
PATIENTS TREATED WITH RADIOSURGERY FOR GLIOMA

Study	No. of Patients	Complications*	
		Acute (%)	Chronic (%)
Shrieve et al[22]	86	12	22
Alexander et al[27]	37	—	19
Hall et al[25]	36	0	19
Buatti et al[24]	11	0	27
Mehta et al[23]	31	0	13
Larson et al[19]	189	9	17†

*Acute and chronic complications defined variably.
†Chronic complications were seen in 17% of patients followed up for at least 1 year.

REFERENCES

1. Leksell L: The stereotaxic method and radiosurgery of the brain. Acta Chir Scand 1951; 102:316–319.
2. Larson DA, Bova F, Eisert D, et al: Current radiosurgery practice: Results of an ASTRO survey. Task Force on Stereotactic Radiosurgery, American Society for Therapeutic Radiology and Oncology. Int J Radiat Oncol Biol Phys 1994; 28:523–526.
3. Larson DA, Bova F, Eisert D, et al: Consensus statement on stereotactic radiosurgery quality improvement. The American Society for Therapeutic Radiology and Oncology, Task Force on Stereotactic Radiosurgery and the American Association of Neurological Surgeons. Int J Radiat Oncol Biol Phys 1994; 28:527–530.
4. Walker MD, Strike TA, Sheline GE: An analysis of dose-effect relationship in the radiotherapy of malignant gliomas. Int J Radiat Oncol Biol Phys 1979; 5:1725–1731.

5. Bleehen NM, Stenning SP: A Medical Research Council trial of two radiotherapy doses in the treatment of grades 3 and 4 astrocytoma. The Medical Research Council Brain Tumour Working Party. Br J Cancer 1991; 64:769–774.

6. Scharfen CO, Sneed PK, Wara WM, et al: High activity iodine-125 interstitial implant for gliomas. Int J Radiat Oncol Biol Phys 1992; 24:583–591.

7. Loeffler JS, Alexander E III, Wen PY, et al: Results of stereotactic brachytherapy used in the initial management of patients with glioblastoma. JNCI 1990; 82:1918–1921.

8. Green SB, Shapiro WR, Burger PC, et al: A Randomized Boost Trial of Interstitial Radiotherapy (RT) Boost for Newly Diagnosed Malignant Glioma: Brain Tumor Cooperative Group (BTCG) Trial 8701. Proceedings of the American Society of Clinical Oncology, Dallas, 1994, p 174.

9. Shrieve DC, Gutin PH, Larson DA: Brachytherapy. *In* Mauch PM, Loeffler JS (eds): Radiation Oncology: Technology and Biology. Philadelphia, WB Saunders, 1994, pp 216–236.

10. Phillips MH, Stelzer KJ, Griffin TW, et al: Stereotactic radiosurgery: A review and comparison of methods. J Clin Oncol 1994; 12:1085–1099.

11. Lutz W, Winston KR, Maleki N: A system for stereotactic radiosurgery with a linear accelerator. Int J Radiat Oncol Biol Phys 1988; 14:373–381.

12. Winston KR, Lutz W: Linear accelerator as a neurosurgical tool for stereotactic radiosurgery. Neurosurgery 1988; 22:454–464.

13. McGinley PH, Butker EK, Crocker IR, et al: A patient rotator for stereotactic radiosurgery. Phys Med Biol 1990; 35:649–657.

14. Podgorsak EB, Olivier A, Pla M, et al: Dynamic stereotactic radiosurgery. Int J Radiat Oncol Biol Phys 1988; 14:115–126.

15. Hall EJ, Brenner DJ: The radiobiology of radiosurgery: Rationale for different treatment regimes for AVMs and malignancies [see comments]. Int J Radiat Oncol Biol Phys 1993; 25:381–385.

16. Goldsmith BJ, Wara WM, Wilson CB, et al: Postoperative irradiation for subtotally resected meningiomas: A retrospective analysis of 140 patients treated from 1967 to 1990. J Neurosurg 1994; 80:195–201.

17. Kondziolka D, Lunsford LD, Coffey RJ, et al: Gamma knife radiosurgery of meningiomas. Stereotact Funct Neurosurg 1991; 57:11–21.

18. Pozza F, Colombo F, Chiergo G, et al: Low-grade astrocytomas: Treatment with unconventionally fractionated external beam stereotactic radiation therapy. Radiology 1989; 171:565–569.

19. Larson DA, Gutin P, McDermott M, et al: Experience with Gamma Knife Radiosurgery in the United States. Proceedings of the US-Japan Radiation Oncology Conference, San Francisco, 1995.

20. Sneed PK, Larson DA, Prados MD, et al: Lack of a Dose-Response Relationship for Survival of Patients With Glioblastoma Treated With Brain Implant Boost. Proceedings of the 62nd Annual Meeting of the American Association of Neurological Surgeons, San Diego, 1994, pp 558–559.

21. Flickinger JC, Schell MC, Larson DA: Estimation of complications for linear accelerator radiosurgery with the integrated logistic formula. Int J Radiat Oncol Biol Phys 1990; 19:143–148.

22. Shrieve DC, Alexander E III, Wen PY, et al: Comparison of stereotactic radiosurgery and brachytherapy in the treatment of recurrent glioblastoma multiforme. Neurosurgery 1995; 36:275–284.

23. Mehta MP, Masciopinto J, Rozental J, et al: Stereotactic radiosurgery for glioblastoma multiforme: Report of a prospective study evaluating prognostic factors and analyzing long-term survival advantage. Int J Radiat Oncol Biol Phys 1994; 30:541–549.

24. Buatti JM, Friedman WA, Bova FJ, et al: Linac radiosurgery for high grade gliomas: The University of Florida experience. Int J Radiat Oncol Biol Phys 1995; 32:205–210.

25. Hall WA, Djalilian HR, Sperduto PW, et al: Stereotactic radiosurgery for recurrent malignant gliomas (abstract). J Neurosurg 1995; 82:355.

26. Sneed PK, Prados MD, McDermott MD, et al: Large effect of age on survival of patients with glioblastoma treated with radiotherapy and brachytherapy boost. Neurosurgery 1995; 36:898–903.

27. Alexander EI, Coffey R, Loeffler JS: Radiosurgery for gliomas. *In* Alexander EI, Loeffler JS, Lunsford LD (eds): Stereotactic Radiosurgery. New York, McGraw-Hill, 1993, pp 207–219.

28. Dempsey PK, Kondziolka D, Lunsford LD, et al: The role of stereotactic radiosurgery in the treatment of glial tumors. *In* Lunsford LD (ed): Stereotactic Radiosurgery Update. Amsterdam, Elsevier, 1992, pp 407–410.

29. Chamberlain MC, Barba D, Kormanik P, et al: Stereotactic radiosurgery for recurrent gliomas. Cancer 1994; 74:1342–1347.

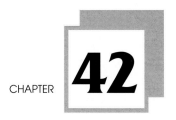

CHAPTER **42**

Radiosensitizers

Enhancement is needed of the differential effect of radiation on tumor and on normal tissues that are included in the radiation volume during radiotherapy of malignant gliomas. Chemical modifiers of radiation response should increase the damage to the tumor without increasing the damage to normal tissues. Radiosensitizers are compounds that, when combined with radiation, produce greater tumor cell kill than would have been expected from a simple additive effect (Fig. 42–1).

Most cancer chemotherapeutic agents have an additive effect that is equivalent to an incremental increase in the radiation dose. Their use in combination with radiation offers no differential effect between tumor and normal tissues. Because the toxicities of the chemotherapeutic agent and the radiation overlap, no major gain is achieved.[1] This is the case with the most commonly used cancer chemotherapeutic agents such as Adriamycin, vincristine, cisplatin, carmustine, and procarbazine (Fig. 42–2).

The addition of a chemical radiosensitizer to a course of radiation should only be considered in for tumor sites that already offer evidence that an increase in dose intensity will translate into an increase in tumor control, particularly tumors with a steep radiation dose-response curve.

CHEMICAL SENSITIZERS OF HYPOXIC CELLS

Tumor cell radioresistance is a multifactorial problem. The tumor microenvironment (notably the presence of hypoxia)

has been known for several years to be one of the factors contributing to radioresistance. In addition, tumor cell kinetics and inherent radioresistance may play important roles. More information on the complexity of the tumor microenvironment has become available. For example, some areas of the tumor may be chronically hypoxic, whereas others are only intermittently (acutely) hypoxic.

Hypoxia may induce molecular changes, such as induction of stress response genes. These new concepts in the tumor microenvironment are also of interest to the cancer chemotherapy field because of their implications for drug resistance.[2–5]

Nitroimidazole Compounds (Metronidazole, Misonidazole, and Etanidazole)

Under hypoxic conditions, nitroimidazole compounds bind to cellular macromolecules and act as electron donors, thus mimicking the effects of oxygen in the fixation of radiation-induced DNA damage (Fig. 42–3).

METRONIDAZOLE

The first compound to be investigated clinically was metronidazole (a 2-nitroimidazole). Its dose-limiting toxic effects were gastrointestinal symptoms (nausea and vomiting) and peripheral sensory neuropathy, allowing this compound

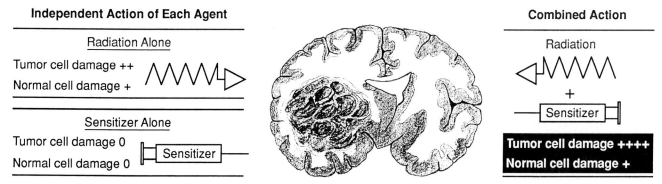

Figure 42–1 Tumor enhancement/sensitization (truly radiosensitizer). Greater tumor inactivation than would have been expected from the additive effect.

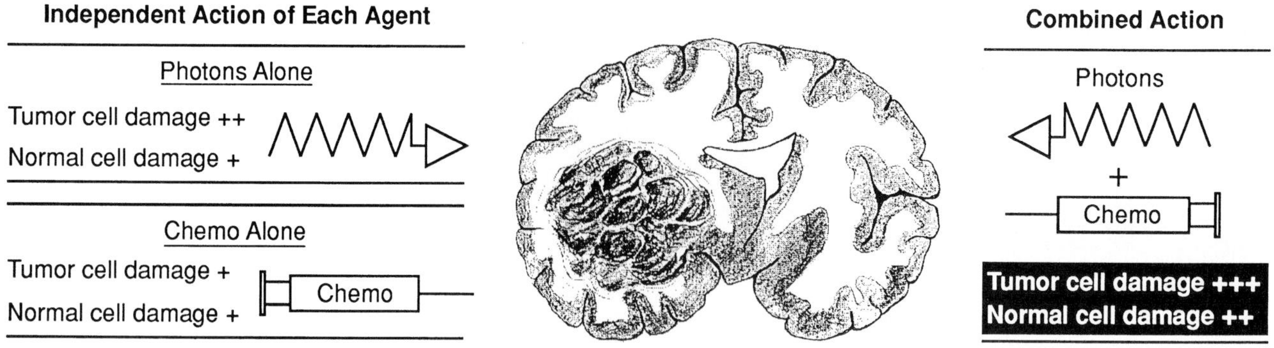

Independent Action of Each Agent

Combined Action

Photons Alone

Tumor cell damage ++

Normal cell damage +

Chemo Alone

Tumor cell damage +

Normal cell damage +   Chemo

Photons

+

Chemo

Tumor cell damage +++
Normal cell damage ++

Figure 42–2 Simple addition of antitumor effects (not truly a radiosensitizer). Toxic effects of chemicals and radiation could overlap with no major gain.

to reach an estimated sensitizer enhancement ratio (SER) of only 1.2.[6] The first efficacy study with metronidazole was done on patients with glioblastoma. In this randomized study, a less than optimal radiation fractionation schedule was imposed by the need to administer the radiosensitizer on an every-other-day schedule because of its toxicity. The addition of metronidazole improved the relatively poor survival of the control arm to the level of survival previously obtained with conventional fractionation. This improvement in survival demonstrated the relevance of tumor hypoxia.[7]

MISONIDAZOLE

This initial investigation prompted a search for new and better nitroimidazole compounds with less toxicity, which

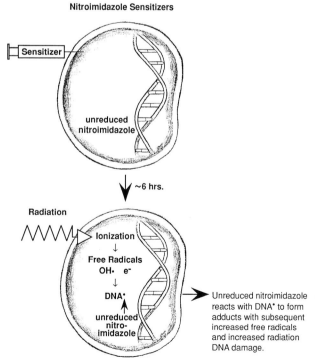

Figure 42–3 Cellular mechanisms of hypoxic cell radiosensitizers. Nitroimidazole compounds.

would allow them to be delivered with each daily fraction of radiation. During the early 1980s, the first clinical studies on the second-generation compound, misonidazole (a 2-nitroimidazole), were initiated in both Europe and North America in patients with anaplastic astrocytoma and glioblastoma. In the oral form, the dose-limiting toxic effects were, again, peripheral sensory neuropathy and gastrointestinal symptoms, which thus limited the delivery of a dose sufficient to obtain an effective SER. Pharmacokinetic studies demonstrated evidence of good tumor drug concentration relative to plasma.[8] However, the results from both small pilot studies and large randomized clinical trials that compared conventional fractionated radiation with or without misonidazole in more than 1,500 patients with malignant glioma failed to demonstrate any benefit from the addition of misonidazole (Table 42–1).[9–14]

Several possible reasons may explain why nitroimidazole compounds (metronidazole and misonidazole) generally failed to demonstrate an advantage when combined with radiation in patients with malignant gliomas. They include the following:

1. An effective drug dose is not delivered due to the limiting toxic effects related to the gastrointestinal tract and peripheral neuropathies.

2. Malignant gliomas lack a steep radiation dose-response curve beyond 5,500 cGy, previously noted as a necessary condition to show benefit.

3. Substantial tumor hypoxia necessary to demonstrate an effect with nitroimidazoles is absent or, alternatively, effective reoxygenation occurs during fractionated radiotherapy.

ETANIDAZOLE

Phase I pharmacokinetic and toxicity studies of a third-generation compound, etanidazole demonstrated that higher doses of sensitizers could be delivered with lower incidences of neuropathy.[15] Based on pharmacokinetic studies with brain tumor biopsies that demonstrated etanidazole penetration into brain tumors,[16] a pilot phase I study to assess the tolerance and logistics of administering a continuous infusion of etanidazole with external radiation (twice-daily fractionation), as well as during interstitial ^{125}I implants, is being conducted. The dose-limited toxic effects of the continuous infusion are cramping and arthralgia, and the cumulative

TABLE 42–1
RESULTS OF HYPOXIC CELL RADIOSENSITIZERS IN PATIENTS WITH MALIGNANT GLIOMA

Compound	No. of Studies With Mixed Population Anaplastic Astrocytoma and Glioblastoma	No. of Studies With Glioblastoma	No. of Studies Showing Benefit in TTP/Survival		No. of Randomized Studies		Total No. of Patients
			Yes	No	Yes	No	
Metronidazole[7]	1	—	1*	—	1	—	33
Misonidazole[9–14]	8	1	—	9	5	4	1,500
Etanidazole[17]	1	—	Too early to assess (ongoing study)		—	1	70

*Within the constraints of the study. No benefit when compared to conventional treatment.
TTP, time to tumor progression.

maximum tolerated dose is 26 g/m^2.[17] Based on these studies, a Radiation Therapy Oncology Group (RTOG) study has been proposed to use etanidazole in combination with stereotactic radiosurgery in malignant gliomas.

Current and Future Directions With Sensitizers of Hypoxic Tumor Cells

During all these years of work with hypoxic cell radiosensitizers, we have learned that tumor hypoxic cell resistance to conventional radiation fractionation in humans is a more complex problem that it appeared to be in the mid-1970s, when these compounds were first tested in experimental models and the first clinical investigations were initiated. Results of recent studies suggest that radiobiologic tumor hypoxia is not a universal phenomenon in glioblastomas despite the presence of areas of necrosis.[18] Beginning in 1992 the first results of assessment of tumor hypoxia in patients with glioblastoma have been reported. These studies used either the microelectrode Eppendorf histograph,[19] positron emission tomography (PET)[20] with fluoromisonidazole or single-photon emission computed tomography (SPECT) with ^{123}I-iodoazomycin ([^{123}I]-IAZA),[21] an azomycin nucleoside. Contrary to expectations, the [^{123}I]-IAZA SPECT scan was positive in only one out of 11 patients with histologic diagnosis of glioblastoma, despite the fact that these tumors, by definition, have areas of necrosis.[18, 21, 22] However, using the invasive computer-driven Eppendorf microelectrode, a high percentage of low pO$_2$ values (<2.5 mm Hg) have been recorded in patients with glioblastoma.[23] The possibility that higher levels of chronic tumor hypoxia are needed for the binding of [^{123}I]-IAZA could explain the disparity between the two methods. Evidence from animal experimental models with transplanted human cell lines suggests that gliomas have an adaptive mechanism for low oxygen consumption, and have altered cell cycles, and that radiobiologic hypoxic cells may not always be found in proximity to areas of necrosis.[24]

INCREASED OXYGEN-CARRYING CAPACITY OF THE BLOOD AND USE OF FLUOSOL

Clinical studies have been completed using hyperbaric oxygen,[25] carbogen,[26] packed red blood cell transfusions,[27, 28] and oxygen-carrier assistance, such as perfluorocarbons (Fluosol).[29, 30] Although the use of the hyperbaric oxygen chamber at three atmospheres presented technical difficulties, such as barotrauma and the limitation of its use to only a few high-dose fractions of radiation, three out of ten clinical trials show significant positive results, particularly in patients with advanced cancer of the cervix.[31] The use of perfluorocarbons (Fluosol) was investigated in a pilot phase I and II trial in patients with malignant gliomas. The results of this study indicated that Fluosol/oxygen added to conventional radiation therapy did not enhance survival of patients with malignant gliomas.[32]

BIOREDUCTIVE AND HYPOXIC CELL CYTOTOXIC AGENTS

It has been recognized that hypoxia can be one of the causes of chemotherapy resistance. Therefore, the use of bioreductive agents that are cytotoxic to hypoxic tumor cells has been proposed.[4, 5] Tirapazamine (SR–4233), the first member of a new class of bioreductive agents (benzotriazine-di-N-oxides) has been developed and tested in animal tumor systems.[33, 34] It is thought that under hypoxic conditions, reduction of tirapazamine results in the production of a highly reactive free radical that can attack DNA. This mechanism makes the combined use of tirapazamine and radiation particularly attractive, as radiation mainly inactivates oxygenated cells, whereas tirapazamine is selectively cytotoxic for hypoxic radioresistant cells. Laboratory data indicate that glioblastomas contain bioreductive enzymes (e.g., diaphorase and cytochrome reductase) capable of reducing hypoxic cytotoxic agents such as tirapazamine.[23] Primary brain tumors may therefore be one of the suitable targets for bioreductive therapy. Considerable clinical activities are expected in the near future with these bioreductive agents.

GLUTATHIONE DEPLETION

Sulfhydryl compounds are scavengers of free radicals, protecting against chemical damage induced by either ionizing radiation or alkylating agents via glutathione-S-transferase. It has been demonstrated in the laboratory that one approach to increasing the efficiency of nitroimidazoles in combination with radiation is to decrease the levels of endogenous sulfhydryls. Glutathione (GSH) is one of the major endogenous sulfhydryls. Buthionine-SR-sulfoximine (BSO) is a specific inhibitor of GSH synthesis. It has been shown to deplete GSH levels in both in vitro and in vivo systems, therefore making misonidazole a more effective sensitizer.[35] Laboratory studies have shown that pretreatment with BSO resulted in little or no increase in the toxic effects of misonidazole in normal tissues; however, an increased sensitizing efficacy was observed in the tumor.[36] Several investigators have demonstrated that GSH depletion can enhance effectiveness of misonidazole and etanidazole[37] as well as increase the effectiveness of bioreductive agents that are cytotoxic to hypoxic cells.[38] Therefore, the use of BSO as a modulator of hypoxic cell sensitizers in combination with radiation, or as a modulator of chemotherapeutic drugs (such as alkylating agents) and bioreductive hypoxic cytotoxic agents is of interest and is being investigated actively.[39, 40] However, controversy exists as to whether depletion of GSH alone will be effective in enhancing the radiation effect. In one experimental model using a human glioma xenograft, it was reported that administration of BSO to radiation alone did not influence duration of animal survival.[41] However, in another experimental animal tumor model system using intracerebral glioma xenografts, the administration of BSO enhanced the activity of interstitial radiotherapy without concomitant increase in toxic effects, which suggests possible future application of BSO to brain tumor brachytherapy.[42]

In the future, patients with malignant glioma could be selected for therapeutic manipulation of the tumor microenvironment, particularly targeting the problem of tumor hypoxia. Selection parameters could include determination of tumor metabolic parameters by (1) oxygen utilization, (2) glucose metabolic rate, and (3) adduct formation using fluorinated misonidazole and PET[20] or radioiodinated azomycin nucleosides, and SPECT.[21, 22]

NONHYPOXIC TUMOR CELL SENSITIZERS

Halogenated Pyrimidine Analogs

5-BROMODEOXYURIDINE (BUdR) AND 5-IODODEOXYURIDINE (IUdR)

The pyrimidine analogs BUdR and IUdR are considered cell-cycle specific radiosensitizers acting independently of the oxygen effect. As previously discussed, the radioresistance of human solid tumors could be multifactorial, where in addition to the microenvironment, tumor cell kinetics play an important role. The presence of rapidly proliferating clonogens may substantially influence the control of tumors by irradiation. Because BUdR and IUdR are incorporated only into rapidly proliferating cells, such tissues, either normal or tumor, could be effectively sensitized. Rapidly proliferating tumor cells surrounded by slowly dividing normal tissue cells constitute the ideal situation for an improved therapeutic ratio. This is theoretically the case for malignant gliomas. The agents, however, require prolonged exposure times to allow for the necessary incorporation into DNA during DNA synthesis.

Pyrimidine analogs substitute for thymidine in DNA through the thymidine salvage pathway. This substitution

alters the physicochemical properties of DNA, resulting in a radiosensitizing effect. The basic mechanisms of radiosensitization are controversial and are not clearly understood. Recent evidence from "in vitro" work suggests two components. One component (decreased repair) is related to the increase in the amount of DNA strand breakage induced by radiation in the presence of IUdR/BUdR substitution. The second component (increased damage) is related to the production of a non-scavengeable hydrated electron at sites of multiple damage. Together, these two component mechanisms support the multiple damage site theory[43] (Fig. 42–4).

Importance of Cell Labeling and DNA Incorporation

Clinical Investigations

The means of achieving an optimal cell incorporation of these compounds in the clinic has been extensively explored over the years, with particular emphasis on the route of administration and length of drug exposure. Initially, BUdR was administered intra-arterially to avoid both dehalogenation by the liver and to increase the drug tumor concentration.[44] However, the prolonged use of this route in patients over several weeks was laborious and was associated with a high incidence of complications. Although reports have been made of rapid debromination of halopyrimidines occurring after IV therapy, Goffinet and Brown[45] showed that following IV infusion enough halopyrimidine apparently passes the hepatic vessels to permit tumor radiosensitization despite dilution of the drug by the systemic circulation. This has also been shown in human studies.[46] A renewed interest has

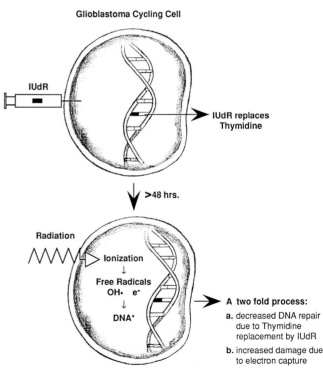

Cellular Mechanisms of Sensitizers Specific for Proliferating Cells

Glioblastoma Cycling Cell

IUdR

IUdR replaces Thymidine

>48 hrs.

Radiation

Ionization
↓
Free Radicals
OH· e⁻
↓
DNA·

A two fold process:
a. decreased DNA repair due to Thymidine replacement by IUdR
b. increased damage due to electron capture

Figure 42–4 Cellular mechanisms of halogenated pyrimidine analogs.

taken place since the mid-1980s in the use of continuous intravenous infusion of halopyrimidines. It has been observed that adequate steady-state arterial plasma levels could be maintained with this route of administration with acceptable systemic toxic responses.[47] Although the generally accepted method of administering halogenated pyrimidines is IV infusion, controversy exists over both the length of the infusion and the dose intensity. Some investigators propose giving these drugs at relatively high doses with short infusions in an attempt to achieve maximum thymidine replacement in DNA.[48] However, others recommend using prolonged low doses of halopyrimidines, not only because the prolonged infusion could be better tolerated, but also because more cells would be exposed to the drug.[49, 50] Theoretically, the proportion of IUdR/BUdR labeled cells should exceed 90%, because the number of cells that are not labeled, and are therefore not sensitized, would limit tumor control. However, results of a study using in vivo tumor xenografts and a mathematical model of continuous exposure to halogenated pyrimidines to assess the kinetics of cell labeling and DNA replacement suggest that a relatively small DNA IUdR replacement can result in significant sensitization and cell kill. Therefore, a modest concentration of halogenated pyrimidines, such as is achievable with use of a long infusion, may result in radiosensitization, provided that all or a high proportion of cells are labeled.[51]

Clinical Experience In 1987, continuous infusion of halopyrimidines in combination with radiation was tested in patients with malignant glioma (mixed population of glioblastomas and anaplastic astrocytomas), and a median survival of 13 months was reported (Tables 42–2 and 42–3).[52] The median survival for a group of 45 patients with glioblastoma treated with continuous intravenous infusion of IUdR at 1 g/m^2 for 14 days' infusion in combination with hyperfractionated radiotherapy was 11 months, with 9% surviving 24 months.[53] A larger series was reported by the Northern California Oncology Group (NCOG)/University of California, San Francisco (UCSF) in 160 patients with glioblastoma treated with 96-hour infusion of BUdR at 800 m/m^2 a day for a total of 6 weeks, in combination with 60 Gy irradiation. In this series, after radiotherapy, the patients received chemotherapy with procarbazine, CCNU and vincristine (PCV) for 1 year. The median survival was 12.8 months.[54] These results are not significantly different from those of other series using radiation with or without chemotherapy (most commonly nitrosureas). However, of interest is the striking improvement observed in the NCOG/UCSF study, in which

TABLE 42–3

HALOGENATED PYRIMIDINE ANALOGS (IUdR AND BUdR) IN PATIENTS WITH ANAPLASTIC ASTROCYTOMA

Compound	Randomized		Benefit in TTP/Survival		Total No. of Patients
	Yes	No	Yes	No	
BUdR[55, 56]		X	X		148
IUdR[57]		X	X		21

148 patients with anaplastic astrocytoma had a median survival of almost 5 years.[55, 56] This observation, along with a recent study utilizing IUdR in anaplastic astrocytoma,[57] indicates that the use of pyrimidine analogs in combination with radiation may be of greater benefit in patients with anaplastic astrocytoma. So far, no evidence has been found of an improvement in time to tumor progression or survival in patients with glioblastoma.

The use of an implantable infusion pump has rekindled interest in the use of intra-arterial BUdR. A small pilot study utilizing intra-arterial BUdR in combination with external radiotherapy reported a median survival of 14 months for glioblastoma patients.[58] However, these results are not significantly better than those achievable with the standard radiation/chemotherapy protocols.

To answer, in part, the controversy over the use of prolonged low-dose infusions vs. short high-dose infusions, a phase I and II clinical study in patients with malignant gliomas was recently completed in which the toxic effects and tumor efficacy of a ''long'' 96-hour IV infusion were compared with two ''short'' schedules of 24 and 48 hours at high-dose intensity. Despite hepatic and bone marrow toxic effects, and the fact that few patients received a minimum of 80% of the targeted dose, a trend to improved survival was seen in patients with anaplastic astrocytomas who received the long 96-hour infusion. It was concluded that the standard use of IUdR with radiation was not warranted in patients with glioblastoma at the dose schedules used in the study.[57] Interest has been aroused in much longer schedules of 6 to 8 weeks' continuous infusion at very low doses, to aim at a possible cell labeling index of more than 90%. This could be a difficult task to achieve, particularly in glioblastomas, as they are known to have lower labeling indices than other tumors, such as squamous cell carcinoma of the head and neck.

Future Directions The degree of incorporation and/or thymidine replacement and the SER are intimately related.[43, 56] Therefore, a need has been demonstrated for measurements of thymidine replacement in individual human brain tumors by flow cytometry and for measurements of the SER as a function of thymidine replacement. This assessment should be performed after short and long infusions and as part of the design of clinical trials with these cell-cycle specific drugs. From previous studies, a clear relationship has been established between the percent of thymidine replacement and the SER.[56]

Modulation of the incorporation of halogenated pyrimidines has been achieved in vitro with the use of 5-fluoroura-

TABLE 42–2

HALOGENATED PYRIMIDINE ANALOGS (IUdR AND BUdR) IN PATIENTS WITH GLIOBLASTOMA

Compound	Randomized		Benefit in TTP/Survival		Total No. of Patients
	Yes	No	Yes	No	
BUdR[52]		X		X	60
IUdR[53]		X		X	45
BUdR[54]		X		X	160
IUdR[57]		X		X	56

cil.[59] This drug increases analog incorporation by blocking the de novo synthesis of thymidine from pyrimidine, which results in increased analog incorporation through the thymidine salvage pathway. This strategy was already attempted in a phase I clinical trial without any therapeutic gain, but with greater systemic toxic effects.[60] Methotrexate also blocks the de novo synthesis of thymidine and has also been considered as a modulator.[51] Another approach to increase the incorporation of these compounds into DNA is to combine them with leucovorin. Efficacy of this combination has recently been demonstrated in vitro, resulting in an enhanced IUdR incorporation and radiosensitization without increased cytotoxic responses.[61]

Chemical Inhibitors of Radiation-Induced DNA Repair

HYDROXYUREA

Hydroxyurea is a cell cycle phase–specific agent that inhibits DNA synthesis. After oral administration, it readily enters the cerebrospinal fluid (CSF), is transported by diffusion into cells, and finally is converted to a free radical. Hydroxyurea also inhibits the repair of DNA damage (unscheduled DNA synthesis) induced by irradiation and chemicals (e.g., alkylating agents, bleomycin, and etoposide).

Since 1976, hydroxyurea has been subject to extensive clinical use to potentiate radiation-induced DNA damage in patients with malignant gliomas. However, only one randomized clinical study, which was published in 1979,[62, 63] has demonstrated an improvement in median time to tumor progression (4 months' improvement in hydroxyurea-plus-radiation-therapy group compared with radiation-therapy-only group). This effect was seen only in patients with supratentorial glioblastoma. Other studies, published between 1984 and 1989, of patients with brainstem gliomas[64] and medulloblastomas,[65] failed to show a potentiating effect and improvement in survival.

Hydroxyurea has, therefore, been widely used in the treatment of primary brain tumors, either with radiation therapy alone or with radiotherapy plus chemotherapy, and although no clearcut evidence of benefit has been seen (except for the abovementioned randomized study conducted in 1977), its use is being continued because of the low level of toxic effects and, concomitantly, because of the clinical judgment that possible benefits outweigh the risks of drug-related toxic effects.[66]

It should be pointed out that in the majority of studies hydroxyurea was administered concomitantly with radiotherapy; however, some evidence suggests that the use of hydroxyurea immediately after radiation or chemotherapy could be of equal or greater benefit.[67]

Polyamine Inhibitors and Difluoromethylornithine

Polyamines (putrescine and spermidine) are involved in the maintenance of DNA structure and function. DNA damage repair is initiated immediately after exposure to radiation. The use of polyamine depletors (alpha-difluoromethylornithine, DFMO) can inhibit these repair processes, which suggests that the depletion of tumor polyamine content may be an effective method of enhancing the sensitivity of human

tumors to irradiation.[68] A clinical randomized trial utilizing conventional and hyperfractionated radiotherapy, with or without DFMO, in patients with glioblastoma was initiated by the Brain Tumor Research Center, University of California, San Francisco. As of Nov 1, 1993, 93 patients had been entered into the study. Only toxicity data have been published.[69]

2-Deoxyglucose Repair and fixation of radiation-induced DNA damage requires metabolic energy supplied by the glycolytic pathways. It has been postulated from in vitro studies that the repair process in cancer cells can be altered by regulating the rate of glycolysis. Glucose analogs, such as 2-deoxyglucose (2-dG), inhibit glucose transport and glycolysis and enhance the radiation damage in cellular systems. Exposure of brain tumor cell line to 2-dG resulted in enhanced radiation damage.[70] A study evaluating the feasibility of utilizing this approach in patients with anaplastic astrocytoma and glioblastoma has been initiated. The toxic effects have been acceptable. The 2-dG was administered orally at a total dose of 200 mg/kg of body weight after overnight fasting, 30 minutes prior to brain irradiation, in a once-a-week schedule with large fractions of radiation. The toxic responses to this approach were acceptable, and a phase II and III clinical trial has been planned.[71]

CONCLUSIONS ON HYPOXIC AND NONHYPOXIC CELL RADIOSENSITIZERS

After two decades of clinical investigations, the goal of using hypoxic cells or cell-cycle specific radiosensitizers with standard radiotherapy of malignant gliomas remains elusive. However, a better understanding has developed of the multifactorial causes of radiation resistance, and efforts are concentrated into the selection of patients in whom one, two, or more factors of resistance have been uncovered. A better understanding of the tumor microenvironment and the effect of modulators, such as glutathione depletors, bioreductive drugs, and modulators of halogenated pyrimidines (methotrexate and leucovorin), are being considered in the clinic. The practical application of radiosensitizers will not be universal in all solid tumors, but they could be specifically directed to tumor sites according to characteristic cell kinetics and presence or absence of hypoxia.

CANCER CHEMOTHERAPEUTIC AGENTS BEING USED AS POSSIBLE RADIOSENSITIZERS IN MALIGNANT GLIOMAS

Paclitaxel

Paclitaxel is being considered as a potentially promising chemotherapeutic agent that has demonstrated activity against breast and ovarian tumors. Evidence suggests that its cytotoxic effects are due to stabilization of microtubules, and that it blocks cell cycle at G2 and M.

Because G2 and M are the most radiosensitive phases of the cell cycle, it was proposed that paclitaxel be used to block human astrocytoma cells at G2/M, thereby making them more radiosensitive. The results from this early in vitro work suggested that the combination of paclitaxel and radiation had a greater than additive effect.[72] However, further in vitro studies using six different human tumor cell lines demonstrated only a modest radiosensitizer effect in some cell lines, with no effect in others, despite the fact that most cells were blocked at G2/M.[73] Similar results were observed in human cervical carcinoma cells when combining paclitaxel and radiation in vitro. These combined treatments were either additive or less than additive.[74] In a summary, Hall reported that the results of most studies suggest that the radiation and the paclitaxel effects are strictly additive, and in only a few instances was a greater than additive radiosensitizer effect observed.[75] However, most of the experimental evidence was based on a 24-hour exposure to paclitaxel. A phase I and II clinical trial has been initiated in patients with glioblastoma, in which a 6-week continuous intravenous infusion of paclitaxel was administered in combination with conventional brain irradiation; this study remains ongoing (Gladstein E: Personal communication, 1994).

Platinum Compounds

Platinum drugs (e.g., cisplatin and carboplatin) interact with radiation effects in cells. This interaction was described in 1976,[76] and reviewed during 1985.[77, 78] These compounds are known to inhibit recovery from radiation-induced sublethal and potentially lethal damage. This interaction with radiation can be observed in vitro and in vivo with both preradiation and postradiation administration.[77] They are weakly electron-affinic, and because of their toxic effects in normal tissues, they are not ideal hypoxic cell radiosensitizers. In addition, because toxic drug dosages are usually necessary for the interaction with DNA-induced damage, critical analysis is needed before any claim of a true radiation-enhancement effect, rather than an additive effect, is accepted. However, in animal tumor models, the combined use of continuous low-dose-rate radiation (such as in brachytherapy) with concurrent and continuous infusion of the cisplatin resulted in supra-additive anti-tumor effect.[79] The timing and schedule of administration (infusion vs. bolus) are therefore of great importance in its use as the modifier of radiation response.

A pilot study using a short intravenous infusion of concomitant cisplatin with conventional radiation in malignant gliomas (glioblastomas and anaplastic astrocytomas) was reported in 1983.[80] In this study, cisplatin was administered at a dose of 40 mg/m[2]/week, IV, during a 6-week course of cranial irradiation. In the 22 eligible patients, the median survival of 53 weeks and the median time to tumor progression of 21 weeks was not considered an improvement; furthermore, a high incidence of auditory toxic effects occurred over and above the 30% observed in patients given cisplatin alone. A study has been completed to evaluate carboplatin in a 2-hour IV infusion combined with accelerated fractionation radiation. The radiation was administered three times a day with 2-hour infusions for two 5-day courses of treatment separated by 2 weeks, with repeat of two 5-day courses. An

8% incidence was seen of toxic effects in the form of focal brain radiation necrosis, which, according to the authors, was no different from that of other published studies that used radiation alone. There was no clear dose-dependent benefit for carboplatin potentiation of radiation therapy in this group of patients.[81]

A phase I study reported by the Pediatric Oncology Group (POG) utilized hyperfractionated radiation and concurrent cisplatin administration in children with brainstem tumors. Cisplatin was infused continuously over 120 hours on weeks 1, 3, and 5 of a 6-week radiotherapy course. This was an escalating dose study, starting at 50 mg/m[2]/120 hours. Sixteen children completed therapy. No excessive renal or ototoxic effects were encountered.[82] In view of the acceptable toxic response levels, a randomized phase III study in children with brainstem tumors was initiated by the same group in June 1992, using continuous intravenous infusion of 100 mg/m[2] of cisplatin for 120 hours on every other week of a 6-week course of radiation. The radiation is being administered either as conventional fractionation or as hyperfractionation. The accrual rate has been excellent, but no results are yet available (Mandell LR: Personal communication, 1994).

In summary, up to the time of this writing, the clinical use of platinum compounds in combination with radiation in patients with malignant glioma has not shown evidence for radiopotentiation.

REFERENCES

1. Steel GG: Combined radiotherapy-chemotherapy: Principles. *In* Steel GG, Adams GE, Horwich E (eds): The Biological Basis of Radiotherapy, ed 2. Amsterdam, Elsevier, 1989, pp 267.
2. Young SD, Hill RP: Effect of re-oxygenation of cells from hypoxic regions of solid tumors: An anti-cancer drug sensitivity on metastatic potential. JNCI 1990; 82:371.
3. Luk CK, Veinot-Drevot L, Jan TE, et al: Effect of transient hypoxia on sensitivity to doxorubicin in human and murine cell lines. JNCI 1990; 82:684.
4. Tannock I, Guttman P: Responsive Chinese hamster ovary cells to anti-cancer drugs under aerobic and hypoxic conditions. Br J Cancer 1991; 43:245.
5. Teicher BA, Lazoj S, Sartorelli C: Classification of anti-neoplastic agents by their selective toxicity towards oxygenated and hypoxic tumor cells. Cancer Res 1991; 41:73.
6. Rabin HR, Urtasun RC, Partington J, et al: Pharmacokinetics and bioavailability using an IV preparation and application of its use as a radiosensitizer. Cancer Treat Rep 1980; 64:1087.
7. Urtasun RC, Band P, Chapman JD, et al: Radiation and high dose metronidazole in supratentorial glioblastomas. N Engl J Med 1976; 294:1364.
8. Urtasun RC, Chapman JD, Feldstein L, et al: Peripheral neuropathy related to misonidazole: Incidence and pathology. Br J Cancer 1978; 271:274.
9. Medical Research Council: A study of the effect of misonidazole in conjunction with radiotherapy for the treatment of grades 3 and 4 astrocytomas: A report from the MRC Working Party on Misonidazole in Gliomas. Br J Radiol 1983; 56:673.
10. EORTC Brain Tumor Group: Misonidazole in radiotherapy of supratentorial malignant brain gliomas in adult patients: A randomized double-blind study. Eur J Cancer Clin Oncol 1983; 19:39.
11. Nelson DF, Schoenfeld D, Weinstein, et al: Misonidazole sensitized radiotherapy plus BCNU compared to radiotherapy plus BCNU for treatment of malignant glioma in a randomized clinical trial: Update report. Int J Radiat Oncol Biol Phys 1983; 9:89.
12. Urtasun RC, Feldstein ML, Partington J, et al: Radiation and nitroimidazoles in supratentorial high grade gliomas: A second clinical trial. Br J Cancer 1982; 46:101.

13. Stadler B, Karcher KH, Kogelnik HD, et al: Misonidazole and irradiation in the treatment of glioblastoma multiforme: Preliminary report of the Vienna study group. Int J Radiat Oncol Biol Phys 1984; 10:1713.

14. Hatlevoll R, Lindegaard KF, Hagen S, et al: Combined modality treatment of operated astrocytomas grade III & IV: Stage II of a prospective multicenter trial of the Scandinavian Glioblastoma Study Group. Cancer 1985; 56:41.

15. Wasserman TH, Lee DJ, Cosmatos D, et al: Clinical trials with etanidazole (SR–2508) by the Radiation Therapy Oncology Group (RTOG). Radiother Oncol 1991; 20:129.

16. Hurwitz SJ, Coleman NC, Riese N, et al: Distribution of etanidazole into human brain tumors: Complications for treating high grade gliomas. Int J Radiat Oncol Biol Phys 1992; 22:573.

17. Reise N, Loeffler J, When P: Results of a phase I trial using radiotherapy and etanidazole in malignant glioma patients. Proceedings of the 8th International Conference of Chemical Modifiers of Cancer Treatment, Kyoto, Japan, 1993, p 345.

18. Urtasun RC, Parliament MB, McEwan AJ, et al: Necrosis and poor blood perfusion but not binding of iodine 123–IAZA in human glioblastomas. Proceedings of the 41st Annual Meeting of the Radiation Research Society, Dallas, 1993, p 164.

19. Vaupel P, Mueller-Klieser: Oxygenation and bioenergetic status of human tumors. In Dewey WC, Edington M, Fry MRG, et al (eds): Radiation Research: A 20th Century Perspective, vol. 2. New York, Academic Press, 1992, p 772.

20. Koh WH, Rasey JS, Evans ML, et al: Imaging of hypoxia in human tumors with (F-18) fluoromisonidazole. Int J Radiat Oncol Biol Phys 1992; 22:199.

21. Parliament MB, Chapman JD, Urtasun RC, et al: Non-invasive assessment of human tumor hypoxia with ^{123}I-iodoazomycin arabinoside: Preliminary report of a clinical study. Br J Cancer 1992; 65:90.

22. Groshar D, McEwan AJB, Parliament MB, et al: Imaging tumor hypoxia and tumor perfusion. J Nucl Med 1993; 34:885.

23. Rampling R, Cruickshank G, Lewis AD, et al: Direct measurements of pO2 distribution and bioreductive enzymes in human malignant brain tumors. Proceedings of the 8th International Conference on Chemical Modifiers of Cancer Treatment, Kyoto, Japan, 1993, p 151.

24. Parliament MB, Turner J, Franko A, et al: Oxygen consumption, cell cycle distribution and misonidazole labeling in human malignant xenografts. Proceedings of the Annual Meeting of the Radiation Research Society, 1994, p 145.

25. Hank JM: Does hyperbaric oxygen have a future in radiation therapy? Int J Radiat Oncol Biol Phys 1981; 7:1125.

26. Rubin P, Hanley J, Keys HM, et al: Carbogen breathing during radiation therapy: Radiation Oncology Group study. Int J Radiat Oncol Biol Phys 1979; 5:1963.

27. Bush RS: The significance of anemia in clinical radiation therapy. Int J Radiat Oncol Biol Phys 1986; 12:2047.

28. Dische S, Saunders MI, Warvurton MF: Hemoglobin, radiation, morbidity and survival. Int J Radiat Oncol Biol Phys 1986; 12:1335.

29. Rose C, Lustig R, McIntosh LN, et al: A clinical trial of fluosol-DA 20% in advanced squamous cell carcinoma of the head and neck. Int J Radiat Oncol Biol Phys 1988; 12:1325.

30. Lustig R, McIntosh LN, Rose C, et al: Phase I/II, study of fluosol-DA and 100% oxygen as adjuvant to radiation in the treatment of advanced squamous cell tumors of the head and neck. Int J Radiat Oncol Biol Phys 1989; 16:1587.

31. Dische S. Hypoxia in local tumor control: Part 2. Radiother Oncol 1991; 20:9.

32. Evans RG, Kimler BF, Morantz RA, et al: Lack of complications in long term survivors after treatment with fluosol and oxygen as an adjuvant to radiation therapy for high grade brain tumors. Int J Radiat Oncol Biol Phys 1993; 26:649.

33. Minchinton AI, Brown JM: Enhancement of the cytotoxicity of SR 4233 to normal or malignant tissues by hypoxic breathing. Br J Cancer 1992; 66:1053.

34. Minchinton AI, Lemmon MJ, Tracey, M, et al: Second generation 1,2,4-benzotriazine 1, 4-DI-N-oxide bioreductive anti-tumor agents: Pharmacology and activity in vitro and in vivo. Int J Radiat Oncol Biol Phys 1992; 22:701.

35. Brown MJ: Sensitizers in radiotherapy. In Withers HR, Peters LJ (eds): Innovations in Radiation Oncology. Berlin, Springer-Verlag, 1988, pp 247, 264.

36. Yu NY, Brown MJ: Depletion of glutathione in vivo as a method of improving the therapeutic ratio of misonidazole and SR 2508. Int J Radiat Oncol Biol Phys 1984; 10:1265.

37. Kramer RA, Soble M, Howes AE: The effect of glutathione (GSH) depletion in vivo by buthionine sulfoximine (BSO) in the radiosensitization SR2508. Int J Radiat Oncol Biol Phys 1989; 16:1325.

38. Giaccia AJ, Biedermann KA, Tosto LM, et al: Characterization of a CHO cell line resistant to killing by the hypoxic cell cytotoxin SR 4233. Int J Radiat Oncol Biol Phys 1992; 22:681.

39. Allalunis-Turner MJ, Barrone GM, Day RS, et al: Heterogeneity in response to treatment with buthionine or sulfoximine or interferon in human malignant glioma cells. Int J Radiat Oncol Biol Phys 1992; 22:765.

40. Britten RA, Warenius HM, White R: BSO-induced reduction of glutathione levels increases the cellular radiosensitivity of drug-resistant human tumor cells. Int J Radiat Oncol Biol Phys 1992; 22:769.

41. Halperin EC, Brizel DM, Honor EG, et al: The radiation dose response relationship in a human glioma xenograft and evaluation of glutathione depletion by buthionine sulfoximine. Int J Radiat Oncol Biol Phys 1992; 24:103.

42. Lippitz BE, Halperin EC, Griffith OW, et al: L-Buthionine-sulfoximine mediated radiosensitization in experimental interstitial radiotherapy of intracerebellar D–54 MG glioma xenograft in athymic mice. Neurosurgery 1990; 26:225.

43. Webb CF, Jones GDD, Ward JF, et al: Mechanisms of radiosensitization in bromodeoxyuridine substituted cells. Int J Radiat Biol 1993; 64:695.

44. Bagshaw MA, Doggett RSL, Smith KC, et al: Intra-arterial 5-bromodeoxyuridine and x-ray therapy. Radiology 1967; 99:886.

45. Goffinet DR, Brown JM: Comparison of intravenous and intra-arterial pyrimidine infusion as a means of radiosensitizing tumors. Radiology 1977; 124:819.

46. Kinsella TJ, Mitchell JB, Russo A: Continuous intravenous infusion of bromodeoxyuridine as a clinical radiosensitizer. J Clin Oncol 1984; 2:1144.

47. Kinsella TJ, Collins J, Rowald J, et al: Pharmacology in phase I/II study of continuous infusions of iododeoxyuridine and hyperfractionated radiotherapy in patients with glioblastoma multiforme. J Clin Oncol 1988; 6:871.

48. Lawrence TS, Davis MA, Maybaum J, et al: The dependence of halogenated pyrimidine incorporation and radiosensitization on the duration of drug exposure. Int J Radiat Oncol Biol Phys 1990; 18:1393.

49. Speth PA, Kinsella TJ, Chang AE: Selective incorporation of iododeoxyuridine (IUdR) into DNA of human hematopoietic cells, normal liver and hepatic metastases in man: As a radiosensitizer and a marker for cell kinetic studies. Int J Radiat Oncol Biol Phys 1989; 16:1247.

50. Uhl V, Phillips TL, Ross GY: Iododeoxyuridine incorporation and radiosensitization in treating human tumor cell lines. Int J Radiat Oncol Biol Phys 1992; 22:489.

51. Rodriguez R, Ritter MA, Fowler JF: Kinetics of cell labeling and thymidine replacement after the continuous infusion of halogenated pyrimidines in vivo. Int J Radiat Oncol Biol Phys 1994; 29(1):105–113.

52. Jackson D, Kinsella TJ, Rowlan J: Halogenated pyrimidines as radiosensitizers in the treatment of glioblastoma multiforme. Am J Clin Oncol 1987; 10:437.

53. Goffman TE, Dachowski JJ, Bobo H, et al. Long term follow up on National Cancer Institute phase I/II study of glioblastoma multiforme treated with iododeoxyuridine and hyperfractionated irradiation. J Clin Oncol 1992; 10:264.

54. Phillips TL, Levin VA, Ahn DK: Evaluation of bromodeoxyuridine in glioblastoma multiforme: A NCOG phase II study. Int J Radiat Oncol Biol Phys 1991; 21:709.

55. Levin VA, Wara WM, Gutin P, et al: Initial analysis of NCOG 6G82–1: Bromodeoxyuridine (BUdR) during irradiation followed by CCNU, procarbazine, and the increasing (PCV) chemotherapy for malignant gliomas. Proc Am Soc Clin Oncol 1990; 9:91.

56. Phillips TL, Prados MD, Bodell WJ, et al: Rationale for and experience with clinical trials with halogenated pyrimidines in malignant gliomas: The UCSF/NCOG experience. In Dewey WC, Edington M, Fry RJ, et al (eds): A 20th Century Perspective, vol 2. New York, Academic Press, 1992, p 601.

57. Urtasun RC, Cosmatos D, DelRowe J, et al: Iododeoxyuridine (IUdR) combined with radiation in the treatment of malignant glioma: A comparison of short vs long intravenous dose schedules (RTOG 86–12). Int J Radiat Oncol Biol Phys 1993, 27:207.

58. Hegarty TJ, Thornton AF, Diaz RF, et al: Intra-arterial bromodeoxyuridine radiosensitization of malignant gliomas. Int J Radiat Oncol Biol Phys 1990,19:421.

59. Lawrence TS, Davis MA, Maybaum J, et al: Modulation of iododeoxyuridine: Mediated radiosensitization by 5-fluorouracil in human cancer cells. Int J Radiat Oncol Biol Phys 1992; 22:499.

60. Speth PA, Kinsella TJ, Belanger K, et al: Fluorodeoxyuridine modulation of the incorporation of iododeoxyuridine into DNA granulocytes: Phase I and clinical pharmacological study. Cancer Res 1988; 48:2933.

61. Miller EM, Kunugi KA, Kinsella TJ: Effects of 5′-aminothymidine and leucovorin on the radiosensitization of iododeoxyuridine in human colon cancer cells. Clin Cancer Res 1995; 1:407–416.

62. Levin VA, Wilson CB, Davis R, et al: Preliminary results of a phase III comparison study of BCNU, hydroxyurea and radiation to BCNU and radiation. Int J Radiat Oncol Biol Phys 1979; 5:1573.

63. Levin VA, Wilson CM, Davis RL, et al: Phase III comparison of BCNU, hydroxyurea and radiation therapy for treatment of primary malignant gliomas. J Neurosurg 1985; 63:218.

64. Levin VA, Edwards MS, Wara WM, et al: 5-Fluorouracil and 1-(2-chlorethyl)-3-cyclohexyl-1-nitrosourea (CCNU) followed by hydroxyurea, misonidazole, and irradiation for brain stem gliomas: A pilot study of the Brain Tumor Research Center and the Children's Cancer Group. Neurosurgery 1984; 14:679.

65. Levin VA, Rodriguez LA, Edwards MS, et al: Treatment of medulloblastoma with procarbazine, hydroxyurea, and reduced radiation doses to whole brain and spine. J Neurosurg 1988; 68:383.

66. Levin VA: The place of hydroxyurea in the treatment of primary brain tumors. Semin Oncol 1992; 19(suppl 9):34.

67. Yarboro SW: Mechanisms of action of hydroxyurea. Semin Oncol 1992; 19(suppl 9):1.

68. Gerner EW, Tome ME, Frye ES: Inhibition of ionizing radiation recovery process in polyamine-depleted Chinese hamster cells. Cancer Res 1988; 48:4881.

69. Phillips TL, Prados MD, Deen DF: Update on clinical trials with chemical modifiers in the treatment of CNS neoplasm at UCSF. Proceedings of the 8th International Conference on Chemical Modifiers of Cancer Treatment. Kyoto, Japan, 1993, p 328.

70. Dwarakanath BS, Jain V: Effects of gamma rays and glucose analogs on the energy metabolism of cell lines derived from human cerebral glioma. Indian J Biochem Biophys 1991; 28:203.

71. Anantha N, Jain V, Cannan V, et al: Improving cancer radiotherapy with 2-deoxyglucose (2-dG) phase II clinical trial on human cerebral gliomas. Proceedings of the 8th International Conference on Chemical Modifiers of Cancer Treatment, Kyoto, Japan, 1993, p 326.

72. Tishler RB, Geard CR, Hall EJ, et al: Taxol sensitized human astrocytoma cells to radiation. Cancer Res 1992; 52:3495.

73. Mitchell JB, Cook JA, Libamann J: Taxol mediated G2/M cell cycle blocks and radiosensitization: Differences among human tumor cell types. Proceedings of the 8th International Conference on Chemical Modifiers of Cancer Treatment, Kyoto, Japan, 1993, p 208.

74. Geard CR, Jones JM: Taxol and radiation effects on human cervical carcinoma cells. Proceedings of the 8th International Conference on Chemical Modifiers of Cancer Treatment, Kyoto, Japan, 1993, p 282.

75. Hall E: Summary and highlights. Proceedings of the 8th International Conference on Chemical Modifiers of Cancer Treatment, Kyoto, Japan, 1993, p 7.

76. Richmond RC, Powers EL: Radiation sensitization of bacterial spores by cis-dichlorodiammineplatinum (II). Radiat Res 1976; 68:20.

77. Douple EB, Richmond RC, O'Hara JA, et al: Carboplatin as a potentiator of radiation therapy. Cancer Treat Rev 1985; 12(suppl A):111–124.

78. Nias AHW: Review: Radiation and platinum drug interaction. Int J Radiat Biol 1985; 48:297.

79. Fu KK, Kitty NL, Rayner PA: The influence of time sequence of cisplatin administration and continuous low dose rate irradiation on the combined effects on a murine squamous cell carcinoma. Int J Radiat Oncol Biol Phys 1985; 2:2119.

80. Feun LG, Stewart JD, Maor M, et al: A pilot study of cis-diamminedichloroplatinum and radiation therapy in patients with high grade astrocytoma. J Neuro Oncol 1983; 1:109.

81. Levin VA, Maor MH, Thall PF, et al: Phase II study of accelerated fractionation radiation therapy with carboplatin followed by PCV chemotherapy for the treatment of glioblastoma multiforme. Int J Radiat Oncol Biol Phys 1995; 33(2):357–364.

82. Kadota RP, Mandell LR, Fontanesy J, et al: Hyperfractionated irradiation and concurrent cis-platin in brain stem tumors: A pediatric oncology group pilot study (9139). Pediatr Neurosurg 1994; 20:221–225.

CHEMOTHERAPY

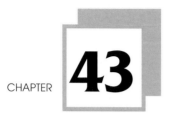

CHAPTER **43**

Pharmacology of Glioma Therapy

The therapeutic efficacy of antineoplastic agents is dependent on three fundamental considerations. First, the agent must have prominent cytotoxic activity that is efficient and selective. Second, it must be delivered to the tumor target in sufficiently high concentrations to ensure cytotoxic activity. Third, it must be able to overcome or circumvent the intrinsic and acquired drug resistance mechanisms that reduce cytotoxic activity. Despite the complexity of these different factors, many physicians continue to attribute the fundamental problems of drug therapy for brain tumors to a highly restrictive blood-brain barrier. In this regard, the comments of Vick and colleagues[1] are as relevant now as they were when they were published two decades ago.

> Most oncologists assume that to be useful for brain tumor chemotherapy, a drug must be lipid soluble, be un-ionized at physiological pH, and be of relatively small size in order to enter the brain from the blood vascular compartment. . . . In experiments with Walker-256–induced carcinomatous meningitis in rats, treatment with cyclophosphamide clearly increased lifespan of the animals. Were lipid solubility the critical factor in therapeutic effectiveness in this model, this drug, whose active metabolites are water soluble, should have been ineffective. . . . We believe, therefore, that there is compelling evidence to suggest that the ''blood-brain barrier,'' as it is generally conceived, is not one of the factors impeding the success of brain tumor chemotherapy. . . . This means that factors other than molecular size, lipid solubility, and ionization must be considered in the design and administration of drugs to treat brain tumors.[1]

The efficient delivery of antineoplastic agents to brain tumors may pose greater challenges now than it has during the past several decades. Most conventional antineoplastic agents with demonstrated activity against gliomas are relatively small compounds whose molecular weights range from approximately 150 to 825 daltons. Despite a wide range in the lipid solubility of these drugs, most are accessible to

brain and brain tumors.[2] However, conventional chemotherapeutic agents yield only marginal improvements in survival for glioma patients when compared to treatment with radiation therapy alone.[3, 4] Accordingly, newer glioma therapeutic strategies are being developed, including monoclonal antibodies,[5] immunotoxins,[6–8] recombinant toxins,[9, 10] and gene transfer therapy,[11, 12] all of which involve the delivery of molecules several orders of magnitude larger than conventional chemotherapeutic agents. The pharmacologic and physiologic restrictions to the delivery of protein or nucleic acid macromolecules to brain tumors are often quantitatively and qualitatively different than those for conventional antineoplastic drugs and require separate consideration.

This chapter examines the major factors involved in drug delivery to brain tumors. General pharmacologic principles of antitumor therapy, including drug distribution, metabolism, and clearance, are not discussed in detail and are the subject of excellent reviews and monographs.[13–17] However, the pharmacology of selected antineoplastic drugs will serve as a model of the principal pharmacokinetic considerations and as a basis of comparison with the delivery of macromolecules into brain tumors. In addition, newer approaches to drug delivery, including the use of drug-impregnated sustained-release polymers, chimeric drugs, and convection-enhanced delivery of macromolecules, are reviewed. As noted, factors in addition to drug delivery play critical roles in the determination of antineoplastic drug efficacy and it is not the objective of this chapter to rank the importance of drug delivery, intrinsic cytotoxic activity, and treatment resistance for brain tumor therapy. Mechanisms of resistance for antineoplastic drugs that are active against gliomas are addressed separately elsewhere in this book.

BLOOD-TO-TUMOR DRUG DELIVERY
General Pharmacologic Considerations

The delivery of intravenously administered drug to brain tumors involves the distribution of drug within the intravascular compartment, transfer of drug through the tumor vascular endothelium, passage across the interstitial compartment, and penetration through the tumor cell membrane and into the intracellular space. Two major forces determine the multicompartmental blood-to-tumor transfer of drugs: (1) diffusion (i.e., the movement of drug along a concentration gradient) and (2) convection (i.e., the movement of drug by bulk solute flow).

PHYSICOCHEMICAL FACTORS

The physicochemical properties of antineoplastic drugs have significant effects on transcapillary drug transfer in the intact blood-brain barrier and in relatively intact regions of blood-tumor barrier. Of these, the most important determinants of brain capillary permeability are lipid solubility, molecular weight, and molecular charge. In general, polar compounds are more highly restricted in their transcapillary diffusion than are uncharged compounds. The lipid permeability of various drugs can be expressed as the octanol-water partition coefficient; for low-molecular-weight compounds, this is closely correlated with the capillary permeability coefficient.[18] The relationship between rat brain capillary permeability to various antineoplastic drugs and their lipid solubility and molecular weight has been described by Levin[19] in the following formula:

$$P_c \propto K (M)^{1/2}$$

in which P_c is the capillary permeability, K is the lipid-water partition coefficient, and M is the molecular weight. Levin further concluded that below drug molecular weights of 400 daltons, increasing lipophilicity significantly improves P_c; however, above 400 daltons, little significant transcapillary transfer occurs regardless of lipophilicity.[19] It is important to recognize that these estimates are obtained from blood-to-brain drug transfer through the normal, intact blood-brain barrier. The importance of physicochemical properties in blood-to-brain tumor transfer through heterogeneously abnormal tumor vasculature is overshadowed by the tumor physiology factors described below.

TUMOR PHYSIOLOGY FACTORS

The rate of drug transfer from the intravascular to the tumor interstitial space is determined primarily by the tumor vascular characteristics and tumor pressure and is driven by the forces of drug diffusion (i.e., concentration gradient) and convection (i.e., bulk flow). The vasculature of malignant gliomas is extremely heterogeneous and represents a combination of blood vessels recruited from normal brain vessels and those generated in response to angiogenic factors.[20, 21] The morphology of tumor vessels, including the length, diameter, number, and spatial distribution, also varies considerably between different gliomas and within the same tumor. In contrast to normal brain vessels, tumor vessels are often tortuous and dilated and may contain anastomoses or venous shunts. The frequent absence of pentilaminar tight junctions and presence of large pores or endothelial fenestrae further distinguish glioma vasculature from normal brain capillary endothelium.[1, 22–24]

The rate of drug transfer from blood to tumor can also be evaluated in terms of the interrelationships between blood flow (F), fractional blood volume (V_c), an extraction fraction (E) or unidirectional transfer constant (K), and the permeability surface area product (PS). As noted by Groothuis and others,[25] the extraction fraction and transfer constant can be measured under experimental conditions and are related by the following equation:

$$K = FV_c E$$

The PS product (expressed in units of volume per units of tissue mass per units of time) cannot be measured directly under experimental conditions but can be calculated from a knowledge of K and FV_c in the following manner[23, 26]:

$$PS = FV_c \ln(1 - K/FV_c)$$

This means that when PS/FV_c is small (e.g., 0.1 or less) the blood-to-tumor drug transfer (K) is dependent mainly on the PS value of the capillaries. By contrast, when PS/FV_c is relatively large (e.g., 2.0 or greater) K is primarily determined by blood flow and blood volume factors.[27]

Regional blood flow and unidirectional transfer constant values have been estimated for experimental brain tumor models by use of quantitative autoradiography[27, 28] and for human gliomas by use of positron emission tomography (PET) techniques.[29–31] For experimental brain tumor models, several observations have important implications for cancer chemotherapy. Blood flow values for tumors are generally lower than for normal cortex, but they higher than normal corpus callosum white matter values. Within malignant gliomas derived from the same cell line, larger tumors tend to have lower blood flow values. And for most experimental gliomas studied, there is continuous increase in blood flow rates from the tumor center to the periphery. However, the most significant observation may be that the capillary permeability and surface area of experimental brain tumors are more likely than blood flow to limit the delivery of conventional chemotherapeutic agents.[32] Similar conclusions can be derived from PET studies of blood flow and tumor permeability in the clinical setting.[33–35]

Once a drug has passed beyond the intravascular compartment, it must cross the interstitial space before reaching the tumor cell membrane. Studies of experimental tumor physiology indicate that the interstitial space in tumors is larger than that in normal tissue.[36] A major factor opposing the passage of drug through the interstitial space is the high interstitial fluid pressure (IFP) measured in tumors.[37, 38] Interstitial fluid pressure is elevated in large tumors that are rigidly confined to a compartmental space and are highest in the center of these tumors. The effect of this interstitial fluid pressure gradient is to maintain an outward convection of interstitial fluid toward the periphery of the tumor. Other factors that influence drug passage through the interstitial compartment include the drug concentration gradient, which in turn is partially determined by drug dose, administration schedule, and clearance (e.g., half-life).

Entry of drug into the intracellular compartment is determined by physicochemical and cell membrane considerations. As noted above, transmembrane passage of most hydrophilic drugs is more rapid in the un-ionized state.

However, quantitative autoradiography and PET studies indicate that the interstitial and intracellular pH of brain tumors may be significantly lower than that of normal brain or systemic organs.[39] These regional acidic conditions may promote a shift in drug equilibrium to favor charged species, thereby reducing intracellular drug concentrations. The intracellular drug concentration may also be reduced by efflux pumps, such as the p170 glycoprotein that is responsible for the multidrug resistance (MDR1) phenotype. Although p170 expression is clearly demonstrable in normal brain capillary endothelial cells,[40, 41] it is expressed in comparatively low concentration in malignant glioma cell membranes.[42] Furthermore, few of the most important brain tumor chemotherapeutic agents are substrates for this efflux pump.

Effective therapy requires the delivery of *active* drug to the tumor. Therefore, factors in addition to those that determine drug transfer must be considered. Systemic or intracerebral drug metabolism may reduce the intravascular or interstitial concentration of active drug. The degree of drug-protein binding not only reduces drug diffusion rates but may also result in functional inactivation of the drug. Intrinsic drug stability is also a factor. For example, a drug that undergoes rapid hydrolysis to an inactive metabolite will have difficulty achieving therapeutic concentrations in the tumor if intercapillary diffusion distances are great. Finally, the interstitial and intracellular compartments may contain high concentrations of molecules that functionally inactivate drug. For malignant gliomas, in which alkylating agents have been shown to be the most active class of antineoplastic drugs, examples of functionally inactivating molecules include glutathione and other thiols, metallothioneins (e.g., platinum drugs), aldehyde dehydrogenase (e.g., cyclophosphamide) and O^6-alkyl guanyl-DNA-alkyltransferase (e.g., nitrosoureas).[43]

PHARMACOLOGY OF REGIONAL DRUG ADMINISTRATION

Intravenous (IV) drug administration is the most common route of drug delivery for conventional glioma chemotherapy. However, two regional routes of drug administration, intracarotid and intratumoral, have been evaluated in gliomas, and their pharmacokinetics differ sufficiently from those of IV administration to warrant further discussion. Intrathecal drug administration is clinically indicated for the treatment of leptomeningeal tumor dissemination. However, it is an ineffective and inappropriate route for intracerebral glioma therapy and therefore is not addressed in this chapter. The pharmacology of intrathecal drug administration has been the subject of comprehensive reviews.[44, 45]

Direct intracarotid artery administration of various antitumor drugs, including nitrosoureas, cisplatin, and methotrexate, achieve high intratumoral drug concentrations and acceptably low systemic drug exposure. The relative advantage of intracarotid vs. IV administration is based on a comparison of the ratios of the brain and systemic drug concentration multiplied by the time integral (i.e., area under the concentration multiplied by the time curve or AUC). The intra-arterial advantage can be expressed quantitatively by the following equation developed by Eckman and co-workers[46]:

$$R d = CL_{TB}/Qi + 1$$

in which Rd is the intra-arterial advantage, CL_{TB} is the total body clearance after IV administration, and Qi is the arterial flow rate entering the tumor. This equation indicates that the greatest intra-arterial advantage will be achieved when local flow rates are low and when total body clearance rates are high.

Despite the theoretical advantages of this approach, several problems have limited its therapeutic efficacy. For many gliomas, arterial blood is not supplied by a single intracerebral artery. Therefore, one region of the tumor may receive inadequate drug concentrations. Sequential infusion through more than one artery carries a significant risk of neurotoxicity. Furthermore, intra-arterial administration may reduce, but does not eliminate, the limitations on drug distribution posed by poorly diffusible drugs. Low intra-carotid infusion rates may produce laminar flow and lead to drug streaming effects, nonhomogenous drug distribution within tumor, and an increased risk of neurotoxicity.[47, 48] An important but obvious issue concerning drug selection for intra-arterial therapy is that prodrugs—that is, agents that require metabolic conversion to a cytotoxically active metabolite (e.g., cytosine arabinoside or cyclophosphamide)—are not candidates for intra-arterial therapy. However, the synthesis of 4-hydroperoxycyclophosphamide, an activated form of cyclophosphamide, has permitted preclinical intra-arterial studies of this agent in human malignant glioma xenografts.[49]

There is a compelling rationale for intratumoral administration of drugs in glioma therapy. With recognition that the primary cause of glioma treatment failure is the inability to control local tumor, any strategy that delivers high concentrations of drug to tumor yet reduces the potential toxic effects to systemic organs has strong potential advantages. The earliest approaches involved intratumoral drug injection or catheter implantation in experimental tumor models and, later, limited clinical trials. However the greatest obstacle to the success of these treatments is the large distance required for diffusion and the significant clearance of drug by leaky brain tumor capillaries. Levin modeled the effects of the size of an intratumoral drug source on regional tumor concentrations of drug and estimated a 1000-fold difference in drug concentration from the center of a 4.0 cm tumor, into which a 1.0-cm-diameter intratumoral drug source has been inserted, to the tumor periphery.[50] Drug concentration gradients are significantly reduced and intratumoral therapy made more effective by higher drug diffusion coefficients and larger drug source surface area. The relatively low stability of many antineoplastic drugs after intratumoral administration, caused either by protein binding or by biotransformation, also reduces the concentration of active drug at the tumor periphery. However, some of these difficulties may be overcome by newer approaches to intratumoral administration.

PHARMACOLOGY OF ANTINEOPLASTIC DRUGS

An examination of preclinical experimental models and phase II clinical trials clearly indicates that classical and nonclassical alkylating agents and platinum compounds are the most active classes of antineoplastic drugs for the treatment of malignant gliomas.[51] These groups of drugs have several characteristics in common. First, alkylating agents and platinum compounds are cell-cycle nonspecific and exert their cytotoxic effects primarily by the formation of covalent cross-links between strands of DNA (interstrand cross-links) or within a single DNA strand (intrastrand cross-links). Second, these drugs show a steep cytotoxicity dose-response curve without evidence of a plateau at higher concentrations.[52] This characteristic represents a fundamental rationale for the use of alkylating agents and platinum compounds in high-dose chemotherapy and autologous bone marrow rescue protocols. Third, the mechanisms of drug resistance tend to be different and non-overlapping in these drug classes.[43] This characteristics facilitates the use of multi-alkylator chemotherapy as an effective clinical strategy.

The pharmacology of each antineoplastic agent has important consequences for its therapeutic efficacy. It is beyond the scope of this chapter to discuss the pharmacology of all chemotherapeutic agents with demonstrated activity against brain tumors; detailed reviews of these agents can be found in several excellent monographs.[15, 16] However, the pharmacology of nitrosoureas is summarized as an example of lipophilic drugs and the pharmacology of cisplatin and cyclophosphamide as examples of hydrophilic drugs, each with significant activity against gliomas.

Nitrosoureas

The first nitrosourea to undergo clinical trial, bis-chloroethyl-nitrosourea (BCNU, or carmustine), is a lipophilic drug with significant activity against malignant gliomas.[53, 54] Subsequently, structural analogs were synthesized with higher lipid solubilities (e.g., chloroethyl-cyclohexyl-nitrosourea [CCNU], or lomustine) or lower lipid solubility (piperidyl-chloroethyl-nitrosourea [PCNU]. Preclinical studies in experimental tumor models predicted higher clinical activity for several of the structural analogs than for carmustine[55]; however, these observations have generally not been borne out in clinical trials.[56] The mechanism of nitrosourea cytotoxicity is based on the production of DNA-DNA cross-links by the alkylation of DNA nucleotides by one of several processes[1]: these include alkylation by the diazonium ion[2] or alkylation of cytidylate and guanylate nitrogen, which forms chloroethylamino groups that undergo dehalogenation to produce a second DNA alkyl cross-link.[57]

The high lipid solubility of nitrosoureas, indicated by its high octanol-water partition coefficient (log $P = 1.5$), predicts that transmembrane transfer occurs by passive diffusion rather than by active transport. This has been confirmed by experimental studies.[58] Furthermore, these agents are neither accumulated within the cell against a concentration gradient nor are they substrates for a multidrug resistance efflux pump. The clinical pharmacology of the nitrosoureas emphasizes that these are highly unstable compounds with a relatively short half-life. Nitrosoureas spontaneously decompose in aqueous solutions to form the chloroethyldiazonium hydroxide alkylating species. They are also denitrosated by hepatic microsomes. In fact, upregulation of hepatic microsomal enzymes by various drugs, including phenobarbital,

may have a clinically significant effect of reducing nitrosourea half-life.[59]

An accurate assessment of nitrosourea pharmacokinetics is made difficult by its instability, large number of metabolites, and technical complexities associated with the assay of nitrosourea metabolites. Peak blood levels of carmustine range from approximately 0.75 to 1.2 μg/mL after a 60 to 80 mg/m^2 dose administered over 30 to 45 minutes[60] to 85 μg/mL after a 600 mg/m^2 dose administered over 120 minutes. Cerebrospinal fluid (CSF), brain, or brain tumor concentrations of carmustine after IV injection have not been measured directly in patients. Levin and associates[61] measured the uptake of ^{14}C-labeled carmustine and lomustine in rat brain and a 9L rat brain gliosarcoma. They reported brain-plasma partition coefficient ratios of 0.8 for both drugs; however, the brain concentration multiplied by time values for carmustine was slightly higher than for lomustine (2.8 μmol and 2.6 μmol $\times$ 40 minutes, respectively.) The concentration of total ^{14}C-labeled carmustine in the rat 9L intracranial tumors 30 minutes after drug injection ranged from 15 to 110 nmol/g of tumor tissue for carmustine doses ranging from 20 to 80 μmol/kg. Clinical pharmacokinetics for the nitrosoureas may be affected by body fat content, which increases the volume of drug distribution and serum lipid content, which may reduce the rate of nitrosourea degradation in serum.

Regional carmustine pharmacokinetics have been studied in human brain and brain tumors using ^{11}C-labeled carmustine and PET methods.[62] Image analysis showed that the ^{11}C-labeled compounds were cleared from tumor three times more slowly than from normal brain; however, the rate of ^{11}C-labeled carmustine decomposition was faster in brain tumor than in normal brain.

Cyclophosphamide

Cyclophosphamide, an analogue of nitrogen mustard, is a classical bifunctional alkylating agent. Unlike nitrogen mustard, however, cyclophosphamide is a prodrug, and the parent compound is inactive. Unlike carmustine, which is also a prodrug, cyclophosphamide requires microsomal oxidation in the liver to initiate a cascade of reactions leading to the production of the active bifunctional alkylator, phosphoramide mustard. This requirement has been circumvented by the synthesis of 4-hydroperoxycyclophosphamide (4-HC), an activated prodrug that spontaneously hydrolyzes to 4-hydroxycyclophosphamide and proceeds to the formation of phosphoramide mustard. The development of 4-HC has enabled preclinical studies of regional therapy including intrathecal[63] and intra-arterial administration.[49] Clinical activity of cyclophosphamide against malignant gliomas has been demonstrated in pediatric and adult phase II trials.[63, 64]

The mechanism of cyclophosphamide antineoplastic action is based on the formation of interstrand DNA cross-links by nuclear substitution reaction of each of its alkylating arms.[57] The N-7 position of deoxyguanylic acid is the preferred alkylation site for nitrogen mustards. Cyclophosphamide has two active metabolites: phosphoramide mustard, which is the most active, and 4-hydroxycyclophosphamide, which has approximately 75% to 90% lower activity. The aldophosphamide intermediate is a substrate for aldehyde dehydrogenase, which converts this compound to the inactive nornitrogen mustard.

Cyclophosphamide and its active metabolites are hydrophilic compounds; their passage across cell membranes occurs by passive diffusion. Whereas phosphoramide mustard is a highly polar molecule and its intracellular transport is slow, the transmembrane transfer of 4-HC is considerably more rapid. There is evidence to suggest that activation of hepatic microsomal enzymes by phenobarbital or other drugs results in increased cyclophosphamide clearance.[65] The half-life for cyclophosphamide appears to be shortened by repeated cyclophosphamide doses, suggesting that cyclophosphamide itself may upregulate hepatic microsomal oxidation. Unfortunately, little published data have evaluated brain or brain tumor concentrations of the active metabolites of cyclophosphamide after parenteral administration.

Cisplatin

Platinum analogues, including *cis*-diamminedichloroplatinum (CDDP), or cisplatin, and CBDCA, or carboplatin, are important components of clinical therapy for many solid tumors. Experimental brain tumor studies in glioma[66] and medulloblastoma cell lines[67] demonstrate cytotoxicity at relatively low cisplatin concentrations. In the clinical setting, cisplatin has shown activity against gliomas when administered by IV or intracarotid routes.[48, 68–70]

The chemical structure of platinum complexes has important stereospecificity. In the 2+ oxidation state (i.e., Pt(II)), the platinum atom has four ligand atoms arranged as the corners of a square. The *cis* isomer has high antitumor activity, whereas the *trans* isomer has no cytotoxicity. Cisplatin and other Pt(II) complexes have chemical and biological similarities to the alkylating agents in that one or both of the chlorine ligands may participate in a nucleophilic substitution reaction and form a covalent bond or bonds with nucleic acid proteins.

Cisplatin is cytotoxic in its native dichloro form; however, its ability to form ligands with DNA, protein, or other target biomolecules is enhanced by its reaction with water. The chloride atoms are displaced by water and diaquo platinum intermediates are formed. These intermediates react with nitrogen sites in DNA and other biomolecules more quickly than do the dichloro forms. The rate of cisplatin aquation in vivo is determined by the relative concentrations of water and chloride in the tissues.[71] The high chloride concentration in plasma favors the dichloro form, whereas the low intracellular chloride concentration favors the aquated species. The primary mechanism of cisplatin cytotoxicity is the formation of DNA cross-links, and the N-7 positions of guanine and adenine represent preferential binding sites. Unlike classic bifunctional alkylators such as cyclophosphamide or nitrogen mustard, which form interstrand cross-links, more than 90% of the total platinum binding to DNA forms intrastrand cross-links. Intrastrand cisplatin-DNA adducts cause a major distortion of DNA conformation and contribute to its cytotoxicity.

The intracellular transport of cisplatin occurs primarily by passive diffusion, but experimental evidence suggests that active transport may also occur. The clinical importance of these observations is that transport defects may represent a mechanism of cisplatin resistance, and human cell lines resistant to cisplatin have been shown to have cisplatin transmembrane transport defects[43] Furthermore, Teicher and others[72] found significant differences between in vivo and in vitro tumor resistance to cisplatin in which the rate of cisplatin transport was reduced in in vivo tumors but not when cells from these tumors were grown in vitro.

Clinical pharmacokinetic studies of intravenously administered cisplatin show a triphasic clearance from the systemic circulation. The first phase ($t\frac{1}{2}_\alpha \cong 20$ minutes) represents drug distribution and clearance of non–protein-bound drug. Under conditions of high-dose cisplatin administration (e.g., 200 to 800 mg/m^2) the $t\frac{1}{2}_\alpha$ may exceed 30 minutes.[73] The second phase of drug elimination represents renal clearance, and the $t\frac{1}{2}_\beta$ ranges from 1.3 to 1.7 hours. The third phase represents clearance of protein-bound cisplatin and ranges from 22 to 40 hours.[71] More than 90% of the total cisplatin clearance is by renal excretion and occurs within the first 24 hours after administration. Biliary excretion accounts for less than 10% of the total drug clearance. However, regional brain pharmacokinetics and brain tissue cisplatin concentrations after IV administration are poorly understood.[74]

PHARMACOKINETICS OF MACROMOLECULAR DRUGS

Development of new strategies for malignant glioma treatment extends the range of therapeutic agents beyond the conventional cytotoxic drugs described above to include other classes of biomolecules. Virtually all of these new strategies involve antitumor agents that are considerably larger than conventional antineoplastic drugs. Examples of these range from antisense DNA oligomers to bivalent monoclonal antibodies (MW range, 200 to 240 kD). Furthermore, glioma clinical trials have been conducted in which anti-tumor agents such as activated lymphocytes (e.g., LAK cells, TIL cells) or viruses (e.g., retroviral vectors, adenoviral vectors, or mutant cytotoxic herpes viruses) that are orders of magnitude larger than monoclonal antibodies must be efficiently delivered to a large brain tumor volume. Delivery of macromolecular drugs to brain tumors poses problems which are quantitatively and qualitatively different from those of the conventional cytotoxic drugs discussed earlier.

Studies of parenterally administered protein distribution in brain and brain tumors indicate that the differences in blood-to-tumor and blood-to-brain transfer are determined by molecular size and diffusion characteristics. Nakagawa and colleagues[75] compared the normal brain and rat RG-2 experimental glioma distribution of IV ^{125}I-labeled albumin (69 kD) to aminoisobutyric acid (AIB; 0.1 kD). Whereas the ^{125}I-labeled albumin extracellular distribution space in normal brain regions was relatively homogenous (mean = 0.53 mL/mg), the extracellular distribution space in tumors was more than 25-fold higher and ranged from 9.4 mL/hg in the dense cellular regions of large tumors to 22.0 in hypocellular regions. Calculation of the regional influx constant (K1) for ^{125}I-labeled albumin demonstrated a 140- to 2000-fold higher influx in tumor regions than in normal brain. Regional inhomogeneities in tumor ^{125}I-labeled albumin transfer constants have important implications for therapeutic drug delivery. ^{125}I-labeled albumin was 50% lower in peripheral tumor than at the tumor center and was 5-fold lower in densely cellular regions than in hypocellular regions. The ratio of ^{125}I-labeled albumin to AIB diffusion constants and transfer constants is nearly identical (i.e., 17 and 16, respectively), suggesting that movement of these molecules in brain tumors occurs by unrestricted diffusion through relatively large pores or channels. Based on the size of the albumin molecule, they estimated that the minimum pore diameter is at least 36 nm. However, it should be emphasized that the total pore area represents a very small fraction of the total vascular surface area of RG-2 rat gliomas. These observations indicate that for mid-sized proteins delivered by the IV route, the periphery of tumors will have lower drug concentrations than the central regions. In addition, the findings that ^{125}I-labeled albumin transfer is much lower under conditions of dense cellularity supports the observations of Jain and others that high tumor interstitial pressures and convective forces represent a barrier to drug delivery.[17]

The delivery of monoclonal antibodies, immunotoxins and other immunoconjugates, and recombinant toxins adds complexity to the problems of macromolecular drug transfer.[76] Considerations of molecular size and vascular sieve effect are as relevant to antibodies as to albumin. However, extracerebral vascular permeability is only three-fold lower for fibrinogen (MW, 340 kD) than for albumin despite a five-fold lower molecular weight for the latter protein. High expression of antigens or receptors and high binding affinities represent important mechanisms of drug clearance for targeted proteins and can significantly reduce the distribution of antibodies throughout the tumor.[77] Antigen-specific binding by antibodies, immunotoxins and recombinant toxins additionally contributes to heterogenous drug distribution. Nearly all studies of antibody delivery to tumors demonstrate a heterogenous distribution of antibodies and/or antigens within the tumor. A heterogenous expression of antigen within the tumor may contribute to heterogenous pharmacokinetics for the targeted proteins.[78] Heterogenous distribution of antibody may be seen as a perivascular or peripheral localization despite uniform distribution of the antigen.[79]

Blood-to-brain and blood-to-tumor transfer rates have been estimated for various antibodies in different experimental tumor systems, and various pharmacokinetic models have been developed. Blasberg and colleagues estimated the influx constant (K1) for 81C6 IgG2 monoclonal antibody transfer to be 1.8 $\mu L/g \cdot$ min in intracranially implanted D54 human malignant glioma xenografts, but only 0.007 $\mu L/g \cdot$ min in normal brain.[80] Their analysis (based on graphic analysis equations developed by Fenstermacher and colleagues[14]) as well as the analyses of others,[81] assumes an essentially unidirectional transfer and may be described as a single-pore model. Recently, Baxter and colleagues[82] proposed a two-pore model to account for solute efflux by convective forces. In this model, fluid that has passed through blood vessels may be recirculated by filtration from large pores or absorbed by the small pores. This recirculation of fluid leads to net drug efflux by convection. A comparison of pharmacokinetic analyses using a one-pore vs. a two-pore model indicates a significantly better fit of experimental data for the transfer of antibodies or antibody fragments from blood

to tumors and normal tissue (normal brain was not studied). Extension of this modeling approach to brain and brain tumor may have significant implications for the development and analysis of new delivery approaches.

Wrobel and colleagues evaluated the brain and brain tumor distribution of diphtheria toxin (MW, 62 kD) and immunotoxins (MW, 210 kD), and these studies serve as an excellent example of the factors that must be addressed to optimize the therapeutic applications of immunotoxins and other targeted proteins. Because rat (but not human) tissues lack a diphtheria toxin receptor, diphtheria toxin is nontoxic to rats but tumoricidal to human xenograft tumors borne by the rats. Using an N417D human small cell lung carcinoma model specifically selected for its relatively intact blood-tumor barrier, the tumor influx constants for diphtheria toxin (0.5 $\mu L/g \cdot$ min) were estimated to be 13- to 18-fold higher than normal brain regions.[7] Furthermore, the half-life of diphtheria toxin is relatively short: approximately 6 hours. These parameters might predict a poor distribution within tumors after IV administration and a consequently negligible therapeutic effect.

In separate studies by Sung and others, an immunotoxin created by the fusion of CRM-107 binding-deficient diphtheria toxin to a monoclonal antibody directed against the human transferrin receptor (454A12) was found to have a 2.2-fold lower influx constant than diphtheria toxin, an observation that might have been predicted based on molecular size considerations alone.[81] However, the cumulative tumor exposure to immunotoxin was more than 80% higher for the immunotoxin than for diphtheria toxin, suggesting that the longer half-life and higher binding parameters for the immunotoxin may be more important than molecular size for determining intratumoral distribution.[81] In fact, when the distribution of immunotoxin and diphtheria toxin was compared by quantitative autoradiography methods, it was found that for tumors treated with diphtheria toxin, more than 80% of the tumor area was above a predefined threshold, whereas less than 20% of the tumor area was above this threshold for tumors treated with immunotoxin.[79] These observations parallel the markedly higher therapeutic response for diphtheria toxin *vs.* the 454A12-107 immunotoxin. The high binding parameters for 454A12-107 immunotoxin, in contrast to the absence of specific binding for diphtheria toxin, result in reduced tumor penetration and heterogenous drug distribution for the former. This effect, termed a ''binding-site barrier''[77] is a critical determinant of the therapeutic efficacy of immunotoxins and other targeted proteins.

STRATEGIES TO IMPROVE DRUG DELIVERY

Various approaches have been used to improve drug delivery to brain tumors. These can be generally classified as modifications in the antineoplastic agents themselves to optimize the physiochemical properties that influence drug distribution or changes in the way that antineoplastic agents are administered. These strategies are not mutually exclusive, and both have been used to improve the delivery of conventional antineoplastic drugs, monoclonal antibodies, and recombinant toxins. However, interest is growing in the development of local delivery systems that may significantly improve the delivery of macromolecules to brain tumors yet reduce systemic exposure to toxic effects of these agents.

Physicochemical Modifications

This approach forms the basis of rational drug development and includes efforts (1) to increase lipophilicity by reducing drug polarity or adding lipophilic substituent groups or (2) to improve the stability of active drug by reducing drug the spontaneous decomposition, inactivation by protein binding, or clearance by local or systemic metabolism. Modification in the lipophilic properties of nitrosoureas is an excellent example of rational drug synthesis. Unfortunately, preclinical and clinical studies of nitrosoureas with higher or lower lipophilicity did not produce therapeutic results that were superior to those of carmustine. Similar efforts are under active development for topoisomerase I inhibitors, including the camptothecin analogues topotecan (less lipophilic than camptothecin) and irinotecan (more lipophilic than camptothecin).

Three innovative strategies have been developed to deliver peptides and other antineoplastic agents to brain. Although they have not been evaluated extensively for use in brain tumors, the fundamental concepts are clearly applicable. Peptide prodrugs can be synthesized that are lipophilic amides or esters of the parent drug. Once transported into the brain, they are converted to their native polar forms by nonspecific tissue esterases.[83] These prodrugs are not protected from proteolytic degradation by aminopeptidases in the vascular endothelium. As a second strategy, chimeric peptides have been synthesized in which a nontransportable peptide is covalently linked to large proteins, such as insulin-like growth factor, insulin, or transferrin, which are transported into cells by receptor-mediated transcytosis systems. The larger proteins function, therefore, as a transport vector. Unfortunately, this approach is not specific for drug delivery to brain, and problems of systemic toxicity as well as difficulty in the release of drug from its protein vector have been noted. A alternative approach has been developed for the delivery of peptides into the CNS that addresses several of the problems noted above. Modification of the NH_2- and COOH-terminal peptide ends results in increased lipid solubility and protection against proteolytic degradation by aminopeptidases. In addition, the peptide is attached to a redox targeter molecule that is lipid soluble on administration but is enzymatically oxidized to its hydrophilic salt in brain. This effectively traps the peptide-targeter complex behind restrictive blood-brain or blood-tumor barrier.[83]

Recombinant toxins represent excellent candidates for rational drug design. Site-specific mutations or deletions yield fundamental changes in molecular weight, topologic conformation, intrinsic stability, and receptor-binding characteristics. Changes in any of these parameters may favorably alter the transport and intratumoral distribution of recombinant toxins.[84] Structural modifications of monoclonal antibodies and immunotoxins, including the use of Fab fragments, have also been made to improve delivery and distribution in tumors.[85]

Parenteral Drug Administration

Parenteral drug delivery is the most commonly used route of administration in conventional glioma therapy; however, important modifications can or have been used to improve therapeutic results. Increasing the drug dose, either in conjunction with hematopoietic stem cell stimulatory factors or in the context of high-dose chemotherapy with bone marrow rescue, increases the drug concentration diffusion gradient and improves drug exposure in brain tumors. Alterations in drug administration schedule may also improve drug transfer. For example, hydrophilic drugs with short half-lives may have more homogenous blood-to-brain transfer when administered by prolonged IV infusions than by rapid IV bolus.[27, 86] In addition to dose and schedule modifications, administration of drug by the intra-arterial route has theoretical advantages, which have been reviewed above. Clinical translations of theoretical intra-arterial advantages include direct intra-arterial infusion with modifications to reduce the effect of laminar flow[47] and the concurrent use of osmotic blood-brain barrier disruption.

Sterically stabilized lysosomes have been developed to improve the distribution and sustained release of drug into tumors. Preclinical therapeutic studies suggest that liposomes improve the distribution of drugs within tumors and may increase the therapeutic activity of various antineoplastic agents.[12, 38, 87, 88] Sterically stabilized liposomes range from 60 to 100 nm in size, and pharmacokinetic comparisons with albumin indicate that their blood-to-tumor transfer rates are approximately six-fold lower than those of albumin.[38] The regional tumor distribution of sterically stabilized liposomes shows an accumulation in tumor perivascular regions. The liposomes protect the packaged antitumor agent from metabolic degradation and release their contents over the course of several days. It remains to be determined if this strategy will improve the distribution of drug to tumor periphery or whether it represents an approach best suited to antiangiogenic therapies.

Convection-Enhanced High-Flow Intratumoral Drug Delivery

Direct administration of antineoplastic agents into brain tumor has been evaluated in several clinical settings, including intratumoral injection of LAK cells and viral vectors as well as implantation of sustained-release polymers. However, most intratumoral injection strategies are ineffective because of large diffusion distances, poor diffusibility, drug instability, and rapid clearance. Earlier studies evaluated a low-flow microinfusion (0.05 μL/hour × 12 hours) of cisplatin directly into rat brain and confirmed that only a small brain volume had significant drug exposure.[89] More recently, Morrison and co-workers[90] modeled the pharmacokinetics of high-flow microinfusion (3.0 μL/hour × 12 hours). This technique makes use of convective flow rather than diffusion flow and results in a significant increase in the volume and homogeneity of drug delivered to brain. Their model predicts that a slowly degraded macromolecule (e.g., MW, 180 kD) delivered at a constant flow rate (3.0 μL/hour) into central gray matter regions would penetrate to a 1.5 cm radius within 12 hours.[90] Furthermore, the predicted concentration profile does not show a steep gradient from the point of infusion to the 1.5 cm margin. When low-flow and high-flow infusion rates were modeled using slow drug degradation rates (e.g., 34-hour half-life), the high-flow microinfusion resulted in a 5- to 10-fold increase in treated volume, and total treatment volumes were estimated as being larger than 10 cm³.[90]

These modeled predictions were confirmed by Bobo and colleagues using high-flow microinfusion of radiolabeled transferrin or sucrose in the normal cat brain.[91] By incrementally increasing the infusion rates from 0.5 to 4.0 μL/min no backleakage from the catheter insertion site occurred and the tracers were homogeneously distributed 1.5 to 2.0 cm from the infusion source. Experimental brain edema is produced by this technique; however, symptoms of lethargy and weakness resolved within 24 hours. The potential advantage of this approach is that extremely large areas of brain or brain tumor may be uniformly exposed to clinically significant concentrations of drug. Furthermore, this technique may be applicable to a broad range of antineoplastic agents, including low-molecular-weight chemotherapeutic drugs, macromolecules (e.g., recombinant toxins), and viral vectors for use in gene transfer therapy.

REFERENCES

1. Vick NA, Khandekar JD, Bigner DD: Chemotherapy of brain tumors. Arch Neurol 1977; 34:523–526.
2. Mellett LB: Physiocochemical considerations and pharmacokinetic behavior in delivery of drugs to the central nervous system. Cancer Treat Rep 1977; 61:527–531.
3. Janus, TJ, Kyritsis, AP, Forman AD, et al: Biology and treatment of gliomas (review). Ann Oncol 1992; 3:423–433.
4. Kornblith PK, Welch WC, Bradley MK: The future of therapy for glioblastoma (review). Surg Neurol 1993; 39:538–543.
5. Hopkins K, Kemshead JT: Progress review: Intrathecal and intratumoral injection of radiolabelled monoclonal antibodies (MoAbs) for the treatment of central nervous system (CNS) malignancies (review). J Drug Target 1993; 1:175–183.
6. Hall WA, Myklebust A, Godal A, et al: In vivo efficacy of intrathecal transferrin—*Pseudomonas* exotoxin a immunotoxin against LOX melanoma. Neurosurgery 1994; 34:649–656.
7. Wrobel CJ, Wright DC, Dedrick RL, et al: Diphtheria toxin effects on brain tumor xenografts. J Neurosurg 1990; 72:946–950.
8. Chatel M, Lebrun C, Frenay M: Chemotherapy and immunotherapy in adult malignant gliomas (review). Curr Opin Oncol 1993; 5:464–473.
9. Pastan I, Fitzgerald D: Recombinant toxins for cancer treatment. Science 1991; 254:1173–1178.
10. Phillips PC, Levow C, Catterall M, et al: Transforming growth factor-a-*Pseudomonas* exotoxin fusion protein (TGF-a-PE38) treatment of subcutaneous and intracranial human glioma and medulloblastoma xenografts in athymic mice. Cancer Res 1994; 54:1008–1015.
11. Chen SH, Shine HD, Goodman JC, et al: Gene therapy for brain tumors: Regression of experimental gliomas by adenovirus-mediated gene transfer in vivo. Proc Natl Acad Sci USA 1994; 91:3054–3057.
12. Martuza RL: Molecular neurosurgery for glial and neuronal disorders (review). Stereotact Funct Neurosurg 1992; 59:92–99.
13. Donelli MG, Zucchetti M, D'Incalci M: Do anticancer agents reach the tumor target in the human brain (review)? Cancer Chemother Pharmacol 1992; 30:251–260.
14. Fenstermacher JD, Blasberg RG, Patlak CS: Methods for quantifying the transport of drugs across brain barrier systems. Pharmacol Ther 1981; 14:217–248.
15. Chabner BA, Collins JM: Cancer Chemotherapy: Principles and Practice. Philadelphia, JB Lippincott, 1990.
16. Carter SK, Hellmann K: Fundamentals of Cancer Chemotherapy. New York, McGraw-Hill, 1987.
17. Jain RK: Haemodynamic and transport barriers to the treatment of solid tumors. Int J Radiat Biol 1991; 60:85–100.
18. Rapoport SI, Ohno K, Pettigrew KD: Drug entry into the brain. Brain Res 1979; 172:354–359.
19. Levin VA: Relationship of octanol/water partition coefficient and molecular weight to rat brain capillary permeability. J Med Chem 1980; 23:682–684.
20. Abe T, Okamura K, Ono M, et al: Induction of vascular endothelial tubular morphogenesis by human glioma cells: A model system for tumor angiogenesis. J Clin Invest 1993; 92:54–61.
21. Goldman CK, Kim J, Wong WL, et al: Epidermal growth factor stimulates vascular endothelial growth factor production by human malignant glioma cells: A model of glioblastoma multiforme pathophysiology. Mol Biol Cell 1993; 4:121–133.
22. Deane BR, Papp MI, Lantos PL: The vasculature of experimental brain tumours: III. Permeability studies. J Neurol Sci 1984; 65:47–58.
23. Preston E, Haas N: Defining the lower limits of blood-brain barrier permeability: Factors affecting the magnitude and interpretation of permeability-area products. J Neurosci Res 1986; 16:709–719.
24. Hirano A, Matsui T: Vascular structures in brain tumors. Hum Pathol 1975; 6:611–621.
25. Groothuis DR, Fischer JM, Vick NA, et al: Experimental gliomas: An autoradiographic study of the endothelial component. Neurology 1980; 30:297–301.
26. Levin VA, Landahl HD, Freeman-Dove MA: The application of brain capillary permeability coefficient measurements to pathological conditions and the selection of agents which cross the blood-brain barrier. J Pharmacokinet Biopharm 1976; 4:499–519.
27. Groothuis DR, Molnar P, Blasberg RG: Regional Blood flow and blood-to-tissue transport in five brain tumor models. Prog Exp Tumor Res 1984; 27:132–153.
28. Blasberg RG, Patlak CS, Shapiro WR: Distribution of methotrexate in the cerebrospinal fluid and brain after intraventricular administration. Cancer Treat Rep 1977; 61:633–641.
29. Dillon WP: Imaging of central nervous system tumors (review). Curr Opin Radiol 1991; 3:46–50.
30. Tomura N, Kato T, Kanno I, et al: Increased blood flow in human brain tumor after administration of angiotensin II: Demonstration by PET. Comput Med Imaging Graph 1993; 17:443–449.
31. Mineura K, Sasajima T, Kowada M, et al: Perfusion and metabolism in predicting the survival of patients with cerebral glioma. Cancer 1994; 73:2386–2394.
32. Blasberg RG, Groothuis D, Molnar P: Application of quantitative autoradiographic measurements in experimental brain tumor models. Semin Neurol 1981; 1:203–221.
33. Jarden JO, Dhawan V, Moeller JR, et al: The time course of steroid action on blood-to-brain and blood-to-tumor transport of 82Rb: A positron emission tomographic study. Ann Neurol 1989; 25:239–245.
34. Baba T, Fukui M, Takeshita I, et al: Selective enhancement of intratumoral blood flow in malignant gliomas using intra-arterial adenosine triphosphate. J Neurosurg 1990; 72:907–911.
35. Yue NC: Advances in brain tumor imaging (review). Curr Opin Neurol 1993; 6:831–840.
36. Boucher Y, Jain RK: Microvascular pressure is the principal driving force for interstitial hypertension in solid tumors: Implications for vascular collapse. Cancer Res 1992; 52:5110–5114.
37. Sevick EM, Jain RK: Measurement of capillary filtration coefficient in a solid tumor. Cancer Res 1991; 51:1352–1355.
38. Yuan F, Leunig M, Huang SK, et al: Microvascular permeability and interstitial penetration of sterically stabilized (stealth) liposomes in a human tumor xenograft. Cancer Res 1994; 54:3352–3356.
39. Rottenberg DA, Ginos JZ, Kearfott KJ, et al: In vivo measurement of brain tumor pH using [¹¹C]DMO and positron emission tomography. Ann Neurol 1985; 17:70–79.
40. Tanaka Y, Abe Y, Tsugu A, et al: Ultrastructural localization of P-glycoprotein on capillary endothelial cells in human gliomas. Virchow Arch 1994; 425:133–138.
41. Cordon-Cardo C, O'Brien JP, Boccia J, et al: Expression of the multidrug resistance gene product (P-glycoprotein) in human normal and tumor tissues. J Histochem Cytochem 1990; 38:1277–1287.
42. Nabors MW, Griffin CA, Zehnbauer BA, et al: Multidrug resistance gene (MDR1) expression in human brain tumors. J Neurosurg 1991; 75:941–946.
43. Phillips PC: Antineoplastic drug resistance in brain tumors. Neurol Clin 1991; 9:383–404.

44. Collins JM: Pharmacokinetics of intraventricular administration. J Neurooncol 1983; 1:283–291.

45. Reiselbach RE, Di Chiro G, Freireich EJ, et al: Subararachnoid distribution of drugs after lumbar injection. N Engl J Med 1962; 267:1273–1278.

46. Eckman WW, Patlak CS, Fenstermacher JD: A critical evaluation of the principles governing the advantages of intra-arterial infusions. J Pharmacokinet Biopharm 1974; 2:257–285.

47. Saris SC, Blasberg RG, Carson RE, et al: Intravascular streaming during carotid artery infusions: Demonstration in humans and reduction using diastole-phased pulsatile administration. J Neurosurg 1991; 74:763–772.

48. Newton HB, Page MA, Junck L, et al: Intra-arterial cisplatin for the treatment of malignant gliomas. J Neurooncology 1989; 7:39–45.

49. Schuster JM, Friedman HS, Archer GE, et al: Intraarterial therapy of human glioma xenografts in athymic rats using 4-hydroperoxycyclophosphamide. Cancer Res 1993; 53:2338–2343.

50. Levin VA: Clinical anticancer pharmacology: Some pharmacokinetic considerations. Cancer Treat Rev 1986; 13:61–76.

51. Mahaley MS: Neuro-oncology index and review (adult primary brain tumors). J Neurooncology 1991; 11:85–147.

52. Frei E, Cannellos GP: Dose: A critical factor in cancer chemotherapy. Am J Med 1980; 69:585.

53. Shapiro WR, Green SB, Burger PC, et al: Randomized trial of three chemotherapy regimens and two radiotherapy regimens in postoperative treatment of malignant glioma: Brain Tumor Cooperative Group Trial 8001. J Neurosurg 1989; 71:1–9.

54. Walker MD, Gehan EA: Clinical studies in malignant gliomas and their treatment with the nitrosoureas. Cancer Treat Rep 1976; 60:713–716.

55. Schabel FM: Nitrosoureas: A review of experimental antitumor activity. Cancer Treat Rep 1976; 60:665–678.

56. Levin VA, Liu J, Weinkam RJ: Comparative pharmacokinetics of PCNU in rats and patients and extrapolation to clinical trials. Cancer Res 1981; 41:3475–3477.

57. Colvin M, Chabner BA: Alkylating agents. In Chabner BA, Collins JA (eds): Cancer Chemotherapy: Principles and Practice. Philadelphia, JB Lippincott, 1990, pp 276–313.

58. Begleiter A, Lam HP, Goldenberg GJ: Mechanism of uptake of nitrosoureas by L5178Y lymphoblasts. Cancer Res 1977; 37:1022–1027.

59. Levin VA, Stearns J, Byrd A, et al: The effect of phenobarbital pretreatment on the antitumor of BCNU, CCNU, and PCNU, and on the plasma pharmacokinetics and biotransformation of BCNU. J Pharmacol Exp Ther 1979; 208:1–6.

60. Levin VA, Hoffman W, Weinkam RJ: Pharmacokinetics of BCNU in man: A preliminary study of 20 patients. Cancer Treat Rep 1978; 62:1305–1312.

61. Levin VA, Kabra PA, Freeman-Dove MA: Relationship of BCNU and CCNU pharmacokinetics of uptake, distribution, and tissue/plasma partitioning in rat organs and intracerebral tumors. Cancer Chemother Pharmacol 1978; 1:233–242.

62. Diksic M, Sako K, Feindel W, et al: Pharmacokinetics of positron-labeled 1,3-bis(2-chloroethyl)nitrosourea in human brain tumors using positron emission tomography. Cancer Res 1984; 44:3120–3124.

63. Fuchs HE, Archer GE, Colvin OM, et al: Activity of intrathecal 4-hydroperoxycyclophosphamide in a nude rat model of human neoplastic meningitis. Cancer Res 1990; 50:1954–1959.

64. Allen JC, Helson L: High-dose cyclophosphamide chemotherapy for recurrent CNS tumors in children. J Neurosurg 1981; 55:749–756.

65. Alberts DS, van Daalen Wetters T: The effects of phenobarbital on cyclophosphamide antitumor activity. Cancer Res 1976; 36:2785–2789.

66. Aida T, Bodell WJ: Cellular resistance to chloroethylnitrosoureas, nitrogen mustard, and cis-diamminedichloroplatinum(II) in human glial-derived cell lines., Cancer Res 1987; 47:1361–1366.

67. Friedman HS, Oakes WJ, Bigner SH, et al: Medulloblastoma: Tumor biological and clinical perspectives. J Neurooncol 1991; 11:1–15.

68. Rogers LR, Purvis JB, Lederman RJ, et al: Alternating sequential intracarotid BCNU and cisplatin in recurrent malignant glioma. Cancer 1991; 68:15–21.

69. Madajewicz S, Chowhan N, Iliya A, et al: Intracarotid chemotherapy with etoposide and cisplatin for malignant brain tumors. Cancer 1991; 67:2844–2849.

70. Feun LG, Savaraj N, Lee YY, et al: A pilot clinical and pharmacokinetic study of intracarotid cisplatin and bleomycin. Select Cancer Ther 1991; 7:29–36.

71. Reed E, Kohn KW: Platinum analogues. In Chabner BA, Collins JA (eds): Cancer Chemotherapy: Principles and Practice. Philadelphia, JB Lippincott, 1990, pp 465–490.

72. Teicher BA, Herman TS, Holden SA, et al: Tumor resistance to alkylating agents conferred by mechanisms operative only in vivo. Science 1990; 247:1457–1461.

73. Ozols RF: Cisplatin dose intensity (review). Semin Oncol 1989; 16:22–30.

74. Stewart DJ, Leavens M, Maor M: Human central nervous system distribution of cis-diamminedichloroplatinum and use of a radiosensitizer in malignant brain tumors. Cancer Res 1982; 42:2472–2479.

75. Nakagawa H, Groothuis DR, Owens ES, et al: Dexamethasone effects on [^{125}I]albumin distribution in experimental RG-2 gliomas and adjacent brain. J Cereb Blood Flow Metab 1987; 7:687–701.

76. Jain RK: Physiological barriers to delivery of monoclonal antibodies and other macromolecules in tumors. Cancer Res 1990; 50:814s–819s.

77. Fugimori K, Covell DG, Fletcher JD, et al: Modeling analysis of the global and microscopic distribution of immunoglobulin G1F9(ab')2 and Fab in tumors. Cancer Res 1989; 46:5656–5663.

78. DePalatis LR, Johnson KA, Kaplan DA: Combined immunohistochemical and autoradiographic analyses of antigen/antibody interactions in tumor xenograft models. Lab Invest 1991; 65:111–120.

79. Sung C, Dedrick RL, Hall WA, et al: The spatial distribution of immunotoxins in solid tumors: Assessment by quantitative autoradiography. Cancer Res 1993; 53:2092–2099.

80. Blasberg RG, Nakagawa H, Bourdon MA: Regional localization of a glioma-associated antigen defined by monoclonal antibody 81C6 in vivo: Kinetics and implications for diagnosis and therapy. Cancer Res 1987; 47:4432–4443.

81. Sung C, Youle RJ, Dedrick RL: Pharmacokinetic analysis of immunotoxin uptake in solid tumors: role of plasma kinetics, capillary permeability, and binding. Cancer Res 1990; 50:7382–7392.

82. Baxter LT, Zhu H, Mackensen DG, et al: Physiologically based pharmacokinetic model for specific and nonspecific monoclonal antibodies and fragments in normal tissues and human tumor xenografts in nude mice. Cancer Res 1994; 54:1517–1528.

83. Bodor M, Prokai L, Wu W-M, et al: A strategy for delivering peptides into the central nervous system by sequential metabolism. Science 1992; 257:1698–1699.

84. Theuer CP, Buchner J, FitzGerald D, et al: The N-terminal region of the 37-kDa translocated fragment of Pseudomonas exotoxin A aborts translocation by promoting its own export after microsomal membrane insertion. Proc Natl Acad Sci USA 1993; 90:7774–7778.

85. Covell DG, Barbet J, Holton OD, et al: Pharmacokinetics of monoclonal immunoglobulin G1 F(ab')2 and Fab' in mice. Cancer Res 1986; 46:3969–3978.

86. Lesser GJ, Grossman S: The chemotherapy of high-grade astrocytomas (review). Semin Oncol 1994; 21:220–235.

87. Riondel J, Jacrot M, Fessi H, et al: Effects of free and liposome-encapsulated taxol on two brain tumors xenografted into nude mice. In Vivo 1992; 6:23–27.

88. Wowra B, Cremer K, Stricker H, et al: Intraneoplastic application of metrizamide-containing liposomes: Kinetic studies with computed tomography. J Neurooncol 1992; 14:9–18.

89. Morrison PF, Dedrick RL: Transport of cisplatin in rat brain following microinfusion: An analysis. J Pharm Sci 1986; 75:120–128.

90. Morrison PF, Bungay PM, Hsiao JK, et al: Quantitative microdialysis: Analysis of transients and application to pharmacokinetics in brain. J Neurochem 1991; 57:103–117.

91. Bobo RH, Laske DW, Akbasak A, et al: Convection-enhanced delivery of macromolecules in the brain. Proc Natl Acad Sci USA 1994; 91:2076–2080.

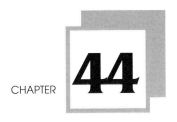

CHAPTER **44**

Intra-arterial Chemotherapy for Malignant Gliomas

Intra-arterial (IA) chemotherapy for the treatment of malignant gliomas, like other "focal" therapies, such as brachytherapy, is based on the *fact* that local recurrence is the most common mode of treatment failure for patients, and on the *premise* that, at least in the majority of patients, the bulk of the tumor can be delineated as a treatment target. The simple goal of IA chemotherapy is to maximize delivery of drug into the tumor for a given amount of systemic exposure. This chapter reviews what has been learned since the mid-1980s in studies of IA chemotherapy given to more than 1,200 patients with malignant gliomas. Despite this impressive number, it is difficult to draw sweeping conclusions regarding IA chemotherapy because of several factors: (1) Most of the published reports are phase I or II studies; the small patient numbers mean wide confidence intervals in response rates and survival outcomes. (2) Differing demographic characteristics of patients in small studies, especially patient age and tumor histology, make comparison of studies somewhat hazardous. (3) Wide variation exists among IA chemotherapy studies in methods of tumor evaluation, definition of tumor response, and definition of patients' response status. (4) Almost no studies directly address what is perhaps the most crucial question, namely, does IA chemotherapy offer a worthwhile therapeutic advantage over systemically administered therapy?

THEORETICAL CONSIDERATIONS

Mathematical modeling of IA chemotherapy for brain tumors predicts up to a fivefold tumor delivery advantage, defined as an increase in the concentration-time integral for a given dose of drug administered by IA vs. intravenous (IV) infusion.[1, 2] In addition, IA infusion is predicted to produce as much as a tenfold increase in peak drug concentration in brain. The rate of IA drug infusion greatly affects peak intratumoral drug concentration but does not affect the total drug exposure.

The entire delivery advantage for IA chemotherapy occurs in the first pass of the drug through the tumor circulation. Favorable drug characteristics for IA use include (1) high capillary permeability (which for brain tumors means lipid solubility); (2) high extraction fraction (first-pass effect) in the target organ; and (3) rapid metabolism and/or excretion, resulting in fewer systemic toxic effects per a given dose.[2–4] According to these criteria, carmustine and other nitrosoureas appear to be well-suited for IA therapy of brain tumors. Intracarotid infusion of ^{14}C-labeled carmustine provided a 2.5-fold delivery advantage over IV infusion in monkeys.[5] Positron emission tomographic (PET) scans in patients receiving "superselective" infusion of carmustine into the middle cerebral artery showed a delivery advantage of up to 50-fold over IV infusion, although considerable variability was found in the first-pass concentration of carmustine in the tumor.[6] Increased peak drug concentration provided by IA infusion may be especially advantageous for nitrosoureas, in light of their steep dose-response curves in experimental systems.[7, 8]

Cisplatin is theoretically not as ideally suited for IA therapy as are nitrosoureas, but studies in animals[9, 10] and humans[11, 12] have demonstrated increased delivery of IA cisplatin compared with IV infusion. A PET study of intravertebral cisplatin in patients found a 2.5-fold delivery advantage over IV infusion.[13] This may be at least partially explained by the ability of IA cisplatin to partially open the blood-brain barrier.[14] IA administration of etoposide can also disrupt the blood-brain barrier in a dose-related manner.[15] The lipid solubility of diaziquone probably contributes to a twofold delivery advantage seen in animal studies.[16]

As is discussed later, considerable variation exists in the reported response rates to IA chemotherapy and in the reported incidence and severity of toxic effects to the eye or brain. A potential source for at least some of this variability is laminar *streaming,* or the inhomogeneous flow of drug into arterial branches and the resulting heterogeneity of drug delivery into tumor and into brain tissue surrounding tumor. Inadequate drug delivery into portions of tumors could theoretically explain some IA chemotherapy treatment failures, and focally excessive drug delivery into the brain surrounding tumor could contribute to neurotoxic effects.

Using quantitative autoradiography, Blacklock and coworkers[17] demonstrated striking non-uniformity of cerebral delivery of ^{14}C-iodoantipyrine following internal carotid infusion in rhesus monkeys, with up to tenfold differences in adjacent regions of cerebral cortex. The streaming effect was more prominent at slower rates of IA infusion. Streaming has also been reported in an in vitro flow model of infusion into the infra-ophthalmic human carotid artery.[18] In that study, the precise position of the catheter tip greatly influenced the pattern of dye distribution. There is doubt, however, as to whether streaming occurs to an important degree in patients receiving intracarotid chemotherapy. In a PET study of the cerebral distribution of ^{15}O-H_2O in patients following infusion at the common carotid bifurcation, Junck and colleagues[19] found homogeneous delivery in the distribution of the ophthalmic artery, major cerebral arteries, and their branches over a 20-fold range of infusion rates (0.5 to 10 mL/min).[19] A similar PET study by Saris and associates[20] reported only a small degree of delivery heterogeneity with continuous intracarotid infusion at the level of the C2 vertebra, unaffected by altering the infusion rate.[20] A likely explanation of the discrepancy between human and animal studies is that the larger diameter of the human internal carotid artery, its greater tortuosity, and the increased distance between the infusion site and the branch points of the carotid all serve to increase flow turbulence and mixing, and thereby reduce the streaming effect.

Streaming is probably a more important phenomenon in patients receiving supraophthalmic carotid or selective intracerebral artery infusion. PET scanning demonstrated markedly inhomogeneous delivery of ^{15}O-H_2O in three of four patients following supraophthalmic intracarotid infusion.[20] The pattern of delivery varied ''markedly'' between repeat infusions in the same patient and between different patients. A similar degree of streaming occurred in eight of ten patients receiving supra-ophthalmic chemotherapy and studied by Tc-99m hexamethyl-propyleneamine oxime (HMPAO) single-photon emission computed tomographic (SPECT) scanning.[21] In both studies the streaming effect was more prominent at slower infusion rates. Diastole-phased pulsatile infusion via a specially designed pump provided more homogeneous delivery than did continuous infusion in a quantitative autoradiography study in monkeys[22] and in a small PET study of patients receiving supra-ophthalmic infusion of cisplatin.[20]

INTRA-ARTERIAL CHEMOTHERAPY FOR RECURRENT TUMORS

Studies of single-agent IA therapy for recurrent malignant gliomas are summarized in Table 44–1. The response rate of patients with recurrent tumors to single-agent intracarotid carmustine in two relatively small studies was 47%[23] and 40%.[25] In another study of IA carmustine, by Hochberg and co-workers,[24] the radiographic response rate was not measured but patients had an encouraging median survival of 50 weeks. Similar response rates are reported for single-agent PCNU,[27] HECNU,[28] and nimustine (ACNU)[29]; the latter two drugs are more water soluble than carmustine and do not require an ethanol diluent. A single study of selective infusion of carmustine into intracerebral arteries in 17 patients yielded an encouraging combined responder/stable disease rate of 64%.[26] In some studies the response rate was better for patients with anaplastic astrocytoma than with glioblastoma.[26, 28]

The most encouraging study of single-agent intracarotid cisplatin is that of Mahaley and colleagues,[32] who reported objective tumor response in 34% of patients and disease stabilization in another 40%. Feun and associates[30] reported a combined responder/stable disease rate of 55%. In contrast, Newton and co-workers[31] observed a radiographic response in only 1 of 12 patients with recurrent tumors who had previously failed IA carmustine therapy. The response rate to intracarotid carboplatin also varies widely,[34, 35] with no obvious therapeutic advantage over cisplatin.

The only randomized study of single-agent IA chemotherapy for recurrent malignant gliomas has been conducted by the Brain Tumor Cooperative Group (BTCG), in which patients were randomized to receive IA cisplatin or IV PCNU.[33] The median survival of 9.4 months for the IA cisplatin group did not differ from 11.8 months for patients receiving IV PCNU. Radiographic tumor response rate was not measured.

Single-agent intracarotid infusion of diaziquone[36] or etoposide[37] for recurrent tumors has yielded rather disappointing response rates, not greater than the published results for the drugs given IV.[38]

Studies utilizing multiple IA agents or combined IA plus IV chemotherapy are summarized in Table 44–2. Most such regimens utilized IA carmustine given sequentially with IA cisplatin at the same treatment session. The exception was the study by Rogers and associates,[43] in which patients received two cycles of intracarotid carmustine followed by two infusions of intracarotid cisplatin. Response rates of 50% or more were seen in several studies,[40–42, 44] but these encouraging results have not been uniform. It is curious that Stewart and others[40] reported a 62% response rate with combined IA carmustine plus cisplatin plus teniposide, but then reported a zero response rate (31% stable disease) with the same combination plus the addition of IV cytarabine.[45] In the few studies in which it was measured, the time to treatment failure was rather short, generally less than 5 months.[40, 42, 46]

More encouraging results were observed in three small studies using supra-ophthalmic carotid or selective cerebral artery infusions. Kapp and Vance[41] reported a response in 8 of 13 patients treated with supra-ophthalmic carotid carmustine plus cisplatin (then oral lomustine), with a median time to failure of 9 months. Some patients underwent surgical modification of the cerebral vasculature to result in the perfusion of the tumor by a single internal carotid artery.[50] Five of the 13 patients (38%), however, manifested postinfusion neurologic deterioration (see following). The same group subsequently reported a 52% response rate to supra-ophthalmic carotid carmustine plus cisplatin with a 12% incidence of neurologic deterioration.[44] In that study, a higher response rate and a higher incidence of neurotoxic effects were seen with cisplatin doses of 150 to 200 mg vs. doses of 110 to 120 mg. Each of the 13 patients treated by

TABLE 44-1

SINGLE-AGENT INTRA-ARTERIAL (IA) CHEMOTHERAPY FOR RECURRENT MALIGNANT GLIOMAS

Study	IA Regimen	Route	No. of Patients Evaluated	% Responders	% Stable	Median TTF (wk)*	Median Survival (wk)*	Toxic Effects (% of Patients)
Greenberg et al[23]	Carmustine, 200–300 mg/m², q 6–8 wk	IC	19	47	21	20†	26 + †	Leukoencephalopathy (10)
Hochberg et al[24]	Carmustine, 240–600 mg/m², q 6 wk	IC or SO	30	NR	NR	NR	50	Seizures (7)
Johnson et al[25]	Carmustine, 150 mg/m², q 6 wk	IC	20	40	NR	NR	35	Vision loss (10)
Bradac et al[26]	Carmustine, 120–180 mg/m², q 6–8 wk	Sel	17	29	35	NR	23†	Neurologic deterioration (24)
Stewart et al[27]	PCNU, 60–110 mg/m², q 7 wk	IC	16	44	NR	20†	NR	Vision loss (19), neurologic deterioration (71)
Poisson et al[28]	HECNU, 120 mg/m², q 6–8 wk	IC	53	49	NR	40†	34	Vision loss (11), neurologic deterioration (7) leukoencephalopathy (11)
Vega et al[29]	Nimustine, 150 mg q 6–8 wk	IC	18	44	NR	24	32	Vision loss (6%)
Feun et al[30]	Cisplatin, 60–120 mg/m², q 4 wk	IC	20	30	25	33†	NR	Vision loss (20), hearing loss (15), seizures (20), neurologic deterioration (40), cerebral herniation (5)‡
Newton et al[31]	Cisplatin, 60–100 mg/m², q 4–6 wk	IC	12	8	0	14	NR	Vision loss (17), seizures (25), neurologic deterioration (33)
Mahaley et al[32]	Cisplatin, 60 mg/m², q 4 wk	IC	34	34	40	20†	35†	Vision loss (3), cerebral herniation (3)
Green et al[33]	Cisplatin, 60 mg/m², q 4 wk§	IC	NR	NR	NR	NR	38	Encephalopathy (4)
Saris et al[20]	Cisplatin, 70–100 mg/m², q 6 wk	IC or SO	10	10	30	NR	NR	Neurologic deterioration (10)
Follezou et al[34]	Carboplatin, 400 mg/m², q 4 wk	IC	23	22	22	NR	NR	Vision loss (4), neurologic deterioration (4)
Stewart et al[35]	Carboplatin, 200–400 mg/m², q 4 wk	IC	10	0	10	NR	8	Vision loss (50), neurologic deterioration (20)
Greenberg et al[36]	Diaziquone, 10–30 mg/m², q 4 wk	IC	20	10	20	NR	NR	Vision loss (10), neurologic deterioration (5), seizures (5)
Feun et al[37]	Etoposide, 100–650 mg/m², q 4 wk	IC	15	7	33	NR	NR	Vision loss (4), seizures (7)

*Median time to treatment failure (TTF) and median survival dated from the beginning of IA chemotherapy.
†Reported for responders only.
‡Among a total of 30 treated patients with malignant gliomas *or* brain metastases.
§Randomized comparison of IC cisplatin vs. IV PCNU.
Abbreviations: IC, cervical internal carotid infusion; SO, supra-ophthalmic carotid infusion; Sel, selective intracerebral infusion; NR, not reported.

TABLE 44–2
COMBINATION INTRA-ARTERIAL (IA) CHEMOTHERAPY FOR RECURRENT MALIGNANT GLIOMAS

Study	Regimen	No. of Patients Evaluated	% Responders	% Stable	Median TTF (wk)*	Median Survival (wk)*	Toxic Effects (% of Patients)
West et al[39]	IC carmustine, 100 mg/m², + VCR, PCB, CCNU	9	22	NR	NR	20	NR
Stewart et al[40]	IA carmustine, 100–125 mg/m², + IA cisplatin, 60 mg/m², + IA teniposide, 150–175 mg/m²	16	62	6	15	NR	Vision loss (19), hearing loss (5), neurologic deterioration (19)†
Kapp et al[41]	SO carmustine, 300 mg, + SO ciplatin, 150–200 mg, q 8 wk × 2, then PO lomustine	13	62	23	36	44	Neurologic deterioration (38)
Stewart et al[42]	IA carmustine, 100 mg/m², + IA cisplatin, 60 mg/m², + IA teniposide, 150 mg/m², + IV bleomycin, VCR, MTX, PCB, q 6 wk	22	52	9	19†	21	Vision loss (5), hearing loss (5), neurologic deterioration (31), seizures (5)
Rogers et al[43]	IC carmustine, 300–400 mg, q 4–6 wk × 2	42 (Carmustine)	10	55	NR	NR	Vision loss (38), hearing loss (12), neurologic deterioration (26), seizures (2)
	Then IC cisplatin, 150–200 mg, q 4–6 wk × 2	27 (Cisplatin)	0	33	NR	36 (All)	
Bobo et al[44]	SO carmustine, 300 mg, + SO cisplatin, 110–200 mg, q 8 wk	25	52	NR	NR	108§	Neurologic deterioration (12)
Stewart et al[45]	IC carmustine, 100 mg/m², + IC cisplatin, 60 mg/m², + IC teniposide, 150 mg/m², + IV cytarabine q 4 wk	16	0	31	NR	NR	Vision loss (12), hearing loss (8), neurologic deterioration (38), seizures (19), neutropenic sepsis (25)
Nakagawa et al[46]	Sel cisplatin, 50–100 mg/m², + Sel etoposide, 50–100 mg/m², q 2 wk × 2	13	23	77	14	24	Neurologic deterioration (23), seizures (23)
Bonstelle et al[47]	IC 5-FU,¶ 900 mg, + IC doxorubicin,¶ 90 mg, + IV carmustine, q 6 wk	18	50	33	NR	NR	Seizures (11), cerebral herniation (11)
Neuwelt et al[48]	IA MTX,¶ 1–5 g, + IV cyclophosphamide, + PCB, q 4–6 wk	35	23	11	NR	70§	Vision loss (3), neurologic deterioration (66), seizures (55)
Gumerlock et al[49]	IA MTX,¶ 1–5 g, + IV cyclophosphamide, + PCB, q 4 wk	37	46	35	NR	88§	Vision loss (5), neurologic deterioration (46), seizures (51), cerebral herniation (3)

*Median time to treatment failure (TTF) and median survival dated from the beginning of IA chemotherapy unless otherwise noted.
†Reported for responders only.
‡Includes patients treated for cerebral metastases.
§From time of initial tumor diagnosis.
¶After hyperosmolar blood-brain barrier disruption.
Abbreviations: IC, cervical internal carotid infusion; SO, supra-ophthalmic carotid infusion; Sel, selective intracerebral infusion; NR, not reported; 5-FU, fluorouracil; MTX, methotrexate; PCB, procarbazine; VCR, vincristine.

Nakagawa and colleagues[46] had tumor response or stabilization after selective cerebral artery infusion of cisplatin plus etoposide[46]; six of the patients (46%) had seizures or neurologic deterioration after IA chemotherapy.

INTRA-ARTERIAL CHEMOTHERAPY FOR NEWLY DIAGNOSED TUMORS

Studies of single-agent IA chemotherapy administered prior to or in conjunction with radiotherapy for patients with newly diagnosed malignant gliomas are outlined in Table 44–3. The median survival times for patients receiving single-agent intracarotid nitrosoureas cluster around 1 year (see Table 44–3), ranging from 32 weeks[29] to 64 weeks.[24] Studies of single-agent intracarotid cisplatin[55-57] or fluorouracil[58] have yielded similar survival times. Clayman and co-workers[52] reported a median survival time of 73 weeks for 13 patients receiving supra-ophthalmic carotid or selective cerebral artery carmustine.[52] Greenberg and others[59] administered fluorouracil as a continuous intracarotid infusion (via an implantable pump) together with the radiosensitizing agent bromodeoxyuridine (BUdR) during and after radiotherapy.[59] The median survival time did not differ from their previous study of radiotherapy and intracarotid BUdR without the fluorouracil.

TABLE 44–3
SINGLE-AGENT INTRA-ARTERIAL (IA) CHEMOTHERAPY FOR NEWLY DIAGNOSED MALIGNANT GLIOMAS

Study	IA Regimen*	Route	No. of Patients Evaluated	% Responders	% Stable	Median TTF (wk)*	Median Survival (wk)*	Toxic Effects (% of Patients)
Greenberg et al[23]	Carmustine, 200–300 mg/m², q 6–8 wk (pre-RT)	IC	12	75	8	25	54	Vision loss (50), seizures (33)
Hochberg et al[24]	Carmustine, 240 mg/m², q 4–6 wk	IC	25	NR	NR	NR	64	Neurologic deterioration (17), seizures (8)
		SO	18	NR	NR	NR	50	
Bashir et al[51]	Carmustine, 400 mg, q 4 wk × 4 (pre-RT)	IC	28	44	NR	NR	37	Vision loss (15), neurologic deterioration (7), leukoencephalopathy (7)
Clayman et al[52]	Carmustine, 150 mg/m², q 6 wk	Sel	13	38	NR	NR	73	Neurologic deterioration (7)
Roosen et al[53]	Nimustine, 100 mg, q 6 wk	IC	35	69 (or stable)		NR	56	Vision loss (6), neurologic deterioration (9), seizures (3)
Vega et al[29]	Nimustine, 150 mg, q 6–8 wk × 3 (pre-RT)	IC	22	26	NR	12	32	Vision loss (9)
Fauchon et al[54]	HECNU, 120 mg/m², q 6–8 wk × 3 (pre-RT)	IC	40	15	55	32	48	Vision loss (15), leukoencephalopathy (10)
Calvo et al[55]	Cisplatin, 40–60 mg/m², q 1 wk × 3–5	IC	11	45	55	NR	42	Vision loss (9), seizures (18)
Dropcho et al[56]	Cisplatin, 75 mg/m², q 4 wk × 4 (pre-RT)	IC	22	45	18	23	63	Vision loss (5), hearing loss (9), seizures (9), neurologic deterioration (4), cerebral herniation (4)
Mortimer et al[57]	Cisplatin, 150 mg, q 3 wk × 2 (½ patients pre-RT)	IC	27	22	NR	NR	41	Neurologic deterioration (5)
Larner et al[58]	5-FU, 200–600 mg, q 1 wk × 4	Sel	25	NR	NR	NR	44	Neurologic deterioration (16)
Greenberg et al[59]	5-FU, 5 mg/m²/day† × 8 wk + BUdR†	IC	39	NR	NR	NR	68	Vision loss (5), neurologic deterioration (2), focal dermatitis or iritis (77)

*Medial time to treatment failure (TTF) and median survival dated from the time of initial tumor diagnosis; IA chemotherapy begun during RT unless otherwise noted.
†Continuous infusion.
Abbreviations: IC, cervical internal carotid infusion; SO, supra-ophthalmic carotid infusion; Sel, selective intracerebral infusion; NR, not reported; 5-FU, fluorouracil; BUdR, bromodeoxyuridine; RT, radiotherapy.

The study of pre-radiotherapy intracarotid cisplatin by Dropcho and colleagues[56] is unique in that it was restricted to patients who underwent biopsy without any tumor resection, allowing an assessment of the sensitivity of untreated malignant gliomas to intracarotid cisplatin without the confounding influence of prior surgery or radiotherapy. Objective tumor response occurred in 45% of patients, with disease stabilization in another 18%. Despite continued intracarotid cisplatin treatments after radiotherapy in the responders, the median time to tumor progression and survival were not dramatically lengthened.

As noted in the introductory paragraph, a basic premise of IA chemotherapy for malignant gliomas is that, at least in selected patients, the tumor is localized to a circumscribed area. If these tumors are ever truly "localized," it would most likely be at the time of initial diagnosis. Few studies of IA chemotherapy have specifically addressed the issue of "local" vs. "distant" treatment failure. In the study of pre-radiotherapy intracarotid cisplatin by Dropcho and associates,[56] tumor progression occurred at the initial tumor site in

80% of patients, still within the distribution of the infused internal carotid artery; only two patients had extension of contrast-enhancing tumor outside the internal carotid territory in the setting of stable tumor at the initial site. Similarly, tumor recurred within the original tumor area in each of the patients treated with pre-radiotherapy intracarotid cisplatin by Recht and co-workers.[60]

Studies of combination therapy, including IA chemotherapy for patients with newly diagnosed tumors, are summarized in Table 44–4. Median survival times, again, hover around 1 year, ranging from 40 weeks among patients with grade 4 tumors treated with intracarotid carmustine plus systemic vincristine and procarbazine[62] to 64 weeks in ten patients treated with intracarotid cisplatin plus etoposide.[63] Watne and colleagues[62] reported a median survival time of more than 4 years in patients with grade 3 tumors.

In the only phase III comparison of IA vs. IV chemotherapy for in patients with newly diagnosed gliomas, the BTCG study randomized more than 300 patients to receive IV or IA carmustine, with or without the addition of IV fluoroura-

TABLE 44–4
COMBINATION INTRA-ARTERIAL (IA) CHEMOTHERAPY FOR NEWLY DIAGNOSED MALIGNANT GLIOMAS

Study	Regimen	No. of Patients Evaluated	% Responders	% Stable	Median TTF (wk)*	Median Survival (wk)*	Toxic Effects (% of Patients)
West et al[39]	IC carmustine, 100 mg/m², + VCR, PCB, lomustine × 4 (pre-RT)	15	75	NR	NR	50	Seizures (7)
Shapiro et al[61]	IA carmustine,† 200 mg/m², q 8 wk, ± IV 5-FU	153	NR	NR	NR	45	Vision loss (17) leukoencephalopathy (10)
Bobo et al[44]	SO carmustine, 300 mg, + SO cisplatin, 110–200 mg, q 8 wk	14	50	NR	NR	50	Neurologic deterioration (14)
Watne et al[62]	IC carmustine, 160 mg, + IV VCR and PCB, q 4 wk × 4	35 (grade 3)	NR	NR	NR	228	NR
		138 (grade 4)	NR	NR	NR	40	NR
Recht et al[60]	IC cisplatin, 90 mg/m², × 2 (pre-RT), then IV carmustine	25	16	52	53	60	Hearing loss (8), neurologic deterioration (8)
Madajewicz et al[63]	IC cisplatin, 40 mg/m², + IC etoposide, 20 mg/m², q 3 wk × 2 (pre-RT)	20	60	0	NR	64‡	Seizures (10)
Williams et al[64]	IA§ MTX, 2.5 g, + IV cyclophosphamide, + PCB q 4 wk (pre-RT)	10	40	NR	100‡	52	Seizures (58)
Iwadate et al[65]	IC nimustine, 100 mg, + IC cisplatin, 100 mg¶, q 8–9 wk × 3	34	54	23	33	52	Leukoencephalopathy (8)

*Median time to treatment failure (TTF) and median survival dated from the time of initial diagnosis; IA chemotherapy begun during RT unless otherwise noted.
†Randomized vs IV carmustine; accrural stopped due to neurotoxicity.
‡Reported for responders only.
§After hyperosmolar blood-brain barrier disruption.
¶Half of patients randomized to hyperosmolar blood-brain barrier disruption.
Abbreviations: IC, cervical internal carotid infusion; SeI, selective intracerebral infusion; NR, not reported; VCR, vincristine; PCB, procarbazine; 5-FU, fluorouracil; MTX, methotrexate; RT, radiotherapy.

cil.[61] The median survival time for the IA carmustine group was 11.2 months and the 24-month survival was 13%, compared with 14.0 months and 25% for the IV carmustine group; the addition of fluorouracil had no impact on survival. Most of the survival difference between the two groups was accounted for by poorer survival times for the ''non-glioblastoma'' IA patients, most of whom had anaplastic astrocytoma. Accrual to the study was halted early because of the development of severe leukoencephalopathy in 10% of patients receiving IA carmustine (see following).

TOXIC EFFECTS OF INTRA-ARTERIAL CHEMOTHERAPY

Vision Loss

Nearly all patients given intracarotid carmustine have ipsilateral periorbital erythralgia during the drug infusion; this often limits the IA infusion rate, despite administration of analgesics. If data from all the relevant studies in Tables 44–1 through 44–4 are pooled, an incidence of ipsilateral vision loss of approximately 10% is seen among 465 patients receiving chemotherapy with a single-agent intracarotid nitrosourea (with or without additional systemic chemotherapy). This figure includes vision loss in 17% of 153 patients randomized to intracarotid carmustine in the phase III BTCG study.[61] Overall the risk of vision loss is not markedly different in patients with recurrent tumors vs. patients with newly diagnosed tumors, although Greenberg and co-workers[23] observed vision loss in none of 19 patients with recurrent tumors and in 6 of 12 patients with newly diagnosed tumors. The risk of vision loss is low following administration of 100 mg/m^2 of carmustine[66]; the risk increases at higher doses, but a strict linear correlation has not been demonstrated. Vision loss seems to be more frequent with intracarotid PCNU[27] or HECNU[28, 54] than with carmustine.

Funduscopic examination in affected patients usually shows retinal arteriolar narrowing, hemorrhages, nerve fiber layer infarctions, and arterial phase leaks on fluorescein angiograms. These findings indicate a toxic retinal vasculitis as the most common substrate of nitrosourea toxic response.[23] In some patients, especially those receiving HECNU, the findings are more consistent with anterior ischemic optic neuropathy.[28, 67, 68]

Selective infusion of carmustine into the internal carotid artery above the origin of the ophthalmic artery greatly reduces, but does not eliminate, toxic effects to the visual system. Visual field deficits consistent with injury to the optic chiasm and subclinical changes in visual evoked potentials have occurred after supra-ophthalmic nitrosourea infusions.[69–71]

The incidence of ipsilateral vision loss following infra-ophthalmic intracarotid cisplatin is approximately 8% among 190 patients pooled from the studies in Tables 44–1 and 44–3. Symptomatic vision loss occurred in only 1 of 35 patients treated with 60 mg/m^2 by Mahaley and colleagues[32] and in none of 25 patients treated with 90 mg/m^2 by Recht and others,[60] but it occurred in 3 of 5 patients treated by Kupersmith and co-workers.[70] A wide range of incidence of vision loss has also been seen following intracarotid car-

boplatin administration.[34, 35] As with the nitrosoureas, acute vision loss can occur in patients who received multiple prior cisplatin infusions without incident. No clear correlation has been shown between the risk of vision loss and the intracarotid cisplatin or carboplatin dose, infusion rate, or cumulative dose. Combining intracarotid cisplatin with carmustine does not appear to result in additive toxic effects; again, marked differences occur in the reported incidence of vision loss, ranging from 5%[42] to 38%.[43]

Most patients with vision loss after intracarotid cisplatin have retinal infarctions, periarteritis, and pigmentary epithelial changes,[72] whereas other patients are believed to have retrobulbar optic neuropathy.[70] Several patients developed bilateral loss of visual acuity and/or abnormal visual evoked potentials following multiple cycles of unilateral intracarotid cisplatin infusion.[30, 73] Symptomatic vision loss has not been reported following supra-ophthalmic carotid infusion of cisplatin[70] or of cisplatin plus carmustine.[41, 44]

Hearing Loss

Bilateral symptomatic hearing loss has been reported in 0% to 15% of patients following intracarotid cisplatin administration (see Tables 44–1 and 44–3). Serial audiometry reveals a much higher incidence of cisplatin ototoxic effects. For example, Dropcho and others[56] observed a >10 dB loss in 45% of the entire patient group and in 62% of patients who received two or more cisplatin infusions.[56] Ototoxic effects following intracarotid cisplatin administration are bilateral, dose-related, mainly limited to the 4000- to 8000-Hz frequency range (although loss at 2000 Hz occurs after high cumulative doses), and irreversible. Because the frequencies most often affected are higher than those used in conversational speech, only a small fraction of patients with hearing loss detectable by audiometry actually notice any deficit. In these respects, the ototoxic effects of intracarotid cisplatin are identical to those caused by IV cisplatin. In contrast, acute bilateral deafness has occurred following intravertebral cisplatin administration.[30]

Neurotoxic Effects

Acute neurotoxic effects of IA nitrosoureas include seizures, confusion, and/or worsening of focal deficits occurring within 24 to 48 hours of treatment. Based on the studies in Tables 44–1 and 44–3, the approximate risk of acute neurotoxic effects is slightly less than 10%. There is no obvious explanation for outliers, such as the 33% incidence of seizures after IA carmustine administration in the study by Greenberg and co-workers[23] or the 71% incidence of transient neurologic deterioration after IA PCNU administration reported by Stewart and associates.[27] Supra-ophthalmic carotid or selective intracerebral artery carmustine infusion probably carries a higher risk of acute neurotoxic effects than does infra-ophthalmic carotid infusion.[24, 26]

Hypodensity of the ipsilateral hemispheric white matter occurs in at least 20% of patients within several weeks following IA carmustine administration; this has occurred after as little as 415 mg/m^2 of carmustine was given in two infusions.[23, 24] This apparent leukoencephalopathy remains subclinical in the majority of patients.[23] Unfortunately, some patients manifest subacute, progressively worsening hemiparesis and mental status changes, often with seizures.[61, 74, 75] The syndrome does not improve with corticosteroids and often results in shortened survival. In a phase III BTCG study, 11 of the 16 patients with leukoencephalopathy also had ipsilateral vision loss.[61] Serial computed tomographic (CT) or magnetic resonance (MR) scans show hypodense white matter, mass effect, and ipsilateral gyral enhancement, which subsequently resolves and is replaced by punctate calcifications.[61, 74] PET scans show diffusely decreased fluorodeoxyglucose uptake in the perfused territory.[76] The toxic effects are not unique to carmustine, as they have also occurred following IA HECNU administration.[28, 54]

The histopathologic findings of delayed neurotoxic effects from IA carmustine administration include confluent areas of coagulative necrosis of edematous white matter within the infused hemisphere, foci of petechial hemorrhages, and axonal swellings and/or calcifications. Fibrinoid necrosis of small vessels, fibrin thrombi, and telangiectasias are often prominent.[74, 75, 77] The overlying gray matter is relatively, but not totally, preserved. These changes closely resemble the pathologic findings of ''radiation necrosis''[78] and of fatal neurotoxic effects of ''megadose'' IV carmustine given without cranial radiotherapy.[79] Animal studies[80] support the neuropathologic findings in humans, implicating injury to small blood vessels as the primary pathogenetic event, although direct damage to myelinated fibers may also occur. Incidentally, the diffuse and widespread neuropathologic changes after intracarotid infusion argue against streaming as an important factor in leukoencephalopathy.

The risk of delayed neurotoxic effects following IA carmustine is related to the cumulative exposure of the brain to the drug. Most reported cases of symptomatic leukoencephalopathy occurred after cumulative intracarotid doses of 300 to 600 mg/m² of carmustine.[61, 74] The incidence of leukoencephalopathy in the BTCG phase III study fell when the intracarotid carmustine dose was reduced from 200 to 100 mg/m².[61] Supra-ophthalmic carmustine infusion probably carries an increased risk of delayed leukoencephalopathy relative to infusions below the ophthalmic artery, presumably due to increased drug delivery to the brain.[24, 26, 41] Progressive clinical deterioration and hyperlucency of ipsilateral hemispheric white matter on CT scans have been reported after a single supra-ophthalmic carotid infusion of 200 mg/m².[81]

The incidence of delayed neurotoxic effects is probably higher in newly diagnosed patients receiving IA carmustine prior to or in conjunction with radiotherapy than in patients treated at time of tumor recurrence after radiotherapy, suggesting a synergistic effect between radiotherapy and the focally high brain concentrations of carmustine achieved by IA infusion.[24, 74] The reported incidence of severe neurotoxicity in ''new'' patients ranges from 10% to 33% after a cumulative IA carmustine dose of 400 mg/m².[51, 61, 74] Severe neurotoxic effects have been observed even when several cycles of IA carmustine are given prior to any radiation therapy.[51] A possible explanation for a carmustine-radiotherapy synergistic effect is the inhibition by carmustine of glutathione reductase-mediated mechanisms to protect cells from radiotherapy injury.[82]

Seizures and/or acute neurologic deterioration (generally manifesting as transient or permanent worsening of pre-existing focal deficits) occurring within 72 hours after single-agent IA cisplatin or carboplatin administration have been reported in a range of 3%[32] to 60%[30] of patients. Pooling data from the studies in Tables 44–1 and 44–2 yields a 6% incidence of postinfusion seizures and a 12% incidence of neurologic deterioration. Seizures or neurologic deterioration after cisplatin are not unique to the IA route, as similar events have been reported in patients receiving IV cisplatin for brain tumors or for extraneural neoplasms.[83, 84] Some studies noted a higher incidence of neurotoxic effects, including permanent deficits, after supra-ophthalmic cisplatin[41, 44] (unpublished observations, 1995) or after infra-ophthalmic carotid doses greater than 60 mg/m².[85] A low incidence of neurotoxic effects in other similar studies[44, 60] refutes a strict dose correlation. Similarly, a correlation between IA cisplatin neurotoxic effects and faster rates of drug infusion has been observed in some studies,[46] but not in others.

The pathophysiology of IA cisplatin neurotoxic effects is probably multifactorial and varies among individual patients. Some patients with acute neurotoxic effects had hyponatremia or hypomagnesemia, whereas other patients appeared to have increased cerebral edema, possibly caused by the administration of high volumes of pretreatment and posttreatment IV fluids. In some but not all patients, the acute neurotoxic effects are reversible with corticosteroids, and they can be ameliorated by boosting the corticosteroid dose immediately before and for several days after IA cisplatin infusions. Another potential cause of seizures is a drop in serum levels of phenytoin or other anticonvulsants, which can occur in the 48 to 72 hours following IV[86, 87] or IA[56] cisplatin, unrelated to emesis. Finally, cisplatin itself may be toxic to the CNS.[56] The rather weak correlation between neurotoxic responses and IA cisplatin dose could theoretically be explained by unpredictable intravascular streaming and focally injurious drug concentrations, but this has not been supported by firm evidence.

The most serious toxic effect of IA cisplatin is cerebral herniation, which has been reported in 3 of 146 patients receiving single-agent IA cisplatin for newly diagnosed or recurrent tumors (see Tables 44–1 and 44–3). These patients showed clinical signs of transtentorial herniation and increased edema on post-infusion CT scans within 72 hours after IA cisplatin administration. Cerebral herniation in brain tumor patients has also been reported several hours after IV cisplatin was given,[88] sometimes but not always in the setting of hyponatremia and/or seizures. Despite this potential for IA cisplatin to cause acute and sometimes life-threatening neurotoxic effects, no reports have been published of single-agent IA cisplatin causing delayed leukoencephalopathy or necrotizing encephalopathy, as has been seen after IA carmustine administration.

BLOOD-BRAIN BARRIER DISRUPTION

The major determinant of delivery of drugs with small, lipid-soluble molecules, such as the nitrosoureas, is local blood flow to the tumor, whereas the entry of larger, water-soluble molecules into brain (and brain tumors) depends mainly on the degree of breakdown of the blood-brain barrier. This has led to efforts at increasing the delivery of drugs into gliomas by transient disruption of the blood-brain barrier with intra-arterial hyperosmolar mannitol immediately prior to IA drug infusion. The relative importance of the blood-brain barrier as a cause of restricted drug entry and consequent chemotherapeutic failure in patients with malignant gliomas, and the practical clinical value of hyperosmolar blood-brain barrier disruption, have been matters of considerable controversy.[89-91] The arguments regarding blood-brain barrier disruption have revolved around three key questions: (1) How much does hyperosmolar blood-brain barrier disruption increase drug delivery into the central tumor and into tumor cells infiltrating the surrounding brain? (2) Will increased drug delivery into the tumor, if it occurs, translate into improved antitumor efficacy? (3) What is the risk of neurotoxic effects from increased drug delivery into normal brain tissue?

The blood-brain barrier (more precisely, the blood-tumor barrier) is at least partially opened in malignant gliomas. In experimental brain tumors, the integrity of the blood-brain barrier varies significantly between different tumor models and between different regions of a given tumor.[92] This variability is often especially prominent in the periphery of a tumor and in the edematous brain adjacent to the tumor (BAT). Quantitative autoradiography studies in animals have verified the ability of IA mannitol or arabinose to increase the permeability of normal brain capillaries. The ability of hyperosmolar blood-brain barrier disruption to increase the capillary permeability of animal tumor models, however, varies greatly between different models and different regions of a given tumor.[93-95] Animal studies indicate that the chemotherapy drug delivery advantage afforded by hypersomolar blood-brain barrier disruption would vary among individual tumors and would be very difficult to predict in advance.

Another limitation to IA chemotherapy with blood-brain barrier modification is the potential for serious neurotoxic effects. Several potentially active agents (including fluorouracil and cisplatin) have produced necrosis and hemorrhagic infarction in dogs when administered after osmotic blood-brain barrier disruption.[14] This clearly limits the number of agents that can be administered in this fashion. In addition, quantitative autoradiographic studies of the entry of radiolabeled methotrexate or aminoisobutyric acid into animal tumors have consistently shown that hyperosmolar blood-brain barrier disruption produces a much greater proportional increase in drug entry into the normal brain surrounding a tumor than into the tumor itself.[94, 96, 97]

Several studies have used IA chemotherapy preceded by hyperosmolar blood-brain barrier modification as part of combination treatment regimens. Bonstelle and others[47] reported a 50% response rate among 18 patients with recurrent tumors following intracarotid flurouracil and doxorubicin plus IV carmustine (see Table 44–2).[47] Combined responder/stabilization rates of 34%[48] and 81%[49] were reported with very similar regimens of IA methotrexate plus systemic cyclophosphamide and procarbazine. Williams and co-workers[64] administered an IA methotrexate-based regimen prior to radiotherapy in ten patients with newly diagnosed tumors,

with four responders and a median survival time of 52 weeks (see Table 44–4). From these studies it is impossible to determine whether blood-brain barrier modification provided any therapeutic benefit over and above that derived from the IA-based chemotherapy regimen itself. In the only published randomized study to date, Iwadate and associates[65] performed blood-brain barrier modification in 18 of 34 patients receiving intracarotid nimustine and cisplatin for newly diagnosed tumors.[65] In this small number of patients, blood-brain barrier modification did not significantly affect the tumor response rate, time to tumor progression, or survival duration.

The reported incidence of acute neurotoxic effects following IA chemotherapy and blood-brain barrier modification varies widely. Seizures occurring during or shortly after treatment were seen in more than 50% of patients in three studies of IA methotrexate.[48, 49, 64] Two studies of IA methotrexate reported the occurrence of neurologic deterioration, which was usually but not always reversible, in half of patients within 24 to 48 hours of treatment.[48, 49] These effects were mainly attributed to a temporary increase in peritumoral cerebral edema. Acute neurotoxic response was much less common following IA fluorouracil plus doxorubicin[47] or nimustine plus cisplatin,[65] although 2 of 17 patients in the latter study developed leukoencephalopathy. The incidence of leukoencephalopathy or other delayed neurotoxic effects following blood-brain barrier modification plus IA methotrexate has been low, as assessed by neuropsychological testing[64] or autopsy[48] in a limited number of patients.

SUMMARY

As stated in the opening paragraph, the simple goal of IA chemotherapy is to deliver a greater amount of drug into the tumor. For several drugs, IA infusion is clearly capable of doing that, and IA chemotherapy has demonstrated antitumor activity in numerous study designs, both for patients with newly diagnosed malignant gliomas and for patients with recurrent tumors. It is also apparent, however, that simply getting more cytotoxic drug into the tumor does not necessarily translate into a therapeutic benefit for patients. The reasons for this are multiple and include therapeutic resistance of tumor cells at a molecular level, inhomogeneous drug delivery within the tumor and in areas in which tumor has infiltrated normal brain, and heightened neurotoxic effects of IA chemotherapy. Much more work needs to be done to determine the role that IA chemotherapy should play in the multimodality treatment of patients with malignant gliomas and to determine whether the therapeutic ratio of IA chemotherapy can be improved by novel delivery methods, combination drug regimens, or blood-brain barrier modification.

ACKNOWLEDGMENTS

Support was provided by grant P20 NS31096 from the National Institute for Neurological Disorders and Stroke and by grant P30 CA13148 from the National Cancer Institute.

REFERENCES

1. Eckman WW, Patlak CS, Fenstermacher JD: A critical evaluation of the principles governing the advantages of intra-arterial infusion. J Pharmacokinet Biopharmacokinet 1974; 2:257.

2. Fenstermacher JD, Cowles AL: Theoretic limitations of intracarotid infusions in brain tumor chemotherapy. Cancer Treat Rep 1977; 61:519.

3. Fenstermacher J, Gazendam J: Intra-arterial infusions of drugs and hyperosmotic solutions as ways of enhancing CNS chemotherapy. Cancer Treat Rep 1981; 65(suppl 2):27.

4. Collins JM: Pharmacologic rationale for regional drug delivery. J Clin Oncol 1984; 2:498.

5. Levin VA, Kabra PM, Freeman-Dove MA: Pharmacokinetics of intracarotid artery ^{14}C-BCNU in the squirrel monkey. J Neurosurg 1978; 48:587.

6. Tyler JL, Yamamoto L, Diksic M, et al: Pharmacokinetics of superselective intra-arterial and intravenous ^{11}C-BCNU evaluated by PET. J Nucl Med 1986; 27:775.

7. Rosenblum ML, Dougherty DA, Wilson CB: Rational planning of brain tumor therapy based on laboratory investigation: Comparison of single and multiple-dose BCNU schedules. Br J Cancer 1980; 41(suppl 4):253.

8. Rosenblum ML, Gerosa MA, Dougherty DV, et al: Improved treatment of a brain tumor model: Advantages of single- over multiple-dose BCNU schedules. J Neurosurg 1983; 58:177.

9. Madajewicz S, Kanter P, West C, et al: Plasma, spinal fluid, and organ distribution of cisplatinum following intravenous and intracarotid infusion (abstract). Proc Am Assoc Cancer Res 1981; 22:176.

10. Ichimura K, Ohno K, Aoyagi M, et al: Capillary permeability in experimental rat glioma and effects of intracarotid CDDP administration on tumor drug delivery. J Neurooncol 1993; 16:211.

11. Stewart DJ, Benjamin RS, Zimmerman S, et al: Clinical pharmacology of intraarterial cisdiamminedichloroplatinum (II). Cancer Res 1983; 43:917.

12. Shani J, Bertram J, Russell C, et al: Noninvasive monitoring of drug biodistribution and metabolism: Studies with intraarterial Pt-195m-cisplatin in humans. Cancer Res 1989; 49:1877.

13. Rottenberg DA, Dhawan V, Cooper AJ, et al: Assessment of the pharmacologic advantage of intra-arterial versus intravenous chemotherapy using ^{13}N-cisplatin and positron emission tomography (PET) (abstract). Neurology 1987; 37(suppl 1):335.

14. Neuwelt EA, Glasberg M, Frenkel E, et al: Neurotoxicity of chemotherapeutic agents after blood-brain barrier modification: neuropathological studies. Ann Neurol 1983; 14:316.

15. Spigelman MK, Zappulla RA, Strauchen JA, et al: Etoposide induced blood-brain barrier disruption in rats: Duration of opening and histological sequelae. Cancer Res 1986; 46:1453.

16. Feun LG, Savaraj N, Lu K, et al: The pharmacologic fate of AZQ by intracarotid or intravenous administration in beagles. J Neurooncol 1983; 1:219.

17. Blacklock JB, Wright DC, Dedrick RL, et al: Drug streaming during intra-arterial chemotherapy. J Neurosurg 1986; 64:284.

18. Lutz RJ, Dedrick RL, Boretos JW, et al: Mixing studies during intracarotid artery infusions in an in vitro model. J Neurosurg 1986; 64:277.

19. Junck L, Koeppe RA, Greenberg HS: Mixing in the human carotid artery during carotid drug infusion studied with PET. J Cereb Blood Flow Metab 1989; 9:681.

20. Saris SC, Blasberg RG, Carson RE, et al: Intravascular streaming during carotid artery infusions: Demonstration in humans and reduction using diastole-pulsatile administration. J Neurosurg 1991; 74:763.

21. Aoki S, Terada H, Kosuda S, et al: Supraophthalmic chemotherapy with long tapered catheter: Distribution evaluated with intraarterial and intravenous Tc-99m HMPAO. Radiology 1993; 188:347.

22. Saris SC, Shook DR, Blasberg RG, et al: Carotid artery mixing with diastole-phased pulsed drug infusion. J Neurosurg 1987; 67:721.

23. Greenberg HS, Ensminger WD, Chandler WF, et al: Intra-arterial BCNU chemotherapy for treatment of malignant gliomas of the central nervous system. J Neurosurg 1984; 61:423.

24. Hochberg FH, Pruitt AA, Beck DO, et al: The rationale and methodology for intra-arterial chemotherapy with BCNU as treatment for glioblastoma. J Neurosurg 1985; 63:876.

25. Johnson DW, Parkinson D, Wolpert SM, et al: Intracarotid chemotherapy with BCNU in 5% dextrose in water in the treatment of malignant glioma. Neurosurgery 1987; 20:577.

26. Bradac GB, Soffietti R, Riva A, et al: Selective intra-arterial chemother-

apy with BCNU in recurrent malignant gliomas. Neuroradiology 1992; 34:73.

27. Stewart DJ, Grahovac Z, Russel NA, et al: Phase I study of intracarotid PCNU. J Neurooncol 1987; 5:245.

28. Poisson M, Chiras J, Fauchon F, et al: Treatment of malignant recurrent glioma by intra-arterial, infra-ophthalmic infusion of HECNU: A phase II study. J Neurooncol 1990; 8:255.

29. Vega F, Davila L, Chatellier G, et al: Treatment of malignant gliomas with surgery, intraarterial chemotherapy with ACNU and radiation therapy. J Neurooncol 1992; 13:131.

30. Feun LG, Wallace S, Stewart DJ, et al: Intracarotid infusion of cis-diammine-dichloroplatinum in the treatment of recurrent malignant brain tumors. Cancer 1984; 54:794.

31. Newton HB, Page MA, Junck L, et al: Intra-arterial cisplatin for the treatment of malignant gliomas. J Neurooncol 1989; 7:39.

32. Mahaley MS, Hipp SW, Dropcho EJ, et al: Intracarotid cisplatin chemotherapy for recurrent gliomas. J Neurosurg 1989; 70:371.

33. Green SB, Shapiro WR, Burger PC, et al: Randomized comparison of intra-arterial cisplatin and intravenous PCNU for the treatment of primary brain tumors (BTCG Study 8420A) (abstract). Proc Am Soc Clin Oncol 1989; 8:86.

34. Follezou JY, Fauchon F, Chiras J: Intraarterial infusion of carboplatin in the treatment of malignant gliomas: A phase II study. Neoplasma 1989; 36:349.

35. Stewart DJ, Belanger JM, Grahovac Z, et al: Phase I study of intracarotid administration of carboplatin. Neurosurgery 1992; 30:512.

36. Greenberg HS, Ensminger WD, Layton PB, et al: Phase I-II evaluation of intra-arterial diaziquone for recurrent malignant astrocytomas. Cancer Treat Rep 1986; 70:353.

37. Feun LG, Lee Y, Yung A, et al: Intracarotid VP-16 in malignant brain tumors. J Neurooncol 1987; 4:397.

38. Dropcho EJ, Mahaley MS: Chemotherapy for malignant gliomas in adults. *In* Thomas DGT (ed): Neuro-Oncology: Primary Malignant Brain Tumours. London, Edward Arnold, 1990, p 222.

39. West CR, Avellanosa AM, Barua NR, et al: Intraarterial BCNU and systemic chemotherapy for malignant gliomas: a follow-up study. Neurosurgery 1983; 13:420.

40. Stewart DJ, Grahovac Z, Benoit B, et al: Intracarotid chemotherapy with a combination of BCNU, cisplatin, and VM-26 in the treatment of primary and metastatic brain tumors. Neurosurgery 1984; 15:828.

41. Kapp JP, Vance RB: Supraophthalmic carotid infusion for recurrent glioma: Rationale, technique, and preliminary results for cisplatin and BCNU. J Neurooncol 1985; 3:5.

42. Stewart DJ, Grahovac Z, Hugenholtz H, et al: Combined intraarterial and systemic chemotherapy for intracerebral tumors. Neurosurgery 1987; 21:207.

43. Rogers LR, Purvis JB, Lederman RJ, et al: Alternating sequential intracarotid BCNU and cisplatin in recurrent malignant gliomas. Cancer 1991; 68:15.

44. Bobo H, Kapp JP, Vance R: Effect of intra-arterial cisplatin and BCNU dosage on radiographic response and regional toxicity in malignant glioma patients: Proposal of a new method of intra-arterial dosage calculation. J Neurooncol 1992; 13:291.

45. Stewart DJ, Grahovac Z, Hugenholtz H, et al: Feasibility study of intraarterial vs intravenous cisplatin, BCNU, and teniposide combined with systemic cisplatin, teniposide, cytosine arabinoside, glycerol and mannitol in the treatment of primary and metastatic brain tumors. J Neurooncol 1993; 17:71.

46. Nakagawa H, Fujita T, Kubo S, et al: Selective intra-arterial chemotherapy with a combination of etoposide and cisplatin for malignant gliomas: Preliminary report. Surg Neurol 1994; 41:19.

47. Bonstelle CT, Kori SH, Rekate H: Intracarotid chemotherapy of glioblastoma after induced blood-brain barrier disruption. AJNR 1983; 4:810.

48. Neuwelt EA, Howieson J, Frenkel EP, et al: Therapeutic efficacy of multiagent chemotherapy with drug delivery enhancement by blood-brain barrier modification. Neurosurgery 1986; 19:573.

49. Gumerlock MK, Belshe BD, Madsen R, et al: Osmotic blood-brain barrier disruption and chemotherapy in the treatment of high grade malignant glioma: Patient series and literature review. J Neurooncol 1992; 12:33.

50. Kapp JP: Vascular diversion in chemotherapy of brain tumors. Surg Neurol 1986; 25:33.

51. Bashir R, Hochberg FH, Linggood RM, et al: Pre-irradiation internal

carotid artery BCNU in treatment of glioblastoma multiforme. J Neurosurg 1988; 68:917.

52. Clayman DA, Wolpert SM, Heros DO: Superselective arterial BCNU infusion in the treatment of patients with malignant gliomas. AJNR 1989; 10:767.

53. Roosen N, Kiwit JC, Lins E, et al: Adjuvant intraarterial chemotherapy with nimustine in the management of World Health Organization grade IV gliomas of the brain. Cancer 1989; 64:1984.

54. Fauchon F, Davila L, Chatellier G, et al: Treatment of malignant gliomas with surgery, intra-arterial infusions of 1-(2-hydroxyethyl) chloroethylnitrosourea, and radiation therapy: A phase II study. Neurosurgery 1990; 27:231.

55. Calvo FA, Dy C, Henriquez I, et al: Postoperative radical radiotherapy with concurrent weekly intra-arterial cis-platinum for treatment of malignant glioma: A pilot study. Radiother Oncol 1989; 14:83.

56. Dropcho EJ, Rosenfeld SS, Morawetz RB, et al: Pre-radiation intracarotid cisplatin treatment of newly diagnosed anaplastic gliomas. J Clin Oncol 1992; 10:452.

57. Mortimer JE, Crowley J, Eyre H, et al: A phase II randomized study comparing sequential and combined intra-arterial cisplatin and radiation therapy in primary brain tumors. Cancer 1992; 69:1220.

58. Larner JM, Kersh CR, Constable WC, et al: Phase I/II trial of superselective arterial 5-FU infusion with concomitant external beam radiation for patients with either anaplastic astrocytoma or glioblastoma multiforme. Am J Clin Oncol 1991; 14:514.

59. Greenberg HS, Chandler WF, Ensminger WD, et al: Radiosensitization with carotid intra-arterial bromodeoxyuridine + 5-fluorouracil biomodulation for malignant gliomas. Neurology 1994; 44:1715.

60. Recht L, Fram RJ, Strauss G, et al: Preirradiation chemotherapy of supratentorial malignant primary brain tumors with intracarotid cis-platinum and IV BCNU. Am J Clin Oncol 1990; 13:125.

61. Shapiro WR, Green SB, Burger PC, et al: A randomized comparison of intra-arterial versus intravenous BCNU, with or without intravenous 5-fluorouracil, for newly diagnosed patients with malignant glioma. J Neurosurg 1992; 76:772.

62. Watne K, Hannisdal E, Nome O, et al: Prognostic factors in malignant gliomas with special reference to intra-arterial chemotherapy. Acta Oncol 1993; 32:307.

63. Madajewicz S, Chowhan N, Iliya A, et al: Intracarotid chemotherapy with etoposide and cisplatin for malignant brain tumors. Cancer 1991; 67:2844.

64. Williams JA, Roman-Golstein S, Crossen JR, et al: Preirradiation osmotic blood-brain barrier disruption plus combination chemotherapy in gliomas: Quantitation of tumor response to assess chemosensitivity. In Drewes LR, Betz AL (eds): Frontiers in Cerebral Vascular Biology: Transport and its Regulation. New York, Plenum Press, 1993, p 273.

65. Iwadate Y, Namba H, Saegusa T, et al: Intra-arterial mannitol infusion in the chemotherapy for malignant brain tumors. J Neurooncol 1993; 15:185.

66. Bremer AM, Kleriga E, Nguyen TQ, et al: Complications associated with intra-arterial BCNU administered in combination with vincristine and procarbazine for the treatment of malignant brain tumors. J Neurooncol 1984; 2:129.

67. Pickrell L, Purvin V: Ischemic optic neuropathy secondary to intracarotid infusion of BCNU. J Neuroophthalmol 1987; 7:87.

68. Defer G, Fauchon F, Schaison M, et al: Visual toxicity following intra-arterial chemotherapy with hydroxyethyl-CNU in patients with malignant gliomas. Neuroradiol 1991; 33:432.

69. Kapp JP, Parker JL, Tucker EM: Supraophthalmic carotid infusion for brain chemotherapy: Experience with a single-lumen catheter and maneuverable tip. J Neurosurg 1985; 62:823.

70. Kupersmith MJ, Frohman LP, Choi IS, et al: Visual system toxicity following intra-arterial chemotherapy. Neurology 1988; 38:284.

71. Shimamura Y, Chikama M, Tanimoto T, et al: Optic nerve degeneration caused by supraophthalmic carotid artery infusion with cisplatin and ACNU. J Neurosurg 1990; 72:285.

72. Miller DF, Bay JW, Lederman RJ, et al: Ocular and orbital toxicity

following intracarotid injection of BCNU and cisplatin for malignant gliomas. Ophthalmology 1985; 92:402.

73. Maiese K, Walker RW, Gargan R, et al: Intra-arterial cisplatin-associated optic and otic toxicity. Arch Neurol 1992; 49:83.

74. Mahaley MS, Whaley RA, Blue M, et al: Central neurotoxicity following intracarotid BCNU chemotherapy for malignant gliomas. J Neurooncol 1986; 3:297.

75. Rosenblum MK, Delattre JY, Walker RW, et al: Fatal necrotizing encephalopathy complicating treatment of malignant gliomas with intra-arterial BCNU and irradiation: A pathological study. J Neurooncol 1989; 7:269.

76. Di Chiro G, Oldfield E, Wright DC, et al: Cerebral necrosis after radiotherapy and/or intraarterial chemotherapy for brain tumors: PET and neuropathologic studies. AJR 1988; 150:189.

77. Kleinschmidt-DeMasters BK, Geier JM: Pathology of high-dose intraarterial BCNU. Surg Neurol 1989; 31:435.

78. Sheline GE, Wara WM, Smith V: Therapeutic irradiation and brain injury. Int J Radiat Oncol Biol Phys 1980; 6:1215.

79. Burger PC, Kamenar E, Schold SC, et al: Encephalomyelopathy following high-dose BCNU therapy. Cancer 1981; 48:1318.

80. Omojola MF, Fox AJ, Auer RN, et al: Hemorrhagic encephalitis produced by selective nonocclusive intracarotid BCNU injection in dogs. J Neurosurg 1982; 57:791.

81. Foo SH, Choi IS, Berenstein A, et al: Supraophthalmic intracarotid infusion of BCNU for malignant glioma. Neurology 1986; 36:1437.

82. Stewart DJ: Intraarterial chemotherapy of primary and metastatic brain tumors. In Rottenberg DA (ed): Neurological Complications of Cancer Treatment. Boston, Butterworth-Heinemann, 1991, p 143.

83. Berman IJ, Mann MP: Seizures and transient cortical blindness associated with cis-platinum therapy in a 30-year-old man. Cancer 1980; 45:764.

84. Bellin SL, Selim M: Cisplatin-induced hypomagnesemia with seizures: A case report and review of the literature. Gynecol Oncol 1988; 30:104.

85. Kapp JP, Sanford RA: Neurological deficit after carotid infusion of cisplatin and BCNU for malignant glioma: An analysis of risk factors. Neurosurgery 1986; 19:779.

86. Neef C, van der Straaten I: An interaction between cytostatic and anticonvulsant drugs. Clin Pharmacol Ther 1988; 43:372.

87. Grossman SA, Sheidler VR, Gilbert MR: Decreased phenytoin levels in patients receiving chemotherapy. Am J Med 1989; 87:505.

88. Walker RW, Cairncross JG, Posner JB: Cerebral herniation in patients receiving cisplatin. J Neurooncol 1988; 6:61.

89. Fishman RA: Is there a role for osmotic breaching of the blood-brain barrier? Ann Neurol 1987; 22:298.

90. Rapoport SI: Osmotic opening of the blood-brain barrier. Ann Neurol 1988; 24:677.

91. Stewart DJ: A critique of the role of the blood-brain barrier in the chemotherapy of human brain tumors. J Neurooncol 1994; 20:121.

92. Groothuis DR, Molnar P, Blasberg RG: Regional blood flow and blood-to-tissue transport in five brain tumor models: Implications for chemotherapy. Prog Exp Tumor Res 1984; 27:132.

93. Nakagawa H, Groothuis D, Blasberg RG: The effect of graded hypertonic intracarotid infusions on drug delivery to experimental RG-2 gliomas. Neurology 1984; 34:1571.

94. Hiesinger EM, Voorhies RM, Basler GA, et al: Opening the blood-brain and blood-tumor barriers in experimental rat brain tumors: The effect of intracarotid hyperosmolar mannitol on capillary permeability and blood flow. Ann Neurol 1986; 19:50.

95. Warnke P, Groothuis D, Nakagawa H, et al: Capillary permeability of experimental brain tumors after hyperosmotic blood-brain barrier disruption (abstract). J Neurooncol 1986; 4:105.

96. Warnke PC, Blasberg RG, Groothuis DR: The effect of hyperosmotic blood-brain barrier disruption on blood-to-tissue transport in ENU-induced gliomas. Ann Neurol 1987; 22:300.

97. Shapiro WR, Voorhies RM, Hiesinger EM, et al: Pharmacokinetics of tumor cell exposure to ¹⁴C-methotrexate after intracarotid administration without and with hyperosmotic opening of the blood-brain and blood-tumor barriers in rat brain tumors: A quantitative autoradiographic study. Cancer Res 1988; 48:694.

IRA J. DUNKEL

JONATHAN L. FINLAY

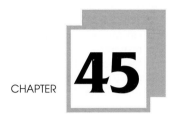

CHAPTER **45**

High-Dose Chemotherapy Followed by Autologous Bone Marrow Rescue for High-Grade Gliomas

The prognosis for patients with newly diagnosed high-grade gliomas remains poor, with few long-term survivors despite treatment with surgery, radiation therapy (RT), and conventional chemotherapy. The prognosis for patients with recurrent disease is dismal, with palliation being the only realistic goal with conventional modalities. Innovative approaches are required for patients with these diseases, and one new strategy undergoing evaluation is the administration of high-dose chemotherapy in conjunction with autologous bone marrow rescue.

Chemotherapy is active against high-grade gliomas, but it has only produced marginal improvements in long-term survival when used at conventional doses.[1] The barrier to dose escalation of many chemotherapeutic agents in use clinically is their hematopoietic toxic effects. One way to overcome this barrier is via autologous bone marrow rescue, the reinfusion of previously harvested and cryopreserved bone marrow after the administration and clearance of high-dose chemotherapy. More recently, autologous hematopoietic stem cells have also been harvested from the peripheral blood after priming with chemotherapy or hematopoietic growth factors. Regardless of the method of harvest, stem cell rescue allows chemotherapeutic agents to be used at doses that are limited only by nonhematopoietic toxic effects. High-grade gliomas rarely metastasize outside of the neuraxis, which therefore allows harvesting of autologous stem cells that are free of contaminating tumor in the vast majority of cases.

Phase II trials in the 1970s indicated that vincristine and the nitrosoureas were active in recurrent brain tumors. Because vincristine does not have hematopoietic toxic effects, but it does have marked neurotoxic effects, even at conventional doses, its dose could not be escalated in conjunction with autologous bone marrow rescue. However, the nitrosoureas did appear to be suitable candidates for dose escalation, and they have been the major drugs evaluated in brain

tumors at marrow-ablative doses. This chapter reviews the published experience with high-dose chemotherapy (primarily with single-agent carmustine [BCNU], but also with other single agents and with multi-agent combinations) in conjunction with autologous bone marrow rescue in children and in adults with high-grade gliomas. A review of the trials in adults has been published.[2]

HIGH-DOSE NITROSOUREAS

In the early 1980s, reports from several centers began to appear in the literature describing the treatment of high-grade gliomas with high-dose BCNU and autologous bone marrow rescue. Hochberg and co-workers[3] described 11 patients with recurrent glioblastoma multiforme after surgery and RT who received 600 to 1,400 mg/m^2 of BCNU and then underwent autologous bone marrow rescue 24 to 36 hours after the completion of the chemotherapy.[3] They noted that the dose of 1,400 mg/m^2 was associated with acute and permanent central nervous system (CNS) toxic effects, which consisted of seizures and memory loss in one patient each. Clinical improvement was seen in four patients, and two demonstrated response on computed tomographic (CT) scanning. The median survival for the 10 patients who could be evaluated (one died of toxic effects) was 7 months, and three patients were alive at 1 to 19 months. These investigators subsequently published their expanded experience in 28 patients with high-grade gliomas (25 biopsy-proved) cases utilizing the same therapeutic approach.[4] Twenty had failed conventional therapy; of these, 11 had evidence of clinical and CT response, and five were alive at 9 to 24 months. Eight patients were treated at the time of diagnosis; in this group, four had response noted on CT, and the median survival was more than 6 months.

Carella and colleagues[5] briefly described four patients

with glioblastoma multiforme, two of whom were in "first remission" following initial surgery and RT, and two of whom were in "second remission." They received 800 mg/m² of BCNU followed by autologous bone marrow rescue, and all were alive at 1 to 12 months. No toxic effects were encountered.

Phillips and associates[6] described 143 patients with refractory cancer, 28 of whom had primary CNS tumors, who were treated on a phase I and II study of BCNU (600 to 2,850 mg/m²) followed by autologous bone marrow rescue. Serious toxic effects consisting of fatal interstitial pneumonitis (9.5%) and fatal hepatic necrosis (3.0%) were encountered at 1,200 mg/m², and higher doses produced unacceptably high rates of toxic mortality. One patient with a glioblastoma multiforme had a complete response and three with glioblastoma multiforme were alive at 134 to 249 weeks. The authors concluded that 1,200 mg/m² was the maximum tolerated dose of BCNU. The same authors later published a report describing 36 patients with malignant gliomas treated with BCNU (1,050 to 1,350 mg/m² in three daily divided doses) and autologous bone marrow rescue.[7] Twenty-seven had progressive disease and nine were treated prior to progression. All had surgery and RT, and five had also received prior chemotherapy. Toxic mortality occurred in 17% due to pulmonary, hepatic, and CNS causes. Two surviving patients also had late unexplained neurologic deterioration. Of the patients with progressive disease, 44% responded to therapy documented by CT, and two of the 27 patients were progression-free at 60 and 84 months. Of the nine patients treated in an adjuvant setting, three were progression-free at 27 to 70 months.

Mortimer and co-workers[8] treated 11 patients with malignant gliomas that recurred after surgery and RT with BCNU (1,050 to 1,200 mg/m² in three daily divided doses) and autologous bone marrow rescue. Four also received fluorouracil. One early toxic death occurred owing to sepsis. Eight of the 10 patients who could be evaluated responded to therapy, with two attaining complete response. Median time to progression was 7.3 months, with a range of 78 to 366 days. One patient received a second course of treatment but died as a result of complications of myelosuppression. Three of the patients were alive at 97 to 263 days.

Hara and colleagues[9] treated four children with "brainstem tumors" (three unbiopsied diffuse pontine lesions, one thalamic low-grade astrocytoma) with another nitrosourea, ACNU (1-(4-amino-2-methyl-5-pyrimidinyl) methyl-3-(2-chloroethyl)-3-nitrosourea hydrochloride). All had received RT and three had also received prior chemotherapy. The dose used was 5 to 7 mg/kg (two patients also received vincristine concurrently) and was followed by autologous bone marrow rescue. One patient experienced seizures, but no other major toxic effects were seen with this regimen. Two patients had response documented by CT (one thalamic, one pontine lesion), and all four were alive at the short follow-up period of 3 to 11 months after autologous bone marrow rescue.

Johnson and associates[10] treated 25 consecutive patients with newly diagnosed high-grade gliomas with BCNU (1,050 mg/m² in three daily divided doses) and autologous bone marrow rescue. After recovery of the absolute neutrophil count, the patients received RT (6,000 cGy). Four pa-

tients died from toxic effects as a result of seizure-related aspiration, pulmonary hemorrhage, bacterial sepsis, and *Candida* pneumonia, in one case each, respectively. Three other patients later died of non–tumor-related causes (one of lupus nephritis and two of *Pneumocystis carinii* pneumonia). Ten patients (40%) attained complete response, and projected median survival was 26 months. This appeared promising, but in a subsequent analysis, the Southwest Oncology Group (SWOG) performed a retrospective comparison between the patients of Johnson and others[10] and patients on SWOG 7703 protocol who were matched for age, degree of resection, and histologic findings.[11] The SWOG patients received conventional-dose BCNU (240 mg/m² in three daily divided doses every 3 weeks) followed by RT (6,000 cGy). The median survival for conventionally treated patients was 14.5 months compared with 14 months for patients treated with high-dose chemotherapy. The SWOG authors concluded that there was no advantage for high-dose BCNU with marrow rescue followed by RT in comparison with conventionally administered BCNU and RT.

Wolff and co-workers[12] reported that 18 patients were treated adjuvantly with BCNU (900 to 1050 mg/m² divided daily over 3 days) and autologous bone marrow rescue after surgery and RT.[12] Six patients suffered BCNU pulmonary toxic effects 1 to 4 months post-treatment (which were fatal in four) and two had development of non–tumor-related diffuse encephalomyelopathy that occurred as long as 4 years after BCNU administration. Two patients remained progression-free (one with severe encephalomyelopathy) at 60 and 77 months.

Mbidde and colleagues[13] treated 22 patients with newly diagnosed glioblastoma multiforme with BCNU (800 to 1,000 mg/m² as one daily dose) and autologous bone marrow rescue in conjunction with RT (5,500 cGy). Three patients received two courses of BCNU (800 mg/m²) 4 to 6 weeks apart, both with autologous bone marrow rescue. Interstitial pneumonitis developed in three patients (fatal in two) and severe hepatic toxic effects occurred in two (fatal in one). Irreversible late marrow failure occurred in four patients whose autologous bone marrow rescue had been reinfused less than 48 hours after BCNU administration. The authors claimed four treatment-related deaths, but two other early deaths occurred owing to herpes simplex encephalitis and pulmonary embolus (one case each). Clinical improvements were noted in all cases, and all patients who had CT scans after autologous bone marrow rescue reportedly had improvement, but none had a complete response. Median survival time was 17 months, with a 25% actuarial probability of survival at 2 years. Four patients were progression-free at 11 to 42 months. In comparison with historical experience within the institution, a small, but not statistically significant, prolongation of survival occurred without an increase in the proportion of long-term survivors.

Finally, the most recent and largest experience utilizing single-agent high-dose BCNU was reported by Biron and co-workers.[14] Ninety-eight patients (89 newly diagnosed, nine experiencing relapse) with high-grade gliomas were treated with BCNU (800 mg/m² as a single dose) and autologous bone marrow rescue, and then received RT (4,500 cGy) beginning on approximately day 45 after autologous bone marrow rescue. The toxic mortality rate was 6.1% and overall survival was only 10% at 36 months, with a median survival of 11 months after autologous bone marrow rescue. The authors thought that age and histologic findings were important predictors of success, and that this strategy was worth continuing only in young patients with completely resected anaplastic astrocytoma.

Summary

The cumulative experience with high-dose BCNU in high-grade glioma demonstrates that this single agent produces responses, including complete response, in an impressive proportion of patients treated, but that this is achieved at the expense of substantial pulmonary, hepatic, and neurologic toxic effects, particularly at doses greater than 1,200 mg/m². Exposure to prior RT and/or prior nitrosourea therapy may increase the risk for BCNU-associated pulmonary toxic effects.[6] The neurotoxic effects include irreversible dementia and encephalopathy, which can be either acute or delayed. Unfortunately, not only has the toxicity of high-dose BCNU proven to be substantial, but, despite the encouraging response data, the median survival for both recurrent and newly diagnosed patients with glioblastoma multiforme does not appear to have been improved with the use of high-dose BCNU as a single agent. However, no randomized trial has been performed comparing this strategy with conventional therapy.

OTHER SINGLE AGENTS

Although most of the literature involves high-dose single-agent BCNU therapy, some investigators have also evaluated other single agents at high doses with autologous bone marrow rescue in patients with high-grade gliomas.

Aziridinylbenzoquinone

Aziridinylbenzoquinone (AZQ) is an alkylating agent with some evidence of activity in brain tumors, but it is highly toxic to marrow even at conventional doses. Abrams and co-workers[15] evaluated high-dose AZQ therapy in patients with refractory CNS neoplasms but found no radiographic response in recurrent high-grade astrocytomas. Stiff and associates[16] treated 49 patients with high-dose AZQ (50 to 295 mg/m² continuous infusion over 24 hours) and autologous bone marrow rescue. They noted only one partial response in the 10 patients with primary CNS tumors (types not specified), six of whom were previously untreated. Dose-limiting nephrotoxic effects were seen, including proteinuria, azotemia, and proximal tubular damage.

Etoposide

Giannone and Wolff[17] treated 16 patients with progressive gliomas (13 high-grade) with etoposide (1,800 to 2,400 mg/m² divided daily over 3 days) followed by autologous bone marrow rescue. Nonhematologic toxic effects were mild.

Three patients (two with high-grade gliomas) had objective responses, and these three patients lived 9, 10, and more than 54 months.

Leff and colleagues[18] treated 13 patients with progressive tumors post-RT (nine with high-grade gliomas, four with low-grade astrocytomas) with etoposide (2,400 mg/m² divided daily over 3 days) followed by autologous bone marrow rescue).[19] They reported severe, but transient, acute neurologic toxic effects, including confusion, papilledema, somnolence, exacerbation of motor deficits, and increased seizure activity, in six patients. Two patients died of sepsis and one died of pulmonary hemorrhage. Clinical improvement was seen in two of 11 patients who could be evaluated for response, but no patient demonstrated significant radiologic improvement. Median survival for all 13 patients was 101 days (range, 8 to 591 days).

In summary, etoposide appears free of significant non-hematopoietic toxic effects at doses up to 2,400 mg/m². However, at these doses, it does not appear to be as active in recurrent brain tumors as is BCNU.

Thiotepa

Thiotepa was one of the earliest anti-cancer drugs discovered, but it rapidly fell into disuse in the 1960s because of unacceptable toxicity to marrow and marginal activity at conventional doses. Due to its properties as an alkylator with minimal nonhematopoietic toxicity at marrow-ablative doses, however, interest was rekindled and resulted in a phase I/II evaluation of high-dose thiotepa in refractory non-CNS cancer.[20]

Because thiotepa is an extremely lipophilic drug, it also appeared to be an excellent candidate for penetrating the putative blood-brain barrier and having an impact on brain tumors. Intravenous administration of thiotepa rapidly produces a plasma-to-cerebrospinal fluid (CSF) ratio of 1:1.[21] Studies in dogs have indicated not only excellent penetrance into the CSF, but also into normal and tumor-bearing brain tissue.[22] Additionally, thiotepa at conventional doses was recently evaluated in a phase II trial in children with CNS malignancies and demonstrated an ability to stabilize disease in patients with high-grade gliomas.[23] Thus, thiotepa appeared to be an excellent agent for use in high-dose chemotherapy regimens for malignant brain tumors.

Ascensao and co-workers[24] and Ahmed and colleagues[25] reported the treatment of 16 adults with newly diagnosed high-grade glioma with thiotepa (600 to 900 mg/m²) followed by autologous bone marrow rescue and RT (6,000 cGy). Toxic effects were described as minimal. Four patients attained a complete response and five a partial response, but survival data were not clearly presented.

In addition, a single case report describes a patient with a multiply recurrent anaplastic oligodendroglioma treated with thiotepa (1,125 mg/m² divided daily over 3 days) followed by autologous bone marrow rescue.[26] No severe toxic effects were encountered, and a complete response was noted. A second course of the high-dose therapy was administered, which resulted in a toxic death from visceral candidiasis.

Summary

AZQ, etoposide, and thiotepa are other drugs that have been evaluated as single agents in small clinical trials at high doses in patients with brain tumors. The results with AZQ were disappointing. Etoposide produced some responses, but was not promising as a single agent. Thiotepa has appealing pharmacologic properties for use in high-grade gliomas and also produced responses as a single agent used at high doses.

MULTIDRUG REGIMENS

Although most of the single-agent investigations described previously have dealt with adult patients, several pediatric neuro-oncology groups have explored multidrug regimens in conjunction with autologous bone marrow rescue to treat high-grade gliomas in children and young adults.

Finlay and others[27] first reported the use of combination high-dose chemotherapy in 10 patients younger than 21 years with recurrent malignant astrocytomas (nine with glioblastoma multiforme).[27] Five received thiotepa (900 mg/m^2) and etoposide (1,500 mg/m^2), both divided daily over 3 days. Another five patients received the same two drugs followed by BCNU (600 mg/m^2 divided into 12 doses over 96 hours). All patients received autologous bone marrow rescue after the completion of chemotherapy. One patient died of *Salmonella* septicemia acquired from a contaminated blood transfusion. No pulmonary toxic effects were seen. One patient manifested liver toxic effects due to acute graft-vs.-host disease (despite irradiation of all blood products), and three manifested neurotoxic effects (encephalopathy, basal ganglia infarction, and transient spinal myoclonus in one case each). Four complete responses and two partial responses were noted radiographically. Two patients were progression-free at 440 and 448 days.

This initial work has been continued at the Memorial Sloan-Kettering Cancer Center, New York, in conjunction with other institutions and partially under the auspices of the Children's Cancer Group (CCG). From 1986 to 1994, a total of 47 patients with recurrent high-grade gliomas have been treated using three high-dose chemotherapy regimens.[28] All had received RT and/or chemotherapy prior to their recurrence (six, RT alone; four, chemotherapy alone; 37, both RT and chemotherapy). Seventeen patients received the thiotepa/etoposide regimen described previously; 11 received BCNU (600 mg/m^2 divided in six doses over 3 days) either prior or following thiotepa (900 mg/m^2) and etoposide (750 to 1,500 mg/m^2), both divided daily over 3 days; and 19 received carboplatin (1,500 mg/m^2 divided daily over 3 days) followed by the thiotepa/etoposide regimen. A mortality rate of 21.3% from toxic reactions (10/47) has been encountered. Event-free survival is 23.4%, with a median follow-up of 38.7 months (range, 12.7 to 64.0 months) from relapse for the survivors. Prognostic factors for improved survival include histologic findings of anaplastic astrocytoma and minimal disease present at the time of autologous bone marrow rescue, achieved by neurosurgical resection of the recurrent disease. Despite the substantial mortality due to toxic effects, this cohort of long-term survivors of recurrent high-grade glioma is noteworthy.

These promising data prompted the initiation of a trial of the BCNU/thiotepa/etoposide regimen plus involved field RT in 26 patients with newly diagnosed high-grade glioma, all of whom have had glioblastoma multiforme.[28] These patients have suffered a mortality rate of 15.4% (4/26) due to toxic effects, with three of the four deaths occurring in patients aged 32, 42, and 42 years, representing three of the five patients older than 30 years. Event-free survival is 50% (13/26), but with a relatively short median follow-up of 8 months (range, 3 to 50 months; mean, 17 months). This strategy has been adopted in a national multicenter trial for children (CCG–9922), which opened in October 1993, but the regimen is thought to be excessively toxic in adults, for whom alternative courses are being developed.

Seventeen children with brainstem tumors have not fared well with these strategies.[29] Eleven were previously treated, all having received RT, four additionally having received chemotherapy, and one having received interferon-β. Six cases were newly diagnosed. Six patients received the thiotepa/etoposide regimen; eight, the BCNU/thiotepa/etoposide regimen; and three, the carboplatin/thiotepa/etoposide regimen. All patients with newly diagnosed disease received the BCNU/thiotepa/etoposide regimen and were consolidated post-autologous bone marrow rescue with hyperfractionated RT (7,200 to 7,800 cGy). Two deaths occurred from toxic effects (12%), both in previously treated patients, due to multisystem organ failure and *Candida* septicemia in one case each. Overall median survival from the time of autologous bone marrow rescue was 7 months (range, 0 to 18 months). Median survival for patients with newly diagnosed disease was 11 months (range, 7 to 17 months). This did not represent any advantage compared with conventional strategies and did not cure any of the children. Kedar and co-workers[30] also treated six patients with brainstem glioma with a similar strategy. They administered cyclophosphamide (3,000 to 3,900 mg/m^2 divided into four daily doses) and thiotepa (750 to 900 mg/m^2 divided into three daily doses), followed by hyperfractionated RT (7,560 cGy) beginning on day 45 to 50 post-autologous bone marrow rescue. One death from toxic effects was encountered, and the median survival was 12.5 months. One patient achieved a complete response post-RT and was disease-free at 24 months.[30]

Other groups have also treated small numbers of patients with high-grade gliomas with multiagent high-dose chemotherapy and autologous bone marrow rescue. Wiley and associates[31] reported the treatment of 41 patients younger than 25 years old with refractory solid tumors with carboplatin (600 to 2,400 mg/m^2 divided daily over 3 days), etoposide (1,800 to 2,400 mg/m^2 continuous infusion over 72 hours), and cyclophosphamide (60 mg/kg/day for 2 days) followed by autologous bone marrow rescue. No transplant-related mortality was encountered. Six of nine patients with brain tumors (types unspecified) who could be evaluated for response attained a partial response.

Kalifa and co-workers[32] treated 20 children (all younger than 16 years) with recurrent malignant brain tumors (including four brainstem tumors and two hemispheric malignant gliomas) with busulfan (600 mg/m^2 divided into 16 oral doses over 4 days) and thiotepa (1,050 mg/m^2 divided into three daily doses) followed by autologous bone marrow rescue.[32] Toxicity was thought to be high, with severe neurotoxic effects (drowsiness, hallucinations, coma) encountered in six patients. Although the overall response rate was 26%, neither of the glioma patients responded, and although one of the four brainstem tumor patients had an objective (25% to 50%) response, the patient died of progressive disease only 3 months after autologous bone marrow rescue.

Graham and colleagues[33] reported the treatment of eight patients with recurrent or high-risk CNS tumors with cyclophosphamide (6,000 mg/m² divided into four daily doses) and melphalan (75 to 120 mg/m² divided into three daily doses) followed by autologous bone marrow rescue or peripheral blood stem cell rescue. Two of these patients had glial tumors. No serious toxic effects were encountered. Response and survival data of the patients with glial tumors were not specified. Pediatric Oncology Group investigators used these same agents in 19 children with recurrent or progressive malignant brain tumors, two of whom had malignant gliomas. The cyclophosphamide dose ranged from 3,000 to 6,000 mg/m² divided into four daily doses, and the melphalan dose was 180 mg/m² divided into three daily doses. Neither patient with malignant glioma responded.[34]

Heideman and associates[35] treated 11 children with newly diagnosed malignant gliomas and two children with recurrent malignant gliomas with thiotepa (900 mg/m²) and cyclophosphamide (6 g/m²), both divided daily over 3 days, followed by autologous bone marrow rescue. Surgery for six of the patients, including five with newly diagnosed disease, was biopsy only. Response was evaluated on day 30, and on day 60 patients with stable disease or better received RT. Interstitial pneumonitis developed in two patients (one fatal). No severe hepatic or neurologic toxic effects were encountered. One complete response and three partial responses were attained. Median progression-free survival was 9 months, and one patient was progression-free at 30 months. Two others, who were progression-free at 23 and 24 months, died of pneumonia and shunt failure.

Summary

Small trials have demonstrated the feasibility of combining multiple agents at high doses prior to autologous bone marrow rescue. Impressive response rates have been noted, and long-term survival of recurrent high-grade gliomas has been documented. Further studies are indicated in research settings, and several trials are currently in progress, both at institutional and in collaborative multi-institutional settings.

CONCLUSIONS

The experience with high-dose chemotherapy and autologous bone marrow rescue in patients with high-grade gliomas has demonstrated that single agents can produce impressive responses, but that these responses have not translated into meaningful improvement in long-term survival. The use of high-dose multiple drug regimens more recently has produced long-term event-free survival in a subset of patients with recurrent high-grade gliomas. Historical experience suggests that this is an improvement in comparison to conventional retrieval strategies, though a prospective randomized trial has not been performed. The patients with recurrent disease enjoying event-free survival are more likely to have had histologic findings of anaplastic astrocytoma and to have had a smaller tumor burden at the time of high-dose chemotherapy/autologous bone marrow rescue due to aggressive surgery post-recurrence. The use of high-dose multiple-drug regimens in patients with newly diagnosed high-grade glioma is under investigation, and though the results are promising, the median follow-up time is still short.

Future efforts must address both the need for more effective therapy, by employing either new agents or new combinations, and the need to decrease toxic effects. This, again, may be accomplished via the use of new regimens or, perhaps, by the increased use of peripheral blood stem cells as an alternative or supplement to autologous bone marrow, which may allow faster hematopoietic reconstitution. Further investigations of these strategies are indicated only in the setting of clinical research studies.

REFERENCES

1. Fine HA, Dear KBG, Loeffler JS, et al: Meta-analysis of radiation therapy with and without adjuvant chemotherapy for malignant gliomas in adults. Cancer 1993; 71:2585.
2. Fine HA, Antman KH: High-dose chemotherapy with autologous bone marrow transplantation in the treatment of high grade astrocytomas in adults: Therapeutic rationale and clinical experience. Bone Marrow Transplant 1992; 10:315.
3. Hochberg FH, Parker LM, Takvorian T, et al: High-dose BCNU with autologous bone marrow rescue for recurrent glioblastoma multiforme. J Neurosurg 1981; 54:455.
4. Takvorian T, Parker LM, Hochberg FH, et al: Autologous bone-marrow transplantation: Host effects of high-dose BCNU. J Clin Oncol 1983; 1:610.
5. Carella AM, Giordano D, Santini G, et al: High dose BCNU followed by autologous bone marrow infusion in glioblastoma multiforme. Tumori 1981; 67:473.
6. Phillips GL, Fay JW, Herzig GP, et al: Intensive 1,3-bis(2-chloroethyl)-1-nitrosourea (BCNU), NSC #4366650 and cryopreserved autologous marrow transplantation for refractory cancer: A phase I–II study. Cancer 1983; 52:1792.
7. Phillips GL, Wolff SN, Fay JW, et al: Intensive 1,3-bis(2-chloroethyl)-1-nitrosourea (BCNU) monochemotherapy and autologous marrow transplantation for malignant glioma. J Clin Oncol 1986; 4:639.
8. Mortimer JE, Hewlett JS, Bay J, et al: High dose BCNU with autologous bone marrow rescue in the treatment of recurrent malignant gliomas. J Neurooncol 1983; 1:269.
9. Hara T, Miyazaki S, Ishii E, et al: High-dose 1-(4-amino-2-methyl-5-pyrimidinyl) methyl-3-(2-chloroethyl)-3-nitrosourea hydrochloride (ACNU) with autologous bone marrow rescue for patients with brain stem tumors. Childs Brain 1984; 11:369.
10. Johnson DB, Thompson JM, Corwin JA, et al: Prolongation of survival for high-grade malignant gliomas with adjuvant high-dose BCNU and autologous bone marrow transplantation. J Clin Oncol 1987; 5:783.
11. Goodwin W, Crowley J: A retrospective comparison of high-dose BCNU with autologous marrow rescue plus radiotherapy vs. IV BCNU plus radiation therapy in high grade gliomas: A Southwest Oncology Group review. Proceedings of the Annual Meeting of the American Society of Clinical Oncology, San Francisco, 1989, abstract 352.
12. Wolff SN, Phillips GL, Herzig GP: High-dose carmustine with autologous bone marrow transplantation for the adjuvant treatment of high-grade gliomas of the central nervous system. Cancer Treat Rep 1987; 71:183.
13. Mbidde EK, Selby PJ, Perren TJ, et al: High dose BCNU chemotherapy with autologous bone marrow transplantation and full dose radiotherapy for grade IV astrocytoma. Br J Cancer 1988; 58:779.
14. Biron P, Vial C, Chauvin F, et al: Strategy including surgery, high

dose BCNU followed by ABMT and radiotherapy in supratentorial high grade astrocytomas: A report of 98 patients. *In* Dicke KA, Armitage JO, Dicke-Evinger MJ (eds): Autologous Bone Marrow Transplantation: Proceedings of the Fifth International Symposium. Omaha, University of Nebraska Medical Center, 1991, pp 637–645.

15. Abrams RA, Casper J, Kun L, et al: High-dose aziridinylbenzoquinone for patients with refractory central nervous system neoplasms: A preliminary analysis. *In* Dicke KA, Spitzer G, Zander AR, et al (eds): Autologous Bone Marrow Transplantation: Proceedings of the First International Symposium. Houston, University of Texas M. D. Anderson Hospital and Tumor Institute, 1985, pp 227–230.

16. Stiff P, Weidner M, Potempa L, et al: Phase I trial of high dose aziridinylbenzoquinone (AZQ) with autologous bone marrow transplantation. Proceedings of the Annual Meeting of the American Society of Clinical Oncology, San Francisco, 1989, abstract 83.

17. Giannone L, Wolff SN: Phase II treatment of central nervous system gliomas with high-dose etoposide and autologous bone marrow transplantation. Cancer Treat Rep 1987; 71:759.

18. Leff RS, Thompson JM, Daly MB, et al: Acute neurologic dysfunction after high-dose etoposide therapy for malignant glioma. Cancer 1988; 62:32.

19. Long J, Leff R, Daly M, et al: Phase II trial of high-dose etoposide and autologous bone marrow transplantation for treatment of progressive glioma. Proceedings of the Annual Meeting of the American Society of Clinical Oncology, San Francisco, 1989, abstract 360.

20. Lazarus HM, Reed MD, Spitzer TR, et al: High-dose IV thiotepa and cryopreserved autologous bone marrow transplantation for therapy of refractory cancer. Cancer Treat Rep 1987; 71:689.

21. Heideman RL, Cole DE, Balis F, et al: Phase I and pharmacokinetic evaluation of thiotepa in the cerebrospinal fluid and plasma of pediatric patients: Evidence for dose-dependent plasma clearance of thiotepa. Cancer Res 1989; 49:736.

22. Finlay JL, Knipple J, Turski P, et al: Pharmacokinetic studies of thiotepa in dogs following delivery by various routes (abstract). J Neurooncol 1986; 4:110.

23. Heideman RL, Packer RJ, Reaman GH, et al: A phase II evaluation of thiotepa in pediatric central nervous system malignancies. Cancer 1993; 72:271.

24. Ascensao J, Ahmed T, Feldman E, et al: High-dose thiotepa with autologous bone marrow transplantation and localized radiotherapy for patients with astrocytoma grade III–IV: A promising approach. Proceedings of the Annual Meeting of the American Society of Clinical Oncology, San Francisco, 1989, abstract 353.

25. Ahmed T, Feldman E, Helson L, et al: Phase 1–2 trial of high dose thiotepa with autologous bone marrow transplantation and localized radiotherapy for patients with astrocytoma grade III–IV. Proceedings of the Annual Meeting of the American Association of Cancer Research, Washington, D.C., 1990, abstract 1023.

26. Saarinen UM, Pihko H, Makipernaa A: High-dose thiotepa with autologous bone marrow rescue in recurrent malignant oligodendroglioma: A case report. J Neurooncol 1990; 9:57.

27. Finlay JL, August C, Packer R, et al: High-dose multi-agent chemotherapy followed by bone marrow ''rescue'' for malignant astrocytomas of childhood and adolescence. J Neurooncol 1990; 9:239.

28. Dunkel IJ, Finlay JL: High-dose chemotherapy with autologous bone marrow rescue for high-grade astrocytomas. Bone Marrow Transplant 1994; 14(suppl 1):S64.

29. Dunkel I, Garvin J, Goldman S, et al: High-dose chemotherapy with autologous bone marrow rescue does not cure children with brain stem tumors. Pediatric Neurosurg 1994; 21:219.

30. Kedar A, Maria BL, Graham-Pole J, et al: High dose chemotherapy with marrow reinfusion and hyperfractionated irradiation for children with brain stem glioma. Proceedings of the Annual Meeting of the American Society of Clinical Oncology, Dallas, 1994, abstract 498.

31. Wiley J, Fresia A, Strauss L, et al: High-dose carboplatin, etoposide and cyclophosphamide with autologous bone marrow rescue in children and young adults with refractory solid or brain tumors. Proceedings of the Annual Meeting of the American Society of Clinical Oncology, San Diego, 1992, abstract 1292.

32. Kalifa C, Hartmann O, Demeocq F, et al: High-dose busulfan and thiotepa with autologous bone marrow transplantation in childhood malignant brain tumors: A phase II study. Bone Marrow Transplant 1992; 9:227.

33. Graham ML, Chaffee S, Kurtzberg J, et al: A phase I–II study of high-dose melphalan and cyclophosphamide with autologous bone marrow and/or stem cell rescue for patients with high-risk CNS tumors. Proceedings of the Annual Meeting of the American Society of Clinical Oncology, Orlando, Fla, 1993, abstract 523.

34. Mahoney D, Strother D, Bowen T, et al: High dose melphalan and cyclophosphamide with autologous bone marrow rescue for recurrent/progressive malignant brain tumors in children: A phase I–II pediatric oncology group study. Proceedings of the Annual Meeting of the American Society of Clinical Oncology, Dallas, 1994, abstract 484.

35. Heideman RL, Douglass EC, Krance RA, et al: High-dose chemotherapy and autologous bone marrow rescue followed by interstitial and external-beam radiotherapy in newly diagnosed pediatric malignant gliomas. J Clin Oncol 1993; 11:1458.

REID C. THOMPSON

HENRY BREM

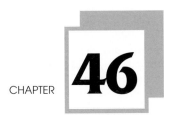

CHAPTER **46**

Treatment of Gliomas Using Polymer-Drug Delivery

Controlled delivery of chemotherapeutic agents by biodegradable polymers is a technique that allows direct exposure of tumor cells to an active therapeutic agent for prolonged periods of time. The use of polymers for local drug delivery expands the spectrum of chemotherapeutic drugs available for the treatment of neoplasms in the central nervous system and facilitates the use of novel biologic approaches for the treatment of gliomas. This chapter discusses the rationale and background for the use of these polymers and reviews examples of the various agents that have been used to treat gliomas.

RATIONALE FOR LOCAL DELIVERY

The potential usefulness of chemotherapy for the treatment of gliomas has been limited by restrictions of drug delivery. The traditional regimens of intravenous (IV) or oral drug delivery are not targeted to the brain and, thus, unnecessarily expose systemic organs to the drugs. Moreover, for a chemotherapeutic agent to be effective, tumor cells must be exposed to sufficient concentrations of drug for adequate amounts of time without local or systemic toxic effects; the constraints imposed by the blood-brain barrier often require administration of high doses of chemotherapeutic agents to achieve these high levels in the brain. Certain classes of drugs that are effective for other tumors have been excluded from clinical use for treating gliomas because they do not cross the blood-brain barrier. The development of a therapeutic strategy designed to deliver a high concentration of drug directly to the site of a tumor in the CNS may obviate both the limitation of the blood-brain barrier and the problem of systemic toxic effects. Local delivery of chemotherapeutic agents may be particularly well suited to the treatment of malignant gliomas, as 80% of these tumors recur within 2 cm of the original tumor site, and metastases are exceedingly rare.[1]

Several strategies for bypassing the blood-brain barrier and delivering drugs directly to the brain have been devel-oped, including administration of agents by direct injection or infusion of a drug through a catheter system. The Ommaya reservoir is an example of a device that allows intermittent, controlled administration of a drug via a catheter implanted directly into a tumor or cyst. Implantable pumps have also been developed that can be placed subcutaneously and allow the constant infusion of agents directly into a tumor.[2–4] These devices have the advantage of attaining high tissue concentrations of drug; nevertheless, their clinical use is complicated by infection, mechanical failure, and obstruction.

Implantable polymers for local drug delivery were developed by Langer and Folkman, who discovered that macromolecules could be incorporated into a non-biodegradable ethylene-vinyl acetate co-polymer (EVAc), and released in a controlled and predictable fashion.[5, 6] A drug incorporated into the polymer matrix is released from the polymer by a process of diffusion, and the release profile can be tailored to provide either a slow or a rapid release. Once released from the polymer, the drug retains its biologic activity. Furthermore, very small amounts of a drug, even microgram or nanogram quantities, can be effectively incorporated into and released from a polymer.

Techniques have been developed to incorporate and release a wide variety of complex, biologically active agents from polymers. For example, proteins,[6] antibodies,[7, 8] and growth factors,[9] as well as chemotherapeutic agents,[10–14] have been successfully incorporated into and released from polymers. Current clinical applications of polymer-mediated drug delivery include treatment of glaucoma, prevention of dental caries, asthma therapy, contraception, and cancer chemotherapy.[15]

The direct delivery of agents to the brain offers many potential therapeutic opportunities to the neurosurgical patient. In particular, the patient with a malignant glioma may benefit from local polymeric delivery of chemotherapeutic drugs, corticosteroids, anticonvulsants, anti-angiogenesis agents, and a variety of complex macromolecules, including immunotoxins (Table 46–1). In this chapter, we review the

TABLE 46–1
CLASSES OF DRUGS FOR CONTROLLED RELEASE BY POLYMER

Drug Class	Example	Study
Chemotherapeutic agents	Carmustine	Brem et al[23]
	Taxol	Walter et al[10]
	Camptothecin	Weingart et al[11]
	Carboplatin	Olivi et al[13]
Modified chemotherapeutic agents	4-HC	Judy et al[14]
	Methotrexate-dextran	Dang et al[31]
Steroids	Dexamethasone	Tamargo et al[33]
Anti-angiogenesis agents	Heparin and cortisone	Tamargo et al[36]
	Minocycline	Weingart et al[38]
Anticonvulsants	Diphenylhydantoin	Tamargo et al[34]
Biologic agents	Immunotoxins	Phillips et al[39]
	Antisense oligonucleotides	Simons et al[42]

4-HC, 4-hydroxyperoxycyclophosphamide.

types of polymer systems available for controlled release and the preclinical and clinical studies that have demonstrated the efficacy of polymer-drug delivery to the brain, and we specifically highlight the potential applications of controlled-release polymers for the treatment of malignant gliomas.

POLYMER SYSTEMS FOR CONTROLLED RELEASE

Both biodegradable and non-biodegradable polymer systems have been investigated as potential means for controlled, local delivery of drugs. EVAc, described by Langer and Folkman,[6] is an example of a non-biodegradable polymer. The EVAc polymer system provides a consistent drug-release profile that is highly predictable and reproducible. A drug that has been incorporated into the polymer matrix is released by a process of diffusion that is governed by the physicochemical properties of the drug itself, including molecular weight, charge, and water solubility. Molecules of low molecular weight, for example, are generally released quite rapidly, whereas the release rate of larger molecules is slower. EVAc has proved to be a useful polymer system in the laboratory for exploring the efficacy of local drug delivery. Although EVAc is extremely inert and non-inflammatory, its chief limitation is that after implantation it does not degrade, and it therefore remains a foreign body.

In contrast to EVAc, biodegradable polymer systems provide controlled local delivery from a polymer that degrades over time. Polyanhydride co-polymers, such as poly[bis(*p*-carboxyphenoxy)propane–sebacic acid] (PCPP-SA) are biodegradable polymers that release drug by surface erosion. In vitro and in vivo release studies have demonstrated that the polyanhydride polymer reacts with water and spontaneously hydrolyzes to form dicarboxylic acids.[16] The degradation of the polyanhydride bond leads to a predictable release of the incorporated drug. As the polymer degrades, active drug is concomitantly released into solution or into the local tissue in vivo. An advantage of the PCPP-SA polymer is that the polymer breakdown rate, and therefore the drug release rate, can be tailored by altering the ratio of carboxyphenoxypro-

pane (CPP) to sebacic acid (SA) in the polymer formulation. It has been estimated that a 1-mm disk of pure PCPP would require 3 years to degrade completely in solution. This rate of degradation can be increased significantly by co-polymerization with increasing percentages of SA. Thus, by altering the CPP-to-SA ratio, nearly any degradation rate between 1 day and several years can be achieved.[17] Drugs can be readily incorporated into the matrix of PCPP-SA at low temperatures (<37°C). The drug is combined with PCPP-SA and the homogeneous solid mixture is compressed under high pressure. The resulting drug–co-polymer mixture can be fabricated into any configuration, including sheets, disks, rods, microspheres, and nanospheres.

The spectrum of drugs that are amenable to controlled release has been extended with the development of additional biodegradable polymers. Whereas the PCPP-SA co-polymers are designed to release hydrophobic drugs, a fatty acid dimer-sebacic acid (FAD-SA) co-polymer was specifically developed to release hydrophilic compounds.[18] The processes governing drug release from the FAD-SA polymer are similar to those of PCPP-SA. In particular, by altering the ratio of FAD to SA, the release profile of a drug may be tailored to yield either a slow or rapid release rate.

An advantage of polymer-mediated delivery of drugs is that the release is continuous. By incorporating a drug in a polymer matrix, the drug is protected from breakdown. Consequently, the bioavailability of the drug is increased, particularly in the case of an agent with a short in vivo half-life. For example, after systemic (IV) administration, the chemotherapeutic agent carmustine is degraded to its inactive metabolite within 15 minutes; however, it can be released in an active form from the PCPP-SA co-polymer over a period of weeks.[19]

BIOCOMPATIBILITY STUDIES

The biodegradable polymer PCPP-SA has been tested extensively in vitro and in vivo for biocompatibility. The degradation products of PCPP-SA have been shown to be nonmutagenic, noncytotoxic, and nonteratogenic.[16] Endothelial and smooth muscle cells showed no adverse effects when plated on a layer of the polyanhydride polymer, and only a minimal inflammatory reaction was observed when such polymers were implanted into the rabbit cornea.[16] In a series of experiments comparing the inflammatory response of PCPP-SA implants in the rat and the rabbit brain with implants of Surgicel and Gelfoam, both of which are standard agents used commonly in the brain to achieve hemostasis, the inflammatory reaction to the polymer was found to be similar in intensity to that of the hemostatic agents. Furthermore, the inflammatory response was found to subside as the polymer degraded in vivo over a period of 1 month. None of the animals treated with PCPP-SA in the brain showed any signs of behavioral change or of neurologic deficits suggestive of toxic effects.[20]

Before the polymers were tested in clinical trials, toxicity studies were carried out in monkey brain. PCPP-SA polymers were implanted in the frontal lobe of cynomolgus monkeys. No adverse behavioral or neurologic changes were noted in any of the animals, and serial serum chemical analyses and hematologic profiles were normal, indicating no evidence of systemic toxic effects from the intracranial polymer implants, with or without carmustine. Subsequent autopsies of these animals showed only a localized reaction at the implant site. Additionally, in this study, the efficacy of combining local carmustine with radiation therapy was evaluated. The combination therapy was found to have no adverse effects. These studies demonstrated that the technique of polymer implantation in the brain of a nonhuman primate was safe.[21]

IMAGING CHARACTERISTICS OF INTRACRANIAL POLYMERS

Computed tomography (CT) and magnetic resonance imaging (MRI) have been used to determine whether the PCPP-SA polymer can be detected in the monkey brain.[21] The polymer was found to be readily identifiable on both CT and MRI. CT showed no evidence of mass effect or edema associated with the polymer implants. MRI scans showed a hyperintense ring around the implant sites, but as the polymers degraded, these abnormalities resolved, and the polymers could no longer be detected. These studies indicated that the polymer implants could be followed radiologically by CT or MRI.

IN VIVO DRUG DISTRIBUTION STUDIES

A critical issue in polymer-mediated local delivery of a drug to the brain is the fate of the drug after release from the polymer. Consequently, the pharmacokinetics of carmustine after release from the PCPP-SA polymer in the rabbit brain was investigated by quantitative autoradiography. The intracerebral distribution of tritium-labeled carmustine released from the polymer was evaluated and compared to the distribution of labeled drug delivered by direct stereotactic intracranial injection. These studies showed that by the third day after polymer implantation, radioactivity associated with carmustine was dispersed throughout the ipsilateral hemisphere, with a minimal amount detectable in the contralateral hemisphere. At 21 days after implantation, the brain tissue immediately surrounding the degrading implant showed drug concentrations 2 SD above background. By contrast, such levels of drug activity were no longer detectable 48 hours after direct injection. Tissue analysis by high-pressure liquid chromatography confirmed that the radioactivity was associated with intact carmustine, and that polymer disks containing 600 μg of carmustine generated 6 mM concentrations of carmustine in brain tissue 10 mm from the polymer at 3 and 7 days.[19] This study established that local delivery of carmustine to brain tissue with a PCPP-SA polymer delivery system achieved a high, sustained, local concentration of carmustine in the brain.

The intracranial distribution of agents released from biodegradable polymers implanted in the brain has been evaluated with radiolabeled agents. By autoradiography, the distribution of tritiated carmustine, dextran, and iodoantipyrine was measured at 6, 24, and 72 hours after implantation. For all of the agents studied, the majority of the radioactivity was found to be within the region 1 to 2 mm from the surface of the polymer. Dextran, however, penetrated farther into the brain than either iodoantipyrine or carmustine. These results demonstrate that agents delivered into the brain by polymers penetrate into the tissue within 1 to 2 mm of the implant and that the size of the treated region depends on the physicochemical properties of the agent.[22]

The preliminary preclinical studies discussed to this point provided evidence that the polyanhydride co-polymer PCPP-SA could be implanted safely into the brain; the polymers were biocompatible; the degradation products were nontoxic; and, notably, a high tissue concentration of drug could be achieved in the brain. By use of an experimental tumor model in Fisher 344 rats, the efficacy of local polymer-mediated drug delivery was investigated.[12] Local delivery of carmustine by polymer was found to be superior to systemic (intraperitoneal) administration of carmustine in controlling tumor growth in a flank model of the rat 9L gliosarcoma. These observations were extended to treatment of animals bearing intracranial 9L gliosarcoma. The 9L was implanted into the brains of Fisher 344 rats and treatment was initiated 4 days later with either (1) local PCPP-SA polymer containing carmustine implanted directly at the tumor site, (2) blank PCPP-SA polymer, or (3) systemic (intraperitoneal) administration of carmustine. Local delivery of carmustine by polymer was found to be more effective than systemic administration in extending survival. Animals in the polymer-treated group had a mean survival of 62.3 ± 9.9 days (mean ± SEM). Moreover, two animals (17%) treated with the intracranial carmustine polymer survived more than 125 days. This was in contrast to animals treated with systemic carmustine, among whom no long-term survivors were seen (mean survival, 27.3 ± 3.1 days). The untreated controls had a mean survival of 10.9 ± 0.8 days.

Preclinical dose response studies with the polymers have demonstrated that loading doses of carmustine as low as 1.9% consistently improved survival in the 9L intracranial model. The most effective loading dose of carmustine has proved to be in the range of 20% to 30%. Clinical trials were initiated on the basis of these preclinical laboratory studies, which demonstrated (1) the biocompatibility and safety of the polymers in the brain, (2) the kinetics of polymer degradation and drug distribution, and (3) the improved efficacy of local delivery as compared with systemic delivery of carmustine.

CLINICAL STUDIES

Phase I–II Trial With BCNU Polymer Implants for Treatment of Recurrent Gliomas

The safety of the PCPP-SA co-polymer (20:80 formulation) has been established in humans in a number of clinical trials. The first of these was a phase I–II study of PCPP-SA loaded with carmustine in 21 patients with a diagnosis of recurrent malignant glioma.[23] Enrollment criteria included patients with malignant glioma in whom standard therapy had failed. All patients had undergone a craniotomy for debulking and all had a diagnosis of glioma. Patients were required to have an indication for reoperation, namely a unilateral single focus of tumor in the cerebrum showing at least 1.0 cm³ enhancing volume on CT or MRI; a Karnofsky performance scale score of at least 60; completion of external-beam radiation therapy; and no nitrosoureas during the 6 weeks before enrollment. Polymers containing carmustine were implanted directly into the tumor resection cavity during reoperation for tumor debulking. Figures 46–1 and 46–2 show intraoperative photographs of the polymer being placed in the resection cavity.

Three increasing concentrations of carmustine were studied: 25 μg of carmustine per square millimeter of polymer (1.93% of carmustine loading dose) yielded 3.85 mg of carmustine per polymer disk; 50 μg of carmustine per square millimeter of polymer (3.85% of carmustine loading dose) yielded 7.7 mg of carmustine per polymer disk; and 82.5 μg of carmustine per square millimeter of polymer (6.35% of carmustine loading dose) yielded 12.7 mg of carmustine per polymer disk. Most of the patients received a total of 8 polymer disks; therefore, the maximum dose of carmustine for the patients in each of the three groups was 31, 62, and 102 mg, respectively. Patients were divided into three groups: 5 patients received the low dose; 5 received the middle dose; and 11 were treated with the highest dose. In the first two treatment groups, 60% had glioblastomas, whereas all of the patients in the third treatment group initially had glioblastomas. Overall, 17 (81%) of the 21 patients had a diagnosis of glioblastoma. Tumor volumes were not significantly different among treatment groups. The treatment was well tolerated at all three doses. After implantation, all patients were able to function independently as measured by the Karnofsky performance scale score. No untoward neurologic events occurred that were attributable to the intracranial polymers. Additionally, no significant reduction in blood counts was found, which would have suggested bone marrow suppression from carmustine. Frequent urinalysis and serum chemical analysis showed no evidence of renal or of hepatic toxic effects.

In 13 of 21 patients, CT imaging obtained on days 14 and 49 of the study showed a distinct area of contrast enhancement adjacent to the implant site. These areas were often intensely enhancing, although it was rare to see significant mass effect. The areas of enhancement generally resolved within 7 weeks, and clinical and neurologic evaluation did not reveal any correlation between development of these radiographic findings and any sign of toxic response. The enhancement presumably reflects disruption of the blood-brain barrier at the site of drug delivery. The polymers could be identified on most of the postoperative imaging studies, and vague outlines of the polymers were detectable by CT imaging at the implant site for up to 49 days following surgery. The polymers were visible on MRI scans as areas of decreased signal intensity on T1 imaging, as shown in Figure 46–3.

The overall median survival times for each of three dosage groups postimplant were 65, 47, and 23 weeks, respectively. The reduced survival in the third group in part reflects the fact that all of the patients in the group had glioblastoma, compared with 60% of patients in the first two groups. The overall median survival for the 21 patients was 46 weeks postimplantation and 87 weeks from initial surgery. Eighteen (86%) of 21 patients lived more than 1 year from the time of initial diagnosis. Eight (38%) of 21 patients lived more than 1 year after having failed standard or other experimental

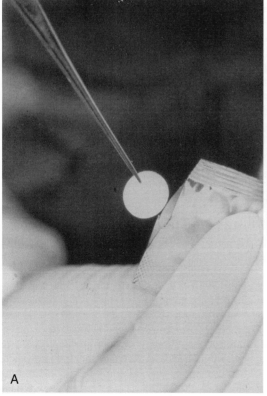

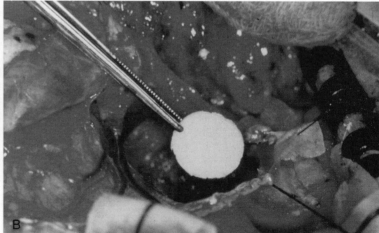

Figure 46–1 *A,* Intraoperative photograph showing removal of a carmustine-polymer disk from sterile packaging prior to implantation. *B,* Intraoperative photograph showing placement of the carmustine-polymer disk in the tumor resection cavity.

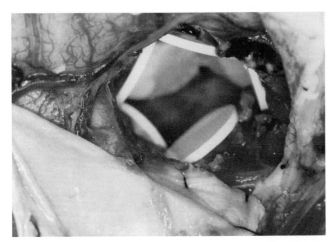

Figure 46–2 Intraoperative photograph of carmustine-polymer disks lining the resection cavity following tumor resection.

therapy. This initial study demonstrated that polymer-mediated release of a chemotherapeutic agent directly to the site of a malignant glioma was safe and well tolerated by patients, and also that there was some improvement, albeit modest, in efficacy. Therefore, a phase III study was initiated.

In a separate clinical trial, 22 patients were treated with carmustine-carrying polymers at the time of initial craniotomy: 21 patients had a diagnosis of glioblastoma, 1 had an anaplastic astrocytoma. The average age was 60 years. Entry criteria included a single, unilateral tumor focus larger than 1 cm³, age greater that 18 years, and a Karnofsky performance scale score of at least 60. Patients were treated by implantation of seven or eight polymer disks (PCPP-SA ratio, 20:80), each of which contained 7.7 mg of carmustine, directly into the tumor resection cavity. All patients received standard radiation therapy averaging 5,000 rad. None re-

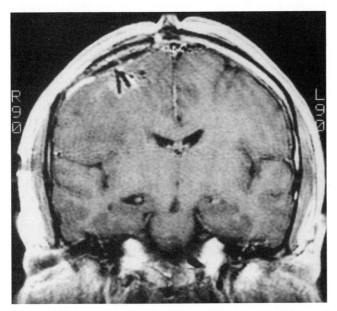

Figure 46–3 T1-weighted coronal MRI scan showing areas of decreased signal intensity corresponding to carmustine-polymer disks.

ceived additional chemotherapy in the first 6 months following polymer implantation. No perioperative mortality was seen and no morbidity was directly attributable to the polymers. Median survival was 44 weeks, and four patients survived more than 18 months. This study demonstrated that chemotherapy with carmustine-polymer appears to be safe as an initial therapy for gliomas. Furthermore, the combination of local chemotherapy and standard radiation therapy was well tolerated by patients.[24]

Prospective, Randomized, Placebo-Controlled, Phase III Clinical Trial of Carmustine-Polymers for Treatment of Recurrent Gliomas

To evaluate further the efficacy of this treatment method for patients with malignant glioma, a multicenter, prospective, randomized, double-blind, placebo-controlled study was initiated.[25] In 27 medical centers, 222 patients with recurrent malignant brain tumors requiring reoperation were randomly assigned to receive surgically implanted biodegradable PCPP-SA polymer disks, with or without 3.85% carmustine. The 3.85% loading dose was selected for further study based on results from the Phase I–II trial. A loading dose of 50 µg of carmustine per square millimeter of polymer (3.85% carmustine loading dose) yielded 7.7 mg of carmustine per polymer disk, for a maximum dose of 62 mg/patient. The patients were followed clinically and radiologically.

Inclusion criteria for patients were the same as in the Phase I–II study in that the patients had recurrent malignant gliomas, had failed standard therapy, and were candidates for reoperation. Prior chemotherapy was allowed, but none during the 4 weeks before enrollment. All patients were eligible to receive systemic chemotherapy 2 weeks after polymer implantation. Of 222 patients, 145 (65.3%) had a diagnosis of glioblastoma multiforme at the time of implantation, 31 (14.0%) had anaplastic astrocytoma, 9 (4.1%) had anaplastic oligodendroglioma, 4 (1.8%) had oligodendroglioma, and 32 (14.4%) had other glial neoplasms. Randomization effectively balanced the treatment groups for all prognostic factors examined. Median survival of the 110 patients who received carmustine-polymers was 31 weeks. By contrast, the 112 patients who underwent reoperation but who received placebo polymers had a median survival of 23 weeks. The effect of treatment was found to be significant (hazard ratio = 0.69, P = 0.005). The 6-month mortality for those treated with placebo was 53%, as compared with the carmustine-polymer group, in which only 40% had died. The results were more striking in the glioblastoma group, with 50% greater survival at 6 months in patients treated with carmustine-polymers compared with placebo controls (P = 0.020). No clinically significant adverse reactions were attributable to the carmustine-polymer. The intracranial infection rate was 2.2% overall, and it was not significantly different between groups.

This is the first study to demonstrate, in a randomized, controlled manner, a statistically significant prolongation of survival due to carmustine in patients with recurrent glioma. To date, 325 patients have undergone intracranial polymer implants with carmustine. These studies demonstrate that biodegradable polymers can be used safely and effectively to treat brain tumor.

Delivery of Other Chemotherapeutic Agents for the Treatment of Experimental Intracranial Tumors

The preclinical and clinical studies with carmustine-polymers have served as a model for the investigation of other potentially promising agents for the treatment of gliomas. One of the important aspects of polymer-mediated, controlled delivery in the treatment of gliomas is the potential to bring to clinical use a variety of chemotherapeutic agents that have shown considerable promise in preclinical investigation but that have not been effectively utilized clinically because of high levels of systemic toxic effects. Following are examples of different classes of antineoplastic agents that have been successfully incorporated into polymers and utilized in experimental models of gliomas.

Taxol

Taxol is a microtubule binding agent that has shown considerable efficacy in clinical trials against several human tumors, including ovarian, breast, and non–small-cell lung cancer. Gliomas have been shown to be sensitive to taxol in vitro.[26] Pharmacokinetic evidence from animal studies and clinical trials, however, indicates that taxol penetrates the intact blood-brain barrier poorly, if at all.[27] Therefore, to exploit taxol's potential as an agent to treat malignant intracranial tumors, a delivery system capable of providing a high local concentration of taxol directly to the site of a brain tumor was developed.

Taxol was incorporated into the biodegradable polymer PCPP-SA (20:80), and was tested for efficacy in extending survival in the rat intracranial 9L gliosarcoma model. The taxol-loaded polymers doubled (38 days with 40% taxol loading dose, $P < 0.02$) to tripled (61.5 days with 20% taxol loading dose, $P < 0.001$) the median survival of rats bearing 9L gliosarcoma compared to controls (19.5 days). Polymer-release kinetic studies showed that drug loadings of 20% to 40% taxol by weight released intact taxol for up to 1,000 hours in vitro. Furthermore, the taxol polymers maintained tumoricidal concentrations of taxol within the brain for more than 1 month after implantation.[10]

Camptothecin

Camptothecin is a naturally occurring inhibitor of the DNA replicating enzyme topoisomerase I. Camptothecin showed promising antitumor activity in preclinical testing against a variety of experimental tumors in vitro. However, because of unexpected toxic effects and low antitumor effects in initial clinical trials in patients with melanoma and advanced gastrointestinal carcinoma, further testing was discontinued. In vitro data, which demonstrated that gliomas are highly sensitive to camptothecin, suggested that this drug may be an effective agent for the treatment of malignant brain tumors. Again, poor bioavailability and high levels of systemic toxic effects have prevented camptothecin from being investigated as a treatment for patients with gliomas.

This raised the possibility that use of a polymer to deliver camptothecin directly to the brain might be an effective treatment strategy, providing a high concentration of drug to the tumor and minimizing systemic side effects.

To evaluate the feasibility of using camptothecin to treat gliomas, the drug was incorporated into the nonbiodegradable polymer EVAc. Local delivery of camptothecin by polymer was compared with systemic (intraperitoneal) delivery in the rat 9L intracranial gliosarcoma model. Local controlled delivery by the polymer significantly extended survival: 59% of the treated animals were long-term survivors (>120 days), whereas none of the controls survived longer than 32 days. Systemic administration did not extend survival compared with that of controls.[11]

Carboplatin

Carboplatin is a second-generation, platinum-based chemotherapeutic agent. It has been shown to exhibit significantly fewer neurotoxic effects than its parent compound, cisplatin.[28] The efficacy of local delivery of carboplatin was investigated using the biodegradable polyanhydride polymer fatty acid dimer-sebacic acid (FAD-SA). In an experimental intracranial model of F98 glioma, rats treated with intracranial FAD-SA polymer containing 5% carboplatin had a median survival of 52 days, in contrast with a median survival of 16 days in animals treated with polymer containing no chemotherapeutic drug.[29]

4-Hydroxyperoxycyclophosphamide

4-Hydroxyperoxycyclophosphamide (4-HC) is a hydrophilic derivative of cyclophosphamide. The advantage of 4-HC is that it does not require hepatic activation and therefore may be well suited for local chemotherapy. The efficacy of polymer-mediated release of 4-HC was investigated in an experimental animal model. Animals were treated with stereotactic intracranial injections of F98 glioma cells. Five days after tumor injection, the animals were treated by implantation of polymer alone or of polymer containing either 10% or 20% 4-HC in FAD-SA directly at the site of the intracranial tumor. Animals treated with blank polymer had a median survival of 22 days, whereas the median survival of animals treated with 10% and 20% 4-HC was extended to 28 and 35 days, respectively.[14]

In vivo release studies demonstrated that 4-HC–loaded FAD-SA polymer implants gave peak drug concentrations in the brain, as measured by HPLC, between 5 and 20 days after intracranial polymer implantation. This was in contrast to cerebral levels of 4-HC after systemic administration, which fell rapidly 48 hours after injection. Furthermore, brain levels of 4-HC achieved with the intracranial implants were found to be substantially higher than blood levels at all time points.[14] This study highlights the advantage of polymer delivery of drugs in achieving and maintaining a high concentration of drug in the brain while minimizing systemic exposure to the drug. The efficacy of polymer-drug delivery was demonstrated in a study that compared the delivery of 4-HC to the brain by two local methods: direct intralesional injection and polymer-mediated drug release.[30] Direct intralesional injection was less effective than controlled release via polymers for the treatment of 9L gliosarcoma in the rat.

Methotrexate-Dextran

Drugs may be specifically modified for local delivery to enhance their therapeutic effect. For example, coupling dextran to a chemotherapeutic agent may increase penetrance into the brain. Dang and co-workers[31] showed that covalently coupling methotrexate to dextran enhanced the penetration of cytotoxic effects into a tissue-like matrix. In an in vitro assay against a human glioma line (H80), the methotrexate-dextran conjugates were shown to have equivalent cytotoxic effects when compared with unmodified methotrexate. Methotrexate-dextran conjugates were then tested for efficacy in an in vivo model. The modified drug, when delivered by the FAD-SA biodegradable polymer, produced modest but significant increases in survival in rats with intracranial 9L gliosarcoma. Furthermore, conjugation of methotrexate to dextran appeared to shift the dose-response curve to a lower dosage, suggesting increased effectiveness at lower concentrations, presumably due to increased retention of methotrexate-dextran conjugates in the brain.

Use of Polymer-Mediated Drug Delivery to Control Cerebral Edema

The principles of local delivery of drugs to the brain may be useful in treating a variety of problems encountered in the management of gliomas, including vasogenic cerebral edema. The use of corticosteroids in the treatment of brain tumors has had a significant beneficial impact on neurosurgical practice. Unfortunately, systemic administration of high- dose steroids has many adverse side effects, including glucose intolerance, immunosuppression, weight gain, gastrointestinal ulceration, skin atrophy leading to poor wound healing, myopathies, osteoporosis, and pathologic fractures.[32] The use of a polymer to deliver steroids directly to the brain may control cerebral edema directly while minimizing the systemic side effects seen with high doses of steroids.

To investigate whether steroids could be delivered locally by polymer, dexamethasone was incorporated into EVAc and its in vitro release was measured by HPLC. Dexamethasone was found to be released from the polymer in a sustained fashion. To test the in vivo release properties of dexamethasone in the brain, dexamethasone-loaded EVAc polymers were implanted intracranially in rats. Dexamethasone levels, as determined by HPLC, were measured in the blood and in both cerebral hemispheres up to 12 hours after implantation of the polymer; these levels were compared with levels attained with intraperitoneal administration of dexamethasone. Compared with systemic administration of the drug, dexamethasone delivered by the intracranial polymer achieved higher, prolonged levels in the brain, with almost negligible plasma levels.[33]

The efficacy of controlled-release dexamethasone polymers in reversing cerebral edema in the brain was evaluated in the rat 9L intracranial tumor model. Vasogenic edema was produced by intracranial implantation of the 9L gliosarcoma. Five days after tumor implantation, animals were treated with either intracranially implanted dexamethasone-loaded EVAc polymers or intraperitoneal injections of dexamethasone. The total dose of steroids was equivalent in the two groups. Animals were sacrificed 8 days after tumor implantation and the water content of the brain was assessed as a measure of cerebral edema. Additionally, dexamethasone levels in the brain and plasma were measured by HPLC. The intracranial dexamethasone polymer resulted in a significant decrease in cerebral edema compared with levels in controls. Indeed, dexamethasone delivered by polymer was found to be as effective in controlling cerebral edema as systemic treatment, while attaining only a fraction of the plasma steroid concentration.[33] These experimental studies suggest that polymer-mediated delivery of steroids may provide an important advantage over systemic therapy in treating cerebral edema in patients with brain tumors.

Controlled Release of Diphenylhydantoin for Seizure Management

Other classes of drugs that may aid in the management of patients with brain tumors have been explored for local delivery by polymer. Anticonvulsants, for example, have been successfully incorporated into and released from polymers. Diphenylhydantoin was loaded into EVAc and in vitro kinetic studies demonstrated that diphenylhydantoin was released in a controlled, sustained fashion. Diphenylhydantoin released from EVAc polymer in this manner was shown to be effective in controlling seizure activity in a rat model of cobalt-induced epileptic activity.[34] No behavioral toxic effects were detected with the intracerebral release of diphenylhydantoin over a period of 11 months. The local administration of an anticonvulsant directly to the brain may prove to be an effective means of achieving long-term seizure control while minimizing the systemic drug side effects in patients with brain tumors.

Controlled Release of Angiogenesis Inhibitors

Angiogenesis inhibition has been shown to restrict the growth of tumors by inhibiting new vessel growth.[35] As angiogenesis appears to be a prerequisite for exponential tumor growth, the control of this process holds potential as a therapy for the treatment of gliomas. Angiogenesis inhibitors have been incorporated into sustained-release polymers and, when delivered in this fashion, have been found to be effective in controlling tumor growth. Early experimental studies investigated whether heparin and cortisone co-released from EVAc polymer could inhibit angiogenesis induced by the VX2 carcinoma in the rabbit cornea.[36] Polymers containing the drugs were implanted adjacent to the tumor and were found to reduce the neovascularization induced by the tumor. Additionally, PCPP-SA polymers containing heparin and cortisone were shown to retard growth of the 9L gliosarcoma in the rat flank.[36] These studies showed that the polymers could simultaneously release two biologically active agents.

Recently, the anti-angiogenesis properties of the semisynthetic tetracycline minocycline have been investigated.[37] Minocycline was incorporated into a controlled-release polymer and its efficacy in inhibiting neovascularization was assessed in the rabbit cornea angiogenesis assay. Tumor angiogenesis was significantly inhibited by the controlled release of minocycline. Local treatment with minocycline delivered by polymer placed at the time of tumor implantation was shown to significantly extend median survival in the 9L intracranial model compared with that seen in controls. This effect was found to be time dependent; when treatment was begun 5 days after tumor implantation, local minocycline had no effect on survival. Treatment with a combination of local minocycline at the tumor site and systemic carmustine 5 days after tumor implantation resulted in a 93% extension of median survival compared to use of carmustine alone. In contrast, treatment with a combination of systemic minocycline and carmustine did not increase survival compared to carmustine alone. These results demonstrate that angiogenesis inhibitors can be delivered effectively by a sustained-release polymer to control neovascularization in an animal model and that the timing of delivery of the anti-angiogenesis agent is a critical variable. Moreover, this study shows that a combination of local and systemic therapy may optimize the potential of these drugs.[38]

Other Classes of Agents Amenable to Local Delivery in the Treatment of Malignant Glioma

Immunotoxins

The design of rational therapeutic treatment strategies for gliomas is evolving as our understanding of the biology of these lesions improves. New classes of drugs for the treatment of gliomas are emerging that are both potent and specific. Immunotoxins are examples of such agents. Immunotoxins are chimeric molecules that are composed of an antibody that is specific for a receptor that is expressed selectively on cancer cells, and which are chemically linked to a potent toxin. The most common immunotoxins combine ligands for either growth factor receptors or transferrin receptor, both of which are overexpressed on glial cells, with a variety of toxins such as ricin A, *Pseudomonas* exotoxin, or diphtheria toxin. These are large, complex molecules that may not cross the blood-brain barrier. The clinical use of these agents for the treatment of gliomas may well be dictated by issues of drug delivery.

The issue of immunotoxin delivery was investigated in an experimental model of intracranial human glioblastoma and medulloblastoma xenographs in nude mice. Treatment with a single intratumoral injection of transforming growth factor α–*Pseudomonas* exotoxin fusion protein (TGFA-PE38) was more effective in prolonging survival than was continuous intraperitoneal administration of the drug.[39] Similarly, using two different immunotoxins, Laske and co-workers[40] demonstrated the efficacy of direct intratumoral therapy of human gliomas in a flank model. These results suggest that local delivery of an immunotoxin may potentiate its efficacy. Clinical studies with a stereotactic delivery method for these potentially toxic agents are under way. The incorporation of these complex macromolecules into a polymer for local, controlled delivery is feasible and may indeed prove to be a safe and effective means of using these agents to treat patients with malignant glioma.

FUTURE APPLICATIONS OF CONTROLLED-RELEASE POLYMERS

Future applications of polymer-mediated drug delivery to the brain include the co-release of two or more agents for combination therapy. For example, the concomitant local delivery of more than one antineoplastic agent may improve efficacy over single-agent therapy. Anti-angiogenesis agents may be synergistic with chemotherapeutic agents, and these may be optimally co-delivered via polymer.[38, 41] The development of polymers to deliver genetically modified cells or antisense oligonucleotides that could be incorporated into cells in the CNS suggests a novel means of gene therapy for the treatment of intracranial neoplasms.[42] New polymer formulations are currently being developed in microsphere- or nanosphere-sized particles,[43] which may be amenable to stereotactic injection or intra-arterial infusion. These cell-sized polymers may be particularly useful for delivering chemotherapeutic agents directly to deep-seated lesions in the brain. Additionally, techniques to modulate drug release from biodegradable polymers by use of ultrasound are being evaluated. This strategy is potentially advantageous in that ultrasound can trigger the release of a drug from certain polymers; hence, the timing of drug delivery can be controlled.[44] By modulating the drug's release in this way, an agent may be delivered long after implantation, depending on the clinical situation.

CONCLUSIONS

The development of controlled-release polymers for local drug delivery to the brain has broad application to the treatment of patients with malignant gliomas. Polymers may be adapted to deliver high concentrations of chemotherapeutic drugs directly to the site of a brain tumor, thus optimizing the tumor levels of the drug while minimizing the systemic side effects. This approach potentially broadens the range of drugs that are available to treat brain tumors. Drugs that may never have been utilized clinically because of toxic effects or inability to cross the blood-brain barrier may become useful therapeutic options for treating gliomas. Moreover, management of patients with gliomas may be improved by intracranial local delivery of steroids to control cerebral edema and of anticonvulsants to control seizures. New classes of therapeutic agents, such as anti-angiogenesis agents, immunotoxins, and antisense oligonucleotides, are all amenable to local delivery to the brain with controlled-release polymers. The application of local, controlled drug delivery to the brain holds considerable promise for the field of neurosurgery in general and the treatment of patients with gliomas in particular.

ACKNOWLEDGMENTS

We would like to thank our numerous co-investigators for their contributions. We appreciate the review of the manuscript by Drs. Matt Ewend, Robert Langer, Pamela Talalay, Rafael Tamargo, Al Sills, Eric Sipos, and Lorraine Ware. The work described was partially funded by the National Cancer Institute grant UO1–CA52857. The clinical trials were funded by Scios-Nova Corporation, Mountain View, Calif, and Guilford Pharmaceutical Inc., Baltimore.

REFERENCES

1. Hochberg F, Pruitt A: Assumptions in the radiotherapy of glioblastoma. Neurology 1980;30:907–911.
2. Heruth K: Medtronic synchromed drug administration system. Ann NY Acad Sci 1988;531:72–75.
3. Lord P, Allami H, Davis M, et al: Minimed technologies programmable implantable infusion system. Ann NY Acad Sci 1988;531:66–71.
4. Johnston J, Reich S, Bailey A, et al: Shiley infusaid pump technology. Ann NY Acad Sci 1988;531:57–65.
5. Langer R: New methods of drug delivery. Science 1990;249:1527–1533.
6. Langer R, Folkman J: Polymers for the sustained release of proteins and other macromolecules. Nature 1976;263:797–800.
7. Saltzman WM, Sheppard NF, McHugh MA, et al: Controlled antibody release from a matrix of poly(ethylene-co-vinyl acetate) fractionated with a supercritical fluid. J Appl Polymer Sci 1993;48:1493–1500.
8. Saltzman WM: Antibodies for treating and preventing disease: The potential role of polymeric controlled release (review). Crit Rev Ther Drug Carrier Syst 1993;10:111–142.
9. Murray J, Brown L, Langer R, et al: A micro sustained release system for epidermal growth factor. In Vitro 1983;19:743–748.
10. Walter K, Cahan M, Gur A, et al: Interstitial taxol delivered from a biodegradable polymer implant against experimental malignant glioma. Cancer Res 1994;54:2207–2212.
11. Weingart J, Thompson R, Tyler B, et al: Local delivery of the topoisomerase I inhibitor camptothecin prolongs survival in the rat intracranial 9L gliosarcoma model. Int J Cancer 1995;62:605–609.
12. Tamargo RJ, Myseros JS, Epstein JI, et al: Interstitial chemotherapy of the 9L gliosarcoma: Controlled release polymers for drug delivery in the brain. Cancer Res 1993;53:329–333.
13. Olivi A, Lenartz D, Domb A, et al: Treatment of F98 rat glioma with local controlled-release of carboplatin from biodegradable polymer. International symposium on Advances in Neurooncology. September, 1990, Saremo, Italy.
14. Judy K, Olivi A, Buahin K, et al: Effectiveness of controlled release of a cyclophosphamide derivative with polymers against rat gliomas. J Neurosurg 1995;82:103–108.
15. Langer R, Wise D (eds): Medical Applications of Controlled Release, vol. I and II. Boca Raton, Fla, CRC Press, 1986.
16. Leong K, D'Amore P, Marletta M, et al: Bioerodable polyanhydrides as drug-carrier matrices: II. Biocompatibility and chemical reactivity. J Biomed Mater Res 1986;20:51–64.
17. Chasin M, Domb A, Ron E, et al: Polyanhydrides as drug delivery systems. In Chasin M, Langer R (eds): Biodegradable Polymers as Drug Delivery Systems. New York, Marcel-Dekker, 1990, pp 43–70.
18. Domb A, Bogdansky S, Olivi A, et al: Controlled delivery of water soluble and hydrolytically unstable anticancer drugs from polymeric implants. Polymer Preprints 1991;32:219–220.
19. Grossman SA, Reinhard C, Colvin OM, et al: The intracerebral distribution of BCNU delivered by surgically implanted biodegradable polymers. J Neurosurg 1992;76:640–647.
20. Tamargo RJ, Epstein JI, Reinhard CS, et al: Brain biocompatibility of a biodegradable, controlled-release polymer in rats. J Biomed Mater Res 1989;23:253–266.
21. Brem H, Tamargo R, Olivi A, et al: Biodegradable polymers for controlled delivery of chemotherapy with and without radiation therapy in the monkey brain. J Neurosurg 1994;80:283–290.
22. Strasser J, Fung L, Eller S, et al: Distribution of 1,3-bis(2-chloroethyl)-1-nitrosourea (BCNU) and tracers in the rabbit brain following interstitial delivery by biodegradable polymer implants. J Pharmacol Exp Ther 1995;275:1647–1655.
23. Brem H, Mahaley MJ, Vick NA, et al: Interstitial chemotherapy with drug polymer implants for the treatment of recurrent gliomas. J Neurosurg 1991;74:441–446.
24. Brem H, Ewend M, Greenhoot J, et al: The safety of interstitial chemotherapy with BCNU-loaded polymer in the treatment of newly diagnosed malignant gliomas: Phase I trial. J Neurooncol 1995;26:111–123.
25. Brem H, Piantadosi S, Burger P, et al: Intraoperative chemotherapy using biodegradable polymers in a prospective, multi-institutional placebo-controlled clinical trial for safety and effectiveness. Neurosurgery 1994;35:574.
26. Cahan MA, Walter KA, Colvin OM, et al: Cytotoxicity of taxol in vitro against human and rat malignant brain tumors. Cancer Chemother Pharmacol 1994;33:441–444.
27. Klecker R, Jamis-Dow C, Egorin M, et al: Distribution and metabolism of 3H-taxol in the rat. Proc Am Assoc Cancer Res 1992;34:381.
28. Olivi A, Gilbert M, Duncan K, et al: Direct delivery of platinum based antineoplastics to the central nervous system: A toxicity and ultrastructural study. Cancer Chemother Pharmacol 1992;31:449–454.
29. Brem H, Walter K, Tamargo R, et al: Drug delivery to the brain. In Domb AJ (ed): Polymer Site-Specific Pharmacotherapy. New York, John Wiley & Sons, 1994, pp 117–139.
30. Buahin K, Brem H: Interstitial chemotherapy of experimental brain tumors: Comparison of intratumoral injection versus polymeric controlled release. J Neurooncol 1995;26:103–110.
31. Dang W, Colvin O, Brem H, et al: Covalent coupling of methotrexate to dextran enhances the penetration of cytotoxicity into a tissue-like matrix. Cancer Res 1994;54:1729–1735.
32. Melby J: Systemic corticosteroid therapy. Ann Intern Med 1974; 81:505–512.
33. Tamargo RJ, Sills AJ, Reinhard CS, et al: Interstitial delivery of dexamethasone in the brain for the reduction of peritumoral edema. J Neurosurg 1991;74:956–961.
34. Tamargo RJ, Rossell LA, Tyler BM, et al: Interstitial delivery of diphenylhydantoin in the brain for the treatment of seizures in a rat model. J Neurosurg 1994;80:372.
35. Guerin C, Tamargo RJ, Olivi A, et al: Brain tumor angiogenesis: Drug delivery and new inhibitors. In Maragoudakis ME (ed): Angiogenesis in Health and Diseases. New York, Plenum Press, 1992, pp 265–274.
36. Tamargo RJ, Leong KW, Brem H: Growth inhibition of the 9L glioma using polymers to release heparin and cortisone acetate. J Neurooncol 1990;9:131–138.
37. Tamargo RJ, Bok RA, Brem H: Angiogenesis inhibition by minocycline. Cancer Res 1991;51:672–675.
38. Weingart J, Sipos E, Brem H: The role of minocycline in treatment of intracranial 9L glioma. J Neurosurg 1995;82:635–640.
39. Phillips P, Levow C, Catterall M, et al: Transforming growth factor-α-Pseudomonas exotoxin fusion protein (TGF-α-PE38) treatment of subcutaneous and intracranial human glioma and medulloblastoma xenografts in athymic mice. Cancer Res 1994;54:1008–1015.
40. Laske D, Ilercil O, Akbasak A, et al: Efficacy of direct intratumoral therapy with targeted protein toxins for solid human gliomas in nude mice. J Neurosurg 1994;80:520–526.
41. Teicher BA, Holden SA, Ara G, et al: Potentiation of cytotoxic cancer therapies by TNP-470 alone and with other anti-angiogenic agents. Int J Cancer 1994;57(6):920–925.
42. Simons M, Edelman E, DeKeyser J, et al: Antisense c-myb oligonucleotides inhibit intimal arterial smooth muscle cell accumulation in vitro. Nature 1992;359:67–70.
43. Gref R, Minamitake Y, Peracchia MT, et al: Biodegradable long-circulating polymeric nanospheres. Science 1994;263:1600–1603.
44. Liu L-S, Kost J, D'Emanuele A, et al: Experimental approaches to elucidate the mechanism of ultrasound-enhanced polymer erosion and release of incorporated substances. Macromolecules 1992;25:511–515.

LESLIE D. McALLISTER

KURT A. JAECKLE

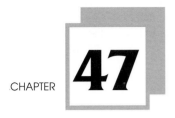

CHAPTER **47**

Intratumoral Administration

Malignant gliomas usually progress owing to failure of local tumor control,[1] which provides a rationale for local application of therapeutic agents. By convention, the term *intratumoral chemotherapy* has been applied to treatment that is directly introduced into a tumor or a postoperative cavity. The technique was first used extensively in 1958 by Bateman[2] for the treatment of breast cancer. Intratumoral chemotherapy was first investigated as a therapeutic modality for brain tumors in 1968 by Heppner and Diemath.[3] These authors applied chemotherapy with a gelatin sponge to the tumor bed following resection. Since then, a number of reports have been published of intratumoral chemotherapy for human gliomas.[3-16] This chapter discusses intratumoral application of liquid-phase chemotherapeutic agents. Techniques involving implantation of agents in solid-phase media, such as biodegradable wafers or rods, are discussed elsewhere in this volume.

The main advantages of intratumoral chemotherapy over conventional systemic chemotherapy administration include the following: (1) increased intratumoral concentration and duration of drug exposure (area under the curve, AUC); (2) effective evasion of the blood-brain barrier, which is of particular importance when using agents of low lipid solubility; (3) drug delivery to relatively avascular areas within the tumor; and (4) lower total drug dose, which minimizes systemic toxic effects. The increased AUC associated with local drug application may be advantageous for cell cycle–specific agents, as only 5% to 10% of cells in most glioblastomas are undergoing DNA synthesis at any given time,[17] and may decrease the development of drug resistance.[18]

The main disadvantages of intratumoral chemotherapy include the following: (1) inadequate drug delivery to the advancing irregular margin of the tumor, which may be quite distant from the main tumor bulk; (2) ineffective distribution in the case of multifocal or multicentric glioma; (3) difficulties with predictive pharmacokinetic modeling of a given drug within tumor and brain tissue; and (4) local brain tissue toxic effects associated with the prolonged intensive tissue drug concentration.

Toxic effects associated with intratumoral chemotherapy may be related to several different aspects of the treatment. The introduction and maintenance of synthetic delivery systems can cause infection, bleeding, and focal injury to the brain.[10] Neurologic morbidity may also accompany mass effect resulting from large injection volumes or from direct tissue necrosis and edema produced by the chemotherapeutic agents and solvent vehicles. Garfield and co-workers[10] described signs and symptoms of increased intracranial pressure and worsening of focal deficits following intratumoral chemotherapy with BCNU in seven of 10 patients treated. Bosch and colleagues[5] described a similar complication in one of three patients treated with intratumoral bleomycin. Systemic toxic effects may result from absorption of the drug into the circulation.

Consequently, important therapeutic considerations involving intratumoral chemotherapy include choice and dosage of agents, mode of drug delivery, timing of treatments, propensity for the drug to distribute within the tumor and adjacent brain, expected local toxic responses, and predictable effects of systemic absorption of agents into the circulation.

DRUG SELECTION

Characteristics of the ideal agent for intratumoral chemotherapy for malignant gliomas would include minimal local neurotoxic effects; predictable local diffusion characteristics; demonstrated in vitro and in vivo activity; limited systemic toxic effects; optimal solubility in biocompatible vehicles at small volumes; stability at physiologic pH and body temperature; and no requirement for initial hepatic activation. As blood-brain barrier penetration is not a significant factor in intratumoral chemotherapy, the characteristics of lipid solubility, protein binding, plasma half-life, and extent of ionization become less relevant. Agents that are relatively water-soluble can often be administered in a smaller volume of fluid, and they have greater distribution in the extracellular fluid (ECF) than do relatively lipid-soluble agents. However, these agents egress from the ECF into blood less freely than do lipid-soluble agents, which may result in an increased local tissue half-life[19] and enhanced local toxic effects.

Agents that have been used for intratumoral chemotherapy in humans and/or animal models include methotrexate, cyclophosphamide, fluorouracil, bleomycin, cisplatin, aziridinyl benzoquinone, acivicin, 1,3-bis(2-chloroethyl)-1-nitrosourea (BCNU, or carmustine), 1-(2-chloroethyl)-3-cyclohexyl-1-nitrosourea (CCNU, or lomustine), 1-(4-amino-2-methyl-5-pyrimidinyl)methyl-3-(2-chloroethyl)-3 nitrosourea (ACNU), and methyl 6-(3-(2-chloroethyl-3-nitrosourea))-6 deoxy-α-D-glucopyranoside (MCNU).[3–16, 20–26]

DRUG DELIVERY

Several techniques have been described for delivery of chemotherapeutic agents into brain tumors; these include freehand direct injection, administration via single catheters, implanted combined catheter/Ommaya systems, and multiple implanted catheters.[3–5, 7–9, 11, 13, 14, 16, 27, 28] Direct injection without stereotactic guidance via a burr hole or skull defect was primarily utilized in earlier studies, but this is less precise and may carry additional risks of bleeding or focal injury. Single-catheter[9, 10] and implanted Ommaya reservoir systems[15, 28] have the advantages of accurate drug delivery, ease of repetitive administration, and reduction of patient discomfort. Nierenberg and others[13] recently described a method of continuous intratumoral chemotherapy using an implanted slotted ventricular catheter and reservoir attached to an implanted infusion pump.

Limited drug diffusion, irregular tumor geometry, and multifocal tumor sites remain the major problems associated with intratumoral chemotherapy. To address these issues, Bouvier and colleagues[7] developed a system for intratumoral drug delivery using multiple chronically implanted catheters and treated three patients with malignant glioma.

PHARMACOKINETICS OF INTRATUMORAL CHEMOTHERAPY

Conclusive data and predictive modeling regarding intratumoral chemotherapy in brain tumors are limited. With systemic chemotherapy, bone marrow toxic response often determines the dosing interval. This factor is relatively less important in intratumoral chemotherapy because systemic drug exposure is minimized. With intratumoral chemotherapy, the dosing interval may be a direct function of the tissue half-life of the administered agent.

A few investigations of drug distribution following intratumoral administration have been conducted. Nierenberg and co-workers[13] measured cerebrospinal fluid (CSF) and serum methotrexate concentrations following intratumoral administration in five recurrent glioblastoma patients. Large variations between patients were noted in CSF methotrexate levels. Methotrexate serum levels appeared to increase linearly as the intratumoral dosage was increased. At steady state, serum methotrexate levels were greater than CSF levels in two patients, but lower in the other two. Brain tissue methotrexate levels were studied in two patients and were highest near the tumor bed; lower levels were identified throughout the brain. Studies on systemic tumors are also limited. In a study of intratumoral oil bleomycin vs. intravenous (IV) bleomycin for treatment of head and neck tumors,[29] tissue concentrations of bleomycin were much higher in intratumorally treated patients than in IV-treated patients.

In addition, high levels of bleomycin were found in regional lymph nodes 3 weeks after intratumoral treatment. Another study in intra-abdominal tumors[30] demonstrated varying amounts of methylene blue in tumors injected at the time of surgery, depending on the consistency of the tissue and the amount of necrosis.

PRECLINICAL STUDIES

Tator and colleagues[22–24] performed the first series of experimental investigations of intratumoral chemotherapy using a murine intracerebral ependymoblastoma model. Escalating doses of intratumoral methotrexate were ineffective, and high doses were associated with significant neurotoxic effects, including convulsions and death.[22, 23] Intratumoral CCNU was less toxic than intraperitoneal (IP) CCNU, and a single intratumoral dose of 40 mg/kg was highly effective in increasing survival.[24] Intratumorally administered agents may also augment the activity of systemically administered chemotherapy, although the mechanisms responsible are poorly defined. Using the murine ependymoblastoma model, Muller and Tator[31] demonstrated increased efficacy of IP administered CCNU in mice pretreated with intratumorally administered amphotericin B, a membrane-active polyene, compared with mice pretreated with IP administered amphotericin B.

Kroin and Penn[11] studied the distribution of cisplatin following chronic intracerebral infusion in a rat model; they used small stainless steel cannulas connected to a subcutaneous pump system and applied this technique to a rat brain tumor model using cisplatin or fluorouracil.[21] The median survival of rats treated with cisplatin or fluorouracil by continuous infusion was extended to 19 and 28 days, respectively, compared with 15 days in a control group of rats injected with saline.

In a study by Zeller and colleagues[26] of mice subcutaneously implanted with T 406 human glioblastoma xenografts, intratumoral administration of three alkyllysophospholipid derivatives produced tumor regression.

Using a 9L gliosarcoma rat model,[25] Vats and colleagues applied intratumoral bleomycin at weekly doses of 1.5 mg/kg and produced longer survivals than with IV bleomycin at weekly doses of 1.5 or 2.5 mg/kg; larger intratumoral doses were associated with drug-related toxic effects and death. Using the same model, Kimler and others[20] studied the effects of IV, IP, and intratumorally administered BCNU, bleomycin, aziridinyl benzoquinone, cisplatin, and acivicin. The activity of IV carmustine and intratumoral bleomycin was confirmed. Intratumoral, but not IP or IV, aziridinyl benzoquinone was effective in increasing mean survival to 35 days compared with 26 days in control animals. Intratumoral chemotherapy with cisplatin at higher doses was associated with severe neurologic toxic effects, as well as with a decreased mean survival compared with controls. However, at lower doses, an increase in survival over the controls was noted. Acivicin failed to improve mean survival when it was given IP or intratumorally.

Morantz and associates[12] treated 9L tumors in Fischer 344 rats with intratumoral bleomycin at doses of 0.1 to 5.0 mg/kg, and compared this method to systemic administration.

The greatest median survival (29 days) was observed with an intratumoral bleomycin dose of 1.0 mg/kg, as compared with 19 days in control animals injected with saline. However, a statistically significant increase in survival over that of rats treated with IP bleomycin (25 mg/kg) was not observed. Intratumoral doses of 5 mg/kg produced seizures in all rats within hours of administration. These studies demonstrated that intratumoral bleomycin enhanced the survival of rats treated with carmustine at a dose of 12 mg/kg IP, an improvement over results observed with bleomycin or carmustine.

CLINICAL STUDIES

A summary of selected clinical experiences with intratumoral chemotherapy is presented in Table 47–1. The reports are uncontrolled and involve relatively small patient numbers. In addition, results are not statistically controlled for other known prognostic factors, such as age, Karnofsky scale status, tumor grade, and prior or concomitant therapy.

After initial characterization in guinea pigs of the toxic effects produced by intracerebral application of sponges soaked with investigational chemotherapeutic agents, Heppner and Diemath[3] performed one of the early studies of intratumoral chemotherapy for the treatment of human brain tumors. Following maximum surgical cytoreduction in 41 patients with a variety of primary brain tumors (primarily high-grade astrocytomas), cyclophosphamide at a dose of 100 to 200 mg proved to be the best of several experimental compounds when instilled in the tumor bed in single doses. Furthermore, the procedure was accomplished with acceptable levels of toxic effects.

Ringkjob[14] treated 40 patients with newly diagnosed and recurrent brain tumors, (32 high-grade astrocytomas), by implanting Surgicel embedded with fluorouracil, with or without a methylenhydrazine derivative, following tumor resection. Five patients had a catheter placed in the tumor for repeated treatments. Other than two patients in whom edema and focal brain softening with hemorrhage occurred, the treatment was well tolerated. However, outcomes were uniformly poor, with no appreciable treatment effect.

Weiss and Raskind[16] treated nine patients (seven with glioblastoma, one with neuroblastoma, one with meningeal carcinomatosis) with methotrexate by means of an Ommaya reservoir placed into the tumor bed at surgery. Doses were repeated every 5 days. Toxic response was limited to transient neutropenia in two patients. Postoperative survival ranged from 12 hours to 10 months. Garfield and Dayan[9] treated nine patients with newly diagnosed, subtotally resected tumors (eight with gliomas, one with metastasis) using intratumoral chemotherapy with methotrexate and folinic acid; however, no benefit was shown. These investigators later treated 10 patients with newly diagnosed supratentorial high-grade gliomas (Kernohan's grade III and IV) with repeated injections of carmustine through a catheter implanted into the tumor bed following subtotal or gross total resection.[10] Total carmustine doses ranged from 200 to 1,050 mg and were given in 100- to 300-mg increments every 2 to 3 days; no patient received concomitant radiotherapy. In seven patients, treatment was complicated by signs of acute increased intracranial pressure and/or worsening of focal neurologic deficits. These complications were transient and reversible in five patients; serious neurologic deterioration occurred in two. This effect was presumed to be due to the volume of fluid injected (10 to 200 mL). Staphylococcal ventriculitis developed in one patient; no renal, hepatic, or hematologic toxic effects were noted. Survival ranged from 1 week to 199 weeks (mean, 44 weeks) from the initial surgery.

Bosch and co-workers[5] treated three newly diagnosed high-grade astrocytomas (Kernohan's grade III or IV) with intratumoral bleomycin via an indwelling catheter following stereotactic biopsy. Five milligrams of bleomycin was administered over 5 hours every 2 days for a total of three treatments. In one patient, a sudden increase in intracranial pressure developed that required surgical debulking, and the patient died of tumor progression 5 months later. The second patient died at 3 months owing to tumor progression. The third patient was alive 2 years post-treatment and had received a second course of treatment at 1 year.

Using an Ommaya reservoir placed into the tumor bed following maximal resection, Morantz and associates[12] evaluated intratumoral bleomycin administration in eight patients

TABLE 47–1
SELECTED CLINICAL REPORTS USING INTRATUMORAL CHEMOTHERAPY IN BRAIN TUMORS

Drug	Delivery	No. of Patients	Response	Toxic Effects	Reference
Cyclophosphamide	Chemotherapy-soaked sponges	41	Unclear	None	3
Fluorouracil	Surgicel	40	No effect	None	14
Methotrexate	Ommaya reservoir	9	Unclear	Transient neutropenia in 2	16
	Catheter	9	None	None	9
	Continuous infusion by catheter	5	No responses	Necrosis at autopsy	13
BCNU	Catheter	10	Possible	Infection; intracranial pressure, 7	10
Bleomycin	Catheter	3	Possible	Intracranial pressure, 1	5
	Ommaya reservoir	8	Unclear	Intracranial pressure	12
Cisplatin	Multiple catheters	3	Minimum survival 6 mo	None	7
Nitrosoureas	Catheter and basket device	20	Average survival 15–17 mo	Necrosis, cranial nerve deficits	15

with recurrent malignant brain tumors. Bleomycin, 2.5 to 10 mg, was injected weekly for 6 weeks, followed by a 4-week rest. Patients received between three and 30 treatments. Headache and vomiting developed in one patient 3 days following injection; this was attributed to cerebral edema. All other patients tolerated the treatments well, with no pulmonary toxic effects observed.

Using 10- to 14-day intratumoral infusions of cisplatin through multiple implanted catheters, Bouvier and colleagues[7] treated three patients with recurrent malignant glioma without performing additional resection. No significant systemic toxic response was noted, and minimum survival was 6 months.

Yamashima and colleagues[15] used intratumoral nitrosoureas to treat 20 patients with malignant gliomas. Thirteen patients received ACNU, and seven received MCNU via an Ommaya reservoir connected to a Silastic catheter and basket device in the tumor cavity. Toxic effects included cerebral edema (which appeared more often with MCNU than with ACNU), focal brain necrosis adjacent to the basket device, cranial nerve deficits associated with pathologically verified demyelination, and hemiparesis associated with narrowing of the anterior cerebral artery. Toxic effects were more common when baskets either were placed near a ventricle or communicated with a cistern. Patients survived an average of 15.3 months following ACNU and 17.1 months following MCNU.

Nierenberg and co-workers[13] treated five recurrent glioblastoma patients with escalating doses of methotrexate by continuous intratumoral infusion via an implanted ventricular catheter and continuous infusion pump. Patients survived from 7 to 49 weeks, but no clinical or radiographic responses were observed. No patient manifested clinical signs of methotrexate neurotoxic effects. Autopsies in four patients revealed liquefactive necrosis, but neither necrotizing leukoencephalopathy nor mineralizing microangiopathy was present.

DISCUSSION

Although intratumoral chemotherapy for malignant gliomas has been in clinical use for nearly 30 years, experience remains limited to small, uncontrolled series. Preclinical data suggest superiority over systemically administered chemotherapy, and available clinical data reveal a surprising lack of local toxic effects. However, several factors have tempered enthusiasm for this mode of chemotherapy delivery; therefore, intratumoral chemotherapy has not been evaluated in large clinical trials. Adequate drug delivery to the peripheral advancing edge of the neoplasm is perhaps the greatest limitation, particularly in diffusely infiltrating or multicentric neoplasms. In addition, intratumoral chemotherapy by definition requires a surgical procedure. Relatively few quantitative data are available for any of the agents regarding diffusion from the tumor or the tumor cavity into the surrounding brain, extracellular fluid, and CSF. Because of small numbers in available clinical trials to date, it is difficult to determine the frequency and spectrum of potential complications of prolonged local exposure of surrounding normal brain to the chemotherapeutic agents.

The limited effectiveness of this modality has raised questions about the logic of application of this technique in future trials. However, it should be noted that most studies have been performed in patients with recurrent, largely unresponsive tumors, and have used agents of marginal efficacy. The potential advantages of this method, including increased drug concentration at the tumor site, avoidance of the blood-brain barrier, delivery of drug to avascular areas of tumor, and minimization of systemic toxic effects, suggest that further research utilizing new agents is warranted. It is theoretically possible that the most practical application of intratumoral chemotherapy will be for delivery of agents that produce high levels of systemic (e.g., hematologic) toxic effects; intratumoral chemotherapy could potentially allow the use of multiple agents that, if administered in combination systemically, would produce unacceptable toxic effects. In addition, patients with multifocal or diffusely invasive disease could potentially receive intratumoral chemotherapy to the most symptomatic site in addition to one or more concomitant systemically administered agents for the invasive disease component. Potentially, intratumoral chemotherapy might allow selective chemoradiosensitization of tumor cells and spare adjacent uninvolved brain parenchyma.

Future research investigations of intratumoral chemotherapy via prospective trials involving larger patient cohorts should adequately define the diffusion characteristics in the tumor and the surrounding brain, improve the drug delivery systems, and quantify the activity and toxic effects of the therapeutic agents.

REFERENCES

1. Hochberg FH, Pruit A: Assumptions in the radiotherapy of glioblastomas. Neurology 1980; 30:907–911.
2. Bateman JC: Palliation of cancer in human patients by maintenance therapy with NN′N′-triethylene thiophosphoramide and N-(3-oxapentamethylene)-N′N′′-diethylene phosporamide. Ann NY Acad Sci 1958; 68:1057–1071.
3. Heppner F, Diemath HE: Local chemotherapy of brain tumors. Acta Neurochir 1963; 11:287–293.
4. Avellanosa A, West C, Barua N, et al: Intracavitary combination chemotherapy of recurrent malignant glioma via Ommaya shunt: A pilot study. Proc Am Soc Clin Oncol 1984; 2:234.
5. Bosch DA, Hindmarsch T, Larsson S: Intraneoplastic administration of bleomycin in intracerebral gliomas: A pilot study. Acta Neurochir 1980; 30(suppl):441–444.
6. Bouvier G, Penn RD, Kroin JS, et al: Intratumoral chemotherapy with multiple sources. Ann NY Acad Sci 1988; 531:213–214.
7. Bouvier G, Penn R, Kroin JS, et al: Stereotactic administration of intratumoral chemotherapy of recurrent malignant gliomas. Appl Neurophysiol 1987; 50:223–226.
8. Bouvier G, Penn RD, Kroin JS, et al: Direct delivery of medication into a brain tumor through multiple chronically implanted catheters. Neurosurgery 1987; 20:286–291.
9. Garfield J, Dayan AD: Postoperative intracavitary chemotherapy of malignant gliomas: A preliminary study using methotrexate. J Neurosurg 1973; 39:315–322.
10. Garfield J, Dayan AD, Weller RO: Post-operative intracavitary chemotherapy of malignant supratentorial astrocytomas using BCNU. Clin Oncol 1975; 1:213–222.
11. Kroin JS, Penn RD: Intracerebral chemotherapy: Chronic microinfusion of cisplatin. Neurosurgery 1982; 10:349–354.
12. Morantz RA, Kimler BF, Vats TS, et al: Bleomycin and brain tumors: A review. J Neurooncol 1983; 1:249–255.
13. Nierenberg D, Harbaugh R, Maurer LH, et al: Continuous intratumoral

infusion of methotrexate for recurrent glioblastoma: A pilot study. Neurosurgery 1991; 28:752–761.

14. Ringkjob R: Treatment of intracranial gliomas and metastatic carcinomas by local application of cytostatic agents. Acta Neurol Scand 1968; 44:318–322.
15. Yamashima T, Yamashita J, Shoin K: Neurotoxicity of local administration of two nitrosoureas in malignant gliomas. Neurosurgery 1990; 26:794–800.
16. Weiss SR, Raskind R: Treatment of malignant brain tumors by local methotrexate: A preliminary report. Int Surg 1969; 51:150–155.
17. Hoshino T, Barker M, Wilson CB, et al: Cell kinetics of human gliomas. J Neurosurg 1972; 37:15–26.
18. Levin VA, Patlak CS, Landahl HD: Heuristic modeling of drug delivery to malignant tumors. J Pharmacokinet Biopharm 1980; 8:257–296.
19. Rall DP, Zubrod CG: Mechanisms of drug absorption and excretion: Passage of drugs in and out of the central nervous system. Ann Rev Pharmacol 1962; 2:109–128.
20. Kimler BF, Liu C, Evans RG, et al: Intracerebral chemotherapy in the 9L rat brain tumor model. J Neurooncol 1992; 14:191–200.
21. Penn RD, Kroin JS, Harris JE, et al: Chronic intratumoral chemotherapy of a rat tumor with cisplatin and fluorouracil. Appl Neurophysiol 1983; 46:240–244.
22. Tator CH, Wassenaar W, Day A, et al: Therapy of an experimental glioma with systemic or intraneoplastic methotrexate or radiation. J Neurosurg 1977; 46:175–184.
23. Tator CH, Wassenaar W: Intraneoplastic injection of methotrexate for experimental brain tumor chemotherapy. J Neurosurg 1977; 46:165–174.
24. Tator CH: Intraneoplastic injection of CCNU for experimental brain tumor chemotherapy. Surg Neurol 1977; 7:73–77.
25. Vats TS, Morantz RA, Wood GW, et al: Study of effectiveness of bleomycin in rat brain tumor model intravenously and intracerebrally. Int J Radiat Oncol Biol Phys 1979; 5:1527–1529.
26. Zeller WJ, Bauer S, Remmele T, et al: Interstitial chemotherapy of experimental gliomas. Cancer Treat Rev 1990; 17:183–189.
27. Ommaya AK, Rubin RC, Henderson ES, et al: A new approach to the treatment of inoperable brain tumors. Med Ann DC 1965; 34:455–458.
28. Rubin RC, Ommaya AK, Henderson ES, et al: Cerebrospinal fluid perfusion for central nervous system neoplasms. Neurology 1966; 16:680–691.
29. Marincic D: Bleomycin in oliger Suspension und lokoregionare Kombinationstherapie der augedenhnten Plaatenepithelkarzinome im ORL-Berieic. Beitr Onkol 1982; 12:63–68.
30. Livraghi T, Bajetta E, Matricardi L, et al: Fine needle percutaneous intratumoral chemotherapy under ultrasound guidance: A feasibility study. Tumori 1986; 72:81–87.
31. Muller PJ, Tator CH: The effect of amphotericin B on the survival of brain-tumor-bearing mice treated with CCNU. J Neurosurg 1978; 49:579–588.

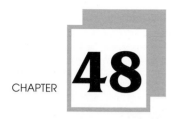

48

Hyperosmolar Disruption of the Blood-Brain Barrier as a Chemotherapy Potentiator in the Treatment of Brain Tumors

Several observations have been cited as evidence that the blood-brain barrier reduces the effectiveness of chemotherapy drugs against brain tumors, and some authors have proposed that the use of agents to transiently disrupt the blood-brain barrier during chemotherapy might augment chemotherapy uptake into and activity against brain tumors. In this chapter, the role of the blood-brain barrier in brain tumor chemotherapy is discussed, as are the prospects of blood-brain barrier disruption as an adjunct to brain tumor chemotherapy.

Most chemotherapy drugs penetrate poorly into the normal central nervous system (CNS) due to the blood-brain barrier and blood–cerebrospinal fluid (CSF) barrier.[1] As a result, opposition has often been put forth to the testing in brain tumor patients of antineoplastic agents that did not readily cross the intact blood-brain barrier, as it was assumed that they would be ineffective due to poor penetration into brain tumors.

The blood-brain barrier is usually disrupted to a variable degree in intracranial tumor deposits.[2–4] Despite this, many clinicians feel that it is important in the treatment of human brain tumors. In arguing for a role of the blood-brain barrier, they point out that the intratumor disruption of the blood-brain barrier may be incomplete, that it may be variable from one part of the tumor to another, and that the degree of blood-brain barrier disruption is considerably less in the brain adjacent to tumor (where one can readily find viable tumor cells) than it is within the tumor itself.

INHOMOGENEITY OF BLOOD-BRAIN BARRIER INTEGRITY IN TUMORS

Animal studies have demonstrated that blood-brain barrier disruption may vary both within and between brain

tumors,[2, 5] and that distribution of some chemotherapy drugs in brain tumors is less homogeneous than it is in subcutaneous tumors,[5, 6] possibly as a result of inhomogeneous disruption of the blood-brain barrier within the brain tumor. Certainly, inhomogeneous distribution of a variety of antineoplastic agents in human brain tumors has been reported.[1] However, this has occurred with agents that readily cross the blood-brain barrier to as great an extent as with agents that do not cross it,[1] and in human and large animal tumors, drug distribution also varies within and between extracerebral tumor deposits.[7–10] Moreover, this author has found average tumor chemotherapy concentrations to be comparable in intracranial and extracranial tumors for a variety of drugs that penetrate poorly across the intact blood-brain barrier.[1] The fact that average drug concentrations are comparable in human intracranial and extracranial tumors strongly suggests that the degree of variability of drug distribution is also comparable in intracranial vs. extracranial tumors: if brain tumors had more areas of low drug concentrations than did extracerebral tumors, then they would also need more areas of unusually high drug concentrations to maintain the same average drug concentration. If brain tumors did have an augmented degree of variability in drug distribution, with areas of unusually low drug concentrations, it would be difficult to explain how they would also have the areas of unusually high drug concentrations that would be needed to maintain an average drug concentration comparable to that in extracranial tumors.

BRAIN ADJACENT TO TUMOR

Some authors have argued that the major problem is with inadequate penetration of drug into the brain adjacent to tumor. Large numbers of tumor cells may be found in the brain adjacent to tumor, but the blood-brain barrier is more intact and capillary permeability and chemotherapy concentrations are lower than in the tumor itself.[2, 5, 11, 12] However, little evidence exists that tumor progression with chemotherapy occurs more frequently in brain adjacent to tumor than in the tumor itself. Moreover, local blood-brain barrier leakiness may be induced by very small numbers of tumor cells,[13] raising the possibility that chemotherapy exposure of tumor cells in the brain adjacent to tumor could far exceed that of most nonneoplastic cells in the brain adjacent to tumor. As with the blood-brain barrier itself, it remains uncertain whether the brain adjacent to tumor significantly limits the effectiveness of chemotherapy against brain tumors.

BLOOD-BRAIN BARRIER AND DRUG UPTAKE AND EFFICACY IN ANIMAL BRAIN TUMORS

Several observations in animal studies of brain tumor therapy have been interpreted as being supportive of an important role of the blood-brain barrier in limiting uptake of lipid-insoluble drugs into brain tumors. A variety of animal studies have reported reduced chemotherapy concentrations,[5, 6, 14, 15] capillary permeability,[5] and anti-tumor efficacy[16–24] in intracranial tumors compared with extracranial tumors. In addition, within classes of antineoplastic agents, efficacy in rodent brain tumors varies with lipid solubility.[23, 24] Several problems arise, however, with the interpretation of these observations.[1] First, differences in drug concentrations have not been found in all studies comparing animal intracranial and extracranial tumors.[25] Second, chemotherapy concentrations in animal intracranial tumors have generally been compared only with those in subcutaneous tumor deposits, and subcutaneous tumors may not be comparable to those in other extracranial sites; for example, soft tissue (i.e., subcutaneous and lymph node) metastases in human cancers often respond better to chemotherapy than do metastases to other extracranial sites,[26–28] which implies that they may also achieve higher drug concentrations than do other extracranial metastases. Moreover, in animal studies, tumor deposits in different extracranial locations also vary in chemotherapy responsiveness[16, 29] and uptake,[29, 30] and chemotherapy agents that penetrate relatively poorly into the CNS are, nevertheless, active against murine brain tumors.[31] Furthermore, lipid-soluble chemotherapy agents (which should easily enter the CNS) are, in some cases, more effective against extracranial than intracranial tumors.[19] At the same time, within a class of chemotherapy drugs, efficacy against brain tumors does not vary directly with lipid solubility,[23] and the optimal lipid solubility for brain tumor therapy differs among classes of chemotherapy agents[23, 24] and among different types of intracranial tumors.[23] Hence, other events clearly occur, besides blood-brain barrier phenomena, that might explain any differences between intracranial and extracranial tumors with respect to chemotherapy uptake and efficacy.

Other potential explanations include the fact that cell membrane characteristics may differ for intracranial and extracranial tumor cells,[32, 33] that intrinsic tumor cell chemo-

sensitivity may vary with tumor site,[34–36] that specific clones of tumor cells (possibly with different drug sensitivities) metastasize preferentially to brain or other specific organs,[37–39] and that the local organ milieu may affect tumor growth characteristics.[40] A number of potentially important methodological differences in treatment of animals with intracranial vs. extracranial tumors have also complicated interpretation of comparisons of drug uptake and efficacy.[1]

BLOOD-BRAIN BARRIER AND CHEMOTHERAPY EFFICACY AGAINST HUMAN BRAIN TUMORS

Clinical observations have also been interpreted as supporting a role of the blood-brain barrier in brain tumor therapy. For example, both acute leukemia[41] and small cell lung cancer[42] often recur in the CNS before they do so at other sites. However, several factors argue against this being a function of the blood-brain barrier.[1] First, chemotherapy that readily penetrates into the CNS has little effect on the rate of CNS recurrence.[42–45] Second, effective CNS prophylaxis has had minimal (if any) impact on survival in small cell lung cancer[46–49] or in most studies of acute leukemia.[50–52] Third, several sites besides brain may house isolated surviving deposits of small cell lung cancer[53] and acute leukemia cells[54–56] following chemotherapy. Fourth, isolated brain recurrences are very uncommon in several other malignancies in which chemotherapy that does not readily cross the blood-brain barrier either results in cure or increases the long-term survival rate when given as adjuvant treatment with surgery or radiation. This is true for acute myelogenous leukemia, diffuse large cell lymphoma, Hodgkin's disease, gestational choriocarcinoma, embryonal rhabdomyosarcoma, Wilms' tumor, Ewing's sarcoma, osteogenic sarcoma, and carcinomas of the testicle, ovary, breast, and colon. Although postoperative adjuvant chemotherapy of non–small cell lung cancer with the blood-brain barrier–excluded agents cyclophosphamide, doxorubicin, and cisplatin does not substantially increase survival times, it does result in a reduction in brain metastases that is comparable to the reduction in metastases to other organs.[57] Fifth, blood-brain barrier–excluded agents are active in the treatment of brain metastases from breast cancer,[58, 59] small cell lung cancer,[60, 61] and non–small cell lung cancer.[61, 62] Sixth, in lung and breast cancer patients treated with blood-brain barrier–excluded chemotherapy, survival times[28, 63–70] and tumor response rates[71, 72] are not significantly different in patients with brain metastases at the time of diagnosis than in those with metastases to most other organs.

The resistance of primary CNS lymphomas[73] and glioblastomas to chemotherapy has also been blamed on limitation of drug uptake by the blood-brain barrier. However, as is the case with brain metastases, this interpretation is fraught with a number of problems.[1] A number of chemotherapy agents or regimens are capable of causing regression of CNS lymphomas[74, 75] and gliomas[76–90] despite poor penetration across the blood-brain barrier. Moreover, primary CNS lymphomas are more resistant to radiotherapy[73, 91–93] than are extracranial lymphomas,[94] and glioblastomas are among the most radioresistant of malignancies. Hence, one does not need to invoke the putative impenetrability of the blood-brain to explain the resistance of these neoplasms to chemotherapy: they appear to be intrinsically resistant to cytotoxic therapy. This conclusion is supported by the observation that glioblastomas are more resistant to chemotherapy than are lower-grade gliomas,[95–97] despite more extensive disruption of the blood-brain barrier in glioblastomas.[98–103]

UPTAKE OF ANTINEOPLASTIC AGENTS INTO HUMAN BRAIN TUMORS

Further questions have been raised regarding the role of the blood-brain barrier in brain tumor chemotherapy by the observation of both this author[1] and others[104–113] that a variety of chemotherapy agents attain potentially cytotoxic concentrations in human brain tumors, despite achieving only low concentrations in the normal CNS. In fact, drug concentrations attained in human brain tumors bear no discernible relationship to those found in normal brain and CSF, and for the majority of drugs tested, concentrations in brain tumors are comparable to those in extracranial tumors.[1]

Should the blood-brain barrier be taken into consideration when choosing new therapies to investigate in the treatment of brain tumors? In answering this question, it must be borne in mind that some drugs that do not cross the blood-brain barrier are active against brain tumors, and that placing undue emphasis on the importance of the blood-brain barrier has probably excessively delayed and biased the investigation in brain tumor therapy of some promising new agents.[1] Furthermore, complete elimination of the blood-brain barrier within a tumor would not make a non-cytotoxic drug active, and a highly cytotoxic agent might only have to achieve low concentrations in a tumor to prove effective. Nevertheless, for agents or regimens that are only moderately cytotoxic, it is possible that residual barrier elements within brain tumors could make the difference between therapeutic success and failure. Hence, although promising new agents should be tested against brain tumors irrespective of whether they cross the intact blood-brain barrier, it remains possible that strategies designed to increase penetration of drugs across the blood-brain barrier could result in augmentation of efficacy.

BLOOD-BRAIN BARRIER STRUCTURE

The blood-brain barrier is formed by the endothelial cells that line brain capillaries. These capillary endothelial cells have relatively few fenestrations and pinocytotic vesicles, and have relatively tight intercellular junctions compared with those of endothelial cells that line the capillaries in most other organs. The endothelial cell basement membrane and astrocytic foot processes probably also contribute to the structure of the blood-brain barrier. In addition to these physical factors, there is probably also a biochemical component to the blood-brain barrier: for example, brain capillary endothelial cells are very rich in P-glycoprotein, a membrane pump that is capable of actively pumping back out various organic substances (including many chemotherapy agents) after they have gained entry to the cell.[114] Tumor cell membrane P-glycoprotein is thought to be an important mechanism by which many cancers are resistant to several chemotherapy agents.[114] P-Glycoprotein also probably helps protect some types of normal cells from various toxins, and it may also perform other physiologic functions.[114]

Blood vessel structure is often very abnormal within brain tumors, and this is partially responsible for the breakdown of the blood-brain barrier that is often seen in tumors.[13, 99–101] In addition, tumor cells produce a diffusible substance that is capable of making local blood vessels leaky.[115] Only a very small number of tumor cells are required to make adjacent vessels leaky.[13]

THERAPEUTIC DISRUPTION OF THE BLOOD-BRAIN BARRIER

Methodology

As noted previously, the degree of blood-brain barrier disruption in tumors can vary both between tumors and within tumors.[2, 5] If one wished to further disrupt the blood-brain barrier one might explore several mechanisms. The topic of therapeutic disruption of the blood-brain barrier has been reviewed in detail.[116] Examples of factors that may transiently disrupt the blood-brain barrier in normal brain include intracarotid infusion of various substances such as mannitol,[14, 117] arabinose,[117] dehydrocholate,[118] and etoposide.[119]

Most therapeutic trials of blood-brain barrier disruption in patients with brain tumors have been conducted with the hyperosmolar agent mannitol. It is hypothesized that a bolus intracarotid infusion of a hyperosmolar agent results in rapid diffusion of fluid across endothelial cell membranes out of endothelial cells into the more hyperosmolar vascular lumen. The resultant sudden shrinkage of the endothelial cells results in a pulling apart of endothelial tight intercellular junctions, thereby rendering the blood-brain barrier leaky in the distribution of the artery receiving the intracarotid mannitol.[120] For the mannitol to be effective in transiently disrupting the blood-brain barrier, the intracarotid infusion must be very rapid.[120] Infusion of the mannitol into the internal carotid artery results in more consistent blood-brain barrier disruption than does infusion into the larger common carotid artery.[121] Vertebral artery infusions result in blood-brain barrier disruption in the area of the posterior circulation.[122] One may monitor and confirm the degree of blood-brain barrier disruption following intra-arterial mannitol infusion by performing contrast-enhanced CT scans,[123, 124] or radionuclide scans,[125, 126] following the disruption procedure. Such studies in animals[124] and humans[125, 126] suggest that in a high proportion of cases, the blood-brain barrier is extensively disrupted in the area of distribution of the artery. Some studies also suggest increased contrast or radionuclide delivery to the tumor itself.[126] The blood-brain barrier disruption is rapid in onset and is fully reversible after a period of about 30 minutes to 2 hours.[120, 124]

EFFECT OF HYPEROSMOLAR BLOOD-BRAIN BARRIER DISRUPTION ON DRUG UPTAKE

With this transient blood-brain barrier disruption, it is generally agreed that penetration of the chemotherapy agent methotrexate into normal ipsilateral brain[127, 128] and brain adjacent to tumor is increased.[127] An increase may also occur in penetration of methotrexate into contralateral brain[121] and CSF.[128, 129] (Augmentation of CSF concentrations of some high-molecular-weight compounds is greater with vertebral artery mannitol infusion than with carotid artery mannitol infusion.[129]) Intracarotid mannitol may also result in a significant increase in brain tumor methotrexate concentration, but the enhancement of uptake into tumor is less than in the surrounding brain.[14, 127, 130, 131] Because the blood-brain barrier is already partially disrupted in brain tumors, the extent of further disruption by intracarotid mannitol is less in tumors than in normal brain.[132] Because hyperosmolar blood-brain barrier disruption augments uptake of methotrexate and other substances to a greater extent in brain tissue than in intracranial tumors, some authors have questioned whether this procedure would result in a favorable therapeutic index.[130–132]

Intra-arterial mannitol has also been demonstrated to increase uptake of bleomycin,[133] fluorouracil,[133] doxorubicin,[134] and various monoclonal antibodies[129, 135–137] (but not cyclophosphamide[133]) into normal brain tissue. Effect on uptake into intracranial tumor has also been tested for one monoclonal antibody: intracarotid mannitol infusion resulted in a modest augmentation of antibody uptake into the tumor.[137] As with methotrexate, the effect on uptake into tumor was much less than the effect on uptake into normal brain and brain adjacent to tumor.

As the blood-brain barrier is already largely disrupted in brain tumors, does any other mechanism exist by which intracarotid mannitol might augment tumor drug uptake than blood-brain barrier disruption? This question has not been investigated thoroughly. First, might the mannitol exert a concentration-dependent effect at the level of the tumor cell membrane to augment drug uptake? This could be tested in vitro. Second, might the intra-arterial mannitol exert a vascular effect that is independent of the blood-brain barrier itself, or could it alter the tumor interstitium to facilitate drug diffusion? These possible alternate explanations are important because if they proved to be correct, it might also be the case that intra-arterial mannitol augments drug uptake into localized extracranial tumors as well as into brain tumors. This could be easily tested in animal models. Although *intracarotid* mannitol did not augment uptake of a monoclonal antibody into a subcutaneous tumor,[137] local drug uptake has not been tested after infusion of mannitol into an artery supplying a tumor in an extracranial site.

HYPEROSMOLAR BLOOD-BRAIN BARRIER DISRUPTION AND CHEMOTHERAPY NEUROTOXIC EFFECTS

Somewhat limiting the potential therapeutic applicability of hyperosmolar blood-brain barrier disruption is the fact that with some important chemotherapy agents, neurologic toxic effects are substantially augmented if the blood-brain barrier is disrupted. This is true for cisplatin, bleomycin, fluorouracil,[133] and doxorubicin.[134] However, animal and clinical studies suggest that it is relatively safe to use hyperosmolar blood-brain barrier disruption with methotrexate, procarbazine,[125, 126] cyclophosphamide,[125, 126] carboplatin, etoposide,[138] and monoclonal antibodies.[136] In clinical studies of some of the latter agents, sequential neuropsychological testing has failed to reveal any significant long-term toxic effects in the majority of patients.[139] However, transient neurologic deterioration and seizures are common during and immediately after the blood-brain barrier disruption procedure: 10% to 30% of patients have transient neurologic deterioration, 7% to 50% suffer seizures in the peritreatment period, and about 7% to 14% have permanent neurologic sequelae, such as hemiparesis or hemiplegia.[125, 126, 139] Fatal neurologic toxic effects are uncommon, but they have been reported.[126]

HYPEROSMOLAR BLOOD-BRAIN BARRIER DISRUPTION AND CHEMOTHERAPY EFFICACY IN GLIOMAS

With respect to therapeutic efficacy, no randomized studies have compared outcome in patients with chemotherapy during hyperosmolar blood-brain barrier disruption to that with the same chemotherapy alone. However, median survival times of 17.5 to 21 months have been obtained in glioblastoma patients (most of whom had recurrent tumor following radiation) treated with blood-brain barrier disruption combined with intracarotid methotrexate, intravenous (IV) cyclophosphamide, and oral procarbazine.[125, 126] This is superior to the outcome in historical controls. In a small series, four of ten patients treated with this approach prior to cranial radiation also had a greater than 50% decrease in tumor volume on CT scan.[140]

In addition, in some cases, tumor has regressed in areas where blood-brain barrier disruption was documented to have occurred, while tumor simultaneously progressed in areas outside of the blood-brain barrier disruption.[141] Although the authors thought that the greater efficacy within the area of disruption was due to enhanced drug delivery made possible by the blood-brain barrier disruption, at least one other explanation is possible: the patients were receiving intra-arterial methotrexate as part of their therapy, and the distribution of the artery into which the methotrexate was infused would probably have matched the area of blood-brain barrier disruption. Hence, it is difficult to be certain whether the important component was the blood-brain barrier disruption or the intra-arterial administration of methotrexate.

Despite the animal evidence that hyperosmolar blood-brain barrier disruption would substantially augment neurotoxic effects of both fluorouracil and doxorubicin,[133, 134, 142] a study of intracarotid fluorouracil plus doxorubicin following blood-brain barrier disruption produced an acceptable level of toxic effects and somewhat encouraging therapeutic results in glioblastomas: of seven comatose patients who were treated, five became fully functional for a period of 3 to 12 months.[143] Because the rate of intracarotid mannitol infusion in this study was somewhat less than that thought to be required for optimal blood-brain barrier disruption,[120] it is possible that the blood-brain barrier disruption procedure had little to do with the therapeutic efficacy, and it is possible that the neurologic toxic effects would have been much greater in the presence of a greater degree of blood-brain barrier disruption. However, other studies using combinations of intra-arterial cisplatin, doxorubicin, and bleomycin or intra-arterial cisplatin plus cytarabine following blood-brain barrier disruption with a more rapid intracarotid mannitol infusion have also produced acceptable levels of toxic effects (20% incidence of transient neurologic deterioration and 3% incidence of seizures) and evidence of efficacy.[144]

Other studies in gliomas have combined intracarotid mannitol with intracarotid ACNU. In two studies, hyperosmolar blood-brain barrier disruption resulted in augmentation of human brain tumor ACNU concentrations.[145, 146] In studies using intracarotid diatrizoate meglumine (Renografin) in place of mannitol as a hyperosmolar agent, intracarotid carmustine (BCNU) and thiotepa were associated with moderate efficacy, with a mean survival time after recurrence of 41 weeks, and CT scan improvement in nine of ten patients.[147]

HYPEROSMOLAR BLOOD-BRAIN BARRIER DISRUPTION AND CHEMOTHERAPY EFFICACY IN OTHER TUMOR TYPES

In other tumor types, hyperosmolar blood-brain barrier disruption resulted in substantial antitumor activity when combined with intracarotid carboplatin and etoposide in the treatment of a small number of patients with CNS germinomas,[138, 148] primitive neuroectodermal tumors, and CNS lymphomas.[138] Patients with brain metastases and gliomas were also included in this series.

In primary CNS lymphomas, hyperosmolar blood-brain barrier disruption combined with intra-arterial methotrexate, IV cyclophosphamide, and oral procarbazine resulted in a 17.8-month median survival time when given after cranial radiation (which was comparable to that given in a historical control group), whereas the same chemotherapy administered initially (with subsequent radiation only for progression or recurrence) resulted in a median survival time of 44.5 months.[139] This survival time is longer than that of most other series of patients with CNS lymphomas. However, because there are no data on the efficacy of this chemotherapy regimen without hyperosmolar blood-brain barrier disruption, it is uncertain what role is played by the blood-brain barrier disruption. The same drug combination has also been tested in a small number of patients with brain metastases, with occasional evidence of therapeutic benefit.[149]

Hence, hyperosmolar blood-brain barrier disruption appears to have a reasonable safety profile with selected chemotherapy agents, and it substantially augments chemotherapy penetration into normal brain tissue and brain adjacent to tumor (where one may locate isolated viable tumor cells that may possibly be protected from chemotherapy by the blood-brain barrier). Hyperosmolar blood-brain barrier disruption may also augment uptake of some chemotherapy agents into brain tumors themselves, although because the blood-brain barrier is already largely disrupted in many brain tumors, the degree of augmentation of drug uptake is substantially less for tumors than it is for normal brain. Suggestive evidence also indicates that therapeutic efficacy of chemotherapy may be augmented for some chemotherapy regimens in the treatment of glioblastomas, primary CNS lymphomas, and CNS germinomas.

FUTURE DIRECTIONS

Despite its apparent promise, the technical complexity of hyperosmolar blood-brain barrier disruption demands that a number of questions be answered before hyperosmolar blood-brain barrier disruption is widely adopted in the treatment of brain tumors. Of paramount importance is the fact that little or no data have been gathered on the efficacy in comparable patient populations of the same chemotherapy regimens (intracarotid methotrexate with IV cyclophosphamide and oral procarbazine, or the intracarotid combination of etoposide and carboplatin) without intracarotid mannitol. Such data are essential. Randomized studies of identical chemotherapy regimens with vs. without intracarotid mannitol could be particularly helpful. Of some concern is a study in rats with transplantable intracerebral osteogenic sarcomas that showed reduced survival (possibly due to toxic effects) when IV or intracarotid methotrexate was combined with hyperosmolar blood-brain barrier disruption.[151]

If comparative studies in humans did confirm the therapeutic utility of hyperosmolar blood-brain barrier disruption, the next question would be whether the same outcome could be obtained more easily by administering higher doses of chemotherapy without blood-brain barrier disruption. For example, in the methotrexate, cyclophosphamide, procarbazine regimen, the total methotrexate dose is 2.5 to 5 g per course, whereas one may administer up to 25 g of methotrexate intravenously with proper attention to urine alkalinization, hydration, and folinic acid rescue. Similarly, the cyclophosphamide dose used is 600 to 1,200 mg/m² per course with blood-brain barrier disruption, whereas in other settings it is possible to use cyclophosphamide doses of up to 6,000 mg/m² as part of combination chemotherapy without requiring bone marrow transplantation.[150] In the intracarotid carboplatin plus etoposide regimen, doses of both drugs were 100 to 400 mg/m² per course. Intravenous etoposide doses of up to 1,500 mg/m² per course are tolerable.[150] Would hyperosmolar blood-brain barrier disruption regimens be superior to maximum tolerable chemotherapy doses administered without blood-brain barrier disruption? If not, which would be least toxic and easiest to administer?

As noted in the first section of this chapter, some pharmacologic questions can be added to the previous ones. Is drug distribution really less uniform or are drug concentrations really lower in brain tumors than in most extracranial tumors? Because very small numbers of tumor cells can induce leakiness in local blood vessels, are tumor cells in the brain adjacent to tumor and in normal-appearing brain really exposed to lower drug concentrations than are cells within the main body of the tumor? Finally, if hyperosmolar blood-brain barrier disruption does indeed prove to be advantageous, is it really due to disruption of the blood-brain barrier, or might the same methodology also prove useful for some locally advanced extracranial tumors?

It may be several years before these questions are answered. In the interim, the preliminary results with hyperosmolar blood-brain barrier disruption are sufficiently positive to justify continued investigation of this therapeutic modality.

REFERENCES

1. Stewart DJ: A critique of the role of the blood-brain barrier in the chemotherapy of human brain tumors. J Neurooncol 1994; 20:121–139.
2. Blasberg RG, Groothuis DR: Chemotherapy of brain tumors: Physiological and pharmacokinetic considerations. Semin Oncol 1986; 13:70–82.
3. Ushio Y, Posner J, Shapiro W: Chemotherapy of experimental meningeal carcinomatosis. Cancer Res 1977; 37:1232–1237.
4. Siegal T, Sandbank U, Gabizon A, et al: Alteration of blood-brain-CSF barrier in experimental meningeal carcinomatosis. J Neurooncol 1987; 4:233–242.
5. Groothuis DR, Fischer JM, Vick NA, et al: Comparative permeability of different glioma models to horseradish peroxidase. Cancer Treat Rep 1981; 65(suppl 2):13–18.
6. Tator CH: Retention of tritiated methotrexate in a transplantable mouse glioma. Cancer Res 1976; 36:3058–3066.
7. Rowe-Jones D: Cytotoxic penetration and concentration in human malignant tumors. Br J Surg 1969; 56:774–778.
8. Straw J, Hart M, Klubes P, et al: Distribution of anticancer agents in spontaneous animal tumors: I. Regional blood flow and methotrexate distribution in canine lymphosarcoma. JNCI 1974; 52:1327–1331.
9. Stewart DJ, Mikhael NZ, Nair RC, et al: Platinum concentrations in human autopsy tumor samples. Am J Clin Oncol 1988; 11:152–158.
10. Stewart DJ, Green RM, Mikhael NZ, et al: Human autopsy tissue concentrations of mitoxantrone. Cancer Treat Rep 1986; 70:1255–1261.
11. Levin VA: A pharmacologic basis for brain tumor chemotherapy. Semin Oncol 1975; 2:57–61.
12. Levin VA, Freeman-Dove W, Landahl HD: Permeability characteristics of brain adjacent to tumors in rats. Arch Neurol 1975; 32:785–791.
13. Stewart PA, Hayakawa K, Farrell CL, et al: Quantitative study of microvessel ultrastructure in human peritumoral brain tissue: Evidence for a blood-brain barrier defect. J Neurosurg 1987; 67:697–705.
14. Neuwelt EA, Frenkel EP, D'Agostino AN, et al: Growth of human lung tumor in the brain of the nude rat as a model to evaluate antitumor agent delivery across the blood-brain barrier. Cancer Res 1985; 45:2827–2833.
15. Levin VA, Clancy TP, Ausman JI, et al: Uptake and distribution of ³H-methotrexate by the murine ependymoblastoma. JNCI 1972; 48:875–883.
16. Wodinsky I, Merker PC, Venditti JM: Responsiveness to chemotherapy of mice with L1210 lymphoid leukemia implanted in various anatomic sites. JNCI 1977; 59:405–408.
17. Schabel FM Jr, Griswold DP Jr, Corbett TH, et al: Curative chemotherapy of advanced ²³⁹Pu-induced osteosarcoma (²³⁹PU OS) in mice with 2-β-D-ribofuranosylthiazole-4-carboxamide (T-CAR) and of advanced L1210 with T-CAR plus BCNU. Proc Am Assoc Cancer Res 1983; 24:265.
18. Chirigos MA, Humphreys SR, Goldin A: Duration of effective levels of three antitumor drugs in mice with leukemia L1210 implanted intracerebrally and subcutaneously. Cancer Chemother Rep 1965; 49:15–19.
19. Freidman HS, Schold SC Jr, Bigner DD: Chemotherapy of subcutaneous and intracranial human medulloblastoma xenografts in athymic nude mice. Cancer Res 1986; 46:224–228.
20. Merker PC, Wodinsky I, Geran RI: Review of selected experimental brain tumor models used in chemotherapy experiments. Cancer Chemother Rep 1975; 59:729–736.
21. Schabel FM Jr, Trader MW, Laster WR Jr, et al: Studies with 2,5-piperazinedione,3,6-bis(5-chloro-2-piperidyl)-dihydrochloride: III. Biochemical and therapeutic effects in L1210 leukemias sensitive and resistant to alkylating agents: Comparison with melphalan, cyclophosphamide, and BCNU. Cancer Treat Rep 1976; 60:1325–1333.
22. Shapiro WR: The chemotherapy of intracerebral vs subcutaneous murine gliomas: A comparative study of the effect of VM-26. Arch Neurol 1974; 30:222–226.
23. Levin VA, Kabra P: Effectiveness of the nitrosoureas as a function of their lipid solubility in the chemotherapy of experimental rat brain tumors. Cancer Chemother Rep 1974; 58:787–792.
24. Levin VA, Crafts D, Wilson CB, et al: Imidazole carboxamides: Relationship of lipophilicity to activity against intracerebral murine glioma 26 and preliminary phase II trial of 5-[3,3-bis(2-chloroethyl)-1-triazeno]imidazole-4-carboxamide (NSC-82196) in primary and secondary brain tumors. Cancer Chemother Rep 1975; 59:327–331.
25. Ushio Y, Hayakawa T, Mogami H: Uptake of tritiated methotrexate by mouse brain tumors after intravenous and intrathecal administration. J Neurosurg 1974; 40:706–716.
26. The French Epirubicin Study Group: A prospective randomized phase III trial comparing combination chemotherapy with cyclophosphamide, fluorouracil, and either doxorubicin or epirubicin. J Clin Oncol 1988; 6:679–688.
27. Henderson IC, Harris JR, Kinne DW, et al: Cancer of the breast: Identifying chemotherapy-responsive patients. In DeVita VT Jr, Hellman S, Rosenberg SA (eds): Cancer: Principles and Practice of Oncology, ed 3. Philadelphia, JB Lippincott, 1989.
28. Sorensen JB, Badsberg JH, Hansen HH: Response to cytostatic treatment in inoperable adenocarcinoma of the lung: Critical implications. Br J Cancer 1989; 60:389–393.
29. Donelli MG, Colombo T, Broggini M, et al: Differential distribution of antitumor agents in primary and secondary tumors. Cancer Treat Rep 1977; 61:1319–1324.
30. Broggini M, Colombo T, D'Incalci M: Activity and pharmacokinetics of teniposide in Lewis lung carcinoma-bearing mice. Cancer Treat Rep 1983; 67:555–559.
31. Mellet LB: Physicochemical considerations and pharmacokinetic behaviour in delivery of drugs to the central nervous system. Cancer Treat Rep 1977; 61:527–531.
32. Volpe JJ, Fujimota K, Marasa JC, et al: Relation of C-6 glial cells in culture to myelin. Biochem J 1975; 152:701–703.
33. Pfeiffer SE, Wechsler W: Biochemically differentiated neoplastic clone of Schwann cells. Proc Natl Acad Sci USA 1972; 69:2885–2889.
34. Zaffaroni N, Silvestrini R, Sanfilippo O, et al: Tumor heterogeneity: Analysis of the chemosensitivity of different tumor sites of the same patient. Proceedings of the 13th International Congress on Chemotherapy, Vienna, 1983, pp 143–146.
35. Tanigawa N, Mizuno Y, Hashimura T, et al: Comparison of drug sensitivity among tumor cells within a tumor, between primary tumor and metastases, and between different metastases in the human tumor colony-forming assay. Cancer Res 1984; 44:2309–2312.
36. Schlag P, Schreml W: Heterogeneity in growth pattern and drug sensitivity of primary tumor and metastases in the human tumor colony-forming assay. Cancer Res 1982; 42:4086–4089.
37. Talmadge J, Fuller I: Metastatic cancer and its biological heterogeneity. Rev Endocrine Rel Cancer 1982; 11:21–27.
38. Ro J, Ro JY, El-Nagger A, et al: Brain metastasis initial presentation of breast cancer: DNA flow cytometric comparison of two sites. Breast Dis 1990; 3:35–38.
39. Nicolson G: Metastatic phenotypic diversity and brain metastasis. Cancer Bull 1986; 38:32–38.
40. Horak E, Darling DL, Tarin D: Analysis of organ-specific effects on metastatic tumor formation by studies in vitro. JNCI 1986; 76:913–922.
41. Aur RJA, Simone J, Hustu HO, et al: Central nervous system therapy and combination chemotherapy of childhood lymphocytic leukemia. Blood 1971; 37:272–281.
42. Aroney RS, Aisner J, Wesley MN, et al: Value of prophylactic cranial irradiation given at complete remission in small cell lung carcinoma. Cancer Treat Rep 1983; 67:675–682.
43. Nugent JL, Bunn PA Jr, Matthews MJ, et al: CNS metastases in small cell bronchogenic carcinoma: Increasing frequency and changing pattern with lengthening survival. Cancer 1979; 44:1885–1893.
44. Alexander M, Glatstein EJ, Gordon DJ, et al: Combined modality

treatment for oat cell carcinoma of the lung: A randomized trial. Cancer Treat Rep 1977; 61:1–6.

45. Hande KR, Oldham RK, Fer MF, et al: A randomized trial of high-dose (HD) vs low dose (LD) methotrexate (MTX) in the treatment of extensive stage small cell lung cancer. Proc Am Assoc Cancer Res Am Soc Clin Oncol 1981; 22:505.

46. Seydel HG, Creech R, Pagano M, et al: Prophylactic versus no brain irradiation in regional small cell lung carcinoma. Am J Clin Oncol 1985; 8:218–223.

47. Baglan RJ, Marks JE: Comparison of symptomatic and prophylactic irradiation of brain metastases from oat cell carcinoma of the lung. Cancer 1981; 47:41–45.

48. Komaki R: Prophylactic cranial irradiation for small cell carcinoma of the lung. Cancer Treat Symposia 1985; 2:35–39.

49. Maurer LH, Tulloh M, Weiss RB, et al: A randomized combined modality trial in small cell carcinoma of the lung. Cancer 1980; 45:30–39.

50. Muriel FS, Pavlovsky S, Penalver JA, et al: Evaluation of induction of remission, intensification, and central nervous system prophylactic treatment in acute lymphoblastic leukemia. Cancer 1974; 34:418–426.

51. Working Party on Leukemia in Childhood: Treatment of acute lymphoblastic leukemia: Effect of ''prophylactic'' therapy against central nervous system leukemia. Br Med J 1973; 2:381–384.

52. Nesbit ME, Sather H, Robison LL, et al: Sanctuary therapy: A randomized trial of 724 children with previously untreated acute lymphoblastic leukemia. A report from Childrens Cancer Study Group. Cancer Res 1982; 42:674–680.

53. Lininger TR, Fleming TR, Eagen RT: Evaluation of alternating chemotherapy and sites and extent of disease in extensive small cell lung cancer. Cancer 1981; 48:2147–2153.

54. Nies BA, Bodey GP, Thomas LB, et al: The persistence of extramedullary leukemic infiltrates during bone marrow remission of acute leukemia. Blood 1965; 26:133–141.

55. Simone JV, Holland E, Johnson W: Fatalities during remission of childhood leukemia. Blood 1972; 39:759–770.

56. Mathe G, Schwarzenberg L, Mery AM, et al: Extensive histological and cytological survey of patients with acute leukemia in ''complete remission.'' Br Med J 1966; 1:640–642.

57. Sadeghi A, Payne D, Rubinstein L, et al, and the Lung Cancer Study Group: Combined modality treatment for resected advanced non-small cell lung cancer: Local control and local recurrence. Int J Radiat Oncology Biol Phys 1988; 15:89–97.

58. Kolaric K, Roth A, Jelicic I, et al: A preliminary report on antitumorigenic activity of cis-dichlorodiammineplatinum in metastatic brain tumors. Tumori 1981; 67:483–486.

59. Rosner D, Nemoto T, Pickren J, et al: Management of brain metastases from breast cancer by combination chemotherapy. J Neurooncol 1983; 1:131–137.

60. Kantarajian H, Farha PAM, Spitzer G, et al: Systemic combination chemotherapy as primary treatment of brain metastases from lung cancer. South Med J 1984; 77:426–430.

61. Lee JS, Murphy WK, Glisson BS, et al: Primary chemotherapy of brain metastasis in small-cell lung cancer. J Clin Oncol 1989; 7:916–922.

62. Maroun JA, Stewart DJ, Young V, et al: Effectiveness of VM-26 in non-small cell carcinoma of the lung (NSCCL) with central nervous system (CNS) metastases: Preliminary results. Proc Am Soc Clin Oncol 1982; 1:140.

63. Robin E, Bitran JD, Golomb HM, et al: Prognostic factors in patients with non–small cell bronchogenic carcinoma and brain metastases. Cancer 1982; 49:1916–1919.

64. Casimir M, Yap H, Atkinson N, et al: Prognostic factors for survival of breast cancer (BC) patients (PTS) with central nervous system (CNS) metastases. Proc Am Soc Clin Oncol 1983; 2:105.

65. van Hazel GA, Scott M, Eagen RT: The effect of CNS metastases on the survival of patients with small cell cancer of the lung. Cancer 1983; 51:933–937.

66. Lanzotti VJ, Thomas DR, Boyle LE, et al: Survival with inoperable lung cancer: An integration of prognostic variables based on simple clinical criteria. Cancer 1977; 39:303–313.

67. Goldhirsch A, Gelber RD, Castiglione M, for the Ludwig Breast Cancer Study Group: Relapse of breast cancer after adjuvant treatment in premenopausal and perimenopausal women: Patterns and prognoses. J Clin Oncol 1988; 6:89–97.

68. Minna JD, Pass H, Glatstein E, et al: Cancer of the lung: Prognostic factors. In DeVita VT Jr, Hellman S, Rosenberg SA (eds): Cancer: Principles and Practice of Oncology, ed 3. Philadelphia, JB Lippincott, 1989, p 632.

69. Shinaki T, Eguchi K, Sasaki Y, et al: A prognostic-factor risk index in advanced non–small-cell lung cancer treated with cisplatin-containing combination chemotherapy. Cancer Chemother Pharmacol 1992; 30:1–6.

70. O'Connell JP, Kris MG, Gralla RJ, et al: Frequency and prognostic importance of pretreatment clinical characteristics in patients with advanced non–small-cell lung cancer treated with combination chemotherapy. J Clin Oncol 1986; 4:1604–1614.

71. Kennealey GT, Boston B, Mitchell MS, et al: Combination chemotherapy for advanced breast cancer: Two regimens containing Adriamycin. Cancer 1978; 42:27–33.

72. Rosner D, Nemoto T, Pickren J, et al: Management of brain metastases from breast cancer by combination chemotherapy. J Neurooncol 1983; 1:131–137.

73. Neuwelt EA, Balaban E, Diehl J, et al: Successful treatment of primary central nervous system lymphomas with chemotherapy after osmotic blood-brain barrier opening. Neurosurgery 1983; 12:662–671.

74. Stewart DJ, Russell N, Quarrington A, et al: Cyclophosphamide, doxorubicin, vincristine, and dexamethasone in primary lymphoma of brain. Cancer Treat Rep 1983; 67:287–291.

75. Stewart DJ, Russell N, Dennery J, et al: Cyclophosphamide, Adriamycin, vincristine, and dexamethasone in the treatment of bulky central nervous system lymphoma. In Walker MD, Thomas DGT (eds): Biology of Brain Tumor. Boston, Martinus Nijhoff, 1986, pp 433–436.

76. Stewart DJ: The role of chemotherapy in the treatment of gliomas in adults. Cancer Treat Rev 1989; 16:129–160.

77. Bertolone SJ, Baum ES, Krivit W, et al: A phase II study of cisplatin therapy in recurrent childhood brain tumors. J Neurooncol 1989; 7:5–11.

78. Rosenstock JG, Packer RJ, Bilaniuk L, et al: Chiasmatic optic glioma treated with chemotherapy. J Neurosurg 1985; 63:862–866.

79. Mahaley M, Urso M, Whaley R, et al: Malignant glioma treatment with interferon. Proc Am Soc Clin Oncol 1984; 3:65.

80. Sklansky BD, Mann-Kaplan RS, Reynolds AF, et al: 4'-Demethyl-epipodophyllotoxin-β-D-thenylidene-glucoside (PTG) in the treatment of malignant intracranial neoplasms. Cancer 1974; 33:460–467.

81. Takeuchi K: A clinical trial of intravenous bleomycin in the treatment of brain tumors. Int J Clin Pharmacol 1975; 12:419–426.

82. Rosenstock JG, Evans AE, Schut L: Response to vincristine of recurrent brain tumors in children. J Neurosurg 1976; 45:135–140.

83. Newlands ES: VP-16 in combinations for first-line treatment of malignant germ-cell tumors and gestational choriocarcinoma. Semin Oncol 1985; 12(suppl 2):37–41.

84. Carey RW, Davis JM, Zervas NT: Tamoxifen-induced regression of cerebral metastases in breast carcinoma. Cancer Treat Rep 1981; 65:793–795.

85. Allen JC, Bosl G, Walker R: Chemotherapy trials in recurrent primary intracranial germ cell tumors. J Neurooncol 1985; 3:147–152.

86. Taylor SG IV, Nelson L, Baxter D, et al: Treatment of grade III and IV astrocytoma with dimethyl triazeno imidazole carboxamide (DTIC, NSC-45388) alone and in combination with CCNU (NSC-79037) or methyl CCNU (MeCCNU, NSC-95441). Cancer 1975; 36:1269–1276.

87. Kida Y, Kobayashi T, Yoshida J, et al: Chemotherapy with cisplatin for AFP-secreting germ-cell tumors of the central nervous system. J Neurosurg 1986; 65:470–475.

88. Stewart DJ, O'Bryan M, Al-Sarraf M, et al: Phase II study of cisplatin in recurrent astrocytomas in adults. J Neurooncol 1983; 1:145–147.

89. Stewart DJ, Richard M, Hugenholtz HN, et al: Cisplatin plus cytosine arabinoside in adults with malignant gliomas. J Neurooncol 1984; 2:29–34.

90. Allen JC, Helson L: High-dose cyclophosphamide chemotherapy for recurrent CNS tumors in children. J Neurosurg 1981; 55:749–756.

91. Socie G, Pipot-Chauffat C, Schlienger M, et al: Primary lymphoma of the central nervous system: An unresolved therapeutic problem. Cancer 1990; 65:322–326.

92. Hochberg FH, Miller DC: Primary central nervous system lymphoma. J Neurosurg 1988; 68:835–853.

93. Murray K, Kun L, Cox J: Primary malignant lymphoma of the central nervous system: Results of treatment of 11 cases and review of the literature. J Neurosurg 1986; 65:600–607.

94. DeVita VT Jr, Jaffe ES, Mauch P, et al: Lymphocytic lymphomas: Treatment of localized aggressive lymphomas. *In* DeVita VT Jr, Hellman S, Rosenberg SA (eds): Cancer: Principles and Practice of Oncology, ed 3. Philadelphia, JB Lippincott, 1989, pp 1776–1777.

95. Fine HA, Dear KBG, Loeffler JS, et al: Meta-analysis of radiation therapy with and without adjuvant chemotherapy for malignant gliomas in adults. Cancer 1992; 71:2585–2597.

96. Gutin PH, Wilson CB, Kumar ARV, et al: Phase II study of procarbazine, CCNU, and vincristine combination chemotherapy in the treatment of malignant brain tumors. Cancer 1975; 35:1398–1404.

97. Eagen RT, Scott M: Evaluation of prognostic factors in chemotherapy of recurrent brain tumors. J Clin Oncol 1983; 1:38–44.

98. Tachibana H, Meyer JS, Rose JE, et al: Local cerebral blood flow and partition coefficients measured in cerebral astrocytomas of different grades of malignancy. Surg Neurol 1984; 21:125–131.

99. Hirano A, Matsui T: Vascular structures in brain tumors. Hum Pathol 1975; 6:611–621.

100. Long DM: Capillary ultrastructure and the blood brain-barrier in human malignant brain tumors. J Neurosurg 1970; 32:127–144.

101. Coomber BL, Stewart PA, Hayakawa K, et al: Quantitative morphology of human glioblastoma multiforme microvessels: Structural basis of blood-brain barrier defect. J Neurooncol 1987; 5:299–307.

102. Nir I, Kohn S, Doron Y, et al: Quantitative analysis of tight junctions and the uptake of ^{99m}Tc in human gliomas. Cancer Invest 1986; 4:519–524.

103. Long D: Capillary ultrastructure and the blood brain barrier: Human brain tumors. Proceedings of the 6th International Congress on Neuropathology, Paris, 1970, pp 994–996.

104. Walker MD, Hilton J: Nitrosourea pharmacodynamics in relation to the central nervous system. Cancer Treat Rep 1976; 60:725–728.

105. Eckhardt S, Csetenyi J, Horvath IP, et al: Uptake of labelled dianhydrogalactitol into human gliomas and nervous tissue. Cancer Treat Rep 1977; 61:841–847.

106. Ojima Y, Sullivan RD: Pharmacology of methotrexate in the human central nervous system. Surg Gynecol Obstet 1967; 125:1035–1040.

107. Hayakawa T, Ushio Y, Morimoto K, et al: Uptake of bleomycin by human brain tumors. J Neurol Neurosurg Psychiatry 1976; 39:341–349.

108. Simon G, Graul EH, Hundeshagen H: Tracer-studien mit radioactiv markiertem cyclophosphamid bei hirntumoren. Acta Neurochir Wien 1965; 13:441–456.

109. Graul EH, Schaumloffel E, Hundeshagen H, et al: Metabolism of radioactive cyclophosphamide: Animal tests and clinical studies. Cancer 1967; 20:896–899.

110. Haranda K, Kiya K, Uozumi T: Pharmacokinetics of a new water-soluble nitrosourea derivative (ACNU) in human gliomas. Surg Neurol 1980; 15:410–414.

111. Sziklai I, Afra D, Ordogh M, et al: The distribution of bromine content of dibromodulcitol in the central nervous system of patients with malignant gliomas. Eur J Cancer 1990; 26:79–82.

112. Savaraj N, Feun LG, Lu K, et al: Central nervous system (CNS) penetration of homoharringtonine (HHT). J Neurooncol 1987; 5:77–81.

113. Lien EA, Wester K, Lonning PE, et al: Distribution of tamoxifen and metabolites into brain tissue and brain metastases in breast cancer patients. Br J Cancer 1991; 63:641–645.

114. Endicott JA, Ling V: The biochemistry of P-glycoprotein-mediated multidrug resistance. Annu Rev Biochem 1989; 58:137–171.

115. Ohnishi T, Sher PB, Posner JB, et al: Capillary permeability factor secreted by malignant brain tumor: Role in peritumoral brain edema and possible mechanism for anti-edema effect of glucocorticoids. J Neurosurg 1990; 72:245–251.

116. Neuwelt EA (ed): Implications of the Blood-Brain Barrier and Its Manipulation. New York, Plenum, 1989.

117. Bullard DE, Bigner DD: Blood-brain barrier disruption in immature Fischer 344 rats. J Neurosurg 1984; 60:743–750.

118. Spigelman MK, Zappulla RA, Malis LI, et al: Intracarotid dehydrocholate infusion: A new method for prolonged reversible blood-brain barrier disruption. Neurosurgery 1983; 12:606–612.

119. Spigelman MK, Zappulla RA, Strauchen JA, et al: Etoposide induced blood-brain barrier disruption in rats: Duration of opening and histological sequelae. Cancer Res 1986; 46:1453–1457.

120. Neuwelt EA, Rapoport SI: Modification of the blood-brain barrier in the chemotherapy of malignant brain tumors. Fed Proc 1984; 43:214–219.

121. Neuwelt EA, Hill SA, Frenkel EP, et al: Osmotic blood-brain barrier disruption: Pharmacodynamic studies in dogs and a clinical phase I trial in patients with malignant brain tumors. Cancer Treat Rep 1981; 65:39–43.

122. Neuwelt EA, Glasberg M, Diehl J, et al: Osmotic blood-brain barrier disruption in the posterior fossa of the dog. J Neurosurg 1981; 55:742–748.

123. Neuwelt EA, Specht HD, Howieson J, et al: Osmotic blood-brain barrier modification: Clinical documentation by enhanced CT scanning and/or radionuclide brain scanning. AJR 1983; 141:829–835.

124. Neuwelt EA, Maravilla KR, Frenkel EP, et al: Use of enhanced computerized tomography to evaluate osmotic blood-brain barrier disruption. Neurosurgery 1980; 6:49–56.

125. Neuwelt EA, Howieson J, Frenkel EP, et al: Therapeutic efficacy of multiagent chemotherapy with drug delivery enhancement by blood-brain barrier modification in glioblastoma. Neurosurgery 1986; 19:573–582.

126. Gumerlock MK, Belshe BD, Madsen R, et al: Osmotic blood-brain barrier disruption and chemotherapy in the treatment of high grade malignant glioma: Patient series and literature review. J Neurooncol 1992; 12:33–46.

127. Neuwelt EA, Barnett PA, Bigner DD, et al: Effects of adrenal cortical steroids and osmotic blood-brain barrier opening on methotrexate delivery to gliomas in the rodent: The factor of the blood-brain barrier. Proc Natl Acad Sci USA 1982; 79:4420–4423.

128. Hasegawa H, Allen JC, Mehta BM, et al: Enhancement of CNS penetration of methotrexate by hyperosmolar intracarotid mannitol or carcinomatous meningitis. Neurology 1979; 29:1280–1286.

129. Neuwelt EA, Barnett PA, McCormick CI, et al: Osmotic blood-brain barrier modification: Monoclonal antibody, albumin, and methotrexate delivery to cerebrospinal fluid and brain. Neurosurgery 1985; 17:419–423.

130. Shapiro WR, Voorhies RM, Hiesiger EM, et al: Pharmacokinetics of tumor cell exposure to [^{14}C]methotrexate after intracarotid administration without and with hyperosmotic opening of the blood-brain and blood-tumor barriers in rat brain tumors: A quantitative autoradiographic study. Cancer Res 1988; 48:694–701.

131. Hiesiger EM, Voorhies R, Basler GA, et al: Opening the blood-brain and blood-tumor barriers in experimental rat brain tumors: The effect of intracarotid hyperosmolar mannitol on capillary permeability and blood flow. Ann Neurol 1986; 19:50–59.

132. Warnke PC, Blasberg RG, Groothuis DR: The effect of hyperosmotic blood-brain barrier disruption on blood-to-tissue transport in ENU-induced gliomas. Ann Neurol 1987; 22:300–305.

133. Neuwelt EA, Barnett PA, Glasberg M, et al: Pharmacology and neurotoxicity of cis-diamminedichloroplatinum, bleomycin, 5-fluorouracil, and cyclophosphamide administration following osmotic blood-brain barrier modification. Cancer Res 1983; 43:5278–5285.

134. Neuwelt EA, Pagel M, Barnett P, et al: Pharmacology and toxicity of intracarotid Adriamycin administration following osmotic blood-brain barrier modification. Cancer Res 1981; 41:4466–4470.

135. Neuwelt EA, Barnett PA, Hellstrom I, et al: Delivery of melanoma-associated immunoglobulin monoclonal antibody and fab fragments to normal brain utilizing osmotic blood-brain barrier disruption. Cancer Res 1988; 48:4725–4729.

136. Neuwelt EA, Specht HD, Barnett PA, et al: Increased delivery of tumor-specific monoclonal antibodies to brain after osmotic blood-brain barrier modification in patients with melanoma metastatic to the central nervous system. Neurosurgery 1987; 20:885–895.

137. Neuwelt EA, Barnett PA, Ramsey FL, et al: Dexamethasone decreases the delivery of tumor-specific monoclonal antibody to both intracerebral and subcutaneous tumor xenografts. Neurosurgery 1993; 33:478–484.

138. Williams PC, Neuwelt EA, Hogan RL, et al: Toxicity and efficacy of carboplatin and etoposide in conjunction with blood-brain barrier modification in the treatment of intracranial neoplasms. Proc AACR 1992; 33:A1527.

139. Neuwelt EA, Goldman DL, Dahlborg SA, et al: Primary CNS lymphoma treated with osmotic blood-brain barrier disruption: Prolonged survival and preservation of cognitive function. J Clin Oncol 1991; 9:1580–1590.

140. Williams JA, Roman-Goldstein S, Crossen JR, et al: Preirradiation osmotic blood-brain barrier disruption plus combination chemotherapy in gliomas: Quantitation of tumor response to assess chemosensitivity. Adv Exp Med Biol 1993; 331:273–284.

141. Neuwelt EA, Hill SA, Frenkel EP: Osmotic blood-brain barrier modification and combination chemotherapy: Concurrent tumor regression in areas of barrier opening and progression in brain regions distant to barrier opening. Neurosurgery 1984; 15:362–366.

142. Neuwelt EA, Glasberg M, Frenkel E, et al: Neurotoxicity of chemotherapeutic agents after blood-brain barrier modification: Neuropathological studies. Ann Neurol 1983; 14:316–324.

143. Bonstelle CT, Kori SH, Rekate H: Intracarotid chemotherapy of glioblastoma after induced blood-brain barrier disruption. Am J Neuroradiol 1983; 4:810–812.

144. Fauchon F, Chiras J, Poisson M, et al: Intra-arterial chemotherapy by cisplatin and cytarabine after temporary disruption of the blood-brain barrier for the treatment of malignant gliomas in adults. J Neuroradiol 1986; 13:151–162.

145. Miyagami M, Kagawa Y, Tsubokawa T: ACNU delivery to malignant glioma tissue by osmotic blood brain barrier modification with intracarotid infusion of hyperosmolar mannitol. No Shinkei Geka 1985; 13:955–963.

146. Hori T, Muraoka K, Saito Y, et al: Influence of modes of ACNU administration on tissue and blood drug concentration in malignant brain tumors. J Neurosurg 1987; 66:372–378.

147. Li V, Levin AB, Turski P: Intra-arterial chemotherapy following blood-brain barrier disruption in patients with recurrent high grade astrocytomas. Proc Am Assoc Neurol Surg 1988; 404:274.

148. Neuwelt EA, Williams PC, Mickey BE, et al: The role of blood-brain barrier disruption in platinum-based chemotherapy of disseminated CNS germinoma. Proc ASCO 1992; 11:155.

149. Neuwelt EA, Dahlborg SA: Chemotherapy administered in conjunction with osmotic blood-brain barrier modification in patients with brain metastases. J Neurooncol 1987; 4:195–207.

150. Huan SD, Yau JC, Dunphy F, et al: Impact of autologous bone marrow infusion on the hematopoietic recovery following high dose cyclophosphamide, etoposide, and cisplatinum. J Clin Oncol 1991; 9:1609–1617.

151. Cosolo W, Christophidis N: Blood-brain barrier disruption and methotrexate in the treatment of a readily transplantable intracerebral osteogenic sarcoma of rats. Cancer Res 1987; 47:6225–6228.

IMMUNOTHERAPY

MITSUHIRO TADA

NICOLAS DE TRIBOLET

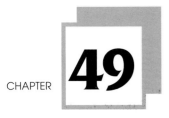

CHAPTER **49**

Tumor Immunobiology

The first recognition of a host immune cell infiltration in malignant gliomas dates to 1960 when Bertrand and Mannen[1] noticed lymphoid cellular infiltrates in these tumors. Eventually, the lymphocyte infiltration was discussed as a phenomenon indicative of a host-mediated immune response,[2] which positively correlates with patient survival.[3, 4] At the same time, various attempts to treat glioma patients with immunologic intervention began, including vaccination with glioma cells, lymphocyte transfer, and use of nonspecific immunopotentiators. From the early 1980s, two important technologies, hybridoma technique and recombinant DNA technique, contributed to the understanding of immunologic aspects and to the advance in immunotherapy of gliomas. The hybridoma technique brought about monoclonal antibodies, which have been used both to analyze the antigenic profile of glioma cells and for their diagnosis and treatment. The recombinant DNA technique enabled the production of recombinant cytokines used for cytokine therapy and adoptive immunotherapy. It also enabled gene level analyses of immunobiologic characteristics of malignant gliomas. Although no real breakthrough in the treatment of malignant gliomas has been achieved so far, considerable knowledge on the immunobiology of malignant gliomas has been accumulated. Especially since the late 1980s, a series of immunomodulatory molecules (cytokines) were found to be produced by glioblastoma cells. Some of these are chemoattractants and immunostimulatory cytokines, which act on the host immune cells. Potent immunosuppressive factors, such as transforming growth factor-β (TGFB) and prostaglandin E$_2$ were also found in glioblastomas, which accounts for the peculiar immunosuppression in patients with glioblastoma. The reasons for the failures of previous immunotherapy protocols have been discussed in the light of the depressed functional immune status of the patients or the immunologic ''evasion'' of the host's immune surveillance by tumor cells. In this chapter, we review the present knowledge on immunobiology of glioblastomas for possible therapeutic intervention.

IMMUNE REACTIONS IN THE CENTRAL NERVOUS SYSTEM

The CNS has been recognized as a peculiar site in regard to the immune response. Its limited immunoreactivity was sometimes overemphasized under the term of *immune privilege,* which was based mainly on the structural isolation from the immune system by the absence of lymphatic drainage and the presence of the blood-brain barrier. However, this concept of immune privilege is becoming ambiguous. Active communication between the immune system and the CNS has been shown to exist. Endothelial cells send signals to the immune system by expressing adhesion molecules and producing cytokines that allow trafficking of immune cells through the blood-brain barrier. Interstitial and cerebrospinal fluids serve as a molecular transport system draining to the cervical lymphatics (for large molecules) and dural sinuses (for smaller molecules).[5] The limited immunoreactivity in the CNS is attributable to certain factors secreted by brain cells. TGFB is a major immunosuppressive factor in the normal CNS that minimizes the antigen-specific cell-mediated immunity and keeps the antibody response within a certain range. This protects the CNS cells, which possess a set of potentially antigenic molecules—such as myelin basic protein (MBP)—because the T cells have not previously been exposed to these molecules in the thymus. Also, the tapered immune reaction is substantiated by the minimal expression of class I major histocompatibility complex (MHC) molecules in brain cells, on which processed antigens are presented for recognition by T cells. A failure in this immunosuppression may cause an autoimmune disease of the CNS, such as multiple sclerosis.

The first-line defense to a non-self in the CNS is initiated with antigen presentation by microglial cells and, perhaps, astrocytes. They process a foreign antigen and present it on the groove of an MHC class II molecule to helper T cells attracted by chemokines. According to co-stimulatory molecules and cytokine signals, the helper T (Th) cells activate either the antibody-mediated immune reaction, the cell-mediated response, or both of them. Thereafter, the full orchestration of immune reactions takes place; bloodborne granulocytes, T cells, B cells, natural killer (NK) cells, and monocytes/macrophages participate on the battlefield. In gliomas, this overall immune reaction is not fully active. Most malignant gliomas have a disrupted blood-brain barrier (due to aberrant neovascularization and vascular permeability factors), which is responsible for contrast enhancement and edema in computed tomographic (CT) scans or magnetic resonance images (MRIs). The reason for the deficient immune reaction is thus not attributed to an anatomic isolation of gliomas from the immune system, but to an abnormality in the patient's immune system, which consists of a scarcity of antigenicity of glioma cells and active immunosuppressive factors produced by glioma cells. These are discussed in the following sections.

THE IMPAIRED CELLULAR IMMUNE FUNCTION OF MALIGNANT GLIOMA PATIENTS

Patients with malignant gliomas have a decreased cellular immunity as assessed by delayed-type cutaneous reactions.[6] This may be a result of suppressed T-cell functions observed by several ex vivo studies, including the following: (1) decreased number of peripheral blood T lymphocytes, (2) impairment of mitogen- and antigen-induced T-cell reactivity, (3) decreased response of T cells to phytohemagglutinin (PHA), (4) decreased production of interleukin 2 (IL2), and (5) decreased expression of the IL2 receptor p55 chain (α-chain).[6] More recently, it was reported that the reduced numbers of circulating T cells in patients with glioblastoma were due to a selective depletion of CD4+ Th cells.[7] Th cells are developmentally categorized into three classes: naive, memory, and effector Th cells. Naive Th cells are resting Th cells that are characterized by a marker CD45RA+ and comprise most of the population of peripheral blood and lymph node Th cells. Effector Th cells (CD45RO+) are subclassified into Th1 and Th2 cells, which are generated from naive Th cells by stimulation with IL12 and IL4, respectively, in the presence of antigen-presenting cells. Th1 cells are capable of producing IL2 and interferon-γ (IFN-γ) and of executing a cell-mediated immune response, whereas Th2 cells produce IL4, IL5, and IL10 and assist in antibody production for humoral immunity. Memory Th cells differentiate from the effector Th cells and serve as quick responders to the second antigenic exposure. Glioblastoma patients have been reported to be deficient in CD45RA+ naive Th cells, which accounts for both the impaired delayed-type hypersensitivity reaction and decreased helper function for immunoglobulin production.[8]

THE IMPAIRED HUMORAL IMMUNE FUNCTION

Despite normal counts of B cells and a normal amount of serum immunoglobulins, patients with glioblastomas are deficient in the ability to produce antibody against tetanus, influenza, or other antigens. This may be due to the impaired Th2 functions, which normally assist in antibody production. Recently, it was demonstrated that antibodies found in the diseased CNS do not come from the bloodstream but are produced in the CNS in situ by migrating B cells.[5] In the tumor-infiltrating lymphocyte population, however, the number of B cells is quite small. Thus, the clinical significance of the systemic production of antiglioma antibodies detected in the patient's serum is probably low, although it indicates that the antigen-recognition system is working at least in part.[9] A relatively large quantity of immunoglobulin is found in glioma cyst fluid, but it is not specific to tumor cells; rather, it is reactive to normal brain.[10] It is noteworthy that glioblastoma cells produce IL6, a potent B-cell stimulator, but also that they produce TGFB2, which has a potent ability to suppress secretion of IgG and IgM by B cells.[11] Moreover, the low concentrations of complement components in brain extracellular fluids diminish the possibility of antibody-mediated inflammatory reactions to the tumor cells in the CNS. Certain glioma cell lines produce complement components in vitro, but their in vivo significance is obscure.[12]

TUMOR-ASSOCIATED ANTIGENS

A tumor-associated antigen is defined as an antigen that is expressed on tumor cells and is potentially recognizable for rejection of the tumor in immunized hosts. When it actually provokes an immunologic reaction that leads to tumor rejection, it is called a *tumor-rejection antigen*. We have not yet come across a tumor-rejection antigen in gliomas. The T-cell repertoire that recognizes self-antigens is shaped down when lymphocytes develop within the thymus. Thymic *educator cells* present self-proteins with MHC class I molecules, which leads to the elimination of the recognition of self-antigens by the T cells. This process is called the *establishment of tolerance*. Extensive efforts have been made to detect a *tumor-specific antigen* in glioma cells using immunization of mice and production of monoclonal antibodies. However, most of these antigens are not exclusively specific to glioma cells, or they are probably already tolerated by the host T cells. Candidate tumor-associated antigens for glioma cells may be classified into three groups on the basis of T-cell tolerance.[13, 14] The first includes tumor antigens encoded by normal genes that are expressed during ontogeny but not (or only at low levels) after birth. These antigens, designated as *oncofetal antigens,* may not be tolerated in the thymic education during early childhood. One good example is MZ2E antigen encoded by melanoma associated antigen (MAGE1) gene. This antigen was initially discovered in human melanoma cells, eventually also in glioblastoma cells, and proved to be recognized by autologous CD8+ cytotoxic T cells with a restriction of HLA-A1 (class I MHC).[15] The second group includes antigens resulting from mutations in the genes of tumor cells. For instance, glioblastoma cells often express mutant p53 proteins and mutant epidermal growth factor receptor (EGFR). Whether these mutant proteins can serve as rejection targets, however, remains unknown.[13, 14] The third group comprises antigens resulting from quantitatively abnormal production of proteins that are expressed by normal adult cells. In human melanoma cells, one overexpressed antigen related to tyrosinase is demonstrated to be recognized by autologous cytotoxic T cells restricted by HLA-A2 (class I MHC). Glioblastoma cells are known to overexpress certain genes, such as wild-type EGFR and tenascin.[16, 17] Although these antigens are not recognized by the patient's cytotoxic T cells, the use of these antigens as targets for immunotherapy is still possible.

CELL-MEDIATED IMMUNE RESPONSES

The cellular immunity against tumor cells is mediated by two major mechanisms: (1) antigen-specific cytotoxicity through MHC-restricted T-cell receptors (TCR), which depends on specific MHC molecules in the recognition of target cells; and (2) non-MHC restricted cytotoxicity.

MHC-Restricted Cellular Immunity

The first type of response—MHC-restricted cellular cytotoxicity—is a rather complicated process. First, microglia/macrophages that have phagocytosed tumor cells, present tumor-associated antigen on their MHC class II molecules. The T-cell receptors of Th cells (naive or memory), coupled with the CD4 molecule, then recognize the presented antigen after an initiation signal by IL12, which has been produced by macrophages. The activated effector Th1 cells produce IL2 and IFN-γ to activate CD8+ cytotoxic T cells. The activated cytotoxic T cells recognize the tumor cells by an interaction between their T-cell receptor coupled with the CD8 molecule and the antigen presented by the tumor cells on class I MHC molecules; then they exert cytotoxic effects against the tumor cells. Certain critical defects in these processes have been demonstrated in gliomas. As the T lymphocytes in peripheral blood, tumor-infiltrating lymphocytes in gliomas are predominantly CD8+, but CD4+ Th cells are scarce.[18, 19] This is in contrast to active inflammatory processes of the CNS, in which CD4+ Th cells predominate.[20] The relative lack of Th cells in tumor-infiltrating lymphocytes of gliomas indicates that the first stimulation by tumor-associated antigen on glioma cells hardly occurs, and that subsequent cytotoxic T-cell activation does not take place.

Furthermore, the in vivo expression of MHC class I molecules (HLA-ABC) is very low on glioma cells,[21, 22] although these cells express MHC molecules when they are grown in culture. Even though cytotoxic T cells are activated, the lack of expression of MHC class I molecules does not allow CTL to recognize the tumor cells as targets for their attack.[23] However, glioblastoma cells express MHC class II molecules (HLA-DR) and are capable of presenting antigens,[24] although antigen presentation on class II molecule to Th cells without proper co-stimulatory signals (B7 or B70 molecules and IL12) can result in a T-cell inactivation called *T-cell anergy*.[25] In malignant melanoma, a high expression of MHC class I indicates a good prognosis, whereas a high expression of MHC class II appears to indicate a poor prognosis.[26] Similarly, the expression of MHC class II is a negative prognostic factor in gliomas.[27]

A recent study of T-cell receptor variable gene usage (which provides the antigen-specific binding site of T-cell receptors) in tumor-infiltrating lymphocytes of gliomas demonstrated a limited use of specific variable gene segment (Vα/β) gene in some cases; in most cases, however, usage was identical to that in the peripheral blood lymphocyte population, which suggests nonspecificity of the tumor-infiltrating lymphocyte population.[28] A cytolysis of autologous glioma cells by tumor-infiltrating lymphocytes has been described, but it is nonspecific in the majority of cases and is even weaker than that of peripheral blood lymphocytes.[29]

Non–MHC-Restricted Cellular Immunity

The second type of cellular immune response against tumor cells is a non–MHC-restricted killing of tumor cells by NK cells. NK cells (CD2+CD3−) recognize tumor cells through NK receptors by a mechanism that is not clearly understood. The actual presence of this type of killing in tumor tissue is quite doubtful.[30] The number of NK cells found in glioma tissue is small.[19, 31] Glioma cells are generally resistant to NK cytolysis.[32] Non–MHC-restricted cytotoxicity can also be mediated by certain T cells.[33, 34] Cell lysis of NK resistant cells might be mediated by this population. However, the presence of these particular cells in glioma tissue has not been demonstrated. Previous adoptive immunotherapy using IL2 and/or PHA in the presence or absence of mixed autologous tumor cells resulted in the generation and expansion of these activated NK cells and of non–MHC-restricted cytotoxic T cells. However, a number of studies have failed to demonstrate a specific tumor cell kill, and no clinical efficacy was observed.

TUMOR-ASSOCIATED MACROPHAGES

Macrophages have been estimated to account for 20% to 75% of the mononuclear cell population in gliomas.[35] More recent studies suggest that the macrophage infiltration in glioma tissue is not so predominant.[19, 31] Because most of the macrophage markers for immunohistochemistry are also expressed more or less by glioma cells, overestimation might occur. Whether the macrophages found in glioma tissue are derived from bloodborne monocytes or brain-derived microglia remains unknown. Bloodborne macrophages and microglial cells are not distinguishable by any means presently available, as they share the same characteristics. The functional role of the tumor infiltrating microglia/macrophages in gliomas is still unclear. If fully activated, they could directly kill tumor cells or initiate tumor cell rejection through their antigen-presenting cell function. However, they also may stimulate neoplastic proliferation, either by producing growth factors or by inducing neovascularization.[36]

PRODUCTION OF IMMUNOMODULATORY MOLECULES BY GLIOMA CELLS

Glioma cells produce a variety of cytokines that modulate the host's immune reactions (Table 49–1). Some of them have potent immunosuppressive activities, which probably account for the previously discussed immunosuppression in

TABLE 49–1
IMMUNOREGULATORY CYTOKINE EXPRESSION BY GLIOMA CELLS

| Cytokine | In Vitro† | | In Vivo |
	Stimulation (−)	Stimulation (+)	
IL1A	±	+ *	+
IL1B	±	+ *	+
IL1RA	+	+ +	+
IL2 ~ 5	−	−	−
IL6	+	+ + *	+
IL7	−	?	−
IL8	+	+ + *	+
IL10	−	?	+
IL9, 11 ~ 13	?	?	?
TNFA	−	+ *	±
LTA, LTB	?	?*	?
IFN-α, -β	−	± *	−
IFY-γ	−	−	−
TGF1 ~ 3	+	+ *	+
SCF	?	?	?
CSF2	+	+ + *	−
CSF3	+	+ + *	?
CSF1	?	?*	+
MCP1	+	+ +	+
MCP2, 3	?	?	?
MIP1A, B	?	?	?
RANTES	?	?	?
LIF	?	?	?

†Stimulation with TNF, IL1, and lipopolysaccharide.
∗, expression in activated normal astrocytes is known; ?, presently unknown; LIF, leukemia inhibitor factor; and LT, lymphotoxin, member of TNF family.

patients with glioblastomas. Some of them, however, have immunostimulatory activities, attracting and activating host immune cells. However, it appears that glioblastoma cells do not suffer from a self-demolishing effect through the activation of the host's immune system. The overlapping immunosuppression probably cancels the overall immune activation. Moreover, glioblastoma cells might utilize the accessory biologic activities of the immunostimulatory cytokines, such as angiogenic activity, by trading off self-demolishment. Attracted host immune cells may help tumor growth through production of cytokines and growth factors that are beneficial to the tumor cells. Normal astrocytes are capable of producing the same set of cytokines when they are activated. The contrasting difference in glioma cells, however, is that they produce the cytokines *constitutively,* without any stimulation. Certain de-repression mechanisms in the gene expression are probably present in glioma cells, inducing the set of the cytokine genes constitutively through activation of transcriptional factors such as nuclear factor of kappa light chain gene enhancer in B cells (NFKB) and c-fos. It is unknown whether the de-repression of gene induction is common in immunosuppressive and immunostimulatory cytokines. The relation between the loss of tumor suppressor genes and induction of cytokines in glioma cells is an interesting question.

Immunosuppressive Factors

TRANSFORMING GROWTH FACTOR-β

TGFB is a family of 25-kD multifunctional dimeric polypeptides that act on a broad spectrum of target cells. TGFB2

produced by glioma cells was first recognized as a soluble factor in the culture supernatant that suppressed the generation of cytotoxic T cells and lymphokine-activated (LAK) cells. Other members of the TGFB family, TGFB1 and TGFB3, which have indistinguishable functions, have also been reported to be present in glioma cells.[37] However, the major isoform detected in glioblastoma cells in vitro and in vivo is TGFB2. TGFB2 is demonstrated in all grades of gliomas without a demonstrable correlation to the degree of malignancy.[38] Normal astrocytes secrete TGFB1 and TGFB2 in a latent form, which harbors an additional peptide chain (latent TGFB-binding protein, LTBP or 210 kD peptide) and must be proteolytically cleaved to have biologic activity. In contrast, glioma cells secrete both latent and active forms of TGFB and produce a factor that activates LTBP.[39] TGFB has a variety of immunomodulatory functions (Table 49–2),[11, 40–44] which are considered to be a major cause of immunosuppression in glioblastomas. Besides immunoregulatory functions, TGFB has multiple functions for tissue repair, which may help tumor growth.[45] TGFB is a potent inducer of many components of the extracellular matrix, including collagen, fibronectin, and cell-surface integrins. It decreases synthesis of enzymes, such as collagenase and transin/stromelysin, that degrade extracellular matrix components. TGFB increases the levels of inhibitors of these enzymes, such as plasminogen-activator inhibitor 1. TGFB can promote angiogenesis by promoting extracellular matrix formation and by directly acting on endothelial cells.[46] Although glioma cells apparently express functional TGFB receptors and normal astrocytes express three types of TGFBR (types I, II, III), the receptor types on glioma cells are yet to be determined. It is interesting that TGFB enhances the growth of glioblastoma cells, which is in contrast with its growth-inhibiting action on normal astrocytes.[47, 48] This suggests that a certain change in the TGFBR system is present in glioblastoma cells. Because TGFB interacts with certain tumor suppressor genes, such as *Rb* and p53,[49, 50] such a change in the signal transduction under TGFBRs may be related to the process of carcinogenesis.

TABLE 49–2
MULTIPLE IMMUNOREGULATORY FUNCTIONS OF TGFB

Cells	Actions
T cells	↓ proliferation
	↓ IL1 receptor expression
CTL	↓ generation of allogeneic CTL
Th cells	↓ production of IFN-γ, TNFA and TNFB
	↓ IL1-driven proliferation
	↓ IL2 receptor expression
B cells	↓ proliferation
	↓ secretion of IgG and IgM
	↑ secretion of IgA
NK cells	↓ activation and activity
LAK cells	↓ in vitro generation
Macrophage	↑ chemotaxis
	↑ expression of IL1, PDGF, FGF, TNFA, TGFB
	↓ production of IL1 by LPS
	↓ release of oxygen radicals
	↓ release of nitric oxide
	↓ respiratory burst
	↓ induction of IL1 receptor antagonist

Symbols: ↓, down-regulation; ↑, up-regulation

INTERLEUKIN 10

IL10 is an immunoregulatory cytokine produced by Th cells (predominantly by Th2 clone). IL10 acts on Th1 cells to inhibit their ability to produce other cytokines and shifts the prevailing immune response in favor of the Th2 side (antibody production rather than delayed-type hypersensitivity).[42, 51] It also acts on monocytes/macrophages to inhibit the expression of MHC class II and cytokine production, such as IL1 and tumor necrosis factor (TNF), resulting in the inhibition of antigen-specific T-cell proliferation and suppression of IL1-driven T-cell proliferation. In contrast, IL10 enhances the viability and class II molecule expression of B cells, stimulating antibody production. It is known that glioblastoma cells express the IL10 gene in vitro and in vivo.[52, 53] Although the production of the IL10 protein by glioblastoma cells in vivo remains to be determined, it is probable that IL10 acts as an immunosuppressive factor in glioblastomas.

PROSTAGLANDIN E₂

Glioblastoma cells secrete a significant amount of prostaglandin E_2 (PGE_2) in vitro and in vivo.[54] PGE_2 profoundly suppresses the production of IL2 and IFN-γ by the Th1 subset and the IL2 receptor expression in T cells. PGE_2 does not affect IL4 synthesis by Th2 cells and promotes IL5 production. This pushes the balance in favor of antibody production (IgG and IgE) and against antigen-specific cellular cytotoxicity, as in the case of IL10.[55] In gliomas, PGE_2 with TGFB2 and IL10 may synergistically suppress cellular immunity.

Immunostimulatory Cytokines

TUMOR NECROSIS FACTOR-α

Macrophages or microglial cells are considered to be the main source of TNF in the CNS, although normal astrocytes produce TNF IL1 stimulation.[56] Production of TNF after appropriate stimulation has been reported in several glioma cell lines.[57, 58] However, these cell lines do not constitutively secrete TNF. Although TNF gene expression has been reported in glioblastomas,[53] we have demonstrated that no TNF bioactivity was detectable in the CSF and tumor-cyst fluids before intracranial administration of TNF to malignant glioma patients.[59] Thus, production of TNF in significant amounts in vivo is not likely. Tumor necrosis factor-α (TNFA) is a member of the large TNF family, but production of other TNF family cytokines by gliomas is not known.[60]

However, glioma cells do express receptors for TNF. Although most glioma cells are resistant to the cytotoxic effect of TNF, TNF stimulation can cause G1-arrest of proliferation and increases or induces the production of a variety of cytokines and cell surface molecules.[61] Two distinct TNF receptors are known, which are referred to as p55 and p75 TNF receptors, according to their molecular size. Glioma cells predominantly express the p55 TNF receptor,[62] and this type of receptor transduces many of the known activities of TNFA.[63] TNF receptors are known to be enzymatically cleaved at the base of the extracellular domain to form soluble TNF receptors. Soluble receptors can compete for the binding to the ligand and thus act as antagonists. It is unknown whether glioma cells produce soluble TNF receptors.

INTERLEUKIN 1 FAMILY

IL1 is a pleiotropic cytokine that plays a key role in inflammatory and immune responses. The three molecular species of IL1 are IL1A, IL1B, and IL1 receptor antagonist (IL1RA).[64] IL1 bioactivity can be demonstrated in glioma culture supernatants, and mRNA transcripts for both IL1A and IL1B are found in glioblastoma cells.[53, 58, 65] An immunohistochemical study also demonstrated IL1A immunoreactivity in glioblastoma tissues.[65] A study using enzyme-linked immunosorbent assay (ELISA) has shown the presence of IL1B in the cyst fluid or CSF of glioma patients.[66] However, whether IL1A or IL1B is the predominant species in gliomas remains to be established.

Various responses of glioma cells to IL1 are known, including growth promotion, up-regulation of intercellular adhesion molecules, down-regulation of MHC class II, and increase in cytokine production. Two distinct molecules have been recognized as the major IL1 receptors; p80 IL1R (type I) and p68 IL1R (type II). Glioblastoma cells predominantly express type I receptors.[62] It is possible that glioblastoma cells form an autocrine loop through this receptor. However, the functional role of IL1 in glioblastomas is not known. An IL1 autocrine loop may induce secondary cytokines that favor tumor growth. IL1 can act as a paracrine angiogenic factor to induce neovascularization of the tumor.[67] It may also increase protease production in tumor cells to facilitate the invasive process.[68]

Recently, we have found that glioblastoma cells can produce IL1RA in vitro and in vivo.[69] IL1RA is a potent suppressor of IL1 actions by its competitive binding to IL1 receptors. It is possible that glioblastoma cells regulate the immune-potentiating actions or hazardous direct actions to themselves of IL1 by producing IL1RA.

INTERFERONS

IFN-γ/β bioactivity was found in glioblastoma culture supernatants,[70] whereas IFN-γ production has not been reported. However, it has not been confirmed by mRNA analysis or by the identification of immunoreactive proteins. Moreover, glioblastoma cell lines frequently lack IFN-α and -β genes.[71] Thus the production of IFN-α/β by glioblastoma cells is questionable. The lack of detection of IFN genes in glioblastoma cells is interesting, because they may act as tumor suppressor genes. Glioma cells express both IFN-α/β receptors and IFN-γ receptors. Certain biologic activities of IFNs on glioma cells are known; IFN-β suppresses MHC class II expression, and IFN-α and IFN-β inhibit their growth. The wider range of IFN-γ action on glioma cells includes intercellular adhesion molecule 1 (ICAM1) induction, MHC class I and II induction, and growth modulation.

INTERLEUKIN 6

Glioblastoma cells produce IL6 in vitro and in vivo.[72] Although IL6 production seems to be a general characteristic of glioblastoma cells, its functional significance remains unknown. The fact that IL6 expression is not seen in benign astrocytomas suggests a potential role of IL6 in glioblastomas.[53] It may be initiated by an autocrine stimulation through IL1 and/or de-repression of the IL6 gene by the p53 gene product,[73] which is often deleted or is anomalous in glioblastoma cells. Although radioreceptor assays have demonstrated IL6 binding sites on glioblastoma cells, it has not been demonstrated that these cells possess functional IL6 receptors.[62] However, certain neuronal cells possess IL6 receptors. IL6 is known to act as a neurotropic factor, as do leukemia inhibitory factor (LIF) and ciliary neurotropic factor (CNTF), which share a common signal transducer (gp130).[74] IL6 can activate the hypothalamic-pituitary-adrenal axis through induction of corticotropin-releasing hormone. It is thus possible that IL6, which is present at high levels in the CSF of patients with glioblastoma, may contribute to immunosuppression through this pathway. It is also known that IL6 may play a role in angiogenesis.[75]

INTERLEUKIN 8

Glioblastoma cells produce IL8 in vitro and in vivo.[76] IL8 is found in the CSF of glioma patients. IL8 produced by glioblastoma cells is a 77-amino acid form. It has an additional 5 amino acids at N-terminal to the 72-amino acid form, which is produced by monocytes.[77] IL8 has a potent chemotactic activity to neutrophils.[78] It was also claimed to be a chemoattractant to T cells, but recently this has been denied. The reason for the scarcity of neutrophil infiltration in gliomas is unclear. It is probable that neutrophil trafficking needs stimulation by some other factor(s) or that it could be inhibited by TGFB2.[49, 79] Radioreceptor assays of IL8 binding on glioblastoma cells have failed to demonstrate significant binding sites, and an autocrine loop involving IL8 is therefore unlikely. However, IL8 acts as a potent angiogenic factor.[80] Thus, IL8 may act as a paracrine growth factor for endothelial cells.

MONOCYTE CHEMOATTRACTANT PROTEIN 1

Monocyte chemoattractant protein 1 (MCP1) is a cytokine that induces chemotaxis to monocytes/macrophages. Glioblastoma cell lines are known to produce MCP1.[81] In vivo production of MCP1 in glioblastomas has recently been demonstrated.[82] MCP1 may be a cause of the macrophage infiltration found in the glioma tissue as well as of other macrophage chemoattractants that are found in glioma tissue, such as TGF-B, vascular endothelial growth factor, and macrophage colony-stimulating growth factor (CSF1).[36] MCP1 has been shown to be chemotactic to T lymphocytes[78] and may therefore account for the T-lymphocyte infiltration in gliomas. Other C-C chemokine family members, such as RANTES and macrophage inflammatory protein 1 (MIP1), might also be chemotactic factors for monocytes/macrophages and T lymphocytes in gliomas.

Colony-Stimulating Factors

Granulocyte-macrophage CSF (CSF2) is known to be produced by astrocytoma or glioblastoma cells in vitro, but not in vivo.[66] The absence of CSF2 in glioma tissue may be explained by the presence of TGFB2 and PGE$_2$, which suppress CSF2 production by glioma cells.

Granulocyte CSF (CSF3) has been shown to be produced by glioma cells in vitro,[83] but it remains unknown whether CSF3 is produced by gliomas in vivo.

CSF1 bioactivity is found in the cerebrospinal fluid of patients with astrocytomas.[84] It is interesting to note that a majority of glioma cells express the CSF1 receptor (CSF1R) gene.[62] CSFR1 is identical to the c-fms proto-oncogene product, and belongs to the tyrosine kinase receptor family. CSF1 may act in an autocrine or paracrine fashion on glioma cells. Like other members of the tyrosine kinase receptor family (fibroblast growth factor [FGF], platelet-derived growth factor [PDGF]), CSF1 may potentially play a substantial role in the growth and progression of malignant gliomas. CSF1 can also act as a chemoattractant to monocyte/macrophages, and it down-modulates both basal and cytokine-induced MHC class II expression on macrophages.[85]

The stem cell factor receptor (SCFR) is known to be expressed in two glioblastoma cell lines.[86, 87] It is also expressed in glioblastomas in vivo.[62] SCFR is the c-kit proto-oncogene product and is also a member of the tyrosine kinase receptor family. It would therefore be interesting to know whether SCF is produced by glioma cells in vivo.

CYTOKINE NETWORK

The cytokines that are produced by glioma cells and by host immune cells can interact with each other through the receptor system on the cells. For instance, several interactions are known to occur between IL1 and TGFB. TGFB can enhance gene expression of IL1A and IL1B, and, reciprocally, IL1 can induce TGFB gene expression.[88] However, TGFB has the ability to antagonize the biologic action of IL1. TGFB inhibits IL1-dependent lymphocyte proliferation, blocks IL1 receptor expression,[40] and induces the expression of the IL1 RA.[41] How the interactions between IL1 and TGFB come into play in neoplastic growth is an interesting question. However, TNF and IL1 can increase many of the cytokine expressions of glioma cells, including IL6, IL8, and MCP1. Several cytokines (IL1, TNF, TGFB, and IL6) appear to be expressed with marked parallelism in gliomas.[31, 53] A complex cytokine network may exist in gliomas that regulates immune and other parenchymal reactions, such as angiogenesis.

THERAPEUTIC IMPLICATIONS

The major immunomodulations in gliomas that have been discussed in this chapter are summarized in Table 49–3. Although some of the proposed immune alterations have yet to be proved, it is quite certain that the immune response to gliomas is characterized by the lack of antigen-specific recognition by the host immune cells. This should be taken into consideration when constructing a new strategy of immunotherapy for patients with gliomas. For *active immunization* (vaccination), two different approaches can be considered.[25] One approach is to identify a tumor-associated

TABLE 49–3
POSSIBLE IMMUNE MODULATIONS CAUSED BY GLIOMAS

Modulations	Consequence
Systemic and regional depletion of Th cells	Lack of antigen-specific recognition of tumor cells
Lack of MHC class I molecules on tumor cells	Loss of recognition by cytotoxic T cells
MHC class II expression on tumor cells	Regional depletion of Th 1 cells (T-cell anergy)
TGFB production by tumor cells	Profound suppression of T-, b-, and NK-cells and macrophages
Prostaglandin E$_2$ and IL10 production by tumor cells	Suppression of Th1 and professional APC functions
Production of colony-stimulating factors	Activation of macrophages
Chemokine production by tumor cells	Chemotaxis of T cells and macrophages into tumor tissue
Presence of IL1 autocrine loop in tumor cells	Potential activation of T cells and macrophages
Production of IL1RA by tumor cells	Regulation of IL1 autocrine loop; suppression of IL1-mediated immune cascade reaction
Lack of IFN-α/β genes in tumor cells	Suppression of MHC molecules and induction of cytokines

antigen that could be utilized by the host T-cell system in an MHC-restricted manner. The antigen encoded by MAGE1 on tumor cells may be a good example. However, the lack of MHC class I expression on glioma cells may be a major obstacle. The MHC class I expression should be induced using certain cytokines, such as IFNs, or the repressive factors of the MHC expression, such as TGFB, should be antagonized. Another approach is to let the immune cells choose a tumor-associated antigen for rejection of the tumor, rather than to specify the tumor-associated antigen. For this, the patient's compromised Th cell system should be corrected. An appropriate environment for a full function of professional antigen-presenting cells (APC) should be made. Alternatively, the class II MHC expression on glioma cells would be useful to directly sensitize the Th1 cells, in the absence of assistance from the macrophages, provided they are given an artificial co-stimulation to mimic professional APC.[89] For *adoptive immunotherapy*, expansion of tumor antigen-specific T-cell populations should be achieved, as previous trials using nonspecific adoptive cells failed to prove effective. A combination of active immunization and adoptive expansion of committed (sensitized) T cells may be useful for this task. However, direct linkage between tumor cell surface antigens and part of the T-cell receptor on cytotoxic T lymphocytes using bispecific monoclonal antibodies, such as anti-EGF receptor/anti-CD3, may be useful. Adoptive cells can be armed by gene transfer of certain cytokines. For *biologic response modification* using cytokines, the overall effects on the cytokine network in gliomas should be understood. Cancellation of the evasion of tumor cells from host immunity, rather than stimulation of the immune cells, would be the ultimate goal of this mode of therapy TGFB, which is the most abundant and most potent

immunosuppresive factor in glioblastomas, may be a target for immunotherapy. Gene therapies, such as gene transfer or usage of antisense oligonucleotides, will be useful for this purpose.[90]

REFERENCES

1. Bertrand J, Mannen H: Etude des reactions vasculaires dans les astrocytomes. Rev Neurol 1960; 102:3.
2. Ridley A, Cavanagh JB: Lymphocytic infiltration in gliomas: Evidence of possible host resistance. Brain 1971; 94:117.
3. Brooks WH, Markesbery WR, Gupta GD, et al: Relationship of lymphocyte invasion and survival of brain tumor patients. Ann Neurol 1978; 4:219.
4. Palma L, Di Lorenzo N, Guidetti B: Lymphocytic infiltrates in primary glioblastomas and recidivous gliomas: Incidence, fate, and relevance to prognosis in 228 operated cases. J Neurosurg 1978; 49:854.
5. Cserr HF, Knopf PM: Cervical lymphatics, the blood-brain barrier and the immunoreactivity of the brain: A new view. Immunol Today 1992; 13:507.
6. Roszman T, Elliott L, Brooks W: Modulation of T-cell function by gliomas. Immunol Today 1991; 12:370.
7. Bhondeley MK, Mehra RD, Mehra NK, et al: Imbalances in T cell subpopulations in human gliomas. J Neurosurg 1988; 68:589.
8. Menage P, Thibault G, Lebranchu Y, et al: Deficiency of CD4 + CD45RA + lymphocytes in patients with glioblastoma multiforme. Eur J Med 1992; 1:362.
9. Dan MD, Schlachta CM, Guy J, et al: Human antiglioma monoclonal antibodies from patients with astrocytic tumors. J Neurosurg 1992; 76:660.
10. Brunet J-FM, Berger F, Gustin T, et al: Characterization of normal brain-reactive antibodies in glioma cyst fluids. J Neuroimmunol 1993; 47:63.
11. Roberts AB, Sporn MB: The transforming growth factor-βs. *In* Sporn MB, Roberts AB (eds): Peptide Growth Factors and Their Receptors, vol I. New York, Springer Verlag, 1990, p 419.
12. Gasque P, Ischenko A, Legoedec J, et al: Expression of the complement classical pathway by human glioma in culture: A model for complement expression by nerve cells. J Biol Chem 1993; 268:25068.
13. Parmiani G: Tumor immunity as autoimmunity: Tumor antigens include normal self proteins which stimulate anergic peripheral T cells. Immunol Today 1993; 14:536.
14. Klein G, Boon T: Tumor immunology: present perspectives. Curr Opinion Immunol 1993; 5:687.
15. Rimoldi D, Romero P, Carrel S: The human melanoma antigen-encoding gene, MAGE-1, is expressed by other tumour cells of neuroectodermal origin such as glioblastomas and neuroblastomas. Int J Cancer 1993; 54:527.
16. Hall WA, Fodstad Ø: Immunotoxins and central nervous system neoplasia. J Neurosurg 1992; 76:1.
17. Higuchi M, Ohnishi T, Arita N, et al: Expression of tenascin in human gliomas: Its relation to histological malignancy, tumor dedifferentiation and angiogenesis. Acta Neuropathol 1993; 85:481.
18. Paine JT, Handa H, Yamasaki T, et al: Immunohistochemical analysis of infiltrating lymphocytes in central nervous system tumors. Neurosurgery 1986; 18:766.
19. Stevens A, Klöter I, Roggendorf W: Inflammatory infiltrates and natural killer cell presence in human brain tumors. Cancer 1988; 61:738.
20. Iwasaki Y, Sako K, Tsunoda I, et al: Phenotypes of mononuclear cell infiltrates in human central nervous system. Acta Neuropathol 1993; 85:653.
21. Lampson LA, Hickey WF: Monoclonal antibody analysis of MHC expression in human brain biopsies: Tissue ranging from ''histologically normal'' to that showing different levels of glial tumor involvement. J Immunol 1986; 136:4054.
22. Morioka T, Baba T, Black KL, et al: Immunophenotypic analysis of infiltrating leukocytes and microglia in an experimental rat glioma. Acta Neuropathol 1992; 83:590.
23. Main EK, Monos DS, Lampson LA: IFN-treated neuroblastoma cell lines remain resistant to T cell mediated allo-killing and susceptible to non-MHC restricted cytotoxicity. J Immunol 1988; 141:2943.

24. Couldwell WT, de Tribolet N, Antel JP, et al: Adhesion molecules and malignant gliomas: Implications for tumorigenesis. J Neurosurg 1992; 76:782.

25. Lanzavecchia A: Identifying strategies for immune intervention. Science 1993; 260:937.

26. Maudsley DJ, Pound JD: Modulation of MHC antigen expression by viruses and oncogenes. Immunol Today 1991; 12:429.

27. Jennings MT, Ebrahim SAD, Thaler HT, et al: Immunophenotypic differences between normal glia, astrocytomas and malignant gliomas: Correlation with karyotype, natural history and survival. J Neuroimmunol 1989; 25:7.

28. Merlo A, Filgueira L, Zuber M, et al: T-cell receptor V-gene usage in neoplasms of the central nervous system: A comparative analysis in cultured tumor infiltrating and peripheral blood T cells. J Neurosurg 1993; 78:630.

29. Grimm EA, Bruner JM, Carinhas J, et al: Characterization of interleukin-2-initiated versus OKT3-initiated human tumor-infiltrating lymphocytes from glioblastoma multiforme: Growth characteristics, cytolytic activity, and cell phenotype. Cancer Immunol Immunother 1991; 32:391.

30. Klein E, Mantovani A: Action of natural killer cells and macrophages in cancer. Curr Opinion Immunol 1993; 5:714.

31. Black KL, Chen K, Becker DP, et al: Inflammatory leukocytes associated with increased immunosuppression by glioblastoma. J Neurosurg 1992; 77:120.

32. Myers RL, Whisler RL, Stephens RE, et al: Sensitivity of human glioma and brain cells to natural killer cell lysis. J Neurosurg 1992; 76:986.

33. Phillips JH, Lanier LL: Dissection of the lymphokine-activated killer phenomenon: Relative contribution of peripheral blood natural killer cells and T lymphocytes to cytolysis. J Exp Med 1986; 164:814.

34. Ruijs TCG, Louste K, Brown EA, et al: Lysis of human glial cells by major histocompatibility complex-unrestricted CD4+ cytotoxic lymphocytes. J Neuroimmunol 1993; 42:105.

35. De Micco C: Immunology of central nervous system tumors. J Neuroimmunol 1989; 25:93.

36. Mantovani A, Bottazzi B, Colotta F, et al: The origin and function of tumor-associated macrophages. Immunol Today 1992; 13:265.

37. Constam DB, Philipp J, Malipiero UV, et al: Differential expression of transforming growth factor-β1, -β2, and -β3 by glioblastoma cells, astrocytes, and microglia. J Immunol 1992; 148:1404.

38. Samuels V, Barrett JM, Bockman S, et al: Immunocytochemical study of transforming growth factor expression in benign and malignant gliomas. Am J Pathol 1989; 134:895.

39. Huber D, Fontana A, Bodmer S: Activation of human platelet-derived latent transforming growth factor-β1 by human glioblastoma cells. Biochem J 1991; 277:165.

40. Dubois CM, Ruscetti FW, Palaszynski EW, et al: Transforming growth factor β is a potent inhibitor of interleukin 1 (IL-1) receptor expression: Proposed mechanism of inhibition of IL-1 action. J Exp Med 1990; 172:737.

41. Wahl SM, McCartney-Francis N, Mergenhagen SE: Inflammatory and immunomodulatory roles of TGF-β. Immunol Today 1989; 10:258.

42. Bogdan C, Paik J, Vodovotz Y, et al: Contrasting mechanisms for suppression of macrophage cytokine release by transforming growth factor-β and interleukin-10. J Biol Chem 1992; 267:23301.

43. Ding A, Nathan CF, Graycar J, et al: Macrophage deactivating factor and transforming growth factors-β1, -β2, and -β3 inhibit induction of macrophage nitrogen oxide synthesis by IFN-γ. J Immunol 1990; 145:940.

44. Wahl SM, Costa GL, Corcoran M, et al: Transforming growth factor-β mediates IL-1-dependent induction of IL-1 receptor antagonist. J Immunol 1993; 150:3553.

45. Lin HY, Lodish HF: Receptors for the TGF-β superfamily: Multiple polypeptides and serine/threonine kinases. Trend Cell Biol 1993; 3:14.

46. Iruela-Arispe ML, Sage EH: Endothelial cells exhibiting angiogenesis in vitro proliferate in response to TGF-β1. J Cell Biochem 1993; 52:414.

47. Morganti-Kossmann MC, Kossmann T, Brandes ME, et al: Autocrine and paracrine regulation of astrocyte function by transforming growth factor-β. J Neuroimmunol 1992; 39:163.

48. Jennings MT, Maciunas RJ, Carver R, et al: TGFβ1 and TGFβ2 are potential growth regulators for low-grade and malignant gliomas in vitro: Evidence in support of an autocrine hypothesis. Int J Cancer 1991; 49:129.

49. Sporn MB, Roberts AB: Transforming growth factor-β: Recent progress and new challenges. J Cell Biol 1992; 119:1017.

50. Reiss M, Vellucci VF, Zhou Z-L: Mutant p53 tumor suppressor gene causes resistance to transforming growth factor β1 in murine keratinocytes. Cancer Res 1993; 53:899.

51. Holland G, Zlotnik A: Interleukin-10 and cancer. Cancer Invest 1993; 11:751.

52. Paulus W, Roggendorf W: Messenger RNA expression of the immunosuppressive cytokine IL–10 in human gliomas. Am J Pathol 1995; 146:317.

53. Merlo A, Juretic A, Zuber M, et al: Cytokine gene expression in primary brain tumours, metastases and meningiomas suggest specific transcription patterns. Eur J Cancer 1993; 29A:2118.

54. Sawamura Y, Diserens A-C, de Tribolet N: In vitro prostaglandin E₂ production by glioblastoma cells and its effect on interleukin-2 activation of oncolytic lymphocytes. J Neurooncol 1990; 9:125.

55. Phipps RP, Stein SH, Roper RL: A new view of prostaglandin E regulation of the immune response. Immunol Today 1991; 12:349.

56. Lee SC, Liu W, Dickson DW, et al: Cytokine production by human fetal microglia and astrocytes: Differential induction by lipopolysaccharide and IL-1β. J Immunol 1993; 150:2659.

57. Bethea JR, Chung IY, Sparacio SM, et al: Interleukin-1β induction of tumor necrosis factor-α gene expression in human astroglioma cells. J Neuroimmunol 1992; 36:179.

58. Valasco S, Tarlow M, Olsen K, et al: Temperature-dependent modulation of lipopolysaccharide-induced interleukin-1β and tumor necrosis factor α expression in cultured human astroglial cells by dexamethasone and indomethacin. J Clin Invest 1991; 87:1674.

59. Tada M, Sawamura Y, Sakuma S, et al: Cellular and cytokine responses of the human central nervous system to intracranial administration of tumor necrosis factor α for the treatment of malignant gliomas. Cancer Immunol Immunother 1993; 36:251.

60. Smith CA, Farrah T, Goodwin RG: The TNF receptor superfamily of cellular and viral proteins: Activation, costimulation, and death. Cell 1994; 76:959.

61. Sakuma S, Sawamura Y, Tada M, et al: Responses of human glioblastoma cells to human natural tumor necrosis factor α: Susceptibility, mechanism of resistance and cytokine production studies. J Neurooncol 1993; 15:197.

62. Tada M, Diserens A-C, Desbaillets I, et al: Analysis of cytokine receptor mRNA expressions in human glioblastoma cells and normal astrocytes by reverse transcriptase polymerase chain reaction. J Neurosurgery 1994; 80:1063.

63. Barna BP, Barnett GH, Jacobs BS, et al: Divergent responses of human astrocytoma and non-neoplastic astrocytes to tumor necrosis factor α involve the 55 kDa tumor necrosis factor receptor. J Neuroimmunol 1993; 43:185.

64. Dinarello CA: Interleukin-1 and interleukin-1 antagonism. Blood 1991; 77:1627.

65. Gauthier T, Hamou M-F, Monod L, et al: Expression and release of interleukin-1 by human glioblastoma cells in vitro and in vivo. Acta Neurochir (Wien) 1993; 121:199.

66. Frei K, Piani D, Malipiero UV, et al: Granulocyte-macrophage colony-stimulating factor (GM-CSF) production by glioblastoma cells: Despite the presence of inducing signals GM-CSF is not expressed in vivo. J Immunol 1992; 148:3140.

67. Giulian D, Woodward J, Young DG, et al: Interleukin-1 injected into mammalian brain stimulates astrogliosis and neovascularization. J Neurosci 1988; 8:2485.

68. Opdenakker G, Van Damme J: Cytokine and proteases in invasive processes: Molecular similarities between inflammation and cancer. Cytokine 1992; 4:251.

69. Tada M, Diserens A-C, Desbaillets I, et al: Production of interleukin-1 receptor antagonist by human glioblastoma cells in vitro and in vivo. J Neuroimmunol 1994; 50:187.

70. Larsson I, Landstroem LE, Larner E, et al: Interferon production in glia and glioma cell lines. Infect Immun 1978; 22:786.

71. Godbout R, Miyakoshi J, Dobler KD, et al: Lack of expression of tumor-suppressor genes in human malignant glioma cell lines. Oncogene 1992; 7:1879.

72. Van Meir E, Sawamura Y, Diserens A-C, et al: Human glioblastoma cells release interleukin 6 in vivo and in vitro. Cancer Res 1990; 50:6683.

73. Santhanam U, Ray A, Sehgal PB: Repression of the interleukin 6 gene

promoter by p53 and the retinoblastoma susceptibility gene product. Proc Natl Acad Sci USA 1991; 88:7605.

74. Lotz M: Interleukin-6. Cancer Invest 1993; 11:732.

75. Motro B, Itin A, Sachs L, et al: Pattern of interleukin 6 gene expression in vivo suggests a role for this cytokine in angiogenesis. Proc Natl Acad Sci USA 1990; 87:3092.

76. Van Meir E, Ceska M, Effenberger F, et al: Interleukin-8 is produced in neoplastic and infectious diseases of the human central nervous system. Cancer Res 1992; 52:4297.

77. Tada M, Suzuki K, Yamakawa Y, et al: Human glioblastoma cells produce 77 amino acid interleukin-8 (IL-8$_{77}$). J Neurooncol 1993; 16:25.

78. Springer TA: Traffic signals for lymphocyte recirculation and leukocyte emigration: The multistep paradigm. Cell 1994; 76:301.

79. Andersson P-B, Perry VH, Gordon S: Intracerebral injection of proinflammatory cytokines or leukocyte chemotaxins induces minimal myelomonocytic cell recruitment to the parenchyma of the central nervous system. J Exp Med 1992; 176:255.

80. Koch A, Polverini P, Kunkel S, et al: Interleukin-8 as a macrophage-derived mediator of angiogenesis. Science 1992; 258:1798.

81. Yoshimura T, Takeya M, Takahashi K, et al: Production and characterization of mouse monoclonal antibodies against human monocyte chemoattractant protein-1. J Immunol 1991; 147:2229.

82. Desbaillets I, Tada M, Diserens A-C, et al: Monocyte chemoattractant protein-1 (MCP-1) is secreted by human astrocytic tumors in vivo and in vitro. Int J Cancer 1994; 58:240.

83. Tweardy DJ, Glazer ED, Mott PL, et al: Modulation by tumor necrosis factor α of human astroglial cell production of granulocyte colony stimulating factor (G-CSF). J Neuroimmunol 1991; 32:269.

84. Gallo P, Pagni S, Giometto B, et al: Macrophage-colony stimulating factor (M-CSF) in the cerebrospinal fluid. J Neuroimmunol 1990; 29:105.

85. Lee SC, Liu W, Roth P, et al: Macrophage colony-stimulating factor in human fetal astrocytes and microglia. J Immunol 1993; 150:594.

86. Berdel WE, de Vos S, Maurer J, et al: Recombinant human stem cell factor stimulates growth of a human glioblastoma cell line expressing c-*kit* protooncogene. Cancer Res 1992; 52:3498.

87. Yarden Y, Kuang W-J, Yang-Feng T, et al: Human proto-ongogene c-kit: A new cell surface receptor tyrosine kinase for an unidentified ligand. EMBO J 1987; 6:3341.

88. Da Cunha A, Jefferson JA, Jackson RW, et al: Glial cell-specific mechanisms of TGF-β1 induction by IL-1 in cerebral cortex. J Neuroimmunol 1993; 42:71.

89. Pardoll DM: Cancer vaccines. Trend Pharmacol Sci 1993; 14:202.

90. Jachimczak P, Bogdahn U, Schneider J, et al: The effect of transforming growth factor-β$_2$-specific phosphorothioate-anti-sense oligodeoxynucleotides in reversing cellular immunosuppression in malignant glioma. J Neurosurg 1993; 78:944.

GLOSSARY

Adhesion molecules A group of cell surface molecules that function in cell-to-cell adhesion and interaction. Adhesion molecules mediate leukocyte trafficking across vessels. They are also relevant in the processes of metastasis and invasion of tumor cells.

Antibodies, immunoglobulins A group of peptides produced by plasma cells whose molecular sizes range from 146 to 970 kD. Each Ig unit consists of an F(ab′)$_2$ portion, which binds to an antigen, and an Fc portion, which binds to the first complement component (C1q) and to the Fc receptor expressed on immune cells. Immunoglobulins are grouped into six main classes: IgG, IgA, IgM, IgA, IgD, and IgE.

Antigen A molecule that induces the formation of an antibody. Antigen is a target of antibody and of T-cell receptor.

Antigen presenting cells (APCs) Cells that present antigens in a form that can stimulate T cells. Antigen presentation is done with restriction of MHC molecules. In the CNS, microglia, astrocytes, endothelial cells, bloodborne macrophages, and B cells are potential APCs.

Autocrine A mode of cytokine action in which the cytokine produced by a cell acts on the same cell.

B cell A population of lymphocytes that can be activated to differentiate into plasma cells and to produce antibodies.

Biologic response modifiers A group of substances that either by themselves or in combination with the host's immune system evoke some type of beneficial biologic response. They include nonspecific immunopotentiators and cytokines.

Cluster of differentiation (CD) A group of cell surface molecules of leukocytes that may be used to differentiate different cell populations. Each CD has a distinct function.

CD4 One of the helper T-cell markers. A receptor of class II MHC, it couples with the antigen-specific T-cell receptor and recognizes an antigen processed and presented on class II MCH molecules.

CD8 One of the cytotoxic T-cell markers. A receptor of class I MHC molecule, it couples with the antigen-specific T-cell receptor and recognizes an antigen processed and presented on class I MHC molecules.

Cellular immunity Immunologic reactions that are mediated by T lymphocytes, natural killer (NK) cells, and phagocytes, rather than by antibody (humoral immunity).

Chemoattraction/chemotaxis Increased directional migration of cells, particularly in response to concentration gradients of certain chemotactic factors or chemoattractants.

Chemokine A group of cytokines that have chemotactic activities to leukocytes. Chemokines are subclassified into two families depending on the amino acid (cystein) sequence adjacent to the N-terminal: C-X-C chemokine and C-C chemokine. C-X-C chemokines include IL8, GRO gene products, neutrophil activating protein 2, and IP10. C-C chemokines include MCP1, MIP-1α and β, and RANTES.

Complement A group of proteins that cause inflammatory cascade reactions following antibody attachment to antigen, leading to the activation of phagocytes and to the lytic attack on cell membrane.

Co-stimulation Assistant signaling in the process of antigen presentation, which is required for proper differentiation and activation of T cells. Co-stimulation is mediated by co-stimulatory molecules (B7, B70), certain adhesion molecules, and cytokines.

Colony-stimulating factor (CSF) A group of cytokines that control the differentiation and activation of hematopoietic stem cells. Granulocyte-macrophage CSF (CSF2) acts on granulocytes, monocytes/macrophages, and their precursor cells. Macrophage CSF (CSF1) acts on monocytes/macrophages. Stem cell factor (SCF) acts on hematopoietic stem cells.

Cytotoxic T lymphocytes (CTL) A population of T cells that has the ability to kill cells directly.

Cytokine A generic term for soluble molecules (peptides) that mediate interactions between cells. The short-term and short-range actions of cytokines differ from those of peptide hormones.

Cytokine network Complex interactive signaling among

cells that involves multiple cytokines. Autocrine and paracrine loops of cytokines form the network.

Epidermal growth factor (EGF) A 6-kD protein that is produced by various tissues and acts on various cells as a growth-promoting factor. Transforming growth factor-α (TGFA) shares the same receptor with EGF.

Gene therapy Therapy of aberrant genetic conditions by introduction (transduction) of a new gene into cells. A gene is introduced to the cells either to express the new gene or to suppress a target gene (antisense technique).

Helper T (Th) cells A functional subclass of T cells that can help to generate cytotoxic T cells and cooperate with B cells in the production of the antibody response. Helper T cells recognize antigens in association with class II MHC molecules.

Human leukocyte antigen (HLA) Human major histocompatibility complex (MHC). HLA-DR equals MHC class I; HLA-A, B, C equals class II.

Humoral immunity Immunity that occurs by humoral factors, including antibodies and complement components.

Hybridoma An artificial immortalized cell line that is usually generated by the hybridization of a myeloma cell and an antibody-producing B-cell of murine origin. Cloned hybridoma cells produce monoclonal antibodies.

Interferon (IFN) A group of mediators that increase the resistance to viral infection, and act as cytokines. Lymphoid cells, particularly B cells, produce IFN-α (lymphoblastoid IFN), fibroblasts produce IFN-β, and helper T cells produce IFN-γ (immune IFN).

Interleukin (IL) A generic term for molecules involved in signaling between cells of the immune system. Cytokines that are mainly (originally) secreted from leukocytes.

Immunotherapy A tumor therapy that manipulates the host's immune reaction or that adds immune components. Immunotherapy is classified into four groups: (1) active immunotherapy (vaccination), (2) passive immunotherapy (administration of antibodies), (3) adoptive immunotherapy (administration of ex vivo adopted immune cells), and (4) biologic response modification (administration of immune or other bioactive molecules).

Lymphokine-activated killer (LAK) cells A functional population of peripheral blood mononuclear cells that are activated and expanded with IL2 and have cytotoxic activities against tumor cells. They consist of heterogeneous sets of cells derived from natural killer (NK) cells, cytotoxic T cells, and large granular lymphocytes.

Macrophages Phagocytic and antigen-presenting cells that originate from bloodborne monocytes.

Monocyte chemoattractant protein 1 (MCP1) A cytokine that was originally cloned from glioma cells and has chemotactic and activating effects on monocytes. Lymphocytes, smooth muscle cells, endothelial cells, and fibroblasts are known as its sources.

Major histocompatibility complex (MHC) A genetic region found in mammals, the products of which are primarily responsible for the rejection of grafts between individuals; they function in signaling between lymphocytes and cells expressing antigen. MHC encodes three major classes of MHC molecules: I, II, and III. A processed antigen is presented on the groove of different MHC class I and II molecules, depending on the amino acid sequence.

MHC restriction A characteristic of many immune reactions in which immunologically active cells cooperate effectively with other cells when they share the same MHC types at either the class I or II loci.

Microglia A group of glial cells in the CNS that have functions similar to those of macrophages.

Neurotropic factors A group of peptide factors that can support survival and cause differentiation of neurons. They include a variety of cytokines and growth factors, such as nerve growth factor, platelet-derived growth factor, ciliary neurotropic factor, IL6, and stem cell factor.

Natural killer (NK) cells A group of lymphocytes that have the intrinsic ability to recognize and destroy some virally infected cells and some tumor cells.

Non–MHC-restricted cells Not restricted by class I or II MHC, but utilizing other unknown cell-recognition systems. NK cells and some cytotoxic T cells mediate cytotoxicity against tumor cells by this mode of recognition.

p53 One of the tumor suppressor genes on chromosome 17 whose product has a molecular weight of 53 kD and which suppresses an unlimited cell growth through interacting with transcriptional factors. A functional loss of this gene product can cause a tumor.

Paracrine A mode of cytokine action in which the cytokine produced by a cell acts on different cells in the neighbourhood.

Prostaglandin E$_2$ One of the end products of the arachidonic acid pathway in cells. It acts on immune cells through a receptor as a potent inhibitor of immune responses.

Recombinant Generated by (artificial) rearrangement of genetic information with DNA insertion into genes. DNA is recombined in plasmid vectors and put into *Escherichia coli* to produce recombinant proteins.

Soluble receptor A special form of cytokine receptor that lacks transmembrane and intracellular domains. A soluble receptor is formed by enzymatic cleavage and is shed from the cells to serve as an antagonist by competing with ligand binding.

T cells A population of lymphocytes that are derived from thymocytes and that function through interacting with B-cells (humoral immunity) and macrophages (cell-mediated immunity) through T-cell receptors and cytokines. T cells are functionally subclassified into helper T cells, suppressor T cells, suppressor-inducer T cells, and cytotoxic T cells.

T-cell receptor (TCR) Receptor on T cell that can specifically bind antigen presented on the MHC molecule. Similar to immunoglobulin, the TCR has a variable region that recognizes a specific antigenic epitope. TCR works in association with CD3 and CD4 or CD8 molecule.

Transforming growth factor-β (TGFB) A group of three cytokines (TGFB1, 2, and 3) that can stimulate growth (transformation) of some cells. TGFB inhibits the proliferation and functions of all classes of lymphocytes, causing immunosuppression.

Tumor necrosis factor-α (TNFA) A multifunctional cytokine released by activated macrophages that can initiate inflammatory reactions. It is structurally related to other members of the TNF family, including lymphotoxin (LT), which is produced by lymphocytes. The name is derived from the fact that its activity causes necrosis of certain tumors.

Tolerance Exclusion of T cells that can react to self-antigens during early development in the thymus.

Transcriptional factors Intracellular peptides that can bind to the specific DNA sequence in the promoter region of genes to induce or suppress the gene expression. Many oncogenes have been identified as transcriptional factors.

W.K. ALFRED YUNG

SAMER E. KABA

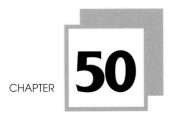

CHAPTER **50**

Biologic Response Modifiers

Biologic response modifiers represent a group of heterogeneous agents (natural or recombinant) that, either by themselves or via the host immune system, can modify the phenotypic characteristics of tumor cells.[1] The rationale for investigating the role of biologic response modifiers in the treatment of brain tumors includes the following: (1) the immune status of patients with brain tumors has been shown to be abnormal; (2) a concept has been put forth that tumor cell growth may represent an escape of the tumor cells from the immune surveillance system; and (3) many biologic response modifiers, such as cytokines, can directly modulate the biologic environment of tumor cells.

Biologic response modifiers in general can be divided into four classes:

1. Agents that trigger active immune response: These agents activate the host immune system to recognize and destroy the tumor cells as foreign substances.

2. Agents or substances that provide passive immunity to the host: These substances, such as specific antibodies, can seek out and destroy the tumor cells.

3. Activated or sensitized immune cells: These can transfer specific cell-mediated cytotoxic capabilities to the patient to fight against the tumor cells.

4. Agents or substances that can elicit various nonspecific immune responses or directly modulate cellular growth mechanisms of the tumor cells: These include interferons, interleukins, and other cytokines (Table 50–1).[1]

Because antibody therapy and adoptive immunotherapy are discussed in other chapters, only active immunotherapy and cytokine therapies are discussed in this chapter.

HOST IMMUNITY OF BRAIN TUMOR PATIENTS

Although patients with malignant brain tumors do not have gross impairment in immune responses, deficits in humoral and cellular immunity have been demonstrated.[2] Decreased delayed hypersensitivity to antigens has also been demonstrated in patients with brain tumors. Although the role of a defective cellular immunity in the development and progression of malignant gliomas is not certain, an immune sup-

pressive factor, transforming growth factor-β (TGFB2), has been isolated from blood samples and from cystic fluid obtained from patients with glioblastoma multiforme.[3, 4] The immunosuppressive effect of TGFB2 has been found to vary among different glioma cell lines, and its effect could be potentiated by retinoic acid or TNF.[5]

Lack of immune response to brain tumor cells may be secondary to inadequate presentation of glioma-associated antigens to macrophages and T-lymphocytes. Recognition of tumor cell antigens by cytotoxic T-cells is in fact dependent on expression of HLA class I antigens,[6] but a decreased expression of class I and II antigens has been shown to occur in many malignant gliomas.[7]

Despite the presence of immunosuppressive factor TGFB2 and a decrease in antigen recognition, evidence of an immune reaction has been noted in many malignant gliomas. Lymphocytic infiltrate can be demonstrated in 30% to 60% of glioblastomas.[8, 9] Peripheral blood lymphocytes from many malignant glioma patients can be stimulated to proliferate by exposure to autologous tumor cells or to interleukin 2.[10, 11]

INTERFERON AND BRAIN TUMORS

Interferons, first described by Isaac and Lindenmann in 1957,[12] represents a family of naturally occurring proteins

TABLE 50–1
BIOLOGIC RESPONSE MODIFIERS IN MALIGNANT BRAIN TUMOR THERAPY

Cytokines
   Interferons (IFN-α, IFN-β, IFN-γ)
   Interleukins (IL2, IL4)
   Tumor necrosis factor (TNF-A)
Passive immunotherapy
   Monoclonal antibodies
   Immunoconjugates
Adoptive immunotherapy
   IL2/lymphokine-activated killer cells
   Tumor infiltrating lymphocyte cells
Active immunotherapy
   Bacille Calmette-Guérin
   Corynebacterium parvum
   Serratia marcescens (Immunert)
   Autologous tumor cells

that constitute the body's defenses against viral, microbial, and neoplastic insults. Interferons in general are divided into three classes (Table 50–2). Interferon-α, synthesized by leukocytes, and IFN-β, synthesized by fibroblasts, are called type I interferons. They are encoded by a cluster of IFN-αβ genes on the short arm of chromosome 9. IFN-α and IFN-β bind to the same receptor. IFN-γ, synthesized by a specific class of immune lymphocytes, is called type II interferon, and binds to its own receptor. Only one IFN-γ gene is located on chromosome 12,[13] whereas the receptor gene is located on chromosome 6. Although viruses are potent inducers of interferons, other chemical/biologic agents and cytokines can also induce interferon synthesis. These include bacterial and mycoplasmal infection, platelet-derived growth factor (PDGF), colony-stimulating factor 1 (CSF1), interleukin 1 (IL1), interleukin 2 (IL2), and TNF.[14–16] Interferon synthesis is regulated both in the transcriptional and translational levels. Activation of specific transcriptional factors that bind to regulatory regions of the interferon genes initiates the process of transcription, whereas translational regulation is mediated by messenger ribonucleic acid (mRNA) stabilization.

The biologic effects of interferons are very species specific. The three main biologic activities of interferons—antiviral, antiproliferative, and immunomodulatory—are mediated by interferon-inducible proteins. Interferon-inducible genes are activiated via a membrane-receptor signaling mechanism, which results in translocation of cytoplasmic signaling factors to the nucleus, where a cascade of transcriptional and translational activities is initiated.[17–19]

Interferons play an important role in defending against virus infection.[20, 21] Interferons are produced early in large quantity, and the level of interferon correlates with the severity and the length of the infection. The mechanism by which interferons inhibit viral replication has not been fully worked out, but it is believed to involve activation of the enzyme, 2′5′-oligoadenylate synthetase by double-stranded ribonucleic acid (ds-RNA).[22, 23]

The antiproliferative or antitumor effect of interferons was discovered after their antiviral effects were known.[24, 25] The mechanism of action may include direct growth inhibitory activity mediated by direct cell cycle regulation, activation of the 2′5′-oligo synthetase pathway, and inhibition of polyamine synthesis by inhibition of induction of ornithine decarboxylase, which is a key rate-limiting step in polyamine synthesis that correlates tightly with cellular proliferation.[26, 27]

The immunomodulating effects of IFN-γ have been better studied than have those of type I IFN-αβ.[28, 29] IFN-γ has a marked effect on modulation of major histocompatibility complex (MHC) antigen expression on the cell surface of many cell types, whereas IFN-αβ may have antagonistic immunomodulatory effects. The interaction between interferons and other immune cytokines is complex and is just beginning to be understood. It has been noted that IFN-γ activates macrophages by inducing production of TNF. Activation of natural killer (NK) cells by IL2 may involve IFN-γ, and TNF exerts antiviral and antitumor effects via induction of IFN-β. All of these examples suggest important cooperation and interaction between interferons and various intracellular signaling cytokines.

IFN-α has been used in cancer therapy for many years. It has been proved to be effective in hairy cell leukemia, chronic myelogeneous leukemia, and renal cell carcinoma. Interferons have been widely used in Japan for the treatment of malignant gliomas. Initial studies in Japan and in America showed better activity of IFN-β against gliomas compared with that of IFN-α. When recombinant interferon-β was given to 65 patients with malignant gliomas, either intratumorally or intravenously, an overall response rate of 26% was seen. Patients with newly diagnosed and those with recurrent disease responded equally well.[30] In a subsequent study, IFN-β was added to 1-(4-amino-2-methyl-5-pyrimidinyl)methyl-3-(2-chloroethyl)-3 nitrosourea (ACNU) as initial chemotherapy. The group that received IFN-β and ACNU had a much higher response rate (41.2%) than the group that received ACNU alone.[31] Since then, IFN-β plus ACNU has become a standard combination initial therapy following radiation therapy for patients with malignant gliomas in Japan. In this country, Mahaley and co-workers[32, 33] pioneered the use of interferons in brain tumor patients in the early 1980s. In several studies, they demonstrated that IFN-α had modest activity in patients with recurrent malignant gliomas, whereas IFN-γ had little or no activity.

It has been shown that, although IFN-α and IFN-β are active in inhibiting glioma cell growth, IFN-β is more active than IFN-α.[34] The mechanism behind this differential sensitivity is not known, as both IFN-α and IFN-β bind onto the same type I receptor.[35] Yung and colleagues[36] had reported results of a phase I study of a recombinant IFN-β (Betaseron), which is non-glycosolated and has a serine substitution in position 17, in 10 patients with recurrent malignant gliomas; a 50% response and stabilization rate was demonstrated. A subsequent multicenter study with the same recombinant IFN-β molecule again demonstrated modest activity in 65 patients with a combined response (23%) and stabilization (28%) rate of 51% and a time to tumor progression of 20 weeks among the responders.[37] In this study, dose-limiting neurotoxic effects, including apathy and acute psychosis, developed in several patients. In most patients, IFN-β was well tolerated. Common side effects of interferon therapy include fever, myalgia, and malaise. These symptoms usually become progressively better during the second and third weeks of therapy. More chronic toxic responses include fatigue, apathy, and Parkinson-like syndrome. Severe apathy and seizure are often associated with higher-dose interferon therapy and require dose reduction or withdrawal.

In a separate study,[38] IFN-β (Betaseron) was administered to 29 pediatric patients with recurrent malignant brain tumors, including brainstem glioma, anaplastic astrocytoma, ependymoma, and medulloblastoma. Fourteen patients showed various degrees of response to the treatment, and the toxic response profile was similar to that seen in adult patients.

TABLE 50–2
CLASSIFICATION OF INTERFERONS

Type	Cell	Chromosome Location
α	Leukocyte	9
β	Fibroblast	9
γ	T-lymphocyte	12

So far, only modest activity has been seen in patients with recurrent malignant gliomas when interferon was used as single agent. It may be more effective when used in combination with other agents.[39] It may also be more effective when used in an adjuvant therapy setting immediately after surgery and radiation, when the tumor burden is lowest. To this end, IFN-α has been combined with carmustine (BCNU) and fluorouracil as chemobiologic therapy in patients with newly diagnosed or recurrent glioblastomas.[40, 41]

INTERLEUKINS AND BRAIN TUMOR THERAPY

Interleukins represent a large family of cytokines with the ability to activate lymphocytes and leukocytes. In the laboratory, interleukin 2 (IL2) has been shown to have a growth inhibitory effect on human glioma cell lines.[42] Systemic injection of IL2 has been associated with acute cerebral edema and seizures due to the capillary leak syndrome. This is believed to be a direct cytotoxic effect of IL2 on endothelial cells, as demonstrated by Merchant and associates.[43] Clinically, IL2 has primarily been administered intratumorally by itself or in combination with lymphokine-activated killer (LAK) cells or tumor infiltrating lymphocyte (TIL) cells.[44] High levels of IL2 can be detected in the CSF when IL2 is given intrathecally.[45] When given intrathecally to patients with meningeal metastases, IL2 (with or without LAK cells) induced a rapid increase in several cytokines, including tumor necrosis factor-α (TNFA), interleukin 1β (IL1B), IL6, IFN-γ.[46] Merchant and colleagues,[47] in a small study of nine patients, showed that intraventricular IL2 and subcutaneous IFN-α can be given safely as long as less than 50,000 IU of IL2 was injected. More recently, IL4 (another interleukin) was demonstrated to inhibit 9L glioma cell growth when it was given with TNFA and IFN-γ. IL4 alone was not effective in this model, which suggests that IL4 is capable of modulating glioblastoma growth only when other cytokines, TNFA, or IFN-γ are present.[48]

TUMOR NECROSIS FACTOR-α IN THE TREATMENT OF BRAIN TUMORS

Tumor necrosis factor-α, a cytokine derived from activated macrophages and astrocytes, was discovered by Carswell and associates in 1975.[49] Several biologic effects of this cytokine were identified in vivo and in vitro. Two major effects were described early: the ability to induce hemorrhagic necrosis in murine tumors and a cytotoxic/cytostatic activity against tumor cell lines, but not against normal cells.[49, 50] Other biologic activities were reported, including stimulation of granulocytes, proliferation of fibroblasts,[51, 52] antiviral activity,[53] and cytotoxic activity toward endothelial cells.[54–56] This cytokine is released within the central nervous system (CNS) in several pathologic processes, including multiple sclerosis and AIDS myelopathy. However, it is found in detectable amounts in the cerebrospinal fluid (CSF) only in bacterial meningitis.

The TNFA gene was cloned in 1985,[57] and large amounts of purified recombinant human TNFA could be produced and used in many laboratories. Multiple phase I and II clinical trials were conducted to evaluate the effectiveness of TNFA in systemic cancers.[58–63] This was followed by a number of studies to assess its potential use in brain tumors.

Using malignant glioma cell cultures, many authors were able to show a cytotoxic or cytostatic effect on certain cell lines.[64, 66] However, others found the majority of human glioma cells to be resistant to TNFA.[67, 68] In 1993, Iwasaki and colleagues[69] showed significant antiproliferative and anti-invasive effects of TNFA on four glioblastoma cell lines in a three-dimensional model. An increase in the percentage of cells resting in G0/G1 phase after treatment with TNFA was illustrated by Cheng and colleagues.[65] TNFA was also shown to reduce the size of established intracranial rat gliomas, especially when it was given via the carotid artery.[70, 71]

The immunobiologic effects of TNFA on malignant gliomas were also studied in vitro and in vivo. At low doses, TNFA stimulated the production of prostaglandin E2, manganese superoxide dismutase, IL6, and IL8 by glioblastoma cells.[72] A differential effect was suggested by Chen and others,[73] who found that different cell lines expressed different cell surface antigens and produced different cytokines when treated with TNFA. Expression of TNFA genes was found in brain tumors of astrocytic lineage including astrocytomas, glioblastomas, mixed oligoastrocytomas, and primitive neuroectodermal tumors.[74] Nitta and associates[75] analyzed the expression of cytokine genes in malignant gliomas and found expression of TNFA genes in tumor and surrounding brain tissue, but not in normal tissue. They concluded that TNFA may participate in local immune reactions of the brain in an autocrine and paracrine fashion.

Tada and co-workers[76] reported on serial CSF and regional fluid (RF) samples of six patients with malignant glioma who received repeated intratumoral TNFA injections. Recruitment of neutrophils in the CSF occurred first, and was followed with less remarkable migration of CD4+ T-lymphocytes and monocytes/macrophages. This leukocytosis lasted for 48 hours and was associated with increased neutrophil chemotactic activity. Increased levels of activity of IL6, IL1B, prostaglandin E2, and TGFB were noted in the CSF and RF. The authors concluded that TNFA is effective in inducing the migration of immune cells and in generating multiple cytokine responses in the human CNS. All of these studies suggest the possibility that the antineoplastic effects of TNFA are mediated by two mechanisms: a direct cytostatic effect and an immunomodulatory effect.

Few reports are available on the use of TNFA in the treatment of glial tumors in humans. Maruno and colleagues reported the complete regression of a recurrent anaplastic astrocytoma in one patient treated with multiple intraventricular doses of TNFA over an 8-month period. No recurrence was seen for 2 years. The side effects were limited to fever and chills during and immediately after infusion and mild thrombocytopenia.[77] Yoshida and associates[78] used intra-arterial injections of TNFA to increase the concentration of TNFA in the tumor without increasing the systemic side effects. Two of ten patients whom it was possible to evaluate had clinical and radiologic response, one complete and one partial. Both had glioblastoma multiforme. Some patients showed marked, rapid neurologic improvement without radiologic changes. Narrowing of tumor-feeding arteries immediately and 1 week after injection, as well as decreased staining ability, was noted on angiogram. Necrosis in the center of the tumor was noted on computed tomographic (CT) scan.[78] Another approach was described by Yamasaki and co-workers,[79] who used multiple intratumoral TNFA injections in two patients with malignant gliomas over a period of 3 to 5 months. Partial response was obtained and was maintained for 28 and 36 months with no significant neurotoxic effects.

Because of its antineoplastic activity and its relatively low toxic effect profile, TNFA, alone or in combination with other cytokines, may play an important role in the treatment of malignant gliomas in some patients. Further controlled studies on larger numbers of subjects are needed for final evaluation of this role.

ACTIVE IMMUNOTHERAPY FOR MALIGNANT GLIOMA

Malignant gliomas are usually associated with minimal inflammatory response. This is due mainly to the limited ability of the brain to generate a cytotoxic immune response and to the ability of gliomas to suppress the immune response in surrounding tissue,[80] and probably systemically.[81-83] The goal of active immunotherapy is to enhance the cytotoxic immune response of the brain, using nonspecific or specific methods to induce a delayed hypersensitivity reaction against the tumor antigens.

Nonspecific or restorative immunotherapy involves a broad enhancement of host immunosurveillance mechanisms. Bacille Calmette-Guérin (BCG) vaccine,[84, 90] and levamisole[89, 91] are the most commonly used agents. Mahaley and others[84] noted an increased survival in rats with avian sarcoma virus–induced gliomas after combined treatment with BCNU and intraperitoneal injection of BCG and sarcoma cells. In a later experiment, BCG cell-wall preparations were injected simultaneously with avian sarcoma virus in the brain of rats with avian sarcoma virus, and a significant reduction in glioma induction by the virus was noted.[85]

Albright and associates[86] injected purified protein derivative (PPD) intratumorally in patients with malignant gliomas after inoculation with BCG. A mild to moderate inflammatory response was induced in four of five patients, but it did not encompass the whole tumor and did not cause detectable tumor regression. Similar results were reported by Knerich and co-workers[89] and DeCearvalho and colleagues,[90] who demonstrated definite increases in immunologic response with no significant effect on survival. *Corynebacterium parvum*,[92] an α_1-thymosin,[93] and OK-432,[94] were also used with no significant benefits. Positive response was reported with mumps virus[95] and with rabies vaccine.[96]

Specific immunotherapy is based on inoculation of malignant glioma patients with live or irradiated tumor cells. These trials started with Bloom's work in the 1960s, and continued until the late 1980s. Trouillas[97] conducted a randomized controlled trial using saline extracts of autologous tumor with Freund's adjuvant. Sixty-five patients were randomized to receive radiation alone, immunotherapy alone, radiation and immunotherapy, or supportive treatment only.

Twenty-four of the 28 patients treated with immunotherapy developed a delayed hypersensitivity reaction, and survival was increased in the group who received radiation and immunotherapy (10.1 months) as compared with the group who received radiation alone (7.5 months). Bloom and colleagues[98] used irradiated tumor cells and reported no increase in survival. In a pilot study on 19 patients, Mahaley and co-workers[99] reported a longer survival in patients inoculated with U251 mg glioma cell line as compared with patients inoculated with D54 mg cell line. All patients received BCG cell-wall preparation and levamisole in conjunction with inoculation and were treated with radiation and BCNU. These results could not be reproduced in a subsequent full-scale study of 50 patients.[100] Several other reports with similar results are available.[101, 102]

When used as adjuvant therapy, active immunotherapy was shown to produce specific hypersensitivity against glioma and to increase survival in some patients. However, no convincing evidence has been documented to suggest that this treatment can play a significant role in treatment of malignant gliomas in humans.

FUTURE DIRECTIONS

The future of biologic therapy for malignant brain tumors depends on several factors. Combination of cytokines, such as interferons and interleukins or interferon and TNFA, need further exploration. Combination of cytokines and chemotherapeutic agents is already being studied in clinical trials. Dose scheduling is a critical issue. Should cytokines be given before or after the chemotherapeutic agents? Interferon may cause growth arrest, rendering the tumor cells less responsive to drugs that kill cycling cells. However, interferon or TNFA may modulate the chemosensitivity of tumor cells, making them more vulnerable to cytotoxic agents. In vitro modeling studies may be crucial to the rational design of the optimal dosing schedule.

Molecular approaches will definitely constitute the next generation of biologic therapy. Yagi and others[103] demonstrated that the IFNB gene can be transfected into U251-SP cells in nude mice by a plasmid pSV2 IFNB. Human IFNB was produced by the tumor and completely disappeared when tumor transfection was performed shortly after the transplantation. The survival of the tumor-bearing mice was markedly prolonged, even when the tumor did not completely disappear. In another study by Yu and co-workers,[104] IL4 gene was transfected into LT-1, a plasmacytoma cell line, which then expressed a high level of IL4. When U87 glioma cells were implanted with the LT-1 cells, significant inhibition of subcutaneous tumor growth was demonstrated. Prolongation of survival was also observed in animals implanted intracranially with U87 and LT-1 cells in a 1:1 ratio. Eosinophilic infiltration and inflammatory response were seen in the implanted site, which suggests that the local high level of IL4 secreted by the LT-1 cells was able to induce cytotoxic lymphocytic activity, which in turn eliminated the U87 tumor cells.

More sophisticated vector design, better mode of vector delivery, and more specific genetic targets, in combination with the recent progress made in molecular therapeutic approaches, will provide a broad field of research in molecular biologic/immunologic therapies for malignant brain tumors.

REFERENCES

1. Gillespie GY, Mahaley MS: Biological response modifier therapies for patients with malignant gliomas. *In* Thomas DGT (ed): Neuro-oncology: Primary Malignant Brain Tumors. London, Edward Arnold, 1990, p 242.
2. Jaeckle K: Immunotherapy of malignant gliomas. Semin Oncol 1994; 21:249.
3. Kuppner MC, Hamou MF, Bodmer S, et al: The glioblastoma-derived T-cell suppressor factors/transforming growth factor β inhibits the generation of lymphokine-activated killer (LAK) cells. Int J Cancer 1988; 42:562.
4. Ruffini PA, Rivoltini L, Silvani, et al: Factors including transforming growth factor β, released in the glioblastoma residual cavity, impair activity of adherent lymphokine-activated killer cells. Cancer Immunol Immunother 1993; 36:409.
5. Helseth E, Ungaard G, Dalen A, et al: Effects of type β transforming growth factor in combination with retinoic acid or tumor necrosis factor on proliferation of a human glioblastoma cell line and clonogenic cells from freshly resected brain tumors. Cancer Immunol Immunother 1988; 26:273.
6. Townsend A, Bodmer H: Antigen recognition by class I restricted T lymphocytes. Annu Rev Immunol 1989; 7:601.
7. Akbasak A, Oldfield EH, Saris C: Expression and modulation of major histocompatibility antigens on murine primary brain tumor in vitro. J Neurosurg 1991; 75:922.
8. Stevens A, Kloter I, Roggendorf W: Inflammatory infiltrates and natural killer cell presence in human brain tumors. Cancer 1988; 61:738.
9. Brooks WH, Markesbery WR, Gupta GD, et al: Relationship of lymphocyte invasion and survival of brain tumor patients. Ann Neurol 1978; 4:219.
10. Yoshida S, Tanaka R, Ono M, et al: Analysis of mixed lymphocyte-tumor culture in patients with malignant brain tumor. J Neurosurg 1989; 71:398.
11. Bosnes V, Hirshberg H: Comparison of in vitro glioma cell cytotoxicity of LAK cells from glioma patients and healthy subjects. J Neurosurg 1988; 69:234.
12. Isaac A, Lindenmann J: Virus interference: I. The interferon. Proc R Soc Lond Biol Soc 1957; 43:655.
13. Weissman C, Weber H: The interferon genes. Prog Nucleic Acid Res Mol Biol 1986; 33:251.
14. Sen GC, Lengyel P: The interferon system, a bird's eye view of its biochemistry. J Biol Chem 1992; 8:5017.
15. Young HA, Hardy KJ: Interferon: Gamma producer cells, activation, stimuli, and molecular genetic regulation. Pharmacol Ther 1990; 45:137.
16. Fields AK, Tytell AA, Lampson GP, et al: Inducers of interferon and host resistance II multistranded synthetic polynucleotide inducers. Proc Natl Acad Sci USA 1967; 58:1004.
17. Hardy KJ, Manger B, Newton M, et al: Molecular events involved in regulating human interferon gamma gene expression during T cell activation. J Immunol 1987; 138:2353.
18. Taylor JL, Grossberg SE: Recent progress in interferon research: Molecular mechanism of regulation, action and virus circumvention. Virus Res 1990; 15:1.
19. Kerr JM, Stark GR: Mini review: The control of interferon-inducible gene expression. FEBS Lett 1991; 285:194.
20. Friedman RM: Antiviral activity of interferons. Bacteriol Rev 1977; 4:543.
21. Lengyel P: Biochemistry of interferons and their actions. Annu Rev Biochem 1982; 51:251.
22. Greenberg SB: Human interferon in viral diseases. Infect Dis Clin North Am 1987; 1:383.
23. Faltyneck CR, Kung H: The biochemical mechanisms of action of the interferons. Biofactors 1988; 1:227.
24. Paucker K, Cantell K, Henle W: Viral influence and suspended L cells: Effect of interfering viruses and interferon on the growth rate of cells. Virology 1962; 17:324.
25. Svet-Moldavski GJ, Nemiroskay BM, et al: Interfero-genicity and antigen recognition. Nature 1974; 247:205.
26. Borden EC: Interferons: Pleiotropic cellular modulators. Clin Immunol Immunopathol 1992; 62:518.
27. Sekar V, Atmar VJ, Joshi AR, et al: Inhibition of ornithine decarboxylase in human fibroblast cells by type I and type II interferons. Biochem Biophys Res Commun 1983; 114:950.
28. De Maeyer D, De Maeyer-Guignard J: Interferon and other regulatory cytokinesis. New York, John Wiley, 1988.
29. Inaba K, Kitaura M, Kato T, et al: Contrasting effects of alpha/beta and gamma-interferons on expression of macrophage Ia antigens. J Exp Med 1986; 163:1030.
30. Nagai M: Clinical effect of human fibroblast interferon (BM532) on malignant brain tumors—with special reference to gliomas. Nippon Gan Chiryo Gakkai Shi 1989; 24:638.
31. Nagai M: Advances of BRM therapy of malignant brain tumors. Gan To Kagaku Ryoho 1991; 18:188.
32. Mahaley MS, Urso MB, Whaley RA, et al: Immunobiology of primary intracranial tumors: X. Therapeutic efficacy of interferon in the treatment of recurrent gliomas. J Neurosurg 1985; 63:719.
33. Mahaley MS, Bertsch L, Cush S: Systemic gamma interferon therapy for recurrent gliomas. J Neurosurg 1988; 69:826.
34. Yung WKA, Steck PA, Kellcher PJ, et al: Growth inhibitory effect of recombinant alpha and beta interferon on human glioma cells. J Neurooncol 1987; 5:323–330.
35. Rosenblum MG, Yung WKA, Kellcher PJ, et al: Growth inhibitory effect of interferon-β but not interferon-α on human glioma cells: Correlation of receptor binding 2′,5′oligodemylate synthetase and protein kinase activity. J Interferon Res 1990; 10:141.
36. Yung WK, Castellanos AM, Van Tassel P, et al: Pilot study of recombinant interferon beta (IFN-beta ser) in patients with recurrent glioma. J Neurooncol 1990; 9:29.
37. Yung WKA, Prados M, Levin VA, et al: Intravenous recombinant interferon beta in patients with recurrent malignant gliomas: A phase I/II study. J Clin Oncol 1991; 9:1945.
38. Allen J, Packer R, Bleyer A, et al: Recombinant interferon beta: A phase I-II trial in children with recurrent brain tumors. J Clin Oncol 1991; 9:783.
39. Nakamura O, Maruo K, Ueyama Y, et al: Interactions of human fibroblast interferon with chemotherapeutic agents and radiation against human gliomas in nude mice. Neurol Res 1986; 8:152.
40. Fine HA, Wen P, Alexander E, et al: Alpha-interferon, BCNU and 5FU in the treatment of recurrent high grade astrocytomas. Proc Am Soc Clin Oncol 1993; 12:174.
41. Buckner JC, Brown LD, Kugler JW, et al: Phase II evaluation of recombinant interferon alpha and BCNU in recurrent glioma. J Neurosurg 1995; 82:430.
42. Benveniste EN, Tozawa H, Gasson JC, et al: Response of human glioblastoma cells to recombinant interleukin-2. J Neuroimmunol 1988; 17:301.
43. Merchant RE, Ellison MD, Young HF: Immunotherapy for malignant glioma using human recombinant interleukin-2 inactivated autologous lymphocytes: A review of preclinical and clinical investigations. J Neurooncol 1990; 8:173.
44. Sawamura Y, DeTribolet N: Immunotherapy of brain tumors. J Neurosurg Sci 1990; 34:265.
45. Miyatake S, Yamashita J, Tokuriki Y, et al: Pharmacokinetics and toxicity of intrathecal administration of recombinant interleukin-2. Gan To Kagaku Ryoho 1986; 13:2393.
46. List J, Moser RP, Steuer M, et al: Cytokine responses to intraventricular injection of interleukin 2 into patients with leptomeningeal carcinomatosis: Rapid induction of tumor necrosis factor alpha, interleukin 1 beta, interleukin 6, gamma-interferon and soluble interleukin 2 receptor (Mr 55,000 protein). Cancer Res 1992; 52:1123.
47. Merchant RE, McVicar DW, Merchant LH, et al: Treatment of recurrent malignant glioma by repeated intracerebral injections of human recombinant interleukin-2 alone or in combination with systemic interferon-α: Results of phase I clinical trial. J Neurooncol 1992; 12:75.
48. Iwasaki K, Rogers LR, Estes ML, et al: Modulation of proliferation and antigen expression of a cloned human glioblastoma by interleukin-4 alone and in combination with tumor necrosis factor-alpha and/or interferon-gamma. Neurosurgery 1993; 33:489.
49. Carswell EA, Old LJ, Kassel RI, et al: An endotoxin-induced serum factor that causes necrosis of tumors. Proc Natl Acad Sci USA 1975; 72:3666–3670.

50. Old LJ: Tumor necrosis factor (TNF). Science 1985; 230:630–632.

51. Beutler B, Cerami A: Chacetin: More than a tumor necrosis factor. N Engl J Med 1985; 316:379–385.

52. Vilcek J, Palombella VJ, Henriksen-DeStefano D, et al: Fibroblast growth enhancing activity of tumor necrosis factor and its relationship to other polypeptide growth factors. J Exp Med 1986; 163:632–643.

53. Mestan J, Digel W, Mittnachant S, et al: Antiviral effects of recombinant tumor necrosis factor in vitro (letter). Nature 1986; 323:816–819.

54. Goldblum SE, Hennig B, Jay M, et al: Tumor necrosis factor alpha-induced pulmonary vascular endothelial injury. Infect Immunol 1989; 57:1218–1226.

55. Sato N, Goto T, Haranaka K, et al: Actions of tumor necrosis factor on cultured vascular endothelial cells: Morphologic modulation, growth inhibition, and cytotoxicity. JNCI 1986; 76:1113–1121.

56. Watanabe N, Niitsu Y, Umeno H, et al: Toxic effect of tumor necrosis factor on tumor vasculature in mice. Cancer Res 1988; 48:2179–2183.

57. Shirai T, Yamaguchi H, Ito H, et al: Cloning and expression on *Escherichia coli* of the gene for human tumor necrosis factor (letter). Nature 1985; 313:803–806.

58. Blick M, Sherwin SA, Rosenblum M, et al: Phase I study of recombinant tumor necrosis factor in cancer patients. Cancer Res 1987; 47:2986–2989.

59. Creagan EG, Kovach JS, Moertel CG, et al: A phase I clinical trial of recombinant human tumor necrosis factor. Cancer 1988; 62:2467–2471.

60. Creaven PJ, Brenner DE, Cowens JW, et al: A phase I clinical trial of recombinant human tumor necrosis factor given daily for five days. Cancer Chemother Pharmacol 1989; 23:186–191.

61. Feinberg B, Kurzrock R, Talpaz M, et al: A phase I trial of intravenously administered recombinant human tumor necrosis factor-alpha in cancer patients. J Clin Oncol 1988; 6:1328–1334.

62. Kemeny N, Childs B, Larchian W, et al: Phase II trial of recombinant tumor necrosis factor in patients with advanced colorectal carcinoma. Cancer 1990; 66:659–663.

63. Kimura K, Taguchi T, Urushizaki I, et al: A-TNF Cooperative Study Group: Phase I study of recombinant human tumor necrosis factor. Cancer Chemother Pharmacol 1987; 20:223–229.

64. Helseth E, Torp S, Dalen A, et al: Effects of interferon-gamma and tumor necrosis factor-alpha on clonogenic growth of cell lines and primary cultures from human gliomas and brain metastasis. APMIS 1989; 97:569–574.

65. Cheng K, Swamura Y, Sakuma S, et al: Antiproliferative effect of tumor necrosis factor-alpha on human glioblastoma cells linked with cell cycle arrest in G1 phase. Neurol Med Chir (Tokyo) 1994; 34:274–278.

66. Rutka JT, Giblin JR, Berens ME, et al: The effects of human recombinant tumor necrosis factor on glioma-derived cell lines: Cellular proliferation, cytotoxicity, morphological and radioreceptor studies. Int J Cancer 1988; 41:573.

67. Zuber P, Acolla RS, Carrel S, et al: Effects of tumor necrosis factor-alpha on the surface phenotype and the growth of human malignant glioma cell lines. Int J Cancer 1988; 42:780.

68. Helseth E, Unsgaard G, Dalen A, et al: Effects of type beta transforming growth factor in combination with retinoic acid or tumor necrosis factor on proliferation of a human glioblastoma cell line and clonogenic cells from freshly resected human brain tumors. Cancer Immunol Immunother 1988; 26:273–279.

69. Iwasaki K, Rogers LR, Barnett GH, et al: Effect of recombinant tumor necrosis factor-alpha on three-dimensional growth, morphology, and invasiveness of human glioblastoma cells in vitro. J Neurosurg 1993; 78:952–958.

70. Liu SK, Jakowatz JG, Pollack RB, et al: Effects of intracarotid and intravenous infusion of human TNF and LT on established intracerebral rat gliomas. Lymphokine Cytokine Res 1991; 10:189–194.

71. Kido G, Wright JL, Merchant RE: Acute effects of human recombinant tumor necrosis factor-alpha on the cerebral vasculature of the rat in both normal brain and in an experimental glioma model. J Neurooncol 1991; 10:95–109.

72. Tada M: In vitro and in vivo immunobiological responses of glioblastoma to human natural tumor necrosis factor-alpha. Hokkaido Igaku Zasshi 1992; 67:498–511.

73. Chen TC, Hinton DR, Apuzzo ML, et al: Differential effects of tumor necrosis factor-alpha on proliferation, cell surface antigen expression, and cytokine interactions in malignant gliomas. Neurosurgery 1993; 32:85–94.

74. Liberski PP, Mirceka B, Alwasiak J, et al: Expression of tumor necrosis factor-alpha cachectin in primary brain tumors of astrocytic lineage. Neuropatol Pol 1992; 30:35–42.

75. Nitta T, Ebato M, Sato K, et al: Expression of tumor necrosis factor-alpha, -beta and interferon-gamma genes within human neurological tumor cells and brain specimens. Cytokine 1994; 6:171–180.

76. Tada M, Swamura Y, Sakuma S, et al: Cellular and cytokine responses of the human central nervous system to intracranial administration of tumor necrosis factor-alpha for the treatment of malignant gliomas. Cancer Immunol Immunother 1993; 36:251–259.

77. Maruno M, Yoshimine T, Nakata H, et al: Complete regression of anaplastic astrocytoma by intravenous tumor necrosis factor-alpha (TNF-α) after recurrence: A case report. Surg Neurol 1994; 41:482–485.

78. Yoshida J, Wakabayashi T, Masaaki M, et al: Clinical effect of intra-arterial tumor necrosis factor-alpha for malignant glioma. J Neurosurg 1992; 77:78–83.

79. Yamasaki T, Moritake K, Paine JT, et al: Intratumoral administration of tumor necrosis factor-alpha for malignant glioma: Two case reports. Neurol Med Chir (Tokyo) 1994; 34:216–220.

80. Swamura Y, de Tribolet N: Immunobiology of brain tumors. Adv Tech Stand Neurosurg 1990; 17:3–64.

81. Jaeckle KA: Immunotherapy of malignant gliomas. Semin Oncol 1994; 21:249–259.

82. Tada M, deTribolet N: Recent advances in immunobiology of brain tumors. J Neurooncol 1993; 17:261–271.

83. Rozman T, Elliott L, Brooks W: Modulation of T-cell function by gliomas. Immunol Today 1991; 12:370–374.

84. Mahaley MS Jr, Gentry RE, Binger DD: Immunobiology of primary brain tumors. J Neurosurg 1977; 47:35–43.

85. Mahaley MS Jr, Aronin PA, Michael AJ, et al: Prevention of glioma induction in rats by simultaneous intracerebral inoculation of avian sarcoma virus plus bacillus Calmette-Guérin cell-wall preparation. Surg Neurol 1983; 19:453–455.

86. Albright L, Seab JA, Ommaya AK: Intracerebral delayed hypersensitivity reactions in glioblastoma multiforme patients. Cancer 1977; 39:1331–1336.

87. Bergquist BJ, Mahaley MS Jr, Steinbok P: Treatment of a brain tumor with BCG wall preparation. Surg Neurol 1980; 13:197–201.

88. Tanaka R, Sekiguchi K, Suzuki Y, et al: Local immunotherapy of malignant brain tumors. Evaluation of intratumoral injection of BCG and a *Streptococcus pyogenes* preparation. Neurol Med Chir (Tokyo) 1984; 24:376–384.

89. Knerich R, Robustelli della Cuna G, Butti G, et al: Chemotherapy plus immunotherapy for patients with primary and metastatic brain tumors. J Neurosurg Sci 1985; 29:19–24.

90. DeCearvalho S, Kaufman A, Pineda A: Adjuvant chemo-immunotherapy in central nervous system tumors. *In* Salmon J (ed): Adjuvant Therapy of Cancer. Amsterdam, Elsevier/North Holland, 1977, pp 495–502.

91. Fisher SWP, Lindermuth J, Hash C, et al: Levamisole in the treatment of glioblastoma multiforme. J Surg Oncol 1985; 28:214–216.

92. Selker RG, Wolmark N, Fisher B, et al: Preliminary observation on the use of *Corynebacterium parvum* in patients with primary intracranial tumors: Effects on intracranial pressure. J Surg Oncol 1978; 10:299–303.

93. Baskies AM, Chretien PB: Thymosine α-1 in malignant gliomas: Augmentation of immune reactivity in a phase I study. Surg Forum 1982; 33:522–524.

94. Shibata S, Mori K, Moryiama T, et al: Randomized control study of the effect of adjuvant immunotherapy with picibanil on 51 malignant gliomas. Surg Neurol 1987; 27:259–263.

95. Yumitori K, Handa H, Yamashita J, et al: Treatment of malignant glioma with mumps virus. No Shinkei Geka 1982; 10:143–147.

96. Filipo FV: A trial of rabies vaccine treatment of patients with glioblastoma multiforme. Zh Vopr Neirokhir Im N N Burdenko 1988; 3:38–40.

97. Trouillas P: Immunologie et immunotherapie des tumeurs cerebrales. Rev Neurol 1973; 128:23–28.

98. Bloom HJG, Peckham MJ, Richardson AE, et al: Glioblastoma multiforme: A controlled trial to assess the value of specific active immunotherapy in patients treated by radical surgery and radiotherapy. Br J Cancer 1973; 27:253–267.

99. Mahaley MS Jr, Steinbok P, Aronin P, et al: Immunobiology of

primary intracranial tumors: VII. Active immunization of patients with anaplastic glioma cell: A pilot study. J Neurosurg 1983; 59:201–207.

100. Mahaley MS Jr: Neuro-oncology index and review (adult primary brain tumors). J Neurooncol 1991; 11:85–147.

101. Bullard DE, Thomas DGT, Darling JL, et al: A preliminary study utilizing viable HLA mismatched cultured glioma cells as adjuvant therapy for patients with malignant gliomas. Br J Cancer 1985; 51:2839.

102. Eggers AE, Tarmin L, Gamboa ET: In vivo immunization against autologous glioblastoma-associated antigens. Cancer 1985; 19:43–45.

103. Yagi K, Hayashi Y, Ishida N, et al: Interferon-beta endogenously produced by intratumoral injection of cationic liposome-encapsulated gene: Cytocidal effect on glioma transplanted into nude mouse brain. Biochem Mol Biol Int 1994; 32:167.

104. Yu JS, Wei MX, Chiocca EH, et al: Treatment of glioma by engineered interleukin 4-secreting cells. Cancer Res 1993; 53:3125.

RANDALL E. MERCHANT

HAROLD F. YOUNG

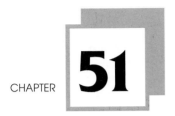

CHAPTER **51**

Intracavitary Immunotherapy

Despite the numerous advances in surgery, radiation, and chemotherapy, survival for patients with a malignant glioma from time of diagnosis is short. As no treatment regimen at this time can be considered curative, numerous laboratories have examined a variety of immunotherapeutic approaches to determine their potential clinical usefulness when applied alone or in conjunction with conventional cytoreductive modalities. In this review, we concentrate our attention on immunotherapies for malignant brain tumors that have involved the intracavitary or intratumoral injection of lymphocytes and/or recombinant cytokines in an attempt to restore and/or to enhance reactivity of the patient's immune system to the tumor. The reasons why many investigators have taken this direct route versus a systemic one for applying immunotherapy are summarized in Table 51–1. Basically, the rationale for intracavitary immunotherapy is based on retrospective histopathologic observations that the greatest concentration of glioma cells that escape surgical extirpation lie within a 2-cm margin around the resection cavity, recurrence invariably occurs at or near the site of the original tumor, and survival correlates with the degree of lymphocytic infiltration into glioma.[1–4]

In the clinical trials outlined in this chapter, therapies were usually applied following operation for gross total tumor removal. In some cases, therapy was applied immediately, either by injection into the neuropil immediately surrounding the resection site or by placement of cells within

TABLE 51–1
RATIONALE FOR INTRALESIONAL IMMUNOTHERAPY FOR GLIOBLASTOMA

Majority of glioma cells that escape surgical resection lie in the tumor margin
Fewer effector cells and/or less cytokine required
Attain high concentrations of cytokines/effector cells in the tumor site
Activation of lymphoid cells already present in and around the tumor site
Increase recruitment and infiltration of host effector cells into the tumor site
Cytokines/effector cells directed at tissue containing tumor cells
Spares normal brain and lowers systemic toxic effects

---

the cavity. In other trials, installation of an Ommaya reservoir allowed for therapy to be repeatedly applied subsequent to craniotomy. In these cases, the head of the reservoir was seated in the skull, and the stem extended into the tumor cavity or one of the cerebral ventricles.

ADOPTIVE IMMUNOTHERAPY

Adoptive immunotherapy for any form of cancer involves the transfer of autologous or allogeneic lymphocytes to the tumor-bearing host with the hope that those cells will directly or indirectly mediate the regression of tumor.[5] In the case of malignant glioma, a large number of clinical trials involving the direct intracavitary injection of autologous peripheral blood lymphocytes or lymphokine-activated killer (LAK) cells have been performed.

Peripheral Blood Lymphocytes

Trouillas and Lapras[6] were the first to transfer autologous leukocytes directly into the postsurgical tumor cavity. They treated three glioma patients with 6 to 22 million cells. None of the tumors responded to treatment. At about the same time, Takakura and co-workers[7] treated ten glioma patients with recurrent disease by intracavitary injection of lymphocytes activated with phytohemagglutinin. Patients received from two to 12 treatments. Significantly prolonged survival rates than were expected were observed in seven subjects.

During the mid-1970s, one of the authors (H.F.Y.) and co-workers[8] developed a clinical program for the treatment of recurrent glioblastoma with autologous leukocyte infusions directed into the tumor bed via an Ommaya reservoir. Autologous leukocytes (buffy coat) were obtained by leukapheresis, washed, and concentrated, and 10 million to 1 billion leukocytes (lymphocyte-to-granulocyte ratio, 1:1) were immediately injected intracavitarily via an Ommaya reservoir. No neurotoxic effects ascribable to the procedure were observed. Survival appeared to be longer than expected in eight of the 17 patients. One patient had a remarkable clinical improvement and long survival. Autopsies performed in six patients revealed extensive tumor necrosis, although there were no histopathologic effects that could be definitely ascribed to the immunotherapy.

Later investigations by Ishizawa,[9] who treated nine glioma patients, and by Steinbok and others,[10] who treated four, also demonstrated that intratumoral immunotherapy with autologous lymphocytes could be performed safely but with little apparent therapeutic benefit. From these early attempts at cellular immunotherapy, no conclusive judgments could be made with regard to the therapeutic efficacy, because all were non-randomized trials involving only small pools of patients. Soon after the latter studies were published, dramatic inroads were made in methodologies relevant to lymphocyte activation and culture. Also, the availability of purified, natural, and recombinant cytokines led directly to greater experimentation and understanding of the actions in biologic systems in vitro and in vivo. As described subsequently, the availability of purified cytokines and improved culture methods have encouraged continued investigation of this immunotherapeutic modality.

Lymphokine-Activated Killer Cells

Beginning in the mid-1980s, when human recombinant interleukin 2 (rIL2) became available, we and a number of other groups conducted laboratory experiments and clinical trials of rIL2 alone or in combination with "activated" lymphocytes, to define its toxic effects and potential efficacy in patients with high-grade glioma. IL2 is a 15-kD glycoprotein that mediates a wide array of biologic functions (Table 51–2). What is most important from an oncology perspective is the capacity of IL2 to amplify the tumoricidal activity of natural killer (NK) cells such that they express what became known as lymphokine-activated killer (LAK) activity.[11–14] These cells express non–major histocompatibility complex–restricted cytotoxicity for tumor cell lines in vitro and some experimental tumors in vivo. For human studies and clinical trials, lymphocytes demonstrating LAK activity are usually produced by culture of peripheral blood mononuclear cells for 3 to 7 days in complete media containing 1,000 to 1,500 units of human rIL2 per milliliter and autologous or AB serum.[11–14]

When administered intravenously (IV), LAK cells tend to get trapped in the first capillary bed they encounter. Therefore, because tumor-specific homing of LAK cells apparently does not occur, the optimal route of administration of LAK cells appears to be directly into the body compartment that contains the tumor.[15] In fact, intralesional treatment with

LAK cells alone or combined with rIL2 was shown to be a safe treatment and to be occasionally effective in cases of melanoma, bladder, and breast cancers, and it avoided the toxic effects, large cell numbers, and rIL2 needed for systemic administration.[15–17] Based on these studies, all of the clinical trials of LAK therapy for malignant glioma have chosen a direct route; infusing cells directly into tumor beds and cystic cavities via indwelling catheters and/or injection into neural parenchyma surrounding tumor during craniotomy.

Grimm's laboratory was the first to show that LAK activity could be generated in vitro from peripheral blood mononuclear cells of glioma patients.[18] These authors also conducted a phase I clinical trial using autologous LAK cells and/or rIL2, injected intracerebrally into the tissue immediately surrounding the cavity that remained following resection for recurrent glioma.[19] Five patients were injected with only LAK effectors (5×10^7 to 5×10^{10}), four others with rIL2 alone (up to 10^6 units, Cetus), and one patient received 3×10^9 LAK cells plus 10^6 units of rIL2. The authors observed no severe toxic effects attributable to any of these treatments. Three months following treatment, nine of the patients showed a stable clinical course and no CT evidence of tumor progression.[19]

In early 1986, we[20, 21] began a clinical trial in patients with malignant glioma of adoptive immunotherapy using human rIL2 plus varying numbers of autologous lymphocytes expressing LAK activity. The number and concentration of activated lymphocytes in the vicinity of any residual tumor was maximized by directly injecting cells and rIL2 into the neuropil surrounding the excision site. All 29 patients who participated in our study had a supratentorial tumor; 27 had glioblastoma and two had a high-grade oligodendroglioma. Five patients had newly diagnosed lesions and 24 had malignant gliomas that had recurred after an average of 13 months from diagnosis. Among the patients, Karnofsky ratings were quite variable, and most patients were taking corticosteroids for control of cerebral edema.

Three times before their craniotomy, our patients underwent leukapheresis to obtain the necessary numbers of peripheral blood mononuclear cells for the therapy. Cells were cultured 3 to 5 days in serum-free RPMI-1640 medium supplemented with 1,000 units of rIL2 (Cetus) per milliliter and human albumin. On the day of surgery, between 1×10^9 and 15×10^9 cells along with 10^6 units of rIL2 were randomly distributed by injection up to 1 cm into areas of brain tissue immediately surrounding the cavity created by surgical debulking. Daily injections of 10^6 units of rIL2 were made into the tumor cavity via Ommaya reservoir for 3 days. The rIL2 injections were given to potentiate and maintain the tumoricidal activity of the injected cells. Ten of the 24 patients with recurrent disease underwent a second round of immunotherapy 2 to 3 weeks after the first. In this case, LAK cells and rIL2 were injected via the Ommaya reservoir.

In our patients, craniotomy combined with immunotherapy triggered a variety of side effects; headache and lethargy, both symptoms of increased intracranial pressure, were probably caused by cerebral edema in those areas of brain where cells and rIL2 had been injected. For most patients, adverse effects of treatment spontaneously disappeared within a few days of the last rIL2 injection, whereas some patients re-

---

TABLE 51–2
IMMUNOLOGIC ACTIVITIES OF INTERLEUKIN-2

Induces the proliferation of antigen-activated T cells
Augments the tumoricidal activity of NK cells and cytotoxic T lymphocytes
Activates NK cells such that they express lymphokine-activated killer activity
Induces and enhances the secretion of cytokines from NK cells, activated T helper cells, cytotoxic T lymphocytes, and activated macrophages

quired acetaminophen (Tylenol) and/or an increase in the daily dexamethasone dose. MRI and CT scans made within a couple of weeks of treatment consistently indicated greater than expected amounts of edema around the surgery site. Three patients who had been among those who received the greatest numbers of adoptively transferred lymphocytes demonstrated a decline in clinical status within 6 weeks of immunotherapy.[22] On MRI, these patients had pronounced edema and an encapsulated mass. All three underwent craniotomy to remove this tissue, which had the histologic characteristics of a chronic sterile abscess. Similar observations were made a few years later by Thomas and co-workers[23] who examined a 5-year-old child with an anaplastic astrocytoma who died 6 weeks after immunotherapy with LAK cells and rIL2. The child's glioma was necrotic and gelatinous at the site of the reservoir and contained a large number of T cells.

Although it was the purpose of our clinical trial[20, 21] to judge efficacy of LAK cell immunotherapy for glioma, patients were followed up by serial evaluation by CT scan or MRI and we were able to determine a time to tumor progression and/or recurrence. In the group of 29 patients, tumor recurrence at the site of surgical resection or somewhere distant from the original site occurred in 20 patients. With regards to the other nine patients, only two patients from the recurrent group are alive, and they have yet to show any evidence of recurrence. Seven patients died at various times following craniotomy and therapy without CT or MRI indications of an enlarging intracranial tumor.[20, 21]

By defining time to tumor recurrence (TTR) as a tumor recurrence on CT scan or death, the 24 patients with recurrent tumor had median TTRs of 5 months and median survival of 9 months. As just mentioned, two patients of this group have yet to show any new tumor and have remained free of recurrent disease for more than 7 years. Median TTR for the five patients who received immunotherapy at the time of first craniotomy was 12 months. Although all of the patients of this group are dead, two had remained free of tumor recurrence for more than 2 years.

The group of Yoshida and colleagues[24] treated 23 patients with recurrent glioma with multiple intracavitary injections of autologous LAK cells plus rIL2. LAK cells were produced by culturing peripheral blood mononuclear cells for 4 to 6 days in media containing 200 units of rIL2 (Shionogi Chemical) per milliliter. Using an Ommaya reservoir, patients received 20 to 170 million LAK cells and 50 to 400 units of rIL2 directly into tumor tissue or its cystic core. The therapy was administered two to three times per week for 5 to 7 weeks; in a few patients it was continued once or twice per month for several months. Patients, therefore, received 1.2 to 324 × 10⁸ LAK cells and 0.8 to 5.4 × 10³ units of rIL2 after all treatments. The authors reported no marked side effects; CT scans demonstrated tumor stabilization in more than half of the patients and showed tumor regression in six.

Barba and colleagues[25] treated nine patients who had undergone a recent surgical excision for a recurrent malignant glioma with multiple intracavitary injections of autologous LAK cells and rIL2 (Cetus) over a 5-day period. Approximately 3 weeks following craniotomy, patients received LAK cells (up to 10¹⁰ cells/day) and 10,000 units of rIL2/ kg (Cetus) via Ommaya reservoir on 2 consecutive days. Injections of rIL2 (up to 60,000 units/kg/dose) were continued for up to 3 more days. Five patients received only one treatment, three had two treatments, and one patient had four. Mild systemic toxic effects were observed in three patients, whereas new neurologic deficits occurred or preexisting deficits worsened in all nine patients. These deficits were focal in nature, referable to increased peritumoral edema in regions that underwent therapy. Four patients recovered completely from their neurologic deficits, whereas five were left with new permanent sequelae. The patient who had received four treatments had a partial response (defined as a more than 50% reduction in maximum tumor diameter on CT scan) and remained alive 16 months after treatment. The other eight patients died 2 to 11 months after immunotherapy.

Blancher and co-workers[26] performed a non-randomized clinical trial to evaluate the feasibility of immunotherapy for recurrent glioblastoma by continuous intracavitary perfusion of rIL2 (Eurocetus) with and without LAK cells. Five patients received 18 million units/day of rIL2 for 5 days following tumor debulking. On postsurgery days 1, 3, and 5, LAK cells were also infused. Five other patients received 24 million units of rIL2 per day and three more patients received 54 million units of rIL2 per day. All three therapies induced fever, confusion, and cerebral edema. Tumor progression was diagnosed in the 13 patients by CT scan 4 to 12 weeks after the immunotherapy.

Most recently, Boiardi and colleagues[27] treated nine patients with recurrent glioblastoma with intracavitary injections of autologous adherent LAK (A-LAK) cells and rIL2. The immunotherapy was well tolerated. They observed one complete response and two partial responses. Four patients exhibited stable disease and two showed progressive disease. Survival at 18 months from initial diagnosis, however, did not differ from that reported in the literature for patients treated conventionally.

In a variation of the LAK cell immunotherapy trials just described, the group of Ingram and others[28, 29] activated and expanded blood mononuclear cell populations of glioma patients prior to their adoptive transfer. They stimulated the blood mononuclear cells for 48 hours with phytohemagglutinin P and then incubated the cells in fresh media containing natural human IL2 (Collaborative Research) or human rIL2 (Amgen). Within 2 weeks, the lymphocyte populations were of adequate quantity for therapy. They termed these expanded lymphoid populations *autologous stimulated lymphocytes* (ASLs), and used them to treat 51 patients with a recurrent grade III or IV glioma. On the day of surgery, ASLs were suspended in approximately 15 mL of autologous plasma, and after surgical debulking, the plasma was recalcified with calcium gluconate. A clot formed, which was then placed within to fill the craniotomy site. The cell suspension always contained 10⁵ units of rIL2. Most patients were treated with 1 to 5 × 10⁹ ASLs. The authors reported that the treatment was well tolerated with no significant toxic effects, although a few patients experienced low-grade fever and/or moderate nausea for the first few postoperative days. The authors reported that 15 of 51 patients either had no response to treatment (i.e., CT evidence of tumor progression within 2 months of treatment) or had an early recurrence (within 4 months of therapy). The median survival for the entire group of patients was approximately 60 weeks.

Using a therapeutic approach similar to that of Ingram and colleagues, Lillehei and co-workers[30, 31] administered ASLs and LAK cells to 11 patients with recurrent or persistent high-grade glioma following surgery and radiation therapy. They produced ASLs, as just discussed, by culturing lymphocytes overnight in media containing phytohemagglutinin P followed by 10 days in media with 100 units of rIL2 (Amgen) per milliliter. Fresh peripheral blood mononuclear cells were also cultured for 4 days with 500 units of rIL2/mL to generate cells with LAK activity. Patients underwent tumor resection followed by intracavitary implantation of LAK cells and ASLs along with 2×10^5 units of rIL2 in a plasma clot. Patients received additional intracavitary injections of 2×10^5 units of rIL2 via a Rickham reservoir for the next 4 days. One month later, LAK cells and ASLs were once again infused intracavitarily using the reservoir. The average number of activated lymphocytes injected ranged from 1.9 to 27.5×10^9 (mean, 7.6×10^9). No major side effects to treatment were seen. The median survival time following initiation of immunotherapy was 18 weeks (range, 11 to 93 weeks). Ten patients died from recurrent tumor growth and the remaining one patient showed no evidence of recurrence after 93 weeks. As a group, the median overall survival time was 63 weeks (range, 36 to 201 weeks) and the median survival time following immunotherapy was 18 weeks (range, 11 to 151 weeks).

An interesting trial that combined adoptive immunotherapy with a bispecific antibody was conducted by Nitta and co-workers.[32, 33] They injected autologous LAK cells treated with bispecific antibody into the tumor cavities of ten patients with malignant glioma and compared the effects of specific targeting therapy with the results of therapy with untreated LAK cells alone. The bispecific antibody was a bifunctional hetero-F(ab′)2 fragment containing the Fab portions from anti-CD3 antibody chemically conjugated to an antiglioma monoclonal antibody. Thus, the antibody simultaneously recognized two different molecules: (1) the CD3 complex on T lymphocytes and (2) human glioma-associated antigens on the glioma targets. Four of the ten patients given specific targeting therapy showed regression of tumor, and in another four patients, CT scans and histologic findings suggested tumor lysis. They reported no recurrences in the 10 to 18 months of follow-up. All but one of the patients receiving nontargeted LAK cells had recurrences within 1 year.

In the hope of strengthening the immune response to a malignant brain tumor using LAK cell immunotherapy, Granger's laboratory used intratumor lymphoid allografts to induce local cytokine production, tissue destruction, and inflammation in gliomas in rat models and patients.[34] Into intracranial T9 gliomas of Fischer rats they injected 10 to 40 million spleen cells from Wistar rats that had been immunized with Fischer spleen cells. This produced 1-year survival rates of 50%, whereas untreated control models all died by 28 days. They observed no change in behavior of treated tumor-bearers, nor was any damage to normal brain noted. These studies indicated that the therapy-induced graft-vs.-host and host-vs.-graft allograft reactions within the microenvironment of intracranial glioblastomas led to the eradi-cation of tumor. These studies led to a small phase I clinical trial of eight patients with recurrent glioblastomas. In groups of two, patients were randomly assigned to receive intratumor implants of 2, 5, 10, or 20 billion allogeneic LAK cells from healthy unrelated donors. Patients showed no implant-induced acute effects, although mild nausea, headache, and discomfort developed in all of them. No serious toxic responses occurred. Any potential benefit of the therapy has yet to be determined.

Taking these studies together, the most common adverse effect observed in patients receiving intracerebral or intracavitary immunotherapy with LAK cells, with or without rIL2, was perilesional edema. This presented clinically as fatigue, headache, and/or exacerbation of any pre-existing deficit. For most patients, overt side effects disappeared within a few days of treatment, although signs of CT evidence of cerebral edema often persisted for several weeks. In none of the studies did any MRI or CT scan or any postmortem examinations provide any indication of a secondary disease process that may have developed in the brain as a consequence of the immunotherapy. The results of these clinical trials indicate that single or multiple treatments with autologous or allogeneic LAK cells and/or ASLs alone or in combination with rIL2 are safe, and for small proportion of patients they slow the recurrence and/or progression of tumor at the site of treatment.

Tumor-Infiltrating Lymphocytes

As noted earlier, lymphocyte infiltration in and around gliomas has been noted by a number of histopathologic investigations to correlate positively with prognosis.[1-3] An invasion of the tumor by lymphoid cells would suggest the development of a delayed hypersensitivity reaction to specific glioma cell antigens. Because the infiltrates are composed predominantly of T cells and macrophages, it is plausible that T lymphocytes attracted to a glioma, once in contact with an antigen, differentiate, multiply, and produce lymphokines, which then attract macrophages to the tumor site and activate them. The nature and functional capacity of lymphoid populations within gliomas, however, have been a matter of much debate. Von Hanwehr and others[35] phenotypically characterized lymphocytes that infiltrated gliomas from six patients using specific monoclonal antibodies. Four gliomas demonstrated infiltrating lymphocytes that were small, with dense nuclei and scant cytoplasm. Occasional clusters of larger lymphoblasts were also encountered. In three of the gliomas, CD8+ (suppressor/cytotoxic cell phenotype) cells were predominant, whereas the remaining glioma had mixtures of CD8+ and CD4+ (helper cell phenotype) cells in fairly equal proportions.

Numerous studies have isolated lymphocytes from a variety of animal and human tumors and expanded their number ex vivo in medium supplemented with rIL2.[36, 37] When tumor-infiltrating lymphocytes (TILs) are co-cultured with autologous or allogeneic tumor targets, they exhibit a strong cytotoxic activity against not only syngeneic tumor cells, but against allogeneic ones as well. When autologous TILs are reintroduced IV into patients or into syngeneic animals bearing tumor, they have been found to be 50 to 100 times more potent on a per-cell basis than the adoptive transfer of LAK cells.

Sawamura and colleagues[38, 39] were among the first to examine the feasibility of isolating and growing glioma-infiltrating lymphocytes in vitro as possible effector cells for use in adoptive immunotherapy. They developed a method for in vitro expansion lymphoid cells isolated from human malignant astrocytomas. Briefly, isolated TILs from glioma specimens were cultured in medium containing 50 to 2,000 units of rIL2 per milliliter. In most preparations, 3 to 6 weeks of culture produced at least 5×10^8 to 5×10^9 cells; $90\% \pm 8\%$ CD3+ T-cells including both CD4+ and CD8+ subpopulations. After 4 to 8 weeks of proliferation, IL2 receptor expression decreased and the lymphocytes ceased to grow. Glioma-derived effector lymphocytes could lyse almost all of the autologous tumor targets as well as allogeneic glioma cells.

Using these same methods, Sawamura[40] later reported that the cytotoxic activity of glioma-infiltrating lymphocytes for autologous glioma cells was similar to or less than that of LAK cells produced from the same patients. The glioma-derived effector cells also lysed three-dimensional glioma spheroids, though at a level significantly lower than that of LAK cells. These results and the observation that the effector cells did not infiltrate the spheroids after 24 hours of co-culture led the authors to conclude there that no therapeutic advantage was likely for use of TILs over LAK for adoptive immunotherapy of glioma.

The studies of Sawamura and colleagues represent initial attempts to isolate and produce cytotoxic T cells in vitro in quantities considered sufficient for adoptive transfer into patients. Although many problems related to specificity, dosage, schedule, and route of delivery have yet to be resolved by phase I clinical trials, their experiments have provided important evidence on the potential usefulness of TILs in the treatment of patients with malignant gliomas.

Relying on TILs as the source of lymphocytes for adoptive immunotherapy for glioma, however, poses many theoretical and technical obstacles. The most problematic is the requirement that large numbers of cytotoxic T lymphocytes (CTLs) must be isolated from tumor specimens. In patients with gliomas, tumor-specific killer cells are present in the peripheral blood.[41, 42] Kitahara and co-workers[43] induced autologous brain tumor-specific lymphocytes from patients' peripheral blood mononuclear cells by a mixed lymphocyte-tumor culture. In this study, 5 to 10 million lymphocytes were mixed with 500,000 autologous cultured glioma cells that had been treated with mitomycin and incubated for 5 to 7 days. Lymphocytes were harvested, resuspended in a complete medium containing exogenous IL2 (100 units/mL), and maintained for up to 2 months in culture. Phenotypic analyses of the resultant cell populations showed that most lymphocytes were T helper cells and only a small proportion (3% to 7.5%) had the phenotype of CTLs. They injected five patients with these autologous T cells intracavitarily via an Ommaya reservoir; 50 million cells were injected twice a week for up to 13 weeks. In two cases, tumors regressed more than 50% in diameter. Autologous T cells were safely administered in five cases without any complications or toxic effects. In all patients, autologous T cells were safely administered without complications or toxic effects.

Recently the laboratory of Kruse and others[44–46] reported on methods for the isolation and in vitro generation of tumor-specific allogeneic peripheral blood lymphocytes. Furthermore, they showed that these allogeneic CTLs were an effective and safe therapy when repeatedly injected intratumorally in a rat glioma model. The advantage of using allogeneic CTLs from a normal blood donor for treatment of glioma has the theoretical advantage of circumventing the immunosuppressive influences of gliomas themselves and of the medications used to treat them. A phase I clinical trial employing allogeneic peripheral blood lymphocytes in patients with malignant glioma is now under way. If the therapy can be applied with minimal toxic effects, a large, multicenter trial of adoptive immunotherapy with allogeneic tumor-specific T cells would be warranted.

CYTOKINES

With the development of recombinant DNA technology and large-scale production methods, quantities of purified human cytokines, such as the interferons, IL2, and tumor necrosis factor-α (TNFA) can now be produced economically in quantities needed for clinical applications. To date, systemic treatments involving these ''manufactured'' cytokines, particularly interferon-α (IFN-α) and IL2, have produced significant tumor regressions in animal models and in patients with various types of cancer. In this section, the review is limited to an overview of preclinical studies that have examined the effects of intracerebral injections of human recombinant IL2 and IFN and a few clinical trials that have tested their toxicity and potential efficacy when injected intracavitarily into patients harboring a malignant glioma.

Interleukin 2

In response to mitogenic or antigenic stimuli, T lymphocytes proliferate and release a variety of *interleukins*: proteins that serve as communication links between lymphoid cells themselves and nonlymphocytes. As mentioned earlier, among the many activities of IL2, it is of paramount importance in the proliferation of T cells and in the lymphokine-activated killing phenomenon. As a sole immunotherapeutic agent, both natural and recombinant human IL2 have been shown to reduce tumors in animal models when injected peritumorally.[47–49] Also, xenografts of human carcinoma lines growing in nude mice have been inhibited following intralesional rIL2 administration.[50]

While the LAK plus rIL2 immunotherapy trial was being conducted in patients, laboratory experiments were also performed to examine any histopathologic findings that could occur as a consequence of intracerebral injection of human rIL2. In the first studies, 6×10^4 units of human rIL2 (Cetus) or excipient was stereotactically injected into the parietal lobes of Fischer rats.[51] Animals were followed for up to 8 days; they showed no decline in functional status, remained afebrile, and continued to gain weight. For histopathologic studies, other groups of animals were killed on various days. Horseradish peroxidase was also injected IV 1 hour prior to killing so that the integrity of the blood-brain barrier could be assessed. Excipient-injected controls and rIL2-injected animals demonstrated blood-brain barrier permeability for horseradish peroxidase up to 24 hours following an intracerebral injection. The capacity of horseradish peroxidase to extravasate, however, persisted in the rIL2-injected animals for up to 8 days. These rats also showed greater leukocytic infiltration, perivascular cuffing, and localized edema compared with excipient-injected controls. The authors' impression was that rIL2 helped to maintain an inflammatory state at the site of trauma, sustaining blood-brain barrier permeability.

Based on these studies, it appeared reasonable to propose that a similar response would be observed in the brains of animals with glioma. Because animals bearing glioma exhibit breakdown of the blood-brain barrier attributable to the tumor, it was postulated that an intratumoral injection of rIL2 may help to extend the area of blood-brain barrier compromise. Should rIL2 be responsible for increasing the vascular alterations in malignancies of the brain, then a study of its histopathologic effects on the vasculature of brain tumors when given in combination with chemotherapies would be the next logical step in the development of a novel treatment protocol for patients with primary or metastatic CNS neoplasms. A summary of these results is given in the following text and is detailed in an article by Watts and one of the authors (R.E.M.).[52]

The blood-brain barrier was first examined in a glioma model. The brains of rats with intracerebral gliomas were examined histologically for endogenous IgG extravasation at 7, 10, and 14 days after tumor inoculation. Under normal circumstances, IgG is not found in the brain if the blood-brain barrier is intact; therefore, its presence has been used as a marker for endothelial cell damage.[53] With bloodborne IgG as the tracer, it was demonstrated that the amount of edema and cerebrovascular permeability increased as the tumor enlarged.

In the animal model of malignant glioma, the effects were investigated of an intralesional injection of 7.2×10^4 units of rIL2 on the neurologic status of glioma-bearing animals and of the histopathologic characteristics of the cerebral vessels and neural parenchyma in areas of normal brain and in areas of glioma.[52] No observable neurologic sequelae could be directly attributed to the single intralesional injection of the rIL2. This injection was made on day 7, when the tumor was small; by the time the experiment was terminated on day 13, the tumor had increased in size, indicating that an intralesional injection of rIL2 apparently was not independently antineoplastic and did not induce sufficient production of other cytokines that could inhibit tumor growth. All animals seemed to tolerate the treatment well, as none experienced seizures, lethargy, or paralysis to a greater degree than did the tumor-bearing controls. At the microscopic level, no increase in cerebrovascular permeability was noted within or around the glioma after treatment with a single intralesional injection of rIL2, and no increase was seen in necrosis in the tumor or in normal brain regions, which suggests that this protocol did not produce additional neurotoxic effects or otherwise adversely affect normal areas of the brain adjacent to the tumor. These data verified what had been observed in clinical trials of LAK cells plus rIL2: that the intracavitary or intracerebral injection of rIL2 was

at least partly responsible for the increase in peritumoral edema seen in patients. The part played by secondary cytokine production within the site of treatment in the rIL2-induced histopathologic and blood-brain barrier permeability changes, however, remains to be determined.

As human rIL2 injected into tumor attracts circulating lymphocytes,[54, 55] the underlying mechanism of anti-tumor activity is believed to be mediated by NK and T cells that are chemotactically attracted to the tumor site; once there, the cells are activated by the rIL2 to increase their cytotoxic effects on tumor cells.[55-57] Human rIL2 attracts circulating NK cells,[54, 56] and the authors believe that this may prove relevant to in situ targeting of activated effector cell populations into sites of brain tumor. Repeated injections of rIL2 would also attract lymphocytes into the tumor, where they would be induced to develop LAK activity and further augment tumor destruction. For these reasons, the first clinical trial involving rIL2 alone for malignant brain tumor involved the intracavitary or intracerebroventricular approach for delivery of the cytokine. It was thought that a direct infusion would concentrate the factor in the vicinity of tumor-infiltrating leukocytes and glioma cells, where it would be most needed.

The phase I clinical trial tested the feasibility and potential toxic effects of repeated intracavitary or intracerebroventricular infusions of rIL2 (Hoffmann-La Roche) alone or in combination with subcutaneous injections of human recombinant IFN-α (Roferon-A, Hoffmann-La Roche) in patients with a malignant glioma.[58] Interferon-α was chosen for testing along with rIL2 because by itself, repeated subcutaneous injections of IFN-α have produced objective responses in glioma patients.[59-61] Nine patients were treated; five were given rIL2 only and four were given rIL2 plus subcutaneous IFN-α. Therapy was administered on a Monday-Wednesday-Friday schedule for up to 10 weeks, beginning with a dose of 10,000 units of rIL2 per injection. Doses were escalated every 2 weeks until some toxic response was apparent. The maximum amount of rIL2 any one patient in this group received was 580,000 units. Patients on combination immunotherapy were held at an rIL2 dosage of 10,000 units while IFN-α, which began at 3 million units, was escalated every other week up to 18 million units per dose. That IFN-α dosage was maintained, and rIL2 was increased to 50,000 IU. The total amount of rIL2 and IFN-α that anyone in this group received was 510,000 IU and 417 million IU, respectively. Repeated injections of 10,000 units of rIL2 were well tolerated by all nine patients. At doses of 50,000 units of rIL2, increased edema around the tumor cavity was observed by MRI and/or CT scan in three of five patients, and clinical side effects in the form of somnolence and headache, along with some morbidity specifically associated with tumor location, were also seen. Patients receiving rIL2 plus IFN-α showed progressive fatigue, muscle weakness, and, occasionally, nausea. Two of these patients showed increased peritumoral edema on MRI and/or CT scan. Neither hematologic abnormalities nor changes from baseline values were seen in blood samples from any of the patients. MRI and/or CT scans made at the conclusion of immunotherapy indicated tumor progression in two of the patients treated with rIL2 alone, whereas no tumor growth occurred at the site of treatment in the other two patients or in the four patients treated with the combination of rIL2 and IFN-α. Therefore, although the overall objective of the clinical trial was to provide evidence that immunotherapy with repeated injections of rIL2, alone or combined with IFN-α, was safe, the therapies may have the potential to be proven effective, as gliomas in six of our nine patients showed no growth during the course of treatment. Therefore, it appears that when the therapy is administered three times per week, patients with malignant brain tumor can tolerate repeated intracavitary or intracerebroventricular injection of 50,000 IU of rIL2 plus subcutaneous injections of up to 12 million IU of Roferon-A for at least 4 weeks. Clinical testing of this cytokine combination is continuing at these dosages and schedule.

Interferon

The three classes of IFN are IFN-α, IFN-β, and IFN-γ. The α and β IFNs are approximately 18 kD proteins produced by leukocytes and fibroblasts, respectively. IFN-γ, a homodimeric glycoprotein of approximately 21 kD, is produced by both CD4 + and CD8 + lymphocytes. The principal actions of all three types of IFN are (1) inhibition of viral replication; (2) direct inhibition of tumor cell growth; (3) enhancement of the cytolytic and tumoricidal activity of NK cells; and (4) upregulation of major histocompatibility complex (MHC) class I molecule expression, which enhances the efficiency of CTL-mediated killing. In addition to these activities, IFN-γ also stimulates macrophages and neutrophils, promotes the differentiation of T and B lymphocytes, upregulates MHC class II molecules, and increases adhesion factor expression on endothelial cells.

In culture studies, all three IFNs slow the growth of glioma cells and increase expression of MHC antigens.[62] Clinical trials of all three types of IFN have been conducted in glioma patients. When administered repeatedly systemically, either subcutaneously or IV, IFN-α and IFN-β have produced objective responses in glioma patients.[59–63] Mahaley and colleagues,[64] however, showed no therapeutic benefit of IFN-γ. With systemic administration, the IFN concentration in the residual glioma tissue can be expected to be low due to the insufficient permeability of IFN into the CNS because of the blood-brain barrier[65, 66] and the rapid catabolism of the cytokine. Direct injections of IFN into the glioma, therefore, appear promising, as they would be expected to provide and sustain a concentration sufficiently high to be efficacious.

A number of preclinical studies in animal models have examined the effects of intralesional IFN injections on the growth of gliomas. The group of Hori and colleagues,[67] for example, examined the effect of local injection of IFN-α on human malignant gliomas (one oligodendroglioma and one glioblastoma) transplanted into nude mice. Animals were injected with IFN vehicle, or 1, 3, or 9 million units of IFN-α. Tumor volumes were monitored daily. At the end of the experiment, each animal received an intraperitoneal injection of bromodeoxyuridine to label cells in S phase (i.e., synthesizing DNA), and the labeling indices were determined for each treatment group. They reported that injections of IFN-α into tumor was effective at all doses for both tumors.

Labeling indices of the treated groups were significantly less than those of controls for both tumors.

Wen and co-workers[68] examined the effects of IFN-γ on immune parameters in the 9L gliosarcoma model. They had previously shown that IFN-γ increased class I MHC expression in 9L cells in vitro. In vivo, intratumor injections of IFN-γ led to increased numbers of inflammatory cells within the tumor, class II + mononuclear phagocytes at its periphery, and increased MHC class I or II expression by endothelial and ependymal cells. Class I expression in 9L cells themselves, however, was not increased. More recently, however, Akbasak and colleagues,[69] using a rat glioma model, found that MHC class I and II antigen expression on gliomas could be upregulated in vivo by intratumoral treatment with IFN-γ. Fischer rats bearing a syngeneic glioma line (S 635c15) received 10,000 units of IFN-γ intratumorally for 5 days. Afterward, the tumors were removed, prepared as a single cell suspension, and examined by flow cytometry. Tumor cells of control animals had low constitutive MHC class I antigen expression and undetectable class II expression, whereas IFN-γ moderately increased class I expression and dramatically increased the intensity of class II expression.

Clinical trials of IFN-α[70–72] and IFN-β[73–75] have shown variable activity against malignant glioma when injected via an Ommaya reservoir. In one of the first phase I trials, Salford and others[70] treated two patients with advanced glioma with daily intratumoral injections of 4 million units of IFN-α.[70] The two patients were treated for 2 months. At about the same time, Nakagawa and colleagues[71] administered human IFN-α intracavitarily or intrathecally into eight patients with glioblastoma. Patients received either 1 million units once or twice a week or received it daily for 1 month and then had a month off. A few years later, Duff and co-workers[73] treated 12 patients with recurrent glioblastoma using IFN-β. Ten million units of the cytokine was injected IV daily and 1 million units was administered every other day intracavitarily over three 10-day cycles. In these and other preliminary studies, therapy with IFN-α and -β was always shown to be well tolerated and occasionally produced tumor remissions.[70–75]

Maleci and colleagues[76] examined the pharmacokinetics of human recombinant interferon-α2 (rIFN-α2, Schering Co.) following intracavitary administration into patients with a recently resected malignant glioma. Following craniotomy, 5 million units of rIFN-α2 was injected daily for 2 weeks and then once a week for 10 additional weeks. During the daily and weekly administration, and for up to 5 weeks after the end of therapy, rIFN-α2 was detectable in the cystic fluid of the tumor cavity. The decay of rIFN-α2 after injection was minimal. The treatments were well tolerated, and although mild febrile reactions occurred within 24 hours of treatment, no serious adverse experiences were observed.

Fetell and co-workers[77] administered 5 to 180 million units of IFN-β twice weekly to 20 patients with recurrent malignant glioma. Cytokine was injected intracavitarily via Ommaya reservoir. Adverse effects, which included nausea, vomiting, fever, and chills, occurred in only one patient. Patients received intracavitary injections of IFN-β until either clinical status or CT scan indicated progressive disease. Mean length of treatment was 82 days. Of the 12 patients who could be evaluated, three had stable disease, whereas the tumors of nine patients showed evidence of progression.

As an indication of the direction in which cytokine therapy for glioma may be heading, a number of laboratories are currently conducting experiments transfecting cytokine genes into glioma cells such that they will either secrete the cytokine and/or express desirable surface antigens or receptors. In one study, Mizuno and colleagues[78] evaluated the effect of liposomal transfection of human IFN-γ gene into human glioma cells. Transfection induced the production and secretion of IFN-γ by two human glioma cell lines in vitro. At 4 days post-transfection, the cells produced from 10 to 50 units of IFN-γ per milliliter. By this time, both MHC class I and II antigens, as well as intercellular adhesion molecule 1 (ICAM1), were upregulated on the glioma cell surfaces. Proliferation of the transfected glioma cells was significantly slowed, and the cells were more susceptible to lysis by LAK cells.

SUMMARY

Although patients with a malignant glioma typically have impaired immune function, the observation that the tumors frequently showed infiltration of lymphocytes, which positively correlates with survival, has spawned the testing of immunotherapeutic approaches to the treatment of glioma. Because immunotherapy using human recombinant cytokines alone or in combination with lymphoid effector cells have shown some promise in other malignancies, it was thought that they might also prove effective for glioma. Furthermore, by virtue of the fact that gliomas usually occur as a single, localized lesion that is readily imaged and accessible by stereotaxy or indwelling catheter, they are among the solid tumors best suited for direct intracavitary or intralesional immunotherapy.

In this chapter, many of the clinical trials have been reviewed that have adoptively transferred lymphocytes and/or cytokines directly into the glioma in an attempt to restore and/or enhance reactivity of the immune system to the tumor. Taking these studies together, the most common side effect of immunotherapy protocols involving intracerebral or intracavitary instillation of autologous or allogeneic lymphocytes and/or cytokines have been attributed to increased perilesional edema that presented clinically as fatigue, headache, and exacerbation of a pre-existing deficit. For most patients, overt side effects disappeared within a few days of treatment, although signs of cerebral edema sometimes persisted for several weeks following treatment. Over the course of follow-up, none of the studies reported that any patients showed indications of a secondary disease process that may have developed in the brain as a consequence of the immunotherapy. Overall, the results of the clinical trials presented in this review indicate that although single or multiple intralesional injections of either human recombinant IFN, rIL2, or adoptively transferred lymphocytes are safe, they are noncurative therapies (although indications have come to light that such therapies may occasionally slow tumor recurrence at the site of treatment). Although early attempts to manipulate a patient's immune system with immunotherapy have been disappointing in terms of tumor rejection, the constantly

evolving developments in recombinant DNA technologies and molecular biology are encouraging, and we can reasonably expect the future development of a wider variety of immunotherapeutic options for brain tumors.

REFERENCES

1. Ridley A, Cavenaugh JB: Lymphocytic infiltration in gliomas: Evidence of possible host resistance. Brain 1971; 94:117–124.
2. DiLorenzo N, Palma L, Nicole S: Lymphocytic infiltration in long-survival glioblastoma: Possible host's resistance. Acta Neurochir 1977; 39:27–33.
3. Palma L, DiLorenzo N, Guidetti B: Lymphocytic infiltrates in primary glioblastomas and recidivous gliomas: Incidence, fate, and relevance to prognosis in 228 operated cases. J Neurosurg 1978; 49:854–861.
4. Bashir R, Hochberg F, Oot R: Regrowth patterns of glioblastoma multiforme related to planning of interstitial brachytherapy radiation fields. Neurosurgery 1988; 23:27–30.
5. Rosenberg SA, Lotze MT, Muul LM, et al: A progress report on the treatment of 157 patients with advanced cancer using lymphokine-activated killer cells and interleukin-2 or high-dose interleukin-2 alone. N Engl J Med 1987; 316:889–897.
6. Trouillas P, Lapras CL: Immunotherapie active des tumeurs cerebrales: A propos de 20 cas. Neurochirurgie 1970; 18:143–170.
7. Takakura K, Miki Y, Kubo O, et al: Adjuvant immunotherapy for malignant brain tumours. Jpn J Clin Oncol 1972; 12:109–120.
8. Young H, Kaplan A, Regelson W: Immunotherapy with autologous white cell infusions ("lymphocytes") in the treatment of recurrent glioblastoma multiforme: A preliminary report. Cancer 1977; 40:1037–1044.
9. Ishizawa A: Immunotherapy for malignant gliomas. Neurol Med Chir 1981; 21:179–191.
10. Steinbok P, Thomas JPW, Grossman L, et al: Intratumoral autologous mononuclear cells in the treatment of recurrent glioblastoma multiforme: A phase I study. J Neurooncol 1984; 2:147–151.
11. Herberman RB, Hiserodt J, Vujanovic N, et al: Lymphokine-activated killer cell activity: Characteristics of effector cells and their progenitors in blood and spleen. Immunol Today 1987; 8:178–181.
12. Grimm EA, Mazumder A, Zhang HZ, et al: Lymphokine-activated killer cell phenomenon: Lysis of natural killer-resistant fresh solid tumor cells by interleukin 2–activated autologous human peripheral blood lymphocytes. J Exp Med 1982; 155:1823–1841.
13. Lange A, Ernst M, Jazwiec B, et al: Large granular lymphocytes are central cells in the interleukin-2-dependent differentiation pathway of natural killer cells. Nat Immun Cell Growth Regul 1987; 6:237–249.
14. Ortaldo JR, Mason A, Overton R: Lymphokine-activated killer cells: Analysis of progenitors and effectors. J Exp Med 1986; 164:1193–1205.
15. Ottow RT, Eggermont AMM, Steller EP, et al: The requirements for successful immunotherapy of intraperitoneal cancer using interleukin-2 and lymphokine-activated killer cells. Cancer 1987; 60:1465–1473.
16. Adler A, Stein JA, Kedar E, et al: Intralesional injection of interleukin-2–expanded autologous lymphocytes in melanoma and breast cancer patients: A pilot study. J Biol Resp Modif 1984; 3:491–500.
17. Pizza G, Severini G, Menniti D, et al: Tumor regression after intralesional injection of interleukin 2 in bladder cancer. Int J Cancer 1984; 34:359–367.
18. Jacobs SK, Wilson DJ, Kornblith PL, et al: Killing of human glioblastoma by interleukin-2–activated autologous lymphocytes. J Neurosurg 1986; 64:114–117.
19. Jacobs SK, Wilson DJ, Kornblith PL, et al: Interleukin-2 or autologous lymphokine-activated killer cell treatment of malignant glioma: Phase I trial. Cancer Res 1986; 46:2101–2104.
20. Merchant RE, Grant AJ, Merchant LH, et al: Adoptive immunotherapy for recurrent glioblastoma multiforme using lymphokine activated killer (LAK) cells and recombinant interleukin-2. Cancer 1988; 62:665–671.
21. Merchant RE, Merchant LH, Cook SHS, et al: Intralesional infusion of lymphokine-activated killer (LAK) cells and recombinant interleukin-2 (rIL-2) for the treatment of patients with malignant brain tumor. Neurosurgery 1988; 23:725–732.
22. Atkinson LL, Merchant RE, Ghatak NR, et al: Sterile abscess in glioma patients treated by intraparenchymal injection of lymphokine-activated

killer (LAK) cells and recombinant interleukin-2. Neurosurgery 1989; 25:805–810.

23. Thomas C, Schober R, Lenard HG, et al: Immunotherapy with stimulated autologous lymphocytes in a case of a juvenile anaplastic glioma. Neuropediatrics 1992; 23:123–125.

24. Yoshida S, Tanaka R, Takai N, et al: Local administration of autologous lymphokine-activated killer cells and recombinant interleukin 2 to patients with malignant brain tumors. Cancer Res 1988; 48:5011–5016.

25. Barba D, Saris SC, Holder C, et al: Intratumoral LAK cell and interleukin-2 therapy of human gliomas. J Neurosurg 1989; 70:175–182.

26. Blancher A, Roubinet F, Grancher AS, et al: Local immunotherapy of recurrent glioblastoma multiforme by intracerebral perfusion of interleukin-2 and LAK cells. European Cytokine Network 1993; 4:331–341.

27. Bioardi A, Sivani A, Ruffini PA, et al: Loco-regional immunotherapy with recombinant interleukin-2 and adherent lymphokine-activated killer cells (A-LAK) in recurrent glioblastoma patients. Cancer Immunol Immunother 1994; 39:193–197.

28. Ingram M, Jacques S, Freshwater DB, et al: Salvage immunotherapy of malignant glioma. Arch Neurol 1987; 122:1483–1486.

29. Ingram M, Shelton CH, Jacques S, et al: Preliminary clinical trial of immunotherapy for malignant glioma. J Biol Resp Modif 1987; 6:489–498.

30. Lillehei KO, Kruse CA, Mitchell DH, et al: Adoptive immunotherapy of recurrent glioma using interleukin-2 stimulated lymphocytes. Surg Forum 1989; 40:493–495.

31. Lillehei KO, Johnson SD, McCleary EL, et al: Long-term follow-up of patients with recurrent gliomas treated with adjuvant adoptive immunotherapy. Neurosurgery 1991; 28:16–23.

32. Nitta T, Sato K, Yagita H, et al: Preliminary trial of specific targeting therapy against malignant glioma. Lancet 1990; 335:368–371.

33. Nitta T, Ishizawa K, Ito M, et al: Induction of cytotoxicityfrom human lymphocytes coated with bispecific antibody against human glioma cells. No Shinkei Geka 1990; 18:1001–1006.

34. Ioli G, Jacques D, Yamamoto R, et al: Basic and clinical studies with intratumor immunotherapy of gliomas with allogeneic lymphoid cells. Proc AACR 1994; 35:518.

35. Von Hanwehr RI, Hofman FM, Taylor CR, et al: Mononuclear lymphoid populations infiltrating the microenvironment of primary CNS tumors: Characterization of cell subsets with monoclonal antibodies. J Neurosurg 1984; 60:1138–1147.

36. Rosenberg SA, Spiess P, Lafreniere R: A new approach to the adoptive immunotherapy of cancer with tumor-infiltrating lymphocytes. Science 1986; 233:1318–1321.

37. Nishimura T, Yagi H, Uchiyama Y, et al: Generation of lymphokine-activated killer (LAK) cells from tumor-infiltrating lymphocytes. Cell Immunol 1986; 100:149–157.

38. Sawamura Y, Abe H, Aida T, et al: Isolation and in vitro growth of glioma-infiltrating lymphocytes, and an analysis of their surface phenotypes. J Neurosurg 1988; 69:745–750.

39. Sawamura Y, Hosokawa M, Kuppner MC, et al: Antitumor activity and surface phenotypes of human glioma-infiltrating lymphocytes after in vitro expansion in the presence of interleukin 2. Cancer Res 1989; 49:1843–1849.

40. Sawamura Y: Isolation and expansion of glioma-infiltrating lymphocytes in vitro: An analysis of their surface phenotypes and antitumor activities. Hokkaido Igaku Zasshi 1991; 66:868–878.

41. Levy NL: Specificity of lymphocyte-mediated cytotoxicity in patients with primary intracranial tumors. J Immunol 1978; 121:903–915.

42. Rainbird S, Allwood G, Ridley A: Lymphocyte-mediated cytotoxicity against gliomas. Brain 1981; 104:451–464.

43. Kitahara T, Watanabe O, Yamaura A, et al: Establishment of interleukin 2 dependent cytotoxic T lymphocyte cell line specific for autologous brain tumor and its intracranial administration for therapy of the tumor. J Neurooncol 1987; 4:329–336.

44. Kruse CA, Lillehei KO, Mitchell DH, et al: Analysis of interleukin 2 and various effector cell populations in adoptive immunotherapy of 9L rat gliosarcoma: Allogeneic cytotoxic T lymphocytes prevent tumor take. Proc Natl Acad Sci USA 1990; 87:9577–9581.

45. Redd JM, Lagarde A-C, Kruse CA, et al: Allogeneic tumor-specific cytotoxic T lymphocytes. Cancer Immunol Immunother 1992; 34:349–354.

46. Kruse CA, Schiltz PM, Bellgrau D, et al: Intracranial administrations of single or multiple source allogeneic cytotoxic T lymphocytes: Chronic therapy for primary brain tumors. J Neurooncol 1994; 19:161–168.

47. Fauci AS, Rosenberg SA, Sherwin SA, et al: Immunomodulators in clinical medicine. Ann Intern Med 1987; 106:421–433.

48. Bubenik J, Indrova M: Cancer immunotherapy using local interleukin 2 administration. Immunol Lett 1987; 16:305–310.

49. Forni G, Giovarelli M, Santoni G: Lymphokine-activated tumor inhibition in vivo: I. The local administration of interleukin 2 triggers nonreactive lymphocytes from tumor-bearing mice to inhibit tumor growth. J Immunol 1985; 134:1305–1311.

50. Bubenik J, Kieler J, Trombolt V, et al: Recombinant interleukin-2 inhibits growth of human tumor xenografts in congenitally athymic mice. Immunol Lett 1987; 14:325–330.

51. Watts RG, Wright JL, Atkinson LL, et al: Histopathologic and blood-brain barrier changes in rats induced by an intracerebral injection of human recombinant interleukin-2. Neurosurgery 1989; 49:202–208.

52. Watts RG, Merchant RE: Histopathologic and blood-brain barrier changes in rats induced by an intratumoral injection of human recombinant interleukin-2 in combination with chemotherapeutic agents in a rat glioma model. Neurosurgery 1992; 31:89–99.

53. Ellison MD, Krieg RJ, Merchant RE: Cerebral vasomotor responses after recombinant interleukin-2 infusion. Cancer Res 1990; 50:4377–4381.

54. Bottazzi B, Introna M, Allavena P, et al: In vitro migration of human large granular lymphocytes. J Immunol 1985; 134:2316–2321.

55. Vaage J: Local and systemic effects during interleukin-2 therapy of mouse mammary tumors. Cancer Res 1987; 47:4296–4298.

56. Natuk RJ, Welsh RM: Chemotactic effect of human recombinant interleukin 2 on mouse activated large granular lymphocytes. J Immunol 1987; 139:2737–2743.

57. Phillips JH, Lanier LL: Dissection of the lymphokine-activated killer phenomenon: Relative contribution of peripheral blood natural killer cells and T lymphocytes to cytolysis. J Exp Med 1986; 164:814–825.

58. Merchant RE, McVicar DW, Merchant LH, et al: Treatment of recurrent malignant brain tumor by repeated intralesional injections of human recombinant interleukin-2 alone or in combination with systemic interferon-α: Results of a phase I clinical trial. J Neurooncol 1992; 12:75–83.

59. Mahaley MS, Urso MB, Whaley RA, et al: Immunobiology of primary intracranial tumors: X. Therapeutic efficacy of interferon in the treatment of recurrent gliomas. J Neurosurg 1985; 63:719–725.

60. Nagai M: Clinical use of interferons in the treatment of malignant brain tumors. Dev Med Virol 1988; 4:183–194.

61. Otsuka S, Yamashita J, Keyaki A, et al: Recombinant interferon-alpha A (Ro 22–8181) therapy for patients with malignant brain tumors. Gan To Kagaku Ryoho 1984; 11:1084–1091.

62. Hokland M, Basse P, Justesen J, et al: IFN-induced modulation of histocompatibility antigens on human cells: Background, mechanisms and perspectives. Cancer Metastasis Rev 1988; 7:193–207.

63. Yung WKA, Prados M, Levin VA, et al: Intravenous recombinant interferon beta in patients with recurrent malignant gliomas: A phase I/II study. J Clin Oncol 1991; 9:1945–1949.

64. Mahaley MS, Bertsch L, Cush S, et al: Systemic gamma-interferon therapy for recurrent gliomas. J Neurosurg 1988; 69:826–829.

65. Riccardi R, Kramer RJ, Trown PW, et al: Serum and cerebrospinal fluid (CSF) pharmacokinetics of recombinant leukocyte A interferon (IFNrA) in monkeys. Proc AACR 1982; 23:203–210.

66. Smith RA, Norris F, Palmer D, et al: Distribution of alpha interferon in serum and cerebrospinal fluid after systemic administration. Clin Pharmacol Ther 1985; 37:85–88.

67. Hori T, Inoue Y, Hokama Y, et al: The effect of local injection of interferon against human malignant glioma transplanted into nude mice and the mechanism of its effect. No To Shinkei 1989; 41:911–917.

68. Wen PY, Lampson MA, Lampson LA: Effects of gamma-interferon on major histocompatibility complex antigen expression and lymphocytic infiltration in the 9L gliosarcoma brain tumor model: Implications for strategies of immunotherapy. J Neuroimmunol 1992; 36:57–68.

69. Akbasak A, Laske DW, Oldfield EH, et al: Enhanced expression of major histocompatibility complex antigens in primary brain tumors in vivo with regional cytokine treatment. Proc Am Assoc Neurol Surg, 1994, p 537.

70. Salford LG, Stromblad LG, Nordstrom CH, et al: Intratumoral administration of interferon in malignant gliomas. Acta Neurochir 1981; 56:130–131.

71. Nakagawa Y, Hirakawa K, Ueda S, et al: Local administration of interferon for malignant brain tumors. Cancer Treat Rep 1983; 67:833–835.

72. Obbens EAMT, Feun LG, Leavens ML, et al: Phase I clinical trial of intralesional and intraventricular leukocyte interferon for intracranial malignancies. J Neurooncol 1985; 3:61–67.

73. Duff TA, Borden E, Bay J, et al: Phase II trial of interferon for treatment of recurrent glioblastoma multiforme. J Neurosurg 1986; 64:408–413.

74. Nagai M, Arai T: Clinical effect of interferon in malignant brain tumors. Neurosurg Rev 1984; 7:55–64.

75. Bogdahn U, Fleischer B, Hilfenhaus J, et al: Interferon-β in patients with low grade astrocytomas: A phase I study. J Neurooncol 1985; 3:125–130.

76. Maleci A, Antonelli G, Guidetti B, et al: Pharmacokinetics of recombinant interferon-alpha 2 following intralesional administration in malignant glioma patients. J Interferon Res 1987; 7:107–109.

77. Fetell MR, Housepain EM, Oster MW, et al: Intratumor administration of beta-interferon in recurrent malignant gliomas A phase I clinical and laboratory study. Cancer 1990; 65:78–83.

78. Mizuno M, Yoshida J, Takaoka T, et al: Liposomal transfection of human gamma-interferon gene into human glioma cells and adoptive immunotherapy using lymphokine-activated killer cells. J Neurosurg 1994; 80:510–514.

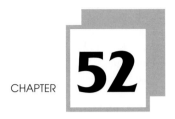

GARY E. ARCHER

MICHAEL R. ZALUTSKY

DARREL D. BIGNER

CHAPTER **52**

Immunoconjugates

It is well documented that gliomas present a formidable problem of diagnosis and treatment. The first line of treatment that has proven to be the best is surgical removal of the tumor mass. Because of the insidious spread of individual tumor cells, no well-defined tumor margins are available for resection. The anatomic location of the tumor may also preclude its complete removal. Adjuvant radiotherapy is a standard treatment protocol that can extend median survival time from 14 to 36 weeks.[1] At this time, adding a single chemotherapeutic agent, 1,3-bis(2-chloroethyl)-1-nitrosourea (BCNU), to the protocol is the most efficacious approach, which extends median survival time by approximately 15 weeks.[2] All adjunct therapies for gliomas are nonspecific and have some component of toxicity to normal tissue. Attempts to circumvent these problems have led to the investigation of immunoconjugates as adjuncts to glioma therapy.

Immunoconjugates are composed of two coupled segments: an antibody and an effector molecule. For our purposes, the targeting agent is an antibody that reacts with a glioma-associated antigen or with a natural ligand to a receptor that may be selectively overexpressed on gliomas. The effector agent may be a radioisotope, a protein toxin, or a drug, any of which can cause tumor cell destruction. The type of effector agent selected is important for efficient tumor destruction; treatment is most effective when the method of action of the effector agent is matched with the antigen being targeted. For example, an immunoconjugate consisting of an antibody and a toxin would not be a good choice for targeting an extracellular matrix antigen. Toxins require that the antigen be internalized into the cell, and extracellular matrix antigens are not internalized.

IMMUNOCONJUGATE EFFECTOR AGENTS

Radioisotopes

Radioisotopes in immunoconjugates have been studied extensively for imaging tumors and for destroying tumor cells. Radioisotopes produce tissue damage by depositing ionizing

energy in the cell. The critical targets within the tumor cell that must be damaged to cause cell death are still largely unknown.[3] Although DNA is almost certainly a critical target, it is postulated that other critical targets exist within the cell. There are two ways in which absorbed energy from isotopes can damage critical cellular targets. The first is through direct contact with critical targets, which causes the target atoms to be ionized or excited and thereby initiates a chain of events that leads to a biologic change. The second method is by indirect action; the radiation comes into contact with a noncritical component, most likely a water molecule. Contact with radiation causes water molecules to become free radicals. When the resulting free radical interacts with another molecule of water, a highly reactive hydroxyl radical is formed that can then diffuse for short distances and interact with DNA. As much as two-thirds of radiation damage can be a result of this indirect mechanism.

Many different isotopes are candidates for use in immunoconjugates. The choice of isotope should be based on the physical half-life and the type of radiation emitted.[4] Most isotopes produce their ionizing radiation by emitting one of three types of radiation: α-particles, β-particles, and γ-rays. The physical characteristics of the three types of radiation vary in terms of energy given off, distance traveled, and biologic effect. The energy released by the different types of radiation is described in terms of linear energy transfer (LET). High LET radiation, such as α-particles, deposits a high level of energy over a short distance. This type of radiation produces most of its cellular damage by direct methods rather than by indirect formation of free radicals. The extent of the biologic effects produced by different types of radiation is expressed in terms of relative biologic effectiveness (RBE), a comparison of the cytotoxic effect of a given type of radiation with that of x-rays. Isotopes that emit radiation with a high LET generally have higher RBE.

To be effective, an immunoconjugate must localize in tumor within the half-life of the isotope, and the isotope must be distributed homogeneously throughout the tumor. In solid tumors, heterogeneous blood supply and antigen distribution can limit immunoconjugate delivery. Therefore, isotopes with a long range are generally used to maximize homogeneous tumor distribution of radiation. The most commonly used isotopes for this purpose are iodine 131 and yttrium 90, which emit long-range β-particles. One drawback of treatment with these isotopes is that they affect untargeted, normal cells.[5] The half-lives of these isotopes correlate well with intravenous administration, because peak monoclonal antibody (MAb) uptake is approximately 1 to 2 days and the half-lives of ^{131}I and ^{90}Y are 8.1 and 2.7 days, respectively.

For α-particle emitters, such as [212]Bi and [211]At, which are of shorter range and possess a high LET, administration within a tumor cyst or within the intrathecal space may be a more fitting method of delivery. The half-lives of [212]Bi and [211]At are 61 minutes and 7.2 hours, respectively, and the more rapid tumor uptake with compartmental administration correlates well with the half-lives of these isotopes. The short penetration of the α-particle suggests that an α-particle emitter would be a good choice for the treatment of thin sheets of tumor cells that lie atop critical tissues (e.g., the spinal cord in cases of neoplastic meningitis) or of tumor cells lining the walls of an intracerebral tumor cyst. α-Particles also have an RBE approximately eight times that of the β-particles emitted from ^{131}I, the most commonly used therapeutic radioisotope.

The labeling methods used to construct radiolabeled immunoconjugates play a significant role in the efficacy of these agents in diagnosis and treatment. Commonly, radiohalogens such as ^{131}I are coupled to targeting agents by electrophilic substitution onto phenyl rings. Unfortunately, the in vivo dehalogenation of radiolabeled immunoconjugates results in an increase in radioactivity accumulation in normal thyroid and stomach. This dehalogenation is most probably due to the action of deiodinases, which are known to be involved in the metabolism of thyroid hormones, and to the similarities of the iodophenyl groups on the immunoconjugate with these thyroid hormones.[6] Alternative methods of labeling have been explored to produce a more stable in vivo radiohalogen. Using a two-step procedure, Zalutsky and Narula[7] radioiodinated the intermediate N-succinimidyl 3-(tri-n-butylstannyl)benzoate (ATE) followed by conjugation of this intermediate to the targeting molecule. In vivo paired-label localization studies of 81C6 (an MAb reactive with the extracellular matrix antigen tenascin, which is associated with gliomas) compared labeling methods using ATE and IODO-GEN and showed a decreased thyroid uptake of 40- to 100-fold for the preparation labeled using the ATE method. A 4- to 12-fold increased tumor uptake resulted when 81C6 was labeled via the ATE method.[8] This method can also be used to label targeting reagents with [211]At without loss of immunoreactivity.[9]

Toxins

Many investigators have attempted to exploit the high efficiency of naturally occurring protein toxins. Immunotoxins are hybrid molecules created by the conjugation of a specific glioma-targeting reagent and a protein toxin. The conjugation of the two moieties can be effected by chemical coupling or by a genetic fusion of the two components. For immunotoxins to be effective, the antigen that is targeted must be internalized. The toxins most commonly used to construct immunotoxins are toxins that are natural by-products of plants or bacteria and that irreversibly inhibit protein synthesis.

Immunotoxins designed for central nervous system (CNS) treatment generally employ *Pseudomonas* exotoxin or diphtheria toxin (from bacteria), or ricin, abrin, pokeweed antiviral protein, gelonin, or saporin (from plants). To be effective, an immunotoxin must bind to the tumor cell and translocate to the cytosol, where it can inhibit protein synthesis. The bacterial toxins from *Pseudomonas* and diphtheria are single-chain proteins with an approximate molecular mass of 60 kD. Structural analysis has shown that the single polypeptide chain of *Pseudomonas* exotoxin can be divided into three domains that are responsible for cell binding (I), translocation into the cytosol (II), and protein synthesis inhibition (III). For diphtheria toxin, the single polypeptide chain requires a proteolytic cleavage within an arginine-rich segment to form the active A and B subunits.[10, 11] Cell binding is facilitated by the B-chain, and the A-chain is responsible for the inhibition of protein synthesis. The plant toxin ricin is a heterodimer composed of two chains of approximately 30 kD linked by a single disulfide bond.[12] The A-chain is responsible for inactivation of cellular ribosomes by binding to the 28S ribosomal subunit; the B-chain is responsible for binding to the cell and may in some way facilitate the translocation of the A-chain into the cytosol.[13–15] The other plant toxins—pokeweed antiviral protein, abrin, saporin, and gelonin—have a mode of action similar to that of ricin, and they inactivate protein synthesis by binding to the 28S ribosomal subunit.[16] These toxins all contain a nonspecific binding domain that can limit their specificity when conjugated to a glioma-reactive targeting agent. Immunotoxins constructed with native toxins such as *Pseudomonas* exotoxin are often effective reagents; however, they can produce normal tissue toxic effects owing to the presence of *Pseudomonas* exotoxin receptors on many normal cells.[17] It is imperative for the production of highly specific and effective immunotoxins that the nonspecific binding of the toxin be eliminated without adversely affecting the toxin's ability to inactivate protein synthesis.

Deletion analysis of the *Pseudomonas* exotoxin has shown that all of domain I can be removed without any loss of toxin activity.[18] Immunotoxins made with either native *Pseudomonas* exotoxin or a truncated form in which all of domain I is missing (PE-40) have antitumor activity in vivo; immunotoxins constructed with PE-40 have a larger therapeutic window than those constructed with native *Pseudomonas* exotoxin.[19] The diphtheria toxin B-chain has been genetically altered at two amino acids to reduce the nonspecific binding 8,000-fold, thereby creating an immunotoxin with tumor specificity that is increased by approximately 10,000-fold.[20, 21] This new form of the diphtheria toxin has been named CRM107 (cross-reacting material 107).

Several approaches have been used to reduce nonspecific binding of ricin. The simplest method is to block nonspecific binding sites on the B-chain by incubating with excess galactose or lactose.[22] A second method is to isolate the A-chain from the B-chain by either biochemical reduction of the disulfide bond or production of pure A-chain through recombinant DNA technology.[23] Immunotoxins made with only the ricin A-chain have shown high specificity, but they possess unpredictable cytotoxicity.[24] The unpredictable nature of these immunotoxins is believed to be a result of the absence of the B-chain and of its function as a facilitator of A-chain entry into the cytosol. Therefore, the cytotoxicity of ricin A-chain immunotoxins becomes dependent on the intracellular processing pathway of the antigen being targeted, and whether the A-chain can gain easy access to the cytosol.

Construction of immunotoxins usually involves a chemical coupling of the MAb and the toxin. This generally involves the use of a heterobifunctional cross-linking agent to introduce a reactive alkyl or sulfhydryl group capable of reacting with a modified toxin. The introduction of chemical modification into one or both of the components creates a heterogeneous mixture of unconjugated, singly conjugated, or multiply conjugated immunotoxin molecules. Further, the chemical modification may also diminish or destroy targeting or toxin function.[25] Once the immunotoxin is constructed, a number of in vivo factors affect its stability. Immunotoxins made by disulphide linking of the MAb and toxin can be broken down in the circulation by glutathione-mediated reduction of the disulphide linkage. Cleavage of the disulfide linkage can be reduced by the use of novel chemical cross-linkers that introduce a hindered disulfide linkage that offers greater resistance to chemical reduction.[26, 27]

IMMUNOCONJUGATE TARGETING AGENTS

The most important part of the immunoconjugate is the targeting agent. Ehrlich[28] was the first to propose the use of specific antibodies to target effector agents; the first actual attempt to use immunoconjugates in human gliomas was made by Day and co-workers.[29] Using radiolabeled rabbit antiglioma antiserum, they showed that there was a preferential localization to human glioma tissue in an amount sufficient for imaging following intra-arterial injection. However, dosimetry calculations indicated that an insufficient dose was delivered for therapeutic purposes. These early attempts to produce specific antibodies to glioma antigens involved the production of polyclonal antibodies using crude heterogeneous glioma extracts for rabbit immunization. The specificity of these early reagents required extensive absorption. The early failure to target a glioma-specific antigen was most likely the result of the limitation of ployclonal antisera and the crude nature of the heterogeneous antigens used for immunization.

The advent of MAb technology by Kohler and Milstein[30] allowed the immune response to be dissected for the production of homogeneous, specific reagents reactive with a single epitope; the MAb reagent could then be conjugated to effector agents for use in imaging and therapy. The nature of the immune response is polyclonal, whether the immunogen is a crude heterogeneous mixture or a highly purified homogeneous preparation. For heterogeneous immunogens, the polyclonal response usually takes the form of antibodies to the different antigens contained within the preparation. In the case of a homogeneous antigen; however, the polyclonal response is represented by antibodies generated to different antigenic epitopes and by antibodies with different immuno-

globulin classes and epitope affinities, rather than to diverse antigen molecules. The MAb process is ideal for use with crude antigens, such as tumor homogenates or even partially purified membrane extracts, in which the target antigen is unknown. Once an MAb-producing clone has been isolated, its specificity can be determined. The only cell-surface–expressed tumor-specific MAbs that have been produced react with a mutated epidermal growth factor receptor (EGFRvIII). Most of the current MAbs can be described as binding to glioma-associated antigens, which are defined as antigens expressed in greater quantities on glioma cells than on normal brain or other normal organ tissue. These may be fetal antigens that are developmentally controlled and not expressed on normal adult tissues, overexpressed normal antigens, or aberrant forms of normal antigens selectively expressed by glioma cells. The glioma-associated antigens that are relevant to immunoconjugate development are those proteins or glycoproteins that are expressed on the cell surface or on the extracellular matrix. Targeting agents may also be normal ligands for receptors that are differentially expressed on tumor cells to a greater extent than on surrounding normal brain. Glioma-associated antigens that have been targeted by immunoconjugates include the extracellular matrix molecule tenascin,[31] the neural cell adhesion molecule,[32] the transferrin receptor, and normal and mutant EGFR.[33]

The vast majority of the MAbs used in the study of human gliomas are of murine origin. The administration of xenogenic antibodies to humans elicits the real possibility of incurring an immune response to the murine MAbs. Current experience in clinical trials of murine MAbs indicates that a human antimouse antibody (HAMA) response is found in 50% of the patients that receive one dose of murine MAb, and it may occur in as many as 90% of patients that receive more than two doses.[34] The consequences of HAMA production are rapid elimination of the immunoconjugate and the potential for a severe allergic reaction, although the latter is rarely seen.[35–38] Originally it was thought that the most immunogenic parts of the molecule were the species-conserved murine-constant regions of the heavy and light chains.[39] Thus, F(ab′)$_2$ or Fab fragments were used to reduce the immunogenicity of the immunoconjugates. A second approach, and the current avenue for generating most immunoconjugates, is the production of chimeric MAbs.

The production of chimeric MAbs has been made possible with recent advances in recombinant DNA technology, permitting the cloning of the individual genes responsible for synthesizing human and murine immunoglobulins.[40] Chimeric MAbs are composed of the constant regions of human immunoglobulins and the antigen-combining variable region of the murine MAb. A second type of chimeric MAb, also referred to as *humanized MAb*, takes only the complementary-determining regions or antigen-binding loops of the murine MAb and places them into the human framework regions.[41, 42]

Patient studies comparing the circulation time of a mouse/human chimeric MAb to a gastrointestinal tumor antigen with its mouse MAb parent showed a sixfold longer circulation time for the mouse/human chimeric than for the murine MAb.[43] A HAMA response was observed in only one of six patients following repeated administration. The amount of antimouse activity directed toward the chimeric MAb was approximately 20-fold less than that of the murine MAb. Studies with other mouse/human chimeric MAbs have indicated a variable HAMA response. These HAMA responses appear to be anti-idiotype antibodies directed against the antigen-combining site of the mouse/human chimeric MAb.[44]

The ability to clone the immunoglobulin-producing genes has also made possible the construction of altered immunoglobulin forms. New single-chain antigen-binding proteins (sFv) can now be constructed by joining, through a flexible linker, only the antigen-binding variable regions of the light and heavy chains of an intact whole IgG murine MAb. The resulting sFv molecules are approximately six times smaller than the intact MAb and retain specific binding activity. The smaller size of the sFv molecules should have better tumor penetration.[45] When sFv molecules are used in immunoconjugates in combination with protein toxins, the immunotoxin can be expressed as one recombinant protein molecule and, therefore, not require the chemical conjugation of the MAb and the toxin; the result is the production of a homogeneous reagent.

PROBLEMS OF IMMUNOCONJUGATE LOCALIZATION

Four main factors affect the homogeneity and level of immunoconjugate to localization in gliomas: heterogeneous distribution of antigen and blood supply, elevated interstitial pressure, and large transport distances.[46, 47] Gliomas have a high degree of antigen heterogeneity in terms of antigens expressed and distribution within the tumor.[48] The heterogeneous antigen expression is further complicated by the existence of relatively antigen-null cells and the tendency for cells to show a cell-cycle variation in antigen density and expression.[49, 50] In intracranial tumors, the delivery of immunoconjugates is further complicated by the blood-brain barrier and the heterogeneous vascular distribution. The blood-brain barrier is formed by tight junctions of the endothelial cells in the cerebral capillaries and limits the entry of most water-soluble compounds into the CNS.[51] Generally, the neovascularization induced by gliomas does not recapitulate the endothelial tight junctions of the blood-brain barrier, which results in the formation of an incomplete barrier with regional variation in permeability.[52] From studies in non-CNS tumors, the normal organization of artery to arteriole to capillary to postcapillary venule to venule to vein is disrupted with the formation of blind-end saccular vessels.[53] As the tumor grows, a decrease in vascularization appears to take place, leaving areas of necrosis and surrounding areas with less perfusion. Once an immunoconjugate has reached the tumor circulation, its extravasation into the tumor occurs by diffusion and convection. Diffusion is proportional to the surface area of the exchange vessel and to the difference in the concentration of immunoconjugate between plasma and the tumor interstitium.[54] Convection is proportional to the rate of fluid extravasation, which is dependent on the differences in the vascular and interstitial pressures. As the tumor grows, the interstitial pressure increases, which further limits the exchange of macromolecules such as immunoconjugates.[55, 56]

The large distances in the interstitium can contribute to the poor distribution of immunoconjugates within the tumor. The movement of macromolecules in the interstitium occurs mainly by diffusion, which is dependent on the size of the molecule; therefore, for large interstitial distances, IgG-containing immunoconjugates can take up to 2 days to diffuse 1 mm.[56] The diffusion of immunoconjugates in the interstitium is further complicated by antigen binding.[57, 58]

The use of compartmental therapy, either by intrathecal delivery or by direct infusion into normally occurring or surgically created cysts, is being investigated to overcome some of these physiological barriers. Compartmental approaches are not influenced by some of the barriers, such as heterogeneous blood distribution and the high interstitial pressure of the tumor, which leaves the distribution to be limited by diffusion of the immunoconjugate. Because diffusion is dependent on the size of the molecule, the use of immunoglobulin fragments such as $F(ab')_2$, Fab, and the newer sFv fragments allow deeper and more uniform tumor penetration. Several studies using tumors other than gliomas have compared the penetration and distribution of the four forms of immunoglobulin: intact IgG, $F(ab')_2$, Fab, and sFv.[59] Using the four immunoglobulin forms of MAb CC49, Yokota and colleagues[45] found that after 6 hours, the IgG had penetrated to a depth of 40 μm, the Fab had penetrated to 70 μm, and the sFv could be found up to 100 μm into the tumor. They also found that the sFv was the most evenly distributed of all of the fragments, and that homogeneous distribution was maintained throughout the 96-hour length of the experiment.

USE OF IMMUNOCONJUGATES TO TARGET GLIOMA-ASSOCIATED ANTIGENS

Glioma-associated antigens are antigens that are differentially expressed in greater quantities on gliomas than in normal tissues. Antigens targeted include extracellular matrix antigens, a heterogeneous group of protein or glycoprotein antigens found on the cell surface of neuroectodermally derived tissues, overexpressed normal receptors, and mutant forms of normal receptors. Table 52–1 gives an overview of the immunoconjugates that have been investigated for glioma therapy. The next section provides a few examples of how different antiglioma immunoconjugates have been used to target glioma-associated antigens.

Extracellular Matrix Antigens

Extracellular matrix antigens provide an abundant target for immunoconjugate therapy. Tenascin is an extracellular matrix antigen that is widely expressed in embryonic development, but its expression is restricted in quantity and in the type of adult normal organ in which it occurs.[60] Tenascin is prevalent in the most anaplastic forms of gliomas and in other tumors, such as fibrosarcoma, osteosarcoma, melanoma, Wilms' tumor, and squamous cell carcinoma of the colon, mammary, and lung. MAb 81C6, originally developed

TABLE 52–1
ANTIGLIOMA IMMUNOCONJUGATES

Targeting MAb(s)	Reactivity	Therapeutic/ Diagnostic Agent	Use	Study
		Normal Receptor Antigens		
454A12	Transferrin receptor	Recombinant ricin A chain	Preclinical	Laske et al[79]
425	Normal EGFR	[131]I	Preclinical	Takahashi et al[85]
		[111]In	Clinical	Dadparvar et al[87]
J2B9 J3F6 L8A4 H10 Y10	Reacts with mutant EGFRvIII; no cross-reactivity with normal EGFR	[131]I	Preliminary immunohistochemistry and in vitro screening	Wikstrand et al[90]
		Extracellular Matrix Antigens		
81C6	ECM tenascin	[131]I	Preclinical and clinical	Bourdon et al[61] Zalutsky et al[31]
BC-2	ECM tenascin	[131]I	Clinical	Riva et al[65]
ERIC-1	NCAM	[131]I	Clinical	Papanastassiou[32]
		Cell Surface Antigens		
Mel-14 F(ab')$_2$	High-molecular-weight proteoglycan	[131]I	Preclinical and clinical	Colapinto et al[70] Zalutsky et al[91]
C12	M_r 160,000–180,000 surface protein	[125]I	Preclinical	Wikstrand et al[92]
D12	M_r 88,000 surface protein	[125]I	Preclinical	Wikstrand et al[92]
MUC2-63	M_r 32,000 surface glycoprotein	[111]In	Clinical	Bergh et al[93]
9.2.27	Core protein of chondroitin sulfate proteoglycan	DAVLBHY	Preclinical	Schrappe et al[76]
ONS-M21	M_r 80,000 cell surface glycoprotein		Preclinical	Moriuchi et al[94]
GA-17	Tyrosine-specific phosphorylated antigens	Neocarzinostatin	Preclinical	Kondo et al[75]
SZ-39	M_r 180,000 cell surface glycoprotein	[131]I	Preclinical	Yang et al[95]
UJ131A	NCAM	[131]I	Clinical	Richardson et al[96]
P96.5	M_r 97,000 cell surface glycoprotein	[90]Y	Preclinical	Williams et al[97]
3H9	Undefined	[125]I	Preclinical	Lee et al[98]
G-22	M_r 67,000 cell surface protein	[123]I	Clinical	Yoshida et al[74]

Abbreviations: EGFR, epidermal growth factor receptor; ECM, extracellular matrix; NCAM, neural cell adhesion molecule; DAVLBHY, 4-desacetylvinblastine-3-carboxyhydrazide.

in our laboratory in 1983,[61] recognizes an alternatively spliced extra repeat in the tenascin structure. Consequently, it does not bind with all tenascin variants, giving it a greater specificity.[62] Preclinical localization studies in xenografts of the tenascin-expressing human tumor line D-54 MG showed that 81C6 had a high degree of localization compared with a nonspecific isotype-matched control immunoglobulin, 45.6.[61] Peak levels were achieved within 24 to 48 hours and persisted for 5 to 7 days. The tumor-to–normal brain ratio for specific MAb 81C6 was 107:1. The selective and specific localization of radiolabeled 81C6 seen in preclinical testing has been confirmed in a preliminary human trial. Tissue biopsy specimens in a clinical paired-label study using ^{131}I-labeled 81C6 and ^{125}I-labeled 45.6 (the isotype-matched nonspecific control MAb) showed biopsy specimens with tumor-to–normal brain ratios for 81C6 ranging from 25:1 to as high as 200:1.[31] The localization index, an indication of specific uptake (ratio of specific to nonspecific MAb in tissue divided by the same ratio in blood), was as high as 5, with an average of 2.83, compared with an average of 1.11 for normal brain.

These studies used an electrophilic substitution method, the IODO-GEN method, for labeling the MAbs. As discussed previously, proteins labeled by this method are subject to dehalogenation. In a preclinical therapy study in D-54 MG human glioma xenografts, Schuster and associates[63] found a greater growth delay when 81C6 labeled with the ATE method was given as compared with an identical amount of 81C6 labeled via the IODO-GEN method. The growth delay associated with the ATE labeling method was statistically significant. Furthermore, the biodistribution data showed a greater radiation dose to tumor delivered by 81C6 labeled using ATE as compared with 81C6 labeled using IODO-GEN (7,723 vs. 5,200 rad). Alternative labeling methods, such as the ATE method, may result in greater delivery of radiation to tumor.

In phase I clinical trials, Bigner and co-workers[64] studied compartmental administration of the 81C6 immunoconjugate as a means of increasing delivery and reducing binding with nontumor tenascin. For intraparenchymal tumors, two groups of patients were treated. In one group of patients the recurrent glioma had a spontaneous cyst, and in the second group a resection cavity was created surgically for the compartmental delivery of 81C6 immunoconjugate. Three of four patients who had recurrent gliomas with spontaneous cysts that were treated with intracavitary ^{131}I 81C6 have had an impressive response. One patient, given 15.2 mCi of ^{131}I-labeled 81C6, had a partial clinical and radiographic response and was able to return to work for 12 months. This patient was re-treated 13 months after initial treatment with a 20-mCi dose of ^{131}I-labeled 81C6 and lived a total of 26 months after initial treatment and a total of 33 months from initial diagnosis. Radiation dosimetry estimated that 12,700 rad was delivered to the cyst wall. In two other patients who had recurrent gliomas with spontaneous cysts that were treated with intracavitary 81C6 immunoconjugate, one had radiographic evidence of stable disease and is alive 31 months after a single treatment with 21 mCi of ^{131}I-labeled 81C6, and the other had a partial radiographic response and is alive 14 months after a single treatment.

The phase I trial of compartmental administration of the 81C6 immunoconjugate into surgically created resection cavities has reached a single dose level of 60 mCi. Of the 17 patients treated, none had evidence of neurologic toxic response. One patient, however, had a seizure following administration of immunoconjugate. This patient had a pre-existing seizure disorder, and the seizure was effectively controlled by an adjustment in the anticonvulsant medication. Of the patients treated, nine of 14 are alive with clinically stable disease, and eight of these also have radiographic evidence of stable disease. Survival times for these patients extend from 1 to 15 months following treatment and from 3 to 41 months since diagnosis. The remaining three patients have not been in the study long enough to determine whether they are responding to treatment.

In phase I trials of intrathecal compartmental therapy with the 81C6 immunoconjugate for neoplastic meningitis, 20 patients with gliomas survived from 2 to 12 months from initial treatment. Seven of these patients are still alive with clinically stable disease. A maximum tolerated single radiation dose of 100 mCi has been established, and a phase II intrathecal study of multiple doses is being written.

Riva and colleagues[65] used two MAbs that also recognize tenascin, BC-2 and BC-4, in intralesional therapy of gliomas. These antibodies bind to a different epitope in the tenascin molecule than does 81C6.[66, 67] Dosimetry calculations showed that 24 hours after direct administration of ^{131}I-labeled MAb into the glioma, the mean tumor-to–normal brain ratio was 16.6:1 and that the percentage of the injected dose per gram of tumor was 2.4%. The mean effective half-life of the immunoconjugate was 74.5 hours. From a 24-patient study, 17 patients were able to be evaluated, and the median survival time was 16 months.

ERIC-1 is a murine MAb that recognizes the human neural cell adhesion molecule. ERIC-1 is positive on all gliomas tested ($n > 50$) and is present on normal neural and astrocytic elements.[68] Direct administration of ERIC-1 into the lesion has been undertaken by Papanastassiou and co-workers,[32] and the degree of normal brain binding is not considered significant by the investigators. Papanastassiou and colleagues studied the therapeutic effect of intralesional ^{131}I-labeled ERIC-1 in a series of seven patients. They found that the tumor-to–normal brain ratios at 300 hours ranged

from 187:1 to 564:1. Radioactivity was confined to the cyst cavity for up to 3 weeks. One patient survived with stable disease 10 months following treatment, and a second patient showed progressive disease 8 months following treatment; two patients remained alive 5 months following treatment. No toxic responses were noted in any of the patients.

These studies indicate that the extracellular matrix is a viable target for immunoconjugate therapy. Intravenously administered immunoconjugates to tenascin showed specific tumor localization that was within the range seen for non-CNS tumors. Compartmental administration was shown to be an effective route for immunoconjugates that react with an antigen expressed on normal brain, rendering them operationally specific, with no apparent CNS toxic effects. Response and survival from single-dose phase I studies are encouraging, as is lack of neurotoxic effects. Repeated treatments using immunoconjugates constructed from chimeric MAbs may increase the survival benefits of targeting extracellular matrix antigens.

Cell Surface Glioma-Associated Antigens

A large number of cell surface proteins and glycoproteins with limited distribution on normal tissues and heterogeneous expression on neuroectodermally derived tumors have been discovered on glioma cells. One of the most extensively studied MAbs directed at the surface molecules is Me1-14. Me1-14 recognizes a high molecular weight proteoglycan antigen found on gliomas and melanomas.[69] Preclinical studies of Me1-14 have demonstrated the delivery advantage of $F(ab')_2$ immunoglobulin fragments as compared with intact IgG. Colapinto and associates[70] showed in a direct paired-label analysis of Me1-$F(ab')_2$ and intact IgG Me1-14 that the two forms had comparable binding affinities; and in intracranial and subcutaneous D-54 MG human glioma xenografts, the $F(ab')_2$ fragment had a higher tumor-to–normal tissue uptake ratio compared with that of intact IgG. In intracranial tumors, the $F(ab')_2$ fragment showed an earlier specific localization and a significantly higher blood-to-tissue transfer constant compared with intact Me1-14. Based on these data, the estimated radiation dosimetry suggested that ^{131}I-labeled Me1-14 $F(ab')_2$ would deliver higher, more favorable tumor-to–normal tissue radiation dose ratios compared with intact IgG. Behnke and co-workers[71] confirmed that radiolabeled Me1-14 $F(ab')_2$ showed a specific localization compared with nonspecific control MAb $F(ab')_2$ when administered to patients with gliomas.

Immunoconjugates are also being investigated for use in imaging, both for diagnostic purposes and to estimate MAb dosimetry for a subsequent therapy study. For example, Me1-14-14 $F(ab')_2$ has been labeled with ^{18}F for use in positron emission tomography (PET).[72] Single-photon emission computed tomography (SPECT) of non-CNS tumors has been successful in tumor detection; however, PET provides superior spatial resolution and more accurate quantitative capabilities. PET can also be correlated with computer-assisted tomography (CT) and magnetic resonance imaging (MRI). Garg and others[73] found that Me1-14 $F(ab')_2$ could be labeled with ^{18}F and maintain immunoreactivity comparable to that of MAb labeled with [131]I. Specific tumor uptake of ^{18}F-labeled Me1-14 F(ab′)$_2$ was seen as early as 4 hours after injection in mice with D-54 MG subcutaneous human glioma xenografts. Preclinical SPECT trials of ^{123}I-labeled MAb G-22 F(ab′)$_2$ in subcutaneous U251 MG xenografts found that tumor images were possible 1 to 7 days after administration; however, the optimal timing was at 3 to 4 days.[74] Although these two trials employ two different targeting agents, this example points out the need for further experimentation and for development of new strategies in the construction of antiglioma immunoconjugates.

Drug-containing immunoconjugates have also been investigated for the treatment of gliomas. Kondo and colleagues[75] conjugated the Fab′ fragment of MAb GA-17, which recognizes a tyrosine-specific phosphorylated cell surface antigen, to neocarzinostatin (NCS), a proteinaceous anticancer antibiotic. Human glioma U-87 MG xenografts were established subcutaneously in athymic mice, and two doses of GA-17-NCS conjugate were given on days 21 and 23 following tumor inoculation. The effect of the GA-17-NCS conjugate on growth delay was compared with that in controls given saline, NCS alone, GA-17 Fab′ alone, and GA-17 Fab′ mixed with, but not conjugated to, NCS. A statistically significant reduction occurred in tumor volume when the animals were treated with intravenous GA-17-NCS compared with any of the controls. Free NCS or GA-17 Fab′ fragments did not produce any significant therapeutic effect on the xenografts.

Recently, a new vinblastine derivative, 4-desacetylvinblastine-3-carboxyhydrazide (DAVLBHY), has been investigated as a potential effector agent in immunoconjugates for the treatment of gliomas. Schrappe and co-workers[76] conjugated DAVLBHY to the MAb 9.2.27, which reacts with the core protein of chondroitin sulfate proteoglycans found in human glioblastomas. The immunoconjugate showed no loss of binding and no increase in nonspecific binding compared with the MAb itself. The therapeutic efficacy of 9.2.27 DAVLBHY was tested on U-87 MG subcutaneous human xenografts in athymic mice and compared with saline, free DAVLBHY, 9.2.27 mixed with but not conjugated to DAVLBHY, and a nonspecific immunoconjugate KS1/4-DAVLBHY. The treatment regimen consisted of four doses given on days 2, 5, 7, and 9 following tumor inoculation. Animals treated with saline or MAb alone reached maximum tumor size by day 28. All treatment groups given DAVLBHY (0.5 mg) (i.e., free drug, nonspecific conjugate, and 9.2.27 DAVLBHY) experienced transiently delayed tumor progression. However, by day 46, tumors in the animals treated with nonspecific conjugate were 50% larger than those in animals treated with specific conjugate. When the dose of DAVLBHY was increased to 2.0 mg per animal, the initial growth delay of the DAVLBHY-containing controls was longer, but the tumor did progress. By day 50, the tumors in the free DAVLBHY and nonspecific conjugate groups had reached maximum volume, whereas those in the animals treated with specific 9.2.27 DAVLBHY conjugate remained tumor free for the duration of the experiment (99 days).

Many of the preclinical and clinical trials of immunoconjugates for glioma therapy have used radioisotopes as effector agents. For antigens that internalize, newer conjugation methods, such as the method using tyramine cellobiose, must be employed. These preclinical studies suggest that for antigens that internalize, immunoconjugates constructed with drugs, toxins, and radioisotopes may be effective agents. The synergy among them remains to be investigated.

Targeting of Normal Receptors

The transferrin receptor is a normal cell surface molecule that is responsible for the transport of iron into cells and is differentially expressed on rapidly dividing cells such as gliomas.[77] Zovickian and colleagues[12] demonstrated a significantly higher level of transferrin receptors on human glioblastoma- and medulloblastoma-derived cell lines as compared with normal brain. The transferrin receptor has been shown to be below detectable levels in normal brain tissues.[78]

Laske and others[79] compared the abilities of transferrin conjugate and an immunoconjugate to accomplish intratumoral targeting of the transferrin receptor. The transferrin conjugate consisted of human transferrin as the targeting agent and CRM107, a genetically engineered diphtheria toxin with a point mutation to eliminate nonspecific binding, as the effector agent (Tf-CRM107). The immunoconjugate was composed of MAb 454A12, which reacts with the human transferrin receptor, and recombinant ricin A-chain (rRA). Both conjugates were reactive in vitro with the human glioblastoma cell line U-251 MG. For in vivo testing, U-251 MG xenografts were established, and a total of four intratumoral injections of the two conjugates were given on days 0, 2, 4, and 6 following tumor inoculation. Controls were saline, MAb 454A12 alone, and the two unconjugated toxins alone. Tf-CRM107 produced a dose-dependent inhibition of tumor growth, with the highest dose (10 μg) causing a 95% regression by day 14. At the termination of the experiment at day 30, no evidence of tumor was seen in three of the five mice treated with Tf-CRM107. The nontargeted CRM107 toxin used alone at a concentration of 10 μg also significantly inhibited tumor growth, but was less potent than Tf-CRM107. The 454A12-rRA immunotoxin also caused significant tumor growth inhibition and regression, but it was less potent than Tf-CRM107. Again, nontargeted rRA alone inhibited growth, but was less effective than targeted immunotoxin 454A12-rRA. Equimolar doses of MAb 454A12 alone were also effective in inhibiting tumor growth, but to a lesser degree than the targeted 454A12-rRA. Martell and co-workers[80] showed that these two toxin conjugates, Tf-CRM107 and 454A12rRA, could inhibit protein synthesis on fresh surgical specimens of glioblastomas multiforme and medulloblastomas. The unconjugated toxins CRM107 and recombinant ricin-A chain (rRA) were less potent in inhibiting protein synthesis than the targeted immunotoxins.

The EGFR has been found to be overexpressed in 30% to 40% of malignant human gliomas.[81–83] The overexpression of EGFR on gliomas has been utilized for imaging and therapy. Takahashi and associates[84] have shown that the F(ab′)$_2$ fragment of MAb 425, a murine IgG$_{2a}$, localizes in tumor tissue in athymic mice containing the EGFR-producing human glioma U-87 MG. No localization in U-87 MG xenografts was observed for an isotype-matched control MAb. MAb 425 failed to localize to a xenograft of a human colorectal carcinoma tumor that does not express the EGFR. Preclinical therapy with ^{131}I-labeled 425 F(ab')$_2$ has shown that two doses given on days 0 and 6 following subcutaneous tumor inoculation of human glioma U-87 MG caused a statistically significant growth delay compared with ^{131}I-labeled isotype-matched control MAb.[85]

In a clinical imaging and therapy trial, Kalofonos and colleagues[86] found that the anti-EGFR MAb EGFR1 localized to tumors in 9 of 12 patients. Using ^{111}In-labeled MAb 425, Dadparvar and co-workers[87] showed that all biopsy-positive gliomas could be imaged. Some uptake of ^{111}In-labeled control antibody and [^{111}In]indium chloride alone was observed; however, the degree of this uptake was less than that seen with specific ^{111}In-labeled 425. In treatment studies, three of five patients receiving ^{131}I-labeled EGFR1 showed clinical improvement lasting from 6 months to 3 years. EGFR-overexpressing cells can be targeted with immunotoxins made with toxins such as PE-40 and natural ligands of the EGFR.

In addition to overexpression, the EGFR gene is often rearranged in a subpopulation of gliomas. The rearranged EGFR gene has deletions involving the coding region for the extracellular domain. Deletions in the extracellular domain can be divided into three classes: type I (EGFRvI) has a deletion of the entire extracellular domain, whereas types II (EGFRvII) and III (EGFRvIII) have only partial in-frame deletions in the extracellular domain.[88] EGFRvIII is the most common, occurring in approximately 17% to 27% of gliomas. In the EGFRvIII, a deletion of 801 nucleotides is present that removes N-terminal amino acid residues 6-273 from the extracellular domain of the intact 170-kD EGFR, resulting in a 145-kD protein. This deletion joins what normally were distant polypeptide sequences in the intact EGFR and creates a new amino acid, glycine, at this fusion junction at position 6 between amino acid residues 5 and 274.[89]

Humphrey and associates[89] produced, in rabbits, polyvalent antisera that were specific for the EGFRvIII mutant protein, as demonstrated by immunohistochemical analysis, and produced specific immunoprecipitation of the EGFRvIII protein from membrane preparations. The production of rabbit polyclonal antisera specifically reactive with EGFRvIII indicates that the generation of a tumor-specific immunologic reagent is possible. However, as mentioned previously, polyclonal reagents are not ideal for use in immunoconjugates. MAbs to EGFRvIII should provide the tumor specificity needed to make effective immunoconjugates.

Until now, producing murine MAbs to the EGFRvIII has proven a difficult task as a result of species-related differences in immunoreactivity. Recently, Wikstrand and co-workers[90] reported the production of five MAbs that were specifically reactive with EGFRvIII. In radioimmunoassay, anti-EGFRvIII MAbs all specifically reacted with the HC cell line, which expresses only the EGFRvIII receptor and does not react with the human A431 line, which overexpresses the wild-type EGFR. Immunoprecipitation studies show that these five anti-EGFRvIII MAbs react only with the 145-kD mutant receptor and do not precipitate the 170-kD wild-type EGFR. Immunohistochemical analysis of human tissues shows reactivity with one of four anaplastic astrocytomas and 15 of 21 glioblastomas. The tumor-specific MAbs failed to react with normal tissues of cerebellum, cerebral cortex, liver, colon, kidney, testes, lung, ovary, skin, peripheral nerves, bone marrow, lymph node, and spleen. The data indicate that the new MAbs are specific for the EGFRvIII epitope and do not possess any cross-reactivity with normal wild-type EGFR. The anti-EGFRvIII MAbs were of varying murine classes and subclasses of varying affinities and should provide excellent reagents for use in immunoconjugates. In addition, the varying properties of the MAbs and their reactivity with the same antigen should allow examination of the effect of affinity on in vivo localization and effector delivery to solid tumors.

CONCLUSION

MAb technology has allowed the production of reagents in unlimited quantities and with homogeneous properties to highly specific epitopes. Not all reagents identified thus far have absolute specificity; however, compartmental administration has been used to render them operationally specific for the treatment of gliomas. Advances in molecular biology have led to the production of chimeric human/mouse antibodies that may reduce the HAMA response and allow repeated administration of immunoconjugates. The same technology has made it possible to generate smaller MAb-based targeting reagents, which have been shown to have a greater penetration into solid tumors. Molecular biology has been used to modify some of the protein toxins to reduce their intrinsic natural binding and thereby create more specific immunoconjugates. Development of different labeling methods can reduce in vivo dehalogenation so that a greater dose of isotope can be delivered to tumor. Experimentation with different isotopes, such as the α-particle emitters, may provide greater therapeutic effectiveness. The most exciting new reagents on the horizon are probably those that are truly tumor specific, such as the anti-EGFRvIII MAbs. The internalization of the anti-EGFRvIII receptor complex makes these MAbs ideal reagents for constructing immunoconjugates with toxins, drugs, or, possibly, radioisotopes.

ACKNOWLEDGMENTS

Editorial assistance was rendered by Ann S. Tamariz, E.L.S.

This work was supported in part by NIH grants NS 20023, CA 56115, CA 42324, and CA 11898, and grants 95ER62021 and 96ER62148 from the Department of Energy.

REFERENCES

1. Walker MD, Alexander E Jr, Hunt WE, et al: Evaluation of BCNU and/or radiotherapy in the treatment of anaplastic gliomas. Neurology 1978; 35:219.
2. Brandes A, Soesan M, Fiorentino MV: Medical treatment of high grade malignant gliomas in adults: An overview. Anticancer Res 1991; 11:719.
3. Hall EJ: The physics and chemistry of radiation absorption. *In* Hall EJ (ed): Radiobiology for the Radiologist, ed 3. Philadelphia, JB Lippincott, 1988, p 1.

4. Mausner LF, Srivastava SC: Selection of radionuclides for radioimmunotherapy. Med Phys 1992; 20:503.

5. Wheldon TE, O'Donoghue JA: The radiobiology of targeted radiotherapy. Int J Radiat Biol 1990; 58:1.

6. Gershengorn MC, Glinoer D, Robbings J: Transport and metabolism of thyroid hormones. In DeVisscher M (ed): The Thyroid Gland. New York, Raven, 1980, p 81.

7. Zalutsky MR, Narula AS: Radiohalogenation of a monoclonal antibody using an N-succinimidyl 3-(tri-n-butylstannyl)benzoate intermediate. Cancer Res 1988; 48:1446.

8. Zalutsky MR, Noska MA, Colapinto EV, et al: Enhanced tumor localization and in vivo stability of a monoclonal antibody radioiodinated using N-succinimidyl 3-(tri-n-butylstannyl)benzoate. Cancer Res 1989; 49:5543.

9. Zalutsky MR, Garg PK, Friedman HS, et al: Labeling monoclonal antibodies and F(ab′)₂ fragments with the alpha-particle-emitting nuclide astatine-211: Preservation of immunoreactivity and in vivo localizing capacity. Proc Natl Acad Sci USA 1989; 86:7149.

10. Pastan I, Willingham MC, FitzGerald DJ: Immunotoxins. Cell 1986; 47:641.

11. Sandvig K, Olsnes S: Rapid entry of nicked diphtheria toxin into cells at low pH: Characterization of the entry process and effects of low pH on the toxin molecule. J Biol Chem 1981; 256:9068.

12. Zovickian J, Johnson VG, Youle RJ: Potent and specific killing of human malignant brain tumor cells by an anti-transferrin receptor antibody-ricin immunotoxin. J Neurosurg 1987; 66:850.

13. Youle RJ, Colombatti M: Hybridoma cells containing intracellular anti-ricin antibodies show ricin meets secretory antibody before entering the cytosol. J Biol Chem 1987; 262:4676.

14. Youle RJ, Murray GJ, Neville DM Jr: Studies on the galactose-binding site of ricin and the hybrid toxin Man6P-ricin. Cell 1981; 23:551.

15. Youle RJ, Neville DM Jr: Kinetics of protein synthesis inactivation by ricin-anti-Thy 1.1 monoclonal antibody hybrids: Role of the ricin B subunit demonstrated by reconstitution. J Biol Chem 1982; 257:1598.

16. Hall WA, Fodstad O: Immunotoxins and central nervous system neoplasia. J Neurosurg 1992; 76:1.

17. Pai LH, Batra JK, FitzGerald DJ, et al: Anti-tumor activities of immunotoxins made of monoclonal antibody B3 and various forms of Pseudomonas exotoxin. Proc Natl Acad Sci USA 1991; 88:3358.

18. Batra JK, Jinno Y, Chaudhary VK, et al: Antitumor activity in mice of an immunotoxin made with anti-transferrin receptor and a recombinant form of Pseudomonas exotoxin. Proc Natl Acad Sci USA 1989; 86:8545.

19. Pai LH, Batra JK, FitzGerald DJ, et al: Antitumor effects of B3-PE and B3-LysPE40 in a nude mouse model of human breast cancer and the evaluation of B3-PE toxicity in monkeys. Cancer Res 1992; 52:3189.

20. Greenfield L, Johnson VG, Youle RJ: Mutations in diphtheria toxin separate binding from entry and amplify immunotoxin selectivity. Science 1987; 238:536.

21. Johnson VG, Wrobel C, Wilson D, et al: Improved tumor-specific immunotoxins in the treatment of CNS and leptomeningeal neoplasia. J Neurosurg 1989; 70:240.

22. Youle RJ, Neville DM Jr: Anti-Thy 1.2 monoclonal antibody linked to ricin is a potent cell-type-specific toxin. Proc Natl Acad Sci USA 1980; 77:5483.

23. O'Hare M, Roberts LM, Thorpe PE, et al: Expression of ricin A chain in Escherichia coli. FEBS Lett 1987; 216:73.

24. Vitetta ES, Fulton RJ, May RD, et al: Redesigning nature's poisons to create anti-tumor reagents. Science 1987; 238:1098.

25. Wawrzynczak EJ: Rational design of immunotoxins current progress and future prospects. Anticancer Drug Des 1992; 7:427.

26. Thorpe PE, Wallace PM, Knowles PP, et al: New coupling agents for the synthesis of immunotoxins containing a hindered disulfide bond with improved stability in vivo. Cancer Res 1987; 47:5924.

27. Goff DA, Carroll SF: Substituted 2-iminothiolanes: Reagents for the preparation of disulfide cross-linked conjugates with increased stability. Bioconjug Chem 1990; 1:381.

28. Ehrlich P: Collected Studies in Immunity. New York, John Wiley & Sons, 1905.

29. Day ED, Lassiter S, Woodhall B, et al: The localization of radioantibodies in human brain tumors: I. Preliminary exploration. Cancer Res 1965; 25:773.

30. Kohler G, Milstein C: Continuous cultures of fused cells secreting antibody of predefined specificity. Nature 1975; 256:495.

31. Zalutsky MR, Moseley RP, Coakham HB, et al: Pharmacokinetics and tumor localization of ¹³¹I-labeled anti-tenascin monoclonal antibody 81C6 in patients with gliomas and other intracranial malignancies. Cancer Res 1989; 49:2807.

32. Papanastassiou V, Pizer BL, Coakham HB, et al: Treatment of recurrent and cystic malignant gliomas by a single intracavity injection of ¹³¹I monoclonal antibody: Feasibility, pharmacokinetics and dosimetry. Br J Cancer 1993; 67:144.

33. Mendelsohn J: The epidermal growth factor receptor as a target for therapy with antireceptor monoclonal antibodies. Semin Cancer Biol 1990; 1:339.

34. Hand PH, Kashmiri SV, Schlom J: Potential for recombinant immunoglobulin constructs in the management of carcinoma. Cancer 1994; 73:1105.

35. Sears HF, Mattis J, Herlyn D, et al: Phase-I clinical trial of monoclonal antibody in treatment of gastrointestinal tumours. Lancet 1982; 1:762.

36. Levy R, Miller RA: Tumor therapy with monoclonal antibodies. Fed Proc 1983; 42:2650.

37. Meeker TC, Lowder J, Maloney DG, et al: A clinical trial of anti-idiotype therapy for B cell malignancy. Blood 1985; 65:1349.

38. Pimm MV, Perkins AC, Armitage NC, et al: The characteristics of blood-borne radiolabels and the effect of anti-mouse IgG antibodies on localization of radiolabeled monoclonal antibody in cancer patients. J Nucl Med 1985; 26:1011.

39. Order SE: Monoclonal antibodies: Potential role in radiation therapy and oncology. Int J Radiat Oncol Biol Phys 1981; 81:193.

40. Morrison SL: Transfectomas provide novel chimeric antibodies. Science 1985; 229:1202.

41. Riechmann L, Clark M, Waldmann H, et al: Reshaping human antibodies for therapy. Nature 1988; 332:325.

42. Hozumi N, Sandhu JS: Recombinant antibody technology: Its advent and advances. Cancer Invest 1993; 11:714.

43. LoBuglio AF, Wheeler RH, Trang J, et al: Mouse/human chimeric monoclonal antibody in man: Kinetics and immune response. Proc Natl Acad Sci USA 1989; 86:4220.

44. Pimm MV: Possible consequences of human antibody responses on the biodistribution of fragments of human, humanized or chimeric monoclonal antibodies: A note of caution. Pharmacol Lett 1994; 55:45.

45. Yokota T, Milenic DE, Whitlow M, et al: Microautoradiographic analysis of the normal organ distribution of radioiodinated single-chain Fv and other immunoglobulin forms. Cancer Res 1993; 53:3776.

46. Dykes PW, Bradwell AR, Chapman CE, et al: Radioimmunotherapy of cancer: Clinical studies and limiting factors. Cancer Treat Rev 1987; 14:87.

47. Jain RK: Physiological barriers to delivery of monoclonal antibodies and other macromolecules in tumors. Cancer Res 1990; 50:814.

48. Wikstrand CJ, Grahmann FC, McComb RD, et al: Antigenic heterogeneity of human anaplastic gliomas and glioma-derived cell lines defined by monoclonal antibodies. J Neuropathol Exp Neurol 1985; 44:229.

49. Wikstrand CJ, Bigner SH, Bigner DD: Demonstration of complex antigenic heterogeneity in a human glioma cell line and eight derived clones by specific monoclonal antibodies. Cancer Res 1983; 43:3327.

50. Lindmo T, Davies C, Rofstad EK, et al: Antigen expression in human melanoma cells in relation to growth conditions and cell-cycle distribution. Int J Cancer 1984; 33:167.

51. Rapoport SI (ed): Sites and Functions of the Blood-Brain Barrier in Physiology and Medicine. New York, Raven, 1976.

52. Vick NA, Weiss L, Gilbert HA, et al (eds): Brain Metastases. Boston, GK Hall, 1980.

53. Jain RK: Determinants of tumor blood flow: A review. Cancer Res 1988; 48:2641.

54. Jain RK, Baxter LT: Mechanisms of heterogeneous distribution of monoclonal antibodies and other macromolecules in tumors: Significance of elevated interstitial pressure. Cancer Res 1988; 48:7022.

55. Wiig H, Tveit E, Hultborn R, et al: Interstitial fluid pressure in DMBA-induced rat mammary tumours. Scand J Clin Lab Invest 1982; 42:159.

56. Jain RK: Transport of molecules across tumor vasculature. Cancer Metastasis Rev 1987; 6:559.

57. van Osdol W, Fujimori K, Weinstein JN: An analysis of monoclonal antibody distribution in microscopic tumor nodules: Consequences of a binding site barrier. Cancer Res 1991; 51:4776.

58. Langmuir VK, Mendonca HL, Woo DV: Comparisons between two monoclonal antibodies that bind to the same antigen but have differing affinities: Uptake kinetics and ¹²⁵I-antibody therapy efficacy in multicell spheroids. Cancer Res 1992; 52:4728.

59. Sutherland R, Buchegger F, Schreyer M, et al: Penetration and binding of radiolabeled anti-carcinoembryonic antigen monoclonal antibodies and their antigen binding fragments in human colon multicellular tumor spheroids. Cancer Res 1987; 47:1627.

60. Erickson HP, Lightner VA: Hexabrachion protein (tenascin, cytotactin, brachionectin) in connective tissues, embryonic brain, and tumors. Adv Cell Biol 1988; 2:55.

61. Bourdon MA, Coleman RE, Blasberg RG, et al: Monoclonal antibody localization in subcutaneous and intracranial human glioma xenografts: Paired-label and imaging analysis. Anticancer Res 1984; 41:33.

62. Ventimiglia JB, Wikstrand CJ, Ostrowski LE, et al: Tenascin expression in human glioma cell lines and normal tissues. J Neuroimmunol 1992; 36:41.

63. Schuster JM, Garg PK, Bigner DD, et al: Improved therapeutic efficacy of a monoclonal antibody radioiodinated using N-succinimidyl-3-(tri-n-butylstannyl)benzoate. Cancer Res 1991; 51:4164.

64. Bigner DD, Brown M, Coleman RE, et al: Phase I studies of treatment of malignant gliomas and neoplastic meningitis with ^{131}I-radiolabeled monoclonal antibodies, anti-tenascin 81C6, and anti-chondroitin proteoglycan sulfate Mel-14 F(ab')₂: A preliminary report. J Neurooncol 1995; 24:109.

65. Riva P, Arista A, Tison V, et al: Intralesional radioimmunotherapy of malignant gliomas: An effective treatment in recurrent tumors. Cancer 1994; 73:1076.

66. Balza E, Siri A, Ponassi M, et al: Production and characterization of monoclonal antibodies specific for different epitopes of human tenascin. FEBS Lett 1993; 332:39.

67. Siri A, Carnemolla B, Saginati M, et al: Human tenascin: Primary structure, pre-mRNA splicing patterns and localization of the epitopes recognized by two monoclonal antibodies. Nucleic Acids Res 1991; 19:525.

68. Bourne SP, Patel K, Walsh F, et al: A monoclonal antibody (ERIC-1), raised against retinoblastoma, that recognizes the neural cell adhesion molecule (NCAM) expressed on brain and tumours arising from the neuroectoderm. J Neurooncol 1991; 10:111.

69. Carrel S, Accolla RS, Carmagnola AL, et al: Common human melanoma-associated antigen(s) detected by monoclonal antibodies. Cancer Res 1980; 40:2523.

70. Colapinto EV, Humphrey PA, Zalutsky MR, et al: Comparative localization of murine monoclonal antibody Mel-14 F(ab')₂ fragment and whole IgG₂ₐ in human glioma xenografts. Cancer Res 1988; 48:5701.

71. Behnke J, Mach JP, Buchegger F, et al: In vivo localisation of radiolabelled monoclonal antibody in human gliomas. Br J Neurosurg 1988; 2:193.

72. Vaidyanathan G, Bigner DD, Zalutsky MR: Fluorine-18-labeled monoclonal antibody fragments: A potential approach for combining radioimmunoscintigraphy and positron emission tomography. J Nucl Med 1992; 33:1535.

73. Garg PK, Garg S, Bigner DD, et al: Localization of fluorine-18-labeled Mel-14 monoclonal antibody F(ab')₂ fragment in a subcutaneous xenograft model. Cancer Res 1992; 52:5054.

74. Yoshida J, Mizuno M, Inoue I, et al: Radioimaging of human glioma xenografts with ^{123}I labeled monoclonal antibody G-22 against glioma-associated antigen. J Neurooncol 1990; 8:221.

75. Kondo S, Nakatsu S, Sakahara H, et al: Antitumour activity of an immunoconjugate composed of anti-human astrocytoma monoclonal antibody and neocarzinostatin. Eur J Cancer 1993; 29A:420.

76. Schrappe M, Bumol TF, Apelgren LD, et al: Long-term growth suppression of human glioma xenografts by chemoimmunoconjugates of 4-desacetylvinblastine-3-carboxyhydrazide and monoclonal antibody 9.2.27. Cancer Res 1992; 52:3838.

77. Gatter KC, Brown G, Trowbridge IS, et al: Transferrin receptors in human tissues: Their distribution and possible clinical relevance. J Clin Pathol 1983; 36:539.

78. Recht LD, Griffin TW, Raso V, et al: Potent cytotoxicity of an antihuman transferrin receptor-ricin A-chain immunotoxin on human glioma cells in vitro. Cancer Res 1990; 50:6696.

79. Laske DW, Ilercil O, Akbasak A, et al: Efficacy of direct intratumoral therapy with targeted protein toxins for solid human gliomas in nude mice. J Neurosurg 1994; 80:520.

80. Martell LA, Agrawal A, Ross DA, et al: Efficacy of transferrin receptor-targeted immunotoxins in brain tumor cell lines and pediatric brain tumors. Cancer Res 1993; 53:1348.

81. Libermann TA, Nusbaum HR, Razon N, et al: Amplification and overexpression of the EGF receptor gene in primary human glioblastomas. J Cell Sci Suppl 1985; 3:161.

82. Wong AJ, Bigner SH, Bigner DD, et al: Increased expression of the epidermal growth factor receptor gene in malignant gliomas is invariably associated with gene amplification. Proc Natl Acad Sci USA 1987; 84:6899.

83. Collins VP: Amplified genes in human gliomas. Semin Cancer Biol 1993; 4:27.

84. Takahashi H, Nakazawa S, Herlyn D: Experimental radioimmunotherapy of a xenografted human glioma using ^{131}I-labeled monoclonal antibody to epidermal growth factor receptor. Neurol Med Chir (Tokyo) 1993; 33:610.

85. Takahashi H, Herlyn D, Atkinson B, et al: Radioimmunodetection of human glioma xenografts by monoclonal antibody to epidermal growth factor receptor. Cancer Res 1987; 47:3847.

86. Kalofonos HP, Pawlikowska TR, Hemingway A, et al: Antibody guided diagnosis and therapy of brain gliomas using radiolabeled monoclonal antibodies against epidermal growth factor receptor and placental alkaline phosphatase. J Nucl Med 1989; 30:1636.

87. Dadparvar S, Krishna L, Miyamoto C, et al: Indium-111-labeled anti-EGFr-425 scintigraphy in the detection of malignant gliomas. Cancer 1994; 73:884.

88. Wong AJ, Ruppert JM, Bigner SH, et al: Structural alterations of the epidermal growth factor receptor gene in human gliomas. Proc Natl Acad Sci USA 1992; 89:2965.

89. Humphrey PA, Wong AJ, Vogelstein B, et al: Anti-synthetic peptide antibody reacting at the fusion junction of deletion-mutant epidermal growth factor receptors in human glioblastoma. Proc Natl Acad Sci USA 1990; 87:4207.

90. Wikstrand CJ, Hale LP, Batra SK, et al: Monoclonal antibodies against EGFRVIII are tumor specific and react with breast and lung carcinomas and malignant gliomas. Cancer Res 1995; 55:3140.

91. Zalutsky MR, Moseley RP, Benjamin JC, et al: Monoclonal antibody and F(ab')₂ fragment delivery to tumor in patients with glioma: Comparison of intracarotid and intravenous administration. Cancer Res 1990; 50:4105.

92. Wikstrand CJ, McLendon RE, Bullard DE, et al: Production and characterization of two human glioma xenograft-localizing monoclonal antibodies. Cancer Res 1986; 46:5933.

93. Bergh J, Nilsson S, Liljedahl C, et al: Radioimaging of human malignant gliomas using indium-labelled monoclonal antibodies. Nucl Med Commun 1990; 11:437.

94. Moriuchi S, Shimizu K, Miyao Y, et al: Characterisation of a new mouse monoclonal antibody (ONS-M21) reactive with both medulloblastomas and gliomas. Br J Cancer 1993; 68:831.

95. Yang WL, Du ZW, Huang Q: Localization of ^{131}I-labelled anti-glioma monoclonal antibody SZ-39 in human brain tumor transplanted in nude mice. Chin Med J (Engl) 1988; 101:919.

96. Richardson RB, Davies AG, Bourne SP, et al: Radioimmunolocalization of human brain tumours: Biodistribution of radiolabelled monoclonal antibody UJ13A. Eur J Nucl Med 1986; 12:313.

97. Williams JA, Wessels BW, Wharam MD, et al: Targeting of human glioma xenografts in vivo utilizing radiolabeled antibodies. Int J Radiat Oncol Biol Phys 1990; 18:1367.

98. Lee WH, Yeh MY, Tu YC: Tumor localization of human brain malignant glioma xenograft in nude mice with a radiolabeled monoclonal antibody. Neurosurgery 1990; 26:381.

Phototherapy

ANDREW H. KAYE

EMIL A. POPOVIC

JOHN S. HILL

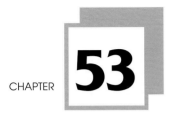

CHAPTER **53**

Photodynamic Therapy

Photodynamic therapy (PDT) is a binary form of local adjuvant tumor treatment. It involves the selective uptake and/or retention of a photosensitizer by tumor tissue followed by treatment of the tissue with light of an appropriate wavelength to penetrate tissue, activate the sensitizer, and cause selective destruction of the tumor. The therapy has been known by a variety of terminologies including *photoradiation therapy, phototherapy,* and *photochemotherapy,* but *photodynamic therapy* is now the accepted term. PDT has been used for the treatment of several different types of malignant tumor, including neoplasms of lung, breast, skin, urinary bladder, and esophagus, and has been shown to be especially useful for the control of local disease, thereby providing a rationale for its further investigation in the treatment of glioma, the most common central nervous system (CNS) tumor.[1] The four-tier grading system of the World Health Organization has been adopted for the classification of the astrocytic gliomas (Table 53–1).[2]

Cerebral glioma is incurable by current therapeutic techniques. The best management regimens for glioblastoma multiforme, which utilize surgery, radiation therapy, and systemic chemotherapy, produce a median survival of less than 1 year.[3, 4] The prognosis for lower grade gliomas is substantially better, but current therapies also fail to control lower grade gliomas in the long term because of recurrence, either in the bed of the original tumor or adjacent to the initial tumor margin.[5, 6] It is evident that an aggressive local adjuvant therapy could be beneficial in the control of cerebral glioma, and this has resulted in numerous adjuvant therapies that have been investigated both in the laboratory and clinically.[7] Any description of PDT in the management of cerebral glioma necessarily involves a discussion of the relevant laboratory studies, brain and tumor biology, and photosensitizer chemistry and light physics, and these topics are discussed in this chapter.

BACKGROUND

History

The goal of PDT research has been the search for a combination of the ideal wavelength of light with the perfect activated photosensitizer. PDT was introduced into clinical neurosurgery by Perria and colleagues in 1980 with a series of nine patients with cerebral glioma who were treated with hematoporphyrin derivative and a helium neon laser.[8] A brief historic account of PDT is summarized in Table 53–2, and a colorful, detailed history of PDT has been reported by Daniell and Hill.[9]

Laboratory Models of Cerebral Glioma

PDT has been used to kill glioma cells in vitro and in vivo. In vitro models have included monolayer cell cultures, single cell suspensions, and multicellular spheroids.[12–14] Animal models have been used to study PDT of cerebral glioma, and although no animal tumor system completely represents the human situation, our laboratory has used a C6 glioma cell line implanted intracerebrally into either rats or mice.[13, 15]

TABLE 53–1
THE WORLD HEALTH ORGANIZATION FOUR-TIER SYSTEM FOR GRADING ASTROCYTOMA

Grade	Name	Synonyms
I	—	Includes juvenile pilocytic, subependymal giant cell, and pleomorphic xanthoastrocytoma
II	Astrocytoma	Diffuse astrocytoma Low-grade glioma
III	Anaplastic astrocytoma	Malignant astrocytoma Intermediate-grade glioma
IV	Glioblastoma multiforme	High-grade glioma

Adapted from Zulch KJ: Histological Typing of Tumours of the Central Nervous System. Geneva, Switzerland, World Health Organization, 1979.

TABLE 53–2
BRIEF HISTORY OF PHOTODYNAMIC THERAPY

Year	Author(s)	Contribution
1841	Scherer	Hematoporphyrin extracted from blood
1900	Raab	Light essential for antimalarial activity of acridine dye
1903	Jesionek & von Tappeiner	Eosin and light used to treat human skin cancer
1904	von Tappeiner & Jodlbauer	Oxygen necessary for photosensitization
1913	Meyer-Betz	Self-injection of hematoporphyrin causes prolonged skin photosensitization
1924	Policard	Fluorescence of animal tumors due to endogenous porphyrin accumulation
1942	Auler & Banzer	Necrosis of animal tumors using hematoporphyrin and quartz lamp
1957	Wise & Taxdal	Exogenous hematoporphyrin concentrated in human brain tumors
1966	Lipson	First use of photodynamic therapy in human breast cancer
1972	Diamond	First use of photodynamic therapy in experimental glioma
1978	Dougherty	First human trial of photodynamic therapy for systemic tumors
1980	Perria	First human trial of photodynamic therapy for glioma

From Popovic EA, Kaye AH, Hill JS: Current status of photodynamic therapy for brain tumors. *In* Salcman M (ed): Current Techniques in Neurosurgery. Philadelphia, Current Medicine, 1994.

Gliomas and the Blood-Brain Barrier

The uptake of photosensitizer into glioma cells is thought to be at least partially dependent on disruption of the barrier between blood and tumor. The selectivity of photosensitizer uptake into tumor cells without uptake into normal brain depends on an intact blood-brain barrier. Gliomas of increasing grade are associated with increasing disruption of the blood-brain barrier and destruction of normal brain parenchyma. Glioblastoma multiforme contains a range of neoplastic cell activity that progresses from the periphery of normal brain parenchyma inward to the mitotically active growing rim, which may surround a necrotic core (Fig. 53–1). In the periphery of a glioblastoma multiforme, isolated tumor cells infiltrate normal parenchyma, where the blood-brain barrier remains essentially intact. The blood-brain barrier is progressively disrupted in the edematous brain-adjacent-to-tumor (BAT) region and is largely absent in the core, where a blood-tumor barrier essentially exists.[6, 16, 17]

Photosensitizers

Photosensitizers are molecules that absorb and re-emit light of specific wavelengths that are unique to the individual

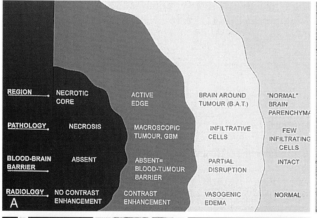
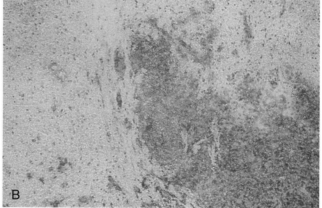
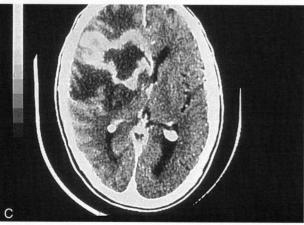

Figure 53–1 *A,* Model of glioblastoma multiforme. *B,* Histopathologic slide of glioblastoma multiforme stained for glial fibrillary acidic protein (GFAP). Note tumor infiltration into brain parenchyma. *C,* Contrast-enhanced head CT scan of a patient with glioblastoma multiforme.

compound. Porphyrins are naturally occurring photosensitizers whose chemical structure is based on the tetrapyrrole ring (Fig. 53–2). The best known examples of porphyrins are the iron-containing molecule protoporphyrin, which binds oxygen in hemoglobin; the series of cytochromes in the mitochondrial respiratory chain of enzymes; and the plant pigment chlorophyll.

The only photosensitizers to have been studied clinically in cerebral gliomas are the first-generation agents hematoporphyrin derivative and Photofrin (the derivative of hematoporphyrin derivative). Numerous other sensitizers have been investigated by laboratory studies.[18] Hematoporphyrin is a complex mixture of porphyrins, the composition of which can vary depending on the method of synthesis and storage.[19] The term hematoporphyrin derivative is confusing because the compound is not a single "derivative," but is rather a series of structurally-related porphyrins.[20] Photofrin is just as complex a mixture as hematoporphyrin derivative but is enriched in the tumor-localizing fraction. The names Photofrin II (Quadralogics, Vancouver, British Columbia, Canada), dihematoporphyrin ether (DHE), and porfimer sodium (Lederle, Pearl River, New York) are synonymous, but Photofrin is now the accepted term. It is highly probable that no single component of hematoporphyrin derivative is active, but a series of related compounds may all be active or may act in synergy to induce a photochemical effect. A description of the chemistry of hematoporphyrin derivative and Photofrin is given by Kessell,[21] and Figure 53–3 outlines their synthetic pathways.

The existence of multiple active compounds in hematoporphyrin derivative and Photofrin has greatly complicated scientific research because of the difficulty of identifying specific molecules with respect to their activity and site of action. The other major disadvantage of hematoporphyrin derivative and other porphyrins is that an activating wavelength of 628 nm must be used to achieve adequate tissue penetration. A wavelength of 628 nm is not ideal to achieve optimal absorbance by a sensitizer; 400 nm is better, but this wavelength penetrates tissue very poorly (Fig. 53–4). A sensitizer with an absorbance maximum in the 650- to 800-nm region would be more desirable because light of these wavelengths penetrates tissue better than does light of 628 nm wavelength.

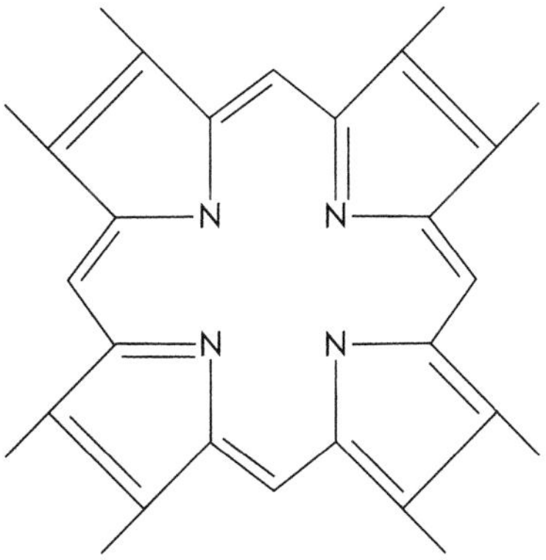

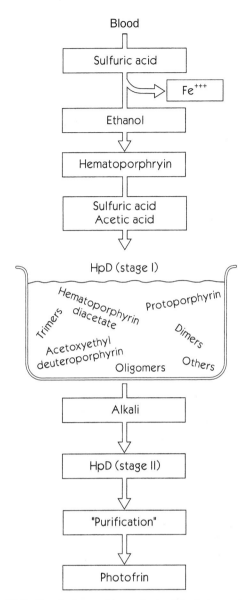

Figure 53–3 Broad schema of the synthesis of the first generation photosensitizers: hematoporphyrin derivative (HpD) and Photofrin.

An ideal photosensitizer for PDT of cerebral tumors should have the following characteristics:

■ Is nontoxic systemically

■ Is a single compound

■ Has maximal tumor-brain selectivity

■ Is able to cross an intact blood-brain barrier to reach infiltrating cells but does not enter normal brain

■ Undergoes peak activation by light of a wavelength capable of maximal tissue penetration (650 to 800 nm)

■ Accomplishes maximal cytotoxic injury to tumor cells with minimal "bystander" injury

■ Is rapidly excreted from systemic tissues to diminish photosensitivity

Figure 53–2 The 20-sided tetrapyrrole ring, the basic structure of porphyrins.

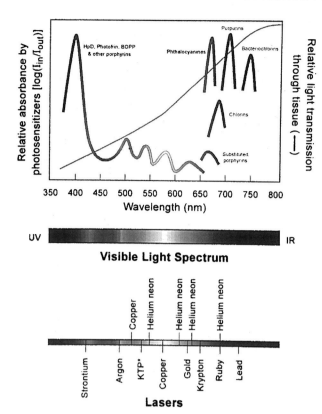

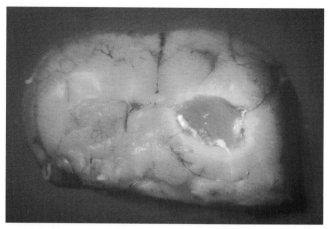

Figure 53–5 Rat C6 glioma fluorescing under ultraviolet light. The animal had been given hematoporphyrin derivative before being killed.

Figure 53–4 Schematic relationship of absorption spectra of photosensitizers to the visible light spectrum and laser wavelengths. Relative light transmission through brain parenchyma is indicated by the *gray line*. Potassium-titanium-phosphate (KTP) laser produces light at 532 or 1064 nm; light can be transduced from 532 to 628 nm by a dye module. Abbreviations: UV, ultraviolet light; IR, infrared light. Reproduced from Popovic EA, Kaye AH, Hill JS: Current status of photodynamic therapy for brain tumors. *In* Salcman M (ed): Current Techniques in Neurosurgery. Philadelphia, Current Medicine, 1994.

Extensive research has pursued the development of numerous second-generation photosensitizers, and although all possess desirable photochemical and spectroscopic properties, much study still needs to be undertaken before they can displace hematoporphyrin derivative and Photofrin from clinical use (Table 53–3).

Tumor Selectivity for Photosensitizers

Tumor selectivity for hematoporphyrin derivative has been demonstrated in various human tumors, and good correlation has been noted between fluorescence and biopsy-proven cancer (Fig. 53–5).[31] Fluorescence microscopy is the most direct method used to determine intracellular localization of photosensitizer, and it has been revolutionized by the introduction of confocal laser scanning microscopy.[24, 32] Microscopy and subcellular fractionation studies have generally shown exclusion of sensitizer from the nucleus with concentration in lysosomes, mitochondria, microsomes, and cytoplasm (Fig. 53–6).

A study of biopsy material from patients undergoing PDT for cerebral glioma in a phase I-II trial at the Royal Melbourne Hospital showed that hematoporphyrin derivative was selectively localized into all glioma grades, with a direct correlation between the grade of the glioma and the hematoporphyrin derivative level in the tumor (Fig. 53–7).[33] The levels were highest in glioblastoma multiforme (hematoporphyrin derivative tumor-to-brain ratio, 30:1) and lower in anaplastic astrocytoma (12:1) and astrocytoma (8:1). Origitano and co-workers[34] have reported a clinical study investigating radioactively labeled Photofrin monitored by single-photon emission computed tomography (SPECT), and they likewise found that the concentration of sensitizer correlated with glioma grade. A separate finding in the Royal Melbourne Hospital study was that hematoporphyrin derivative was selectively localized into the BAT region, in some cases at higher levels than in the tumor bulk[33]; this has also been confirmed by others.[35]

BLOOD-BRAIN BARRIER

Impairment of the blood-brain barrier around a tumor (blood-tumor barrier) almost certainly has a major role in

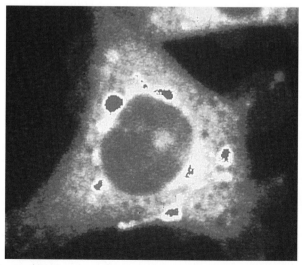

Figure 53–6 Fluorescence confocal microsopy of the photosensitizer hematoporphyrin derivative (HpD) within human astrocytic tumor cells. Note that the HpD stellate cytoplasmic inclusions has been excluded from the nucleus.

TABLE 53–3
CHARACTERISTICS OF THE FIRST- AND SECOND-GENERATION PHOTOSENSITIZERS USED IN PHOTODYNAMIC THERAPY OF BRAIN TUMORS

Photosensitizer	Generation	Porphyrin	Pure Compound	Clinical Studies	Laboratory Studies	Glioma: Brain Uptake Ratio	Comments	Additional References
Hematoporphyrin derivative	1st	+	–	+	+	30:1		
Photofrin	1st	+	–	+	+	?	Low skin photosensitivity	22, 23
Porphyrin C	2nd	+	+	–	+	1000:1		24
Boronated protoporphyrin (BOPP)	2nd	+	+	+†	+	400:1	Potential for combined use of BNCT† with photodynamic therapy	
Purpurins	2nd	–	+	–	+		Better absorption spectra than 1st-generation agents	23
Phthalocyanines Aluminum Chloraluminum	2nd	–	+	–	+			12
Rhodamine-123	2nd	–	+	–	+	Potentially very high	A lipophilic cationic dye that localizes to mitochondria; major disadvantage is blue-green peak absorption (490–515 nm)	25
Merocyanine 540	2nd	–	+	–	+		Phase I trials done in hematologic malignancies	26
Pheophorbide	2nd	–	+	–	+		Minimal skin photosensitization	27
mTHPP	2nd	–	+	–	+		More efficacious at 100% O_2	28
TPP	2nd	–	+	–	+		A lipophilic cationic dye	29
Chlorins	2nd	–	+	–	–		Desirable photochemical and spectroscopic properties*	30
Bacteriochlorins	2nd	–	+	–	–			30
Porphycenes	2nd	–	+	–	–			30
Verdins	2nd	–	+	–	–			30

*See Figure 53–4.
†Studied with boron neutron capture therapy (BNCT), but not photodynamic therapy.
From Popovic EA, Kaye AH, Hill JS: Current status of photodynamic therapy for brain tumors. *In* Salcman M (ed): Current Techniques in Neurosurgery. Philadelphia, Current Medicine, 1994.

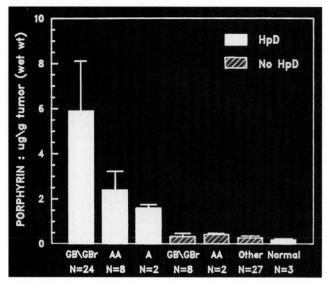

Figure 53–7 Graph of hematoporphyrin derivative (HpD) (porphyrin) concentration in human tissue samples of various grades of astrocytoma. A, diffuse (grade II) astrocytoma; AA, anaplastic (grade II) astrocytoma; GB, glioblastoma multiforme (grade IV astrocytoma); GBr, recurrent glioblastoma multiforme. (From Hill JS, Kaye AH, Sawyer WH, et al: Selective uptake of hematoporphyrin derivative into human cerebral glioma. Neurosurgery 1990; 26:248–254.)

the uptake of photosensitizer. Malignant cerebral tumors in various animal models have demonstrated selective uptake of hematoporphyrin and hematoporphyrin derivative with exclusion of sensitizer from normal brain, and with accumulation in regions known to be outside of the blood-brain barrier, such as the pituitary gland and area postrema.[33, 36, 37] Photofrin, however, has been reported to cross the blood-brain barrier in photoirradiated but otherwise normal brain to enter astrocytes, neurons, and endothelial cells.[38] These results may be encouraging, because photosensitizers are likely to be more effective if they can cross normal blood-brain barrier to reach the more peripheral infiltrating tumor cells, provided that the sensitizer retains the selectivity for tumor cells. In our C6 glioma model, the photosensitizers hematoporphyrin derivative and boronated protoporphyrin (BOPP) have been detected within isolated tumor cells infiltrating the BAT region,[24, 33] and confocal microscopy has identified similar uptake of hematoporphyrin derivative into these nests of cells in human biopsy specimens (Hill JS, Kaye AH: Unpublished results, 1986). This is a critical finding, because it is the first unequivocal evidence that photosensitizer is taken up into the very cells that are thought to be responsible for tumor recurrence after surgery.[6]

SERUM PROTEIN–MEDIATED UPTAKE

Several investigators have suggested that serum proteins play a vital role in photosensitizer transport and cellular uptake. Hematoporphyrin derivative has been shown to bind to serum albumin and to lipoproteins (particularly low-density lipoprotein [LDL], which is the major serum carrier of cholesterol).[39] Cholesterol is in increased demand by proliferating cells, and it is perhaps teleologically understandable that cancer cells should have elevated numbers of LDL receptors compared to those of their normal counterparts.[40]

It has been suggested that the intracellular localization of sensitizer is mediated at least in part by LDL receptors, whereas complexes of hematoporphyrin derivative with albumin or high-density lipoprotein enter tumor by non-receptor–mediated processes to localize in the interstitial stroma.[41]

EXTRACELLULAR pH

Extracellular pH is known to be lower in tumors than in normal tissue and correlates with a tissue's nutrient supply and rate of metabolism. Extracellular acidosis causes an increase in the passive diffusion of porphyrins into cells and may contribute to selective photosensitizer localization.[42]

MITOCHONDRIA-RELATED FACTORS

Mitochondria appear to be a major target for phototoxic damage, and their selective targeting by photosensitizers may be mediated by benzodiazepine receptor binding.[43] The class of lipophilic cationic dyes, of which rhodamine 123 is an example, appears to have selective mitochondrial localization related to the internal negative membrane potential of the mitochondria.[44]

Light and Lasers

LIGHT

Light output is measured in watts (joules per second), recorded at the tip of the delivery fiber. Light dose delivered to a surface is measured as energy delivered per unit area of irradiated surface (joules per square centimeter), and for implanted fibers, light dose is measured as joules per centimeter of length along the delivery fiber.

The penetration depth of light into tissue is defined as the depth at which the incident irradiance is reduced to 1/e, or 37%. In more practical terms, the effective depth of PDT-induced necrosis is approximately three times the penetration depth.[45] Direct tumor cell phototoxicity is not the sole mechanism for necrosis, and PDT-induced vascular ischemic damage certainly plays an additional role.[23, 38]

Light penetration determines the extent of tissue damage, and both increase as a function of the following variables:

■ Wavelength, increasing from between 350 nm to above 800 nm (see Fig. 53–4)

■ Light dose, increasing above a threshold to a maximum value that causes damage to normal blood-brain barrier and cellular elements, with or without preadministered photosensitizer[13, 46 – 48]

■ Cellularity of tissue, increasing with the grade of tumor, up to twofold the penetration depth of normal brain[49]

If a tumor contains sufficient sensitizer to mediate a photochemical reaction, the depth of tumor necrosis should largely be related to the penetration of light. However, some sensitizers are more effective than others in producing a photochemical reaction; increased doses of photosensitizer may not result in greater depth of necrosis, but they could increase the degree of cerebral edema.[13] The optimal wavelength for photoactivation of hematoporphyrin derivative and Photofrin is red light at 628 nm, but the penetration depth is only approximately 1.5 mm for normal brain and 2.9 mm for tumor.[50] The therapeutic depth of activity of 628 nm light is therefore only about 9 mm, three times the penetration depth in tumor, which is a major limitation of PDT in its current form.[51] Our own laboratory studies have shown a selective tumor destruction of up to 1 cm with hematoporphyrin derivative and red light in the rat model.[13] As assessed on computed tomographic (CT) and magnetic resonance imaging (MRI) scans, the crude estimated depth of therapeutic effect of PDT has been up to 18 mm.[35]

Heating of cerebral tissue by microwave light could potentially occur with PDT, but this can be avoided by irrigation with normal saline at body temperature.[13] It has been suggested that hyperthermia is a significant component of PDT's efficacy,[52] but tumor destruction has clearly been shown to occur without significant heating of tissue.[13] Our laboratory has endeavored to study the pure effects of PDT, but in the future it is possible that hyperthermia could be used advantageously to produce a synergistic effect.

LASERS

Lasers produce high doses of light of a single known wavelength and are the most efficient method of light delivery. The power output can be accurately measured and the light can be delivered by a fiberoptic cable to a tumor, either stereotactically or under direct vision.[35, 53, 54] The laser systems used have included the helium neon, argon-ion pumped dye, and gold metal vapor lasers.[53, 55, 56] The argon pumped dye laser produces continuous light but is relatively immobile and has an ineffective coupling mechanism, which results in a significant loss of light during delivery. The gold metal vapor laser is easier to transport, produces a much higher intensity light at 627.8 nm, and has the theoretical advantage of producing a pulsed rather than a continuous beam. Pulsed light may improve sensitizer activation and increase the depth of penetration, but its benefit compared with continuous laser light has not yet been proved experimentally. More recently we have used a frequency-doubled Nd-YAG-KTP (neodymium–yttrium-aluminum-garnet–potassium-titanium-phosphate) laser to pump a tunable dye laser (Fig. 53–8). The KTP laser has the advantage of delivering high doses of light, the wavelength can be varied for use with different photosensitizers in the laboratory, it requires minimal maintenance, and it is easily moved from the laboratory to the operating room.

Physicochemical Basis of Photodynamic Therapy

The photophysical and photochemical properties of photosensitizers vary markedly, but the processes leading to a photosensitizing effect are similar for all of these compounds. Following the absorption of activating light of an appropriate wavelength, the sensitizer is converted from ground state to an excited singlet state, in which no unpaired electrons are present (Fig. 53–9).[57] The sensitizer may de-excite and lose its energy by a variety of competing pathways. From the singlet state the sensitizer can decay back to ground state and emit energy in the form of fluorescence, or it may decay down to an intermediate state from which

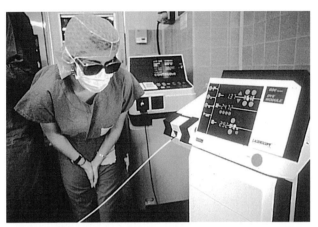

Figure 53–8 The neodymium–ytrium-aluminum-garnet (YAG)–potassium-titanium-phosphate (KTP) laser (background). The dye module (foreground) transduces KTP light into red 628 nm light, which is delivered through an optical diffusion fiber. Note the use of protective glasses.

level the sensitizer can transfer to the metastable triplet state, in which two unpaired electrons are present. From the metastable triplet state the sensitizer can either decay back to ground state, with the emission of energy in the form of long-lived phosphorescence, or it can participate in a series of photochemical reactions, which are designated as type I or II.[18] In a type I reaction, the sensitizer in its metastable triplet state reacts directly with a cellular substrate to yield a radical ion pair. In a type II reaction, the sensitizer reacts directly with oxygen to produce the highly reactive molecular singlet oxygen ($^1O_2$), and this reaction is thought to be the major mechanism of damage to biomolecules and cells following PDT. The type I and II reactions are competitive, with increases in oxygen concentration pushing the equilibrium in favor of the type II reaction; but both cause oxidation of target molecules and have an absolute requirement for oxygen.

Pathologic Effects of Photodynamic Therapy

Damage to sensitized tumor and brain parenchyma by PDT is observed experimentally and clinically within 48 hours of photoirradiation.[35, 46, 47, 54] The controversy surrounding the precise site of action of PDT has yet to be resolved. This confusion is partly due to PDT's powerful ability to induce numerous cellular changes and the fact that hematoporphyrin derivative's heterogeneous nature results in variable localization and subsequent phototoxic damage due to its accumulation in numerous intracellular and extracellular sites.

CYTOTOXIC DAMAGE

Experimental models of photosensitized but otherwise normal rat brain have revealed lethal injury to astrocytes, and later to neurons, occurring within 24 to 48 hours of photoirradiation when high doses of sensitizer and light are used.[46, 47] CT and MRI studies in patients treated with PDT have likewise shown the development of radiologic changes in a similar time frame.[35, 54]

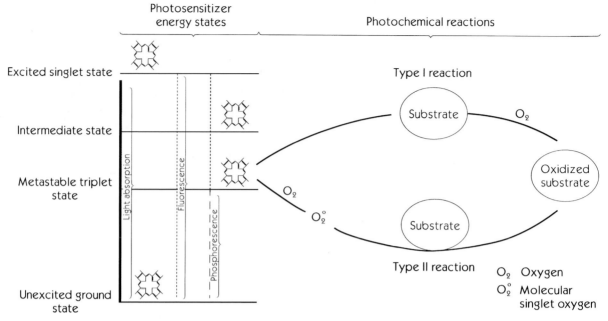

Figure 53–9 Schematic diagram of photosensitizer activation by light. Energy level diagram *(left)* shows activation of the photosensitizer's electron shell from ground state and the various possible subsequent pathways of decay. Photosensitizer in its metastable triplet state *(right)* may undergo release of energy as phosphorescence or may become involved in a type I or type II (molecular singlet oxygen formation) reaction.

VASCULAR INJURY

Histologic evidence of ischemic necrosis by PDT has been reported consistently in experimental and clinical studies.[38, 47, 55] Vascular injury may be a significant component of PDT and appears to explain tissue damage beyond the theoretical reach of phototoxic injury per se.

PHOTODYNAMIC THERAPY IN CLINICAL NEUROSURGERY

The use of PDT to treat gliomas in clinical practice involves consideration of a number of practical and technical problems; this has resulted in a wide variation of treatment techniques used in different series. These include the choice of sensitizer to be used, the dose and timing of its administration, the type of light irradiation system, and the dose of light and mechanism by which it is to be delivered to the tumor. The delivery of PDT must be balanced not only to optimize therapy but also to minimize possible complications, such as cerebral edema. The clinical experience with PDT at the Royal Melbourne Hospital has evolved since 1985.[22, 23, 53, 55] Our current practice is described below and is discussed with reference to other management regimens.

Preoperative Management

Patients are given routine preparation for surgery, which includes administration of dexamethasone, 16 mg/day, and consent is obtained under the auspices of the Hospital Medical Research and Ethics Committee. Hematoporphyrin derivative is administered intravenously 24 hours preoperatively,[53, 55] as our laboratory data have indicated this to

be the optimal time.[37] The principles of hematoporphyrin derivative administration are that it should be well diluted (5 mg/kg in 200 mL of normal saline), protected from light, and given slowly over 30 to 60 minutes through a well-running intravenous cannula. Skin contamination and subcutaneous extravasation must be avoided, because local photosensitivity would persist for months; consequently, hematoporphyrin derivative should never be given in a dorsal hand vein. Patients are considered to be immediately photosensitive and must avoid direct or indirect sunlight for 6 to 8 weeks, but no restriction is placed on exposure to normal indoor lighting.

Other groups have reported the use of hematoporphyrin derivative in doses from 2.5 to 5.0 mg/kg, and Photofrin has usually been given at 2.0 to 2.5 mg/kg. A recent SPECT study of labeled Photofrin has reported that photosensitizer uptake into tumor varies between patients and that the timing of PDT may need to be tailored.[34]

Stereotactic biopsy for preliminary diagnosis of glioma may be necessary if the neurosurgeon is not confident of the diagnosis on the basis of radiologic investigations.

Intraoperative Management

SURGERY

The patient is positioned as for a routine craniotomy, but additional attention is paid to the orientation of the anticipated resection cavity so that it may maximally retain the solution used for light dispersion. The tumor is approached and resected as for any craniotomy. A maximal tumor excision has been performed in all patients, usually with the aid of the CUSA (Cavitron Ultrasonic Surgical Aspirator, Cooper Laboratories, Stanford, Calif).[53, 55] It has been suggested

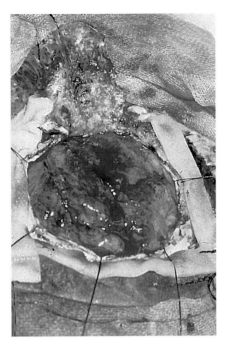

Figure 53–10 · Recurrent cerebral convexity glioblastoma multiforme prior to resection.

that entry into the ventricular system should be avoided, but no theoretical grounds have been established for this practice, and our experience with ventricular entry has not proved to be a problem. After hemostasis is achieved, the resection bed is left in a raw state, without any hemostatic agents in situ that could potentially retard light delivery to tissue (Figs. 53–10 and 53–11).

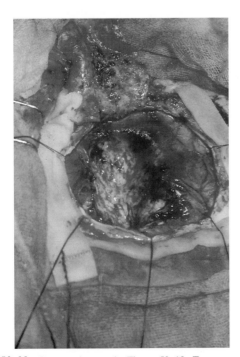

Figure 53–11 Same patient as in Figure 53–10. Tumor resection has resulted in a surgical cavity suitable for Intralipid instillation prior to light irradiation.

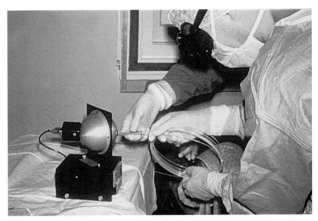

Figure 53–12 Calibrating light output from an optical diffusion fiber.

The surface area to be irradiated is measured, the laser power output at the optical diffusion fiber tip is calibrated (Fig. 53–12), and light from the fiber is directed onto the resection bed by attachment to a fixed retractor arm (Fig. 53–13). An inspired oxygen concentration of 100% may be of value for the duration of photoirradiation,[28] which has been between 12 and 94 minutes (median time, 50 minutes). The fiber is moved at regular intervals to cover the tumor bed and to ensure even distribution of the hot spot emanating from the tip (Fig. 53–14). The optical diffusion fiber used has usually had a "flat cut" delivery end, but more recently we have used cylindrical or spherical ends. Diffuse delivery of light to the resection bed is greatly improved if resection results, as is usually the case, in a cavity that allows use of Intralipid (Tuta Laboratories, Braeside, Melbourne, Australia), diluted to 0.5%, as a light dispersion agent.[56] We no longer measure brain temperature routinely, but this was monitored in the first 40 cases by a thermal diffusion cerebral blood flow monitor on the irradiated surface (Flowtronics Inc., Phoenix, Ariz) and by a thermocouple at 2 mm depth (model RFG-3B Lesion Generator System, Radionics Inc., Burlington, Mass). Brain temperature can easily be kept below 37.5 °C by irrigation with Intralipid or with physiologic saline solutions at room temperature.

In all cases, surgical closure has involved complete dural

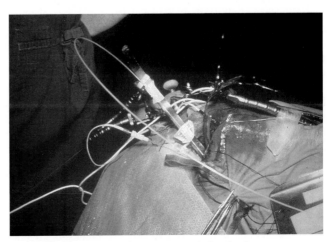

Figure 53–13 Optical diffusion fiber attached to fixed retractor system.

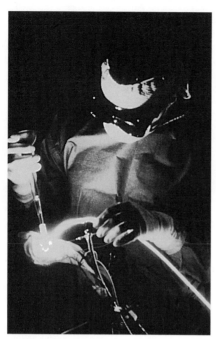

Figure 53-14 Operative photograph of craniotomy showing delivery of red 628 nm laser light through an optical diffusion fiber. The tumor resection cavity is being irrigated with Intralipid.

closure and replacement of the bone flap. The total time for surgery, including PDT, has varied from 2 to 5.5 hours, with a median time of 3 hours.[53]

SURGICAL ISSUES

Stereotaxis Direct intratumoral injection of photosensitizer has been advocated for the treatment of glioma,[57] but this would seem to be inappropriate, as the basis of PDT is its selectivity for tumor cells, especially those infiltrating beyond the margins of the proposed resection. Sensitizer is most likely to be effective if it can localize into infiltrating cells beyond surgical reach, and it is unlikely to do so if injected intratumorally. However, stereotactic delivery of light is particularly suitable for deeper lesions and may be effective when administered to gliomas without resection.[35] Computer-assisted stereotaxy can be applied to guide resection of lesions at all depths[58] and has been reported to predict the theoretical volume of gross phototoxic damage in PDT using implanted fibers.[35, 54] Delayed phototoxic injury to eloquent neural structures, such as has been reported with the optic apparatus, may be reduced with this technology.[35]

Extent of Decompression Cytoreductive issues aside, we believe that a radical decompression minimizes the effects of postoperative cerebral edema that are caused by the effects of PDT on residual tumor. It is probable that PDT-induced cerebral edema increases in proportion to the amount of residual tumor bulk, because more photoirradiated tissue is available to undergo necrosis. Maximal tumor resection should therefore diminish the amount of tissue that undergoes phototoxic reactions and allow more room into which edematous brain may expand. We therefore do not advocate PDT without tumor decompression. The benefits

of maximal tumor resection have been shown in a controlled animal study[59] and by Origitano and Reichman,[54] who monitored postoperative intracranial pressure in 15 patients following PDT. Powers and colleagues[35] reported clinically significant cerebral edema in their patients following stereotactic administration of light; steroids were not used and tumor mass was not resected. The use of PDT in eloquent regions of the CNS would require greater selectivity of the sensitizer-light combination.[11] PDT of posterior fossa tumors would require careful dosimetry and has been reported in pediatric patients, including those with ependymoma.[60] A recent animal study reported the use of PDT in the treatment of posterior fossa tumors.[61] These authors advocated lower light doses than have been used conventionally and recommended the use of intratumoral rather than intracavitary photoradiation. Being cognizant of the need to modify both surgery and photoradiation in eloquent CNS, we recommend maximal tumor resection and agree with the approach of Wharen and co-workers,[60] who performed gross total resections of posterior fossa neoplasms and obtained "their most encouraging results" in this small group of patients. Although not yet described in clinical practice, PDT could also potentially be used to treat spinal cord gliomas, but this would require exquisite sensitizer-light selectivity.[11]

Laser-Tumor Interface Techniques Apart from Intralipid instillation into resection cavities, various surgical techniques have been used to interface light and tumor, including light shone directly onto the resection bed[53, 55] and illumination through an inflatable balloon.[50] The inflatable balloon applicator adopts the shape of the resection cavity to produce a uniform distribution of light, but it is not particularly suited to irradiation of a tumor bed with a flat surface (e.g., such as occurs after a lobectomy). Interstitial laser light has been administered by stereotactic implantation of single[35] or multiple[54] optical diffusion fibers.

LIGHT IRRADIATION SYSTEMS

An argon-rhodamine pumped dye laser (Spectra-Physics, model 164-05,argon laser; Spectra-Physics, model 375 dye laser; Spectra-Physics, Mountain View, Calif) was used to treat our first 18 patients. A gold metal vapor laser (Quentron, Adelaide, South Australia, Australia) was used to treat most of the remaining patients, but more recently a KTP laser (KTP/532 Laserscope Surgical Laser Systems, San Jose, Calif) has been used. A 16 watt light of 532 nm wavelengh is delivered from the KTP laser and transduced to 628 nm by a dye module, which produces light up to 3.2 watts at the fiber tip (Dye Module 600 series, Laserscope Surgical Systems). A flat-cut quartz fiber (600 μm diameter early in the series, and 1 mm in the remainder) has been used as our optical diffusion fiber, but it is unsuitable for stereotactic implantation because of excessive heating and local charring at the tip. This major technical problem has been overcome by the development of a new fiber, which allows safe use of PDT in stereotaxy.[35]

LIGHT DOSIMETRY

The accuracy of light dosimetry requires further improvement and standardization so that results can be optimally compared between study groups. Output from the laser needs to be calibrated (see Fig. 53–12) prior to every use, because minor fluctuations in power output occur. Determination of the exact dose of laser light delivered can be difficult because of inaccuracies in the measurement of the surface area, loss of light from the tumor cavity, and lack of uniformity of light distribution.

Our initial laboratory studies[13] showed that higher light doses could be tolerated than had been used in earlier clinical series (Table 53–4), and we have therefore used a light output up to 5 watts.[22, 53] In our initial experience, treatment commenced with 70 J/cm², and the dose has been elevated to 260 J/cm² without increased toxic effects. We now regularly use 240 to 260 J/cm², which is considerably higher than doses reported in other published series.

Postoperative

RADIOTHERAPY

Initial concerns were present about the possible interaction of postoperative radiotherapy with photosensitizer.[62, 63] Wharen and others[64] studied the in vitro interaction between x-irradiation and hematoporphyrin derivative in a rat glioma model and found potentiation of radiosensitivity only at high intracellular hematoporphyrin derivative concentrations and at large x-irradiation fraction sizes. Although hematoporphyrin derivative does not cross an intact blood-brain barrier, it may remain in small vessels for some time; consequently, it has been our policy not to commence radiotherapy until at least 4 weeks after PDT. In 65 patients treated with conventional radiotherapy (45 Gy in 20 divided doses), no increase

in radiation-related complications was observed.[53] A dose of 45 Gy is the standard dose used to treat cerebral glioma in the state of Victoria (Australia), and it is somewhat lower than that used in North America. Muller and Wilson[65] also reported no increased toxic effects in 17 patients treated with higher doses of postoperative radiotherapy.

SIDE EFFECTS

Cerebral Edema Cerebral edema has been reported as a clinical complication of PDT despite perioperative steroid administration,[65, 66] although, in our experience, this can be easily controlled with steroid therapy.[22, 53] Our patients receive 16 mg/day of dexamethasone preoperatively (32 mg the first postoperative day and then a slowly tapering dose over 2 weeks). It has been suggested that more than 12 mg of dexamethasone per day may affect the blood-tumor barrier and may result in diminished photosensitizer uptake,[34] but in studies of the rat C6 glioma model we have noted no effect of steroids on hematoporphyrin derivative uptake except at very high doses of steroid (Megison PD, Hill JS, Kaye AH: Unpublished observations, 1985). Laws and co-workers[67] suggested that the avoidance of tissue heating during PDT prevented post-therapy cerebral edema, but this has not been confirmed by others.[50, 65]

Skin Photosensitization Hematoporphyrin derivative and Photofrin both accumulate in the skin to cause photosensitization. Our initial instructions to patients are to remain out of direct sunlight for 4 to 6 weeks, depending on the time of year. Skin testing is then performed to determine if direct sunlight can be tolerated, and the patients are instructed to gradually increase their daily exposure to the sun.

TABLE 53–4
SERIES REPORTING PHOTODYNAMIC THERAPY OF CEREBRAL TUMORS

Study	No. of Patients	Power (Watts)	Total Dose to Tumor (J)	Dose per Unit Surface Area (J/cm²)
Perria et al.[8]	9	0.025	—*	0.9–9
Perria et al.[68]	8	0.06–0.4	720–2,400	—*
McCulloch et al.[66]	16	0.280–0.460	1,620–2,520	—*
Laws et al.[67]	5	0.250–0.400	540–1,440	—*
Wharen et al.[69]	3	—*	—*	180†
Muller & Wilson[65]	50	0.175–1.00	439–3,888	8–175
Kostron et al.[70]	20	—*	—*	25–200
Powers et al.[35]	7	—*	658–2,028	400 J/cm‡
Laws et al.[11, 71]	23	≤0.200	500–1000§	150–200¶ 24–180**
Wharen et al.[71]††	31	≤0.200	500–1000§	150–200¶ 24–180**
Origitano & Reichman[54]	15	1.0–4.0‡‡	1,400–14,300§§	50¶¶
Kaye et al.[22, 23, 53]	116	0.75–5.0	3,360–12,613	72–260

*Information not available.
†Derived from 100 mW/cm² for 30 minutes delivered by xenon arc lamp.
‡Refers to J/cm of length of interstitial stereotactic fibers.
§Interstitial stereotactic therapy.
¶To supratentorial resection cavities.
**To infratentorial resection cavities.
††Includes patients from Laws et al.[71]
‡‡1 W/cm for interstitial stereotactic fibers.
§§100 J/cm of fiber for interstitial stereotactic delivery.
¶¶Based on reported 2.5 cm depth of implantation of interstitial fibers.
Modified from Popovic EA, Kaye AH, Hill JS: Current status of photodynamic therapy for brain tumors. *In* Salcman M (ed): Current Techniques in Neurosurgery. Philadelphia, Current Medicine, 1994.

The longest period of significant sensitization has lasted 18 weeks with a median period of 7 weeks. Various strategies have been suggested to reduce skin photosensitivity from the currently available drugs, including administration of lower doses of sensitizer and co-administration of carotene-containing substances. It is likely that the second-generation photosensitizers will produce less skin photosensitization.

IMAGING STUDIES

Radiologic testimony to the efficacy of PDT in malignant glioma has been reported by Powers and co-workers.[35] In this series, light was delivered stereotactically without tumor resection and produced CT and MRI evidence of tumor destruction at 24 hours, evidenced by loss of contrast enhancement of the treated volume. New contrast enhancement appeared peripherally, presumably corresponding to phototoxic damage to the BAT region, and has been reported to persist for up to 3 months on MRI.[54] Of note is that when tumor recurred, it did so outside of the stereotactically targeted volume of treatment.[35, 54]

Clinical Series

PDT has been evaluated as an adjuvant treatment for malignant cerebral tumors by a number of investigators; these series are summarized in Table 53–4 and includes our update of the Royal Melbourne Hospital series.[8, 22, 35, 53, 54, 60, 65–71] Overall assessment of the reported series is difficult because of the wide variation of techniques, doses of photosensitizer and light, and types of cerebral tumor. Most of the series have been small, and length of follow-up has been short. The majority of tumors have been high-grade or recurrent gliomas, but most reports have included small numbers of metastatic tumors, and more recently, our group has been treating patients with low-grade gliomas. The clinical results in the initial series were disappointing because recurrent high-grade gliomas were the predominant tumor treated, and the doses of light used were up to 100 times lower than those used in systemic tumors.[8, 59, 66, 67] Lower light doses were used because of the lack of availability of powerful light-producing sources and also because of the fear of side effects of PDT in high doses, particularly when combined with x-ray therapy.[63]

In the Royal Melbourne Hospital series, 116 patients with cerebral glioma have been treated with 5 mg/kg of hematoporphyrin derivative and up to 260 J/cm^2 of red light at 628 nm, produced by either the argon dye, gold metal vapor, or KTP laser. Table 53–5 shows the tumor grades and the number of patients treated. Initially only patients with glioblastoma multiforme were selected for treatment, but patients with lower-grade tumors have more recently been included following the observation that sensitizer was also selectively retained in astrocytoma and anaplastic astrocytoma.[33] Six patients have had re-treatment with PDT when the tumor recurred. The median survival for 36 patients with glioblastoma multiforme was 24 months, and 50% of patients survived beyond 2 years. The median survival for 39 patients with recurrent glioblastoma multiforme was 10 months, and 37% survived 2 years (Fig. 53–15). A historically matched control group of 100 patients with glioblas-

TABLE 53–5
ROYAL MELBOURNE HOSPITAL SERIES OF PHOTODYNAMIC THERAPY OF CEREBRAL GLIOMAS

Tumor Type	Number of Patients (N = 116)	Median Survival (mo)
Glioblastoma multiforme (grade IV)	36	24
Recurrent glioblastoma multiforme	39	10
Anaplastic astrocytoma (grade III)	24	N
Recurrent anaplastic astrocytoma	10	N
Astrocytoma (grade II)	5	N
Recurrent astrocytoma	2	N

N, median survival not yet reached.
Adapted from Kaye AH: Photoradiation therapy of brain tumors. *In* Photosensitizing Compounds: Their Chemistry, Biology and Clinical Use. Ciba Foundation Symposium No. 146. Chichester, UK, John Wiley & Sons, 1989, pp 209–221; and Kaye AH, Morstyn G, Brownbill D: Adjuvant high-dose photoradiation therapy in the treatment of cerebral glioma: A phase I–II study. J Neurosurg 1987; 67:500–505.

toma multiforme at the Royal Melbourne Hospital had a median survival of 8 months, and no patients survived longer than 3 years. Survival for high-grade glioma has previously been reported as 17 weeks following surgery, 36 weeks following surgery and adjuvant radiotherapy, and 51 weeks if chemotherapy is also given.[3, 4] A median survival has not yet been reached for patients in our series with anaplastic astrocytoma or diffuse astrocytoma. Two patients received PDT for presumptive diagnoses of glioma, but the lesions proved to be a metastasis in one case and a hamartoma in the other. No direct serious complications from PDT occurred in the Royal Melbourne Hospital study, although one patient died from an acute myocardial infarction and another suffered hemiplegia after resection of a medial temporal lobe glioblastoma multiforme.

In the series of Muller and Wilson[65] of patients with malignant supratentorial tumors, median survival time was 6.3 months for 50 patients with newly diagnosed glioblastoma multiforme.[65] This median survival was shorter than that of the Royal Melbourne Hospital series, and it might have been due to the lower doses of light used (8 to 175 J/cm^2; median, 27 J/cm^2). Muller and Wilson noted no significant difference in median survival between the group of patients who received a total dose greater than 1,400 joule and those who received less than 1,400 joule, but the higher light dose group did have a greater proportion of 1- and 2-year survivors.

Wharen and colleagues[60] reported a median survival of 10 months for 6 patients with recurrent malignant glioma treated with interstitial PDT. Sixteen other patients with recurrent malignant glioma had a mean survival of 11 months after resection and intracavitary PDT, but it should be noted that this figure was quoted with respect to 8 patients who have died. This group also described posterior fossa tumors, including ependymoma, that have been treated with lower doses of light than had been used for supratentorial tumors.[60, 71] No complications were noted following gross total resection of tumor, and the therapy was well tolerated.

The initial results of the larger clinical studies of PDT for the treatment of glioma do show a favorable trend, particularly in the percentage of patients with long-term survival.

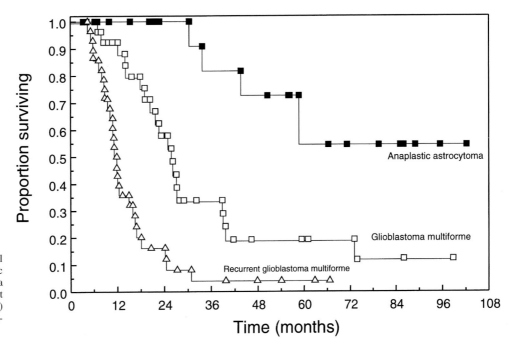

Figure 53–15 Actuarial survival curve for 99 patients with anaplastic astrocytoma (N = 24), glioblastoma multiforme (N = 36), and recurrent glioblastoma multiforme (N = 39) treated at the Royal Melbourne Hospital.

However, no phase III clinical trials have yet been undertaken, and it is therefore not possible to draw absolute conclusions concerning the efficacy of PDT.[72]

FUTURE APPLICATIONS

The clinical application of PDT for the treatment of gliomas is still in its infancy. Improvements in PDT will depend on obtaining a better understanding of tumor biology and of the basic sciences (i.e., physics, chemistry), and it is critical that the development of photosensitizers and lasers proceed together rather than in isolation. It is probable that laser and sensitizer development will focus on wavelengths of less than 900 nm, as the absorption of incident energy by water at longer wavelengths becomes significant, with subsequent decreases in penetration depth of light.[73] The titanium-doped sapphire crystal (Ti:sapphire) and alexandrite lasers are solid-state lasers that operate at 700 to 900 nm and 720 to 800 nm, respectively.[74]

A problem with testing PDT as an adjuvant treatment is that the tumor responses are difficult to measure. Because the depth of tumor kill of PDT is probably only 0.5 to 1.0 cm, it could be expected that PDT has little to offer as a sole treatment of large tumors. At surgery, most glioblastomas consist of approximately 10^{11} cells. Resection and radiotherapy can result in three orders of magnitude of cellular reduction, with the remaining tumor burden still being of the order of 10^8 tumor cells. Further adjuvant therapies need to reduce the tumor burden to at least 10^4 to 10^5 tumor cells, at which level the body's immune system may be able to eliminate the residual tumor cells.[7] In the foreseeable future, the strategies for treating gliomas should be aimed at using multiple adjuvant therapies that have been optimized so as to achieve the maximal reduction of residual tumor cells. This multimodal therapy will also overcome the inherent problems of the state of tumor cell heterogeneity in which

subpopulations of resistant cells may remain following a particular therapy, resulting in tumor recurrence.

The possibility of combining binary treatment systems, such as PDT and boron neutron capture therapy (BNCT),[75] is an exciting development made possible by the synthesis of boronated porphyrins such as BOPP,[24] which may act as a dual sensitizer for both PDT and BNCT. BOPP has the same spectral properties as hematoporphyrin derivative, and it is possible to envisage a treatment protocol of surgery with adjuvant PDT followed several days later by BNCT. BOPP has a long duration of retention in tumor tissue, and the several centimeters' penetration capacity of an epithermal neutron beam would overcome the limited penetration of red light.

The PDT process is now being investigated by molecular biology at the protein and genetic level. Porphyrin photosensitivity has been examined in tumor cell lines that express the multi-drug resistance (MDR) phenotype, and tumor cells with high expression of MDR genes have shown decreased uptake of hematoporphyrin derivative and subsequent resistance to PDT-induced damage.[76]

Techniques in molecular biology involving gene therapies appear to be the most likely avenue to produce the "cure" for gliomas, but in the foreseeable future the strategies for treating gliomas should be aimed at using multiple adjuvant therapies to achieve the maximal reduction of residual tumor and overcoming the inherent problems of tumor cell heterogeneity of subpopulations of resistant cells. Until biologic control of neoplasia is developed, PDT is likely to become one of a number of adjuvant therapies in the treatment armamentarium for cerebral glioma.

ACKNOWLEDGMENTS

The laboratory studies mentioned in this chapter as being performed by the authors were undertaken with the aid of grants from the National Health and Medical Research Council, the Anti-Cancer Council of Victoria, the Royal Australasian College of Surgeons, the Royal Melbourne Hospital Victor Hurley Medical Research Fun, and the Stroke Research Foundation.

The authors thank Dr. Stephen Kahl, UCSF School of Pharmacy, Dr. David Ward, Department of Organic Chemistry, University of Adelaide, and Dr. J. Keith Henderson, Neurosurgeon, for their advice. We also thank Gaye de Boer for secretarial assistance.

REFERENCES

1. Hayata Y, Kato H, Konaka C, et al: Photoradiation therapy in early stage cancer cases of the lung, esophagus and stomach. *In* Andreoni A, Cubeddu R (eds): Porphyrins in Tumor Phototherapy. New York, Plenum Press, 1984, pp 405–412.
2. Zulch KJ: Histological Typing of Tumours of the Central Nervous System. Geneva, Switzerland, World Health Organization, 1979.
3. Walker MD, Alexander E Jr, Hunt WE, et al: Evaluation of BCNU and/or radiotherapy in the treatment of anaplastic gliomas: A cooperative clinical trial. J Neurosurg 1978; 49:333–343.
4. Walker MD, Green SB, Byar DP, et al: Randomized comparisons of radiotherapy and nitrosoureas for the treatment of malignant glioma after surgery. N Engl J Med 1980; 303:1323–1329.
5. Bashir R, Hochberg F, Oot R: Regrowth patterns of glioblastoma multiforme related to planning of interstitial brachytherapy radiation fields. Neurosurgery 1988; 23:27–30.
6. Choucair AK, Levin VA, Gutin PH, et al: Development of multiple lesions during radiation therapy and chemotherapy in patients with gliomas. J Neurosurg 1986; 65:654–658.
7. Kaye AH: Adjuvant treatment of malignant brain tumors. Aust NZ J Surg 1989; 59:831–833.
8. Perria C, Capuzzo T, Cavagnaro G, et al: First attempts at the photodynamic treatment of human gliomas. J Neurosurg Sci 1980; 24:119–129.
9. Daniell MD, Hill JS: A history of photodynamic therapy. Aust NZ J Surg 1991; 61:340–348.
10. Wise BL, Taxdal DR: Studies of the blood-brain barrier utilizing hematoporphyrin. Brain Res 1957; 4:387–389.
11. Laws ER Jr, Wharen RE Jr, Anderson RE: Photoradiation therapy for malignant gliomas. *In* Wilkins RH, Rengachary SS (eds): Neurosurgery Update I. New York, McGraw-Hill, 1990, pp 260–265.
12. Abernathy CD, Anderson RE, Kooistra KL, et al: Activity of phthalocyanine photosensitizers against human glioblastoma in vitro. Neurosurgery 1987; 21:468–473.
13. Kaye AH, Morstyn G: Photoradiation therapy causing selective tumor kill in a rat glioma model. Neurosurgery 1987; 20:408–415.
14. Christensen T, Moan J, Torbjorg S, et al: Multicellular spheroids as an in vitro model system for photoradiation therapy in the presence of HPD. *In* Doiron DR, Gomer CJ (eds): Porphyrin Localization and Treatment of Tumors. New York, Alan R Liss, 1984, pp 381–390.
15. Kaye AH, Morstyn G, Gardner I, et al: Development of a xenograft glioma model in mouse brain. Cancer Res 1986; 46:1367–1373.
16. Yamada K, Ushio Y, Hayakawa T, et al: Quantitative autoradiographic measurements of blood-brain barrier permeability in the rat glioma model. J Neurosurg 1982; 57:394–398.
17. Levin VA, Freeman-Dove M, Landahl HD: Permeability characteristics of brain adjacent to tumors in rats. Arch Neurol 1975; 32:785–791.
18. Mitchell JB, Cook JA, Russo A: Biological basis for phototherapy. *In* Morstyn G, Kaye AH (eds): Phototherapy of Cancer. London, Harwood Academic Publishers, 1990, pp 1–22.
19. Kessel D, Thompson P, Musselman B, et al: Probing the structure and stability of the tumor-localizing derivative of hematoporphyrin by reductive cleavage. Cancer Res 1987; 47:4642–4645.
20. Berenbaum MC, Bonnett R, Scourides PA: In vivo biological activity of the components of haematoporphyrin derivative. Br J Cancer 1982; 45:571–581.
21. Kessel D: Chemistry of photosensitizing products derived from hematoporphyrin. *In* Morstyn G, Kaye AH (eds): Phototherapy of Cancer. Harwood Academic Publishers, London, pp 23–35, 1990.
22. Kaye AH: Photoradiation therapy of brain tumors. *In* Photosensitizing Compounds: Their Chemistry, Biology and Clinical Use, Ciba Foundation Symposium No. 146. Chichester, United Kingdom, John Wiley & Sons, 1989, pp 209–221.
23. Kaye AH, Hill JS: Photodynamic therapy of cerebral tumors. Neurosurg Q 1992; 1:233–358.
24. Hill JS, Kahl SB, Kaye AH, et al: Selective tumor uptake of a boronated porphyrin in animal model of cerebral glioma. Proc Natl Acad Sci USA 1992; 89:1785–1789.
25. Powers SK, Pribil S, Gillespie GY III, et al: Laser Photochemotherapy of rhodamine-123 sensitized human glioma cells in vitro. J Neurosurg 1986; 64:918–923.
26. Whelan HT, Traul DL, Przybylski C, et al: Interactions of merocyanine 540 with human brain tumor cells. Pediatr Neurol 1992; 8:117–120.
27. Fujishima I, Sakai T, Tanaka T, et al: Photodynamic therapy using pheophorbide and Nd:YAG laser. Neurol Med Chir Tokyo 1991; 31:257–263.
28. Lindsay EA, Berenbaum MC, Bonnett R, et al: Photodynamic therapy of a mouse glioma: Intracranial tumours are resistant while subcutaneous tumours are sensitive. Br J Cancer 1991; 63:242–246.
29. Steichen JD, Weiss MJ, Elmaleh DR, et al: Enhanced in vitro uptake and retention of ^{3}H-tetraphenylphosphonium by nervous system tumor cells. J Neurosurg 1991; 74:116–122.
30. Van Lier JE: New sensitizers for photodynamic therapy of cancer. *Photodynamic Therapy* Douglas RH, Moan J, Dall'Acqua F (eds): Light in Biology and Medicine. New York, Plenum, 1988, pp 133–140.
31. Benson RC: Phototherapy of bladder cancer. *In* Morstyn G, Kaye AH (eds): Phototherapy of Cancer. London, Harwood Academic Publishers, 1990, pp 199–214.
32. Woodburn KW, Vardaxis NJ, Hill JS, et al: Sub-cellular localization of porphyrins using confocal laser scanning microscopy (CLSM). Photochem Photobiol 1991; 54:725–732.
33. Hill JS, Kaye AH, Sawyer WH, et al: Selective uptake of haematoporphyrin derivative into human cerebral glioma. Neurosurgery 1990; 26:248–254.
34. Origitano TC, Karesh SM, Henkin RE, et al: Photodynamic Therapy for intracranial neoplasms: Investigations of photosensitizer uptake and distribution using indium-111 Photofrin-ii single photon emission computed tomography scans in humans with intracranial neoplasms. Neurosurgery 1993; 32:357–364.
35. Powers SK, Cush SS, Walstad DL, et al: Stereotactic intratumoral photodynamic therapy for recurrent malignant brain tumors. Neurosurgery 1991; 29:688–696.
36. Goldacre RJ, Sylven V: On the access of blood-borne dyes to various tumor regions. Br J Cancer 1962; 16:306–313.
37. Kaye AH, Morstyn G, Ashcroft RG: Uptake and retention of hematoporphyrin derivative in an in vivo/in vitro model of cerebral glioma. Neurosurgery 1985; 17:883–890.
38. Yoshida Y, Dereski MO, Garcia JH, et al: Photoactivated Photofrin II: Astrocytic swelling precedes endothelial injury in rat brain. J Neuropathol Exp Neurol 1992; 51:91–100.
39. Kongshaug M, Moan J, Brown SB: The distribution of porphyrins with different rumor localizing ability among human plasma lipoproteins. Br J Cancer 1989; 59:184–188.
40. Gal D, McDonald PC, Porter JC, et al: Cholesterol metabolism in cancer cells in monolayer culture. III. Low density lipoprotein metabolism. Int J Cancer 1981; 29:315–319.
41. Jori G: Transport and tissue delivery of photosensitizers. *In* Photosensitizing Compounds: Their Chemistry, Biology and Clinical Use. Ciba Foundation Symposium No. 146. Chichester, United Kingdom, John Wiley & Sons, 1989, pp 78–94.
42. Evenson JF, Moan J, Hindar A, et al: Tissue distribution of ^{3}H-hematoporphyrin derivative and its main components, ^{67}Ga and ^{131}I-albumin in mice bearing Lewis lung carcinoma. *In* Doiron DR, Gomer CJ (eds): Porphyrin Localization and Treatment of Tumors. New York, Alan R Liss, 1984, pp 541–562.
43. Verma A, Nye J, Snyder S: Porphyrins are endogenous ligands for the mitochondrial (peripheral type) benzodiazepine receptor. Proc Natl Acad Sci USA 1987; 84:2256–2260.
44. Oseroff AR, Ohuoha D, Ara G, et al: Intramitochondrial dyes allow selective in vitro photolysis of carcinoma cells. Proc Natl Acad Sci USA 1986; 83:9729–9733.
45. Dougherty TJ, Weishaupt KR, Boyle DG: Photodynamic sensitizers. *In* DeVita VT Jr, Helman S, Rosenberg SA (eds): Cancer: Principles and Practice of Oncology. Philadelphia, JB Lippincott, 1985, pp 2272–2279.

46. Leach MW, Khoshyomn S, Bringus J, et al: Normal brain tissue response to photodynamic therapy using aluminum phthalocyanine tetrasulfonate in the rat. Photochem Photobiol 1993; 57:842–845.

47. Yoshida Y, Dereski MO, Garcia JH, et al: Neuronal injury after photoactivation of Photofrin II. Am J Pathol 1992; 141:989–997.

48. Ji Y, Walstad D, Brown JT, et al: Interstitial photoradiation injury of normal brain. Lasers Surg Med 1992; 12:425–431.

49. Svaasand LO, Ellingsen R: Optical penetration in human intracranial tumors. Photochem Photobiol 1985; 41:73–76.

50. Muller PJ, Wilson BC: Photodynamic therapy: Cavitary photoillumination of malignant cerebral tumors using a laser coupled inflatable balloon. Can J Neurol Sci 1985; 12:371–373.

51. Muller PJ, Wison BC: An Update on the penetration depth of 630 nm light in normal brain and malignant human brain tissue in vivo. Phys Med Biol 1986; 31:1295–1297.

52. Waldow SM, Dougherty TJ: Interactions of hyperthermia and photoradiation therapy. Radiat Res 1984; 97:380–385.

53. Kaye AH, Morstyn G, Brownbill D: Adjuvant high-dose photoradiation therapy in the treatment of cerebral glioma: A phase 1–2 study. J Neurosurg 1987; 67:500–505.

54. Origitano TC, Reichman OH: Photodynamic therapy for intracranial neoplasms: development of an image-based computer-assisted protocol for photodynamic therapy of intracranial neoplasms. Neurosurgery 1993; 32:587–596.

55. Berenbaum MC, Hall GW, Hoyes AD: Cerebral photosensitization by hematoporphyrin derivative: Evidence for an endothelial site of action. Br J Cancer 1986; 53:81–89.

56. Allardice JT, Abulafi AM, Webb DG, et al: Standardization of intralipid for light scattering in clinical photodynamic therapy. Lasers Med Sci 1992; 7:461–465.

57. Doiron DR: Photophysics of an instrumentation for porphyrin detection and activation. In Doiron DR, Gomer CJ (eds): Porphyrin localization and treatment of tumors. New York, Alan R Liss, 1984, pp 41–73.

58. Kelly PJ, Kall BA, Goerss SJ, et al: Computer-assisted stereotaxic resection of intra-axial brain neoplasms. J Neurosurg 1986; 64:427–439.

59. Ji Y, Walstad D, Brown JT, et al: Improved survival from intracavitary photodynamic therapy of rat glioma. Photochem Photobiol 1992; 56:385–390.

60. Wharen RE, Anderson RE, Laws ER Jr: Photoradiation therapy of brain tumors. In Salcman M (ed): Neurobiology of Brain Tumors. Baltimore, Williams & Wilkins, 1991, pp 341–357.

61. Whelan HT, Schmidt MH, Segura AD, et al: The role of photodynamic therapy in posterior fossa brain tumors: A preclinical study in a canine glioma model. J Neurosurg 1993; 79:562–558.

62. Schwartz SK, Absolon K, Vermund H: Some relationships of porphyrins, x-rays and tumors. U Minn Med Bull 1955; 27:7–13.

63. Forbes IJ, Ward AD, Jacka FJ, et al: A multi-disciplinary approach to phototherapy of human cancers. In Doiron DR, Gomer CJ (eds): Porphyrin Localization and Treatment of Tumors. New York, Alan R Liss, 1984, pp 693–708.

64. Wharen RE Jr, So S, Anderson RE, et al: Hematoporphyrin derivative photocytotoxicity of human glioblastoma in cell culture. Neurosurgery 1986; 19:495–501.

65. Muller PJ, Wilson BC: Photodynamic therapy of malignant brain tumors. Can J Neurol Sci 1990; 17:193–198.

66. McCulloch GAJ, Forbes IJ, Lee See K, et al: Phototherapy in malignant brain tumors. In Doiron DR, Gomer CJ (eds): Porphyrin Localization and Treatment of Tumors. New York, Alan R Liss, 1984, pp 709–717.

67. Laws ER Jr, Cortese DA, Kinsey JH, et al: Photoradiation therapy in the treatment of malignant brain tumors: A phase I (feasibility) study. Neurosurgery 1981; 9:672–678.

68. Perria C, Carai M, Falzoi A, et al: Photodynamic therapy of malignant brain tumors: Clinical results of, difficulties with, questions about, and future prospects for the neurosurgical applications. Neurosurgery 1988; 23:557–563.

69. Wharen RE Jr, Anderson RE, Laws ER Jr: Quantitation of hematoporphyrin derivative in human gliomas, experimental central nervous system tumors, and normal tissues. Neurosurgery 1983; 12:446–450.

70. Kostron H, Fritsch E, Grunert V: Photodynamic therapy of malignant brain tumors: A phase I-II trial. Br J Neurosurg 1988; 2:241–248.

71. Laws ER JR, Wharen RE, Anderson RE: The treatment of brain tumors by photoradiation. In Pluchino F, Broggi G (eds): Advanced Technology in Neurosurgery. Berlin, Springer-Verlag, 1988, pp 46–60.

72. Noske DP, Wolbers JG, Sterenborg HJ: Photodynamic therapy of malignant glioma: A review of the literature. Clin Neurol Neurosurg 1991; 93:293–307.

73. Wilson BC: Photodynamic therapy: Light delivery and dosage for second generation sensitizers. In Photosensitizing Compounds: Their Chemistry, Biology and Clinical Use. Ciba Foundation Symposium No. 146. Chichester, United Kingdom, John Wiley & Sons, 1989, pp 60–77.

74. Aimsworth MD, Piper JA: Laser systems for photodynamic therapy. In Morstyn G, Kaye AH (eds): Phototherapy of Cancer. London, Harwood Academic Publishers, 1990, pp 37–72.

75. Barth RF, Soloway AH, Fairchild RG: Boron neutron capture therapy for cancer. Sci Am 1990; 263:100–107.

76. Gomer CJ, Rucker N, Ferrario A, et al: Properties and applications of photodynamic therapy. Radiat Res 1989; 120:1–18.

ADDITIONAL READING

1. Kaye AH, Morstyn G, Apuzzo MLJ: Photoradiation therapy and its potential in the management of neurological tumours: A review. J Neurosurg 1988; 69:1–14.

2. Morstyn G, Kaye AH (eds): Phototherapy of Cancer. London, Harwood Academic Publishers, 1990.

Special Topics

KAREN L. FINK

S. CLIFFORD SCHOLD, JR.

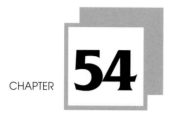

CHAPTER **54**

Tumor Dissemination and Management

Gliomas usually spread by local growth and infiltration, rather than by dissemination and metastasis, despite histologic appearances that may be just as malignant as systemic tumors that metastasize widely. Some gliomas do escape from their primary location, giving rise to cerebrospinal and even extraneural metastases. In this chapter, we review the available literature on the incidence and treatment of both neuraxis and systemic metastases of gliomas.

HISTORY

Traditional wisdom held that gliomas could not spread beyond the intracranial space. In 1926, Bailey and Cushing found no evidence for extracranial spread of gliomas. In fact, they said gliomas "do not form metastases, and rarely if ever inoculate the leptomeninges."[1] Since then, reports of neuraxis and extraneural metastases of gliomas have accumulated. In 1955, Weiss[2] described four criteria that should be met for acceptance of a case as a metastasizing CNS tumor: (1) a histologically characteristic CNS tumor must be proved; (2) initial symptoms must be attributable to this tumor; (3) a complete autopsy must be performed in sufficient detail to rule out other primary sites; and (4) the metastasis and the CNS tumor must be morphologically and histologically similar, allowing for change in the degree of anaplasia over time. These criteria remain largely valid today, though noninvasive imaging techniques and percutaneous biopsies in combination with immunohistochemical techniques (particularly staining for glial fibrillary acidic protein, or GFAP[3, 4] have made complete autopsy less strictly necessary. Application of these "Weiss criteria" to possible cases of metastases from gliomas gives some uniformity to the literature, though the constant revision of classification schemes for CNS tumors makes review and summary of the literature difficult. Nevertheless, it is clear that although they are rare, neuraxis and extracraniospinal metastases of gliomas do occur.

NEURAXIS DISSEMINATION OF GLIOMAS

Frequency of Meningeal Gliomatosis

Gliomas most often spread beyond their primary site via cerebrospinal fluid (CSF) pathways. Autopsy series have revealed leptomeningeal spread in a surprisingly high percentage of patients dying of gliomas. As many as 30% of patients with gliomas have microscopic meningeal tumor deposits at autopsy.[5, 6] Onda and co-workers[6] found histologic evidence of leptomeningeal spread in 14/51 patients (27.5%) dying of glioblastoma, and a review of autopsy cases from Memorial Sloan-Kettering Cancer Center revealed 11 cases of meningeal gliomatosis out of 52 gliomas (21%).[7] Some of the autopsy-detected leptomeningeal metastases are microscopic and are asymptomatic during the patient's lifetime.

The frequency with which leptomeningeal spread of gliomas is detected is affected by how thoroughly a search is made. Even asymptomatic patients may have detectable glioma cells in CSF. Balhuizen and colleagues[8] reported that when CSF was sampled prior to surgery for astrocytomas, 9/53 patients (17%) had positive cytologic findings. The ratio was somewhat higher postoperatively, with 5/21 tested samples (24%) showing positive cytologic findings. The number of patients in whom symptoms of leptomeningeal spread subsequently developed was not stated. Microscopic involvement of the leptomeninges by gliomas is thus relatively frequent, but it may be clinically insignificant. Clinically symptomatic leptomeningeal metastases from gliomas have been reported to occur in 1.5% to 4.0% of glioma patients.[9–12]

The method employed to detect leptomeningeal spread of gliomas affects the apparent incidence of this complication. Magnetic resonance imaging (MRI) with gadolinium, computed tomography (CT), myelography and CSF cytologic findings were compared in a recent study of pediatric patients with miscellaneous CNS tumors and symptoms suggesting leptomeningeal metastases. MRI with gadolinium contrast detected leptomeningeal metastases in 65% of patients, CT-myelography was positive in 47%, and cytologic findings were positive in only 29% of cases. In no cases did MRI imaging fail to detect metastases that were detected by the other two tests. Assuming that MRI had a sensitivity of 100% in the detection of leptomeningeal metastases, CT myelography detected 72% of metastases, and cytology only 45%.[13] GFAP staining may increase the sensitivity of CSF cytologic analysis,[14] but this method alone will miss a significant number of cases of neuraxis spread of gliomas.

MRI is thus the method of choice for detecting leptomeningeal metastases of gliomas, with some caveats: (1) Gadolinium contrast is essential for optimum detection of leptomeningeal seeding, which can be completely undetectable on noncontrasted scans[9, 15]; (2) MRI is very sensitive, but it may not be completely specific. Inflammation of meninges due to non-neoplastic causes can mimic leptomeningeal neoplasm. In the study of Kramer and colleagues, one patient had an MRI consistent with leptomeningeal tumor spread that was proved clinically and on repeated imaging studies to be subarachnoid blood rather than tumor deposits.[13] Despite these limitations, MRI with gadolinium is the most sensitive and least invasive method for detecting leptomeningeal processes and is therefore the modality of choice for detecting neuraxis dissemination of gliomas.[9, 15]

Symptoms of Meningeal Gliomatosis

Symptoms attributable to neuraxis spread of glioma cells parallel those expected in syndromes involving meningeal irritation or spinal cord compromise. Several studies have also found a high incidence of altered mental status. In fact, Yung and others[7] found mental status changes in 100% of one series of patients with meningeal gliomatosis.[7] Data from the literature published from 1978 to 1995 from which clinical information can be compiled reveal that local pain, headache, altered mental status, and paresis or myelopathy are the most frequent symptoms of meningeal gliomatosis (Table 54–1 and Fig. 54–1). The high percentage of patients with headache may reflect the prevalence of hydrocephalus in patients with leptomeningeal dissemination of gliomas. Grant and co-workers[16] found that 8 out of 11 patients (73%) with meningeal gliomatosis had hydrocephalus on MRI or CT, and Yung and associates[7] reported that glioma patients with leptomeningeal dissemination required more ventriculosystemic shunts (58%) than did patients without this complication (5%). Other frequently reported symptoms of meningeal gliomatosis include meningeal signs, cranial nerve palsies, and paresthesias (see Table 54–1). Less frequently cited symptoms included seizures, ataxia, decreased vision, and vomiting.[5, 7, 16, 17] It is difficult to tell from review of published data whether all of these symptoms are due to the leptomeningeal process or whether some might be attributable to the primary tumor.

Factors That Predispose to Meningeal Gliomatosis

LOCATION/STRUCTURAL FEATURES THAT FAVOR NEURAXIS DISSEMINATION

Grant and colleagues[16] asserted that structural features contributed to the likelihood of dissemination of gliomas, as 9 out of the 11 primary gliomas that later developed leptomeningeal dissemination abutted the ventricles or the basal cisterns. In contrast, Grabb and others[17] found that gliomas with and without leptomeningeal spread had an equal frequency of periventricular location on imaging. In this study, it was found that entering the ventricles at surgery was a risk factor for subsequent leptomeningeal spread of gliomas.[17]

Location above or below the tentorium may be an important factor in the frequency of dissemination of gliomas, but this is controversial. Kandt and co-workers[18] found leptomeningeal spread in 4 out of 7 hemispheric glioblastomas (57%), and in only 2 out of 6 brainstem glioblastomas (33%). However, Grant and associates[16] state that 20% of supratentorial and 60% of posterior fossa glioblastomas spread throughout the neuraxis. It is difficult to make a definitive statement regarding frequency of neuraxis dissemination from various locations because the number of patients in each study is small, and the denominator (i.e., patients with gliomas without leptomeningeal spread) is rarely defined.

PATIENT AGE AND SURVIVAL

Patients with meningeal gliomatosis have tended to be younger than glioma patients without leptomeningeal spread.[9, 10] Yung and others[7] found that patients with leptomeningeal dissemination of gliomas were an average age of 40 years, whereas glioma patients without meningeal gliomatosis were an average age of 57 years. Delattre and colleagues[11] reported Brain Tumor Cooperative Group data that showed that clinically symptomatic leptomeningeal spread occurred in 8.8% of glioma patients younger than 45 years and in only 1.3% of patients older than 45 years.

In addition, clinically symptomatic neuraxis spread generally manifests slightly later than the average survival time for similar gliomas, indicating that patients who survive their primary glioma longer may be at higher risk of leptomeningeal spread.[9, 10] The longer survival time enjoyed by these patients may allow leptomeningeal metastases to become clinically evident.

HISTOLOGIC GRADE AS A RISK FACTOR FOR NEURAXIS DISSEMINATION

Tumor type and histologic grade are the most important determinants of whether a given glioma undergoes leptomeningeal dissemination. Anaplastic tumors tend to undergo leptomeningeal spread more often than well-differentiated tumors of the same type.[19] Data regarding the frequency of neuraxis dissemination of individual types of gliomas are difficult to extract from the literature, because most studies group all primary CNS tumors together, and the nomenclature of gliomas is still evolving. Early papers reported meningeal tumors and medulloblastomas as gliomas. In addition, case studies rarely report the population of patients from which the metastatic glioma patients are derived. All of these problems make accurate frequency estimates difficult, but certainly glioblastomas, astrocytomas, ependymomas, ependymoblastomas, oligodendrogliomas, and gangliogliomas have all been reported to spread throughout the neuraxis.

Neuraxis Spread of Astrocytic Tumors   Glioblastomas and astrocytomas may diffusely seed the neuraxis[5, 6] (Fig. 54–2) and are the most frequently reported gliomas with cerebrospinal metastases.[17, 20] This reflects the overall prevalence of astrocytic tumors. Choucair and others[12] found 15 patients with spinal spread out of 1,035 cases of supratentorial glioblastomas and astrocytomas, for a frequency of 1.5%.

TABLE 54-1
FREQUENT SYMPTOMS OF MENINGEAL GLIOMATOSIS*

Study (Year)	No. of Patients	Local Pain	Altered MS	Paresis/ Myelopathy	Headache	Meningeal Signs	Asymptomatic	CNS Palsies	Paresthesia	CT Findings Hydrocephalus	CT Findings Meningeal Enhancement
Dietrich et al (1993)[108]	8	—	7	3	8	4	0	4	—	8	—
Grant et al (1992)[16]	11	7	5	1	2	1	0	2	1	8	—
Grabb et al (1992)[17]	11	4	4	2	4	4	4	—	—	3	8
Vertosick & Selker (1990)[9]	11	9	—	8	—	—	0	1	1	—	—
Onda et al (1989)[6]	14	—	2	2	—	—	7	1	—	1	—
Vincent (1983)[109]	2	1	—	2	—	—	—	1	—	3	5
Civitello et al (1988)[110]	6	1	3	1	2	—	1	1	1	4	—
Delattre et al (1986)[11]	7	6	—	2	5	—	—	—	—	6	5
Awad et al (1986)[10]	13	—	1	4	2	1	5	1	1	—	4
Kandt et al (1984)[18]	6	3	2	2	—	—	1	—	1	—	2
Packer et al (1983)[100]	5	5	—	5	4	—	0	1	2	10	—
Yung et al (1980)[7]	12	—	12	3	1	—	0	3	—	1	—
Erlich & Davis (1978)[5]	5	—	2	2	—	1	1	—	—	—	—
Totals	111	36	38	37	28	11	19	17	6	44	19
% of Total (111 patients)		32.4	34.2	33.3	25.2	9.9	17.1	15.3	5.4	63.8	52.8

*These data are presented as a bar graph in Figure 54-1.

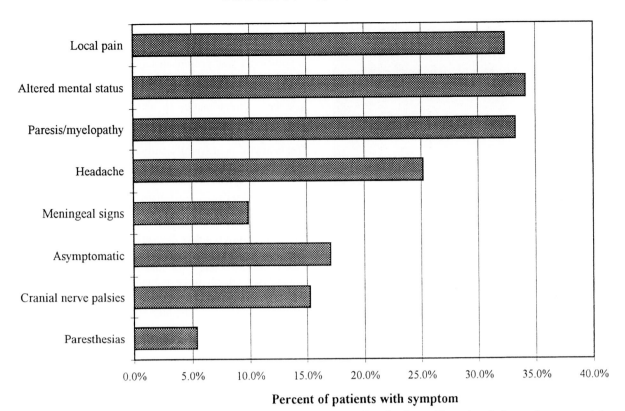

Percent of patients with symptom

Figure 54-1 Frequent symptoms of meningeal gliomatosis. Data from 13 recent studies of patients with meningeal gliomatosis are presented as a bar graph. Most of the 111 cases were diagnosed antemortem, though a few were detected at autopsy only (asymptomatic patients). The most frequently reported symptom was altered mental status, ranging from confusion to stupor. Paresis, myelopathy, and local pain were also reported frequently. (Data from references 5–7, 9–11, 16–18, 100, and 108–110.)

The most important factor determining the likelihood of leptomeningeal spread of a given astrocytic tumor is histologic grade. Lower grade astrocytic tumors metastasize less frequently than do higher-grade tumors. Kandt and co-workers[18] found clinical or cytologic evidence of leptomeningeal spread of high-grade astrocytomas in six out of 13 children (46%), whereas none of 16 low-grade astrocytic tumors spread in this fashion. Typical low-grade childhood cerebel-

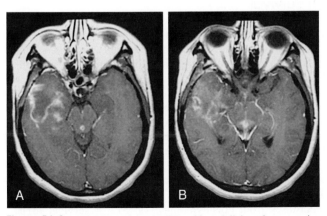

Figure 54-2 Axial T1-weighted MRIs with gadolinium from a patient with leptomeningeal dissemination of glioblastoma multiforme. The right temporal lobe lesion was resected 3 years prior to this study, but has recurred. In addition, diffuse enhancement of the intracranial ependyma and leptomeninges is present, particularly in the cerebral aqueduct *(A)* and in the fourth ventricle *(B)*.

lar astrocytomas spread via CSF in only three out of 72 cases from the literature (4.2%) reviewed by Shapiro and Shulman.[21] Similarly, Rutka and others[22] found only one case of leptomeningeal spread in 25 low-grade childhood astrocytomas (4%). A few cases of leptomeningeal metastasis from childhood pilocytic astrocytomas have been reported (Fig. 54–3), but in general, these tumors are less likely to disseminate than are more anaplastic fibrillary astrocytic tumors.[23–26]

Leptomeningeal dissemination may rarely be present at diagnosis in low-grade astrocytomas, but the lag period between excision of the primary astrocytoma and leptomeningeal spread can be long (up to 6 to 8 years later).[23, 24]

Neuraxis Spread of Ependymomas Ependymomas can also disseminate throughout the neuraxis. Early autopsy series reported micrometastases in the leptomeninges in 12% to 34% of patients with ependymomas.[27–29] Clinically evident leptomeningeal spread is less common, occurring in 3% to 12% of patients.[27, 30] Lyons and Kelly[31] reviewed 729 reported cases of posterior fossa ependymomas in 1991. Clinically evident leptomeningeal dissemination was present in 42/729 (6%) of the patients with posterior fossa ependymomas. Rawlings and co-workers[32] found clinically evident leptomeningeal metastases in five ependymoma patients out of 62 (8%).

Histologic grade strongly influences the likelihood of leptomeningeal spread in ependymomas. Lyons and Kelly[31] found neuraxis spread more often when the primary ependy-

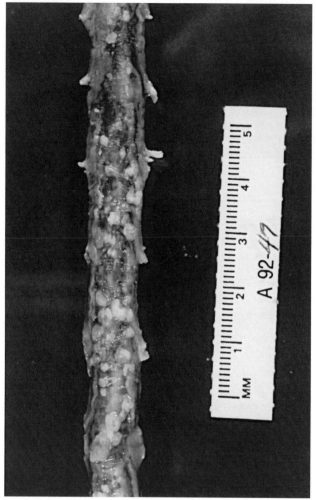

Figure 54-3 Neuraxis dissemination of pilocytic astrocytoma. Postmortem photograph shows extensive involvement of the spinal leptomeninges by nodular deposits from an intracranial pilocytic astrocytoma. (Specimen provided by Dennis K. Burns, M.D., Department of Pathology, University of Texas—Southwestern).

moma was described as high grade (13%) than when it was called low grade (3%). Salazar also found that high-grade ependymomas metastasized more frequently than low-grade tumors. In his review, high-grade ependymomas accounted for 80% of the cases of neuraxis metastases of ependymomas reported in the literature.[30]

Location above or below the tentorium intracranially does not appear to influence the likelihood of leptomeningeal metastases in ependymomas, as 13.6% of supratentorial ependymomas and 9.5% of infratentorial ependymomas underwent neuraxis dissemination in the series of Rawlings and colleagues.[32] No metastases from the 19 spinal ependymomas were seen in this series, but the spinal ependymomas were almost universally low-grade tumors. A few cases of intraspinal and extraspinal metastases have been reported from spinal ependymomas, and these patients may have prolonged survival despite metastatic disease.[2, 33]

Ependymoblastomas are very rare tumors that generally occur in young children. They have a higher frequency of leptomeningeal seeding than ependymomas. Mork and

Rubinstein[34] reviewed the literature in 1985 and found a total of 12 reported cases of ependymoblastoma. Leptomeningeal involvement was present in ten of 12 of these cases (83%). However, neuraxis involvement was described as extensive in only three cases, and it is not stated whether the metastases were symptomatic. In addition to the leptomeningeal dissemination of ependymoblastomas, extraneural metastasis to the lung was noted in one case (8%). Based on the high frequency of neuraxis dissemination of ependymoblastomas, Mork and Rubinstein advocated neuraxis radiation therapy for all ependymoblastomas.

Neuraxis Spread of Oligodendrogliomas Oligodendrogliomas also occasionally spread via the CSF.[35, 36] In fact, a perception exists that oligodendrogliomas metastasize more frequently than other gliomas.[23] In the small series of Grabb and associates[17] of malignant gliomas with leptomeningeal spread, all three patients with malignant oligodendrogliomas had development of leptomeningeal metastases (100%) compared with only four of 14 patients with glioblastomas (29%) and two of nine patients with astrocytomas (22%). However, in the study by Nijjar and others[37] of 72 patients with oligodendroglioma, leptomeningeal metastases developed in only two patients, for a frequency of 2.8%. Much of this discrepancy may be explained by the different histologic grades of the oligodendrogliomas in these two series, as the tumors in the series with the high frequency of neuraxis spread were malignant oligodendrogliomas,[17] whereas the study with the lower incidence of leptomeningeal spread included all grades of oligodendrogliomas.[37] It may be true that oligodendroglial tumors have a greater tendency to spread by CSF pathways, but this is not well documented in the literature.

Neuraxis Spread of Other Gliomas Data regarding neuraxis dissemination of less common gliomas are nearly nonexistent, but reports of leptomeningeal spread of gangliogliomas have been published.[38, 39]

Effect of Leptomeningeal Dissemination on Survival

Leptomeningeal dissemination of gliomas is associated with short survival. In the series of Grant and co-workers,[16] patients with leptomeningeal spread of gliomas survived only 8 weeks. Other studies report somewhat longer survival with leptomeningeal dissemination of glioma: Packer and others[40] reported 3 months survival; Kandt and associates[18] (brainstem gliomas), 7 months; and Vertosick and Selker[9] (glioblastoma), 2.8 months. Grabb and co-workers[17] report a 3-year survival of 9% in patients with leptomeningeal spread of malignant gliomas vs. 41% 3-year survival in patients without neuraxis spread. Similarly, Kim and Fayos[41] reported a 5-year survival rate of 16.7% in patients with neuraxis metastases from ependymomas, vs. 51.3% survival in patients without leptomeningeal dissemination. In the series of Rawlings and colleagues,[32] of ependymomas with leptomeningeal spread, all five patients who developed leptomeningeal metastases died within 12 months of the diagnosis of disseminated disease.

Most patients in whom leptomeningeal metastases of gliomas develop also have recurrence of the primary tumor. In the series of Dropcho and co-workers[42] of 50 children with supratentorial gliomas, leptomeningeal spread developed in 13 patients, and ten of 13 had progression of the primary tumor at the time of diagnosis of neuraxis spread (77%). Ninety percent of the patients in the series of Vertosick and Selker[9] of leptomeningeal spread of glioblastoma died of progressive primary tumor. In contrast, Grabb and colleagues[17] report that in their pediatric series, all of the patients with leptomeningeal dissemination of malignant gliomas died of disseminated disease rather than local progression. Successful prevention of neuraxis spread of gliomas ultimately depends on better therapy for the original tumor.

EXTRANEURAL SPREAD OF GLIOMAS

Rarity of Extraneural Spread of Gliomas

Despite their often malignant histology, gliomas rarely spread beyond the confines of the CNS. A variety of hypotheses have been advanced to explain the rarity of extraneural spread of gliomas.[43] Several anatomic features of the CNS are cited as preventing metastases of gliomas. The venous anatomy of the CNS is thought to be particularly important. The dense dural coats of venous sinuses provide one barrier, and some authors believe that the venous channels in the CNS are too easily collapsed by expanding gliomas to allow egress of tumor cells.[44, 46] Lack of lymphatics in the CNS is also invoked as an explanation of the failure of spread of gliomas.[47]

Pansera and Pansera[48] believe that lack of connective tissue stroma in the CNS represents another barrier to extraneural metastases of CNS tumors. In this model, cells that can invade connective tissue stroma may escape the primary tumor, and can invade other stroma elsewhere in the body. Lack of connective tissue stroma within the CNS means that this selection pressure is absent. Therefore, tumor cells arising in the CNS do not develop the means to invade connective tissue stroma elsewhere in the body, and are confined to local expansion.[48]

Aside from the physical barriers to glioma cell dissemination, Alvord[49] believes that the cytokinetics of CNS tumors make clinically detectable extraneural spread unlikely. In their confined environment, gliomas are detectable for only four to five generations of cell division prior to the death of the patient. This is approximately one half the number of generations for which systemic tumors are detectable. Alvord's model predicts that if metastasis occurs at surgery with a tiny residual tumor volume, the primary tumor will kill the patient before any metastases reach detectable size.[49]

Even if glioma cells escape the CNS, other organs are thought to provide a hostile environment for the growth of glioma masses. Systemic immunologic defenses may be important in preventing the proliferation of metastatic glioma cells.[50] Grace and colleagues[51] showed that normal brain and gliomas provoked delayed hypersensitivity reactions on intradermal testing in some patients, which suggests that immunologic systems might prevent the growth of metastatic glioma masses.

Despite these barriers to dissemination of gliomas, research has accumulated that suggests that gliomas can overcome these hurdles. Kung and others[52] showed that glioma cells can invade veins. Other researchers found tumor cells in blood draining from gliomas.[53] Surgery may also provide the means for extraneural dissemination of glioma cells by creating a negative pressure gradient that allows glioma cells access to systemic venous channels.[54] These studies suggest that hematogenous dissemination of glioma cells is possible.

Other studies suggest that lymphatic dissemination of gliomas is also possible. Prineas[55] described histologic spaces in the CNS that resemble lymphatic capillaries, indicating that the brain has a system of lymphatic drainage. McComb[56] showed that lymphatic drainage occurs from CSF to extraneural tissues. Thus, the longstanding notion that the CNS is isolated from systemic lymphatics may be an oversimplification.

Once they have escaped the primary tumor via lymphatic or hematogenous routes, glioma cells must invade basement membranes in order to form distant metastases. Several investigators have shown that glioblastoma cells can penetrate Matrigel, indicating that they should be able to overcome the basement membrane of other organs in vivo.[57, 58] Other experiments show that gliomas can grow outside of the nervous system, disproving the ''hostile soil'' theory. Zimmerman[59] showed that murine glioma cells can form systemic metastases in pleura and other organs when delivered directly to the systemic circulation. Vecht and co-workers[60] also showed that glioma cells injected intracranially in mice can spread in the subarachnoid space and extraneurally. Grace and others,[51] Mitts and Walker,[61] and Battista and colleagues[62] showed that autotransplants of human primary gliomas placed in subcutaneous locations during initial surgery are able to enlarge and thrive, despite their extraneural location, in 20% to 40% of cases, which proves that glioma cells can survive in tissues other than the CNS. Experimental evidence suggests that extraneural metastasis of gliomas is biologically possible, so the precise explanation for the relative rarity of this phenomenon remains elusive.

Factors That Affect the Frequency of Extraneural Metastases of Gliomas

Extraneural metastases of intracranial tumors are even rarer than neuraxis dissemination, and they occur in fewer than 1% of glioma patients. In 1969, Smith and co-workers[63] found 35 cases of extraneural metastases from 8,000 neuroectodermal tumors, for a rate of 0.4%. A population-based study in Scotland found only four cases of extraneural metastases out of 2,850 neuroectodermal tumors, for a metastasis frequency of 0.14%.[64] These early reports included many tumors that would no longer be classified as gliomas. Despite their rarity, reports of extraneural glioma metastases have continued to appear, and systemic metastases are a well recognized, though extremely rare, complication of glioblastomas,[4, 65–69] astrocytomas,[3, 70] ependymomas,[2, 71–74] ependymoblastomas,[34, 70, 75] and oligodendrogliomas.[76–78] Liwnicz and Rubenstein[66] reviewed the literature regarding extraneural metastases of gliomas in 1979 and compared the number of reported metastases with the frequency of each glioma type in a population study. This analysis showed that the nongliomatous medulloblastomas were the most likely to undergo extraneural metastases, followed by ependymomas, oligodendrogliomas, and astrocytic tumors. Despite the lower tendency of astrocytic tumors to metastasize, this type of tumor makes up the majority of reported cases of extraneural gliomatous metastases because of its higher frequency in the population.

HISTOLOGIC TUMOR TYPE

Extraneural Metastases From Astrocytic Tumors

Extraneural metastases are a rare complication of astrocytic tumors. Choucair and others[12] found only one case of extraneural metastasis out of 1,047 astrocytic tumors, for a metastasis frequency of 0.1%. Nevertheless, astrocytic tumors account for 63% to 79% of reported cases of extraneural glial metastases.[63, 73]

In 1980, Pasquier and co-workers[79] reviewed the literature regarding extraneural metastases of astrocytic tumors, restricting the analysis to autopsied cases that met the Weiss criteria outlined previously. They found 72 cases of extraneural metastases of astrocytic tumors in the literature. Glioblastomas accounted for most of the metastases (51 cases). The most common sites of extraneural spread of astrocytic tumors in this review were lung/pleura in 59.7%, lymph nodes in 51.4%, bone in 30.5%, and liver in 22.2%. The lymph nodes most frequently involved were cervical (62%) or hilar (32%). The most frequently involved bones were vertebrae (72.7%). Miscellaneous involved organs included heart, adrenal medulla, kidney, diaphragm, mediastinum, pancreas, thyroid, and peritoneum.[79]

Most of the extraneural metastases of gliomas in this review occurred in adults (63/72, or 87.5%). Hoffman and Duffner[80] reviewed the literature on extraneural metastases of gliomas in 1985 and found 68 case reports of astrocytic extraneural metastases in adults and only 11 in children. It is difficult to determine whether astrocytic tumors are more likely to metastasize in adults or in children simply by examining the number of case reports in the literature, because the frequency of astrocytic tumors is higher in adults, and studies have not clearly stated the number of glioma patients of different ages from which the metastatic cases derived. Studies that address the frequency of metastases of astrocytic tumors find similar frequencies of this complication in adults and children. In the series of Campbell and others[70] of pediatric brain tumors, 0.3% of patients with astrocytomas or glioblastomas developed extraneural metastases, which is comparable to the 0.1% frequency that Choucair and colleagues[12] found in adults.

Extraneural Metastases From Ependymomas

Ependymomas also metastasize extraneurally.[2, 35, 70–74, 81–83] Wentworth and Birdsell[75] found one case of extraneural metastases out of 72 ependymomas for a frequency of metastasis of 1.4%. Liwnicz and Rubinstein[66] found that although ependymomas accounted for 6.2% of all gliomas in their series, they accounted for 16.4% of the extraneural metastases of gliomas in the literature. Ependymomas thus appear to be more likely to metastasize to extraneural sites than oligodendrogliomas or astrocytic tumors. Ependymomas are most likely to metastasize to lung/pleura, followed by lymph nodes, bone, and liver.[66] In a literature review in 1985, Hoffman and Duffner[80] found 22 cases of extraneural metastases of ependymomas 13 of which occurred in children, and nine of which occurred in adults.

A special case of systemic metastasis of ependymoma was reported by Vagaiwala and co-workers[84] in 1979. The primary ependymoma was located extradurally, in the lumbar area, in association with spina bifida. The patient had a pulmonary nodule, noted on chest x-ray at presentation, that was later confirmed by histologic analysis to be a metastasis from the extradural ependymoma. The patient survived 5 years after initial diagnosis and underwent multiple resections of pulmonary metastases. The authors reviewed the literature on primary extraspinal ependymomas and found only 11 cases; systemic metastases developed in three of these, for a high frequency of 27%.[84] It is likely that the primary extraneural location of the gliomas facilitated metastasis by traditional lymphatic and hematogenous routes.

Ependymoma metastases can occur years after diagnosis of the primary tumor. Usually these cases are low-grade ependymomas, often originating in the spinal cord. Mavroudis and colleagues[33] report a patient in whom a lung metastasis developed 29 years after resection of a low-grade spinal ependymoma. Wight and others[85] report a case of cauda equina ependymoma with metastases to humerus and lung, with patient survival of 32 years after initial surgery.

Extraneural Metastases From Oligodendrogliomas

Oligodendrogliomas also metastasize extraneurally[76–78, 80] (Fig. 54–4). The literature review of Pasquier and others[79] of extraneural metastases of astrocytic tumors in 1980 contained three mixed astrocytomas with oligodendroglial components. The more general review by Liwnicz and Rubenstein of extraneural metastases of gliomas reported seven oligodendrogliomas out of 116 metastasizing gliomas. The oligodendroglioma metastases were most likely to occur in bone, followed by lung/pleura and liver.[66] Some authors believe that oligodendrogliomas are more likely to metastasize than are other gliomas.[23] However, Liwnicz and Rubenstein[66] found that oligodendrogliomas comprised 5.0% of gliomas and 5.2% of reported cases of extraneural metastases of gliomas. Based on these data, oligodendrogliomas are less likely to metastasize than are ependymomas.[66]

EFFECTS OF SURGERY ON THE FREQUENCY OF EXTRANEURAL METASTASES OF GLIOMAS

The Role of Craniotomy in Extraneural Metastases

Surgery may be an important factor favoring spread of gliomas beyond the confines of the primary tumor. Most reported cases of cerebrospinal and extraneural metastases of gliomas have occurred following surgical procedures (e.g., resection, biopsy or shunting).[79, 86, 87] Surgery likely allows entry of glioma cells into the vasculature or lymphatic system, promoting their dissemination. This remains difficult to prove, because most patients with CNS masses require surgery for relief of symptoms or definitive diagnosis; therefore,

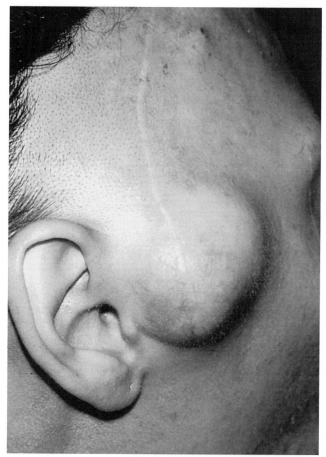

Figure 54–4 Extraneural metastasis of oligodendroglioma. Patient had undergone resection of an oligodendroglioma several months earlier. The mass beneath the craniotomy scar was histologically identical to the primary intracranial oligodendroglioma and likely represented implantation at surgery. This kind of local metastasis may precede further systemic metastases from intracranial gliomas.

the frequency of metastases from gliomas, with and without surgical intervention, will likely never be known.

A few cases have been reported of metastases from gliomas in the absence of surgery. Extraneural metastasis of astrocytic tumors in the absence of prior surgery are reported more frequently than are nonsurgical extraneural metastases from other gliomas.[78, 79, 88–92] Pasquier and colleagues[79] reviewed the available literature in 1980 and reported a total of 72 cases of extraneural metastases of astrocytic tumors, only 8 (11%) of which occurred prior to surgery. These studies show that extraneural spread of astrocytic tumors is infrequent, and that astrocytic metastases in the absence of surgery are rarer still. Table 54–2 summarizes the reported cases of extraneural metastases of astrocytic tumors in the absence of surgery, and Figure 54–5 presents these data as a bar graph. Bone marrow involvement is the most frequent site of extraneural metastases of astrocytic tumors in the absence of surgery and was present in six out of 12 (50%) of the reported cases. Bone marrow involvement was thus more frequent in the nonsurgical cases than in the review of extraneural metastases reported by Pasquier and others,[79] which found bone marrow involvement in only 30.5% of all patients with extraneural metastases. This may indicate that

gliomas spread to the systemic circulation via hematogenous routes in the absence of surgery, whereas surgery promotes lymphatic metastases.

At least one case has been reported of extraneural metastasis of ependymoma prior to surgery, in which a patient had a lung mass on chest x-ray at presentation that was later histologically confirmed as metastatic ependymoma.[84] The primary tumor was located extradurally in this case. Ependymoblastomas are rare tumors with a high frequency of leptomeningeal dissemination. Mork and Rubinstein[34] found only one case of extraneural metastasis (to lung) out of 12 reported cases of ependymoblastoma, and this metastasis was present at diagnosis, prior to any surgery.

Brander and Turner[78] reported a case of pleural metastases from an oligodendroglioma in the absence of surgery. The patient had much longer survival (13 years) than patients with astrocytic tumors. The metastases were discovered only at autopsy. This is the only reported case of oligodendroglioma with extraneural metastases in the absence of surgery.[78]

The Role of Ventriculosystemic Shunts in Extraneural Metastases

The role of ventriculosystemic shunts in systemic metastasis of gliomas is controversial. In 1989, Lovell and co-workers[93] showed that even "normal" glial elements could transfer to the peritoneal cavity following VP shunt. The first report of glioma metastasis via ventricular shunt was reported by Wolf and others[94] in 1954. In the literature review by Pasquier and colleagues,[79] systemic metastases developed after ventriculosystemic shunt placement in eight patients out of 72 with extraneural metastases. The distribution of the systemic metastases suggests a role for dissemination via shunt, because in many of the post-shunt cases, metastases were located in the same body cavity into which the shunt drained.[79] The data are difficult to interpret, because the number of patients with astrocytic tumors and shunt placement in whom extraneural metastases did not develop is unknown. Newton and associates[95] reported two cases of peritoneal metastases from intracranial glioblastomas following vetriculoperitoneal shunting. Other studies have found a similar predilection of systemic metastases of gliomas for the body cavities into which ventricular shunts drain.[94, 96, 97, 80]

A study by Berger and co-workers[98] asserts that shunt placement does not increase the likelihood of systemic metastases from intracranial tumors in pediatric patients. The authors found that systemic metastases from CNS tumors were as likely to occur in patients who did not have shunting procedures as they were in patients with shunts. In the eight patients who had CNS tumors with extraneural metastases, three had ventriculosystemic shunts and five did not. The role of vetriculoperitoneal shunting was nevertheless confirmed in at least one case, in which ascites developed from gliomatosis peritonei while the patient had a ventriculoperitoneal shunt in place, and the patient had no other metastases. The majority of the tumors in this series were medulloblastomas, and all the cases of extraneural metastases were medulloblastomas, so these data may not be applicable to gliomas.

Filter placement in ventriculosystemic shunts may prevent the spread of intracranial tumors, based on data derived from studies on medulloblastomas. Hoffman and Duffner[80] found

TABLE 54–2
SITES OF EXTRANEURAL METASTASES OF ASTROCYTIC TUMORS IN THE ABSENCE OF SURGERY

Study (Year)	Tumor Type	Sites of Metastases					
		Bone Marrow	Lung/ Pleura	Lymph Nodes	Liver	Retroperitoneum	Heart
Gropp (1955)[111]	Glioblastoma, monstrocellular	—	—	—	—	—	1
Bogdanovich (1958)[112]	Spongioblastoma multiforme	—	1	—	—	—	—
Rubinstein (1967)[113]	Malignant astrocytoma	1	—	1	—	1	—
Anzil (1970)[86]	Glioblastoma	1	—	—	1	—	—
Dolman (1974)[88]	Glioblastoma	—	—	1	—	—	—
Brander & Turner (1975)[78]	Mixed astrocytoma-oligodendroglioma	—	1	—	—	—	—
Hulbanni & Goodman (1976)[89]	Glioblastoma	1	1	1	—	—	—
Russell & Rubinstein (1977)[114]	Glioblastoma	—	1	1	—	—	—
Choi et al (1981)[90]	Astrocytoma	1	—	—	—	—	—
Pasquier (1986)[115]	Glioma	1	—	—	—	—	—
Leifer et al (1989)[91]	Glioblastoma	—	—	—	1	—	—
Gamis et al (1990)[92]	Glioblastoma	1	—	—	—	—	—
Total (12 studies)		6	4	4	2	1	1

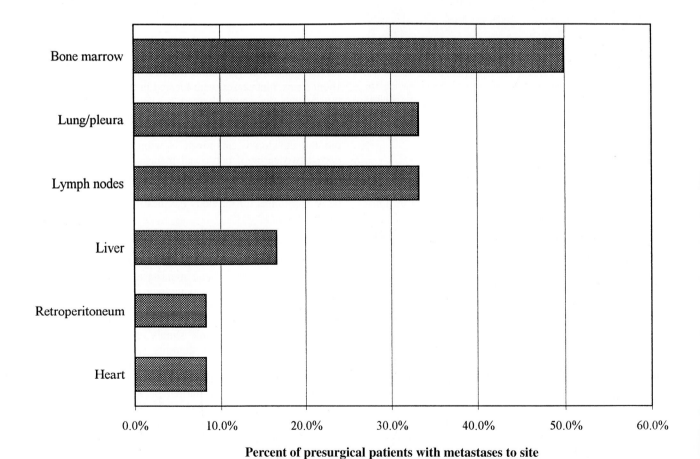

Percent of presurgical patients with metastases to site

Figure 54–5 Sites of extraneural metastases of astrocytic tumors in the absence of surgery. A few cases of extraneural metastases of astrocytic tumors have been reported in patients who did not undergo craniotomy or biopsy of the primary lesion. This bar graph summarizes data from 12 studies reporting patients with astrocytic tumors and extraneural metastases in the absence of surgery. (Data from references 78, 79, 86, 88–92, and 111–114.)

extraneural metastases in one out of 24 patients (4.2%) with ventriculosystemic shunts with filters vs. five out of 25 patients (20%) without filters. They strongly favor the avoidance of shunting when possible and the use of filters when shunts are placed.[80] Unfortunately, ventriculosystemic shunts with filters in place malfunction and require replacement more often than shunts without filters, and even with shunts in place, few glioma patients experience metastases, so the advisability of universal filter usage in ventriculosystemic shunts in glioma patients is uncertain.

Effects of Extraneural Metastases on Survival

The direct effect of extraneural metastases of gliomas on patient survival is usually minimal, but the detection of extraneural metastases predicts short survival. In the review by Liwnicz and Rubenstein[66] of reported cases of extraneural dissemination of gliomas, all of the patients succumbed to progression of the primary tumor rather than to extraneural metastases.

Scattered reports have appeared of prolonged survival despite extraneural metastases of a primary glioma. An exceptional patient with disseminated glioblastoma had a survival of 20 years.[50] Campbell reported a patient with low-grade astrocytoma and extraneural metastases who survived at least 7.5 years.[70] Patients with extraneural metastases from low-grade ependymomas can also have prolonged survival. One patient with an ependymoma originating in the cauda equina developed pulmonary metastases after 32 years and survived at least 1 year following detection of the metastases.[33] Despite these optimistic examples, the majority of patients with extraneural metastases from gliomas die within 12 months.

TREATMENT OF GLIOMA METASTASES

The treatment of neuraxis metastases of intracranial gliomas has not been uniform, and reported cases or trials have always consisted of very few patients. This makes analysis of the effectiveness of radiation therapy and various modes of chemotherapy problematic. Several studies report improvement in symptoms in patients with leptomeningeal or systemic gliomatous metastases with chemotherapy or radiotherapy, but effects on patient survival have generally been minimal.

Treatment of Leptomeningeal Glioma Metastases

CHEMOTHERAPY

Chemotherapy has been of benefit in some patients with gliomatous leptomeningeal metastases. Grant and co-workers[16] treated a series of patients with meningeal gliomatosis with a variety of chemotherapeutic regimens and found that patients with leptomeningeal dissemination of anaplastic astrocytoma had temporary clinical improvement after treat-ment with intrathecal methotrexate. Another patient had prolonged survival when treated with intrathecal methotrexate followed by intrathecal cytosine arabinoside. This patient survived at least 175 weeks. A single patient with neuraxis dissemination of oligodendroglioma improved with intravenous carmustine and craniospinal radiation therapy. Chemotherapy was not effective when the primary tumor was a glioblastoma.[16] Kandt and others[18] reported that symptoms of leptomeningeal dissemination improved in five of six patients treated with intrathecal methotrexate, intrathecal thiotepa, systemic cisplatin, or craniospinal radiation therapy. In the pediatric series of Kellie and co-workers,[99] three patients with leptomeningeal spread of astrocytic tumors were treated with cisplatin and etoposide, and two had stable disease, whereas one patient had complete response of leptomeningeal disease but no change in the primary tumor. Thus, chemotherapy of various types can be useful in the management of leptomeningeal spread of gliomas, but the optimum regimen and delivery route remain uncertain.

RADIATION THERAPY

Radiation therapy of localized neuraxis metastases of systemic tumors and gliomas is often used in patients with local spinal cord compression or pain. Dropcho and colleagues[42] reported improvement in three out of seven patients with intraspinal malignant glioma metastases treated with local radiation therapy. Vertosick and Selker[9] found that radiation therapy improved local pain caused by leptomeningeal metastases of supratentorial glioblastomas, but produced no improvement in neurologic symptoms or signs. In fact, two patients developed radiation-induced esophagitis that decreased their quality of life.

Radiation therapy is also helpful in preventing leptomeningeal metastases from gliomas. Craniospinal irradiation is recommended for infratentorial high-grade astrocytomas in children,[100] and for the rare ependymoblastoma, regardless of location.[34] The need for craniospinal irradiation in ependymomas is less certain. Goldwein and associates[101, 102] studied craniospinal radiation therapy in malignant ependymoma. Age and dose of radiotherapy were the most important prognostic factors. Patients younger than 4 years at diagnosis had a 2-year survival rate of 20% vs. 83% for older children. Patients receiving 4,500 cGy or more had a survival rate of 55% at 2 years as opposed to a survival rate of 0% for patients receiving less than 4,500 cGy. Local relapse was still the most frequent site of relapse and cause of death. Similar prognostic factors were found in ependymomas in general.[103] Kim and Fayos[41] believe that craniospinal radiation therapy is necessary for infratentorial or high-grade ependymomas.

Treatment of Extraneural Metastases of Gliomas

Extraneural metastases of gliomas have been treated systemically with chemotherapy and locally with radiation therapy when they cause symptoms. It has been suggested that chemotherapy that does not affect primary brain tumors may be useful in the treatment of systemic metastases.[74] Theoretically, extraneural metastases might be more sensitive to chemotherapy once they have escaped the confines of the CNS and the blood-brain barrier. Unfortunately, the available literature does not suggest a dramatic response of extraneural metastases to usual chemotherapeutic regimens.

Hoffman and Duffner[80] report improvement in local pain for patients with gliomatous bony metastases treated with chemotherapy that did not affect the primary tumors. Newton and colleagues[95] reported eradication of ascites with intraperitoneal cisplatin in a patient with intraperitoneal metastases of glioblastoma. Pang and Ashmead[68] treated an extraneural metastasis from glioblastoma with vincristine, cyclophosphamide, and dacarbazine with resolution of local pain. The patient of Vagaiwala and others[84] who had extraspinal ependymoma and lung metastases did not improve with cyclophosphamide, vincristine, papaverine, hydroxyurea, cytosine arabinoside, or high-dose methotrexate with leucovorin rescue.

Radiotherapy can also be useful when extraneural metastases of gliomas cause pain. Sadik and co-workers[69] found improvement in bone pain when radiation therapy was used on a vertebral bone metastasis of glioblastoma multiforme. Thus chemotherapy and local radiotherapy can provide some symptomatic relief for patients with extraneural metastases of intracranial gliomas, but complete remission is very unlikely. The best therapy for gliomatous metastases will be effective therapy for primary gliomas, which prevents metastases altogether.

Future Options for Treatment

More aggressive therapeutic options for recurrent or disseminated gliomas are under study. The small numbers of patients with leptomeningeal or extraneural spread makes the effectiveness of any therapy difficult to ascertain. Possibilities for treatment in the future include newer forms of chemotherapy and immunomodulating agents, such as interleukin 2.

One interesting possibility involves gene therapy. A model for neuraxis dissemination of glioma in the rat has been developed, and this may allow trials of chemotherapeutic and genetic therapy regimens for gliomas.[104–106] A mouse model has been developed in which targeted viral vectors are used to deliver genetic material to glioma cells.[107] Some genetic changes have been found to be frequent in gliomas, and these changes may provide a target for future genetic manipulations of both primary gliomas and their disseminated metastases. The development of appropriate and safe vectors and the selection of genetic targets are ongoing, although they are years away from any practical application.

CONCLUSIONS

Neuraxis and extraneural metastases are a rare but well-described complication of gliomas. Most cases of metastases from gliomas have been from astrocytic neoplasms. Ependymomas and oligodendrogliomas may produce metastases slightly more frequently than astrocytic tumors. Within a given glioma type, histologic grade has a strong influence on the tendency to form metastases, with high-grade tumors

disseminating more often than low-grade tumors. Treatment of metastases of gliomas remains as problematic as the treatment of gliomas themselves. Chemotherapy and radiation therapy provide some palliation of symptoms, but they give little lasting benefit. The best therapy for glioma metastases will be better control of gliomas at the sites of origin.

REFERENCES

1. Bailey P, Cushing H: A Classification of Tumors of the Glioma Group on a Histogenic Basis with a Correlated Study of Prognosis. Philadelphia, JB Lippincott, 1926, p 114.
2. Weiss L: A metastasizing ependymoma of the cauda equina. Cancer 1955; 8:161.
3. Sunita IM, Kapila K, Singhal RM, et al: Extracranial metastasis of an astrocytoma detected by fine-needle aspiration: A case report. Diagn Cytopathol 1991; 7:290.
4. Yung WKA, Tepper SJ, Young DF: Diffuse bone marrow metastasis by glioblastoma: Premortem diagnosis by peroxidase-antiperoxidase staining for glial fibrillary acidic protein. Ann Neurol 1983; 14:581.
5. Erlich SS, Davis RL: Spinal subarachnoid metastasis from primary intracranial glioblastoma multiforme. Cancer 1978; 42:2854.
6. Onda K, Tanaka R, Takahashi H, et al: Cerebral glioblastoma with cerebrospinal fluid dissemination: A clinicopathological study of 14 cases examined by complete autopsy. Neurosurgery 1989; 25:533.
7. Yung WKA, Horten BC, Shapiro WR: Meningeal gliomatosis: A review of 12 cases. Ann Neurol 1980; 8:605.
8. Balhuizen JC, Bots GTAM, Schaberg A, et al: Value of cerebrospinal fluid cytology for the diagnosis of malignancies in the central nervous system. J Neurosurg 1978; 48:747.
9. Vertosick FT, Selker RG: Brain stem and spinal metastases of supratentorial glioblastoma multiforme: A clinical series. Neurosurgery 1990; 27:516.
10. Awad I, Bay JW, Rogers L: Leptomeningeal metastasis from supratentorial malignant gliomas. Neurosurgery 1986; 19:247.
11. Delattre JY, Walker RW, Rosenblum MK: Leptomeningeal gliomatosis with spinal cord or cauda equina compression: A complication of supratentorial gliomas in adults. Acta Neurol Scand 1989; 79:133.
12. Choucair AK, Levin VA, Gutin PH, et al: Development of multiple lesions during radiation therapy and chemotherapy in patients with gliomas. J Neurosurg 1986; 65:654.
13. Kramer ED, Rafto S, Packer RJ, et al: Comparison of myelography with CT follow-up versus gadolinium MRI for subarachnoid metastatic disease in children. Neurology 1991; 41:46.
14. Weschler LR, Gross RA, Miller DC: Meningeal gliomatosis with ''negative'' CSF cytology: The value of GFAP staining. Neurology 1984; 34:1611.
15. Rippe DJ, Boyko OB, Fuller GN, et al: Gadopentetate-dimeglumine-enhanced MR imaging of gliomatosis cerebri: Appearance mimicking leptomeningeal tumor dissemination. Am J Neuroradiol 1990; 11:800.
16. Grant R, Naylor B, Junck L, et al: Clinical outcome in aggressively treated meningeal gliomatosis. Neurology 1992; 42:252.
17. Grabb PA, Albright AL, Pang D: Dissemination of supratentorial malignant gliomas via the cerebrospinal fluid in children. Neurosurgery 1992; 30:64.
18. Kandt RS, Shinnar S, D'Souza BJ, et al: Cerebrospinal metastases in malignant childhood astrocytomas. J Neurooncol 1984; 2:123.
19. Bryan P: CSF seeding of intra-cranial tumours: A study of 96 cases. Clin Radiol 1974; 25:355.
20. Polmeteer FE, Kernohan JW: Meningeal gliomatosis: A study of forty-two cases. Arch Neurol Psychiatry 1947; 57:583.
21. Shapiro K, Shulman K: Spinal cord seeding from cerebellar astrocytomas. Childs Brain 1976; 2:177.
22. Rutka JT, George RE, Davidson G, et al: Low-grade astrocytoma of the tectal region as an unusual cause of knee pain: Case report. Neurosurgery 1991; 29:608.
23. Obana WG, Cogen PH, Davis RL, et al: Metastatic juvenile pilocytic astrocytoma: Case report. J Neurosurg 1991; 75:972.
24. Mishima K, Nakamura M, Nakamura H, et al: Leptomeningeal dissemination of cerebellar pilocytic astrocytoma: Case report. J Neurosurg 1992; 77:788.

25. Kocks W, Kalff R, Reinhardt V, et al: Spinal metastasis of pilocytic astrocytoma of the chiasma opticum. Childs Nerv Syst 1989; 5:118.
26. McLaughlin JE: Juvenile astrocytomas with subarachnoid spread. J Pathol 1976; 118:101.
27. Bloom HJG: Intracranial tumors: Response and resistance to therapeutic endeavors, 1970–1980. Int J Radiat Oncol Biol Phys 1982; 8:1083.
28. Svien HJ, Gates EM, Kernohan JW: Spinal subarachnoid implantation associated with ependymoma. Arch Neurol Psychiatry 1949; 62:847.
29. Salazar OM, Rubin P, Bassano D, et al: Improved survival of patients with intracranial ependymomas by irradiation: Dose selection and field extension. Cancer 1975; 35:1563.
30. Salazar OM: A better understanding of CNS seeding and a brighter outlook for postoperatively irradiated patients with ependymomas. Int J Radiat Oncol Biol Phys 1983; 9:1231.
31. Lyons MK, Kelly PJ: Posterior fossa ependymomas: Report of 30 cases and review of the literature. Neurosurgery 1991; 28:659.
32. Rawlings CE III, Giangaspero F, Burger PC, et al: Ependymomas: A clinicopathologic study. Surg Neurol 1988; 29:271.
33. Mavroudis C, Townsend JJ, Wilson CB: A metastasizing ependymoma of the cauda equina: Case report. J Neurosurg 1977; 47:771.
34. Mork SJ, Rubinstein LJ: Ependymoblastoma: A reappraisal of a rare embryonal tumor. Cancer 1986; 55:1536.
35. Eade OE, Urich H: Metastasizing gliomas in young subjects. J Pathol 1971; 103:245.
36. Reggiani R, Solime F, Del Vivo RE, et al: Intracerebral oligodendroglioma with metastatic involvement of the spinal cord. J Neurosurg 1971; 35:610.
37. Nijjar TS, Simpson WJ, Gadella T, et al: Oligodendroglioma: The Princess Margaret Hospital experience (1958–1984). Cancer 1989; 71:4002.
38. Wacker MR, Cogen PH, Etzell JE, et al: Diffuse leptomeningeal involvement by a ganglioglioma in a child: Case report. J Neurosurg 1992; 77:302.
39. Bell WO, Packer RJ, Seigel KR, et al: Leptomeningeal spread of intramedullary spinal cord tumors: Report of three cases. J Neurosurg 1988; 65:295.
40. Packer RJ, Siegel KR, Sutton LN, et al: Leptomeningeal dissemination of primary central nervous system tumors of childhood. Ann Neurol 1985; 18:217.
41. Kim YH, Fayos JV: Intracranial ependymomas. Ther Radiol 1977; 124:805.
42. Dropcho EJ, Wisoff JH, Walker RW, et al: Supratentorial malignant gliomas in childhood: A review of 50 cases. Ann Neurol 1987; 22:355.
43. Ley A, Campillo D, Oliveras C: Extracranial metastasis of glioblastoma multiforme. J Neurosurg 1961; 18:313.
44. Willis RA: Pathology of Tumors, ed 2. London, Butterworth, 1953.
45. Willis RA: The Spread of Tumors in the Human Body, ed 2. London, Butterworth, 1952, p 101.
46. Winkelman NW Jr, Cassel C, Schlesinger B: Intracranial tumors with extracranial metastases. J Neuropathol Exp Neurol 1952; 11:149.
47. Peters A, Palay SL, Webster HF: The Fine Structure of the Nervous System: The Neurons and the Supporting Cells. Philadelphia, WB Saunders, 1976, p 295.
48. Pansera F, Pansera E: An explanation for the rarity of extraaxial metastases in brain tumors. Med Hypotheses 1992; 39:88.
49. Alvord EC: Why do gliomas not metastasize? Arch Neurol 1976; 33:73.
50. Hitchcock MH, Hollinshead AC, Chretien P, et al: Soluble membrane antigens of brain tumors: I. Controlled testing for cell mediated immune responses in a long surviving glioblastoma multiforme patient. Cancer 1977; 40:660.
51. Grace JT Jr, Perese DM, Metzger RS, et al: Tumor autograft responses in patients with glioblastoma multiforme. J Neurosurg 1961; 18:159.
52. Kung PC, Lee JC, Bakay L: Vascular invasion by glioma cells: An electron microscopic study. J Neurosurg 1969; 31:339.
53. Morley TP: The recovery of tumour cells from venous blood draining cerebral gliomas. Can J Surg 1959; 2:363.
54. Abbott KH, Love JG: Metastasizing intracranial tumors. Ann Surg 1943; 118:343.
55. Prineas JW: Multiple sclerosis: Presence of lymphatic capillaries and lymphoid tissue in the brain and spinal cord. Science 1979; 203:1123.
56. McComb JG: Recent research into the nature of cerebrospinal fluid formation and absorption. J Neurosurg 1983; 59:369.
57. Ohnishi T, Arita N, Hayakawa T, et al: Purification of motility factor (GMF) from human malignant glioma cells and its biological significance in tumor invasion. Biochem Biophys Res Comm 1993; 193:518.
58. Paulus W, Tonn JC: Basement membrane invasion of glioma cells mediated by integrin receptors. J Neurosurg 1994; 80:515.
59. Zimmerman HM: The natural history of intracranial neoplasms with special reference to gliomas. Am J Surg 1951; 93:913.
60. Vecht CJ, Van Zwieten MJ, Maat B, et al: Metastasis from the brain of transplanted N-ethyl-N-nitrosourea–induced central nervous system tumors in rats. Eur J Cancer 1981; 17:703.
61. Mitts MG, Walker AE: Autotransplantation of gliomas. J Neuropathol Exp Neurol 1964; 23:324.
62. Battista AF, Bloom W, Loffman M, et al: Autotransplantation of anaplastic astrocytoma into the subcutaneous tissue of man. Neurology 1961; 11:977.
63. Smith DR, Hardman JM, Earle KM: Metastasizing neuroectodermal tumors of the central nervous system. J Neurosurg 1969; 31:50.
64. Jackson AM, Graham DI: Remote metastases from intracranial tumours. J Clin Pathol 1978; 31:794.
65. El Gindi S, Salama M, El Henawy M, et al: Metastases of glioblastoma multiforme to cervical lymph nodes: Report of two cases. J Neurosurg 1973; 38:631.
66. Liwnicz BH, Rubinstein LJ: The pathways of extraneural spread in metastasizing gliomas: A report of three cases and critical review of the literature. Hum Pathol 1979; 10:453.
67. Dietz R, Burger L, Merkel K, et al: Malignant gliomas: Glioblastoma multiforme and astrocytoma III-IV with extracranial metastases: Report of two cases. Acta Neurochir 1981; 57:99.
68. Pang D, Ashmead JW: Extraneural metastasis of cerebellar glioblastoma multiforme. Neurosurgery 1982; 10:252.
69. Sadik AR, Port R, Garfinkel B, et al: Extracranial metastasis of cerebral glioblastoma multiforme: Case report. Neurosurgery 1984; 15:549.
70. Campbell AN, Chan HSL, Becker LE, et al: Extracranial metastases in childhood primary intracranial tumors: A report of 21 cases and review of the literature. Cancer 1984; 53:974.
71. Maass L: Occipital ependymoma with extracranial metastases. J Neurosurg 1954; 11:413.
72. Sherbaniuk RW, Shnitka TK: Metastasizing intracranial ependymoma. Am J Pathol 1956; 32:53.
73. Glasauer FE, Yuan RHP: Intracranial tumors with extracranial metastases: Case report and review of the literature. J Neurosurg 1963; 20:474.
74. Duffner PK, Cohen ME: Extraneural metastases in childhood brain tumors. Ann Neurol 1981; 10:261.
75. Wentworth P, Birdsell DC: Intracranial ependymoma with extracranial metastases: Case report. J Neurosurg 1966; 25:648.
76. James I, Pagel W: Oligodendroglioma with extracranial metastasis. Br J Surg 1951; 39:56.
77. Spataro J, Sacks O: Oligodendroglioma with remote metastases: Case report. J Neurosurg 1968; 28:373.
78. Brander WL, Turner DR: Extracranial metastases from a glioma in the absence of surgical intervention. J Neurol Neurosurg Psychiatry 1975; 38:1133.
79. Pasquier B, Pasquier D, N'Golet A, et al: Extraneural metastases of astrocytomas and glioblastomas: Clinicopathological study of two cases and review of literature. Cancer 1980; 45:112.
80. Hoffman HJ, Duffner PK: Extraneural metastases of central nervous system tumors. Cancer 1985; 56:1778.
81. Fragoyannis S, Yalgin S: Ependymomas with distant metastases: Report of two cases and review of the literature. Cancer 1966; 19:246.
82. Perry RE: Extracranial metastasis in a case of intracranial ependymoma. Arch Pathol 1957; 64:337.
83. Watt V: Ependymoma of the cauda equina with distant metastasis. J Neurosurg 1968; 29:424.
84. Vagaiwala MR, Robinson JS, Galicich JH, et al: Metastasizing extradural ependymoma of the sacrococcygeal region: Case report and review of literature. Cancer 1979; 44:326.
85. Wight DGD, Holley KJ, Finbow JAH: Metastasizing ependymoma of the cauda equina. J Clin Pathol 1973; 26:929.
86. Anzil AP: Glioblastoma multiforme with extracranial metastases in the absence of previous craniotomy: Case report. J Neurosurg 1970; 33:88.
87. O'Connor W, Challa V, Nelson O, et al: Extracranial metastases of

glioblastoma multiforme confirmed by electron microscopy. Surg Neurol 1977; 8:347.

88. Dolman CL: Lymph node metastasis as first manifestation of glioblastoma. J Neurosurg 1974; 41:607.

89. Hulbanni S, Goodman PA: Glioblastoma multiforme with extraneural metastases in the absence of previous surgery. Cancer 1976; 37:1577.

90. Choi BH, Holt JT, McDonald JV: Occult malignant astrocytoma of pons with extracranial metastasis to bone prior to craniotomy. Acta Neuropathol 1981; 54:269.

91. Leifer D, Moore T, Ukena T, et al: Multifocal glioblastoma with liver metastases in the absence of surgery. J Neurosurg 1989; 71:772.

92. Gamis AS, Egelhoff J, Roloson G, et al: Diffuse bony metastases at presentation in a child with glioblastoma multiforme. Cancer 1990; 66:180.

93. Lovell MA, Ross GW, Cooper PH: Gliomatosis peritonei associated with a ventriculoperitoneal shunt. Am J Clin Pathol 1989; 91:485.

94. Wolf A, Cower D, Stewart WB: Glioblastoma with extraneural metastasis by way of ventriculopleural anastomosis. Trans Am Neurol Assoc 1954; 79:140.

95. Newton HB, Rosenblum MK, Walker RW: Extraneural metastases of infratentorial glioblastoma multiforme to the peritoneal cavity. Cancer 1992; 69:2149.

96. Brust JCM, Moiel RH, Rosenberg RN: Glial tumor metastases through a ventriculopleural shunt: Resultant massive pleural effusion. Arch Neurol 1968; 18:649.

97. Wakamatsu T, Matsuo T, Kawano S, et al: Glioblastoma with extracranial metastasis through ventriculopleural shunt: Case report. J Neurosurg 1971; 34:697.

98. Berger MS, Baumeister B, Geyer JR, et al: The risks of metastases from shunting in children with primary central nervous system tumors. J Neurosurg 1991; 74:872.

99. Kellie SJ, Kovnar EH, Kun LE, et al: Neuraxis dissemination in pediatric brain tumors: Response to preirradiation chemotherapy. Cancer 1992; 69:1061.

100. Packer RJ, Allen J, Nielsen S, et al: Brainstem glioma: Clinical manifestations of meningeal gliomatosis. Ann Neurol 1983; 14:177.

101. Goldwein JW, Corn BW, Finlay JL, et al: Is craniospinal irradiation required to cure children with malignant (anaplastic) intracranial ependymomas? Cancer 1991; 67:2766.

102. Goldwein JW, Glauser TA, Packer RJ, et al: Recurrent intracranial ependymomas in children: Survival, patterns of failure, and prognostic factors. Cancer 1990; 66:557.

103. Goldwein JW, Leahy JM, Packer RJ, et al: Intracranial ependymomas in children. Int J Radiat Oncol Biol Phys 1990; 19:1497.

104. Rewers AB, Redgate ES, Deutsch M, et al: A new rat brain tumor model: Glioma disseminated via the cerebral spinal fluid pathways. J Neurooncol 1990; 8:213.

105. Yoshida T, Shimizu K, Ushio Y, et al: Development of experimental meningeal gliomatosis models in rats. J Neurosurg 1986; 65:503.

106. Yoshida TK, Shimizu K, Koulousakies A, et al: Intrathecal chemotherapy with ACNU in a meningeal gliomatosis rat model. J Neurosurg 1992; 77:778.

107. Yamada M, Shimizu K, Miyao Y, et al: Retrovirus-mediated gene transfer targeted to malignant glioma cells in murine brain. Jpn J Cancer Res 1992; 83:1244.

108. Dietrich PY, Aapro MS, Rieder A, et al: Primary diffuse leptomeningeal gliomatosis (PDLG): A neoplastic cause of chronic meningitis. J Neurooncol 1993; 15:275.

109. Vincent FM: Spinal leptomeningeal invasion from intracranial glioblastoma multiforme. Arch Phys Med Rehabil 1983; 64:34.

110. Civitello LA, Packer RJ, Rorke LB, et al: Leptomeningeal dissemination of low-grade gliomas in childhood. Neurology 1988; 38:562.

111. Gropp A: Uber ein metastasierendes "gliom". Z Krebsforsch 1955; 60:590.

112. Bogdanovich NK: Metastatic spreading of cerebral tumors. Arkh Patol 1958; 20:83.

113. Rubinstein LJ: Development of extracranial metastases from a malignant astrocytoma in the absence of previous craniotomy. J Neurosurg 1967; 26:542.

114. Russell DS, Rubinstein LJ: Pathology of Tumors of the Nervous System, ed 4. London, Edward Arnold, 1977, p 344.

115. Pasquier B, Keddari E, Pasquier D, et al: Micrométastase ostéomédullaire spontanée d'un gliome cérébral. Diagnostic immunohistochimique sur un prélèvement biopsique et revue de la littérature. Ann Pathol 1986; 6:130–136.

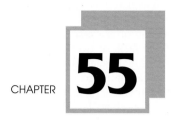

CHAPTER **55**

Management of Recurrent Gliomas

Renewed growth of a mass at the site of a previously treated brain glioma raises the issues of indications for and choices of treatment. Important considerations include the following: (1) is the mass a recurrence of the original tumor; (2) why did the tumor regrow; (3) what threat to the patient's neurologic function and survival does the regrowth pose; and (4) what additional therapy is appropriate?

CONFIRMATION OF RECURRENCE

When recurrent growth of a glioma is suspected clinically or radiographically, the full set of imaging studies should be reviewed with careful notice of change of imaging signals and documentation of lesion size. The original pathology specimen should be reviewed.

Differential Diagnosis

An enlarging lesion at the site of a previously treated glioma likely represents renewed growth of an incompletely eradicated initial tumor rather than the development of a new pathologic entity. Exceptions, as follows, are infrequent:

- A tumor of related histology may supplant the original tumor (e.g., the astrocytic component may replace the oligodendrocytic component as the predominant subtype of a mixed glioma, or a gliosarcoma may arise from a previously treated glioblastoma).
- A distinctly new tumor may arise near the site of an eradicated tumor. This is more likely if a genetic predisposition to tumor development exists that is shared by cells in the area (e.g., multiple gliomas in a patient with tuberous sclerosis or neurofibromatosis).
- Non-neoplastic lesions induced by treatment of the original tumor may mimic tumor growth (e.g., an abscess at the site of tumor resection or radiation necrosis following focal high-dose irradiation).

These alternative diagnoses must be excluded before prognosis is addressed and therapy chosen. Neurodiagnostic imaging usually permits accurate prediction of the diagnosis. Usually, recurrent gliomas have imaging features similar to those of the original lesion. A recurrent malignant glioma will likely have central low intensity, rim enhancement, and hypodense surround components on computed tomographic (CT) scans that are T1 hypointense–T2 hyperintense, rim enhancing, and T1 hypointense–T2 hyperintense, respectively, on magnetic resonance imaging (MRI).[8, 9] In some cases, however, attention to subtle differences may be required: a more spherical, sharply demarcated contrast-enhancing rim may suggest abscess rather than recurrent malignant glioma and a more diffuse, irregularly marginated pattern of surrounding edema may indicate radionecrosis rather than recurrent tumor. Two scenarios, descriptions of which follow, often pose particular diagnostic difficulty. In each case, alternative diagnoses are often unable to be distinguished by imaging criteria alone.

Malignant Progression

The first scenario is the renewed growth of a low-grade tumor. When low-grade gliomas regrow after therapy, approximately half remain non-anaplastic tumors, but the other 50% have progressed to a more malignant form.[29, 35, 45, 46, 69] Molecular analyses have delineated genetic correlates of this progression.[65] Enlarging low-grade tumors are likely to resemble the original tumor on imaging studies. When progression in grade has occurred, the new tumor may also resemble the old one, especially if the original tumor enhanced with contrast. Enhancement is highly predictive of recurrence; low-grade enhancing tumors are 6.8 times as likely to recur as are non-enhancing ones.[45] Most commonly, new malignant growth in a previously non-enhancing glioma enhances, and is thus readily identified. In one study, only 30% (16/42) of low-grade tumors enhanced initially, but 92% (22/24) enhanced at recurrence.[45] Occasionally, however, an enlarging malignant focus may not enhance. It might, however, be apparent as a region of hypermetabolism on a 2-deoxyglucose positron emission tomographic (PET) study or an area of increased cerebral blood volume on a functional MRI scan.[1, 19, 36] Usually, however, histologic analysis after biopsy or resection is warranted to verify malignant transformation.

Radiation Effects

The second scenario that causes diagnostic difficulty is renewed enlargement of a tumor mass following radiation. Often, CT and MRI inadequately distinguish recurrent tumor from radiation-induced necrosis. Radiation can cause tumor enlargement by an early reaction (which is likely to be edema occurring during or shortly after irradiation), by an early delayed reaction that involves edema and demyelination arising a few weeks to a few months after radiation, and by a late delayed reaction that occurs 6 to 24 months after radiation and reflects radiation-induced necrosis.[37] Only large, very malignant tumors grow sufficiently fast to show significant enlargement during, or within 3 months of completing, a course of radiation. In most cases, tumor enlargement from early or early delayed effects represents edema, is transient, and responds to a short course of corticosteroids. In contrast, radiation-induced necrosis appears at about the time malignant tumors might be expected to recur. It is thus more likely to be mistaken for recurrent tumor growth.

The risk of radiation necrosis increases with the volume treated, dose delivered, and fraction size.[44] Regional teletherapy to a dose of 60 Gy is the current standard radiation treatment for most gliomas.[66] It has a low risk of inducing radiation necrosis.[64] Radiation-induced changes following regional teletherapy are relatively diffuse. The CT and MRI enhancement is patchy and irregularly marginated. The low-density, T1 hypointense–T2 hyperintense regions of edema correspond to the area irradiated. Often, delayed late radiation change after regional teletherapy is distinguishable from the more focal appearance of recurrent tumor.

In contrast, radiation necrosis following focal radiation treatments, such as brachytherapy and radiosurgery, is more difficult to distinguish from recurrent tumor. These methods deliver high doses of radiation to relatively small volumes over a short period.[2, 43, 57] A common protocol for brachytherapy is a 60-Gy boost (to 60 Gy of regional external-beam radiotherapy) to a 0- to 5-cm tumor delivered over approximately 1 week. The radiosurgery equivalent is a 10- to 20-Gy boost to a 0- to 3-cm diameter tumor delivered in less than 1 hour.[41] Necrosis occurs in almost all cases. Radiographically, radiation-induced necrosis is a ring contrast–enhancing mass similar to a malignant tumor. It has a CT hypodense, T1 hypointense–T2 hyperintense center, an enhancing annular region, and a hypodense, T1 hypointense–T2 hyperintense surround. The surround corresponds to edema that strikingly conforms to the patterns of white matter tract radiations. The similarity of the appearance to that of recurrent tumors and the time course of its occurrence presents great difficulty in distinguishing radiation-induced necrosis from recurrent tumor. A variety of functional neurodiagnostic imaging techniques are currently being studied for their ability to distinguish between these two possibilities. These include PET scans, thallium studies, and cerebral blood volume mapping. Regions of high activity are thought to distinguish recurrent tumor from relatively metabolically inactive and hypovascular radiation necrosis.[1, 19, 36, 61]

In many cases, the data from these studies is inconclusive and the diagnosis is revealed either by the clinical course or by analysis of a pathology specimen. When an enlarging mass that is either recurrent tumor, radiation necrosis, or both, becomes symptomatic, corticosteroid therapy is required.[20] About half of patients who receive brachytherapy and radiosurgery develop symptoms that either prove refractory to corticosteroids or require debilitating long-term steroid use.[41–43, 57] Surgery for resection of an enlarging, symptomatic mass is needed in 20% to 40% of cases following brachytherapy or radiosurgery of a malignant glioma.[41–43, 57] At reoperation for presumed radiation necrosis following focal radiation treatment of a malignant glioma, necrosis was found in 59% of cases, tumor alone in 20%, and a mixture of radiation necrosis and tumor in 66%.[57] In almost all cases, the tumor that is seen is of reduced viability.[15, 54]

CAUSES OF RECURRENCE

Renewed growth of a brain glioma following surgery and, possibly, radiation and chemotherapy indicates failure of these therapies to reduce the tumor mass to a size that permits eradication by the patient's immune system (Fig. 55–1).[55–58] Failure arises from a number of factors that limit the efficacy of each modality.

Recurrence After Surgery

Surgery may fail because of anatomic considerations, pathologic features, or errors in judgment or technique. The involvement of critical structures may limit the initial resection. Tumor investment of the middle or anterior cerebral arteries; involvement of the optic pathway, the diencephalon, the internal capsule or brainstem; or proximity to eloquent cortex warrants incomplete removal. Tumor recurrence, despite removal of all macroscopically evident tumor, can occur if microscopic infiltration of adjacent structures occurs. Even low-grade cerebral gliomas are usually infiltrative, and microscopic foci of neoplastic cells are frequently found several centimeters from the densely cellular tumor. Anaplastic astrocytomas characteristically are widely invasive.

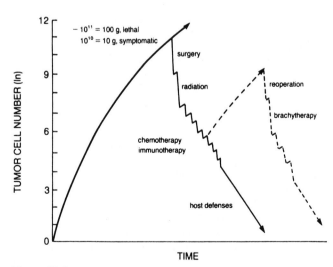

Figure 55–1 Multimodality therapy of malignant gliomas. Combined use of various therapeutic methods, including reoperation, attempts reduction of tumor cell number. (From Harsh GR IV: Surgical management of recurrent gliomas. *In* Schmidek HH, Sweet WH (eds): Operative Neurosurgical Techniques, ed 5. Philadelphia, WB Saunders, 1995, p 536.)

Finally, errors in judgment, such as preoperatively underestimating the amount of tumor that can be safely removed or intraoperatively failing to remove tumor that was targeted, result in leaving potentially resectable tumor as a nidus of regrowth.

Recurrence After Radiation

Radiation therapy may fail because of inadequate targeting, underutilization of tolerable dose, or radiation resistance of the tumor cells. The correlations between imaging abnormality and tumor extent are incomplete. Pathologic studies have shown that individual tumor cells can be found throughout and even beyond CT hypodense and MRI T2 hyperintense areas of malignant glioma.[9, 30] The choice of field size for irradiation of such a lesion is difficult and relies as much on the tradeoff between target volume and tolerable dose as on the accurate delineation of tumor boundaries. Failure to include an adequate annulus of tissue about the tumor to accommodate imaging uncertainty and technical error may leave tumor cells incompletely irradiated. Even if the maximal dose tolerated by infiltrative surrounding brain is delivered, tumor cells may remain viable. Hypoxic, nonproliferating cells are particularly radioresistant; with time or change in the physiologic conditions following therapy, re-entry of cells into the cell cycle permits the proliferation that results in clinically apparent tumor recurrence.[26]

Recurrence After Chemotherapy

Chemotherapy fails as a result of inadequate drug delivery, toxic effects, or cell resistance. The blood-brain barrier is deficient in the contrast-enhancing region of the tumor, but surrounding brain usually has an intact blood-brain barrier; lipid-insoluble drugs thus have limited access to tumor cells infiltrating peripheral regions. The margin between drug efficacy and neurotoxic effects, bone marrow suppression, pulmonary injury, and intestinal side effects is often narrow. Noncycling cells are resistant to cell cycle–specific drugs, and potentially vulnerable cells often rapidly develop biochemical means of resistance to chemotherapeutic agents.[26, 33]

Even if these therapies significantly reduce the tumor burden, the patient's immune response may be rendered ineffective by chemotherapy and by the tumor's secretion of factors antagonistic to immune cytokines.[32] Each of these limitations of each component of multimodality therapy may contribute to failure to prevent tumor regrowth. At the time of tumor recurrence, consideration of these reasons for failure is essential to assessment of prognosis and to the choice of subsequent therapy.

PROGNOSTIC IMPLICATIONS OF RESIDUAL AND RECURRENT TUMOR

In the management of a recurrent glioma, consideration of the prognostic implications of regrowth is essential. The presence of residual tumor and the occurrence of tumor regrowth likely have different prognostic implications.

Residual Tumor

Radiologic demonstration of residual tumor after initial treatment may be consistent with preoperative goals and expectations; the prognosis would be that originally formulated. If, however, residual tumor is identified unexpectedly, the prognosis may need to be altered. The prognostic import of residual tumor is best seen in the relationship between extent of resection and likelihood of tumor recurrence.

Cytoreductive surgery is a fundamental part of the treatment of most systemic malignancies.[17] In most cases, a strong relationship exists between the extent of resection and outcome. For gliomas, the relationship between extent of resection or, more significantly, size of residual tumor, and outcome measures, such as interval to tumor progression and survival, is less clear.

Correlation of survival with extent of resection for low-grade gliomas has been suggested by retrospective uncontrolled reviews and comparisons with historical controls.[35, 45, 63] One study of 461 adult patients with low-grade cerebral gliomas found that gross total surgical removal correlated with length of survival.[35] Another reported a median survival of 7.4 years following maximal surgical resection. The median survival of a subgroup of hemispheric tumors compared favorably (10 years vs. 8 years) with that of a comparable series treated in which treatment consisted of biopsy and radiation alone.[45, 63]

For high-grade gliomas, the correlations between the extent of resection at the initial operation and both the time to tumor recurrence and the duration of patient survival are disputed.[14] Historical reports and reviews of large series have noted the association of survival and extent of resection for both astrocytomas and oligodendrogliomas.[10, 27, 48, 60, 66] Extensive reviews of the literature, however, have failed to locate randomized, controlled clinical trials comparing survival after biopsy with that after radical resection of malignant gliomas.[47, 53] Nevertheless, the benefit of surgical cytoreduction has been strongly suggested:

1. Reviews of multicentered trials have shown that the more complete the resection, the longer the survival time.[58, 71]

2. In another study of 243 patients, multivariate regression analysis identified extent of resection as an important prognostic factor ($P<.0001$) for survival.[62]

3. Single-center studies have confirmed this relationship: in one study that included 21 patients with glioblastoma and 10 with anaplastic astrocytoma, median survival after gross total resection was 90 weeks vs. only 43 weeks following subtotal resection, and the 2-year survival rates were 19% and 0%, respectively, even though the two groups were well matched for other prognostically significant variables;[3, 13] in another study, patients who underwent a gross total resection of malignant glioma lived longer (76 vs. 19 weeks) than those who underwent only a biopsy, even after correction for tumor accessibility and all other prognostically significant variables.[70]

4. In two larger series, patients with resected cortical and subcortical grade IV gliomas lived longer (50.6 vs. 33.0 weeks[18] and 39.5 vs. 32.0 weeks)[34] after surgery and radiation than those who underwent biopsy and radiation.

5. Small postoperative tumor volume has been shown to

correlate with time to tumor progression after surgery[39] and with longer patient survival.[5]

Although less than ideal, the data which exist for gliomas and experience with tumors outside the central nervous system (CNS) suggest the benefit of cytoreduction when a near-total removal (1- to 2-log reduction of tumor cell number) of a glial tumor can be achieved. Thus, failure to identify and remove readily accessible tumor mass at an initial operation might warrant reoperation before regrowth occurs.

Recurrent Tumor

Regrowth of tumors after an initial response (diminution or stability) to surgery and radiation therapy is ominous. This is particularly true if the growth is more rapid or more infiltrative than that of the original tumor. Such growth often manifests changes in the basic biology of the tumor that make it less responsive to subsequent therapy. A short interval between initial treatment and recurrence of symptoms often indicates rapid regrowth and a poor prognosis. Factors to be considered in estimating prognosis include the biology of the tumor (its pathology, growth rate, and invasiveness), its resectability, its prior response to radiation and chemotherapy, and the age and performance status of the patient. Estimates of the recurrent tumor's size, growth rate, invasiveness, and location must be made in assessing its potential for causing both neurologic deficit and death. Reappearance of a slowly growing, well-demarcated frontal oligodendroglioma in a young patient of good neurologic condition after a 10-year interval of postsurgical quiescence clearly carries a much different prognosis than diffuse diencephalic spread of a glioblastoma multiforme in an elderly patient with a poor performance status 3 months after treatment with surgery, radiation, and chemotherapy.

THERAPY OF RECURRENT TUMORS

The choice of therapy of a recurrent glioma is based on a comparison of the natural history of the regrowing tumor with the risk/benefit calculus of potential therapies. Gliomas that recur warrant aggressive multimodality therapy if the patient is in acceptable neurologic and general medical condition and therapeutic options offer a realistic chance for significant palliation of neurologic status or extension of survival.[56]

Patterns of Recurrence

When gliomas recur, most do so locally. More than 80% of recurrent glioblastomas multiforme arise within 2 cm of the original margin of contrast-enhancing tumor.[25, 67] This tendency to recur locally is a function of tumor cell distribution. There is a gradient of tumor cell density in which tumor cell number decreases rapidly at increasing distances from the contrast-enhancing rim of solid tumor. Thus, although individual tumor cells are spread through the brain at great distances from the primary site, there are so many more cells locally that odds favor local reaccumulation of tumor mass.[8, 9, 30] Factors contributing to the likelihood of local recurrence include the following: (1) the relative predominance of tumor cell mass in the region; (2) the statistical likelihood that a local cell will be the cell that first develops a competitive proliferative advantage; and (3) the possibility that the physiologic milieu (hypervascularity, disrupted tissue architecture, and paracrine growth factor stimuli) at the site is particularly conducive to regrowth.

As tumor cell proliferation resumes at the initial tumor site, cells again spread rapidly and diffusely. Tumor cell proliferation resumes at distant sites as a result of the influx of these new, mitotically active cells or the renewed growth of cells that spread before the initial treatment.[12] Consequently, treatments targeting local recurrence alone will, at best, be briefly palliative. Treatment of tumor recurrences thus usually involves a combination of modalities aimed at both local and distant disease.

Multimodality Therapy

An enlarging lesion that was originally a low-grade glioma should undergo biopsy (stereotactically or, if resection is anatomically feasible, by open craniotomy) to confirm histology. If the tumor remains low grade and a majority of the lesion can be resected without inflicting significant neurologic deficit, it should be removed; if previously irradiated to less than maximal tolerable dose, the tumor bed and surrounding area should receive fractionated teletherapy. If the tumor is inaccessible to surgery, radiation alone should be prescribed. If a previously irradiated low-grade tumor recurs as a low-grade glioma, it should be resected, if possible. If inaccessible, stereotactically delivered focal radiation should be given.[50]

If the low-grade tumor recurs as a high-grade tumor or if a high-grade tumor recurs, reoperation should be attempted if the patient has a Karnofsky score of at least 70 and removal of all or almost all of the contrast-enhancing tumor is potentially attainable, or if the tumor mass is causing neurologic symptoms that might be palliated by its reduction. If previously unirradiated, the tumor bed and its annular margin should receive regional teletherapy; a stereotactically delivered focal boost of interstitial brachytherapy or radiosurgery should be given to any contrast-enhancing residual mass, particularly if the recurrent tumor is a glioblastoma.[2, 42, 57]

Brachytherapy has proven valuable in treating glioblastomas both initially and at the time of recurrence.[51] The median survival following brachytherapy was 49 weeks for recurrent glioblastomas but only 52 weeks for anaplastic astrocytomas.[57] Patients receiving brachytherapy were highly selected; only about 20% of recurrent tumors met the criteria of size and focality. Almost 10% of patients suffered severe acute toxic effects and approximately 40% required reoperation for medically refractory neurologic deterioration and intracranial mass effect. Although tumor was identified in 95% of the specimens harvested at reoperation, reoperation was associated with longer survival after brachytherapy (90 vs. 37 weeks for those not undergoing reoperation). The authors suggested that this morbidity was justified by the prolongation of survival achieved in patients with glioblastomas but not by that for those with anaplastic astrocytoma.[57] Stereotactic radiosurgery is a less invasive way of inducing tumor necrosis. Reported median survival following radiosurgery of recurrent glioblastomas is 40 weeks, and for recurrent anaplastic astrocytomas it is at least 16 months. Here, too, patients were highly selected and significant radiation injury was frequent (21% of cases).[2]

Chemotherapy of recurrent astrocytomas is often valuable. Low-grade tumors have generally not been treated by chemotherapy at the time of initial presentation unless a predominant oligodendrocytic component warranted PCV (procarbazine, CCNU [lomustine], vincristine) chemotherapy.[22] Adjuvant chemotherapy of malignant gliomas, in combination with radiation and surgery, increases the percentage of patients surviving at 1 year by 10% (a relative increase of 23.4%) and at 2 years by 8.6% (a 52.4% relative increase).[21, 59] For grade IV tumors, carmustine and PCV chemotherapy provide similar results, but the PCV combination is superior for grade III tumors.[21, 40] At the time of renewed growth of a high-grade tumor, if the tumor has not previously been exposed to a nitrosourea, carmustine or the PCV combination should be tried.[52] If nitrosourea therapy is unsuccessful, non-nitrosourea alternatives, such as carboplatin, cisplatin, or tamoxifen, might be appropriate. The

response rates (partial response or stable disease) to such chemotherapy at the time of recurrence range from 20% to 50%. In a recent study using intravenous carboplatin, a response occurred in 48% of patients (57% of patients with recurrent anaplastic astrocytomas and 40% of patients with glioblastomas multiforme); responders had a median time to tumor progression of 26 weeks compared to a median of 11 weeks for the entire group.[73]

Rationale for Reoperation

Early reoperation, within months of the initial procedure, might be indicated for complications such as intracerebral, subdural, or epidural hematoma, wound dehiscence and infection, or hydrocephalus and CSF leakage. Occasionally, failure to identify and remove readily accessible tumor mass might warrant reoperation. In the Royal Melbourne Hospital experience, five of 200 patients underwent early reoperation.[29]

More frequently, true tumor recurrence after an interval of response to the initial therapy is the reason for considering reoperation (Fig. 55–2). Reoperation is justified if it pro-

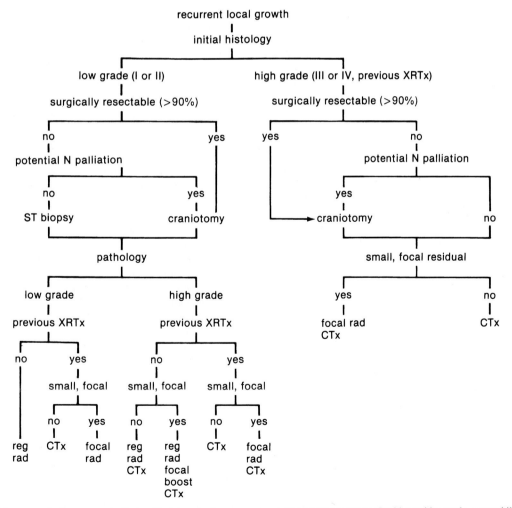

Figure 55–2 Management of a recurrent glioma. Decisions in the management of a recurrent tumor should consider grade, resectability, and previous therapy. Abbreviations: N, neurologic; reg rad, regional fractionated radiation therapy; focal rad/boost, stereotactic radiosurgery, brachytherapy, or radiotherapy; small, focal, <10 cm³, radiographically demarcated; CTx, chemotherapy. (From Harsh GR IV: Surgical management of recurrent gliomas. *In* Schmidek HH, Sweet WH (eds): Operative Neurosurgical Techniques, ed 5. Philadelphia, WB Saunders, 1995, p 540.)

duces sustained improvement of neurologic condition and quality of life and/or significant enhancement of response rates to adjuvant therapy. Palliation of neurologic symptoms by surgery results from reduction of the local mass effect produced by the tumor and tumor-induced edema.

Multiple studies have shown that primary surgical cytoreduction can both improve neurologic deficits and promote maintenance of high performance status. One review of 82 patients examined five categories of neurologic function in each patient. One hundred ninety-one neurologic deficits were noted preoperatively. Postoperatively, 151 deficits were improved or stable, and 40 were worse.[59] Another study showed that patients undergoing gross total resection of malignant gliomas were likely to have improved neurologic condition (on examination, 97% of 36 patients had either improved or stable neurologic findings), improved functional status (mean Karnofsky score improvement of 6.8%), and extended maintenance of good functional status (185 weeks).[3, 13] A third study confirmed that extent of surgery was correlated with better immediate postoperative performance, lower 1-month mortality rate, and longer survival: 43% of patients with malignant gliomas improved, 50% remained unchanged, and 7% suffered deterioration in neurologic condition following resection of at least 75% of the tumor; in contrast, the conditions of 28% improved, 51% were unchanged, and 21% were worse after a more limited resection.[62]

Similar results can be achieved by reoperation. Forty-five percent of patients in one series had an improved Karnofsky score following reoperation.[3, 64] In another reoperation series, when gross tumor resection was achieved, 82% of patients (32/39) had improvement or stability in their Karnofsky score.[68]

The doubling rate of malignant gliomas is so high, however, that the benefit from reoperation is very brief unless adjuvant therapies are able to induce remission of tumor growth. Surgical resection is especially beneficial when reduction of tumor burden improves the response rate to such therapies. Studies from the University of California at San Francisco (UCSF), Memorial Sloan-Kettering Cancer Center, New York, and the University of Washington at Seattle have shown that reoperation followed by chemotherapy leads to stabilization of performance score for significant intervals.[4, 7, 23] At UCSF, 44% of 39 patients with glioblastomas maintained a performance level of at least 70 (a level consistent with self-care and judged to be survival of high quality[28]) for at least 6 months after reoperation; 18% maintained this level for at least a year, and three patients did so for longer than 3 years (Fig. 55-3). Most patients with anaplastic astrocytomas (52% of 31) maintained this performance level for at least 12 months after reoperation; 13% had more than 4 years of high-quality survival. Approximately 90% of the survival after reoperation for anaplastic astrocytoma was of high quality.[23] In the Memorial Sloan-Kettering Cancer Center group, the median duration of maintenance of independent status (Karnofsky score of at least 80) was 34 weeks.[4] In the University of Washington series, patients with a Karnofsky score of at least 70 maintained this high level of function for an average of 37 weeks after reoperation for glioblastoma and for 70 weeks after reoperation for anaplastic astrocytoma.[7]

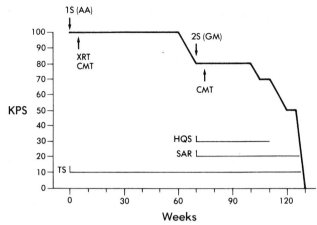

Figure 55–3 Quality-of-life considerations in the management of patients with malignant gliomas. Maintenance of high performance status is a critical feature of outcome. The Karnofsky score (KPS) as a function of time indicates the quality of the survival time that follows each intervention. Abbreviations: 1S, initial surgery; XRT, radiation therapy; CMT, chemotherapy; 2S, reoperation; TS, total survival; HQS, high-quality survival (K = ≥70); SAR, survival after reoperation; AA, anaplastic astrocytoma; GM, glioblastoma multiforme. (From Harsh GR IV: Surgical management of recurrent gliomas. *In* Schmidek HH, Sweet WH (eds): Operative Neurosurgical Techniques, ed 5. Philadelphia, WB Saunders, 1995, p 541.)

Aggressive surgical cytoreduction at the time of recurrence increases the duration as well as the quality of patient survival. Support for reoperation is found in comparisons of the outcomes in cases in which different degrees of tumor removal was accomplished and in comparisons of the survival of patients following reoperation with that of historical controls not receiving reoperation. Patients in whom gross total resection of a glioblastoma is achieved survive longer than do those receiving near total or subtotal resections (45.6 vs. 25.6 weeks); for anaplastic astrocytomas, the effect of extent of resection is similar (87.5 vs. 55.7 weeks).[7] In the Memorial Sloan-Kettering Cancer Center series that grouped glioblastomas and anaplastic astrocytomas together, a similar difference was found (51.2 vs. 23.3 weeks).[4] In the UCSF series, survival of patients undergoing reoperation and chemotherapy for either anaplastic astrocytoma or glioblastoma was longer than that of patients receiving chemotherapy alone at the time of tumor recurrence.[23]

The benefit of reoperative surgery is also suggested by experience with brachytherapy. Patients undergoing reoperation for tumor recurrence and/or radiation necrosis following brachytherapy for glioblastomas either initially or at first recurrence survived longer than those not undergoing reoperation: median total survival of 120 vs. 62 weeks for patients with primary treated tumors and 90 vs. 37 weeks for patients treated with brachytherapy at the time of first recurrence.[57]

Reoperation as a part of the multimodality treatment of recurrent gliomas is further supported by study of long-term survivors of glioblastoma multiforme. A review of the UCSF experience identified 22/449 patients (5%) with glioblastomas who survived at least 5 years after diagnosis. Sixteen of 22 had tumor recurrence that was treated; 9 underwent between one and three reoperations. For 8 of the 16 patients with treated recurrence, survival after treatment of recurrence (median, 4.5 years) was longer than the remission produced by the initial treatment.[11]

Selection of Patients for Reoperation

Case selection is critical to outcome. The patient's profile of prognostic factors, the patient's predicted tolerance for the procedure, and the feasibility of extensive tumor resection without undue risk of new neurologic morbidity must all be considered (Fig. 55–4). Multiple characteristics have been identified as predictive of a good response to reoperation (Table 55–1). Foremost among these are tumor histology, patient age, performance status, interoperative interval, and extent of resection.

The prognostic significance of tumor grade is evident in most series. Median survival after reoperation was 88 weeks for patients with anaplastic astrocytomas but only 36 weeks for those with glioblastomas at UCSF and 61 weeks and 29 weeks, respectively, at Memorial Sloan-Kettering Cancer Center.[4, 24]

The effect of age may overwhelm that of tumor grade. In one series, survival after reoperation was 57 weeks for those younger than 40 years but only 36 weeks for older patients.[56] Other authors found an association between youth and total survival after diagnosis and between youth and quality of

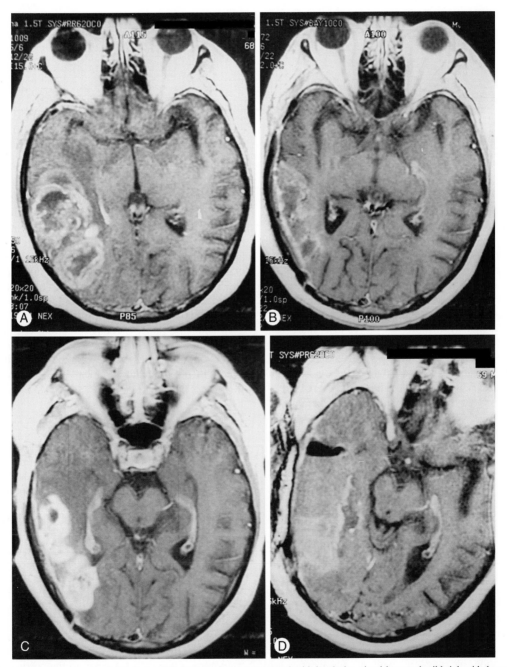

Figure 55–4   Reoperation for recurrent glioblastoma. This 68-year-old man presented with headache, visual loss, and mild right-sided weakness. A series of gadolinium-enhanced axial MR images show his initial right posterior temporal, inferior parietal tumor (*A*), the minimally enhancing tumor bed after craniotomy for resection (*B*), recurrent growth of his tumor six months following surgery and radiation therapy (*C*), and no residual contrast-enhancing tumor following reoperation (*D*). Four months after reoperation, he remains asymptomatic except for his original visual field loss. (From Harsh GR IV: Surgical management of recurrent gliomas. *In* Schmidek HH, Sweet WH (eds): Operative Neurosurgical Techniques, ed 5. Philadelphia, WB Saunders, 1995, p 539.)

TABLE 55–1
REOPERATION FOR RECURRENT GLIOMAS

Study	No. of Patients	Tumor Pathology	SAR	HQS	Morbidity*	Mortality*	↑K*	Complications*	Positive Relations	Weeks of Survival†
Young et al[72]	24	GM	14		52	17	25	25	K≥60→SAR	22 vs. 9
									II>12 mo→SAR	16.5 vs. 8.5
Salcman et al[56]	40	MG	37			0		8	Age<40 yr→SAR	57 vs. 36
Ammirati et al[4]	55	64% GM	36	34	16	1.4	45	18	K>70→SAR	48.5 vs. 19
									Grade→SAR	61 vs. 29
									Ext. resect.→SAR	51.2 vs. 23.3
Harsh[23]	49	GM	36	10	5.7	0	0		Age→SAR	
									K≥70→HQS	
Harsh[23]	21	AA	88	83	5.7	0	0		Age→HQS	
Berger[7]	56	GM	65	31	0	0	0	0	K≥70→SAR	70.7 vs. 36.5
									K≥70→SQE	36.6 vs. 8.4
									Age≤60 yr→SQE	35.1 vs 9.4
									II>12 mo→SAR	150 vs. 48
									II>12 mo→SQE	99.5 vs. 22.4
Berger[7]	14	AA	129	66	0	0	0	0		
Kaye[29]	50	GM			16	0		52	Age→SAR	
									Grade→SAR	
									II→SAR	
									Age→HQS	
									Grade→HQS	
									II→HQS	

*Expressed as a percentage.
†Mean, rather than median, values.
Abbreviations: GM, glioblastoma multiforme; MG, malignant glioma; AA, anaplastic astrocytoma; SAR, survival after resection; HQS, high-quality survival; ↑K, increased performance score; II, interoperative interval; Ext. resect., extent of resection; SQE, same quality of existence.
From Harsh GR IV: Surgical management of recurrent gliomas. In Schmidek HH, Sweet WH (eds): Operative Neurosurgical Techniques, ed 5. Philadelphia, WB Saunders, 1995, p 542.

survival after reoperation, but not between youth and duration of survival after reoperation.[4, 24]

Preoperative performance score significantly affects outcome. At the University of Kentucky, survival after reoperation was 22 weeks for patients with performance scores of at least 70 but only 9 weeks for more disabled patients.[72] In the University of Washington series, for glioblastomas, survival after reoperation was almost twice as long (71 vs. 36 weeks) for patients with Karnofsky scores of at least 70.[7]

The prognostic importance of the interval between initial treatment and recurrence is disputed.[69] The Kentucky series found survival to be twice as long if the interval between operations exceeded 6 months. In the University of Washington study, a threefold difference (150 vs. 48 weeks for glioblastoma and 164 vs. 52 weeks for anaplastic astrocytoma) was noted when the time to progression exceeded 3 years.[7] Others, however, have found either no relation or an inverse relation between the interoperative interval and survival after reoperation.[4, 24, 56]

A more complete resection of recurrent tumor portends longer survival. At Memorial Sloan-Kettering Cancer Center, gross total resection afforded a median survival of 51.2 weeks vs. 23.3 weeks for a more limited resection.[4, 68] Others have noted a strong trend in the correlation between a more complete removal of tumor and survival duration.[7] The ability to remove sufficient tumor mass to be of oncologic benefit depends on the location of the tumor and its physical characteristics. Removal is facilitated by a more superficial location in noneloquent areas; a discrete pseudoencapsulated mass is more easily removed than a less well-marginated diffuse mass; drainage of a cystic component often provides immediate reduction of mass, as well as an avenue for further resection of tumor.

During the interval between initial surgery and tumor recurrence, the patient usually undergoes therapy that might affect tolerance for surgery. The decision to reoperate must consider overall physical condition, tissue viability, blood coagulability, hematologic reserve, and immune function following surgery, radiation, corticosteroids, and chemotherapy. High risk of multisystem failure, failure to thrive, intracranial hemorrhage, anemia, wound infection, pneumonia, and neurologic damage may exist. This risk should be assessed for each patient by obtaining preoperative chemical, hematologic, and radiographic studies.

In choosing patients for reoperation, consideration of the individual patient's profile of these prognostically significant factors permits a reasonable estimate of the likelihood of the benefit of the procedure.

Preparation for Reoperation

Preoperatively the patient is likely to be receiving corticosteroids; these should be continued. At the time of induction of anesthesia, the patient is fitted with elastic stockings and thigh-high intermittent compression airboots. He is given additional steroids, prophylactic antibiotics, an anticonvulsant, and osmotic and loop diuretics and is hyperventilated. In positioning the patient, the likelihood of elevated intracranial pressure makes elevation of the head above the level of the heart particularly important.

Reoperative Exposure

In planning the needed exposure, the location of the tumor can be specified by its relationship to the margins of the craniotomy plate on a CT scan, to the cortical pattern of gyri and sulci on an MRI scan, or by intraoperative stereotactic localization techniques. The procedure should be planned in advance to ensure adequate skin opening, craniotomy, and durotomy to expose the recurrent mass. All may need enlarging because of the increased extent of the tumor or a desire to perform corticography for mapping of motor and/or speech function.

The previous skin incision is usually used. The skin opening can be increased by additional incisions. They should be external to the previous flap, avoid its base and other vascular pedicles, and intersect the previous incision at right angles. The margins of the previous craniotomy flap should be defined. Generally, this is best accomplished with a curet beginning at a prior trephination. Only rarely does the previous curf need to be recut. Dissection in the epidural plane can be begun with a curet followed by a No. 3 and then a No. 2 Penfield dissector. The craniotomy plate is further elevated as the dura is stripped from its inner surface with a periosteal elevator. Epidural adhesions fixing dura to the craniotomy margin should be preserved as prophylaxis against postoperative extension of an epidural fluid collection unless the craniotomy needs to be enlarged. In this case, these adhesions are dissected with a curet and trimmed. After the dura has been stripped from the undersurface of the cranial plate, an additional segment of bone can be removed with a craniotome.

The durotomy may need to be enlarged, but often it can be limited to part of the dural exposure. It should be planned to minimize traverse of cortical adhesions. For instance, in re-exposing a temporal lesion, the durotomy can be placed over the cyst remaining from the prior resection. Flapping the dura superiorly then allows adhesions to be put on traction such that they may be dissected from cortex, coagulated, and sharply divided. Extending a durotomy along an old incision line should be avoided. The prior incision line should be traversed perpendicularly and as infrequently as possible in that it is often the site of the densest adhesions. Microdissection of larger vessels from dural attachments may be necessary.

Once the dura is opened and retracted, the exposed cortex is inspected for the surface presentation of the tumor; its abnormal color, consistency, and vascularity should be apparent.

Localization of the subcortical extent of the tumor is then undertaken. Again, the preoperative imaging studies and stereotactic techniques are of value.[31] Transcortical ultrasonography is often helpful, although this technique tends to overestimate the volume of recurrent tumor.[38] Tumor may also be found by locating a cystic resection cavity or encephalomalacic brain left after the previous operation. In that almost all tumors recur within 2 cm of the original tumor margin, exposure of the surgical bed of the initial tumor usually reveals at least part of the recurrent mass.

Electrocorticographic mapping of motor, sensory, and speech areas may reduce the chance of inflicting neurologic deficit and may encourage a more extensive resection by revealing the relationship of the site of cortical traverse and of the subsequent subcortical dissection to eloquent brain.[6] This technique is often more difficult at the time of reoperation because of cortical disruption by the tumor and prior surgery. An intraoperative photograph from cortical mapping at the time of the initial craniotomy may suffice.

Generally, the appearance of the tumor itself is the best guide to its extent. Tumor-infiltrated cortex is likely to have increased vascular markings, a pink to gray color, and a firm consistency. Its central core may vary from yellow cystic fluid of low viscosity to high-viscosity, soupy white necrosis that resembles pus to a yellow-gray, granular, honeycomb-like material. Generally, the center is relatively avascular, although it may be traversed by thrombosed blood vessels.

Some authors advocate incision into the tumor mass and internal debulking with an ultrasonic aspirator or laser as an initial step. However, this often induces significant hemorrhage. Enucleation by circumferential dissection in the pseudoplane about the rim of solid tumor is usually more satisfactory. Arteries supplying the tumor and veins draining it can be coagulated and divided as they enter the tumor mass much as the vascular supply of an arteriovenous malformation is handled. Particularly in areas of noneloquent brain, the softened, necrotic, highly edematous white matter around the tumor provides an excellent plane of dissection. The use of bipolar cautery forceps and suction together accomplishes this dissection while reducing local mass. Beyond the encephalomalacic brain lies more normal brain that, although edematous and possibly injured by prior retraction and radiation therapy, is often functional and should be preserved.

Often, the tumor can be removed as a single specimen without the need for significant retraction of surrounding brain. In general, gentle, temporary displacement of a cottonoid patty lying on the margin of resection provides sufficient exposure of the dissection plane that fixed self-retaining retractors are unnecessary. Retraction of the tumor mass is preferable to retraction of surrounding brain. Often, identification of the appropriate plane for the circumferential dissection is facilitated by this retraction on the tumor; coherence of the tumor mass helps delineate the plane between solid tumor and tumor-infiltrated brain.

Once the tumor mass has been removed, the margins of resection should be inspected to verify completeness of the excision. The margins should be free of tumor that is more firm, glassy, opaque, and hypervascular. Biopsies of the surrounding edematous brain should be sent for frozen-section analysis to verify absence of tumor. If solid tumor or tumor infiltrating into non-eloquent areas remains, it should be removed. In some cases, extension of tumor into eloquent areas or diencephalic structures will preclude resection of the entire mass. In such cases, the tumor should be divided. This often entails coagulation of numerous strands of small, thin-walled blood vessels. This is particularly true if the extension is in the direction of the vascular supply (for example, extension of a temporal lobe tumor toward the sylvian fissure). Particular care should be taken to coagulate and sharply divide these vessels. Tearing them without prior coagulation leaves a loose end that retracts and continues to bleed. Such loose ends should be directly coagulated rather than tamponaded with hemostatic packing, which may encourage deeper dissection of a hematoma.

After the resection has been completed, hemostasis should be confirmed by filling the tumor cavity with saline and, during a Valsalva maneuver, observing for wisps of continuing hemorrhage. This should be performed with the patient's blood pressure at least as high as his normal pressure. The cavity is then aspirated, lined with a single layer of Surgicel, and filled again with irrigation fluid. Hyperventilation is then discontinued to permit expansion of the brain during closure.

Water-tight dural closure is essential. Often, this can be

attained by primary suturing, given the decompression from the operation. If the dura is incompetent, it may be supplemented by a pericranial graft. Peripheral and central dural tacking sutures are placed. The bone fragments are wired together, and then the craniotomy plate is fixed with either stainless steel wire or nonabsorbable monofilament suture. The wound is irrigated multiple times with antibiotic solution and then closed in layers with 2–0 absorbable suture in muscle, fascia, and galea. The galeal sutures should be inverted and the knots should be cut short to avoid erosion superficially. They should be placed in sufficient proximity that tension-free closure of the skin is possible. Simple running 4–0 nylon skin sutures provide adequate skin closure except at sites of attenuation, where horizontal mattress sutures may be less likely to compromise blood supply.

Postoperatively, the patient should be closely monitored for at least 72 hours for signs of increased intracranial pressure from hematoma or edema. Fluid restriction, dehydration, and corticosteroids should be continued throughout this period. The patient should be mobilized as soon as possible, and a gadolinium-enhanced MRI scan should be obtained as soon as it can be tolerated.

REFERENCES

1. Alavi JB, Alavi A, Chawluk J, et al: Positron emission tomography in patients with gliomas: A predictor of prognosis. Cancer 1988; 62:1074–1078.
2. Alexander EA, Loeffler JS: Radiosurgery using a modified linear accelerator. Neurosurg Clin North Am 1992; 3:174–176.
3. Ammirati M, Vick N, Liao Y, et al: Effect of the extent of surgical resection on survival and quality of life in patients with supratentorial glioblastomas and anaplastic astrocytomas. Neurosurgery 1987; 21:201–206.
4. Ammirati M, Galicich JH, Arbit B: Reoperation in the treatment of recurrent intracranial malignant gliomas. Neurosurgery 1987; 21:607–614.
5. Androeu J, George AE, Wise A, et al: CT prognostic criteria of survival after malignant glioma surgery. AJNR 1983; 4:488–490.
6. Berger MS, Ojemann GA, Lettich E: Neurophysiological monitoring during astrocytoma surgery. Neurosurg Clin North Am 1990; 1:65–80.
7. Berger MS, Tucker A, Spence A, et al: Reoperation for glioma. Clin Neurosurg 1992; 39:172–186.
8. Burger PC, Dubois PJ, Schold SC Jr, et al: Computerized tomography and pathologic studies of the untreated, quiescent, and recurrent glioblastoma multiforme. J Neurosurg 1983; 58:159–169.
9. Burger PC, Heinz ER, Shibata T, et al: Topographic anatomy and CT correlations in the untreated glioblastoma multiforme. J Neurosurg 1988; 68:698–704.
10. Chang CH, Horton J, Schoenfeld O, et al: Comparison of postoperative radiotherapy and combined postoperative radiotherapy and chemotherapy in the multidisciplinary management of malignant gliomas. Cancer 1983; 52:997–1007.
11. Chandler KL, Prados MD, Malec M, et al: Long-term survival in patients with glioblastoma multiforme. Neurosurgery 1993; 32:716–720.
12. Choucair AK, Levin VA, Gutin PH, et al: Development of multiple lesions during radiation therapy and chemotherapy in patients with gliomas. J Neurosurg 1986; 65:654–658.
13. Ciric I, Ammirati M, Vick N, et al: Supratentorial gliomas: Surgical considerations and immediate postoperative results; gross total resection versus partial resection. Neurosurgery 1989; 21:21–26.
14. Coffey RJ, Lunsford LD, Taylor FH: Survival after stereotactic biopsy of malignant gliomas. Neurosurgery 1988; 22:465–473.
15. Daumas-Duport C, Blond S, Vedrenee C, et al: Radiolesion versus recurrence: Bioptic data in 30 gliomas after interstitial implant or combined interstitial and external radiation treatment. Acta Neurochir 1984; 33(suppl):291–299.
16. Deutsch M, Green SB, Strike TA, et al: Results of a randomized trial comparing BCNU plus radiotherapy, streptozotocin, plus radiotherapy, BCNU plus hyperfractionated radiotherapy and BCNU following misonidazole plus radiotherapy in the postoperative treatment of malignant glioma. Int J Radiat Oncol Biol Phys 1989; 16:1389–1396.
17. Devita VT: The relationship between tumor mass and resistance to chemotherapy. Cancer 1983; 51:1209–1220.
18. Devaux BC, O'Fallon JR, Kelly PJ: Resection, biopsy, and survival in malignant gliomas: A retrospective study of clinical parameters, therapy, and outcome. J Neurosurg 1993; 78:767–775.
19. DiChiro G, Brooks R, Bairamian D, et al: Diagnostic and prognostic value of positron emission tomography using [18F]fluorodeoxyglucose in brain tumors. In Reivich M, Alavi A (ed): Positron Emission Tomography. New York, Alan R Liss, 1985, pp 291–309.
20. Edwards MS, Wilson CB: Treatment of radiation necrosis. In Gilbert HA, Kagan AR (eds): Radiation Damage to the Nervous System: A Delayed Therapeutic Hazard. New York, Raven Press, pp 120–143.
21. Fine HA, Dear KBG, Loeffler JS, et al: Meta-analysis of radiation therapy with and without adjuvant chemotherapy for malignant gliomas in adults. Cancer 1993; 71:2585–2597.
22. Glass J, Hochberg FH, Gruber ML, et al: The treatment of oligodendrogliomas and mixed oligodendroglioma-asrocytomas with PCV chemotherapy. J Neurosurg 1992; 76:741–745.
23. Harsh GR, Levin VA, Gutin PH, et al: Reoperation for recurrent glioblastoma and anaplastic astrocytoma. Neurosurgery 1987; 21:615–621.
24. Harsh GR, Wilson CB: Neuroepithelial tumors in adults. In Youmans JR (ed): Neurological Surgery. Philadelphia, WB Saunders, 1990, chap 107.
25. Hochberg FH, Pruitt A: Assumptions in the radiotherapy of glioblastoma. Neurology 1980; 30:409–411.
26. Hoshino TA: A commentary on the biology and growth kinetics of low-grade and high-grade gliomas. J Neurosurg 1984; 61:895–900.
27. Jelsma R, Bucy PC: Glioblastoma multiforme: Its treatment and some factors effecting survival. Arch Neurol 1969; 20:161–171.
28. Karnofsky D, Burchenal JH, Armistead GC Jr, et al: Triethylene melamine in the treatment of neoplastic disease. Arch Intern Med 1951; 87:477–516.
29. Kaye AH: Malignant brain tumors. In Rothenberg RE (ed): Reoperative Surgery. New York, McGraw-Hill, 1992, pp 51–76.
30. Kelly PJ, Daumas-Duport C, Scheithauer B, et al: Stereotactic histologic correlation of computed tomography and magnetic resonance imaging defined abnormalities in patients with glial neoplasma. Mayo Clin Proc 1987; 62:450–459.
31. Kelly PJ: Stereotactic biopsy and resection in thalamic astrocytomas. Neurosurgery 1989; 25:185–195.
32. Kikuchi K, Neuwelt EA: Presence of immunosuppressive factors in brain tumor cyst fluid. J Neurosurg 1983; 59:790–799.
33. Kornblith PL, Walker M: Chemotherapy of gliomas. J Neurosurg 1988; 68:1–17.
34. Kreth FW, Warnke PC, Scheremet R, et al: Surgical resection and radiation therapy in the treatment of glioblastoma multiforme. J Neurosurg 1993; 78:762–766.
35. Laws ER, Taylor WF, Clifton MB, et al: Neurosurgical management of low-grade astrocytoma of the cerebral hemispheres. J Neurosurg 1984; 61:665–673.
36. Le Bihan D, Douek M, Argyropoulou M, et al: Diffusion and perfusion magnetic resonance imaging in brain tumors. Top Magn Reson Imaging 1993; 5:25–31.
37. Leibel SA, Sheline GE: Radiation therapy for neoplasms of the brain. J Neurosurg 1987; 66:1–22.
38. LeRoux PD, Berger MS, Ojemann GA, et al: Correlation of intraoperative ultrasound tumor volumes and margins with preoperative computerized tomography scans. J Neurosurg 1989; 71:691–698.
39. Levin VA, Hoffman WF, Heilbron DC, et al: Prognostic significance of the pretreatment CT scan on time to progression for patients with malignant gliomas. J Neurosurg 1980; 52:642–647.
40. Levin VA, Silver P, Hannigan J, et al: Superiority of post radiotherapy adjuvant chemotherapy with CCNU, procarbozine, and vicriptine (PCV) over BCNU for anaplastic gliomas NCOG 6G 61 final report. Int J Radiat Oncol Biol Phys 1990; 18:321–324.
41. Li A, Shea WM, Wyn, et al: Radiosurgery as part of the initial management of patients with malignant glioma. J Clin Oncol 1992; 10:1379–1385.

42. Loeffler JS, Alexander E III, Hochberg FH, et al: Clinical patterns of failure following stereotactic interstitial irradiation for malignant gliomas. Int J Radiat Oncol Biol Phys 1990; 19:1455–1462.

43. Loeffler JS, Alexander E III, Wen PY, et al: Results of stereotactic brachytherapy used in the initial management of patients with glioblastoma. JNCI 1990; 82:1918–1921.

44. Marks JE, Boylan RJ, Prossal SC, et al: Cerebral radionecrosis: Incidence and risk in relation to dose, time, fractionation, and volume. Int J Radiat Oncol Biol Phys 1981; 7:243–252.

45. McCormich BM, Miller DC, Budzilovich GN, et al: Treatment and survival of low grade astrocytoma in adults, 1977–1988. Neurosurgery 1992; 31:636–642.

46. Muller W, Aftra D, Schroder R: Supratentorial recurrences of gliomas: Morphological studies in relation to time intervals with astrocytomas. Acta Neurochir (Wien) 1977; 37:75–91.

47. Nazzaro J, Neuwelt E: The role of surgery in the management of supratentorial intermediate and high-grade astrocytomas in adults. J Neurosurg 1990; 73:331–344.

48. Nelson DF, Nelson JS, Davis DR, et al: Survival and prognosis of patients with astrocytoma with atypical or anaplastic features. J Neurooncol 1985; 3:99–103.

49. Olmsted WW, McGee TP: Prognosis in meningiomas through evaluation of skull bone patterns. Radiology 1977; 123:375–377.

50. Ostertag CB: Biopsy and interstitial radiation therapy of cerebral gliomas. Ital J Neurol Sci 1983; 2(suppl):121–128.

51. Prados MB, Gutin PH, Phillips TL, et al: Interstitial brachytherapy for newly diagnosed patients with malignant gliomas: The UCSF experience. Int J Radiat Oncol Biol Phys 1992; 24:593–597.

52. Prados MB, Gutin PH, Phillips TL, et al: Highly anaplastic astrocytoma: A review of 357 patients treated between 1977 and 1989. Int J Radiat Oncol Biol Phys 1992; 23:3–8.

53. Quigley MR, Maroon JC: The relationship between survival and the extent of the resection in patients with supratentorial malignant gliomas. Neurosurgery 1991; 29:385–389.

54. Rosenblum ML, Chiu-Liu H, Davis RL, et al: Radiation necrosis versus tumor recurrence following interstitial brachytherapy: Utility of tissue culture studies. Proc Am Assoc Neurol Surg 1985; 53:264.

55. Salcman M, Kaplan RS, Samaras GM, et al: Aggressive multimodality therapy based on a multicompartmental model of glioblastoma. Surgery 1982; 92:250–259.

56. Salcman M, Kaplan RS, Durken TB, et al: Effect of age and reoperation on survival in the combined modality treatment of malignant astrocytomas. Neurosurgery 1982; 10:454–463.

57. Scharfen CD, Sneed PK, Wara WM, et al: High activity iodine-125 interstitial implant for gliomas. Int J Radiat Oncol Biol Phys 1992; 24:583–591.

58. Shapiro WR: Treatment of neuroectodermal brain tumors. Ann Neurol 1982; 12:231–237.

59. Shapiro WR, Green SB, Burger PL, et al: Randomized trial of three chemotherapeutic regimens in postoperative treatment of malignant glioma. J Neurosurg 1989; 71:1–9.

60. Shaw EG, Scheithauer BW, O'Fallon JR, et al: Oligodendrogliomas: The Mayo experience. J Neurosurg 1992; 76:428–434.

61. Valk PE, Budinger TF, Levin VA, et al: PET of malignant cerebral tumors after interstitial brachytherapy: Demonstration of metabolic activity and correlation with clinical outcome. J Neurosurg 1988; 69:830–838.

62. Vecht CJ, Avezaat CJ, van Patten WL, et al: The influence of the extent of surgery on the neurological function and survival in malignant glioma: A retro-operation analysis in 243 patients. J Neurol Neurosurg Psychiatry 1990; 53:466–471.

63. Vertosick FT, Selker RG, Arena VC: Survival of patients with well differentiated astrocytomas diagnosed in the era of computed tomography. Neurosurgery 1991; 28:496–501.

64. Vick NA, Coric IS, Eller TW, et al: Reoperation for malignant astrocytoma. Neurology 1989; 39:430–432.

65. Von Diemling A, Louis DM, Von Ammon K, et al: Subsets of glioblastoma multiforme defined by molecular genetic analysis. Brain Pathol 1993; 3:19–26.

66. Walker MD, Alexander E, Hunt WE, et al: Evaluation of BCNU and/or radiotherapy in the treatment of anaplastic gliomas. J Neurosurg 1978; 49:333–343.

67. Wallner KE, Galicich JH, Krol G, et al: Patterns of failure following treatment for glioblastoma multiforme and anaplastic astrocytoma. Int J Radiat Oncol Biol Phys 1989; 16:1405–1409.

68. Wallner KE, Galicich JH, Malkin MG: Inability of computed tomography appearance of recurrent malignant astrocytoma to predict survival following reoperation. J Clin Oncol 1989; 7:1492–1496.

69. Wilson CB: Reoperation for primary tumors. Semin Oncol 1975; 2:19–20.

70. Winger MJ, Macdonald DR, Cairncross JG: Supratentorial anaplastic gliomas in adults: The prognostic importance of extent of resection and prior low grade glioma. J Neurosurg 1989; 71:487–493.

71. Wood JR, Green SB, Shapiro WR: The prognostic importance of tumor size in malignant gliomas: A computed tomographic scan study by the Brain Tumor Cooperative Group. J Clin Oncol 1988; 6:338–343.

72. Young B, Oldfield EH, Markesberry WR, et al: Reoperation for glioblastoma. J Neurosurg 1981; 55:917–921.

73. Yung WKA, Mechtler L, Gleason MJ: Intravenous carboplatin for recurrent malignant glioma: A phase II study. J Clin Oncol 1991; 9:860–864.

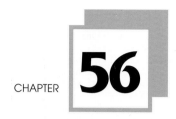

MITCHEL S. BERGER

CHARLES B. WILSON

CHAPTER **56**

Extent of Resection and Outcome for Cerebral Hemispheric Gliomas

Except in the management of intractable epilepsy or symptomatic mass effect, therapy for patients with low-grade glioma of the cerebral hemispheres is controversial. Technological advances in surgical equipment and neurosurgical technique permit resection of a maximum amount of tumor, even in eloquent areas of brain, without detriment to function.[1] Nonetheless, questions regarding efficacy, timing of surgery, and which patients are optimal candidates for radical resection have not been addressed.

RATIONALE FOR AGGRESSIVE RESECTION OF LOW-GRADE AND HIGH-GRADE GLIOMAS

Surgery is recommended in the treatment of low-grade gliomas on the basis that resection of the tumor gains a longer period of survival, improves the patient's quality of life, and delays tumor recurrence and malignant progression. In assessing the potential efficacy, the surgeon must also weigh the risks of radical surgery in the light of other therapeutic options. The reported incidence of surgical mortality and morbidity for low-grade gliomas has dropped dramatically over the years. Laws and co-workers[2] reported a drop in mortality rates from 16.2% to 4.9% to 1.9% from the periods before 1949, 1950–1969, and 1970–1975, respectively. Reported 30-day mortality for patients with low-grade astrocytoma treated since the introduction of computed tomography (CT) has ranged from 0% to 5%, with most being in the 2% to 3% range. Neurologic morbidity is not as well documented, but ranged from none[3] to 4%[4] in two studies; no differences in preoperative and postoperative clinical performance scores were noted in another study.[5] Unfortunately none of these studies evaluated mortality or morbidity relative to extent of resection.

Although it is generally believed that survival rates are higher for patients who undergo gross total resection of tumor than for those who have only biopsy, perhaps the conflict between clinical conscience and research principles accounts for there being no randomized controlled trial to assess the possible influence of extent of resection on recurrence patterns or survival. The well-designed prospective study would call for randomization of patients to conditions requiring different degrees of tumor resection and quantitative analysis of the volume of tumor removed at the time of surgery. Failing such a study, the role of cytoreductive surgery for low-grade gliomas is debated on the basis of retrospective studies of the effect of gross total, nearly total, and subtotal resection and on biopsy alone as determined qualitatively from postoperative CT scans or magnetic resonance imaging (MRI), on the measurement of the tumor's perpendicular diameter on contrast-enhanced images, or on the neurosurgeon's qualitative description in the operative report, which often is not correlated with postoperative imaging studies.[2, 6–8] Because of variability among studies in the definition of tumor, patient, and treatment factors and in the details reported—a drawback intrinsic to retrospective studies—it is difficult to interpret the results or to arrive at any valid determination of efficacy or effect of tumor resection on survival.[3, 9, 10]

The interpretation of surgical results is also confounded by empirical observations that many and diverse types of glial tumors initially diagnosed as low-grade glioma may recur in a histologically more malignant form.[2, 7, 8, 11–15] This transformation, called *de-differentiation* or *upgrading*, may be in part a result of histologic heterogeneity or simply the result of an error in tissue sampling at the time of initial diagnosis.[2, 3, 16, 17] However, a greater tendency toward early, malignant recurrence appears to exist when low-grade gliomas are managed with a conservative approach.[10]

Several investigators have retrospectively examined the relation of extent of resection to outcome. Initial studies showed lobectomy to be associated with longer survival times.[18, 19] Jelsma and Bucy[20, 21] were the first to report that patients who underwent extensive tumor resection had longer survival times. Although some investigators who based the estimated extent of resection on qualitative operative descriptions reported that patients undergoing less extensive resection are at no disadvantage,[22, 23] most reports suggest that this is not the case. Two later studies, done mainly to evaluate the efficacy of postoperative irradiation and chemotherapy,[24, 25] also showed that patients who had total tumor excision survived longer than those who had only biopsy. In treating patients with malignant gliomas, Levin and colleagues[26] observed that the time to tumor progression was longer for those in whom postoperative CT scans showed a smaller area of residual contrast enhancement, as did Andreou and associates.[27] Several more recent studies show a favorable influence on outcome with radical surgical resection in patients with a low-grade glioma, although, again, the estimated extent of resection was based on the surgeons' intraoperative observations as reflected in the operative report or on a qualitative assessment from postoperative CT scans without volumetric analysis.[2, 7, 11, 15, 28, 29] Wood and co-workers[30] reported a clear survival advantage for patients whose CT scans showed lesser amounts of residual tumor. Ammirati and associates,[31] based on contrast-enhanced CT scans, documented significantly longer survival with a good quality of life for patients who had gross total tumor resection. Most recently, in work based on volumetric analysis by using a computerized image analysis technique,[32] Rostomily and others[1, 33] reported that patients who underwent extensive resection had a significantly longer time to tumor progression and survival, and that the benefit of radical surgery was even greater for patients whose initial operation accomplished total resection.

Few studies have specifically addressed whether radical tumor resection increases the risk of neurologic morbidity. One group[31] reported that patients undergoing gross total tumor resection had a significantly increased Karnofsky performance status scores (KPS) postoperatively and that they continued to have a KPS of 80 or greater for a longer period than did patients who had undergone subtotal resection. In another study,[34] 41% of patients with supratentorial gliomas who underwent gross total tumor resection had an improved neurologic status immediately after surgery, and 55% had a stable clinical status. Rostomily and co-workers[1] reported a series of patients, most with a tumor in the dominant hemisphere, who underwent tumor resection with the aid of intraoperative stimulation mapping techniques. In that series, outcome in terms of improved postoperative KPS was significantly correlated with the percentage of resection ($P <$ 0.05) and volume of residual disease ($P <$ 0.05), but not with tumor volume before surgery. Patients who had no apparent residual disease had a slightly better postoperative KPS than did patients undergoing a less than total tumor resection.

Large malignant gliomas are often treated with cytoreductive surgery to alleviate the mass effect associated with symptoms and signs of increased intracranial pressure (ICP). Areas of necrosis are more responsive to surgical aspiration than is firm white matter infiltrated with low-grade glial tumor. A greater willingness to consider the radical approach to malignant gliomas does not imply, however, that surgeons believe the extent of resection always relates to increased survival. A retrospective study evaluating outcome after stereotactic biopsy showed that patients with glioblastoma and those with anaplastic astrocytoma both had a median survival time of less than 30 weeks. When patients with deep midline tumors were excluded, the median survival times improved to 47 weeks for patients with glioblastoma and 129 weeks for those with anaplastic astrocytoma. No statistical difference in outcome was noted between the patients undergoing biopsy and the few patients in the study who underwent aggressive cytoreductive surgery, but extent of resection was not discussed.[35] In another study,[36] patients with glioblastoma who underwent complete stereotactically guided resection survived 48 weeks, whereas those who had a biopsy or a standard craniotomy and resection survived for 30 and 38 weeks, respectively. Many cooperative prospective multimodality trials also show that subtotal and gross total resection provide a survival advantage as compared with biopsy only, and radiographic studies show an inverse relation between the postoperative tumor volume and survival.[26, 30]

Paired with the concept of extensive cytoreductive resection to positively influence outcome[24–26, 37] is the critical issue of the influence of surgery on the patient's quality of life. Biopsy and the removal of very small tumors can result in excessive morbidity from swelling or hemorrhage.[38, 39] In contrast, our and others' experience[31, 34] supports the notion that patients who undergo aggressive tumor removal are usually improved or remain unchanged neurologically. When aggressive cytoreductive resection is combined with current techniques for neurophysiologic cortical and subcortical mapping, the potential for creating permanent deficit should be less than 3% to 5%.[10]

Whereas the role of radical cytoreductive surgery for adults who have a malignant supratentorial glioma has been evaluated quite extensively, relatively few reports concern its role in children. The estimated incidence of cerebral hemispheric tumors in children is 6 to 8 cases per million children per year. These tumors are more common during the first year of life,[40–42] and their relative incidence is also higher after age 8 to 10 years.[43, 44] Although the reports on cytoreductive surgery in children do not relate how extent of resection was determined, they suggest that children who undergo radical resection survive longer than those who have only biopsy.[45, 46] A study from the Children's Cancer Group (CCG–945) that examined the relation of extent of resection to survival showed that the 3-year progression-free survival rate was significantly higher for children undergoing radical resection (50%) than for those who had less aggressive resections (28%).[47] The morbidity rate in this study was 14%, and most of the children benefited from reduced mass effect. Further study of pediatric series is needed to provide documentation on the relation between extent of resection and outcome.

The preponderance of the evidence supports the view that surgeons take an aggressive approach not only to glioblastomas, but also to other forms of glioma in the cerebral hemispheres.[48–50] When compared to a more limited tumor resection, radical tumor resection performed under the proper conditions and with proper technique usually preserves or improves a patient's functional status and affords survival for a longer period.[51–54]

TIMING OF SURGERY FOR LOW-GRADE GLIOMA

Views differ about the timing of surgery after documentation of a low-grade glioma with diagnostic imaging. Some surgeons recommend immediate intervention,[15, 17, 55] whereas others have suggested that patients with low-grade gliomas may be conservatively observed with serial CT or MRI; some even question the need for surgical intervention in treating low-grade glial tumors.[56, 57] Shibamoto and colleagues[58] reported a significant improvement in survival for patients with tumors smaller than 25 cm² who underwent surgery soon after diagnosis, as compared with patients for whom surgery is delayed. We, too, have found that patients who undergo surgery while the tumor is smaller are less at risk for early recurrence and malignant transformation.[3] Moreover, tumors that were less than 10 cm³ in volume when they were resected did not recur. In a retrospective study of patients whose lesions had a classic low-grade appearance on initial imaging study, Recht and others[57] found that of 58% of patients who did not have biopsy and treatment of a suspected low-grade glioma until the time of disease progression, all underwent surgery eventually (median interval, 29 months), and half of the removed tumors had anaplastic features. In contrast, of those patients who underwent surgery at the time of radiographic diagnosis, none had a malignant tumor. No difference in survival was apparent between the two groups, but the patients whose operation was delayed had a shorter time to tumor progression. Controversy will no doubt continue about the timing of surgery, but evidence appears to indicate a trend toward a greater risk of a more rapid and malignant recurrence with conservative management.

TECHNIQUES FOR RESECTION

Biopsy

Before the biopsy, a CT scan or MRI is obtained. An opening is made with a small twist drill or burr. After a tumor sample is taken, another CT scan is made to detect any sign of hemorrhage. Although it appears that no significant difference exists in morbidity and mortality between the freehand method of obtaining biopsy samples and biopsy performed with a stereotactic apparatus, the freehand method was a bit safer and afforded a greater diagnostic yield rate[59]; hemorrhages occurred after biopsy in both groups, and more patients in the stereotactic group incurred symptoms from the clot—although that finding was biased by the larger, more superficial lesions approached with stereotactic biopsy technique.

Ultrasonography through a burr hole provides an alternative approach to biopsy.[60–62] It provides accuracy, can be performed on lesions greater than 7 to 10 mm, and provides immediate feedback after the biopsy to ensure that no hemorrhage has occurred. Diagnostic yield rates for the CT-guided stereotactic technique (94%) and the ultrasound-guided biopsy (91%) were comparable,[63] as were complications. The ultrasound-guided biopsy had a shorter operative time, however, and was substantially more economical.

Astrocytic tumors are subject to the greatest discrepancy rate in assigning tumor grade between the histologic findings for lesions that were biopsied and then resected.[64] Clearly, this presents a serious problem when small samples are obtained, particularly in differentiating between low-grade

glioma and reactive gliosis.[65] Despite the advantages of the alternative methods, stereotactic biopsy technique is the standard against which other techniques for obtaining small tissue samples must be compared. It is the most accurate method for obtaining tissue samples, irrespective of the type of frame used.

Stereotactic-Guided Volumetric Resection

In the innovative stereotactic-guided volumetric resection technique devised by Kelly and others,[66, 67] imaging is coupled with computer-assisted stereotactic resection of tumors. Instrumentation displays reconstructed tumor sections based on CT and MRI scans to the surgeon on a video terminal during surgery. The procedure permits precise stereotactic laser vaporization of any intracranial target. This approach is more useful in treating circumscribed lesions, such as metastasis or pilocytic astrocytoma, than for the more infiltrative glial tumors.[68] Although morbidity associated with this procedure is at an acceptable level, the results for patients with malignant glial tumors are disappointing, as the survival rates approximate those obtained with conventional radical resection.[69]

The infiltrative nature of gliomas tests the limitations of every surgical technique. Any treatment plan must take full account of the infiltrated brain adjacent to the main tumor nidus, and functional white matter tracts must be respected when extending resection into areas of diffuse infiltration to avoid unacceptable morbidity.[10]

Frameless Navigational Resection

For the most part, the stereotactic frame will shortly be obsolete among the systems for image-based computerized localization for tumor resection. New systems have a localizing arm that, during both preoperative planning and surgery, initializes and calibrates fiducial markers attached to the patient's head. In some systems, changes in the position of the localizing arm are updated by using acoustic transit times between the sound sources and the fiducial markers,[70, 71] whereas in others, mechanical sensors[72] or light emitters are used. Irrespective of the system used, this technology is rapidly becoming the standard for the preoperative planning of incisions and bone flaps as well as for guiding the initial phases of resection. Because localization with these systems is based on the preoperative scan, their usefulness during the resection of intra-axial tumors is clearly limited by the shifting of the brain contents. However, this is not a drawback in performing complex skull-base surgery.[10]

Intraoperative Localization of Tumor and Margins

During surgery, normal brain is distinguished from tumor by gross visualization for consistency and color. Low-grade glial tumors differ from the malignant glial tumors both in texture, as they are firmer than normal brain, and in color, as they are somewhat more pale than white matter. Malignant gliomas often are very soft with a necrotic grayish appearance. Glioblastomas almost always contain characteristic thrombosed veins. These tumors are highly vascular in correspondence to the contrast-enhancing rim on imaging studies.[10]

After the dura is opened, the cortex is inspected for expanded gyri and for the red, arterialized veins that are pathognomonic for malignant gliomas. Before resection begins, ultrasound is used to determine the size and depth of the tumor and underlying cystic structures. Tumor volumes as seen on CT and MRI correspond closely to the actual volumes for high-grade and low-grade gliomas that have not been resected or treated before.[73, 74] Gliosis accumulates after the tumor is operated on and irradiated, increasing the echogenic background and thereby tending to overrepresent the tumor's actual size.[10]

Verification of the tumor and of the transition zone between the tumor and adjacent tumor-infiltrated brain is obtained during surgery by means of serial frozen sections or smear preparations.[75] This often time-consuming process is complicated by the need to distinguish reactive astrocytes from infiltrating tumor cells. As an adjunct for documenting the extent of tumor removal during surgery, it may be possible to use dedicated CT and MRI, laser activation of hematoporphyrin,[76] fluorescent dyes,[77] intravenous indocyanine green,[78] and intravenous fluorescein with ultraviolet photoactivation.[79] The latter technique is seldom used at present, and the others are still under development.

Maximum Resection Through Functional Mapping Techniques

The risk of damage to important functional regions of brain is the factor that deters most surgeons who reject radical resective surgery. During the past several years, however, functional mapping of cortical and subcortical brain regions by means of intraoperative and extraoperative techniques has evolved rapidly to become an indispensable adjuvant technique that permits the surgeon to obviate functional morbidity yet perform wide, radical resections of tumor in eloquent brain areas.[10] For patients with tumors involving the posterior frontal, anterior parietal, or temporal lobe in the dominant cerebral hemisphere, language testing is performed to identify brain eloquent for reading, speech, and naming before resection is undertaken. Patients with deficits in these language functions preoperatively may have edema, or there may be tumor infiltration into essential language sites. A preoperative trial of high-dose dexamethasone therapy usually distinguishes between the two causes. The motor cortex is located within 3 to 5 cm behind the coronal suture superiorly and a similar distance posterior to the outer border of the sphenoid wing. The region is flanked posteriorly by the primary somatosensory cortex and, near the vertex, by the supplementary motor area anteriorly. Tumor located on either side of the motor cortex requires functional mapping with bipolar electrical stimulation to identify the cortical motor neurons and their descending motor tracts in the subcortical white matter, including the corona radiata, inter-

nal capsule, cerebral peduncles, and corticospinal pathways to the brainstem and spinal cord. Tumors that involve the insula, thalamus, and basal ganglia often abut the descending motor tracts, which can readily be stimulated. The rationale and techniques for functional brain mapping during glioma surgery are detailed elsewhere in this volume (see Chapter 34).

Because low-grade gliomas tend to have an indolent growth pattern, they are often associated with seizures. Although these seizures are often refractory to medication, neurosurgical approaches adapted from epilepsy surgery can provide improved seizure control. Epileptogenic areas are readily identified with intraoperative mapping of seizure foci by using electrocorticography (ECoG). In combination with the functional brain map, ECoG mapping permits resection of epileptogenic regions without causing neurologic deficit.[10, 39]

Resection of Tumor Alone vs. Electrocorticography-Guided Surgery

Seizure activity that is refractory to medication is particularly characteristic of oligodendrogliomas, gangliogliomas, and astrocytic gliomas.[80–82] The role of intraoperative ECoG guidance during tumor resection to minimize postoperative seizures is not universally accepted.[83–85] It must be noted that several of the reports questioning the need for ECoG during tumor resection do not discuss requirements for antiepileptic therapy after surgery. Seizure control varied between 50% and nearly 90% in those studies, usually after radical resection that often included probable epileptogenic foci (e.g., resection of tumor involving the temporal lobe with adjacent cortex or mesial structures). In one pediatric series,[81] 24% of the patients required continued antiepileptic therapy to remain seizure free, and another 19% continued to have seizures despite the therapy. Only 57% of the children in their patient population were seizure free without antiepileptic therapy. In a study reported from the Mayo Clinic, tumors were resected without adjacent epileptogenic tissue by using the computer-assisted, stereotactic-guided techniques of Kelly and associates.[66, 67] Most patients with intractable seizures in that series improved in regard to their seizure status, but more than 95% of patients required antiepileptic therapy to do so. That study also emphasizes the usefulness of ECoG in maximizing seizure control following surgery without antiepileptic therapy for patients with tumor-associated intractable epilepsy. In such patients, ECoG may avert the necessity of reoperation for seizure control.

The information that the mapping of seizure foci provides about the location of epileptogenic zones at the periphery of the tumor makes a convincing case for the use of ECoG-guided tumor surgery in patients who have epilepsy refractory to medication, and many investigators have advocated this course.[86–88] Other investigators, however, describe excellent seizure results obtained with aggressive temporal lobectomy performed together with tumor resection, without ECoG.[89–91] Several of these retrospective series do not report whether continuing anticonvulsant therapy was used in achieving the seizure control rate. Nonetheless, the results emphasize the need to extend resection beyond the tumor nidus.

For most patients who have intermittent seizures that are well controlled with antiepileptic drugs, removal of the tumor without seizure mapping produces good control of tumor-associated epilepsy.[81, 92–95] For some patients who have low-grade glioma and intractable seizures, however, tumor removal alone may not alleviate seizure activity.[91–93, 96] Because of the infiltrative nature of low-grade astrocytic gliomas of the cerebral hemispheres, gross examination may not provide confirmation that the tumor has been totally resected. In such cases, incomplete removal of the tumor has a better chance of providing seizure control if epileptogenic foci are completely removed.[96] When seizure foci reside in a site that precludes their being removed, a good outcome can be obtained by debulking the tumor as completely as possible, except when the tumor infiltrates the sensorimotor cortex. In such a case, it is difficult to obtain complete control of the persistent rolandic seizures, but tumor resection usually produces improvement.

We advocate the use of ECoG during tumor resection to identify discrete seizure foci near the tumor nidus.[97] Of the adult patients in our series, 88% were seizure free, with (47%) or without (41%) antiepileptic drugs, after surgery. Although a few patients had persistent seizure activity on medication, even they had fewer seizures that were often less intense after the operation. All but two children among the children and adolescents in our series were seizure free without medication. Those two children continued antiepileptic drug therapy after surgery. Others have had similar results with ECoG in this particular patient population.[86, 96, 98–100]

METHODS OF ASSESSMENT FOR EXTENT OF RESECTION

Analysis of the extent of tumor resection should include imaging documentation of calculated tumor volume before and after surgery, because subjective intraoperative assessments of the extent of resection and the residual tumor burden are likely to be inaccurate.[101] Volumetric analysis is accomplished either by actual calculation of the area of tumor on each image slice[3, 32, 102] or by an estimation of the volume of an ellipsoid or sphere based on measurements of the maximum diameters of the tumor on several planes.[103]

Stereotactic biopsy samples from brain adjacent to contrast-enhanced and hypodense areas in low-grade gliomas, as well as in high-grade gliomas, have shown isolated tumor cells well beyond the image-defined tumor mass.[104] Serial stereotactic biopsy studies and autopsy studies of low-grade gliomas confirm the diffuse, infiltrative growth pattern of these tumors,[105, 106] correlating isolated tumor cell invasion with the increased T2-weighted signal abnormalities observed on MRI or with hypodense regions on CT scans.[107–110] The volume represented by the increased T2 signal on MRI or hypodensity on CT scans, then, seems to be the best imaging correlate for tumor volume that includes the infiltrating tumor periphery.[9]

Among the sources of error to be aware of in analyzing tumor volume are the timing of scans obtained after surgery and the use of steroids. Scans should be obtained after surgical trauma has subsided and before other therapy is instituted, but the optimal timing in relation to these events has not been established. Steroids can reduce edema and may decrease the T2-weighted signal on MRI or hypodensity on CT scans, thereby leading to an underestimation of the tumor volume. Reportedly such changes stabilize when the steroid dosage is kept constant for a 14-day period.[111, 112] Another consideration is whether outcome is more heavily dependent on the absolute tumor cell burden or on the volume of brain involved by tumor. Any evaluation of surgical efficacy based on volumetric analyses may not be informative if the tumor cell density is variable within regions of similar increased T2 signal abnormality.[9]

OUTCOME VARIABLES

The outcome for patients undergoing treatment for a low-grade glioma depends on a variety of factors[113] that can confound an attempt to determine the efficacy of surgery. Although the factors most consistently associated with outcome are the age of the patient and the patient's KPS before and after surgery,[2, 4–8, 11, 58, 103, 114, 115] many other factors independently influence outcome, including altered mental status or neurologic deficit[2, 7]; tumor grade,[5, 114] cell type,[103, 116] or proliferative potential[4, 117]; radiologic features, such as contrast enhancement; presence of a cyst, mass effect, or midline shift; tumor location[8, 58, 102, 115, 118]; use of CT or MRI in the course of treatment[8, 16]; and use of adjuvant radiation therapy.[2, 116, 118, 119, 120] Radiation therapy is a particularly important factor because it is often reserved for patients who have had a subtotal resection.[9]

In most series, a greater extent of resection was shown to significantly extend the survival of patients with oligodendroglioma. Patients with mixed oligoastrocytomas have a better prognosis than do those with pure astrocytomas.[121] For patients with astrocytoma, the relation between a greater extent of resection and improved outcome in terms of survival is less certain. Of the several prognostic variables that may influence outcome in patients with astrocytoma, the most important are the patient's age at diagnosis, the patient's functional status, how completely the tumor is resected, and the tumor's histologic characteristics. Youth,[6–8, 15, 116, 122–124] an absence of postoperative performance deficits, alteration of consciousness, personality change,[6–8, 15, 116] and more extensive resection[7, 11, 15, 116, 122] are associated with improved outcome.

Except in relation to tumor-associated epilepsy, the efficacy of radical resection in the treatment of low-grade gliomas has been most thoroughly assessed in regard to survival or tumor progression, and some reports address quality of survival as related to extent of resection.[7, 125] In general, however, the data available at present are inadequate to specifically analyze and stratify outcome for endpoints including time to tumor progression, malignant degeneration, mortality rates, morbidity rates, and duration of high-quality survival by extent of resection.

LOW-GRADE INFILTRATIVE GLIOMAS
Astrocytoma

Seven studies done since the introduction of CT scanning have evaluated the association between the extent of resection and survival by multivariate techniques (Table 56–1). Four studies analyzed ordinary low-grade astrocytomas only or as a discrete group.[5, 7, 8, 117] Among 179 patients reported by Philippon and co-workers,[5] a greater extent of resection was significantly associated with prolonged survival in multivariate analysis ($P < 0.01$). Although this study included patients in all surgical conditions and controlled for a large number of prognostic factors, the analysis of extent of resection was based solely on operative reports, and radiation therapy was not uniformly administered to patients in all groups. North and colleagues[7] reported patients with astrocytoma in Kernohan grades I and II, including nine pilocytic tumors. Patients who had subtotal or gross total resection had better outcomes than those who had only biopsy ($P = 0.002$, multivariate analysis). In the series reported by Peipmeier,[8] no relation was noted between extent of resection and prognosis for a subgroup of 49 patients with astrocytoma, either in univariate testing or when stratified according to the administration of radiation therapy. Extent of resection was determined on the basis of postoperative CT scans and marginal biopsy results in that series, but the number of patients undergoing marginal biopsy, the histologic criteria defining a "positive" margin, and the criteria for CT evaluation were not described. Ito and co-workers[117] also showed a correlation between greater extent of resection and prolonged survival, although the duration of follow-up was short (median, 28 months) and the statistical analysis included relatively few variables and omitted the KPS.

Three studies done since the introduction of CT evaluated heterogeneous populations of low-grade glial tumor types by multivariate analysis.[4, 103, 114] Nicolato and others[4] evaluated 76 patients with a mixture of low-grade tumors, including fibrillary astrocytomas, mixed oligodendrogliomas, and pilocytic tumors, and determined extent of resection by comparison of CT scans obtained before and after surgery. In all patients who underwent subtotal resection (i.e., patients undergoing biopsy only or gross total resection), extent of resection was associated with prolonged survival. Conversely, Miralbell and colleagues[103] found no association between extent of resection or preoperative or postoperative tumor volume and survival in 49 patients with ordinary astrocytoma, oligodendrogliomas, mixed oligoastrocytoma, or pilocytic tumor. Residual tumor volumes of less than 23 cm^3 were associated with a better outcome in univariate analysis, but not significantly so in multivariate analysis. This finding was attributed to the influence of tumor type (oligodendroglioma) instead of extent of resection, although 12 of 16 oligodendrogliomas were completely or nearly completely resected as compared with only 4 of 33 nonoligodendroglial tumors. The lack of association between extent of resection or residual tumor volume and outcome in this study must be taken into account with consideration of the small numbers of patients in each study subgroup and the covariance of histologic type with extent of resection and outcome; moreover, patients with no measureable disease were not analyzed as a separate group.

Rajan and co-workers,[114] analyzing extent of resection based on operative reports, found no association with prolonged survival in multivariate models. Extent of resection was significant when analyzed as a single variable. In contrast, histologic subtype (astrocytoma grades I and II and

oligodendroglioma) was significant only in multivariate models. An analysis of extent of resection by histologic type was not provided and might have elucidated the apparent relation between histology and extent of resection, similar to that noted in the study by Miralbell and others.[103]

Four studies of the effect of extent of resection on survival included patients diagnosed before and after the introduction of CT.[6, 11, 58, 116] In those studies, the patients whose diagnosis was based on CT scan were not analyzed separately, and this lack of stratification may confound interpretation of the results, as may the wide variation in the percentage of patients undergoing radiation therapy after resection. A significant association of extent of resection with survival was found in only one of these studies,[11] an analysis of a large number of potential prognostic factors in patients with "well-differentiated" astrocytoma. Although total tumor resection was shown to correlate significantly with improved outcome by multivariate analysis, extent of resection was determined only on the basis of operative reports, and patients whose diagnosis was based on CT were not treated as a separate group.

Three studies that included patients treated both before and after the introduction of CT showed no association of greater extent of resection with better outcome. Shibamoto and associates,[58] in a separate analysis of 67 irradiated patients with CT-based diagnosis, excluded extent of resection because only 11 of those patients had extensive resection of greater than 80% of tumor. In the overall series, including patients receiving diagnoses before and after CT was introduced, extent of resection was found not to influence outcome, although only 15 patients in the entire series had undergone "extensive" surgery as defined. Extent of resection did not influence outcome in the series of 126 nonpilocytic low-grade gliomas, including 17 gemistocytic astrocytomas reported by Shaw and colleagues.[116] In this study, extent of resection was based on operative reports, but volumetric definitions were not given. Only 23 of 126 patients with nonpilocytic astrocytoma had a gross total or radical subtotal resection, and the number undergoing gross total resection was not specified or analyzed separately.

Gemistocytic astrocytoma as a tumor type had a negative influence on outcome, but the distribution of these tumors by extent of resection was not specified. In a study of 50 irradiated patients, Medbery and associates[6] found no difference in survival between the group that had undergone gross total resection and those that had undergone subtotal resection or biopsy. Although this study showed a significant influence of age, treatment before or after the use of CT, and radiation dose on survival, it included too few patients with different degrees of resection to stratify according to these prognostic factors. The analysis of extent of resection appears to be inadequate, the report does not indicate clearly whether extent of resection was examined in only univariate analysis, the method by which extent of resection was determined is not given, and the use of CT for determining extent of resection is not reported.

Pure Oligodendroglioma or Mixed Oligoastrocytoma

Oligodendrogliomas are less common than other glial neoplasms and often arise during late childhood. The mean age

TABLE 56-1
LOW-GRADE ASTROCYTOMA SURVIVAL AND EXTENT OF RESECTION (EOR): CT ERA* STUDIES WITH MULTIVARIATE ANALYSIS

Study	Total No. of Patients	Pilocytic Tumors	Surgery: EOR—No. of Patients	Survival by EOR	Effect on Survival (Multivariate)	Radiation Therapy
Nicolato[4]	74	8	"Grossly radical"—16 Partial—58	2-yr /5-yr survival 100%/86.5% 60.3%/25.5%	(+)	56/76 (76%); 40–60 Gy
Rajan[114]	82	0	Total—11 Subtotal—30 Partial—22 Biopsy—19	5-yr /10-yr survival 90%/68% 52%/36% 50%/31% 42%/28%	(−)	All: 50–55 Gy
Ito[117]	69	0	Total—19 Subtotal—51 Biopsy—17	NA	(+)	
Miralbell[103]	40/49	5	Complete—6 Almost complete—10 Partial—24 Biopsy—9	5-yr survival—all ≤23 cm³—85% >23 cm³—68% Exclude complete/almost ≤71 cm³—85% >71 cm³—60%	(−)	All: 45–60 Gy; 80%, >54 Gy
Philippon[5]	179	0	Total—45 Subtotal—95 Biopsy—39	5-yr survival 80% 50% 45%	(+)	118/179; 50–60 Gy (67/113 grade I, 51/66 grade II)
North[7]	77	9	Gross total—8 Subtotal—43 Biopsy—26	5-yr survival 85% 64% 43%	(+)	66/77; 50.4–55.8 Gy
Piepmeier[8]	58	0	EOR (all patients/astro I–II) Total—(23/19) Subtotal—(22/17) Biopsy—(13/13)	Mean survival (yr) (all patients/astro I–II) (8.12/8.47) (7.08/7.22) (5.88/6.24)	(−)	31/58; 50–60 Gy
Laws[2]	461	Not specified	Total—57 Radical subtotal—48 Subtotal + biopsy—356	5-yr survival 61% 44% 32%	(+)	For astro I–II 5/19 total EOR 13/17 subtotal EOR 8/13 biopsy None or <40 Gy: 252; Unknown: 135; ≥40 Gy: 74

*All data from CT era except Laws.[2]
Abbreviations: astro I/II, astrocytoma Kernohan's grade I and II; NA, data not available; (+), associated with prolonged survival; (−), not associated with prolonged survival.
From Berger MS, Rostomily RC: Low-grade gliomas: Functional mapping resection strategies, extent of resection, and outcome. J Neurooncol 1997; 34:85–101.

of patients diagnosed with the tumor is 13.5 years.[126] The effect of extensive resection on outcome for patients with oligodendroglioma is not well documented. Although some studies have shown that total tumor resection increased survival,[127–130] another[131] showed no effect. Oligodendroglioma may be more amenable to total resection than other infiltrative low-grade gliomas because of its somewhat circumscribed nature and macroscopically distinct margins.[132] As with all low-grade gliomas, radical tumor removal should be the goal to the maximum extent possible.

Only one of seven series (Table 56–2) that examined the effect of extent of resection on outcome for patients with oligodendroglioma or mixed oligoastrocytoma concerns only patients treated with benefit of CT.[102] Most of those studies showed an association between extent of resection and prolonged survival, and in four studies the effect was shown in multivariate analysis.[118–120, 132] Shaw and co-workers[119] reported a significant association between gross total resection and prolonged survival in 71 patients with mixed oligoastrocytoma. Celli and colleagues[120] analyzed 105 patients, 44 with benign mixed oligoastrocytoma, 35 with benign pure oligodendroglioma, and 26 with anaplastic oligodendroglioma. Patients with benign lesions were analyzed separately, and patients were grouped by clinical presentation as syndrome "A," with seizures only, or syndrome "non-A," which included all others (e.g., increased ICP, neurologic deficit, altered mental status). Prolonged survival was associated with greater extent of resection for the patients with benign tumors and those in the A group, but not for those in the non-A group. Reoperation was also associated with prolonged survival for the A group. Shaw and associates[118] and Lindegaard and colleagues[132] also showed an association between gross total resection and prolonged survival in series of 82 and 170 patients with oligodendroglioma, respectively.

Three studies evaluated extent of resection for oligodendrogliomas without multivariate analysis. Mørk and others[128] showed that gross total resection was somewhat more favorable than subtotal resection in prolonging survival in 194 patients ($P = 0.051$), although most of those patients were included in the series reported by Lindegaard and others,[132] which showed benefit from more extensive resection in multivariate analysis. Whitton and Bloom,[124] evaluating 24 patients with oligodendroglioma as a subset of a larger series of low-grade gliomas, showed that patients undergoing total or subtotal resection did better than patients who had either partial excision or biopsy ($P < 0.05$). Kros and co-workers,[102] in a series of 82 patients with pure oligodendroglioma, analyzed separately a subgroup of 40 patients in whom volumetric calculations were based on preoperative CT scans and reported no association between preoperative volume and outcome. However, the potential role of radical surgery for oligodendroglioma cannot be discounted on the basis of this analysis, as postoperative tumor volume was not assessed, and the criteria and methods of stratification of patients into groups are not detailed.

In a retrospective analysis performed at the University of Washington Medical Center in Seattle,[3] preoperative and postoperative tumor volumes were assessed based on CT

TABLE 56–2
OLIGODENDROGLIOMAS: SURVIVAL AND EXTENT OF RESECTION (EOR)*

Study	Surgical EOR—No. of Patients	Median Survival by EOR	Radiation Therapy	Effect of Greater EOR on Survival
Shaw[119]	Gross total—10 Radical subtotal—5 Subtotal—46 Biopsy—10	~6.5 yr; all others, ~5 yr	66/82; 38 ≥ 50 Gy	(+)—Multivariate analysis
Celli[120]	Total—9 Subtotal—20 Partial—71 Biopsy—5	14.8 yr 7.3 yr 4.8 yr 3.8 yr	77/105 (data on 42/77); 30/42 < 50 Gy	(+)—Multivariate analysis
Kros[102]	"Decompression"—23 Biopsy—17	Not reported	52/82; doses not reported	(−)—Univar *—EOR not quantified or stratified
Shaw[118]	Gross total—19 Subtotal—63	~13 yr ~5.5 yr	63 yes; 19 no (11 GTR); ≥ 50 Gy (33/63)	(+)—Multivariate analysis
Whitton[124]	Total—3 Subtotal—10 Partial—10 Biopsy—1	5-yr survival 　Total/subtotal ~83% 　Partial/biopsy ~40% 　$P = < 0.05$ 　(univariate)	All; 50–55 Gy	(+)—Univariate analysis
Lindegaard[132]	Total (−RT)—9 Total (+RT)—34 Subtotal (−RT)—49 Subtotal (+RT)—72	~6.8 yr ~3.5 yr ~1.75 yr ~2.8 yr 3.8 yr	108 Doses given (65) ≥40 Gy; 41/65	(+)—Multivariate analysis
Mørk[128]	Gross total—47 Subtotal—142 Biopsy—8	Subtotal + biopsy, 2.7 yr	Surgery + RT—107 Surgery only—87 (RT extended survival 11 mo; $P = 0.0092$)	(+)*—Univariate analysis *—Borderline $P = 0.51$

*Includes one report exclusively on mixed oligoastrocytomas.

Abbreviations: EOR, extent of resection; RT, radiation therapy; ~, estimated from survival curves; (+), associated with prolonged survival; (−), not associated with prolonged survival; GTR, gross total resection.

From Berger MS, Rostomily RC: Low-grade gliomas: Functional mapping resection strategies, extent of resection, and outcome. J Neurooncol 1997; 34:85–101.

hypodensity and/or T2 signal hyperintensity on MRI. The series included 53 patients with astrocytoma in Kernohan grades I or II, oligoastrocytoma (mixed glioma), or oligodendroglioma situated in the cerebral hemispheres. These patients were selected from 231 patients with low-grade glial tumors evaluated between January 1977 and June 1990. The extent of resection and tumor volumes were quantified by using a previously described method of computerized volumetric image analysis[32] to eliminate interobserver variability and bias. The study sought to confirm whether the percent of resection and postoperative volume of residual disease influenced the incidence of recurrence, time to tumor progression, and histology of the recurrent tumor. The investigators detected no recurrence in patients with preoperative tumor volumes of less than 20 cm^3, irrespective of percent of resection and volume of residual disease (mean follow-up interval, 41.7 months). Patients with tumors of 10 to 30 cm^3 had a 13.6% incidence of recurrence and a time to tumor progression of 58 months. In contrast, those with tumors measuring greater than 30 cm^3 had a 41.2% incidence of recurrence and a time to tumor progression of 30 months ($P = 0.016$). The 13 patients who had total resection had a mean recurrence-free follow-up interval of 54 months. For the other 40 patients, the incidence of recurrence increased, together with a shorter time to tumor progression, as the percent of resection decreased ($P = 0.03$) (Table 56–3). Patients with a residual tumor volume greater than 10 cm^3 had a higher incidence of recurrence (46.2%) and a shorter time to tumor progression (30 months) than patients who had a residual volume less than 10 cm^3 ($P = 0.002$); the incidence of recurrence was 14.8% and time to tumor progression was 50 months. Of those patients who had a residual tumor volume greater than 10 cm^3, 46% had a tumor that recurred at a higher histologic grade—significantly more than the 3.7% of patients with a residual tumor volume less than 10 cm^3 who had a higher-grade recurrence ($P = 0.0009$). Age, radiation therapy, and the tumor's histologic

subtype were not associated with recurrence patterns. The study population was not observed long enough to evaluate survival.[3]

The findings in that study are similar to those in studies using volumetric measurements of postoperative tumor volume and survival time for low-grade gliomas,[26] which showed that postoperative tumor volumes greater than 10 cm^3 were associated with a 46% chance of recurrence (median time to tumor progression, 30 months), whereas tumor volumes less than 10 cm^3 were associated with a 15% chance of recurrence (median, 50 months). The study showed no recurrences after complete resection after a mean follow-up interval of 54 months (Table 56–4).

The findings from the University of Washington suggest that patients with low-grade gliomas and a tumor volume greater than 10 cm^3 benefit from radical surgery at the time of radiographic diagnosis in terms of the chances of recurrence, the time to tumor progression, and the incidence of malignant transformation.[3] It is possible that the biology of low-grade gliomas larger than 30 cm^3 differs from that of the smaller lesion. Although percent of resection appeared to have a direct influence on the time to tumor progression, all recurrences of the large tumors showed malignant transformation, but that was not the case for tumors of 10 to 30 cm^3. Although patients with tumors less than 10 cm^3 seem to tend not to have a recurrence, the percent of resection appears not to affect the pattern of recurrence for these patients. However, as only 3 of 14 patients had less than a 90% resection, it is difficult to draw any conclusion regarding a less aggressive surgical approach for tumors less than 10 cm^3, which tend to be more amenable to radical resection. As compared with the smaller tumors, it is less likely that an extensive resection can be achieved with the more diffusely infiltrative tumors larger than 10 cm^3. Nonetheless, until the biology and natural history of low-grade gliomas are better understood, we advocate radical resection of all low-grade gliomas, regardless of the tumor's size.[3]

TABLE 56–3

THE EFFECT OF EXTENT OF RESECTION ON RECURRENCE, RECURRENCE AT A HIGHER HISTOLOGIC GRADE, AND TIME TO TUMOR PROGRESSION*

	Resection			
	<50%	50%–89%	90%–99%	≥100%
Patients (No.)	8	18	14	13
Age (yr), (range)	36.4 (12–55)	42.2 (25–70)	39.6 (7–74)	29.8 (6–39)
Follow-up (mo), (range)	42.1 (24–60)	43 (24–124)	53.8 (24–150)	54.4 (24–152)
Preoperative tumor volume (cm³), (range)	41.56 (104–115.86)	28.49 (5.47–58.59)	27.07 (8.03–53.06)	14.16 (1.9–18.95)
Postoperative tumor volume (cm³), (range)	32.54 (0.79–83.18)	14.58 (0.84–28.04)	1.24 (0.12–4.88)	0
Pathology (%)				
Astrocytoma	50	16	14	77
Oligodendroglioma	12	56	50	0
Mixed glioma	38	28	36	23
Radiotherapy (% received)	63	94	86	46
Recurrence (%), patients (No.)	37.5, 3	27.8, 5	14.3, 2	0
Recurrence at higher grade histology (%), patients (No.)	37.5, 3	16.7, 3	7.1, 1	0
Time to tumor progression (mo), (range)	24 (13–31)	36 (12–64)	63 (34–91)	NA

*Age, follow-up, preoperative and postoperative tumor volumes, and time to tumor progression are expressed as a mean value, and ranges are shown in parentheses.

From Berger MS, Keles GE, Ojemann GA, et al: Extent of resection affects recurrence patterns in patients with low-grade gliomas. Cancer 1994; 74:1784–1791.

TABLE 56–4
THE EFFECT OF POSTOPERATIVE TUMOR VOLUMES ON RECURRENCE, RECURRENCE AT A HIGHER HISTOLOGIC GRADE, AND TIME TO TUMOR PROGRESSION*

	Postoperative Tumor Volume		
	0 cm³	*<10 cm³*	*>10 cm³*
Patients (No.)	13	27	13
Age (yr), (range)	29.8 (6–59)	39.6 (7–74)	41.2 (31–55)
Follow-up (mo), (range)	54.4 (24–172)	47.9 (24–150)	44 (24–60)
Preoperative tumor volume (cm³) (range)	14.16 (1.9–48.95)	21.72 (1.04–53.06)	49.07 (18.95–115.86)
Resection (%) (range)	100	83.1 (24.5–98.3)	38.8 (10.7–67.2)
Pathology (%)			
Astrocytoma	77	18	31
Oligodendroglioma	0	56	23
Mixed glioma	23	26	46
Radiotherapy (% received)	46	85	85
Recurrence (%), patients (No.)	0	14.8, 4	46.2, 6
Recurrence at higher histologic grade (%), patients (No.)	0	3.7, 1	46.2, 6
Time to tumor progression (mo), (range)	NA	50 (12–91)	30 (13–45)

*Age, follow-up, preoperative tumor volume, percent of resection, and time to tumor progression are expressed as a mean value, and ranges are shown in parentheses.
From Berger MS, Keles GE, Ojemann GA, et al: Extent of resection affects recurrence patterns in patients with low-grade gliomas. Cancer 1994; 74:1784–1791.

OTHER NONINFILTRATIVE GLIOMAS

Pilocytic Astrocytomas

Although children develop high-grade astrocytomas relatively infrequently, low-grade astrocytomas are in general the most common tumors of the cerebral hemispheres in children.[39, 42, 133–137] They affect children in all age groups, and their peak incidence is in children 8 to 12 years old.[137–139] The supratentorial juvenile pilocytic astrocytoma (JPA) most often occurs in the cerebral hemispheres, and then—in order of decreasing frequency—the optic pathways, hypothalamus, and thalamus.[140, 141] Most children with JPAs develop symptoms during their first three decades of life, in particular between the ages of 10 and 25 years.[140, 142, 143] The duration of symptoms before surgery is usually 3 to 5 years.[10] Most JPAs of the cerebral hemispheres are cystic, with a tumor nidus seen as a mural nodule.[144, 145] A few JPAs are arranged in a plaque-like manner at the margin of a cyst that shows bright contrast enhancement on CT.[146] Not all cystic hemispheric lesions, whether they have the appearance of a mural nodule or not, are astrocytic in nature, however, and a clinical differential diagnosis must include ependymoma, hemangioblastoma, neuroblastoma, meningioma, and primitive neuroectodermal tumor.[10]

Astrocytomas in the region of the third ventricle, optic apparatus, and cerebellum in children have a similar histologic appearance and biologic behavior. They have in common a singular feature in that their cells have spindle-shaped nuclei and long, thin, eosinophilic cytoplasmic processes that extend from the cells in a bipolar array. These elongated spindled astrocytes are called *pilocytes* or "hair-like" cells.[147] Rosenthal fibers, the unique eosinophilic beaded structures derived from astrocytic processes, are found within the tumor or at its margins and at its interface with surrounding brain. The eosinophilic material is ultrastructurally electron dense, and residual intermediate filament can be observed at its periphery. Immunocytochemical studies for glial fibrillary acidic protein (GFAP) usually show peripheral positive reactivity in Rosenthal fibers, with a largely negative reaction in the center.[10]

Besides these features in common, astrocytomas in different sites have distinctive features. Parenchymal pilocytic astrocytomas are cystic, with a mural nodule that grossly appears fleshy and dark red, and is distinguished histologically by its biphasic nature. It is seen as an irregular alternating pattern of pilocytic areas and looser microcystic areas. The microcysts contain eosinophilic, acellular, proteinaceous material. Cells in the looser areas are more stellate and have round nuclei and many short cell processes. The pilocytic areas are usually situated around blood vessels. The abundant blood vessels may demonstrate thickening and hyalinization of the walls with endothelial cell hypertrophy or proliferation, simulating the vascular mural cell proliferation seen in malignant astrocytomas of the cerebral hemispheres. In children with pilocytic astrocytomas, however, these vascular changes do not predict a poor outcome. Some areas of the tumor may contain cells with clear cytoplasm, like the oligodendroglioma. Nuclei of the pilocytes may be enlarged, hyperchromatic, and pleomorphic, but although this nuclear pleomorphism may represent a degenerative change, its presence does not predict a poor outcome. The pilocytic astrocytomas with the biphasic pattern are called *juvenile* pilocytic astrocytomas to distinguish them from the diffuse astrocytomas with a pilocytic growth pattern that occur in the cerebral hemispheres of adults or in the brainstem. These diffuse pilocytic astrocytomas are usually graded according to the usual criteria for malignant astrocytomas and behave in a more aggressive manner.[10]

Pilocytic astrocytomas of the optic apparatus and in the region of the third ventricle are less often biphasic than are hemispheric parenchymal astrocytomas, but they have distinctive pilocytes and lack mitotic activity. The tumor distorts the usual organizational pattern of the optic nerves and chiasm. The tumor shows an increase in glial cellularity but little pleomorphism. The tumor often has Rosenthal fibers and an abundant growth of connective tissue, and it can grow into the leptomeninges of the optic structures. It may metastasize by way of the cerebrospinal fluid, even with no increased histologic anaplasia.[148] Pilocytic astrocytomas are characterized by strong cytoplasmic GFAP immunoreactivity in the pilocytic cells with diffuse reactivity in the stellate cells. Vascular structures do not stain with GFAP, but Mason trichrome stain labels the perivascular collagen, reticulin stain delineates connective tissue fibers, and factor VIII immunostain shows the endothelial cells.[10]

Tuberous sclerosis, or Bourneville's disease, is a phakomatosis associated with supratentorial noninfiltrative gliomas. Typical signs of this syndrome in children and young adults include cognitive retardation, seizures that are often refractory to medication, and dermatologic signs of facial adenoma sebaceum. Cortical hamartomas are characteristic in association with periventricular calcified nodules[149]; these lesions are most often situated near the foramen of Monro and are histologically subependymal giant cell astrocytomas,[150] a lesion that has not been documented in patients who do not have tuberous sclerosis.[151] As the subependymal nodule grows, it blocks the foramen of Monro and causes obstructive hydrocephalus. This frequently very indolent process produces a gradual onset of symptoms.[10]

The goal of surgery for patients with JPA in the cerebral hemispheres is to evacuate the cyst contents and remove all the contrast-enhancing tissue observed on preoperative CT scans or MRI, including the mural nodule and all contrast-enhanced portions of the cyst. If the cyst is simply drained and the lesion is not removed, the cyst contents will reaccumulate. It can be expected that the cyst wall is gliotic and lacking neoplastic cells if it does not show contrast enhancement,[145, 146] but if contrast enhancement is seen, the cyst wall must be resected completely to avert recurrence.[152] The mural nodule is discrete, friable, and moderately bloody, appearing reddish brown. After the resection, adjacent noninfiltrated white matter should be clearly visible. A distinct microscopic margin lies between the tumor and contiguous white matter.[142] Contrary to the views of Mercuri and colleagues[137] and Palma and co-workers,[153] we do not advocate fenestration of the cyst into the ventricle, because the cyst is frequently in continuity with the ependymal surface of the ventricular system.[10] After the tumor is resected, the cyst will not recur, but debris from the resection cavity may seep into the ventricle to cause communicating hydrocephalus.

It can be more difficult to achieve complete resection of solid JPAs, particularly when the tumor is located deep in the brain or is joined to subcortical functional tracts. Solid JPAs should undergo radical resection, however, unless such a course would cause unacceptable complications. Although long-term results of a complete resection are excellent, with no need for irradiation or chemotherapy, careful routine follow-up evaluations should be performed as a precautionary measure every 6 to 12 months for several years after surgery. When complete resection of a hemispheric JPA is confirmed on postoperative imaging studies, the 10-year survival rate for both children[116, 154] and adults[142] approaches 100%. Routine follow-up is mandatory for patients with incompletely resected tumors, however, as recurrence is likely, although it may take years to occur.[144]

Thalamic JPAs are usually well circumscribed and they can be associated with a cyst.[155] For thalamic tumors located anteriorly, the ventricle should be entered anteriorly through a parasagittal incision made in front of the premotor cortex. Such tumors displace the internal capsule laterally. In contrast, because posterior thalamic JPAs push the posterior limb of the internal capsule forward, the best approach to such a tumor is through the posterior ventricle, or atrium. To obviate complications while maximizing the extent of resection, capsular motor fibers must be identified by using subcortical stimulation technique.[156] Alternatively, the JPA can be resected volumetrically by using computer-assisted stereotactic technique.[157] Although this technique is highly effective and precise, it is available in few centers.

Subependymal Giant-Cell Astrocytoma

Although the subependymal giant-cell astrocytoma is usually classified as an astrocytoma, the histogenesis of this tumor has not been established. Although the cells may show histologic pleomorphism to suggest a diagnosis of glioblastoma multiforme, they lack mitotic activity and necrosis. Subependymal giant-cell astrocytomas are localized to the subependymal region. They generally occur in patients who have tuberous sclerosis, but sporadic cases of such tumors have occurred in patients who have no history of that condition.[158] The tumor is highly cellular, with large and bizarre cells. Characteristically, profuse eosinophilic cytoplasm is seen, and the nuclei are very large with prominent nucleoli, possibly suggestive of a neuronal etiology.[159] Ultrastructural study shows numerous intermediate filaments and long, thickened cytoplasmic processes. However, because the neoplastic cells may mark for both glial and neuronal antigens, or may mark poorly for both, immunohistochemical analysis provides no defined histogenesis for this tumor. Subependymal giant-cell astrocytomas are usually considered benign and curable by surgical excision with no additional adjuvant therapy.[151]

As subependymal giant-cell astrocytomas are always found within the anterior horn of the lateral ventricle, the size of the ventricle dictates the optimal surgical approach. Patients who have symptoms must undergo ventricular dilatation because of the relation of the tumor to the foramen of Monro. In most cases, a frontal transventricular approach is appropriate because it provides the necessary exposure, taking advantage of the large ventricles. Some surgeons still advocate a transcallosal approach, however, because it requires less retraction of the brain and because some consider that it may present a smaller risk of postoperative epilepsy.[150] Subependymal giant-cell astrocytomas should be removed only when the patient has symptoms of ventricular obstruction.[10]

Pleomorphic Xanthoastrocytoma

Pleomorphic xanthoastrocytoma is a distinctive, relatively rare, and newly identified astrocytoma variant that affects children and, more frequently, young adults.[160, 161] The lesions are almost always located superficially, situated entirely within the cerebral hemispheres near the arachnoidal spaces, and often adjacent to a leptomeningeal surface.[162] They usually involve the temporal lobe, but may also occur in the parietal lobe. Seizures are usually the presenting symptom in our patients, and a patient may have been symptomatic for several years before the surgical diagnosis. Although generally considered a benign lesion with an indolent clinical course, rapidly progressive tumor growth culminating in death has been reported.[163] The tumor exhibits marked and even bizarre histologic pleomorphism in the absence of significant mitotic activity and necrosis,[162, 164] which can cause difficulty in determining the histologic diagnosis and can result in a mistaken diagnosis of glioblastoma multiforme. The individual tumor cells have a high lipid content, which is observed in frozen sections by staining for neutral fat with oil red O. These foamy, lipidized cells show their astrocytic nature with positive cytoplasmic immunoreactivity for GFAP.[165] It is particularly important to be watchful of the diagnosis and prognosis for patients older than 30 years when the suspected neoplasm demonstrates mitotic activity or necrosis, as some such neoplasms have been reported to behave in a malignant fashion or to transform to glioblastoma.[163] The pleomorphic xanthoastrocytoma is usually surgically curable. This tumor has been associated with von Recklinghausen's disease and, although the association is quite unusual, patients should be evaluated for neurofibromatosis.[166]

Although pleomorphic xanthoastrocytomas grossly appear as an encapsulated mass distinct from the adjacent brain, their frequent contiguous relation with the leptomeninges[167] can make resection difficult, particularly when the tumor lies within the sylvian fissure. A superficial, pial-based attachment indicates that the tumor is circumscribed and amenable to total resection. Even when a pleomorphic xanthoastrocytoma is completely resected, however, the patient must be followed routinely with postoperative imaging studies because there is a 30% chance of recurrence.[168]

Desmoplastic Cerebral Astrocytoma

The desmoplastic cerebral astrocytoma is a rare and distinctive pathologic entity that usually arises during infancy or childhood,[169–171] although it may also occur in adults. Its singular histologic feature is marked spindling of the astrocytes within an extensive collagen matrix. The neoplasm may be located superficially in the cerebral hemisphere, and it has been suggested that the collagen proliferation may arise from pia as it is invaded by neoplastic growth. Desmoplastic cerebral astrocytoma may resemble a sarcoma, but its astrocytic nature is revealed by immunohistochemical studies positive for GFAP. The prognosis is considered good for patients who undergo gross total resection of the tumor.[10]

Ganglioglioma

In contrast to the astrocytic tumors, gangliogliomas more frequently arise in children than in adults. They constitute 1.7% to 7.6% of all tumors of the central nervous system in the pediatric population.[172–174] The duration of symptoms may be as long as 15 to 20 years before a definitive clinical

diagnosis is made.[85, 175] Gangliogliomas most often arise in the temporal[44] and frontal lobes and almost always cause complex partial epilepsy, with or without secondary generalization. Patients who have these lesions frequently have epilepsy refractory to medication and require intraoperative ECoG to improve control of seizures.[82]

The ganglioglioma has a characteristic histologic appearance, and prominent vascular septa divide the tumor into a lobular pattern. A biphasic tumor, it has a mature, atypical neuronal component mixed with a neoplastic glial component. The glial component is usually low-grade and astrocytic with rare or absent mitotic figures.[176] The glial morphology may suggest a pilocytic astrocytoma. The astrocytic component has an intermixed population of neurons that are atypical in their size, shape, arrangement, and histology. There may be multinucleated forms. Because large gemistocytic astrocytes can simulate atypical neurons with their profuse eosinophilic cytoplasm, it may be necessary to confirm the diagnosis by using special immunohistochemical markers of neuronal differentiation, such as synaptophysin or neurofilament protein.[177]

There is universal consensus that cerebral hemispheric gangliogliomas should be treated with gross total resection,[175, 178] but there is none regarding the extent of resection as it relates to optimal control of the tumor. Reports relating seizure control to extent of surgical resection appear to indicate that complete tumor resection reduces the occurrence of seizures in individual patients by 50%—a result that is almost matched by incomplete tumor removal.[176] However, for patients who had gross total resection of tumor, the use of intraoperative ECoG to map epileptogenic foci and inclusion of those foci in the area of resection increased the likelihood of complete seizure control to 92%[82]; even with incomplete resection of the tumor, a 95% reduction in postoperative seizures was obtained. Intraoperative ECoG is an indispensable adjuvant to surgery for patients with intractable epilepsy associated with gangliogliomas or other lesions, such as desmoplastic infantile gangliogliomas and dysembryoplastic neuroepithelial tumors. For the latter two noninfiltrative, circumscribed tumors, complete resection will positively influence control of recurrence as well as seizures.[171, 179]

Desmoplastic Infantile Ganglioglioma

The desmoplastic infantile ganglioglioma is a distinctive and rare tumor that occurs in very young infants, usually those younger than 2 years.[171, 180] They typically are very indolent neoplasms with a long natural history.[179] A distinct, well-demarcated entity, both grossly and radiographically,[181] they closely resemble the superficial cerebral astrocytoma with dural attachment described by Taratuto and colleagues[182] and tend to be located in the frontal and parietal regions. They are often multicystic and contain large volumes of proteinaceous fluid, which produces severe mass effect and intracranial hypertension.[171]

Desmoplastic infantile gangliogliomas may be large with a prominent cystic or multicystic appearance. They often are located superficially in the cerebral hemispheres. Their histologic characteristics resemble those of the desmoplastic cerebral astrocytoma, but they also exhibit primitive small cells and neuronal differentiation. Although they have a firm gross consistency, deriving from a predominant desmoplastic character, they nonetheless infiltrate into brain. The desmoplasia comprises admixed fibrous collagen and glial elements. The astrocytic component may be moderately pleomorphic but is revealed by a positive cytoplasmic immunoreactivity for GFAP. The neuronal elements range from mature neurons to primitive small cells, as detected by immunohistochemical stains for synaptophysin or neurofilament protein. The neuronal elements usually are found in less desmoplastic areas of the tumor, and their number may vary. Mitoses and necrosis are more likely to be seen with the small-cell component. Despite their cellular heterogeneity and primitive small-cell component, a prolonged survival can be achieved if the tumor is radically resected.[10]

HIGH-GRADE GLIOMAS

The prognosis for patients with glioblastoma multiforme has improved very little, even with technological advances that have improved the odds for patients with other tumor types.[25, 35, 101, 183] Adjuvant radiation therapy, either alone or in combination with chemotherapy, can improve survival time,[24, 25, 184, 185] but the role of surgery as a determinant of outcome has not been established.[101, 183, 185] Several series have shown an association between extensive resection and longer survival for patients with malignant glioma,[18–21, 24, 25, 30, 31, 186–188] whereas other studies show no benefit whatever from radical resection.[22, 23, 35, 184, 189, 190]

Studies based on diagnostic imaging and neuroimage-guided stereotactic biopsies of gliomas and their periphery have lately reinforced the concept that most gliomas are infiltrative into adjacent brain. This, together with technological innovations in image-guided neurosurgical instrumentation and techniques that permit precise tissue sampling, has had a substantial impact on the management of patients with a glioma and particularly on the role of surgery.[10]

Correlating the results of CT scans with those of postmortem examination to assess the extent of disease in patients with glioblastoma, Burger[191] detected tumor beyond the contrast-enhancing margin at autopsy in most cases in which hypodense regions had been seen on the scans. A limitation to this study considered significant by the authors was in the methodology used to identify neoplastic cells in adjuvant brains. Moreover, the hiatus between the imaging study and a patient's death was several weeks, and death was directly due to tumor in fewer than 50% of the cases. Daumas-Duport and others[192] improved tissue fixation methodology to define more precisely cells that apparently were neoplastic and were obtained stereotactically from the periphery of a glioma. When these investigators implanted corresponding specimens into nude mice, the implants formed tumors composed of astrocytes. They attempted no correlation between the site from which these isolated tumor cells were taken and the recurrence patterns in the patients based on follow-up imaging studies, and a lack of specific tumor cell markers hinders the qualitative interpretation of neoplastic vs. reactive astrocytes. In MRI studies, biopsies obtained from hyperintense T2-weighted signal regions have also verified the presence of isolated tumor cells outside of the contrast-enhancing margin of high-grade glial tumors.[193]

Although these findings suggest breaches in the histologic limits of infiltrative gliomas, clinical studies have supported a focal origin and localized growth pattern of malignant gliomas.[194–196] Despite improvements in imaging, the conclusions were the same in both of two studies done 10 years apart,[194, 196] which documented recurrences within 2 cm of the contrast-enhancing margin in 85% to 90% of patients. In another study,[197] recurrence in all cases evaluated was within 4 cm of the contrast rim.

It is important to note, however, that assessment of extent of resection in the studies of high-grade gliomas suffers from the same drawbacks as those of low-grade gliomas. They have usually been based on the neurosurgeon's qualitative intraoperative estimation as recorded in the operative report and often have not been correlated with postoperative imaging studies. If radiographic evidence is provided, the amount of tumor removed has often been based on nonvolumetric evaluation of postoperative CT scans.[18, 22, 23, 25, 30, 31, 35, 184, 186, 188] The substantial variability in patient characteristics, in the methods used to determine extent of resection, and in therapeutic modalities among studies also confounds the interpretation of the available data.[101]

Extension of High-Grade Gliomas Beyond the Tumor Mass

In combination with these confounding factors, the evidence that glioblastomas multiforme are diffuse, infiltrative lesions extending beyond the contrast-enhancing area on imaging studies is convincing.[191, 198, 199] In a retrospective study of the extent of resection and high-grade glioma done at the University of Washington in Seattle,[1] attempts were made to minimize the persistent methodologic problems seen in previous studies. The investigators assessed the preoperative and postoperative tumor volumes of patients to define the percentage of resection and the volume of residual disease as it relates to time to tumor progression and overall survival in patients with hemispheric glioblastoma multiforme. The effect of volumetrically calculated percentage of resection on outcome had previously been reported by these investigators for both hemispheric low-grade gliomas[3] and recurrent malignant gliomas treated with chemotherapy.[1, 33]

Only adult patients with hemispheric glioblastomas multiforme who initially had a KPS of 70 or higher were evaluated. All patients were treated with radiation therapy after surgery, and most of those patients also received chemotherapy. To eliminate potential for overestimating the amount of tumor removal and the interobserver variability related to a nonvolumetric assessment, the contrast-enhancing tumor volume documented on both the preoperative and the postoperative scans was quantified by using a volumetric image-analysis technique.[32] As in other retrospective studies,[26, 30, 31, 34, 200, 201] the entire contrast-enhancing volume as observed on CT scans or MRIs were used to document tumor size and to determine the importance of residual tumor in predicting patient outcome.

In all, 417 patients with glioblastoma multiforme of the cerebral hemispheres who were evaluated and treated on the

Neuro-oncology Service at the University of Washington Hospitals in Seattle between January 1980 and June 1991 were analyzed.[1] A histologic diagnosis of glioblastoma multiforme was based on the presence of hypercellularity, mitoses, vascular endothelial proliferation, cellular and/or nuclear pleomorphism, and foci of coagulation necrosis. Multicentric glioblastoma multiforme was excluded from the analysis. Criteria for inclusion comprised the availability of preoperative and postoperative CT scans or MRIs and follow-up data recorded until the time of the patient's death or, if the patient was still alive, until June 1992. The cause of death during the follow-up interval was determined from the death certificate or autopsy report unless the patient was being observed at that time by our service. Patients who died within the first 4 weeks after surgery were excluded from analysis. The study group consisted of 92 patients ranging in age from 15 to 80 years (median, 51 years), who underwent a total of 107 operations. Of those patients, 41 (45%) were female and 51 (55%) were male. The tumors were located predominantly in the frontal lobe (38 patients), and then the temporal lobe (30 patients), parietal lobe (21 patients), and occipital lobe (3 patients). The majority of tumors were located in the left hemisphere (n = 62 [58%]).

VOLUMETRIC MEASUREMENTS

Volumetric measurements were obtained from CT scans or MRIs performed at the time of the initial surgical procedure for 55 patients (60%). There were 52 reoperations (49% of all operations) in patients who had previously had resection or biopsy. For 15 patients, volumetric assessment of the extent of resection was possible for both their initial operation and later reoperation. In each case, contingent on the relation of tumor to functional cortex and subcortical white matter, brain mapping through bipolar electrode stimulation was done intraoperatively to maximize resection, to avoid functional morbidity, and, when applicable, to gain optimal seizure control.[156, 202, 203] After their initial surgical resection, all patients underwent radiation therapy, and 84% of patients also had chemotherapy.

MEASUREMENT OF THE EXTENT OF RESECTION

The preoperative and the first postoperative CT scans or MRIs were digitized. Preoperative and postoperative tumor volumes were measured by using an image-analysis technique.[32] The percentage of resection and volume of residual disease were calculated for each operation. MRIs were used to determine volume measurements for 22 operations (21%) and CT scans for 31 operations (29%). Most measurements (40%) were based on preoperative MRIs and early postoperative CT scans, which at the time of the study were easier to obtain during the first few days after surgery. For the other 11 operations (10%), a preoperative CT scan and a postoperative MRI were used. All tumors showed enhancement with the administration of contrast agent. The tumor volume was the contrast-enhanced area, including any central necrotic region. Preoperative scans were obtained from 0 to 16 days (median, 7 days) before surgery, and postoperative scans were obtained from 0 to 24 days (median, 4 days) after surgery—the variability owing to differing views of the

attending surgeons in regard to appropriate timing of imaging after resection. For totally resected tumors, time to tumor progression was based on a comparison between the first postoperative scan and evidence of recurrence on later scans; for tumors not completely resected initially, time to tumor progression was based on disease progression.[1]

OUTCOME ANALYSIS

The study endpoints were time to tumor progression and overall survival from the initial histologic diagnosis.[1] Variables analyzed by using Kaplan-Meier survival curves with the Mantel-Cox test[204] were patient's age, preoperative and postoperative KPS,[205] tumor histologic type, preoperative tumor volume, volume of residual disease, percentage of resection, and chemotherapy. Kaplan-Meier survival curves were also assessed for different operations to evaluate the variation in shape, if any, between curves. The model also estimated the estimated the relative risk for a unit change in a particular covariate, provided that all other covariates stayed the same.[206]

TIME TO TUMOR PROGRESSION

Time to tumor progression ranged from 4 to 170 weeks (median, 29.5 weeks).[1] Preoperative KPS ($P < 0.05$), chemotherapy ($P < 0.05$), percentage of resection ($P < 0.001$), and volume of residual disease ($P < 0.001$) were significantly associated with time to tumor progression. The median time to tumor progression for patients who had total tumor resection with no residual disease was 53 weeks. As percentage of resection decreased and volume of residual tumor increased, there was a shorter time to tumor progression. There was no significant difference in median age or preoperative KPS for each subgroup (i.e., percentage of resection and volume of residual disease).

Patients were grouped according to each progressive number of operations performed to determine whether the effect of percentage of resection and volume of residual disease on time to tumor progression was influenced by its being the initial as opposed to a subsequent operation. Although percentage of resection was significant in predicting time to tumor progression for the initial operation and for the second, third, or fourth operation, the significance was less for subsequent operations on recurrent lesions. Volume of residual disease also had a highly significant effect on time to tumor progression after the initial operation, but less after the second operation, and the effect was insignificant for the third or fourth operation.

SURVIVAL

Survival ranged from 6 to 188 weeks (median, 61 weeks).[1] Age ($P < 0.05$), preoperative KPS ($P = 0.05$), postoperative KPS ($P < 0.005$), percentage of resection ($P < 0.0005$), and volume of residual disease ($P < 0.0001$) were significantly associated with survival. Total tumor resection with no residual disease produced a median survival of 93 weeks. The least percentage of resection (<25%) and the greatest volume of residual tumor (<20 cm³) gradually shortened survival time to 31 and 50 weeks, respectively. Patient age, which was similar in each subgroup, had no significant effect on survival.

Many of the patients in this study had undergone the initial operation at another hospital and had no pretreatment or postoperative radiographs, which obviated an initial evaluation of percentage of resection and volume of residual tumor. Nonetheless, the patients were evenly distributed into the entire study population, resulting in a statistically significant advantage in terms of time to tumor progression and overall survival. Each patient underwent aggressive tumor removal at some time point in the entire course of treatment. The number of second, third, or fourth operations was clearly higher for patients who had a shorter time to tumor progression and overall lower survival rate, which would exclude repeat operations as a positive influence on outcome in this study.

Gliosarcoma and Gliomatosis Cerebri

The extremely invasive gliosarcoma presents difficult surgical problems because, although it may appear somewhat circumscribed,[207] the tumor is highly vascular and often invades overlying dura.[208] Although patients with gliosarcoma and those with glioblastoma should respond similarly with extensive resection, survival data for this tumor at present are inadequate to support that conclusion. Gliomatosis cerebri, an unusual finding, is an extensive, diffusely infiltrating glioma that usually presents with symptoms and signs of increased ICP. There is no indication for extensive resection of this lesion, but stereotactic biopsy is mandatory and must be directed at any contrast-enhancing tissue, when present, together with MRI sequences.[209] Patients remain for observation in the intensive care unit overnight because intracranial hypertension associated with the large tumor mass may cause rapid neurologic deterioration after biopsy.[210]

RECURRENCE AND MALIGNANT PROGRESSION

Although many patients diagnosed with low-grade or high-grade gliomas die from recurrence and malignant progression, the potential of radical surgery to alter this course of events is debated. Recht and colleagues[57] compared delayed therapy to immediate treatment to find that the time of intervention had no effect on the rates and times to malignant progression; details of the immediate interventions were not provided. Steiger and co-workers[211] found that 38-month progression-free survival was higher, although not significantly so ($P = 0.09$), among patients who had undergone gross total resection of grade II astrocytomas (with pilocytic tumors excluded) than among patients who had had partial resection or biopsy. In this study, no mention was made of use of postoperative CT scans to confirm extent of resection, and radiation therapy was differentially administered to 6 of 18 patients (33%) who had had subtotal resection but to only 4 of 32 patients (13%) undergoing gross total resection, potentially introducing treatment bias into the analysis of extent of resection.

In contrast, Berger and colleagues[3] reported that a greater extent of resection and smaller residual tumor volume sig-

nificantly prolonged the time to recurrence and reduced the malignant transformation rate. The study used volumetric analyses of preoperative and postoperative tumor volumes to assess heterogeneous low-grade glial tumors (19 astrocytomas, 18 oligodendrogliomas, 16 mixed oligoastrocytomas) in 53 patients. Of the 10 patients who had a recurrence during the follow-up interval (mean, 48.7 months; range, 24 to 172 months), 7 had malignant degeneration and all had had tumors greater than 30 cm³ at presentation. No tumor that had been less than 10 cm³ at presentation recurred irrespective of extent of resection, and patients with no residual tumor developed no recurrence. Of the six patients with recurrence in the group with residual tumor greater than 10 cm³, all developed malignant degeneration. In contrast, only one of the four recurrences in the group with residual tumor less than 10 cm³ postoperatively had a higher histologic grade. Both a smaller preoperative and postoperative tumor volume and a greater extent of resection correlated with prolonged mean time to tumor progression in univariate analysis.

This study suggests that greater extent of resection may have an impact on the natural history of low-grade gliomas. As the composition of the three groups with volume analyzed preoperatively or postoperatively may be similar, however, there is no way to know for certain whether the more important factor in determining outcome is the relative influence of preoperative tumor volume or the ability to achieve a particular level of residual tumor through surgical intervention.[9] Greater information would be provided by a larger study that would be performed by using the same design for volumetric analysis, but would be extended to examine survival.

Role of Tumor Volume in Determining Histologic Type of Recurring Tumors

From 13% to as many as 85% of glial tumors initially diagnosed as being low-grade tumors reportedly recur at a higher histologic grade.[2, 7, 8, 11–14, 16, 17] The factors that result in such a change to a malignant phenotype are not clear, nor is it known what role tumor volume may play, either preoperatively or postoperatively, in determining the histologic type of the tumor when it recurs.

A retrospective study from the University of Washington[3] was undertaken to determine if recurrence patterns may be influenced by the amount of tumor initially removed. Because most patients in the series were still alive and the follow-up interval was too brief to permit an evaluation of survival, the study assessed only the effect of extent of resection and that of preoperative and residual tumor volumes on recurrence patterns, including time to tumor progression and histology of the recurrent tumor. Age, radiation therapy, and histologic subtype had no influence on recurrence patterns. No high-grade recurrence was documented in patients who had complete resection and no radiographic evidence of residual tumor postoperatively. Moreover, time to tumor progression was longer in patients who had more extensive resections associated with a smaller residual tumor volume. The findings in this study[3] suggested that the risk of recurrence, either as a low-grade lesion or at a higher histologic grade, is significantly less in patients who have less residual tumor volume after surgery, particularly for patients with tumors greater than 10 cm³. It may be that the amount of residual tumor volume is more important than the percent of resection in influencing the phenotype of the recurrent tumor. It may also be that the biology of larger low-grade tumors differs from that of smaller lesions. If so, radical resection of these tumors may prove mandatory, regardless of their size.[10]

In another study from the University of Washington,[33] 51 adult patients with recurrent malignant gliomas were treated in a phase II trial of multidrug chemotherapy (6-thioguanine, dibromodulcitol, procarbazine, 1-[2-chloroethyl]-3-cyclo-hexyl-1-nitrosourea, 5-fluorouracil, and hydroxyurea). Of those patients, 31 underwent radical resection of the tumor before chemotherapy. Of all patients in the series, 57% either showed an objective radiographic response or disease stabilization after therapy was begun. The median survival time was 79 weeks for patients with anaplastic astrocytomas and 33 weeks for those with glioblastomas. The median time to tumor progression was 32 weeks for patients with astrocytomas and 13 weeks for those with glioblastomas. Overall median survival time was 40 weeks, and overall median time to tumor progression was 19 weeks. The response and disease stabilization rate, median survival time, median time to tumor progression, and toxicity levels in this study were comparable to those for other regimens used in treating recurrent malignant glioma. Several prognostic factors and potentially important treatment factors were revealed by the comprehensive statistical analysis of the factors that affected median time to tumor progression, median survival time, and response to treatment for recurrent malignant glioma. For example, degree of myelotoxicity may have a direct influence on the tumor response and the patient's outcome, and patients who have local and hemispheric lesions fare better than do patients with invasive or diffuse patterns of recurrence and deep, distant, or disseminated lesions. This study also added to the view that prior chemotherapy potentially can exert a negative effect on the tumor's response to subsequent chemotherapy.[33] Evaluation of the role of surgery in this study indicated that the volume of the tumor at the time of recurrence is more critical than the postoperative tumor volume and lessens the potential benefit of cytoreductive surgery. Nonetheless, surgery was influential in prolonging time to tumor progression when other prognostic factors were controlled.

CONCLUSIONS

Methodologic limitations that are intrinsic to retrospective studies of relatively small populations of selected patients that have no uniform prognostic or adjuvant treatment profiles, and in which extent of resection is determined mainly by subjective measures, cannot produce a compelling answer to the question of whether radical surgical resection may improve the outcome for patients with low-grade or high-grade gliomas. Nonetheless, limitations aside, about half of the studies performed with CT or MRI that have analyzed exclusive sets of patients by using multivariate analysis have shown that a greater extent of resection for astrocytoma is significantly associated with longer survival. The studies that show a significant benefit of surgery tend to be those that evaluate a larger population of patients, perhaps because the variance within subgroups is reduced when a larger population is evaluated, permitting more meaningful statistical analysis.[9] Although no large study has been performed with CT or MRI to determine the relation of extent of resection to outcome for patients with oligodendroglioma, as evaluated with multivariate analysis, the studies that have been done in general support a maximum extent of resection. The role of a greater extent of resection in prolonging the time to tumor progression and reducing the frequency of malignant progression, and the duration of high-quality survival are all factors that require rigorous study. The extent of mortality and morbidity relative to extent of resection have not been analyzed, but they must be taken into account when recommending radical surgery over other treatment options.[1]

The extent of tumor resection both for hemispheric glioblastomas multiforme and for anaplastic gliomas significantly affects outcome in relation to postoperative KPS, time to tumor progression, and survival. By prolonging life at the same or a better quality of existence through surgery, the time gained may permit the institution of innovative adjuvant treatment modalities that are now under development and trial, including such new strategies as gene therapy or antisense oligodeoxynucleotides that block mRNA translation of specific regulatory proteins.[1] It is conceivable also that such therapies may act more effectively against a smaller volume of residual tumor.

REFERENCES

1. Rostomily RC, Berger MS, Keles GE: Radical surgery in the management of low grade and high grade gliomas. *In* Yung WKA (ed): Clinical Neurology: International Practice and Research, Cerebral Gliomas Series. London, Baillière Tindall, 1996, pp 345–369.
2. Laws ER, Taylor WF, Clifton MB, et al: Neurosurgical management of low-grade astrocytomas of the cerebral hemispheres. J Neurosurg 1984; 61:665–673.
3. Berger MS, Deliganis AV, Dobbins J, et al: The effect of extent of resection on recurrence in patients with low-grade cerebral hemisphere gliomas. Cancer 1994; 74:1784–1791.
4. Nicolato A, Gerosa GA, Fina P, et al: Prognostic factors in low-grade supratentorial astrocytomas: A uni-multivariate statistical analysis in 76 surgically treated adult patients. Surg Neurol 1995; 44:208–221.
5. Philippon JH, Clemenceau SH, Foncin JF: Supratentorial low-grade astrocytoma in adults. Neurosurgery 1993; 32:554–559.
6. Medbery CA, Straus KL, Steinberg SM, et al: Low-grade astrocytomas: Treatment results and prognostic variables. Int J Radiat Oncol Biol Phys 1988; 15:837–841.
7. North CA, North RB, Epstein JA, et al: Low-grade astrocytomas: Survival and quality of life after radiation therapy. Cancer 1990; 66:6–14.
8. Piepmeier JM: Observations on the current treatment of low-grade astrocytic tumors of the cerebral hemispheres. J Neurosurg 1987; 67:177–181.
9. Berger MS, Rostomily RC: Low grade gliomas: Functional mapping resection strategies, extent of resection, and outcome. J Neurooncol 1997; 34:85–101.
10. Berger MS, Leibel S, Bruner JM, et al: Primary central nervous system tumors of the supratentorial compartment. *In* Levin VA (ed): Cancer in the Nervous System. New York, Churchill Livingstone, 1995, pp 57–126.
11. Soffietti R, Chio A, Giordana MT, et al: Prognostic factors in well-differentiated cerebral astrocytomas in the adult. Neurosurgery 1989; 24:686–692.

12. Afra D, Muller W, Benoist G, et al: Supratentorial recurrences of gliomas: Results of reoperations on astrocytomas and oligodendrogliomas. Acta Neurochir 1978; 43:217–227.

13. Afra D, Muller W, Slowik F, et al: Supratentorial lobar pilocytic astrocytomas: Report of 45 operated cases, including 9 recurrences. Acta Neurochir 1986; 81:90–93.

14. Muller W, Afra D, Schroder R: Supratentorial recurrences of gliomas: Morphological studies in relation to time intervals with astrocytomas. Acta Neurochir 1977; 37:75–91.

15. Laws ER, Taylor WF, Bergstraith EJ, et al: The neurosurgical management of low-grade astrocytoma. Clin Neurosurg 1985; 33:575–588.

16. Vertosick FT, Selker RG, Arena VC: Survival of patients with well-differentiated astrocytomas diagnosed in the era of computed tomography. Neurosurgery 1991; 28:496–501.

17. Weingart J, Olivi A, Brem H: Supratentorial low-grade astrocytomas in adults. Neurosurg Q 1991; 1:141–159.

18. Davis L, Martin J, Goldstein SL: A study of 211 patients with verified glioblastoma multiforme. J Neurosurg 1949; 6:33–44.

19. Frankel SA, German WJ: Glioblastoma multiforme: Review of 219 cases with regard to natural history, pathology, diagnostic methods and treatment. J Neurosurg 1958; 15:489–503.

20. Jelsma R, Bucy P: The treatment of glioblastoma multiforme of the brain. J Neurosurg 1967; 27:388–400.

21. Jelsma R, Bucy P: Glioblastoma multiforme: Its treatment and some factors affecting survival. Arch Neurol 1969; 20:161–171.

22. Weir B: The relative significance of factors affecting postoperative survival in astrocytomas, grades 3 and 4. J Neurosurg 1973; 38:448–452.

23. Gehan EA, Walker MD: Prognostic factors for patients with brain tumors. National Cancer Institute Monograph 1977; 46:189–195.

24. Walker MD, Alexander E Jr, Hunt WE, et al: BCNU and/or radiotherapy in treatment of anaplastic gliomas: A cooperative clinical trial. J Neurosurg 1978; 49:333–343.

25. Chang CH, Horton J, Schoenfeld D, et al: Comparison of postoperative radiotherapy and combined postoperative radiotherapy and chemotherapy in the multidisciplinary management of malignant gliomas: A joint Radiation Therapy Oncology Group and Eastern Cooperative Oncology Group study. Cancer 1983; 52:997–1007.

26. Levin VA, Hoffman WF, Heilbron DC, et al: Prognostic significance of the pretreatment CT scan on time to progression for patients with malignant gliomas. J Neurosurg 1980; 52:642–647.

27. Andreou J, George AE, Wise A, et al: CT prognostic criteria of survival after malignant glioma surgery. AJNR 1983; 4:488–490.

28. Guthrie BL, Laws ER: Supratentorial low-grade gliomas. Neurosurg Clin North Am 1990; 1:37–48.

29. Weir B, Grace M: The relative significance of factors affecting postoperative survival in astrocytomas, grades 1 and 2. Can J Neurol Sci 1976; 3:47–50.

30. Wood JR, Green SB, Shapiro WR: The prognostic importance of tumor size in malignant gliomas: A computed tomographic scan study by the Brain Tumor Cooperative Group. J Clin Oncol 1988; 6:338–343.

31. Ammirati M, Vick N, Liao Y, et al: Effect of extent of surgical resection on survival and quality of life in patients with supratentorial glioblastomas and anaplastic astrocytomas. Neurosurgery 1987; 21:201–206.

32. Duong DH, Rostomily RC, Haynor DR, et al: Measurement of tumor resection volumes from computerized images. J Neurosurg 1992; 77:151–154.

33. Rostomily RC, Spence AM, Duong D, et al: Multimodality management of recurrent adult malignant gliomas: Results of a phase II multiagent chemotherapy study and analysis of cytoreductive surgery. Neurosurgery 1994; 35:378–388.

34. Ciric I, Ammirati M, Vick N, et al: Supratentorial gliomas: Surgical considerations and immediate postoperative results: Gross total resection versus partial resection. Neurosurgery 1987; 21:21–26.

35. Coffey RJ, Lunsford LD, Taylor FH: Survival after stereotactic biopsy of malignant gliomas. Neurosurgery 1988; 22:465–473.

36. Kelly PJ: Image-directed tumor resection. In Rosenblum M (ed): The Role of Surgery in Brain Tumor Management. Neurosurg Clin North Am 1990; 1:81–95.

37. Dinapoli RP, Brown LD, Arusell RM, et al: Phase III comparative evaluation of PCNU and carmustine combined with radiation therapy for high-grade glioma. J Clin Oncol 1993; 11:1316–1321.

38. Fadul C, Wood J, Thaler H, et al: Morbidity and mortality of craniotomy for excision of supratentorial gliomas. Neurology 1988; 38:1374.

39. Berger MS, Keles GE, Geyer JR: Cerebral hemispheric tumors of childhood. Neurosurg Clin North Am 1992; 3:839–852.

40. Fessard C: Cerebral tumors in infancy. Am J Dis Child 1968; 115:302–308.

41. Jooma R, Kendall BE: Intracranial tumours in the first year of life. Neuroradiology 1982; 23:267–274.

42. Hoffman HJ: Supratentorial brain tumors in children. In Youmans JR (ed): Neurological Surgery, vol 5. Philadelphia, WB Saunders, 1982, pp 2702–2732.

43. Childhood Brain Tumor Consortium: A study of childhood brain tumors on surgical biopsies from ten North American institutions: sample description. J Neurooncol 1988; 6:9–23.

44. Walker ML, Fried A, Pattisapu J: Tumors of the cerebral hemispheres in children. In McLaurin RL, Venes JL, Schut L, et al (eds): Pediatric Neurosurgery, ed 2. Philadelphia, WB Saunders, 1989, pp 373–382.

45. Allen JC, Bloom J, Ertel I, et al: Brain tumors in children: Current cooperative and institutional trials in newly diagnosed and recurrent disease. Semin Oncol 1986; 13:110.

46. Artico M, Cervoni L, Celli P, et al: Supratentorial glioma in children: A series of 27 surgically treated cases. Childs Nerve Syst 1993; 9:7.

47. Wisoff JH, Boyett J, Brandt K, et al: Neurosurgical management and influence of extent of resection on survival in pediatric high-grade astrocytomas: A report on CCG 945. Proceedings of the 61st Annual Meeting of the American Association of Neurological Surgeons, Boston, April 24–29, 1993.

48. Krouwer HGJ, Davis RL, Silver P, et al: Gemistocytic astrocytomas: A reappraisal. J Neurosurg 1991; 74:399.

49. Prados MD, Gutin PH, Phillips TL, et al: Highly anaplastic astrocytoma: A review of 357 patients treated between 1977 and 1989. Int J Radiat Oncol Biol Phys 1992; 23:3.

50. Winger MJ, Macdonald DR, Cairncross JG: Supratentorial anaplastic gliomas in adults: The prognostic importance of extent of resection and prior low-grade glioma. J Neurosurg 1989; 71:487.

51. Chandler KL, Prados MD, Malec M, et al: Long-term survival in patients with glioblastoma multiforme. Neurosurgery 1993; 32:716.

52. Kaplan RS: Supratentorial malignant gliomas: Risk patterns and therapy. J Natl Cancer Inst 1993; 85:690.

53. Kornblith PD, Welch WC, Bradley MK: The future of therapy for glioblastoma. Surg Neurol 1993; 39:538.

54. Mornex F, Mayel H, Taillandier L: Radiation therapy for malignant astrocytomas in adults. Radiother Oncol 1993; 27:181.

55. Morantz RA: Radiation therapy in the treatment of cerebral astrocytoma. Neurosurgery 1987; 20:975–982.

56. Cairncross JG, Lapierriere NJ: Low-grade glioma: To treat or not to treat? Arch Neurol 1989; 46:1238–1239.

57. Recht LD, Lew R, Smith TW: Suspected low-grade glioma: Is deferring treatment safe? Ann Neurol 1992; 31:431–436.

58. Shibamoto Y, Kitakabu Y, Takahashi M, et al: Supratentorial low-grade astrocytoma: Correlation of computed tomography findings with effect of radiation therapy and prognostic variables. Cancer 1993; 72:190–195.

59. Wen DY, Hall WA, Miller DA, et al: Targeted brain biopsy: A comparison of freehand computed tomography–guided and stereotactic techniques. Neurosurgery 1993; 32:407.

60. Berger MS: Ultrasound guided stereotaxic biopsies the extent of resection through a burr hole using a newly designed apparatus. J Neurosurg 1986; 65:550.

61. Enzmann DR, Irvin KM, Marshall WH, et al: Intraoperative sonography through a burr hole: Guide for brain biopsy. AJNR 1984; 5:243.

62. Tsutsumi Y, Andoh Y, Sakaguchi J: A new ultrasound-guided brain biopsy technique through a burr hole: Technical note. Acta Neurochir 1989; 96:72.

63. Di Lorenzo N, Esposito V, Lunardi P, et al: A comparison of computerized tomography–guided stereotactic and ultrasound-guided techniques for brain biopsy. J Neurosurg 1991; 75:763.

64. Chandrasoma PT, Smith MM, Apuzzo MLJ: Stereotactic biopsy in the diagnosis of brain masses: Comparison of results of biopsy and resected surgical specimen. Neurosurgery 1989; 24:160.

65. Taratuto AL, Sevlever G, Piccardo P: Clues and pitfalls in stereotactic biopsy of the central nervous system. Arch Pathol Lab Med 1991; 115:596.

66. Kelly PJ, Alker GJ, Goerss S: Computer-assisted stereotactic laser

microsurgery for the treatment of intracranial neoplasms. Neurosurgery 1982; 10:324.

67. Kelly PJ, Kall B, Goerss S, et al: Precision resection of intraaxial CNS lesions by CT-based stereotactic craniotomy and computer monitored CO_2 laser. Acta Neurochir 1983; 68:1.

68. Kelly PJ, Kall BA, Goerss S, et al: Computer-assisted stereotaxic laser resection of intra-axial brain neoplasms. J Neurosurg 1986; 64:427.

69. Kelly PJ: Volumetric stereotactic surgical resection of intra-axial brain mass lesions. Mayo Clin Proc 1988; 63:1186.

70. Barnett GH, Kormos DW, Steiner CP, et al: Use of a frameless, armless, stereotactic wand for brain tumor localization with two dimensions and three-dimensional neuroimaging. Neurosurgery 1993; 33:674.

71. Roberts DW, Strohbehn JW, Hatch JF, et al: A frameless stereotaxic integration of computerized tomographic imaging and the operating microscope. J Neurosurg 1986; 65:545.

72. Watanabe E, Watanabe T, Manaka S, et al: Three-dimensional digitizer (neuronavigator): New equipment for computed tomography-guided stereotaxic surgery. Surg Neurol 1987; 27:543–547.

73. LeRoux PD, Berger MS, Ojemann GA, et al: Correlation of intraoperative ultrasound tumor volumes and margins with preoperative computed tomography scans: An intraoperative method to enhance tumor resection. J Neurosurg 1989; 71:691.

74. LeRoux PD, Winter TC, Berger MS, et al: A comparison between preoperative magnetic resonance and intraoperative ultrasound tumor volumes and margins. J Clin Ultrasound 1994; 22:29–36.

75. Reyes MG, Homsi MF, Mcdonald LW, et al: Imprints, smears and frozen sections of brain tumors. Neurosurgery 1991; 29:575.

76. Perria C, Carai M, Falzoi A, et al: Photodynamic therapy of malignant brain tumors: Clinical results of, difficulties with, questions about, and future prospects for the neurosurgical applications. Neurosurgery 1988; 23:557.

77. Poon WS, Schomacker KT, Deutsch TF, et al: Laser-induced fluorescence: Experimental intraoperative delineation of tumor resection margins. J Neurosurg 1992; 76:679.

78. Hansen DA, Spence AM, Carski T, et al: Indocyanine green (CG) and demarcation of tumor margins in a rat glioma model. Surg Neurol 1993; 40:451.

79. Moore GE: Fluorescein as an agent in the differentiation of normal and malignant tissues. Science 1947; 106:130.

80. Arseni C, Petrovici IN: Epilepsy of temporal lobe tumors. Eur Neurol 1971; 5:201.

81. Hirsch JF, Sainte Rose C, Pierre-Khan A, et al: Benign astrocytic and oligodendrocytic tumors of the cerebral hemispheres in children. J Neurosurg 1989; 70:568.

82. Pilcher WH, Silbergeld DL, Berger MS, et al: Intraoperative electrocorticography during tumor resection: Impact on seizure outcome in patients with ganglioliomas. J Neurosurg 1993; 78:891.

83. Blume WT, Girvin JP, Kaufmann CE, et al: Childhood brain tumors presenting as chronic uncontrolled focal seizure disorders. Ann Neurol 1982; 12:538–541.

84. Goldring S: Pediatric epilepsy surgery. Epilepsia 1987; 28:S82–S102.

85. Kaylan-Raman UP, Olivero WC: Ganglioglioma: A correlative clinicopathological and radiological study of 10 surgically treated cases with follow-up. Neurosurgery 1987; 20:428–433.

86. Gonzales D, Elvidge AR: On the occurrence of epilepsy caused by astrocytomas of the cerebral hemispheres. J Neurosurg 1962; 19:470–482.

87. Penfield W, Jasper H: Epilepsy and the Functional Anatomy of the Human Brain. Boston, Little, Brown, 1954.

88. Penfield W, Erickson TC, Tarlov I: Relation of intracranial tumors and symptomatic epilepsy. Arch Neurol Psychiatr 1940; 44:300–315.

89. Davis PC, Wichman RD, Takei Y, et al: Primary cerebral neuroblastoma: CT and magnetic resonance findings in 12 cases. AJNR 1990; 11:115–120.

90. Falconer MA, Cavanagh JB: Clinico-pathological considerations of temporal lobe epilepsy due to small focal lesions. Brain 1959; 82:483–504.

91. Spencer DD, Spencer S, Mattson RH, et al: Intracerebral masses in patients with intractable partial epilepsy. Neurology 1984; 34:432–436.

92. Cascino GD: Epilepsy and brain tumors: Implications for treatment. Epilepsia 1990; 31S:3.

93. Cascino GD, Kelly PJM, Hirschorn KA, et al: Stereotactic resection of intra-axial cerebral lesions in partial epilepsy. Mayo Clin Proc 1990; 65:1053.

94. Franceschetti S, Binelli S, Casazza M, et al: Influence of surgery and antiepileptic drugs on seizures symptomatic of cerebral tumors. Acta Neurochir 1990; 103:47.

95. Goldring S, Rich KM, Picker S: Experience with gliomas in patients presenting with a chronic seizure disorder. Clin Neurosurg 1986; 33:15.

96. Awad IA, Rosenfeld J, Ahl J: Intractable epilepsy and structural lesions of the brain. Mapping, resection strategies, and seizure outcome. Epilepsia 1991; 32:179–186.

97. Berger MS, Ghatan S, Haglund MM, et al: Low grade gliomas associated with intractable epilepsy seizure outcome utilizing electrocorticography during tumor resection. J Neurosurg 1993; 79:62.

98. Drake J, Hoffman HJ, Kobayashi J, et al: Surgical management of children with temporal lobe epilepsy and mass lesions. Neurosurgery 1987; 21:792.

99. Rasmussen TB: Surgery of epilepsy associated with brain tumors. Adv Neurol 1975; 8:227.

100. Ribaric I: Excision of two and three independent and separate ipsilateral potentially epileptogenic cortical areas. Acta Neurochir Suppl 1984; 33:14.

101. Nazzaro JM, Neuwelt EA: The role of surgery in the management of supratentorial intermediate and high-grade astrocytomas in adults. J Neurosurg 1990; 73:331–344.

102. Kros JM, Pieterman H, Van Eden CG, et al: Oligodendroglioma: The Rotterdam-Dijkzigt experience. J Neurosurg 1994; 34:959–966.

103. Miralbell R, Balart J, Matias-Guiu X, et al: Radiotherapy for supratentorial low-grade gliomas: Results and prognostic factors with special focus on tumour volume parameters. Radiother Oncol 1993; 27:112–116.

104. Kelly PJ: Stereotactic resection and its limitations in glial neoplasms. Stereotact Funct Neurosurg 1992; 59:84.

105. Scherer HJ: Cerebral astrocytomas and their derivatives. Am J Cancer 1940; 40:159–198.

106. Scherer HJ: The forms of growth in gliomas and their practical significance. Brain 1940; 63:1–35.

107. Kelly PJ, Daumas-Duport C, Kispart DB, et al: Imaging-based stereotactic serial biopsies in untreated intracranial glial neoplasms. J Neurosurg 1987; 66:865–874.

108. Kelly PJ, Daumas-Duport C, Scheithauer BW, et al: Stereotactic histologic correlations of computed tomography and magnetic resonance imaging-defined abnormalities in patients with glial neoplasms. Mayo Clin Proc 1987; 62:450–459.

109. Johnson PC, Hunt SJ, Drayer BP: Human cerebral gliomas: Correlation of postmortem MR imaging and neuropathologic findings. Radiology 1989; 170:211–217.

110. Earnest F IV, Kelly PJ, Scheithauer BW, et al: Cerebral astrocytomas: Correlation of postmortem MR imaging and neuropathologic findings. Radiology 1989; 170:211–217.

111. Cairncross JG, Macdonald DR, Pexman JHW, et al: Steroid-induced CT changes in patients with recurrent malignant glioma. Neurology 1958; 38:7224.

112. Watling CJ, Lee DH, Macdonald DR, et al: Corticosteroid-induced magnetic resonance imaging changes in patients with recurrent malignant glioma. J Clin Oncol 1994; 12:1886–1889.

113. Rostomily RC, Halligan JB, Keles GE, et al: Management of adult recurrent supratentorial gliomas. Neurosurg Q 1993; 3:219–252.

114. Rajan B, Pickuth D, Ashley S, et al: The management of histologically unverified presumed cerebral gliomas with radiotherapy. Int J Radiat Oncol Biol Phys 1993; 28:4405–4413.

115. Kreth FW, Fast M, Warnke PC, et al: Interstitial radiosurgery of low-grade gliomas. J Neurosurg 1995; 82:4418–4429.

116. Shaw EG, Daumas-Duport C, Scheithauer BW, et al: Radiation therapy in the management of low-grade supratentorial astrocytomas. J Neurosurg 1989; 70:853–861.

117. Ito S, Chandler KL, Prados MD, et al: Proliferative potential and prognostic evaluation of low-grade astrocytomas. J Neurooncol 1994; 19:1–9.

118. Shaw EG, Scheithauer BW, O'Fallon, et al: Oligodendrogliomas: The Mayo Clinic experience. J Neurosurg 1992; 76:428–434.

119. Shaw EG, Scheithauer BW, O'Fallon JR, et al: Mixed oligodendrogliomas: A survival and prognostic factor analysis. Neurosurgery 1994; 34:577–582.

120. Celli P, Nofrone I, Palma L, et al: Cerebral oligodendroglioma: Prognostic factors and life history. Neurosurgery 1994; 35:1018–1035.

121. Shaw EG, Scheithauer BW, O'Fallon Jr: Management of supratentorial low-grade gliomas. Semin Radiat Oncol 1991; 1:23.

122. Leibel SA, Sheline GE, Wara WM, et al: The role of radiation therapy in the treatment of astrocytomas. Cancer 1975; 35:1551.

123. Marsa GW, Goffinet DR, Rubinstein LJ, et al: Megavoltage irradiation in the treatment of gliomas of the brain and spinal cord. Cancer 1975; 36:1681.

124. Whitton AC, Bloom HJ: Low-grade glioma of the cerebral hemispheres in adults: A retrospective analysis of 88 cases. Int J Radiat Oncol Biol Phys 1990; 18:783–786.

125. Singer JM: Supratentorial low-grade gliomas in adults: A retrospective analysis of 43 cases treated with surgery and radiotherapy. Eur J Surg Oncol 1995; 21:198–200.

126. Dohrmann GJ, Farwell JR, Flannery JT: Oligodendrogliomas in children. Surg Neurol 1978; 10:21–25.

127. Chin HW, Hazel JJ, Kim TH, et al: Oligodendrogliomas: A clinical study of cerebral oligodendrogliomas. Cancer 1980; 45:1458.

128. Mørk SJ, Lindegaard K-F, Halvorsen TB, et al: Oligodendroglioma: Incidence and biological behavior in a defined population. J Neurosurg 1985; 63:881–889.

129. Shaw EG, Scheithauer BW, O'Fallon JR, et al: Oligodendrogliomas: The Mayo Clinic experience. J Neurosurg 1992; 76:428.

130. Varma RR, Crumvine PK, Bergman I, et al: Childhood oligodendrogliomas presenting with seizures and low density lesions on computed tomography. Neurology 1983; 33:806.

131. Sun ZM, Genka S, Shitara N, et al: Factors possibly influencing the prognosis of oligodendroglioma. Neurosurgery 1988; 22:886.

132. Lindegaard K-F, Mørk SJ, Eide GE, et al: Statistical analysis of clinicopathological features, radiotherapy, and survival in 170 cases of oligodendroglioma. J Neurosurg 1987; 67:224–230.

133. Balestrini MR, Zanette M, Micheli R, et al: Hemispheric cerebral tumors in children: Longterm prognosis concerning survival rate and quality of life—considerations on a series of 64 cases operated upon. Childs Nerv Syst 1990; 6:143–147.

134. Farwell JR, Dohrmann GJ, Flannery JT: Central nervous system tumors in children. Cancer 1977; 40:3123–3132.

135. Gjerris F: Clinical aspects and long-term prognosis in supratentorial tumors of infancy and childhood. Acta Neurol Scandinav 1978; 57:445–470.

136. Low NL, Correll JW, Hammed JF: Tumors of the cerebral hemispheres in children. Arch Neurol 1965; 13:547–554.

137. Mercuri S, Russo A, Palma L: Hemispheric supratentorial astrocytomas in children: Long-term results in 29 cases. J Neurosurg 1981; 55:170–173.

138. Dohrmann GJ, Farwell JR, Flannery JT: Astrocytomas in childhood: A population-based study. Surg Neurol 1985; 23:64–68.

139. Palma L, Guidetti B: Cystic pilocytic astrocytomas of the cerebral hemispheres: Surgical experience with 51 cases and long-term results. J Neurosurg 1985; 62:811–815.

140. Clark GB, Henry JM, McKeever PE: Cerebral pilocytic astrocytoma. Cancer 1985; 56:1128.

141. Sutton IN: Current management of low-grade astrocytomas of childhood. Pediatr Neurosci 1987; 13:98.

142. Garcia DM, Fulling KH: Juvenile pilocytic astrocytoma of the cerebrum in adults. J Neurosurg 1985; 63:382.

143. Schisano G, Tovi D, Nordenstam H: Spongioblastoma polare of the cerebral hemisphere. J Neurosurg 1963; 20:241.

144. Palma L, Guidetti B: Cystic pilocytic astrocytomas of the cerebral hemispheres: Surgical experience with 51 cases and long-term results. J Neurosurg 1985; 62:811–815.

145. Tomita T, McLone DF, Naidich TP: Mural tumors with cysts in the cerebral hemispheres of children. Neurosurgery 1986; 19:998.

146. Maiuri F: Cysts with mural tumor nodules in the cerebral hemispheres. Neurosurgery 1988; 22:703.

147. Burger PC, Scheithauer BW, Vogel PS: Surgical pathology of the nervous system and its coverings, 3rd ed. New York, Churchill Livingstone, 1991.

148. Obana WG, Cogen PH, Davis RL, et al: Metastatic juvenile pilocytic astrocytoma. J Neurosurg 1991; 75:972.

149. Pinto-Lord MC, Abroms IF, Smith TW: Hyperdense cerebral lesion in childhood tuberous sclerosis: Computed tomographic demonstration and neuropathologic analysis. Pediatr Neurol 1986; 2:245.

150. McLaurin RL, Towbin RB: Tuberous sclerosis: Diagnostic and surgical considerations. Pediatr Neurosci 1986; 12:43.

151. Shepherd CW, Scheithauer BW, Gomez MR, et al: Subependymal giant cell astrocytoma: A clinical, pathological, and flow cytometric study. Neurosurgery 1991; 28:864.

152. Morota N, Sakamoto K, Kobayashi N, et al: Recurrent low-grade glioma in children with special reference to computed tomography findings and pathological changes. Childs Nerv Syst 1990; 6:155.

153. Palma L, Russo A, Mercuri S: Cystic cerebral astrocytomas in infancy and childhood: Long-term results. Childs Brain 1983; 10:79.

154. Wallner KE, Gonzales MF, Edwards MS, et al: Treatment results of juvenile pilocytic astrocytoma. J Neurosurg 1988; 69:171–176.

155. Wald SL, Fogelson H, McLaurin RL: Cystic thalamic gliomas. Childs Brain 1982; 9:381.

156. Berger MS, Ojemann GA, Lettich E: Neurophysiological monitoring during astrocytoma surgery. Neurosurg Clin North Am 1990; 1:65–80.

157. Lyons MK, Kelly PJ: Computer-assisted stereotactic biopsy and volumetric resection of thalamic pilocytic astrocytomas: Report of 23 cases. Stereotact Funct Neurosurg 1992; 59:100.

158. Boesel CP, Paulson GWK, Kosmik EJ, et al: Brain hamartomas and tumors associated with tuberous sclerosis. Neurosurgery 1979; 4:410.

159. Nakamura Y, Becker LE: Subependymal giant cell tumor: Astrocytic or neuronal? Acta Neuropathol 1983; 60:271.

160. Stuart G, Appleton DB, Cooke R: Pleomorphic xanthoastrocytoma: Report of two cases. Neurosurgery 1988; 22:422–427.

161. Whittle IR, Gordon A, Misra BK, et al: Pleomorphic xanthoastrocytoma: Report of four cases. J Neurosurg 1989; 70:463–468.

162. Kepes JJ, Rubinstein LJ, Eng LF: Pleomorphic xanthoastrocytoma: A distinctive meningocerebral glioma of young subjects with relatively favorable prognosis: A study of 12 cases. Cancer 1979; 44:1839.

163. Weldon-Linne CM, Victor TA, Groothius DR, et al: Pleomorphic xanthoastrocytoma: Ultrastructural and immunohistochemical study of a case with a rapidly fatal outcome following surgery. Cancer 1983; 52:2055.

164. Kepes JJ: Pleomorphic xanthoastroastrocytoma: The birth of a diagnosis and concept. Brain Pathol 1993; 3:269.

165. Grant JW, Gallagher PJ: Pleomorphic xanthoastrocytoma: Immunohistochemical methods for differentiation from fibrous histiocytomas with similar morphology. Am J Surg Pathol 1986; 10:336.

166. Ozek MM, Sav A, Pamir MN, et al: Pleomorphic xanthoastrocytoma associated with von Recklinghausen neurofibromatosis. Childs Nerv Syst 1993; 9:39.

167. Kepes JJ, Runinstein LJ, Ansbacher L, et al: Histopathological features of recurrent pleomorphic xanthoastrocytomas: Further corroboration of the glial nature of this neoplasm. Acta Neuropathol 1989; 78:585.

168. Macaulay RJ, Jay V, Hoffman HJ, et al: Increased mitotic activity as a negative prognostic indicator in pleomorphic xanthoastrocytoma: Case report. J Neurosurg 1993; 79:761.

169. de Chadarevian J-P, Pattisapu JV, Faerber EN: Desmoplastic cerebral astrocytoma of infancy: Light microscopy, immunocytochemistry, and ultrastructure. Cancer 1990; 66:173.

170. Louis DN, Von Deimling A, Dickersin GR, et al: Desmoplastic cerebral astrocytomas of infancy: A histopathological, immunohistochemical, ultrastructural, and molecular genetic study. Hum Pathol 1992; 23:1402.

171. VandenBerg SR: Desmoplastic infantile ganglioglioma and desmoplastic cerebral astrocytoma of infancy. Brain Pathol 1993; 3:275.

172. Garrido E, Becker LF, Hoffman JH, et al: Gangliogliomas in children: A clinicopathological study. Childs Brain 1978; 4:339–346.

173. Johnson JH, Rekate HL, Roessmann U: Gangliogliomas: Pathological and clinical correlation. J Neurosurg 1981; 54:58–63.

174. Sutton LN, Packer RJ, Zimmerman RA, et al: Cerebral gangliogliomas of childhood. Prog Exp Tumor Res 1987; 30:239–246.

175. Silver JM, Rawlings CE III, Rossitch E, et al: Ganglioglioma: A clinical study with long-term follow-up. Surg Neurol 1991; 35:261.

176. Haddad SF, Moore SA, Menezes AH, et al: Ganglioglioma: Thirteen years of experience. Neurosurgery 1992; 31:171.

177. Miller DC, Lang FF, Epstein FJ: Central nervous system gangliogliomas: I. Pathology. J Neurosurg 1993; 79:859.

178. Otsubo H, Hoffman HJ, Humphries RP, et al: Detection and management of gangliogliomas in children. Surg Neurol 1992; 38:371.

179. Daumas-Duport C: Dysembryoplastic neuroepithelial tumours. Brain Pathol 1993; 3:283.

180. VandenBerg SR, May EE, Rubinstein LJ, et al: Desmoplastic supra-

tentorial neuroepithelial tumors of infancy with divergent differentiation potential (''desmoplastic infantile gangliogliomas''). J Neurosurg 1987; 66:58.

181. Koeller KK, Dillon WP: Dysembryoplastic neuroepithelial tumors: MR appearance. AJNR 1992; 13:1319.

182. Taratuto AL, Monges J, Lylyk P, et al: Superficial cerebral astrocytoma attached to dura. Cancer 1984; 54:2505.

183. Salcman M: Supratentorial gliomas: Clinical features and surgical therapy. *In* Wilkins RH (ed): Neurosurgery, vol 1. New York, Mcgraw-Hill, 1985, pp 579–590.

184. Scanlon PW, Taylor WF: Radiotherapy of intracranial astrocytomas: Analysis of 417 cases treated from 1960 through 1969. Neurosurgery 1979; 5:301–308.

185. Shapiro WR: Treatment of neuroectodermal brain tumors. Ann Neurol 1982; 12:231–237.

186. Albert FK, Forsting M, Sartor K, et al: Early postoperative magnetic resonance imaging after resection of malignant glioma: Objective evaluation of residual tumor and its influence on regrowth and prognosis. Neurosurgery 1994; 34:45–60.

187. Jeremic B, Grujicic D, Antunovic V, et al: Influence of extent of surgery and tumor location on treatment outcome of patients with glioblastoma multiforme treated with combined modality approach. J Neurooncol 1994; 21:177–185.

188. Yoshida J, Kajita Y, Wakabayashi T: Long-term follow-up results of 175 patients with malignant glioma: Importance of radical tumor resection and postoperative adjuvant therapy with interferon, ACNU and radiation. Acta Neurochirologica 1994; 127:55–59.

189. Huber A, Beran H, Becherer A, et al: Supratentorial glioma: Analysis of clinical and temporal parameters in 163 cases. Neurochirurgia 1993; 36:189–193.

190. Kreth FW, Warnke PC, Scheremet R, et al: Surgical resection and radiation therapy versus biopsy and radiation therapy in the treatment of glioblastoma multiforme. J Neurosurg 1993; 78:762–766.

191. Burger PC: The anatomy of astrocytomas. Mayo Clinic Proc 1987; 62:527–529.

192. Daumas-Duport C, Scheithauer BW, Kelly PJ: A histologic and cytologic method for the spatial definition of gliomas. Mayo Clin Proc 1987; 62:435.

193. Kelly PJ: Computed tomography and histologic limits in glial neoplasms: Tumor types and selection for volumetric resection. Surg Neurol 1993; 39:458.

194. Hochberg FH, Pruitt A: Assumptions in the radiotherapy of glioblastoma. Neurology 1980; 30:907–911.

195. Gutin PH, Leibel SA: Stereotaxic interstitial irradiation of malignant brain tumors. Neurology Clin 1985; 3:883–893.

196. Liang BC, Thornton AF, Sandler HM, et al: Malignant astrocytomas: Focal tumor recurrence after focal external beam radiation therapy. J Neurosurg 1991; 75:559.

197. Gaspar LE, Fisher BJ, Macdonald DR, et al: Supratentorial malignant glioma: Patterns of recurrence and implications for external beam local treatment. Int J Radiat Oncol Biol Phys 1992; 24:55.

198. Kelly PJ, Daumas-Duport C, Scheithauer BW, et al: Stereotactic histologic correlations of computed tomography and magnetic resonance imaging-defined abnormalities in patients with glial neoplasms. Mayo Clinic Proc 1987; 62:450–459.

199. Halperin EC, Burger PC, Bullard DE: The fallacy of the localized supratentorial malignant glioma. Int J Rad Oncol Biol Phys 1988; 15:505–509.

200. Tsuboi K, Yoshii Y, Nakagawa K, et al: Regrowth patterns of supratentorial gliomas: Estimation from computed tomographic scans. Neurosurgery 1986; 19:946–951.

201. Filipek PA, Kennedy DN, Caviness VS Jr: Volumetric analyses of central nervous system neoplasm based on MRI. Pediatr Neurol 1991; 7:347–351.

202. Berger MS, Ojemann GA: Intraoperative brain mapping techniques. Stereotact Funct Neurosurg 1992; 59:153–161.

203. Berger MS, Ghatan S, Geyer JR, et al: Seizure outcome in children with hemispheric tumors and associated intractable epilepsy: The role of tumor removal combined with seizure foci resection. Pediatr Neurosurg 1992; 17:185–191.

204. Kaplan EL, Meier P: Nonparametric estimation from incomplete observations. J Am Stat Assoc 1958; 53:457–481.

205. Schag CC, Heinrich RL, Gains PA: Karnofsky performance status revisited: Reliability, validity and guidelines. J Clin Oncol 1984; 2:187–193.

206. Breslow NE, Day NE: Statistical Methods in Cancer Research. Lyon, France, International Agency for Research on Cancer Scientific Publications, 1980.

207. Maiuri F, Stella L, Benvenuti D, et al: Cerebral gliosarcomas: Correlation of computed tomographic findings, surgical aspect, pathologic features and prognosis. Neurosurgery 1990; 26:261.

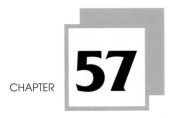

57

Gliomas in the Very Young Child

Central nervous system tumors in the very young child continue to represent one of the major challenges to the pediatric neuro-oncologist. The survival of older children with tumors of the central nervous system has improved significantly during the last several decades. Improvement has been less evident in the very youngest patients, who are less than 2 or 3 years of age at the time of diagnosis. In addition, the adverse late effects of treatment have become increasingly apparent in children who do survive tumors that manifest at an early age. This chapter discusses some of the unique aspects of epidemiology, diagnosis, treatment, and outcome in the very young child with central nervous system tumors.

EPIDEMIOLOGY

Approximately 13% of childhood brain tumors occur in children younger than 2 years.[1] Two population-based studies in North America have examined the incidence of brain tumors in the very young. In the Connecticut Tumor Registry, patient entries were reviewed over a 40-year period from 1935 to 1974.[2] A total of 54 primary intracranial tumors occurred in infants 18 months or younger; 40% were located in the cerebellum and 30% in the cerebral hemispheres; 30% were medulloblastomas and 16% were ependymal neoplasms. The largest population-based study to date was a review of the Surveillance, Epidemiology and End Results (SEER) registry from 1974 to 1980. Of 887 brain tumors in childhood, 112 (13%) occurred in children younger than 2 years.[1] The most common tumor in this group was medulloblastoma (23%), followed by low-grade astrocytoma and ependymoma. Brainstem gliomas, cerebellar astrocytomas, and high-grade gliomas were rare. The histologic frequencies seen in institutional series are shown in Table 57–1.

The youngest children, those younger than 1 year, have a somewhat different distribution of tumor location than older children. In children younger than 1 year at diagnosis, a preponderance of supratentorial tumors is seen.[3, 4] In a series of 100 children younger than 1 year at diagnosis, 60% of tumors were supratentorial, the greatest proportion of which were suprasellar low-grade astrocytomas. In a multicenter retrospective study of 886 infants younger than 1 year with brain tumors, 65.4% of tumors were supratentorial and 29.6% were infratentorial. Of these patients, 254 (29%) had astrocytomas, 101 (11.4%) had ependymomas, and 102 (11.5%) had medulloblastomas.[5]

The distribution of brain tumor types in very young children, those younger than 2 years, is not greatly different than that in older children; medulloblastoma is the single most common tumor type, comprising about 20% to 25% of the total, followed in frequency by low-grade astrocytomas. However, several differences from older children are noteworthy: Ependymal tumors of the posterior fossa are more frequent, and high-grade astrocytomas and brainstem gliomas are less frequent. In children younger than 1 year, a particularly high incidence of supratentorial tumors is seen, primarily optic chiasm tumors.

UNIQUE HISTOLOGIC TYPES

Several central nervous system tumors unique to the very young child have been described. The desmoplastic infantile

TABLE 57–1
TUMOR HISTOLOGIC FINDINGS IN VERY YOUNG CHILDREN WITH BRAIN TUMORS

	DiRocco et al[53]	DiRocco et al[5]	Mapstone & Warf[54]
No. of patients	886	47	22
Age (mo)	<12	<12	<24
Astrocytoma (%)	29	14	4
Chiasmatic/hypothalamic astrocytoma (%)		10	23
Malignant astrocytoma (%)		10	9
Ependymoma (%)	11	11	5
Medulloblastoma (%)	11	26	27
Choroid plexus papilloma (%)	11	6	5
PNET (non-medulloblastoma) (%)	6	6	9
Teratoma (%)	5	4	5
Sarcoma (%)	2	0	0
Meningioma (%)	2	6	0
Ganglioglioma (%)	1	2	5
Choroid plexus carcinoma (%)	<1	2	0
Rhabdoid tumor (%)	0	0	0

PNET, primitive neuroectodermal tumor.

ganglioglioma is a supratentorial embryonal tumor with a good prognosis following surgical removal.[6, 7] This tumor presents within the first 18 months of life and usually occurs within the frontal and parietal lobes. The tumor is usually massive in size, and its histologic features are desmoplasia and differentiating astrocytes and ganglionic cells. In other tumors, a mixture of astrocytes and mature fibroblasts have also been described (i.e., the gliofibroma and the superficial cerebral astrocytoma).[8–10] Rushing and co-workers[11] argued that although histologic differences exist between these tumor types,[11] they might be considered a spectrum of desmoplastic tumors of childhood, particularly because the prognosis for all of these tumors, with adequate surgical intervention, appears to be good.

Another tumor type that is apparently unique to the infant group is the rhabdoid tumor, which consists of cells that exhibit variable morphologic features and which always contain a population of rhabdoid cells (similar to those found in infantile rhabdoid tumors of the kidney); this tumor also displays areas similar in appearance to the primitive neuroectodermal tumors (PNET).[12] Additionally, the tumors may contain neoplastic mesenchyme or other types of ectodermally derived tissue. Recently, abnormalities of chromosome 22 have been described in association with this tumor.[13] Children with this tumor have a very poor prognosis.

SIGNS AND SYMPTOMS

The presenting signs and symptoms of brain tumor in the very young child (Table 57–2), similar to those the older child, are predominantly symptoms of increased intracranial pressure (i.e., vomiting, lethargy, and irritability). The presence of open sutures in this age group, however, frequently results in macrocephaly as a presenting sign of increased intracranial pressure.

Poor weight gain, sometimes despite good appetite, and often not initially associated with vomiting, has been described as the diencephalic syndrome. This syndrome is seen predominantly in children with third ventricular region

TABLE 57–2
SYMPTOMS AND SIGNS IN VERY YOUNG CHILDREN WITH BRAIN TUMORS (% SYMPTOMATIC)

Symptoms and Signs	Mapstone and Warf[54]	DiRiocco et al[5]	DiRiocco et al[53]	Cohen et al[52]
↑ Intracranial pressure	73	75	49	41
Ataxia	18	10		18
Hemiparesis	14		2	
Proptosis	9	4	2	
Optic atrophy	5			
Nystagmus	5	16		14
Developmental delay	9	16		19
CNS palsy	5	12	6	
Seizure	5	16	12	13
↓ Consciousness		16	4	26
Failure to thrive		4	4	
Visual loss				19

*First symptom.

tumors, most commonly chiasmatic gliomas. Nystagmus and poor vision, when noted, further suggest this tumor location.

The ubiquitous presence of gastrointestinal tract symptoms, particularly vomiting, in the very young child often results in an extensive diagnostic workup of the gastrointestinal tract prior to a correct but delayed diagnosis of brain tumor. In one study, done before the advent of the computed tomographic (CT) scan, only 80% of infant brain tumors were diagnosed antemortem. Even in the CT era, diagnosis in half of all patients was delayed for greater than 1 month after onset of symptoms.

PROGNOSIS

Historically, survival of infants with brain tumors has been worse than that of older children. Duffner and colleagues[1] reported a 5-year survival rate of 30% in children younger than 2 years at diagnosis, compared with a 57% 5-year survival rate in children between 10 and 14 years of age. The 12-month survival of patients younger than 2 years with medulloblastomas or ependymomas was less than 30%, and the rate of 5-year survival was less than 12%. Similarly, another study reported a 23% survival rate at 1 year in patients who were 18 months or younger at diagnosis of these tumor types.[14]

These reported low survival rates, however, result in part from a variety of causes that do not necessarily reflect the biologic curability of brain tumors in the very young child. For example, operative mortality in this group of patients has, until recently, been very high. In a single institution study of 68 patients younger than 1 year who were operated on before 1968, the surgical mortality was 33%. In patients with medulloblastoma, 43% died of operative causes.[15] With modern methods of anesthesia and improved neurosurgical technique, however, the operative mortality in very young children has significantly decreased. In a more recent series of infants younger than 1 year at diagnosis, the operative mortality was only 7.3%.[16]

Delay in diagnosis, more common in the very young child, may adversely affect outcome. In addition, in several series, brain tumors diagnosed post mortem have been included in survival statistics.

PRIMITIVE NEUROECTODERMAL TUMORS, INCLUDING MEDULLOBLASTOMA

There are few data concerning the outcome in very young children with medulloblastoma treated with conventional radiotherapy. In a review of patients treated in a single institution from 1955 to 1985, the projected 5-year survival of children younger than 18 months at the time of diagnosis of medulloblastoma was 50%,[17] not significantly different from that of children older than 36 months at diagnosis. Others have reported a 45% event-free survival rate for medulloblastomas in children younger than 2 years at diagnosis who were treated with chemotherapy and craniospinal radiation, compared with a 75% event-free survival overall.[18]

Two large cooperative group studies of medulloblastoma in childhood have recently been published.[19, 20] In both studies, patients were randomized to receive craniospinal radiation only or craniospinal radiation and chemotherapy. Children younger than 2 years were not eligible for the Childrens Cancer Group Study (CCGS), but were included in the International Society of Pediatric Oncology (SIOP) Study. The outcome for the very youngest children in each study (younger than 4 years in the CCGS Study and younger than 2 years in the SIOP Study) were quite similar (i.e., 5-year event-free survival of approximately 40% compared with 5-year event-free survival of greater than 50% for older children, a difference that is significant) (Table 57–3).

In both group studies, chemotherapy appeared to be of benefit to younger children.[21] In the SIOP Study, infants who received only radiation fared poorly, whereas approximately 50% of those treated with both chemotherapy and radiation were long-term survivors. These studies did not include uniform staging of all patients at diagnosis, and it is possible that the poor survival of infants who received only radiation indicates, in part, the greater likelihood of the presence of metastasis in this age group.

As the adverse effects of radiotherapy in the very young child with a malignant brain tumor have become apparent, interest has increased in the use of alternative approaches to treatment. At M.D. Anderson Cancer Center, Houston, children with brain tumors who were younger than 36 months at diagnosis were treated with MOPP chemotherapy (nitrogen mustard, vincristine, prednisone, and procarbazine) as primary therapy, and radiation was reserved for recurrence of tumor following surgery. Of 13 children with medulloblastoma/PNET, 7 who were not given radiation are surviving without evidence of tumor, whereas 4 of the infants who have suffered relapse have survived at a median of 77 months following salvage treatment with cisplatin, radiotherapy, or a combination of the two.[1]

This study and other institutional pilot studies have demonstrated the feasibility of using chemotherapy as a primary adjuvant treatment in the very young child with medulloblastoma/PNET, in an attempt to delay radiotherapy. Neurodevelopmental assessments have suggested that chemotherapy alone may have minimal impact on cognitive function,[22] and several cooperative group studies have reported using postoperative chemotherapy and delaying, or in some cases avoiding, radiotherapy.

In the Childrens Cancer Group Study, children younger than 18 months at the time of diagnosis were treated with eight drugs (lomustine, vincristine, procarbazine, hydroxyurea, prednisone, cisplatin, cytosine arabinoside, and cyclophosphamide chemotherapy). Radiotherapy was to be deferred until the completion of the chemotherapy in an attempt to minimize late sequelae from the radiation.[23] Forty-six children with medulloblastoma, 8 with pinealoblastoma, and 11 with nonpineal supratentorial PNETs were entered. The 3-year progression-free survival for medulloblastoma, pinealoblastoma, and supratentorial nonpineal PNET was 22%, 0%, and 26%, respectively, with a median time to progression of 6 months. The only independent predictors of progression-free survival were metastasis stage and location of the tumor within the pineal region. Twenty-four children completed this chemotherapeutic regimen without tumor progression, and of these, 19 are event-free survivors more than 2 years after diagnosis. Only three of these patients received radiation therapy.

The Pediatric Oncology Group has recently completed a study treating children younger than 36 months with malignant brain tumors with cyclophosphamide, vincristine, cisplatin, and etoposide.[24] Children younger than 24 months at the time of diagnosis were treated for 24 months prior to planned radiation therapy, whereas those 24 to 36 months of age were treated for 12 months. Standard radiation, appropriate to the tumor type, was then administered. Most children received radiation at the completion of chemotherapy.

The 2-year PFS rate on this study for patients with medulloblastoma, 34%, was similar to that noted in the Childrens Cancer Group Study. As in the Childrens Cancer Group Study, disease progression occurred early in treatment in the majority of patients. Thus, treatment of young infants with medulloblastoma or other PNETs using primary chemotherapy can result in event-free survival for between 20% and 40% of such children. A small subset of these children may not require radiotherapy.

The presence of metastases is a known predictor of poor prognosis in medulloblastoma. Several reports have documented a high incidence of metastases in younger children. In patients with medulloblastoma treated in Seattle from 1955 to 1984, 40% of adequately staged children younger than 3 years at diagnosis of medulloblastoma had evidence of metastases (i.e., the finding of tumor cells in the cerebrospinal fluid or a positive myelogram). Another study reported a 50% incidence of metastases in children who were younger than 3 years at the time of diagnosis of medulloblastoma.[25]

However, in the prospective Childrens Cancer Group Study, only 23% of infants had metastatic disease at the

TABLE 57–3
OUTCOME OF VERY YOUNG CHILDREN WITH MALIGNANT BRAIN TUMORS

Study	Radiotherapy Prior to Progression	Chemotherapy	No. of Patients (MB)	Medulloblastoma EFS (%)	No. of Patients (MA)	Malignant Astrocytoma EFS (%)
Tait et al[20]	+	±	26	39 (5 yr)		
Duffner et al[1]	−	+	13	55 (5 yr)		
Duffner et al[24]	+	+	53	34 (2 yr)	18	43 (2 yr)
Geyer et al[23]	−	+	46	22 (3 yr)		
Geyer et al[38]	−	+			39	36 (3 yr)

EFS, event-free survival.

time of diagnosis, a percentage that is the same as that seen in older children. Furthermore, 50% of infants had complete tumor resection; findings, again, not different from those in older children. Thus, although a very young age at diagnosis of medulloblastoma is associated with poorer long-term survival, it is not clear whether infants with this tumor have a significantly worse prospect for cure than do older children of similar stage at diagnosis who are given similar treatment.

EPENDYMOMA

The histopathologic analysis, treatment, and prognosis of patients with ependymal tumors are controversial, and this is all the more true for very young children with this tumor type. Two series have examined the effect of age on outcome of patients with ependymal tumors. One series found a significantly worse 5-year disease-free survival rate in children younger than 4 years as compared with those older than 7 years (64.2% vs. 27%),[26] whereas the other series showed improved 5-year survival (55% vs. 30%) in patients older than 4 years at diagnosis of intracranial ependymoma.[27] Thus, as with medulloblastoma, young age at diagnosis of ependymoma appears to be an indicator of poor prognosis. In both series, the initial site of recurrence was at the site of the primary tumor in almost all cases, regardless of histologic classification (malignant or benign) or field of radiation (involved field or craniospinal). However, the majority of patients with malignant histopathologic classification received craniospinal radiation.

In addition to age at diagnosis of ependymoma, extent of surgical resection has emerged in a number of studies as an important prognostic factor. In one report, all patients with totally resected noninvasive tumors were alive without disease. In another report, although gross total resection as reported by the neurosurgeon was not correlated with a significantly better outcome than less extensive resections, presence or absence of postoperative enhancement was highly correlated with outcome.[28] No patients with postoperative residual tumor survived to age 5 years, whereas in the absence of postoperative enhancement, 75% of patients were living without disease at 5 years.

Because of concerns of the long-term effect of radiotherapy on the very young child, a number of investigators have utilized chemotherapy in an attempt to defer use of radiotherapy in very young children with ependymoma. In the Pediatric Oncology Group Study discussed earlier, the 2-year progression-free survival of children with ependymoma was approximately 40%. In those children without metastasis and with complete surgical resections, it was 80%. In the Childrens Cancer Group Study using "8-drugs-in-1-day" chemotherapy, the progression-free survival at 2 years was less than 40%. However, only children with high-grade ependymomas were eligible for study entry.

Because of the apparently good prognosis associated with complete resection of ependymoma, as well as the lack of unanimity of the value of adjuvant therapy, some have advocated that no adjuvant therapy be utilized in the instance of a completely resected lesion demonstrated on MRI.[29]

Thus, the prognosis overall for ependymoma, with the possible exception of a completely resected nonmetastatic tumor, remains poor, in the very young child. Whether chemotherapy may be useful as primary adjuvant treatment in this age group remains unclear.

CHIASMATIC OPTIC GLIOMA

The natural history and response to therapy of this tumor are not well established. In most series, approximately 50% of children with this tumor have progression of disease, even following radiotherapy, despite having low-grade histologic characteristics.[30] However, prolonged periods without tumor progression are well documented with these tumors, even when they are not treated. The 10-year actuarial survival rate approaches 60%. In a series in Boston, 24 children with chiasmatic gliomas were treated with radiation doses from 4,500 to 5,660 cGy. With a median follow-up of 6 years, the 6-year actuarial disease-free overall survival was 88% and 100%. However, neuropsychiatric and endocrine abnormalities were found in the majority of children.[31]

Two forms of chiasmatic optic glioma have been described. The infant type of tumor is seen in children younger than 1 year at diagnosis; it is often very large and invades the hypothalamus early in the disease. These lesions present with severe loss of vision and hypothalamic dysfunction and have a poor prognosis. The lesions seen in older children are localized to the optic nerves, chiasm, and tracts, and have a good long-term prognosis.

Several reports have documented the feasibility and value of radical resection of exophytic chiasmatic-hypothalamic tumors.[32] Wisoff and co-workers[34] reported on 16 children who underwent significant resection with no mortality and minimum morbidity; six of nine who underwent radical resection (greater than 60%) and no further treatment are stable at a mean of 27 months follow-up. Thus, in selected chiasmatic tumors with a significant exophytic component, resection may be a viable alternative to radiation or chemotherapy,[33, 34] particularly in the very young child.

The timing and modality of treatment of the chiasmatic tumor is controversial. As discussed earlier, these tumors can remain stable, even without treatment, or they can progress despite treatment. Radiotherapy results in at least stabilization of tumor growth in most patients, but it may have adverse long-term effects, particularly in the very young.

Several chemotherapeutic regimens for the treatment of progressive (clinically or radiographically) low-grade gliomas of the optic chiasm and/or hypothalamus in children younger than 5 years have been published (Fig. 57–1). In the first such approach reported,[35] vincristine and dactinomycin were used to treat 24 patients (median age, 1.6 years). At a median follow-up of 4.3 years, all patients were alive, and the projected 70-month event-free survival was 25%. Nine of the 24 patients had developed radiographic or clinical evidence of progressive disease; in two patients, these findings appeared during therapy. In the seven patients who had progressive disease after completion of chemotherapy, progression occurred at a median of 3 years after initiation of treatment. Of seven patients evaluated prior to and after chemotherapy, none showed a sequential decline in cognitive function. Other chemotherapeutic approaches to low-grade gliomas of the young child have been published. Carboplatin

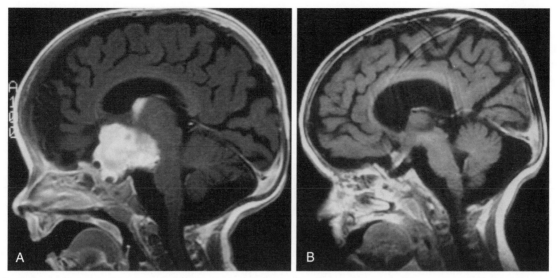

Figure 57-1 *A,* Suprasellar pilocytic astrocytoma before treatment. *B,* Suprasellar pilocytic astrocytoma after treatment with vincristine and carboplatin.

and vincristine resulted in a 40% partial response rate in patients with newly diagnosed chiasmatic hypothalamic tumors.[36] Nitrosourea-based chemotherapy has also been of use in treating young patients, resulting in either tumor shrinkage or stabilization of tumor size in the majority of patients.[37] These results suggest that this chemotherapy regimen can at least delay the need for radiotherapy in many infants and young children with gliomas of the optic chiasm and hypothalamus.

HIGH-GRADE ASTROCYTOMAS IN INFANCY

As noted, high-grade astrocytomas constitute a very small proportion of brain tumors of the very young child (i.e., between 3% and 11%). In a cooperative group study of pediatric patients with high-grade astroctyoma, 17% of 234 patients entered in the study were younger than 24 months at diagnosis.[38] Thirty-nine children were enrolled, of whom 32 had a reviewed pathologic diagnosis consistent with malignant astrocytoma. Twenty patients had anaplastic astrocytoma, nine had glioblastoma multiforme and three had anaplastic mixed gliomas. The primary tumor site was within the cerebral cortex in 14 patients, the midline in 11, the posterior fossa in 3 and the spinal cord in 4. All children were treated with chemotherapy, which per protocol was to have been followed by radiotherapy. In fact, only two children received radiotherapy prior to disease recurrence.

The 3-year progression-free survival rate for patients with anaplastic astrocytoma treated in this fashion was 44%, but all infants with glioblastoma multiforme showed progression of disease by 3 years. The overall progression-free survival for patients with anaplastic astrocytomas is not significantly different than that of older children who received both chemotherapy and radiotherapy. However, the overall progression-free survival is clearly worse for those patients with glioblastoma multiforme than for the older children treated with both modalities.

The Pediatric Oncology Group has recently reported results using cyclophosphamide, vincristine, etoposide, and cisplatin to treat very young children with malignant tumors.[39] Progression-free survival and survival of 18 children with malignant astrocytomas was 43% and 50%, probably not different from the results noted above in view of the small numbers (Table 57–3). Young infants with malignant astrocytomas appear to have an overall prognosis similar to that of the tumors in older children; in some instances, chemotherapy alone can be successful as an adjuvant treatment.

TREATMENT SEQUELAE

In addition to having a worse prognosis for survival, infants are significantly less likely to achieve normal physical and mental development following radiation therapy than are older children. Concern of the late effects of radiotherapy in the very young child has significantly altered the therapeutic approach in this age group.

The most extensive studies documenting the effects of radiation on long-term intellectual function in very young children are those associated with acute lymphoblastic leukemia. It is clear[40] that the combination of whole-brain radiation and chemotherapy, particularly with methotrexate, results in significant decline in cognitive function; this appears to be particularly true in the very young. One study showed a 15 point IQ differential between patients and their siblings following whole-brain radiation and chemotherapy for acute leukemia in children younger than 3 years at the time of diagnosis.[41] Another study found a progressive decline in full-scale IQ, most marked in children between the ages of 2 and 5 years at the time of diagnosis.

Studies of the long-term outcome relating to cognitive function in very young children following treatment for brain tumors are few. Furthermore, many variables, such as tumor location and volume and site of brain radiation, affect later cognitive function in children with brain tumors, making it difficult to assign causality.

A prospective study reported sequential intelligence testing in 43 children treated for brain tumors.[43] Children were tested within 1 month of diagnosis, 3 months after diagnosis (after completion of radiation therapy, if any was given), and at sequential 6-month follow-ups. At all testing points, children with hemispheric tumors showed IQs much lower than those with tumors of either the third or fourth ventricles. Whole-brain radiation was closely associated with decrease in cognitive function; this was especially the case in younger children. Eight of nine patients younger than 7 years who received whole-brain radiation showed IQ loss. All seven children who were given whole-brain radiation before age 5 years had below-average IQs at follow-up, with declines of up to 47 points. The study showed no consistent deficits either in children receiving local radiation or in those who had been given chemotherapy.

Results of a prospective study of cognitive function in children receiving whole-brain radiotherapy for treatment of brain tumors were reported.[44] Patients in this study received 2,400 cGy whole-brain radiotherapy if they were 18 to 36 months of age, and 3,600 cGy if they were older than 36 months; children younger than 18 months were not studied. Children younger than 7 years at diagnosis had a mean decline in full-scale IQ of 25 points at 2 years following treatment. The three youngest children, all of whom received 2,400 cGy, had a fall of 34 to 37 points in full-scale IQ at retesting 2 years after receiving radiation. Children with cerebellar astrocytomas who were not given radiation did not show significant decline over time in any measure of intelligence.

Thus, whole-brain radiotherapy can result in significant cognitive deficits, the severity of which may be proportional to age at diagnosis.[43] The relationship between dose and degree of intellectual impairment is not clear, however. As discussed earlier, the most severe deficits in one study occurred in children who received only 2,400 cGy of whole-brain radiotherapy.[44] However, these children were also the youngest children in the study. A study suggests that factors such as perioperative complications are a better predictor of intellectual deficit than is age.[45] However, early evidence from studies of children with acute lymphoblastic leukemia suggests that lowering the cranial dose of irradiation from 2,400 to 1,800 cGy may decrease the severity of intellectual deficit without adversely affecting survival.

The role of chemotherapy in the development of intellectual deficits is even less clear than is that of radiation. Evidence exists that the addition of chemotherapy, particularly methotrexate, to whole-brain radiotherapy has contributed to intellectual decline both in patients with acute lymphoblastic leukemia and in those with brain tumors,[40] but little evidence is available to suggest that systemic chemotherapy alone is responsible for IQ loss.

In addition to the effects of CNS irradiation of the cognitive function of young children, the effect of such treatment on growth and development has been well documented. Radiation to the pituitary/hypothalamus results in abnormal (decreased) growth hormone responses to provocative stimulation as well as to growth retardation in the majority of patients treated.[46] Some evidence suggests that children younger than 10 years at the time they are given CNS radiotherapy are more vulnerable to these effects.[47, 48] Spinal irradiation can result in impaired spinal growth, the severity of which is directly related to the age at which the radiation was given as well as to the total dose delivered.

NEW TREATMENT STRATEGIES

With few exceptions, the types of brain tumors seen in the very young are the same as those found in the older child; however, important differences in prognosis and a greater vulnerability to the late effects of treatment are both considerations. Because of these differences, investigators have attempted to avoid or to delay radiotherapy in the very young.

Tumor growth at the original tumor site remains the predominant mode of treatment failure in all brain tumor histologic types. Increasing evidence points to the necessity of achieving a complete response, as confirmed by radiologic imaging, as a prerequisite to durable survival in both medulloblastoma and ependymoma. A second-look operation following cytoreductive chemotherapy is being explored in new treatment protocols as a means of improving local control.

Chemotherapy protocols utilized to delay, or perhaps in some cases to obviate, the need for radiation have shown promise, although survival results for infants remain poor in comparison to those obtained in older children, at least for medulloblastoma/PNET. Most infants have tumor progression very early in treatment; thus, new strategies utilizing intensive induction chemotherapy are being explored in conjunction with the introduction of colony-stimulating factors to allow dose intensification of chemotherapy. High-dose chemotherapy with stem cell rescue of bone marrow function has been investigated in the treatment of very young children with malignant brain tumors with some encouraging preliminary results (J.L. Finlay, personal communication, 1994).

Although the long-term consequences of total neuraxis radiation in the very young child are quite clear, the impact of involved field radiation has not been fully assessed. The advent of new technologies allowing very focused radiation may limit late effects while increasing local control, and these should be explored in the treatment of infants with brain tumors.

It is of great importance that laboratory investigation of pediatric brain tumors is accelerating. For example, DNA content and N-myc copy number have both been correlated with prognosis in medulloblastoma,[49, 50] and nude mouse medulloblastoma xenografts have aided in the development of chemotherapeutic strategies.[49, 51] Vital to further advances in this area is the appropriate processing of tumor tissue at the time of surgery; it is an important part of newly developed groupwide protocols for the treatment of infants.

Although infants constitute a minority of all pediatric brain tumor patients, lessons learned in their treatment are potentially broadly applicable. Careful cooperative investigations involving basic researchers and clinical neuro-oncology teams are paramount if progress is to continue.

REFERENCES

1. Duffner PK, Cohen ME, Myers MH, et al: Survival of children with brain tumors: SEER program 1973–1980. Neurology 1986; 36:597–601.

2. Farwell JR, Dohrmann GJ, Flannery JT: Central nervous system tumors in children. Cancer 1977; 40:3123–3132.

3. Kokunai S, Matsumoto S: Congenital brain tumors in Japan (ISPN Cooperative Study): Specific clinical features in neonates. Childs Nerv Syst 1990; 6:86–91.

4. Tomita T, McLone D: Brain tumors during the first 24 months of life. Neurosurgery 1985; 17:913–919.

5. Di Rocco C, Ceddia A, Iannelli A: Intracranial tumours in the first year of life: A report on 51 cases. ACTA Neurochir 1993; 123:14–24.

6. Paulus W, Schlote W, Perentes E, et al: Desmoplastic supratentorial neuroepithelial tumours of infancy. Histopathology 1992; 21:43–49.

7. Vandenberg SR, May EE, Rubinstein LJ, et al: Desmoplastic supratentorial neuroepithelial tumors of infancy with divergent differentiation potential (''desmoplastic infantile gangliogliomas''): Report of 11 cases of a distinctive embryonal tumor with favorable prognosis. J Neurosurg 1987; 66:58–71.

8. Aydin F, Ghatak N, Salvant J, et al: Desmoplastic cerebral astrocytoma of infancy. Acta Neuropathol 1993; 86:666–670.

9. Chadarevian J, Pattisapu J, Faerber E: Desmoplastic cerebral astrocytoma of infancy. Cancer 1990; 66:173–179.

10. Louis D, Deimling A, Dickersin G, et al: Desmoplastic cerebral astrocytomas of infancy: A histopathologic, immunohistochemical, ultrastructural and molecular genetic study. Hum Pathol 1992; 23:1402–1409.

11. Rushing EJ, Rorke LB, Sutton L: Problems in the nosology of desmoplastic tumors of childhood. Pediatr Neurosurg 1993; 19:57–62.

12. Perilongo G, Sutton L, Czaykowski D, et al: Rhabdoid tumor of the central nervous system. Med Pediatr Oncol 1991; 19:310–317.

13. Biegel JA, Burk CD, Parmiter AH, et al: Molecular analysis of a partial deletion of 22q in a central nervous system rhabdoid tumor. Genes Chromosom Cancer 1992; 2:104–108.

14. Farwell JR, Dohrmann GJ, Flannery JT: Medulloblastoma in childhood: An epidemiological study. J Neurosurg 1984; 61:657–664.

15. Jooma R, Hayward R, Grant D: Intracranial neoplasms during the first year of life: Analysis of 100 consecutive cases. Neurosurgery 1984; 14:31–41.

16. Asai A, Hoffman H, Hendrick E, et al: Primary intracranial neoplasms in the first year of life. Childs Nerv Syst 1989; 5:230–233.

17. Geyer JR, Levy M, Berger M, et al: Infants with medulloblastoma: A single institution review of survival. Neurosurgery 1991; 29:707–711.

18. Hirsch JF, Renier D, Czernichow P, et al: Medulloblastoma in childhood: Survival and functional results. Acta Neurochir 1979; 48:1–15.

19. Evans A, Jenkin D, Sposto R, et al: The treatment of medulloblastoma: Results of a prospective randomized trial of radiation therapy with and without CCNU, vincristine and prednisone. J Neurosurg 1990; 72:572–582.

20. Tait D, Thorton-Jones H, Bloom H, et al: Adjuvant chemotherapy for medulloblastoma: The first multi-centre control trial of the International Society of Paediatric Oncology (SIOP I). Eur J Cancer 1990; 26:464–469.

21. Allen JC, Bloom J, Ertel I, et al: Brain tumors in children: Current cooperative and institutional chemotherapy trials in newly diagnosed and recurrent disease. Semin Oncol 1985; 1:110–122.

22. Horowitz M, Mulhern R, Kun L, et al: Brain tumors in the very young child. Cancer 1988; 61:428–434.

23. Geyer JR, Zeltzer PM, Boyett JM: Survival of infants with primitive neuroectodermal tumors or malignant ependymomas of the CNS treated with eight drugs in 1 day: A report from the Childrens Cancer Group. J Clin Oncol 1994; 12:1607–1615.

24. Duffner P, Horowitz M, Krischer J, et al: Postoperative chemotherapy and delayed radiation in children less than 3 years of age with malignant brain tumors. N Engl J Med 1993; 328:1725–1731.

25. Allen J, Epstein F: Medulloblastoma and other primary malignant tumors of the CNS. J Neurosurg 1987; 57:446–451.

26. Lefkowitz I, Evans A, Sposto R, et al: Adjuvant chemotherapy of childhood posterior fossa (PF) ependymoma: Craniospinal radiation with or without CCNU, vincristine and prednisone (abstract). Pediatr Neurosci 1988; 14:149.

27. Goldwein JW, Leahy JM, Packer RJ, et al: Intracranial ependymomas in children (abstract). Pediatr Neurosci 1988; 14:153.

28. Nazar G, Hoffman H, Becker L, et al: Infratentorial ependymomas in childhood: Prognostic factors and treatment. J Neurosurg 1990; 72:408–417.

29. Awaad Y, Allen J, Miller D, et al: Radical surgery as the sole therapy for intracranial low-grade ependymoma (abstract). Ann Neurol 1994; 36:507.

30. Packer R, Savino P, Bilaniuk L, et al: Chiasmatic gliomas of childhood. Childs Brain 1983; 10:393–403.

31. Pierce S, Barnes P, Loeffler J, et al: Definitive radiation therapy in the management of symptomatic patients with optic glioma: Survival and long-term effects. Cancer 1990; 65:45–52.

32. Petronio J, Edwards M, Prados M, et al: Management of chiasmal and hypothalamic gliomas of infancy and childhood with chemotherapy. J Neurosurg 1991; 74:701–708.

33. Moser R, Baram Z, Bruner J, et al: Management of chiasmal gliomas: A surgical perspective. *In* Programs and Abstracts of the 2nd Annual International Symposium on Pediatric Neuro-oncology, Philadelphia, 1990.

34. Wisoff J, Abbott R, Epstein F: Surgical management of exophytic chiasmatic-hypothalamic tumors of childhood. J Neurosurg 1990; 73:661–667.

35. Packer R, Sutton L, Bilaniuk L, et al: Treatment of chiasmatic/hypothalamic gliomas of childhood with chemotherapy: An update. Ann Neurol 1988; 23:79–85.

36. Packer RJ, Lange B, Ater J, et al: Carboplatin and vincristine for recurrent and newly diagnosed low-grade gliomas of childhood. J Clin Oncol 1993; 11:850–856.

37. Petronio J, Edwards MS, Prados M, et al: Management of chiasmal and hypothalamic gliomas of infancy and childhood with chemotherapy. J Neurosurg 1991; 74:701–708.

38. Geyer JR, Finlay JL, Boyett JM, et al: Survival of infants with malignant astrocytomas: A report from the Childrens Cancer Group. Cancer (in press).

39. Duffner P, Kun L, Krischer J, et al: Postoperative chemotherapy and delayed radiation in infants with malignant gliomas: A Pediatric Oncology Group study (abstract). Ann Neurol 1993; 34:480.

40. Bleyer WA, Griffen W: White matter necrosis, mineralizing microangiopathy and intellectual abilities in survivors of childhood leukemia. *In* Gilbert H, Kagen R (eds): Radiation Damage to the Central Nervous System. New York, Raven Press, 1980, pp 155–173.

41. Jannoun L: Are cognitive and educational development affected by age at which prophylactic therapy is given in acute lymphoblastic leukemia? Arch Dis Child 1983; 58:953–958.

42. Meadows AT, Massari DJ, Fergusson J, et al: Declines in IQ scores in children with acute lymphocytic leukemia treated with cranial irradiation. Lancet 1981; 2:1015–1018.

43. Ellenburg L, McComb JG, Siegel SE, et al: Factors affecting intellectual outcome in pediatric brain tumor patients. Neurosurgery 1987; 21:638–644.

44. Packer RJ, Bruce DA, Atkins TA, et al: Factors impacting on neurocognitive outcome in long term survivors of primitive neuroectodermal tumors/medulloblastoma. Ann Neurol 1986; 20:396.

45. Kao GD, Goldwein JW, Schultz DJ, et al: The impact of perioperative factors on subsequent intelligence quotient deficits in children treated for medulloblastoma/posterior fossa primitive neuroectodermal tumors. Cancer 1994; 74:965–971.

46. Duffner PK, Cohen ME, Thomas PRM: The long term effects of cranial irradiation in the central nervous system. Cancer 1985; 56:1841–1847.

47. Oberfield SE, Allen J, Pollack J, et al: Long-term endocrine sequelae after treatment of medulloblastoma: Prospective study of growth and thyroid function. J Pediatr 1986; 108:219–223.

48. Voorhess ML, Breecker ML, MacGillivaray MH, et al: Hypothalamus-pituitary function of children with acute lymphocytic leukemia after three forms of central nervous system prophylaxis. Cancer 1986; 57:1287–1291.

49. Friedman H, Oakes W, Bigner S, et al: Medulloblastoma: Tumor biological and clinical perspectives. J Neurooncol 1991; 11:1–15.

50. Schofield D, Yunit E, Geyer, et al: DNA content and other prognostic features in childhood medulloblastoma: Proposal of a scoring system. Cancer 1992; 69:1307–1314.

51. Friedman H, Burger P, Bigner S, et al: Establishment and characterization of the human medulloblastoma cell line and transplantable xenograft D283 Med. J Neuropathol Exp Neurol 1985; 44:592–605.

52. Cohen BH, Packer RJ, Siegel KR, et al: Brain tumors in children under 2 years: Treatment, survival and long-term prognosis. Pediatr Neurosurg 1993; 19:171–179.

53. Di Rocco C, Iannelli A, Ceddia A: Intracranial tumors of the first year of life. Childs Nerv Syst 1991; 7:150–153.

54. Mapstone TB, Warf BC: Intracranial tumor in infants: Characteristics, management and outcome of a contemporary series. Neurosurgery 1991; 28:343–348.

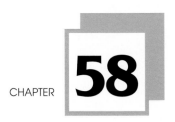

ROGER J. PACKER

GILBERT VEZINA

H. STACY NICHOLSON

WILLIAM M. CHADDUCK

CHAPTER **58**

Childhood and Adolescent Gliomas

Glial tumors comprise well over half of primary central nervous system (CNS) tumors arising in childhood and adolescence.[1] Various classification schema have been used for these malignancies, and the distinction between childhood primitive neuroectodermal tumors with glial differentiation and primary glial tumors, especially in very young patients, is often arbitrary. The World Health Organization (WHO) classification of CNS tumors has recently been modified; it divides astrocytic tumors into various subtypes based predominantly on light microscopic characteristics.[2] Because of the histologic diversity of pediatric brain tumors, including astrocytomas, classification takes on great importance when the effects of treatment on outcome are being evaluated (Table 58–1). Glial tumors with neuronal elements, such as gangliogliomas and gangliocytomas, are classified in the revised WHO schema as neuronal or neuronal-glial tumors. Other tumor types, which occur primarily in infants (e.g.,

desmoplastic infantile ganglioglioma and dysembryonic neuroepithelial tumor), do not fit neatly into older classification systems and are now considered to be separate entities. These difficulties in categorizations of neoplasms are, in great part, the result of a limited understanding of the biology of pediatric glial tumors and associated molecular (genetic) changes. The etiology of the vast majority of pediatric glial tumors remains unknown. Cytogenetic and molecular genetic alterations associated with glial tumors and subsequent malignant transformations have been primarily identified in adult neoplasms.[3] Because pediatric gliomas, especially in infants and very young children, tend to differ from those of their adult counterparts in terms of site of origin, tendency to dedifferentiate from low-grade to high-grade lesions, and, possibly, responsiveness to chemotherapy, the molecular findings in adult lesions may not be representative of those in the pediatric population. Molecular genetic differences between pediatric and adult gliomas have been suggested by chromosomal studies and, more recently, by analysis for mutations of the TP53 gene and loss of heterozygosity for the 17p chromosome.[4–6]

The pediatric brain is rapidly developing, and glial tumors in the same region of brain may present differently in children than in adults. Lesions in young patients may present as an arrest or a deterioration in normal development. The nonspecific nature of symptoms in infants, such as irritability, listlessness, vomiting, and failure to thrive, is discussed primarily in the chapter on infantile gliomas. Preschool and early school-aged children often have difficulty explaining their symptoms, and personality change and school failure may herald the presence of a pediatric glioma, especially a slow-growing midline tumor, in the weeks to months before diagnosis. Diagnosis has been significantly simplified with the advent of computed tomography (CT) and magnetic resonance imaging (MRI). Given the greater predilection of pediatric brain tumors, to disseminate to the neuroaxis early in the course of illness, as compared with adult malignancies, staging studies are often an important component of management.[7]

Treatment of gliomas in children also often differs significantly from that in adults. Due to the immature, developing nature of the pediatric brain, the reluctance to institute neurotoxic treatments is significant. Interest has been in-

TABLE 58–1
TUMORS OF NEUROEPITHELIAL TISSUE

1.1	Astrocytic tumors
1.11	Astrocytoma
1.111	Variant: Fibrillary
1.112	Protoplasmic
1.113	Gemistocytic
1.1.2	Anaplastic (malignant) astrocytoma
1.1.3	Glioblastoma
1.1.4	Pilocytic astrocytoma
1.1.4	Pleomorphic xanthoastrocytoma
1.1.6	Subependymal giant cell astrocytoma
1.2	Oligodendroglial tumors
1.3	Ependymal tumors
1.4	Mixed gliomas
1.5	Choroid plexus tumors
1.6	Neuroepithelial tumors of uncertain origin (includes astroblastoma, polar spongioblastoma, and gliomatosis cerebri)
1.7	Neuronal and mixed neuronal-glial tumors (includes desmoplastic infantile ganglioglioma, dysembryonic neuroepithelial tumor, and ganglioglioma)
1.8	Pineal parenchymal tumors
1.9	Embryonal tumors (inlcudes medulloblastoma, primitive neuroectodermal tumor, and medulloepithelioma)

Adapted from Kleihues P, Burger PC, Scheithauer BW: Histologic Typing of Tumours of the Central Nervous System. Berlin, Springer-Verlag, 1993.

creasing in the use of more extensive surgery and/or chemotherapy to manage deep-seated, large lesions, in an attempt to delay or obviate extensive cranial irradiation. Because pediatric low-grade gliomas tend to remain low-grade throughout the pediatric years, observation is often a reasonable approach to treatment. This is especially true for children with neurofibromatosis and suspected glial neoplasms.

For purposes of this chapter, glial tumors of childhood and adolescence are initially subdivided on the basis of the site of origin and are discussed on the basis of histologic features. Ependymomas of childhood are also reviewed. Clinical presentation is discussed in greater depth when it differs significantly from presentation in adulthood or has an impact on management.

CEREBELLAR ASTROCYTOMAS

Gliomas of the cerebellum are the most frequent type of pediatric glial neoplasm. They constitute approximately 20% of all pediatric primary CNS tumors and 40% of those arising in the posterior fossa.[8, 9] Three fourths or more of all cerebellar pediatric glial tumors are the classic juvenile, or pilocytic, cerebellar astrocytomas, which are composed of fusiform astrocytes loosely interwoven in a fine fibrillary background. These tumors frequently have a microcystic component, Rosenthal's fibers, and tend to have large macrocystic structures that are filled with proteinaceous fluid. One or more mural nodules are usually present in the wall of the cyst. A second variety, the diffuse or Gilles type B lesion, is more histologically similar to low-grade astrocytomas of the cerebral hemisphere, as the tumor is more cellular and infiltrative.[8, 9]

Clinical Presentation

Clinical presentation of these two forms of cerebellar gliomas overlaps; however, the classic juvenile cerebellar astrocytoma, arising in the lateral cerebellar hemispheres, more frequently causes lateralized appendicular symptoms for weeks to months before extending to the midline and obstructing the fourth ventricle. When cerebrospinal fluid (CSF) flow is obstructed, the more nonspecific and nonlocalizing symptoms of increased intracranial pressure, which include headache and vomiting, become preeminent. In the young child, this may be manifest by irritability, apathy, and meningeal irritation. In contradistinction, patients with diffuse cerebellar astrocytomas, which more commonly arise in the midline, are more likely to present with midline cerebellar deficits early in the course of illness, such as truncal unsteadiness, either followed by or concomitant with signs of increased intracranial pressure. Because the diffuse cerebellar astrocytoma frequently abuts, or apparently infiltrates into, the brainstem, cranial nerve palsies are more frequent.

Radiologic Features

Neuroradiographically, the two subvarieties of cerebellar astrocytoma also differ (Fig. 58–1).[10] On CT, low-grade

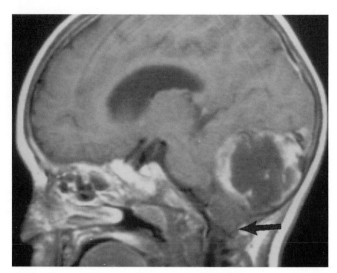

Figure 58–1 Cerebellar pilocytic astrocytoma in a 2-year-old boy with recent-onset vomiting and ataxia. An enhanced parasagittal T1-weighted image reveals a large mass with heterogeneous enhancement and nonenhancing T2 bright center. This appearance is typical of a pilocytic astrocytoma with microcystic features. Note the inferiorly displaced cerebellar tonsils (arrow).

cerebellar astrocytomas usually display a homogeneous low-density pattern associated with a macrocystic component. Within the macrocystic component, a nodule (the so-called mural nodule) is frequently present, which shows marked contrast enhancement. Hydrocephalus is present in most patients at the time of diagnosis. CT of the diffuse cerebellar astrocytoma more commonly discloses an isodense or hypodense lesion that enhances in a variable fashion after contrast. As stated previously, the diffuse cerebellar astrocytoma usually arises in the midline, compressing the fourth ventricle. On MR, the noncystic components of both the juvenile pilocytic and diffuse cerebellar astrocytoma are commonly isointense or hypointense in comparison to adjacent normal cerebellum on T1-weighted images and hyperintense to normal tissue to T2-weighted images. The cyst of the juvenile pilocytic astrocytoma may have intermediate signal intensities, which are dependent on protein content. Hemorrhage may occur within the cyst, but it is relatively uncommon. After injection of gadolinium, the mural nodule of the pilocytic astrocytoma usually readily enhances. Cyst wall enhancement is infrequent, and such enhancement suggests tumor within the wall of the cyst. A major advantage of MRI in the evaluation of the diffuse cerebellar astrocytoma is the demonstration of the infiltrative nature of such lesions, including involvement of the brainstem or cerebellar peduncles. Because low-grade cerebellar gliomas rarely disseminate to the neuroaxis early in illness, staging studies for the extent of spread at diagnosis have not been routinely performed.[7, 11]

Management

The initial management of both types of cerebellar lesions is surgical resection.[8, 9, 11, 12] After gross total resections, survival rates for patients with juvenile pilocytic astrocytoma are excellent, with most series reporting that greater than 95% of patients are alive and free of progressive disease 5 years after treatment; the vast majority are cured of the disease. For those patients with partially resected juvenile astrocytomas, re-resection or close observation followed by re-resection at time of progression is recommended most commonly. Radiotherapy has been used in patients with partially resected lesions and may delay the time to recurrence, but because of potential long-term effects and questionable efficacy, it tends to be used only when re-resection is not feasible.[11–13]

The management of diffuse childhood cerebellar astrocytomas is less straightforward. Five- and 10-year survival rates ranging between 7% and 30% have been reported for patients with such lesions.[8, 9, 12] In general, due to their infiltrative nature, these tumors tend to be less amenable to gross total resection. It is unclear whether the natural history of diffuse cerebellar astrocytoma differs from that of pilocytic cerebellar astrocytoma when the extent of resection is similar. Owing to either their infiltrative nature or, possibly, the tendency of diffuse cerebellar astrocytoma to transform into more histologically malignant lesions, diffuse cerebellar gliomas have been reported to have a greater tendency to disseminate to the neuroaxis.[7, 11] This is especially true for lesions with frank anaplastic areas. In patients with subtotally resected diffuse cerebellar astrocytomas, radiation is frequently recommended, unless further attempts at total resections are feasible.[11–13] It is unclear if such radiation should be delivered only to the primary tumor site or if craniospinal irradiation is indicated.[7, 11–13] Because chemotherapy has been shown to be active in children with low-grade astrocytomas, it may also have a future role in the management of diffuse subtotally resected cerebellar astrocytomas.[14]

MALIGNANT GLIOMAS OF THE CEREBELLUM

Occasionally, histologically anaplastic gliomas of the cerebellum arise in childhood.[8, 11, 15] Considerable overlap occurs between these tumors and the diffuse midline cerebellar astrocytoma. Malignant cerebellar gliomas tend to be diffuse, infiltrating, and are infrequently amenable to total resection. The reported incidence of leptomeningeal dissemination of childhood high-grade cerebellar gliomas is variable.[7, 8, 11, 15] In the experience at Children's Hospital of Philadelphia, five of seven cases disseminated early in the course of illness, whereas in the multi-institutional group experience of the Children's Cancer Group, dissemination was less frequently noted, even after local recurrence.[7] Because of the possibility of neuroaxis dissemination, evaluation for extent of dissemination with whole-spine gadolinium-enhanced MR or CT myelography and CSF fluid cytologic analysis is often recommended at the time of diagnosis or after initial surgery.

The most appropriate management for high-grade posterior fossa gliomas is unclear. Some observers have recommended craniospinal plus local boost radiotherapy, whereas others have contended that local radiotherapy results in comparable disease control.[15] Overall, the reported 5-year survival rates for malignant cerebellar gliomas ranges between 10% and 40%; these rates are similar to survival rates for patients with cerebral malignant gliomas. The role of adjuvant chemotherapy has not yet been defined in this group of patients.

BRAINSTEM GLIOMAS

Glial tumors of the brainstem comprise 10% of childhood CNS neoplasms. Concepts concerning brainstem gliomas have changed remarkably since the advent of MRI.[10, 16] MRI more clearly identifies the extent of lesions and the tendency of some brainstem tumors to be relatively well localized, whereas others appear highly infiltrative, with contiguous involvement of the diencephalon, cervical cord, and even the cerebellum. Upward of 80% of children with brainstem gliomas have tumors that arise in the pons, though subsets of patients have been identified with more caudal or rostral primary lesions.

Although both pure low- and high-grade gliomas of the brainstem probably exist, a mixed glial composition is more commonly seen.[17] It is difficult to make statements concerning the significance of light microscopic findings to outcome because of the relative surgical inaccessibility of most brainstem lesions. Even after biopsy or partial resection is performed (as only a portion of the tumor can be removed), sampling error becomes a significant limitation. For reasons that are unclear, the location of the tumor within the brainstem is often related to histopathologic features, as histologically benign lesions tend to occur more frequently in the mesencephalon and low medulla.[18] This relationship becomes even more confusing when age is factored in, as adults are more likely to have more localized high brainstem (midbrain) tumors and a more favorable outcome.[19] MRI has allowed separation of brainstem gliomas into three relatively distinct, but overlapping, groupings: diffuse pontine gliomas; tectal (focal) mesencephalic lesions; and exophytic cervicomedullary masses (Figs. 58–2 through 58–4).[16, 20–22] Gray areas exist within these subcategories, such as pontine tumors that seem relatively well circumscribed on MRI (possibly focal lesions) and lesions that arise in the cervicomedullary region, but are not primarily exophytic.

Clinical Presentation

As can be expected, clinical presentation is highly dependent on the location of brainstem involvement. Diffuse intrinsic brainstem gliomas classically present with the triad of cranial neuropathies, ataxia, and long tract signs. Sixth and seventh nerve dysfunction are most common, but lower cranial nerve deficits may also occur as the first signs of a diffuse intrinsic brainstem tumor. Very young children often present with unexplained irritability and a change in personality. Hydrocephalus and associated symptoms and signs of increased intracranial pressure are present in approximately a third of patients at diagnosis. A subset of children with brainstem gliomas that tend to have a relatively favorable prognosis are those who present with isolated sixth or seventh nerve palsies due to focal, often juvenile pilocytic, intrinsic pontine gliomas.

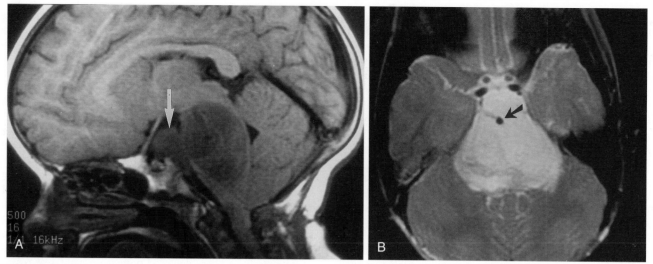

Figure 58–2 Diffuse infiltrating brainstem glioma in a 2-year-old girl with cranial nerve palsies, paraparesis. Enhanced sagittal T1- *(A)* and axial T2-weighted *(B)* images reveal a mass occupying almost the entire brainstem, with a large exophytic prepontine component *(arrow)* that encases the basilar artery.

The presentation of children with cervicomedullary lesions differs from that of patients with diffuse intrinsic tumors.[20, 21] Patients with cervicomedullary lesions often have long histories of nonspecific headaches and vomiting. The headaches and vomiting occur at variable intervals during the day. These patients may have little in the way of focal neurologic deficits and often have swallowing difficulties associated with other lower cranial nerve dysfunction. Infants with such lesions may present with excessive drooling and feeding difficulties.

Recently, a subset of patients with midbrain or tectal lesions have been identified, many of whom have been

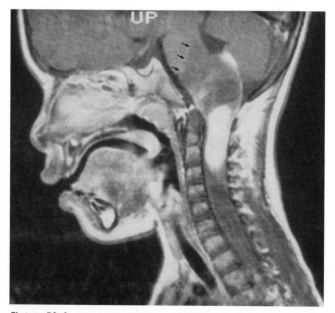

Figure 58–3 Anaplastic cervicomedullary astrocytoma in a 4-year-old boy with ataxia, torticollis. Postcontrast sagittal T1-weighted image reveals a large lesion with a solid component in the medulla and upper cervical cord, a dorsal exophytic component invaginating the inferior fourth ventricle, and invasion into the lower pons (low T1 signal; *arrows*). The cervical spinal cord below the enhancing component is edematous.

diagnosed prior to the availability of MR as suffering from idiopathic aqueductal stenosis.[22, 23] These patients tend to present with hydrocephalus and few, if any, focal neurologic deficits. After diversion of CSF, symptoms may disappear completely. Less frequently, children with tectal lesions have extraocular movement dysfunction, including Parinaud's syndrome (paralysis of upgaze, eyelid retraction, conversion nystagmus, and pupils that react better to accommodation than to light).

Patients with neurofibromatosis and enlarged brainstems require separate consideration.[24] Children with neurofibromatosis may often have areas of abnormal signal intensity within the brainstem, with or without brainstem enlargement. Such patients are often asymptomatic or have nonspecific findings, such as hypotonia and incoordination. It is unclear whether such patients have true brainstem gliomas or if they have hamartomas, which will not grow for prolonged periods.

Radiologic Features

MRI has essentially supplanted other neuroimaging techniques in the diagnosis of brainstem gliomas.[10, 16] CT demonstrates the majority of brainstem lesions; however, detection of small intrinsic lesions, cervicomedullary masses, and tectal tumors is difficult. On CT, brainstem tumors tend to be hypodense or isodense, and approximately a third show some degree of contrast enhancement. Various types of contrast enhancement have been seen, including ring enhancement. Tectal lesions are often not well visualized on CT. A third of patients with primary pontine lesions have ventriculomegaly, whereas the majority of those with tectal gliomas have enlarged ventricles.

On MRI, diffuse intrinsic brainstem gliomas are usually hypointense with respect to surrounding brain on short TR/TE images and are hyperintense compared to surrounding brain on long TR/TE images. Relatively few tumors are limited to one primary anatomic site, with the majority of

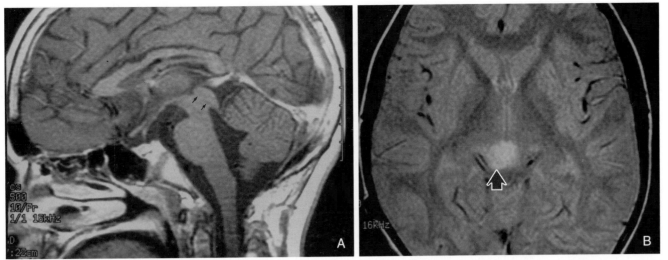

Figure 58–4 A 10-year-old boy with shunted hydrocephalus secondary to a tectal mass (not biopsied). Enhanced sagittal T1-weighted *(A)* and axial proton-density *(B)* images reveal a thickened mid-brain tectum with abnormal T2 signal *(arrow)*. No enhancement was present. The lesion was unchanged over a 4-year follow-up. The appearance is consistent with either a benign tectal glioma or a hamartoma.

tumors involving the pons and at least one other brainstem site. Tumors of the pons are often exophytic, growing ventrally into the prepontine cistern, engulfing the basilar artery, or growing in the cerebellopontine angle cistern. Longitudinal infiltrations into the midbrain or medulla and axial extension into the middle cerebellar peduncles or even the cerebellum are not uncommon. Enhancement patterns of pontine brainstem gliomas on MRI, as on CT, are quite variable; at presentation, the majority of tumors show little, if any, enhancement. Tumors of the cervicomedullary junction often have the same neuroimaging characteristics as pilocytic astrocytomas of the cerebellum. Cervicomedullary tumors may have associated cystic and enhancing solid components. Dorsal midbrain masses tend to be localized within the tectal area; involvement of contiguous mesencephalic regions or the dorsal thalamus is seen on occasion. These lesions may or may not demonstrate contrast enhancement.

Management

The diagnostic evaluation and management of a patient with a radiographically diagnosed diffuse intrinsic brainstem glioma remains somewhat unsettled. A major diagnostic issue is whether surgery, except for diversion of CSF in patients with hydrocephalus, is indicated. Recent series have confirmed the specificity of MRI in the diagnosis of brainstem gliomas.[25] Although differing pathologies have been found in patients with presumed brainstem gliomas in adult series, the finding of anything other than a brainstem glioma on biopsy in a child with radiographically diagnosed brainstem tumor is infrequent.[25–27] Surgical resections have not been shown to be of therapeutic benefit for patients with diffuse intrinsic lesions, although this may not be the case for the rare focal pontine tumor or for the less frequent primary medullary or midbrain lesion. Biopsies, both open and stereotactic, have been performed by multiple groups in patients with pontine gliomas.[26, 27] In a recent nationwide series, nearly 35% of children with diffuse intrinsic brainstem gli-

oma underwent biopsy prior to the initiation of treatment, although the findings on biopsy did not alter treatment.[25] The tissue removed at the time of diagnostic biopsy (stereotactic or open) is usually small, and it may not be representative of the tumor as a whole. Studies performed in the mid-1970s and early 1980s suggested that up to a third of specimens obtained at the time of open biopsy were nondiagnostic and that nearly 30% of patients had increased neurologic dysfunction after such biopsies.[17, 25] With wider utilization of stereotactic approaches, it seems that the diagnostic yield is somewhat higher and that less surgical morbidity is associated with biopsy.[26, 27] However, the information obtained at the time of biopsy infrequently alters therapy for patients with diffuse pontine lesions. If the tissue is found to show areas of anaplasia, prognosis is quite poor. However, in contradistinction, low-grade histologic findings have not been shown to correlate with improved outcome in patients with diffuse intrinsic lesions, either because of sampling error or the tendency of such lesions to dedifferentiate over time. When more effective means become available for the treatment of diffuse intrinsic brainstem gliomas or when biologic studies can be shown to provide more useful prognostic information, it is conceivable that biopsy of brainstem gliomas will take on more clinical importance.

The management of diffuse intrinsic lesions remains suboptimal. After radiographic diagnosis, with or without surgical intervention, radiotherapy has been the most frequently used treatment. Local radiation therapy, in doses ranging between 5,000 and 5,500 cGy, given in once-daily dose fractions of 180 to 200 cGy, results in transient clinical improvement in the majority of patients with a diffuse intrinsic tumor; however, 80% or more of patients die of disease within 18 months of diagnosis.[17, 18] Retrospective series have suggested that disease control is related, at least in part, to the total dose of radiotherapy used. For these reasons, recent attempts have been made to increase the overall dose of local radiotherapy by using hyperfractionated radiation therapy delivery schedules. In theory, larger total doses of radiotherapy are tolerated by the normal surrounding brain if treatment is given in smaller individual dose fractions multiple times per day. Various trials have been undertaken since the mid-1980s that have used doses of radiotherapy ranging between 6,400 and 7,800 cGy, in dose fractions ranging from 100 to 126 cGy, delivered twice daily.[19, 28–34] Initially, results of these studies suggested improved duration and frequency of survival, especially in older (primarily adult) patients and in patients with more localized lesions (Table 58–2).[19, 29] More recent multi-institutional cooperative trials have disclosed that even when treated at these higher doses of radiotherapy, the majority of children with pontine brainstem gliomas develop disease progression within 9 months of completion of radiotherapy and die of disease within 18 months of diagnosis.[30–34] Compared with more conventional radiotherapy studies, hyperfractionated radiotherapy trials have possibly resulted in a higher rate of initial objective initial tumor shrinkage, but this has not translated into improved disease control.[32, 34] In addition, nearly one third of patients treated on the higher-dose radiotherapy studies have been steroid-dependent for weeks following radiotherapy, and development of intralesional tumor necrosis with associated neurologic dysfunction has been noted within 2 months of completion of radiotherapy in nearly 10% of treated patients.[30–34]

Other radiotherapy techniques have been suggested for children with brainstem gliomas, including the use of focused high-dose irradiation. However, no evidence has indicated that focused irradiation benefits patients with brainstem glioma, and given the infiltrative nature of such lesions, it is difficult to understand the biologic rationale for such an approach.

The published experience with chemotherapy for children with diffuse intrinsic brainstem gliomas is scant.[35] A variety of drugs, including cisplatin, carboplatin, different types of nitrosoureas, cyclophosphamide, and ifosfamide have been used singly or in combination for children with recurrent brainstem tumors.[36] The results, to date, are quite disappointing, with most series reporting objective response rates of less than 20%, independent of the agent or agents used. Adjuvant post-radiotherapy chemotherapy has also been used in children with brainstem gliomas without evidence of improved survival.[35] Alternative chemotherapeutic approaches have included the use of chemotherapy prior to radiation therapy, in an attempt to both identify active agents for patients with brainstem glioma and to improve survival. However, because children with brainstem gliomas tend to

be severely neurologically impaired at the time of diagnosis, physicians have been reluctant to utilize pre-radiation and, thus, radiotherapy is delayed. One study using cisplatin and cyclophosphamide demonstrated that such therapy could be delivered prior to radiotherapy, but therapy resulted in a poor response rate and no improvement in survival.[37] Other studies have used chemotherapy concomitantly with radiotherapy, attempting to achieve a synergistic effect of the agents.[36] High-dose multi-agent chemotherapy followed by autologous bone marrow rescue has also been used in patients with brainstem gliomas. Initial attempts to use the high-dose chemotherapy/transplant approach prior to radiotherapy demonstrated significant toxic response; studies are under way to assess feasibility and efficacy of this approach following radiotherapy.

Management of cervicomedullary exophytic brainstem gliomas in children differs from that of diffuse pontine lesions, as reports suggest that such tumors can often be extensively resected.[20, 21] Short-term follow-up studies demonstrate that after extensive resection, the condition of many patients remains stable for months to years without any other forms of specific intervention. However, such resections result in increased neurologic morbidity in a sizable minority of patients, including respirator dependence.[38] It is unclear whether the best management of patients with exophytic cervicomedullary tumors consists of aggressive attempts at total or near total resection followed by observation, or less aggressive partial resections or biopsy followed by either radiotherapy or chemotherapy. Because the majority of patients with such lesions harbor low-grade gliomas, there is a hesitancy to use radiotherapy, especially in very young patients. Chemotherapy, such as the combination of carboplatin and vincristine, may be effective in controlling disease in patients with progressive low-grade brainstem tumors.[39]

The management of children with localized tectal lesions also remains unsettled. Increasing evidence has accumulated that some patients with isolated tectal lesions presenting with hydrocephalus can be treated with CSF diversion and then carefully followed without any specific intervention.[22, 23] In a recent series of 16 patients, progressive disease developed in four children a mean of 4.25 years from diagnosis, and more definitive treatment was required.[23] The remaining 12 patients experienced stable disease without specific intervention. At the time of tumor progression, the majority of patients have been given local radiotherapy. The long-term disease control rate for patients with localized tectal or

TABLE 58–2

RESULTS OF HYPERFRACTIONATED RADIOTHERAPY TRIALS FOR BRAINSTEM GLIOMAS IN CHILDHOOD: DOSE >7,000 cGy

Series	Dose Schedule (cGy)	Total Dose (cGy)	ORR (%)	Outcome
UCSF (N = 20)[19]	100 bid	7,400–7,800	NA	Median survival, 50 wk
UCSF (N = 53)[33]	100 bid	7,200	NA	Median survival, 44 wk
CHOP/NYU (N = 35)[29]	100 bid	7,200	74	PFS, 9 mo; 61%, 1 yr
CCG I (N = 53)[32]	100 bid	7,200	62	PFS, 7 mo
POG II (N = 57)[28]	117 bid	7,020	77	PFS, 6 mo; 40, 1 yr; 33% 2 yr
POG III (N = 39)[31]	126 bid	7,560	17	PFS, 10 mo; 39%, 1 yr; 7%, 2 yr
CCG II (N = 66)[34]	100 bid	7,800	34	PFS, 8 mo; 35%, 1 yr; 11%, 3 yr

UCSF, University of California, San Francisco; CHOP, Children's Hospital of Philadelphia; NYU, New York University; POG, Pediatric Oncology Group; CCG, Children's Cancer Group; ORR, objective response rate; and PFS, progression-free survival.

midbrain lesions after irradiation is poorly documented; however, in older CT-based studies, patients with such lesions had a relatively favorable outcome after radiotherapy, with greater than 50% being alive and free of progressive disease 5 years after treatment.[25]

DIENCEPHALIC GLIOMAS

In total, gliomas of the chiasm, hypothalamus, and thalamus comprise 20% to 30% of all pediatric gliomas. These tumors often are not confined to one anatomic site, and separation of the hypothalamic lesions from thalamic or chiasmatic masses can be arbitrary and misleading, especially in very large lesions with neuroradiographically ill-defined borders.

Clinical Presentation

As in adults, diencephalic tumors in children may present with loss of visual acuity, visual field loss, endocrinologic dysfunction, and hemiparesis; but in children, other more subtle and less specific presentations are also frequent.[40, 41] In infants, a classic presentation is the diencephalic syndrome. This is manifest by failure to thrive (despite apparently adequate caloric intake), apparent euphoria, and overactivity. Diencephalic tumors may also be extremely extensive in very young children at the time of diagnosis, with minimal early overt signs of visual or motor dysfunction. Patients may have histories of delayed development or unexplained irritability, often associated with macrocephaly.

Visual pathway gliomas in children with neurofibromatosis are now being diagnosed at a time when they are asymptomatic or no static visual impairment is apparent.[42] This is primarily a result of screening programs in which MRI is performed on all children with neurofibromatosis, at some institutions, at initial diagnosis. Because neurofibro-

matosis is diagnosed in many cases within the first 3 years of life, the determination of visual impairment, even visual acuity loss, can be difficult. The classic bitemporal field cut is uncommon, and children with neurofibromatosis are more frequently asymptomatic or have documented loss of vision in one eye with some degree of visual impairment in the other (usually partial loss of visual field).[41] Nystagmus, which often has a shimmering quality, may also be present at diagnosis.

Radiographic Features

Neuroradiographically, diencephalic gliomas can usually be distinguished from other types of malignancies (Figs. 58–5 through 58–7).[10, 40, 43] Chiasmatic/hypothalamic tumors are more frequent than thalamic lesions. When the optic nerves are involved, a primary site in the chiasm is inferred. Conversely, when the optic nerves and tracts are spared, especially if the chiasm can be differentiated from the mass, then a hypothalamic origin is likely. Anterior thalamic tumors can be difficult to distinguish from hypothalamic lesions, whereas posterior thalamic lesions can be confused with tumors of pineal origin. Midline thalamic lesions are, at times, difficult to differentiate from primary third ventricular tumors. On CT, glial tumors in this region tend to be hypodense and to show significant contrast enhancement despite their low-grade nature. Cystic components and calcifications are less commonly seen than in pilocytic astrocytomas of the posterior fossa. MRI demonstrates the same signal intensity abnormalities as are seen in other low-grade tumors.[42] However, MRI often shows the widely infiltrative nature of these lesions, with involvement of multiple anatomic sites. Abnormal signal intensities along the optic tracts and optic radiation—at times extending into the temporal, parietal, and/or occipital regions—are not infrequent, especially in children with neurofibromatosis. It is unclear whether such

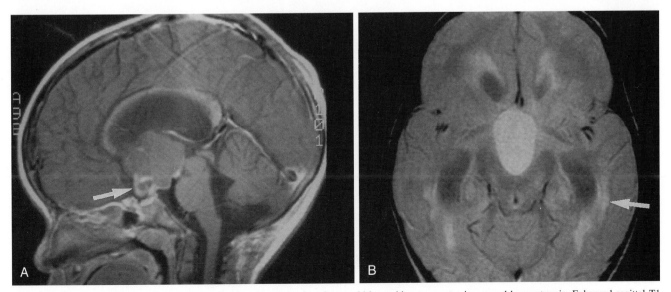

Figure 58–5 Low-grade (nonpilocytic) hypothalamic astrocytoma in a 3-year-old boy with new-onset seizures and hyponatremia. Enhanced sagittal T1-weighted image *(A)* and axial proton-density image through the lower third ventricle *(B)* reveal a mass with minimal enhancement *(arrow, A)*. The lesion did not extend into the optic nerves or optic tracks. Note ventriculomegaly and periventricular interstitial edema *(arrow, B)*.

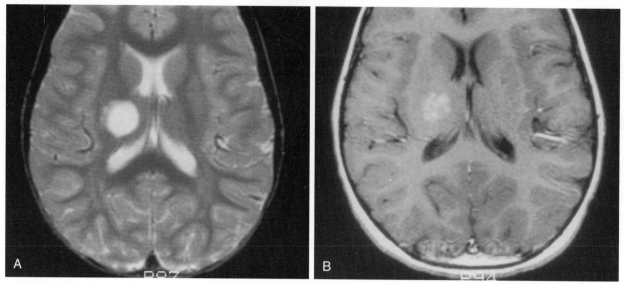

Figure 58–6 Thalamic pilocytic astrocytoma in a 4-year-old girl with headaches. Axial T2-weighted image *(A)* and axial enhanced T1-weighted image *(B)* through the level of the thalamus reveal a well-circumscribed lesion with bright T2 signal and heterogeneous diffuse enhancement.

abnormalities represent tumor, edema, or hamartomatous regions of brain.

Management

The management of diencephalic gliomas is dependent on the size of the tumor, the presence of associated necrotic or cystic areas, clinical manifestations of disease at the time of diagnosis, and whether the tumor occurs in a child with neurofibromatosis. Histologically, greater than 90% of diencephalic lesions in childhood will be low-grade lesions.[40, 42–45] In patients with minimal symptoms or apparently stable disease, especially those with neurofibromatosis,

it is unclear whether any intervention is necessary until tumor progression is demonstrated clinically or radiographically. If the tumor is bulky, necrotic, or partially cystic, extensive surgical resections may be possible and may result in apparent arrest of disease progression for weeks to months.[46]

In children without neurofibromatosis, biopsies or partial resections are usually undertaken to confirm the pathologic diagnosis of the lesion; but more definitive treatment is usually required. Local radiation therapy remains the standard of treatment. Radiotherapy doses ranging between 5,400 and 6,000 cGy result in disease stabilization for months to years in the majority of patients.[44, 47, 48] The frequency of objective tumor shrinkage or clinical improvement

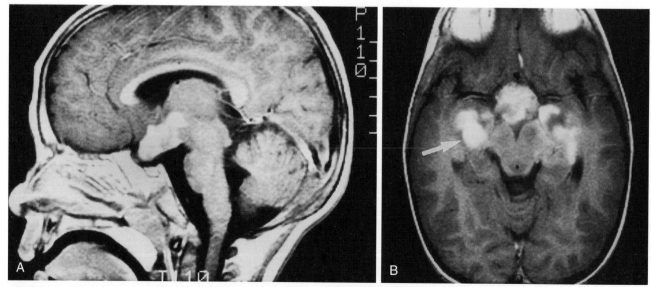

Figure 58–7 Chiasmatic optic glioma with spread into the optic radiations (not biopsied) in a 4-year-old girl with neurofibromatosis type I and decreased vision. Enhanced sagittal *(A)* and axial *(B)* T1-weighted images reveal an enhancing mass within the chiasm extending posteriorly into the optic tracks *(arrow, B)*. Both optic nerves were involved. (From Packer RJ, Vezina G: Pediatric glial neoplasms including brain-stem gliomas. Semin Oncol 1994; 21(2):262.)

after local radiotherapy is poorly defined. Also, after local radiotherapy in patients with low-grade gliomas, MR or CT performed 6 weeks following completion of treatment will sometimes show apparent tumor enlargement; this is often associated with no clinical change at the onset of nonspecific symptoms, such as headache and increased sleepiness. This tumor "swelling" is most commonly a subacute effect of radiotherapy, with improvement in the symptoms and shrinkage of tumor occurring over ensuing weeks to months.

The use of local radiotherapy becomes more problematic in younger children. Given the size of many diencephalic gliomas, adequate local radiotherapy often encompasses large areas of the brain including the subfrontal and temporal region. Some information suggests that this will cause long-term neurocognitive dysfunction.[40] In addition, after local radiotherapy to the diencephalic region, the majority of patients develop growth hormone insufficiency and other endocrinologic dysfunction.[40] Treatment of children with neurofibromatosis is even more difficult, as they often have areas of abnormal signal intensity in regions that are noncontiguous with, but close to, the apparent diencephalic growth.[42] It is unclear whether such patients require radiotherapy only to the diencephalic mass lesion when radiographic or clinical progression is documented, or whether these other areas of MR signal abnormality also need to be included in the radiation portal. Inclusion of such lesions in the local radiotherapy field will result in the delivery of more extensive cranial irradiation. If such lesions are not included in the radiation field, effective treatment in the future, due to technical limitation of field overlap, may be impossible if the noncontiguous regions demonstrate growth.

In an attempt to decrease the potential long-term effect of radiotherapy, chemotherapy has been used in newly diagnosed children, especially those younger than 5 years, with diencephalic lesions.[39, 49–53] Evaluation of the response of such lesions to chemotherapy was less exact until the advent of MR. The widest early experience with chemotherapy was with the combination of actinomycin and vincristine.[49, 50] In a series of 30 patients younger than 5 years with newly diagnosed progressive low-grade visual pathway gliomas, 80% of children were shown to have at least disease stabilization during chemotherapy. This stabilization lasted for a mean of 3 years and resulted in radiation being delivered at a median age of 4.5 years instead of 1.5 years. More recently, other drugs or drug combinations have been used (Table 58–3).[39, 51–53] The largest series to date has utilized the combination of carboplatin and vincristine.[39] In more than 60 patients with newly diagnosed disease, more than half have been shown to have an objective shrinkage of tumor, and more than 90% have either clinical improvement or disease stabilization during treatment. It is presently unknown which regimen is best in controlling disease in children with low-grade diencephalic lesions, but mounting evidence indicates that some patients with low-grade lesions respond to treatment, which delays or obviates the need for radiotherapy.

CEREBRAL LOW-GRADE GLIOMAS

The classification of low-grade gliomas of the cerebrum in children is at times difficult, especially in very young patients. Often included within the category of low-grade childhood cerebral gliomas are such histologically divergent lesions as pleomorphic xanthoastrocytomas, dysembryoplastic neuroepithelial tumors, and desmoplastic infantile gliomas. As stated previously, other tumors, such as gangliogliomas, have significant glial elements although they are classified as neuronal tumors. Biologic differences have been suggested between childhood low-grade tumors and those that arise in adults, because of the infrequent apparent dedifferentiation of childhood tumors into more malignant lesions. The biologic underpinnings, if any, of these differences have not been defined, and it is unclear whether the lack of malignant change is due to molecular differences or other factors, such as age and duration of tumor growth.

Clinical Presentation

Clinical manifestation of childhood low-grade gliomas are, as can be expected, highly dependent on their site of origin within the cortex.[54] Headaches may occur, but they are infrequent early in illness, and are often erratic and of variable severity. The pattern of tumor growth for childhood low-grade neoplasms of the cortex tends to be infiltrative and local. Metastases and leptomeningeal dissemination can occur, but these are rare. Patients with low-grade gliomas of the frontal and temporal lobe may present with months or years of intractable epilepsy, without focal neurologic findings or radiographic evidence of tumor growth. The desmoplastic infantile glioma, which tends to occur in children

TABLE 58–3
SELECTED SERIES OF CHEMOTHERAPY FOR CHILDHOOD LOW-GRADE GLIOMAS IN THE CT/MRI ERA

Study	No. of Patients	Drugs Used	Tumor Location/ Status	Response*	Outcome
Packer et al.[50]	24	ACT/VCR	Diencephalic/ND	9 OR (3 PR)	Median TTP >3 yr
Petronio et al.[39]	15	TG/PCB/DBD/BCNU/VCR	Diencephalic/RD	10 OR	Median TTP >79 wk
Friedman et al.[52]	12	Carbo	All/RD	9 SD	SD 2–68 + mo
Packer et al.[39]	62	Carbo/VCR	All/RD + ND	37 OR (22 PR; 1 CR)	Median TTP >14 mo
Pons et al.[51]	20	VP-16/VCR	All/RD + ND	3 OR (1 PR)	Median TTP >10 mo

ACT, actinomycin; VCR, vincristine; Carbo, carboplatin; ND, newly diagnosed; RD, recurrent; TG, thioguanine; VP-16, etoposide; PCB, procarbazine; BCNU, carmustine; DBD, dibromodulcitol; CR, complete response; PR, partial response; OR, objective response (>25%, <50% shrinkage); SD, stable disease; TTP, time to progression; and NG, not given.
*Radiographically proven.

younger than 2 years, is frequently large at the time of diagnosis, and it may demonstrate histologic features that suggest the potential for rapid growth while growing slowly, if at all.[55] Similarly, the dysembryoplastic neuroepithelial tumor, although having a heterogeneous cellular population, also has an apparently limited growth potential.[56] Pleomorphic xanthoastrocytomas tend to act benign, despite worrisome histologic features. A significant subgroup of low-grade gliomas, up to 10% to 15% in some series, have mixed gliomatous elements, including areas of ependymoma or oligodendroglioma. It is unclear whether they carry a less favorable prognosis, and malignant degeneration has been encountered.

Radiographic Features

Both CT and MRI are sensitive in the detection of cortical low-grade gliomas.[10] These tumors may be quite infiltrative, but some tumors may seem relatively well marginated. This is especially true for gangliogliomas, which tend to show little or no contrast enhancement and have high T2-weighted signal abnormalities on MRI, without associated cystic components. Pleomorphic xanthoastrocytomas typically have an enhancing solid nodule that is cortically based, with slight meningeal involvement and a deeper nonenhancing cystic component. Dysembryonic neuroepithelial tumors often mimic the neuroradiographic findings of gangliogliomas (Fig. 58–8).[56] The more common fibrillary low-grade gliomas have less specific features, and their diagnosis is suggested by the presence of a lesion with a limited amount of associated edema and a modest amount of mass effect when compared with the overall tumor size. This lack of edema and mass effect tends to separate them from higher-grade lesions.

Management

Treatment of choice for childhood low-grade cortical neoplasms is surgical resection.[54] The need for adjuvant therapy

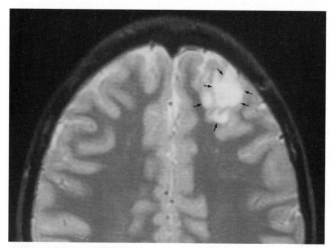

Figure 58–8 Ganglioglioma in a 10-year-old boy with frontal seizures. Axial T2-weighted image through the centrum semiovale reveals a cortically based lesion with mild mass effect, high signal, and heterogeneous borders *(arrows)*.

after total or even partial resection is controversial. Because these neoplasms in childhood usually do not mutate into higher-grade lesions, a period of observation after partial resection is often recommended. The resection of lesions in eloquent areas of brain, such as those abutting speech areas and motor cortex, has been greatly aided by the use of brain mapping techniques.[57] Because many of these lesions have arisen over many years, and are possibly congenital tumors, they have often altered the functional architecture of cortical structures, allowing for more extensive resections than once was believed possible. In addition, such surgical techniques as stereotactic tumor resection and resection aided by stereotactic localization make more aggressive resections possible. An unsettled issue is the degree of preoperative evaluation needed in patients with seizures and radiographically inferred low-grade cortical gliomas.[57, 58] Preoperative electroencephalographic monitoring, including the use of depth electrodes, to determine the electrical site or sites of seizure origin have been used, but it is unclear whether outcome (seizure control and tumor control) in patients undergoing surgery based on these techniques is better than that in patients treated with non-electroencephalographic based ''tumor'' resection (based purely on neuroimaging findings).

Recent attempts have been made to perform randomized prospective studies on children with low-grade neoplasms to determine which patients can be observed and which require adjuvant therapy. Despite the uncertainty of treatment outcome, these studies have been difficult to perform due to inherent biases of the treating physicians.

Based on results obtained primarily in children with diencephalic tumors, a recent interest has been seen in the use of chemotherapy to treat very young children, especially those younger than 5 years, with partially resected low-grade cortical tumors.[39] Once again, the indications for the initiation of chemotherapy in partially resected cortical tumors remains unclear.

HIGH-GRADE CORTICAL GLIOMAS

Anaplastic gliomas and glioblastomas multiforme comprise approximately one quarter of all childhood cortical gliomas.[59, 60] They may occur in the same regions of brain as lower-grade tumors, although a chiasmatic/hypothalamic or cerebellar site of origin is uncommon. Preliminary evidence, in a small number of tissue samples, suggests biologic differences between childhood high-grade gliomas and those occurring in adults.[4–6] Childhood tumors, although frequently showing chromosomal changes, tend to have fewer characteristic abnormalities than adult tumors. The abnormalities on chromosome 17 and the presence of double minute chromosomes, which occur commonly in adult tumors, have only been noted infrequently in childhood studies.[61] Alterations of the TP53 gene were noted in 12 of 27 patients between 18 and 45 years of age with malignant gliomas, whereas only 1 of 6 children with high-grade lesions showed similar abnormalities.[4] Despite these interesting results, given the small number of specimens studied, the significance of the results should be not exaggerated.

Clinical Presentation

High-grade cortical gliomas usually present more explosively than do low-grade glial lesions. Headaches and focal neurologic symptoms are common early in the course of illness.[6, 59] The headache from increased intracranial pressure, due to surrounding tumor edema, is frequent. Approximately one in five patients develop seizures by the time of diagnosis. High-grade childhood gliomas tend to grow locally and involve multiple, contiguous anatomic sites. It is virtually impossible to distinguish the leading edge of the tumor from tumor-related edema. The reported incidence of leptomeningeal dissemination of cortical high-grade gliomas has varied, but few tumors are disseminated at the time of diagnosis.[7, 59, 62]

Radiographic Features

Neuroradiographically, childhood malignant gliomas tend to be identical to similar lesions in adults.[10] Most lesions are hypodense on CT and hypointense, as compared to normal brain, on T1-weighted MRI. On T2-weighted images, these tumors show increased signal intensity, associated with areas of hemorrhage and/or necrosis. High-grade gliomas usually enhance and are associated with surrounding edema with resultant mass effect; the amount of mass effect is a relatively good predictor of the degree of malignancy.

Management

Management of childhood high-grade gliomas remains suboptimal. Evidence indicates that the extent of resection is a determinant of outcome in children. Patients with partially resected or biopsied lesions rarely survive, whereas children who undergo total resection tend to have a better outcome, as up to a third will be alive 3 years following diagnosis.[63]

After treatment with local radiotherapy alone, fewer than 25% of children with high-grade gliomas experience long-term disease control.[59, 60, 63] Although attempts have been made to utilize higher doses of local radiotherapy and focused radiotherapy in children with high-grade gliomas, no information to date has suggested improved disease control. The volume of radiation therapy that is optimal for disease control in children with malignant gliomas is poorly characterized. A survival advantage for whole-brain radiotherapy, as compared with local radiotherapy, has never been shown in prospective randomized trials.[14, 63]

A benefit for adjuvant chemotherapy for children with high-grade malignant gliomas has been suggested by a trial undertaken by the Children's Cancer Group in the late 1970s and 1980s.[14] In this trial, the addition of lomostine and vincristine chemotherapy, during and after radiotherapy, improved survival as compared with treatment with radiotherapy alone. Forty-six percent of children on this randomized trial who received radiotherapy and adjuvant chemotherapy were alive and free of disease 5 years following treatment, as compared with 18% of those treated with postsurgery radiotherapy alone. Surprisingly, the benefit of chemotherapy was seen primarily in children with glioblastoma multi-

forme. The Children's Cancer Group has recently completed a trial comparing pre-irradiation chemotherapy and post-irradiation chemotherapy with the 8-drug-in-1-day regimen to the aforementioned lomustine and vincristine protocol, which had improved survival in the previous Children's Cancer Group trial.[63] No survival advantage was shown for those children treated with preradiation and postirradiation 8-drug-in-1-day as compared with adjuvant lomustine and vincristine in this study.[63] Overall, the survival rates for children with anaplastic gliomas and glioblastomas was somewhat lower in the most recent Children's Cancer Group trial, with approximately 30% of children with anaplastic gliomas and 20% of children with glioblastoma alive and free of disease 5 years following treatment.

The apparent better disease control in children with high-grade gliomas, especially glioblastoma multiforme, compared with adults, and the suggested chemosensitivity of some pediatric malignant glial tumors is further supported by the results of studies performed primarily in infants and young children using drug combinations such as the 8-drug-in-1-day approach and a drug regimen of cyclophosphamide, cisplatin, vincristine, and etoposide.[63, 64] Thirty percent to 40% of children younger than 3 years had prolonged (1 to 2 year) disease control after treatment with surgery and chemotherapy alone.[63, 64] It is unclear whether this difference in response, as compared with that in adult tumors, is due to biologic differences between tumors arising at different ages or related to other factors, such as the aggressiveness of the chemotherapies used, the ability of young patients to better tolerate intensive chemotherapeutic regimens, the extent of resection, or other poorly characterized host factors.

Other approaches are currently under study for children with high-grade cortical gliomas. Based on evidence that at the time of recurrence, 40% of children with anaplastic gliomas or glioblastoma multiforme transiently respond to high-dose carmustine, thiotepa, and etoposide, followed by autologous bone marrow rescue, studies evaluating the efficacy of postsurgery high-dose chemotherapy followed by autologous bone marrow rescue, prior to irradiation, for children with malignant gliomas are being conducted.[65] The utilization of high-dose chemotherapy prior to irradiation, augmented by hemopoietic growth factors or autologous stem cell rescue, in an attempt to intensify treatment without requiring autologous bone marrow rescue, is also being pursued.

EPENDYMOMAS

Approximately two thirds of childhood ependymomas arise in the posterior fossa, and one third arise supratentorially. Overall, ependymomas constitute 5% to 10% of all childhood primary CNS tumors.[66–68] These tumors tend to occur in relatively young children; more than 50% of patients are younger than 5 years at the time of diagnosis. Ependymomas have been separated primarily into benign or anaplastic lesions, although it remains unclear whether such a distinction has any prognostic significance.

Clinical Presentation

Posterior fossa ependymomas have variable clinical manifestations. They most commonly present with ataxia and signs of increased intracranial pressure, mimicking medulloblastomas or cerebellar astrocytomas, but they may also cause cranial nerve palsies. Symptoms and signs of tumors that involve the lateral and third ventricles are highly dependent on involvement of adjacent brain.

Neuroradiographic Features

On CT, ependymomas tend to appear as isodense or hyperdense lesions that show homogeneous contrast enhancement.[10] On MRI, these tumors tend to be isointense or hypointense on T1-weighted images as compared with the surrounding brain. On T2-weighted images, ependymomas tend to be isointense or hyperintense and more heterogeneous than the usually homogeneous medulloblastomas. Most will readily enhance after gadolinium infusion. Despite their origin within or adjacent to the linings of the ventricular system, ependymomas are rarely disseminated early in the course of illness. After multiple relapses, leptomeningeal dissemination is more frequent.[7] In the posterior fossa, ependymomas usually occupy the fourth ventricle and one or both cerebellopontine cisterns. Inferior growth into the foramen magnum is also common.[69]

Management

Recent studies have suggested that surgery is the single most important determinant of outcome for children with ependymomas.[70, 71] Patients with totally or near totally resected lesions have a more favorable prognosis, as 60% or more of patients are alive and free of disease 5 years following diagnosis.[70, 71] After total resection, the most commonly recommended treatment is radiotherapy. The need of prophylactic craniospinal radiation therapy in patients without evidence of subarachnoid disease is a matter of debate.[72, 73] Although local relapse is the dominant mode of failure, at least one series has suggested that the addition of craniospinal radiotherapy improves overall disease control.[72] Other studies have failed to demonstrate this relationship.[66, 73] The local invasive potential of ependymomas has been shown by MRI.[69] Posterior fossa lesions often infiltrate the brainstem and extend along the upper cervical cord. It is conceivable that disease failure occurring after local radiotherapy is due, in part, to the use of inappropriately small radiation volumes.

Disease control for children with subtotally resected tumors is quite poor, with most series suggesting that between 60% and 80% of patients will have progressive disease 5 years from initial treatment. Attempts have been made to improve survival by increasing the overall dose of radiotherapy and/or utilizing chemotherapy. As yet, no evidence shows that such alterations in therapy have improved overall survival.[66, 74]

REFERENCES

1. Young JL Jr, Miller RW: Incidence of malignant tumors in US children. J Pediatr 1975; 86:254–258.
2. Kleihues P, Burger PC, Scheithauer BW: Histologic Typing of Tumours of the Central Nervous System. Berlin, Springer-Verlag, 1993.
3. Schofield DE: Diagnostic histopathology, cytogenetics and molecular markers of pediatric brain tumors. Neurosurg Clin North Am 1992; 3:723–738.
4. Rasheed BKA, McLendon RE, Herndon JE, et al: Alterations of the TP53 gene in human gliomas. Cancer Res 1994; 54:1324–1330.
5. Griffin CA, Hawkins AL, Packer RJ, et al: Chromosome abnormalities in pediatric brain tumors. Cancer Res 1985; 48:175–180.
6. Chadduck WM, Boop FA, Sawyer JR: Cytogenetic studies of pediatric brain and spinal cord tumors. Pediatr Neurosurg 1991–92; 17:57–65.
7. Packer RJ, Siegel KR, Sutton LN, et al: Leptomeningeal dissemination of primary central nervous system tumors of childhood. Ann Neurol 1984; 56:1748–1755.
8. Gilles F: Cerebellar tumors in children. Clin Neurosurg 1983; 30:181–188.
9. Gjerris F, Kliken L: Long-term prognosis in children with benign cerebellar astrocytoma. J Neurosurg 1978; 49:929–933.
10. Barkovich AJ, Edwards MSB: Brain tumors of childhood. *In* Barkovich AJ (ed): Contemporary Neuroimaging, vol. 1, Pediatric Neuroimaging. New York, Raven Press, 1990, pp 149–204.
11. Conway PD, Oechler HW, Kun LE, et al: Importance of histologic condition and treatment of pediatric cerebellar astrocytoma. Cancer 1991; 67:2772–2775.
12. Hayostek CJ, Shaw EG, Scheithauer B, et al: Astrocytomas of the cerebellum. Cancer 1993; 72:856–863.
13. Leibel SA, Sheline GE, Wara WM, et al: The role of radiation therapy in the treatment of astrocytomas. Cancer 1975; 35:1551–1557.
14. Sposto R, Ertel IJ, Jenkin RDT, et al: The effectiveness of chemotherapy for treatment of high grade astrocytoma in children: Results of a randomized trial. A report from the Childrens Cancer Study Group. J Neurooncol 1989; 7:165–177.
15. Salazar OM: Primary malignant cerebellar astrocytomas in children: A signal for postoperative craniospinal irradiation. Int J Radiat Oncol Biol Phys 1981; 7:1661–1665.
16. Barkovich AJ, Krishner J, Kun L, et al: Brainstem gliomas: A classification system based on magnetic resonance imaging. Pediatr Neurosci 1991; 16:73–83.
17. Littman P, Jarret P, Bilanuk L, et al: Pediatric brainstem gliomas. Cancer 1980; 45:2787–2792.
18. Albright AL, Guthkelch AN, Packer RJ: Prognostic factors in pediatric brain-stem gliomas. J Neurosurg 1986; 65:751–755.
19. Edwards MSB, Wara WM, Urtasan RC, et al: Hyperfractionated radiation therapy for brainstem gliomas: A phase I-II trial. J Neurosurg 1989; 70:691–700.
20. Epstein F: Intrinsic brain stem tumors of childhood. Prog Exp Tumor Res 1987; 30:160–169.
21. Stroink AR, Hoffman JH, Hendrick EB, et al: Diagnosis and management of pediatric brain-stem gliomas. J Neurosurg 1986; 65:745–750.
22. Vandertop WP, Hoffman JH, Drake JM, et al: Focal midbrain tumors in children. Neurosurgery 1992; 31:186–194.
23. Pollack IF, Pang D, Albright AL: The long-term outcome in children with late onset aqueductal stenosis resulting from benign intrinsic tectal tumors. J Neurosurg 1994; 80:681–688.
24. Milstein JM, Geyer JR, Berger MS, et al: Favorable prognosis for brainstem gliomas in neurofibromatosis. J Neurooncol 1989; 7:367–371.
25. Albright AL, Packer RJ, Zimmerman R, et al: Magnetic resonance scans should replace biopsies for the diagnosis of diffuse brainstem gliomas: A report from the Childrens Cancer Group. Neurosurgery 1993; 33:1026–1030.
26. Coffey RJ, Lunsford LD: Stereotactic surgery for mass lesions of the midbrain and pons. Neurosurgery 1985; 17:12–18.
27. Franzini A, Allegranza A, Melcarne A, et al: Serial stereotactic biopsy of brain stem expanding lesions: Consideration on 45 consecutive cases. Acta Neurochir Suppl (Wien) 1988; 42:170–176.
28. Freeman CR, Krischer J, Sanford RA, et al: Hyperfractionated radiation therapy in brain stem tumors: Results of treatment at the 7020 cGy dose level of Pediatric Oncology Group Study #8495. Cancer 1991; 68:474–481.
29. Packer RJ, Allen JC, Goldwein JL, et al: Hyperfractionated radiotherapy for children with brainstem gliomas: A pilot study using 7,200 cGy. Ann Neurol 1990; 27:167–173.
30. Packer RJ, Littman PA, Sposto RM, et al: Results of a pilot study of

hyperfractionated radiotherapy for children with brainstem gliomas. Int J Radiat Oncol Biol Phys 1987; 13:1647–1657.

31. Freeman CR, Krischner JP, Sanford A, et al: Final results of a study of escalating doses of hyperfractionated radiotherapy in brain stem tumors in childhood: A pediatric oncology study. Radiat Oncol Biol Phys 1993; 27:197–206.

32. Packer RJ, Boyett JM, Zimmerman RA, et al: Hyperfractionated radiation therapy (72 Gy) for children with brain stem gliomas. Cancer 1993; 72:1414–1421.

33. Shrieve DC, Wara WM, Edwards MS, et al: Hyperfractionated radiation therapy for gliomas of the brainstem in children and in adults. Int J Radiat Oncol Biol Phys 1992; 24:599–610.

34. Packer RJ, Zimmerman RA, Kaplan A, et al: Early cystic/necrotic changes following hyperfractionated radiotherapy in children with brainstem gliomas: Results from a Childrens Cancer Group trial. Cancer 1993; 71:2666–2674.

35. Jenkin RDT, Goesel C, Ertel I, et al: Brainstem tumors in childhood: A prospective randomized trial of irradiation with and without adjuvant CCNU, VCR, and prednisone. J Neurosurg 1987; 66:227–233.

36. Packer RJ, Nicholson HS, Johnson DL, et al: Dilemmas in the management of childhood brain tumors: Brainstem gliomas. Pediatr Neurosurg 1992; 17:37–43.

37. Kretschmar CS, Tarbell NJ, Barnes PD, et al: Preirradiation chemotherapy and hyperfractionated radiation therapy (66 Gy) for children with brain stem tumors. Cancer 1993; 72:1404–1423.

38. Robertson PL, Allen JC, Abbott R, et al: Pediatric cervicomedullary tumors: A distinct subset of brainstem tumors. Neurology 1993; 43: A248.

39. Packer RJ, Lange B, Ater J, et al: Carboplatin and vincristine for progressive low-grade gliomas of childhood. J Clin Oncol 1993; 11:850–857.

40. Packer RJ, Savino PJ, Bilaniuk L, et al: Chiasmatic gliomas of childhood: A reappraisal of natural history and effectiveness of cranial irradiation. Childs Brain 1983; 10:393–402.

41. Glaser JS, Hoyt WF, Corbett J: Visual morbidity with chiasmal glioma. Arch Ophthalmol 1971; 85:3–12.

42. Packer RJ, Bilaniuk LT, Cohen BH, et al: Intracranial visual pathway gliomas in children with neurofibromatosis. Neurofibromatosis 1988; 1:212–222.

43. Fletcher WA, Imes RK, Hoyt WF: Chiasmatic gliomas: Appearance and long-term changes demonstrated by computed tomography. J Neurosurg 1986; 65:154–159.

44. Ellsworth C, Alvord MD, Lofton S: Gliomas of the optic nerve or chiasm. J Neurosurg 1988; 68:85–98.

45. Miller NR, Iliff WJ, Green WR: Evaluation and management of gliomas of the anterior visual pathway. Brain 1975; 97:743–754.

46. Baram TZ, Moser RP, Van Eyes J: Surgical management of progressive visual loss in optic gliomas of childhood. Ann Neurol 1986; 20:398.

47. Rush JA, Young BR, Campbell RJ, et al: Optic glioma, long-term follow-up of 85 histopathologically verified cases. Ophthalmology 1982; 89:1213–1219.

48. Taveras JM, Mont LA, Wood EH: The value of radiation therapy in management of gliomas of optic nerves and chiasm. Radiology 1956; 66:518–528.

49. Rosenstock JG, Packer RJ, Bilaniuk LT, et al: Chiasmatic optic glioma treated with chemotherapy: A preliminary report. J Neurosurg 1985; 63:862–866.

50. Packer RJ, Sutton LM, Bilaniuk LT, et al: Treatment of chiasmatic/hypothalmic gliomas of childhood with chemotherapy: An update. Ann Neurol 1988; 23:79–85.

51. Pons MA, Finlay JL, Walker RW, et al: Chemotherapy with vincristine and etoposide in children with low-grade astrocytoma. J Neurooncol 1992; 14:151–158.

52. Friedman HS, Krischer JP, Burger P, et al: Treatment of children with progressive or recurrent brain tumors with carboplatin or iroplatin: A Pediatric Oncology Group randomized phase II study. J Clin Oncol 1992; 10:249–256.

53. Gajjar A, Heideman RL, Kovnar EH, et al: Response of pediatric low grade gliomas to chemotherapy. Pediatr Neurosurg 1992; 19:113–121.

54. Hirsch JF, Sainte-Rose C, Pierre-Kahn A, et al: Benign astrocytic and oligodendrocytic tumors of the cerebral hemispheres in children. J Neurosurg 1989; 70:568–572.

55. VanderBerg SR, May EE, Rubinstein LJ, et al: Desmoplastic supratentorial neuroepithelial tumors of infancy with divergent differentiation potential (''desmoplastic infantile gangliogliomas''). J Neurosurg 1987; 66:58–71.

56. Daumas-Duport C, Scheithauer BW, Chodkiewicz JP, et al: Dysembryoplastic neuroepithelial tumor: A surgically curable tumor of young patients within intractable partial seizures. Neurosurgery 1988; 23: 545–556.

57. Berger MS, Ghatan S, Haglund MM, et al: Low-grade gliomas associated with intractable epilepsy: Seizure outcome utilizing electrocorticography during tumor resection. J Neurosurg 1993; 79:62–69.

58. Packer RJ, Sutton LN, Patel KM, et al: Seizure control following tumor surgery for children with low-grade gliomas. J Neurosurg 1994; 80:998–1003.

59. Dropcho EJ, Wisoff JH, Walker RW, et al: Supratentorial malignant gliomas in childhood: A review of 50 cases. Ann Neurol 1987; 22:355.

60. Marchese MJ, Chang CH: Malignant astrocytic gliomas in children. Cancer 1990; 65:2771.

61. Sawyer JR, Swanson CM, Roloson GJ, et al: Cytogenetic findings in a case of pediatric glioblastoma. Cancer Genet Cytogenet 1992; 64: 75–79.

62. Kandt RS, Shinnar S, D'Souza BJ, et al: Cerebrospinal metastases in malignant childhood astrocytomas. J Neurooncol 1984; 2:123.

63. Finlay JL, Boyett JM, Yates AJ: Outcome of a phase III trial in childhood high-grade astrocytoma comparing vincristine, CCNU and prednisone with ''eight-drug-in-1-day'' regimen: A report of the Childrens Cancer Group Trial CCG–945. Pediatr Neurosurg (in press).

64. Duffner PK, Horowitz ME, Krishner JP, et al: Postoperative chemotherapy and delayed radiation in children less than 3 years of age with malignant brain tumors. N Engl J Med 1993; 328:1275–1731.

65. Finlay JL: High-dose chemotherapy with marrow rescue in children and young adults with malignant brain tumors. Pediatr Neurosurg 1990–91; 16:116.

66. Goldwein JW, Leahy JM, Packer RJ: Intracranial ependymomas in children. Int J Radiat Oncol Biol Phys 1990; 19:1497.

67. Pierre-Kahn A, Hirsch JF, Roux FX, et al: Intracranial ependymomas in childhood: Survival and function results of 47 cases. Childs Brain 1983; 10:145.

68. Nazar GB, Hoffman JH, Becker LE, et al: Infratentorial ependymomas in childhood: Prognostic factors and treatment. J Neurosurg 1990; 72:408.

69. Spoto GP, Press GA, Hesselink JR, et al: Intracranial ependymoma and subependymoma: MR manifestations. AJNR 1990; 11:83.

70. Tomita T, McLone DG, Das L, et al: Benign ependymomas of the posterior fossa in childhood. Pediatr Neurosci 1988; 14:277.

71. Sutton LN, Goldwein JW, Perilongo G, et al: Prognostic factors in childhood ependymoma. Pediatr Neurosurg 1991; 61:57–65.

72. Salazar OM, Casto-Vita M, Van Houtte D, et al: Improved survival in cases of intracranial ependymoma after radiation therapy: Late report and recommendations. J Neurosurg 1983; 59:652.

73. Goldwein JW, Corn BJ, Finlay JL, et al: Is craniospinal irradiation required to care children with malignant (anaplastic) ependymomas. Cancer 1991; 67:2766–2771.

74. Lefkowitz I, Evans A, Sposto R, et al: Adjuvant chemotherapy of childhood posterior fossa (PF) ependymoma: Craniospinal radiation with or without CCNU, vincristine (VCR) and prednisone (P) (abstract). Pediatr Neurosci 1989; 14:149.

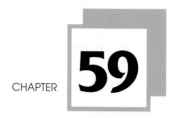

CHAPTER **59**

Pregnancy and Gliomas

The clinical problem of brain tumor during pregnancy is certain to generate interest and opinion. Management considerations are protean, embracing the difficulties of an often recalcitrant disease imposed on a rapidly changing and complex host physiology and immune state. Two lives are at risk, and management depends on what is often anecdotal data and misapprehension. Management strategy is confounded by the diverse biological behaviors of several kinds of brain tumors—pituitary tumors, meningiomas, gliomas, and acoustic neuromas—each with individual sex and age predilection, hormonal responsiveness, and clinical course. Finally, the generalization of the appearance of one brain tumor into a *propensity* for occurrence of brain tumors in pregnant women is misleading.

Reports in the literature have been confusing and sometimes contradictory regarding the coincidence of brain tumor and pregnancy. For example, in 1958 Bickerstaff and coworkers[1] had observed that symptoms in pregnancy occurred "more frequently than can be regarded as purely coincidental." McClure Browne, an obstetrician, stated that "75% of intracranial tumors which appear in women of childbearing age first declare themselves during pregnancy."[2] However, one may read that the coincidence of tumors and pregnancy is *rare*, and that the emergence (and timing) of symptoms is by chance. Because the number of actual cases of brain tumor during pregnancy in the literature is small, it is difficult to reason the relationship statistically. A focus specifically on gliomas further vitiates the ability to draw conclusions based on statistics; gliomas are a small subset of these tumors and are likely to be underreported.

This chapter examines the hypothesis that a special relationship links glioma to pregnancy that is different from the simultaneous occurrence of the two separate entities. The management issues specific to gliomas in pregnancy are discussed with respect to surgery, radiotherapy, chemotherapy, and medical management. Opinions on indications for abortions and for cesarean section are presented. Although some material reviewed elsewhere[3] that pertains to brain tumors in general in pregnancy is introduced here, issues specific to gliomas are emphasized.

HORMONES, CONCEPTION, AND RECEPTORS

If there is a link between pregnancy and glioma, and if that link is attributable to the hormonal milieu in pregnancy, then it might be useful to examine the hormonal differences between the nonpregnant and the pregnant woman. At the time of ovulation, estradiol levels are high, having risen during the follicular phase of the menstrual cycle to peak just before ovulation. Ovulation is heralded by a surge of both follicle-stimulating hormone (FSH) and luteinizing hormone (LH). A release of androgens occurs before and during ovulation.[4]

At the peak of the LH surge, estradiol estrogen levels fall, and progesterone secretion begins; the progesterone nurtures the uterine endometrial lining to secretory state to receive the blastocyst for implantation. If fertilization does not occur, estradiol and progesterone levels fall to normal. If fertilization does occur, then human chorionic gonadotropin (hCG), elaborated by the trophoblast, or the outer shell of the implanted blastocyst, maintains the corpus luteum, which would otherwise degenerate. The corpus luteum, in turn, maintains steroid (estrogen and progesterone) production until the placental steroidogenesis is well established by the ninth to tenth week of gestation. As placental steroidogenesis increases, corpus luteal hormone production declines. Placental progesterone levels continue to rise until the 36th week.

Other hormonal changes of possible significance include a rise in prolactin levels from 40 to 500 ng/mL. The increased prolactin secretion does not cause lactation during pregnancy because estrogen inhibits that function. The estrogen levels increase from baseline just at the end of pregnancy. Triiodothyronine (T_3) and thyroxine (T_4) levels are elevated, as is calcitonin, during pregnancy.

In summary, significant differences between the postovulatory half of the menstrual cycle and pregnancy include the following: (1) increased secretion of progesterone and prolactin; (2) hCG secretion, which peaks at 10 weeks, then slowly drops; and (3) elevated estrogen levels, which increase until near term. The periovulatory pulses of androgen, LH, and FSH do not recur if fertilization takes place.

These specific hormonal differences are compelling in view of recent information regarding steroid receptors on brain tumors. Kornblum and colleagues[5] made the observation that progesterone and androgen receptors were present in 27% of the meningiomas that they examined for receptors. Surprisingly, *no* estrogen receptors were found on the meningiomas, despite a correlation between breast cancer and meningioma in women and the fact that meningiomas are more common in women. Eleven gliomas of various grades were found in their series, including two oligodendrogliomas and an ependymoma. None of these tumors had progesterone receptors. Whittle and associates[6] looked at 16 gliomas as well as at a variety of other tumors, including a large number of meningiomas. Again, progesterone receptors were documented and were confirmed on the meningiomas. Among these 16 tumors were nine glioblastomas, three low-grade astrocytomas, one mixed oligodendroglioma, one pure oligodendroglioma, one ependymoma, and one medulloblastoma. No receptors for estrogen and progesterone were found among these gliomas. In an important paper Sica and co-workers[7] found a difference between male and female subjects regarding the receptor distribution in poorly differentiated neoplasms. Specifically, they looked at 53 neuroepithelial tumors with respect to glucocorticoid receptors, estrogen receptors, progesterone receptors, and androgen receptors. Two thirds of the tumors had progesterone receptors, half had androgen receptors, and one third had estrogen receptors; however, the quantity of receptors was significantly lower than that found on meningiomas. They found a significant difference between men and women. Unexpectedly, this difference was between estrogen and androgen receptors, *not* progesterone receptors. In high-grade (anaplastic and glioblastoma) glial tumors, women had a significantly higher percentage of receptor-positive tumors. This difference was not demonstrated for low-grade gliomas. In a large series specific for neuroepithelial tumors, Paoletti and associates[8] examined 25 glioblastomas, 18 anaplastic astrocytomas, and 14 lower-grade astrocytomas. They found androgen-specific binding proteins in 22% of the cases; 9% were estrogen positive and 4% were progesterone positive.

In summary, although meningiomas may have progesterone receptors, no evidence exists that gliomas have specific sex hormone receptors other than, possibly, androgen receptors. Androgen secretion occurs during ovulation but not during pregnancy.

The putative hormonal influences have been thought to involve not just tumor receptor activation, but the modulation of immunity. Because the fetus is immunologically foreign, it follows that the immune surveillance for antigenic tissue should decrease to maintain the pregnancy.[9] Gleicher and colleagues[10] have ascribed this decrease to immunoglobulin G, and suggest T-cell–mediated suppression. hCG, progesterone, and estrogen hormones have all been implicated in humoral depression of cell-mediated immunity. This consideration should be compelling to support the hypothesis of increased tumor frequency in pregnancy. In a sense, the alteration of one's *own* glial cells to malignant glial cells is less "foreign" than the appearance of a blastocyst and subsequent fetus, which carries paternal transplantation antigens. That is, if the body tolerates a pregnancy, it should certainly tolerate a glioma.

IMMUNE SURVEILLANCE

Donegan[9] has said that a state of immune compromise exists both in pregnancy and in cancer. Despite our sophisticated knowledge of immunology, it remains a mystery why a fetus is not rejected by the mother. After all, the fetus contains paternal antigens in the HLA complex; they are present in the placenta as well. Mills[11] has reviewed numerous explanations, including blocking antibodies that "hide" the paternal antigens from the mother's surveillance, or restriction of the response of the mother to recognized antigens. If one were to try to support the hypothesis that cancer is more common in pregnancy, then these maternal immune responses might affect cancer surveillance as well. Although maternal responses may be a commonality in cancer and pregnancy with respect to abnormal T-cell responses, a significant quantitative difference exists in the extent of these responses in cancer compared with those in pregnancy. Mills[11] has summarized extensive work on the matter: "Although there is a specific non-responsiveness or a blocking response to the conception itself during pregnancy, the immune system is generally intact and able to deal completely with foreign challenges such as infections and tumors."

BLOOD VOLUME/TUMOR VOLUME

Circulating blood volume is increased during pregnancy by as much as 50% in the third trimester. The increased volume is primarily from additional plasma, although red cells are produced to maintain a proper hematocrit level. Although the hypervolemia is said to be greatest in the third trimester, it abates quickly after parturition. During this time, organs indeed become more hyperemic. Almost certainly, vascular tumors and venous malformations enlarge as a result. Meningiomas are likely to become hyperemic, and probably larger, and are consequently more likely to become symptomatic during pregnancy. Michelsen and New[12] first documented a volume reduction from pregnancy to postpartum period in 1967 by angiography. The case, thought to be a meningioma during the pregnancy, turned out to be an astrocytoma on postpartum biopsy. Roelvink and associates[13] noted a definite increase in the number of pregnant women with meningiomas who became symptomatic as the pregnancy progressed. They found that 42% became symptomatic in the third trimester. Conversely, they found that fully half of the women with gliomas became symptomatic in the first trimester. By contrast Depret-Mosser and co-workers[14] found gliomas to be most frequently symptomatic in the third trimester.

This hypervolemia factor alone may have formed the basis for a putative relationship between pregnancy and brain tumors. Because some brain tumors do become symptomatic in pregnancy, and especially because attention tends to be focused on presentation during pregnancy, the author conjectures that an extrapolation may have been made to the unwarranted conclusion that brain tumors actually occur more frequently in pregnancy than at other times.

INCIDENCE DURING PREGNANCY

The assignment of brain tumor risk to the pregnancy period is extremely difficult. The disease must be recognized during

TABLE 59–1
AGE-SPECIFIC RISK FOR GLIOMA*

	Risk	
Age (yr)	*Male*	*Female*
15–19	1.93	1.85
20–24	2.51	1.45
25–29	2.15	2.02
30–34	2.79	2.68
35–39	4.34	2.16
40–44	4.26	3.18

*Estimated for Connecticut based on the Connecticut Tumor Registry's 10-year experience in gliomas and the 1990 Census of Population and Housing, U.S. Department of Commerce, Bureau of the Census.

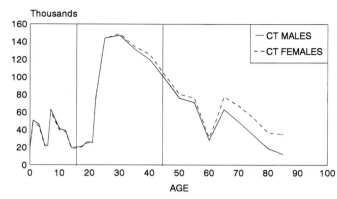

Figure 59–2 Connecticut Tumor Registry data: comparison of Connecticut female and male populations. Age is given in years.

that period or it must be established that the disease began in that period or that some event in that interval caused the disease to be expressed. In the reports of tumors and pregnancy, all three of these situations are found.

Expected Frequency of Brain Tumor in Pregnancy

For the individual woman, the "childbearing years" are the years between menarche and menopause. In statistical treatment this interval is defined as ages 15 to 44 years. This choice alone may seriously affect statistical calculations. Women aged 40 to 44 years are less likely to have children and are slightly more likely to have a brain tumor (Table 59–1). A number of difficulties accompany the assignment of brain tumor risk to pregnancy. Women of childbearing age may become pregnant more than once in the interval spanned by the tumor. The presence of a tumor cannot be counted unless the tumor is identified, either by chance or by symptom. As a result, there is no way to know how many asymptomatic women in childbearing years, pregnant or not, may be harboring a tumor. Once identified, the tumor must then be reported. Not all states require reporting. In formal reporting mechanisms, such as the tumor registry of the German Democratic Republic and of the State of Connecticut, additional pitfalls occur. For example, once a

woman has been enrolled, it is unlikely that later, on recognition of pregnancy, the physician will go back to the registry and amend the entry data. Relative risk cannot be assessed with 100% confidence by comparison with that in males; the epidemiology (and likely the biology) of many tumor types is different. In the final analysis, it is not possible to ascertain the risk for the pregnant woman; only a guess can be made.

This author and other authors have found the Connecticut Tumor Registry[15] to be an excellent source of tumor data to establish background risk. To reason from Connecticut Tumor Registry data, it is necessary to show that Connecticut has demographics similar to those of the entire United States. In comparing the female population of Connecticut with the female population of the United States, using data from the 1990 census (Fig. 59–1), 46% of women were of childbearing age[15] in both Connecticut and the United States, which supports the use of the Connecticut population for projections. In comparing the male and female population of Connecticut (Fig. 59–2), their similarity implies that the irregularities in the population in the under-10-year age groups are not unique to Connecticut females.

In this chapter, *glioma* is used to mean the histologic tumor types of astrocytic tumors (astrocytoma, anaplastic astrocytoma, glioblastoma multiforme), oligodendroglioma, and ependymoma. Medulloblastoma is excluded. This author has queried the Connecticut Tumor Registry for all gliomas by age and sex. The number of these tumors occurring between 1981 and 1991 is shown in Figure 59–3 for both

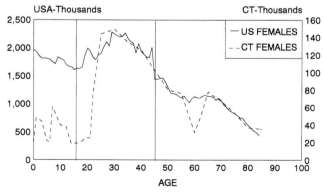

Figure 59–1 Connecticut Tumor Registry data: 1990 female population. Connecticut female population compared with U.S. female population. Age is given in years.

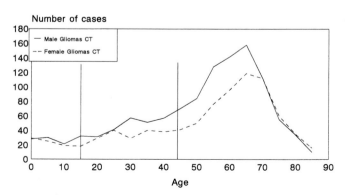

Figure 59–3 Connecticut Tumor Registry data: number of gliomas of all histologic types in Connecticut, 1981–1991. Age is given in years.

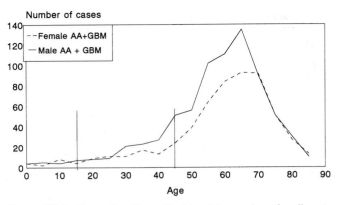

Figure 59–4 Connecticut Tumor Registry data: number of malignant astrocytomas (including anaplastic astrocytomas [AA] and glioblastomas multiforme [GBM]) in Connecticut, 1981–1991. Age is given in years.

males and females by age. Anaplastic astrocytoma and glioblastoma multiforme are shown in Figure 59–4. Anaplastic astrocytomas and glioblastomas were combined because the change from the Kernohan and Sayre to the World Health Organization classifications occurred during the indexed decade. The meaning of both *anaplastic astrocytoma* and *glioblastoma multiforme* changed sufficiently to influence the interpretation of the frequency data for anaplastic astrocytoma and glioblastoma multiforme, taken separately. A computed sex- and age-adjusted risk are given in Table 59–1. We can conclude that specific risk during childbearing years of 0.224 per 100,000 appears to be *lower* than that in other age groups. Note that nonpregnant women have not been separated from pregnant women during childbearing years in these data.

DISTRIBUTION OF TUMOR TYPES

The distributions have been reported by Zulch and Christensen[17] and by Schoenberg.[15] Gliomas are said to represent 37% of all brain tumors. Using a definition of the childbearing years to be ages 20 to 40 years (instead of 15 to 45 years) in their personal series aggregated with another 220 cases, Roelvink and co-workers[13] found the distribution of meningiomas, gliomas, and benign tumors at the base of the brain to be nearly identical to the predicted frequency among the general population as reported by Zulch and Christensen.[17] However, Haas and others[18] found the proportion of meningiomas to be lower than expected. The distribution of tumor types is summarized in Table 59–2.

What about the actual incidence of brain tumors in pregnancy? Haas and others[18] in reviewing the tumor registry for the German Democratic Republic in the years 1961 through 1971 (women aged 15 to 44 years) found the meningioma incidence to be substantially below the expected incidence in age-matched nonpregnant women. They found 1,520 women with malignant brain tumors in that interval. This figure does *not* include meningiomas or other benign intracranial lesions. This represented a risk of 0.232 to 0.238 per 100,000 women, which is comparable to the author's estimate in Connecticut of 0.224 per 100,000. Among the 1,532 women with malignant brain tumors, 17 were women with malignant gliomas (16 astrocytomas) associated with pregnancy. This risk is 0.11 per 100,000. They published corresponding ob-

TABLE 59–2
CLASSIFICATION OF TERATOGENIC DRUGS

Category A:	Controlled studies in women fail to demonstrate a risk to the fetus in the first trimester (and no evidence of a risk is seen in later trimesters), and the possibility of fetal harm appears remote
Category B:	Either animal reproduction studies have not demonstrated a fetal risk, but no controlled studies have been performed in pregnant women, or animal reproduction studies have shown an adverse effect (other than a decrease in fertility) that was not confirmed in controlled studies in women in the first trimester (and no evidence of a risk has been seen in later trimesters)
Category C:	Either studies in animals have revealed adverse effects on the fetus (teratogenic, embryocidal, or other) and no controlled studies have been performed in women, or studies in women and animals are not available; drugs should be given only if the potential benefit justifies the potential risk to the fetus
Category D:	Positive evidence exists of human fetal risk, but the benefits from use in pregnant women may be acceptable despite the risk (e.g., if the drug is needed in a life-threatening situation or for a serious disease for which safer drugs cannot be used or are ineffective)
Category X:	Studies in animals or human beings have demonstrated fetal abnormalities, or evidence of fetal risk has been found based on human experience, or both, and the risk of the use of the drug in pregnant women clearly outweighs any possible benefit. The drug is contraindicated in women who are or who may become pregnant.

From Briggs GG, Freeman RK, Yaffe SJ: Drugs in Pregnancy and Lactation: A Reference Guide to Fetal and Neonatal Risk, ed 4. Baltimore, Williams & Wilkins, 1994.

served vs. expected frequency of approximately .30 for both time intervals 1961–1969 and 1970–1979. Their data would suggest that not only is malignant brain tumor not common in pregnancy, but that there may be some *sparing* effect of pregnancy. (Note that an equally valid interpretation is that the tumor may ''prevent'' the pregnancy with a consequent reduction in frequency of pregnancy in women with tumors.) An alternative explanation, given by Haas and co-workers,[18] relates to underreporting.

The most recent collection of cases has been from Depret-Mosser and others.[14] Isolated cases have been reported since the comprehensive review of Roelvink and co-workers[13] in 1987 that are not included in the 1993 review of Depret-Mosser and colleagues.[19–23] Treatment and histologic verification were subsequent to delivery. These isolated reports appear in the literature either because they are intrinsically interesting or because the presence of the tumor presents certain management problems of interest. In summary, no compelling data support a conclusion that brain tumors are more common in pregnancy, that gliomas specifically are more common in pregnancy, or that tissue type distributions are altered by pregnancy. But this conclusion must be interpreted in the context of assumed underreporting of pregnancy.

MANAGEMENT OF GLIOMAS DURING PREGNANCY

Shift in Philosophy

Although extensive earlier reports have appeared in the literature regarding the management of brain tumors during pregnancy,[24–27] this problem has not gotten a great deal of attention. In the past, when the problem had been recognized late in pregnancy, the strategy had been to hold the symptoms in abeyance, if possible, and to treat the tumor after delivery of the baby. The early literature espoused a philosophy that mothers harboring malignant tumors discovered early during pregnancy should have abortions. Now, different viewpoints in management are in evolution as specific therapeutic risks become more clearly defined. In reality, most of the risks apply to the fetus; very few risks directly apply to the mother beyond those intrinsic to the nature of the tumor and to the possible relationship of delivery to intracranial pressure.

What Are the Risks to the Fetus?

In assessing the occurrence of malformations as a result of treatment, it must be borne in mind that a 3% baseline rate of congenital anomalies occurs among *all* pregnancies.

Most studies of cancer therapy assessing fetal risk consider developmental stage at exposure. The particular kind of risk depends on the stage of fetal development at exposure to the teratogenic treatment agent:

- Mutation (parental germ cell)
- Abortion (preimplantation; 6–7 days, early implantation)
- Teratogenesis (organ formation, 16–90 days)
- Birth abnormalities (low birth weight, prematurity, minor structural abnormalities)
- Functional abnormalities (cognitive)

Briggs and co-workers publish a yearly reference guide to fetal and neonatal risk: *Drugs in Pregnancy and Lactation.*[29] They classify risk from A–D, and X (see Table 59–2). Their data are compiled from the literature and reflect an aggregate experience. Of interest here are categories C, D, and X. It should be borne in mind that humans appear to be more resistant to malformations than do animals.

Although one might think that preconception exposure would logically lead to fetal mutation, it is interesting to note that mutation is rare in humans following cancer treatment of the mother. The oocytes are more likely to die than to mutate.[30] In a definitive study of the mutation issue, Mulvihill[31] examined the offspring of female cancer survivors (born 9 or more months after completion of treatment) and the offspring of their siblings. No significant difference was found in the incidence of cytogenetic or single-gene mutations or of simple malformations.

The most critical time of exposure is during the time of organogenesis. In this period, the fetus is most vulnerable to

the so-called teratogenic agents: surgery, drugs, and radiation.

Surgery and Neurosurgery

Historically, a longstanding perception has persisted that surgery during pregnancy is anathema. Kempers and Miller[24] have recommended that surgery be deferred until the fetus achieves a size that offers a good chance for viability. Current data do not support that viewpoint. Nowadays the attitude regarding surgery is much more aggressive; lesions best managed surgically *should* be managed surgically. General anesthesia itself, by and large, has not been a problem. Appropriate anesthetics can be chosen. The key strategy is to avoid hypoperfusion of the placenta (i.e., uterine ischemia).[32] As a technical point, one should avoid prolonged supine positions for fear of compression of the great vessels, which can compromise uteroplacental circulation.

Chemotherapy

The risks of chemotherapy to the *mother* have not been shown to be any different from the risks to any nonpregnant woman. The risks of cytotoxic drugs to the *fetus* are very definitely related to the time in the fetal development when the drug is given.

When cytotoxic agents are given in the first trimester, the potential for a spontaneous abortion is very high. The incidence of spontaneous abortion depends both on the kind of agent and the specific agent. For example, antimetabolites, such as the folate antagonist aminopterin, have a high rate of abortion. Indeed, aminopterin has been used to induce abortion, and when this drug is given and abortion fails, a high rate of anomalies occurs. Nicholson[33] showed that 34 out of 52 pregnancies aborted spontaneously when aminopterin was given. Zemlickis and colleagues[34] reviewed 13 pregnancies exposed in the first trimester and found four spontaneous abortions.

The overwhelming concern regarding chemotherapy is the risk of major morphologic abnormalities from risk in the first trimester, specifically during organogenesis. With the exception of one major report, the consensus is that risk is high, ranging from 17%[35, 36] to 40%.[34] In a contradictory report from Mexico, Avilés and associates[37] reported a long-term (15- to 19-year) follow-up of children of women treated for lymphoma. Of these 43 cases, 19 had been exposed to chemotherapy in the first trimester, and *no* functional or morphologic abnormalities were seen in these cases. The agents were combination regimens (ABVD, MOPP), busulfan, and/or mercaptopurine.

Chemotherapy given during the second and third trimester appears to bear a substantially lower risk. The babies tend to have lower birth weights[34] and may have granulocytopenia, but they do not appear to carry an increased incidence of anomalies.[36] Doll and colleagues have reviewed much of the older literature and have concluded that ''there is no evidence of increased risk of teratogenicity from chemotherapy in second and third trimesters. Single and combination chemotherapy may be given in the second and third trimesters with low risk of teratogenicity.''[36]

An important consideration is the long-term effect of chemotherapy on *subsequent* pregnancies. During an interesting study of potential teratogenicity from a variety of cancer treatments in a variety of cancers, Mulvihill and co-workers[38] observed that 40% of patients experienced abnormal pregnancy outcomes when pregnancies occurred *after* therapy had been concluded. The specific abnormalities were low birth weight and premature terminations rather than morphologic abnormalities. Three fourths of patients had received radiation alone or in conjunction with chemotherapy. Pajor and co-workers[39] looked at a subset of women with lymphoma who became pregnant during remission. Of the 15 women who continued the pregnancy, one spontaneous abortion occurred (at 10 weeks), and one minor and one major birth defect were seen.

A most remarkable report from Milliken and others[40] discussed three successful pregnancies with *normal* children in two women after bone marrow transplantation. These women were treated before transplantation with melphalan rather than radiation. Despite flagging maternal gonadal function, the children were conceived some years after therapy.

Experience does not touch on the agents of special interest to the neurooncologist. Few data are available regarding the nitrosoureas. As would be expected, multiple-agent regimens that contain procarbazine appear to be teratogenic in the first trimester. In summary of many reports and many drugs, Briggs and colleagues[29] list virtually no drugs as being useful in brain tumors except dactinomycin in group C. In group D they include bleomycin, cisplatin, cyclophosphamide, daunorubicin, doxorubicin, fluorouracil, hydroxyurea, mithramycin, procarbazine, vinblastine, and vincristine. Predictably, aminopterin is in group X.

Radiotherapy

The embryo is particularly sensitive to radiation. There is a high rate of malformation when radiation exposure occurs from the second to the eighth week of the first trimester of pregnancy. Many authors recommend abortion after an fetal exposure of 10 Gy or more. Although no safe doses have been determined, it is suggested that doses below 0.05 Gy delivered at any time during gestation are safe. The effects of therapeutic radiation are very difficult to estimate because of body scatter. Subdiaphragmatic radiation is contraindicated, even with shielding. At 2.5 Gy, significant abnormalities developed in *more than half* of the infants exposed between the third and tenth week. Even after 20 weeks of gestation, although there were no gross abnormalities, exposed infants suffered hematologic and dermatologic disorders.

One must be cautious about superdiaphragmatic radiation; evidently substantial scatter to the fetus does occur. It is suggested that it may be safe to give ionizing radiation to the neck or axilla if absolutely necessary.[41] This is, of course, important in the consideration of treatment of neurosurgical problems. After the first trimester, it is reasonable to begin brain radiotherapy with modification of field and dose and appropriate abdominal shielding.[42] The role of highly focused stereotactic radiosurgery or stereotactic radiotherapy in pregnancy has not been reviewed in the context of fetal risk. At first blush, the control of highly focused areas inherent in radiosurgery would suggest a protective advantage to the fetus. This advantage may be offset by substantial secondary scatter from the target to the fetus during a high single dose with significant radiobiologic effect.

Uterine exposure from radionuclides can be underestimated. Cox and co-workers[43] have reported a spontaneous abortion in a woman who received ^{131}I for a thyroid treatment. The isotope had unexpectedly accumulated in the uterus and remained there. These authors suggested that iodide and pertechnetate might accumulate in the gestating uterus in early pregnancy. This possibility should be kept firmly in mind, because perfusion lung scans with ^{99m}Tc are the most common nuclear studies in pregnant women.

Other Management Issues

The use of antiepileptic drugs in pregnant women has been just as controversial as all the other issues associated with interventions in pregnant women, with beliefs and principles having been founded on few data. Unfortunately, very few definite facts had been established regarding the use of these drugs. The use of anticonvulsants during pregnancy is said to double the usual 3% incidence of abnormalities in a normal pregnancy. Diphenylhydantoin, valproic acid, and trimethadione have been cataloged as teratogenic.[44] Briggs and colleagues[29] classify valproic acid in category D, along with phenytoin, phenobarbital, primidone, and phensuximide. According to Briggs and others,[29] carbamazepine and clonazepam may be used with relatively low risk (category C), as is the case for ethosuximide and mephenytoin.

But the increased risks of phenobarbital, phenytoin, and valproic acid cited by Briggs and co-workers[29] is not so clear in the minds of other authors. In a symposium involving the leading publishers and authors involved in the area of anticonvulsants in pregnancy, the series and data were presented and a consensus established. Delgado-Escueta and Janz[45] have published the guidelines in a comprehensive review of all the current relevant reports. First, it should be noted that the use of antiepileptic drugs might actually triple, rather than double, the baseline rate of 3% of congenital malformations. Second, it was clear that folate supplements should be provided. Phenytoin, phenobarbital, and primidone have antifolate actions; carbamazepine and valproic acid are thought to have similar actions.[46] The four major antiepileptics—carbamazepine, phenytoin, phenobarbital, and valproic acid—were compared for teratogenicity. In essence, no malformation rate in any specific drug in this group could be demonstrated than the other three. The nature of the malformations varied with the use of the drug. For example, Lindhout and others[47] found elevated incidence of midline defects with valproic acid. Certainly all agreed that *polytherapy was the one factor that was associated with the highest rate of malformations*, particularly when valproic acid was one of the elements of the polytherapy. Trimethadione was mentioned as being totally contraindicated, and its use in pregnancy was condemned.

TABLE 59–3
GUIDELINES FOR THE USE OF ANTIEPILEPTIC DRUGS DURING PREGNANCY

1. Use first-choice drug for seizure type and epilepsy syndrome
2. Use antiepileptic drug as monotherapy at lowest dose and plasma level that protects against tonic-clonic seizures
3. Avoid valproate and carbamazepine when a family history of neural-tube defects is present
4. Avoid polytherapy, especially combination of valproate, carbamazepine, and phenobarbital
5. Monitor plasma antiepileptic drug levels regularly and, if possible, monitor free or unbound plasma antiepileptic drug levels
6. Continue folate daily supplement and ensure normal plasma and red cell folate levels during the period of organogenesis in the first trimester
7. In cases of valproate treatment, avoid high plasma levels of valproate; divide doses over 3 to 4 administrations per day
8. In cases of valproate or carbamazepine treatment, offer amniocentesis for α-fetoprotein at 16 weeks and real-time ultrasonography at 18 to 19 weeks, to look for neural tube defects; ultrasonography at 22 to 24 weeks can detect oral clefts and heart anomalies

From Delgado-Escueta AJ, Janz D: Consensus guidelines: Preconception counseling, management, and care of the pregnant woman with epilepsy. Neurology 1992; 42(suppl 5):149–160.

In an interesting prospective study, Gaily and Granström[48] looked at children of mothers with epilepsy in comparison with control children, all of whom had been examined for minor anomalies. They found out that some of the minor abnormalities that had been associated with the use of phenytoin actually were more likely related to inheritance from the mother. Although this observation is made in a context that is a significant departure from any likely neurosurgical clinical situation, it does point out the frailty of the limited observations available.

In later trimesters, it appears that the greatest risk of anticonvulsants is growth retardation. Only transient retardation was associated with the use of barbiturates, probably related to sluggish feeding. The guidelines for treating physicians have been concisely presented in the article by Delgado-Escueta and Janz,[45] and are reproduced in Table 59–3.

Although glucocorticoids cause birth anomalies in animals, no evidence indicates that they are teratogenic in humans. In the context of pulmonary diseases and dermatologic disorders, therapeutic doses have not caused addisonism in children (reviewed in reference 49).

Abortion

After a review of the literature combined with eight personal cases, Depret-Mosser and co-workers[14] recommend abortion if the tumor is inoperable in the first trimester, if the clinical situation is uncontrollable medically or surgically, if the patient has had radiation in the first trimester, if there has been chemotherapy (contrary to other authors), if the maternal prognosis is bad, or if the patient wishes to have one.

Delivery

The management issues at delivery relate primarily to intracranial pressure.[50] The bearing-down reflex, not the uterine contractions, raises the intracranial pressure. The consensus is that pain management is the important strategy to control intracranial pressure during delivery.[22] The timing of delivery can sometimes be a problem. Goroszeniuk and co-workers[51] reported a case of a mother at 28 weeks who had obvious difficulties with intracranial neoplasm. In their report, a decision was made, based on the poor prognosis of the mother, to wait an additional 6 weeks until the child could be safely delivered. Delivery was hastened by worsening of the mother's condition. The modern techniques of steroid-induced fetal lung maturation open up more options for timing of delivery.

Cesarean section is almost never indicated unless it is intended to assuage *obstetric* concerns. Depret-Mosser and associates[14] consider the indications for cesarean section to be a poorly controlled or an uncontrollable clinical course, neurosurgical urgency near term, or the usual obstetric reasons.

Metastasis to Fetus

Care must be taken to distinguish the fetal acquisition of a brain tumor from the mother (metastasis) and the prenatal diagnosis of fetal brain tumor. Pollack and co-workers[52] have reported a metastasis of an intracerebral medulloblastoma to the products of conception (placenta). Spread from the mother to the fetus has not gone unreported; Rothman and colleagues[53] reported 36 cases of cancer spreading to products of conception. But metastasis of gliomas outside of the central nervous system is rare. Finding a way to the uterus would be even rarer; crossing of the placental membrane would be extraordinary. For astrocytomas and oligodendrogliomas this risk is virtually nil. Of the cases reported by Rothman and associates,[53] the 11 instances of fetal involvement were all with lymphoproliferative tumors, and none with glial tumors.

REFERENCES

1. Bickerstaff ER, Small JM, Guest IA: The relapsing course of certain meningiomas in relation to pregnancy and menstruation. J Neurol Neurosurg Psychiatry 1958; 21:89–91.
2. McClure Brown JC, Dixon G: Browne's Antenatal Care, ed 11. Edinburgh, Churchill Livingstone, 1978.
3. Simon RH: Brain tumors in pregnancy. *In* Donaldson JO (ed): Seminars in Neurology. New York, Thieme, 1988, pp 214–221.
4. Brown JS, Crombleholme WR: Handbook of Gynecology and Obstetrics. Norwalk, Conn, Appleton-Lange, 1993.
5. Kornblum JA, Bay JW, Gupta MK: Steroid receptors in human brain and spinal cord tumors. Neurosurgery 1988; 23:185–188.
6. Whittle IR, Hawkins RA, Miller JD: Sex hormone receptors in intracranial tumours and normal brain. Eur J Surg Oncol 1987; 13:303–307.
7. Sica G, Zibera C, Ranelletti FO, et al: Some differences in steroid receptors between meningeal and neuroepithelial tumors. J Neurosurg Sci 1989; 33:71–75.
8. Paoletti P, Butti G, Zibera C, et al: Characteristics and biological role of steroid hormone receptors in neuroepithelial tumors. J Neurosurg 1990; 73:736–742.
9. Donegan WL: Cancer and pregnancy. CA Cancer J Clin 1983; 33:194–214.
10. Gleicher N, Deppe G, Cohen CJ: Common aspects of immunologic tolerance in pregnancy and malignancy. Obstet Gynecol 1979; 54:335–342.

11. Mills GB: Immunology of cancer and pregnancy. *In* Allen HH, Nisker JA (eds): Cancer in Pregnancy: Therapeutic Guidelines. New York, Futura, 1986.

12. Michelsen JJ, New PFJ: Brain tumour and pregnancy. J Neurol Neurosurg Psychiatry 1969; 32:305–307.

13. Roelvink FCA, Kamphorst W, van Alphen AM, et al: Pregnancy-related primary brain and spinal tumors. Arch Neurol 1987; 44:209–215.

14. Depret-Mosser S, Jomin M, Monnier JC, et al: Tumeurs cérébrales et grossesse. J Gynecol Obstet Biol Reprod 1993; 22:71–80.

15. Schoenberg BS: Epidemiology of primary nervous system neoplasms. *In* Schoenberg BS (ed): Neurological Epidemiology: Principles and Clinical Applications. New York, Raven Press, 1978.

16. National Data Book and Guide to Services: Statistical Abstract of the United States. Washington, DC, US Dept. of Commerce, Bureau of the Census, 1993.

17. Zulch KJ, Christensen E: Pathologische Anatomie der Raumbeengenden Intrakraniellen Prozesse. Berlin, Springer-Verlag, 1956.

18. Haas JF, Jänisch W, Staneczek W: Newly diagnosed primary intracranial neoplasms in pregnant women: A population-based assessment. J Neurol Neurosurg Psychiatry 1986; 49:874–880.

19. Shin YK, Chapman CC, Lees DE: Postpartum transient blindness probably related to undiagnosed brain tumor. Southern Med J 1992; 85:760–761.

20. Topliss DJ: Optic-nerve glioma and pregnancy. Med J Aust 1989; 150:287.

21. Ershov VN, Okladnikov GI, Komissarov GM: Delivery in the presence of a brain tumor. Zh Vopr Neirokhir Im N N Burdenko 1987; 1:54–55.

22. Cook HE: Cesarean section in a patient with brain tumor: A clinical report. Mil Med 1989; 154:330–331.

23. Gauna NM, Garcallo Lopez MC, Castells Armenter MV, et al: Anestesia para cirugia de un tumor cerebral durante el embarazo: A propósito de un caso. Rev Esp Anestesiol Reanim 1990; 37:291–293.

24. Kempers RD, Miller RH: Management of pregnancy associated with brain tumors. Am J Obstet Gynecol 1963; 87:858–864.

25. Soutoul JH, Gallier J, Gouazé A, et al: La neuro-chirurgie pendant la grossesse: Problèmes posés par les explorations, les médications et l'anesthésie-réanimation. J Gynecol Obstet Biol Reprod 1972; 1:33–46.

26. Gallier J, Santini JJ, Soutoul JH, et al: Tumeurs cérébrales et grossesses. Semin Hop Paris 1971; 47:2040–2050.

27. Bray RS, Lynch R, Grossman RG, et al: Management of neurosurgical problems in pregnancy. Clin Perinatol 1987; 14:243–257.

28. Tarnow G: Brain tumor and pregnancy. Zentralbl Neurochir 1960; 20:134–158.

29. Briggs GG, Freeman RK, Yaffe SJ: Drugs in Pregnancy and Lactation: A Reference Guide to Fetal and Neonatal Risk, ed 4. Baltimore, Williams & Wilkins, 1994.

30. Ogilvy-Stuart AL, Shalet SM: Effect of radiation on the human reproductive system. Environ Health Perspect Suppl 1993; 101(suppl 2):109–116.

31. Mulvihill JJ: Sentinel and other mutational effects in offspring of cancer survivors. *In* Mendelsohn ML, Albertini RJ (eds): Mutation and the Environment: Part C: Somatic and Heritable Mutation, Adduction, and Epidemiology, volume 340C. New York, Wiley-Liss, 1990, pp 179–186.

32. Rosen MA: Anesthesia for neurosurgery during pregnancy. *In* Shnider SM, Levinson G (eds): Anesthesia for Obstetrics, ed 3. Baltimore, Williams and Wilkins, 1993.

33. Nicholson HO: Cytotoxic drugs in pregnancy. Br J Obset Gynaecol 1968; 75:307–312.

34. Zemlickis D, Lishner M, Degendorfer P, et al: Fetal outcome after in utero exposure to cancer chemotherapy. Arch Intern Med 1992; 152:573–576.

35. Sutcliffe SB: Treatment of neoplastic disease during pregnancy: Maternal and fetal effects. Clin Invest Med 1985; 8:333–338.

36. Doll DC, Ringenberg QS, Yuarbro JW: Management of cancer during pregnancy. Arch Intern Med 1988; 148:2058–2064.

37. Avilés A, Díaz-Maqueo JC, Talavera A, et al: Growth and development of children of mothers treated with chemotherapy during pregnancy: Current status of 43 children. Am J Hematol 1991; 36:243–248.

38. Mulvihill JJ, McKeen EA, Rosner F, et al: Pregnancy outcome in cancer patients. Cancer 1987; 60:1143–1150.

39. Pajor A, Zimonyi I, Koos R, et al: Pregnancies and offspring in survivors of acute lymphoid leukemia and lymphoma. Eur J Obstet Gynecol Reprod Biol 1991; 40:1–5.

40. Milliken S, Powles R, Parikh P, et al: Case report: Successful pregnancy following bone marrow transplantation for leukaemia. Bone Marrow Transplant 1990; 5:135–137.

41. Jacobs C, Donaldson SS, Rosenberg SA, et al: Management of the pregnant patient with Hodgkin's disease. Ann Intern Med 1981; 95:669–675.

42. Woo SY, Fuller LM, Cundiff JH, et al: Radiotherapy during pregnancy for clinical stages IA–IIA Hodgkin's disease. Int J Radiat Oncol Biol Phys 1992; 23:407–412.

43. Cox PH, Klijn JGM, Pillay M, et al: Case report—Uterine radiation dose from open sources: The potential for underestimation. Eur J Nucl Med 1990; 17:94–95.

44. Shepard TH: Catalog of Teratogenic Agents, ed 6. Baltimore, The Johns Hopkins University Press, 1989.

45. Delgado-Escueta AV, Janz D: Consensus guidelines: Preconception counseling, management, and care of the pregnant woman with epilepsy. Neurology 1992; 42(suppl 5):149–160.

46. Dansky LV, Rosenblatt DS, Andermann E: Mechanisms of teratogenesis: Folic acid and antiepileptic therapy. Neurology 1992; 42(suppl 5):32–42.

47. Lindhout D, Omtzigt JGC, Cornel MC: Spectrum of neural-tube defects in 34 infants prenatally exposed to antiepileptic drugs. Neurology 1992; 42(suppl 5):111–118.

48. Gaily E, Granström ML: Minor anomalies in children of mothers with epilepsy. Neurology 1992; 42(suppl 5):128–131.

49. Cherry SH, Merkatz IR (eds): Complications of pregnancy: Medical, surgical, gynecologic, psychosocial, and perinatal. Baltimore, Williams & Wilkins, 1991.

50. Finfer SR: Management of labour and delivery in patients with intracranial neoplasms. Br J Anaesth 1991; 67:784–787.

51. Goroszeniuk T, Howard RS, Wright JT: The management of labour using continuous lumbar epidural analgesia in a patient with a malignant cerebral tumour. Anaesthesia 1986; 41:1128–1129.

52. Pollack RN, Pollak M, Rochon L: Pregnancy complicated by medulloblastoma with metastases to the placenta. Obstet Gynecol 1993; 81:858–859.

53. Rothman LA, Cohen CJ, Astarloa J: Placental and fetal involvement by maternal malignancy: A report of rectal carcinoma and review of the literature. Am J Obstet Gynecol 1973; 116:1023–1034.

54. Potter JF, Schoeneman M: Metastasis of maternal cancer to the placenta and fetus. Cancer 1970; 25:380–388.

FRED G. BARKER II

STEPHEN L. HUHN

MICHAEL D. PRADOS

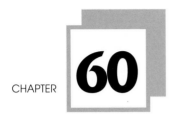

CHAPTER **60**

Clinical Characteristics of Long-Term Glioma Survivors*

Before the clinical characteristics of long-term survivors of glioma can be discussed, the concept of "long-term survival" must first be considered. Long-term survival has a different meaning for each tumor type: patients are much less likely to live 3 years after diagnosis if their tumor is a glioblastoma multiforme than if it is a pilocytic astrocytoma. We will consider prognostic factors separately for each histologic type of tumor.

Examination of the literature shows, however, that even when a histologically homogeneous group is defined, "long-term survival" means something different to different authors. For "malignant gliomas," for example, this may range from 2 years[1,2] to 10 years.[3] Other groups have used multivariate survival analysis to define prognostic factors. In Cox proportional hazards models, it is assumed that the presence or absence of a given prognostic factor has an effect on the chance of mortality that remains constant over time. However, there is no a priori reason to believe that this is true for all types of glioma or for all prognostic factors or clinical situations within a given type of glioma. Factors that predict 2-year survival may not influence median survival, and vice versa. An effect of this type has been postulated for adjuvant chemotherapy in glioblastoma.[4] This type of prognostic factor may be detected more efficiently by studies that compare the presence or absence of a suggested prognostic factor in a certain cohort (e.g., 5-year glioblastoma multiforme survivors) to the overall frequency in a population of patients with a specific type of glioma. We describe both types of prognostic factors in this chapter, and on the basis of our review, we have tabulated those that we consider the most reliable for each tumor type.

When discussing long-term survival with patients it is best to specify what is meant by "long-term." A clinician may think of 5-year survival as "long-term" when talking with a glioblastoma multiforme patient, but a 30-year-old patient will naturally see this as quite short when compared with the lifespan that had previously been expected. The patient will want to know the chances of being cured. What little is known about these chances is also reviewed in this chapter.

GLIOBLASTOMA MULTIFORME

The principal characteristic of long-term survivors of glioblastoma multiforme is their rarity. Harvey Cushing had no 5-year glioblastoma multiforme survivors in his 30-year career.[5,6] In a national survey of glioblastoma multiforme patients diagnosed in 1980, only 5.5% survived 5 years.[7] This proportion is similar to that seen in the University of California, San Francisco (UCSF) series,[8] but the rate in some population-based series has been lower: less than 4% in Georgia, 1977–1981,[9] and zero in the Stockholm region, 1958–1977.[10] To the patient with newly diagnosed glioblastoma multiforme, however, these unusual cases assume a particular importance: each patient with glioblastoma multiforme wants to join the ranks of long-term survivors. A great deal has been learned in recent years that allows the clinician to approximate the chances of a relatively favorable outcome for an individual patient (Table 60–1).

Age and Other Demographic Variables

Age at diagnosis has consistently been found to be an important prognostic factor, both in multivariate analyses of

TABLE 60–1
FAVORABLE PROGNOSTIC FACTORS IN GLIOBLASTOMA MULTIFORME

Younger age
Longer preoperative duration of symptoms
Higher Karnofsky Performance Status score
Extensive surgical resection
Use of postoperative radiation therapy
Use of adjuvant chemotherapy (probable)

*Supported in part by National Cancer Institute Grant 13525 and National Institutes of Health Training Grant CA09291 (Drs. Barker and Huhn).

large series,[11–19] and in specific studies of long-term survivors.[2, 3, 8, 20–22] Age is inversely correlated with survival, and its effect on prognosis is so strong that a series that fails to confirm it is "probably suspect in terms of its design or its analysis."[23]

Long-term survivors of glioblastoma multiforme are typically younger than 40 years at diagnosis. In the UCSF cohort of 22 5-year survivors of glioblastoma multiforme, the median age was 39.2 years (range, 15 to 63 years).[8] In Salcman and co-workers' group of 58 malignant glioma patients surviving more than 3 years, 66% were younger than 40 years at diagnosis.[21] The median age for nine 2-year glioblastoma multiforme survivors was 34 years in a series reported by Phuphanich and others.[2]

The importance of younger age in predicting longer survival is not limited to the relatively small group of long-term survivors; it is apparent in Cox proportional hazards models as well. In 645 patients with glioblastoma multiforme from three pooled Radiation Therapy Oncology Group (RTOG) trials, 66% of patients aged 14 to 39 years survived 1 year, compared with 43% of patients aged 40 to 59 years and just 25% of patients aged 60 to 74 years.[18] Age was the most significant prognostic factor in a multivariate analysis. In another series, patients aged 18 to 44 years survived more than twice as long as those aged 45 to 55 years, and more than three times longer than those older than 55 years.[24] The Brain Tumor Study Group (BTSG) reached similar conclusions in its prospective trials,[11, 25] as have many other groups.[14, 15, 17, 26, 27]

The sex of the patient has not been found to influence survival. Men constituted 45% of 5-year glioblastoma multiforme survivors in the UCSF series[8] and 52% of 3-year malignant glioma survivors in the series by Salcman and colleagues.[21] Neither the BTSG,[11] the Medical Research Council (MRC) Brain Tumour Working Party,[17] nor the European Organization for Research on Treatment of Cancer[28] found any influence of sex on survival in patients with glioblastoma multiforme.

The possible effect of race on survival in glioblastoma multiforme has not been studied extensively. McLendon and associates[9] found no difference in survival between white and black glioblastoma multiforme patients in a population-based study. Other large studies have not addressed this question.

Symptoms and Signs at Time of Diagnosis

Roth and Elvidge[29] noted in 1960 that glioblastoma multiforme patients who survived longer than 18 months were more likely to have presented with seizures and less likely to have been confused or obtunded than shorter-lived patients. Early prospective studies conducted by the BTSG confirmed these impressions: seizures or symptoms related to cranial nerves II, III, IV, or VI predicted longer survival in univariate models.[25, 30] The favorable import of seizures as a first symptom has been noted repeatedly in univariate models.[19, 31, 32] However, in multivariate models that include Karnofsky Performance Status (KPS), the presence of seizures has not been significant. One exception is the analysis

conducted by the MRC Brain Tumour Working Party,[17] which stratified patients by duration of history of seizures. This variable remained significant after adjustment for age, performance status, and extent of surgery.

Duration of preoperative symptoms, as well as their nature, has been examined for prognostic importance. This was noted for seizures by Roth and Elvidge[29] and by the MRC,[17] and for all symptoms by the BTSG.[30] Several other groups have found duration of symptoms to be a valid prognostic factor in multivariate analyses.[19, 31, 32] Reports of cohorts of long-term glioblastoma multiforme survivors have not addressed the nature or duration of symptoms before diagnosis.

Laterality, Location, and Preoperative Size of Tumor

It is plausible to suppose that some factors related to the tumor itself, such as location, laterality, or size, might be of prognostic importance, but, surprisingly, this has not been demonstrated.

Laterality of the tumor (right vs. left hemisphere) made no difference in survival in several BTSG studies, even after adjustment for the handedness of the patient.[11] Of 35 long-term glioblastoma multiforme survivors in two series,[8, 22] 37% had tumors in the left hemisphere.

Tumor location as a prognostic factor has been more controversial. One BTSG study[25] found parietal location to be unfavorable. The RTOG,[18] in three pooled studies, found that patients with frontal lobe tumors survived longer, but this factor was less significant than age, KPS, and extent of surgery. Another study also suggested a relatively favorable prognosis for patients with frontal lobe tumors.[33] Glioblastomas multiforme in the thalamus, brainstem, and cerebellum have a worse prognosis than tumors in the cerebral hemispheres.[29, 34, 35] Fortunately, lesions in these locations are quite rare.

Preoperative tumor size has not been found to be of prognostic importance in large prospective trials. Reeves and Marks[36] reported in 1979 that tumor size (measured by computed tomography [CT] as the area of the enhancing lesion and surrounding hypodensity) failed to predict survival in a cohort of 56 patients with glioblastoma multiforme. This counterintuitive conclusion has been confirmed by other groups using CT or magnetic resonance imaging (MRI)-based estimates of preoperative tumor size. The pooled RTOG trials[18] of 645 patients found a very slight survival advantage for smaller tumors at 1 year after diagnosis, which was not statistically significant. The Brain Tumor Cooperative Group,[37] in a trial with 510 patients, found no survival difference at all between patients with large and small tumors.

These findings are relevant in assessing the efficacy of stereotactic radiation therapy methods, such as brachytherapy and radiosurgery, because these methods are currently only suitable for smaller tumors. Curran and co-workers[38] attempted to quantify the difference in survival between patients who were or were not eligible for radiosurgery in a large RTOG trial. Only patients whose preoperative tumor size was less than 4 cm and whose KPS was 70 or higher were considered eligible. A few patients were excluded because of their tumor's proximity to vital structures. Although there was a significant survival advantage in eligible patients (median survival 14.4 months vs. 11.7 months for ineligible patients), it was attributed predominantly to the difference in KPS. After adjustment for this factor, no significant survival advantage was noted for patients with smaller tumors. Florell and colleagues[39] found a significantly improved prognosis for glioblastoma multiforme patients judged suitable for interstitial brachytherapy. One criterion for eligibility was tumor size (less than 6 cm), but whether size was measured on preoperative or postoperative CT scans was unclear. Imbalances in known prognostic factors were also substantial between brachytherapy-eligible and -ineligible patients; eligible patients were younger, had a higher KPS, and had more complete surgical resections. For these reasons, this study cannot be interpreted as evidence for better prognosis with smaller preoperative tumor size.

Although some reports of cohorts of long-term glioblastoma multiforme survivors have specified tumor location,[8, 22, 23] none has explicitly made comparisons with short-term survivors. No large series of long-term glioblastoma multiforme survivors has included information on preoperative tumor size, with the exception of one report of 19 "malignant glioma" patients who survived more than 700 days.[40] No significant difference in preoperative tumor sizes was found between short- and long-term survivors.

KPS and Related Measures

The KPS,[41] or a similar measure of patient condition, has consistently been found to be an important prognostic indicator, usually second in importance only to age. This effect was noted in early BTSG trials[31, 32, 42] and has been confirmed many times by different groups.[13, 18, 19, 43–46] Although the KPS has been the most widely studied, similar scales have been found to predict survival, such as the Eastern Cooperative Oncology Group performance score[47] and the World Health Organization performance status.[17, 48] A typical estimate of the magnitude of this effect has been provided by the RTOG: 1-year survival was 47% for patients with a KPS of 80 to 100 and 30% for patients with a KPS less than 80.[18] Cohort studies of long-term glioblastoma multiforme survivors have reached similar conclusions.

Extent of Surgical Resection and Postoperative Tumor Size

Extent of surgery as a prognostic factor in gliomas is treated elsewhere in this volume. Controversy has arisen over the suggestion that extensive resection improves prognosis in glioblastoma multiforme.[49–52] Substantial evidence, however, does suggest that patients who have undergone more extensive removal of glioblastoma multiforme survive significantly longer than those who have not. This is true even after adjustment for other prognostically important variables, such as age, KPS, and tumor location. The RTOG[18] found that extent of surgical resection was the third most important prognostic factor in survival, after age and KPS. This result,

based on a relatively large patient group, confirmed similar results in multiple prior studies, all of which used multivariate analysis.[12, 13, 17, 19, 46, 47] An analysis of the UCSF/Northern California Oncology Group (NCOG) series also reached the same conclusion (Barker FG, Prados MD: Unpublished data, June 1994).

Other groups have addressed the same question by measuring postoperative tumor burden on CT scans[37, 40, 53] or MRI.[54, 55] Multivariate analyses[37, 54] demonstrated a significant survival advantage for patients with small postoperative tumor burdens.

Given this strong evidence, it seems that extensive tumor resection would be beneficial if it could be performed without a deleterious effect on the patient's KPS. Three groups have demonstrated that contemporary neurosurgical methods (and judgment) result in no greater morbidity in glioblastoma multiforme patients chosen for extensive resections.[27, 53, 56] Ammirati and others[53] found that postoperative KPS was improved in patients who underwent gross total resection, but not in those who underwent partial resections. Vecht and colleagues[27] has similar results.

Cohort studies of long-term glioblastoma multiforme survivors underscore the prognostic importance of extensive initial surgical resection. Only 2 of 13 long-term glioblastoma multiforme survivors in the series of Vertosick and Selker[22] and none of 22 in the UCSF series[8] had undergone biopsy only.

Radiation Therapy

Since the publication of two randomized trials conducted by the BTSG that established the therapeutic value of external beam radiation therapy in glioblastoma multiforme,[32, 42] nearly all patients have received external beam radiation therapy as the initial portion of the treatment. Thus, all of the long-term survivors in the series of Salcman,[23] Vertosick and Selker,[22] Phuphanich and co-workers,[2] and the UCSF series[8] had undergone external beam radiation therapy.

Many groups have attempted to augment the results of external beam treatment by administering a tightly focused radiation "boost," either by interstitial brachytherapy or with stereotactic radiosurgery. As discussed earlier, patients who meet the eligibility requirements for these treatments have an *ab initio* survival advantage over non-eligible patients.[38, 39] However, these treatments appear to be beneficial even after adjustment is made for this bias. Median survival for glioblastoma multiforme patients treated with interstitial brachytherapy at UCSF was 87 weeks,[57] considerably longer than the median of 60 weeks in comparable patients from another institution who were eligible for, but did not undergo, brachytherapy.[39] Wen and co-workers[58] found that the 34% 2-year survival rate for glioblastoma multiforme patients treated with brachytherapy after initial radiation was significantly higher than the 13% rate for a brachytherapy-eligible historic control group. A similar advantage is seen when patients treated with a radiosurgical boost for glioblastoma multiforme[59, 60] are compared with a group of glioblastoma multiforme patients from an RTOG study who were radiosurgery-eligible but did not undergo radiosurgery.[38]

Cohorts of long-term glioblastoma multiforme survivors include some patients treated with interstitial brachytherapy as a boost after initial radiation treatment,[8, 22, 23] but these reports do not specify the proportion of patients treated with brachytherapy in their overall glioblastoma multiforme population. Consequently, these reports cannot be cited as evidence that brachytherapy promotes long-term survival.

Chemotherapy

Although many randomized trials have been performed in an attempt to gauge the effects of adjuvant chemotherapy for malignant glioma,[61] most grouped anaplastic astrocytomas together with glioblastomas multiforme in reporting the results. This makes evaluating the results of these trials difficult, because a chemotherapy regimen might not be equally beneficial for both glioblastoma multiforme and anaplastic astrocytoma.

A meta-analysis of the results of 16 randomized trials that tested adjuvant chemotherapy for malignant gliomas reported a survival advantage for chemotherapy, although in glioblastoma multiforme patients the maximum advantage was not seen until 18 to 24 months after diagnosis.[4] The benefit after 6 or 12 months was considerably smaller. Younger patients seemed to have a larger treatment effect than older ones, although this part of the meta-analysis was highly indirect.[4]

Cohort studies of long-term survivors of glioblastoma multiforme generally note that the great majority were treated with adjuvant chemotherapy.[2, 8, 21, 22] However, explicit comparison with the proportion of short-term survivors was only made by Salcman and others,[21] who grouped anaplastic astrocytomas together with glioblastomas multiforme and did not perform a multivariate analysis. Chemotherapy with nitrosoureas was the least statistically significant variable in their univariate analysis, after age, repeated surgery, radiation therapy, and tumor histology.

Interaction Between Prognostic Variables

Prognostic variables in glioblastoma multiforme have complex and important interactions, but these have not been studied extensively. For example, tumor location clearly affects the likelihood of achieving an extensive surgical resection. Younger age and greater extent of resection are associated with higher postoperative KPS values. Other variables are less likely to have a significant association: age and extent of resection do not appear to be directly correlated. For these reasons, a given variable should not be accepted as a valid prognostic indicator in glioblastoma multiforme unless it maintains its significance in a multivariate analysis that includes, as a minimum, age, KPS, and extent of surgical resection.

Cure of Glioblastoma

Although nearly all patients with glioblastoma multiforme will die as a direct result of their tumors, the question whether the disease can ever be cured sometimes will arise. For example, when an apparently fit patient with no signs of recurrence after 5 years of treatment asks whether she or he is cured, what should the clinician's answer be?

Remarkably few data are available to help answer this question. Data from the UCSF series suggest that patients who survive 5 years after diagnosis of glioblastoma multiforme with no sign of recurrence have a nearly 90% chance of living another 5 years,[8] although this conclusion is based on a small number of patients. Anecdotal reports[62] indicate that, in a lucky few, glioblastoma multiforme may be cured. Unfortunately, when the original pathology specimens on such patients are reviewed, the original diagnosis is often found to be in error.[3, 10] Our own practice in managing such patients is to recommend a clinical evaluation and an MRI every year until 10 years after diagnosis, and every 2 years thereafter.

ANAPLASTIC ASTROCYTOMA

Less is known about prognostic factor for patients with anaplastic astrocytoma than for those with glioblastoma multiforme. To some degree this is because of the tumor's relative rarity; only 12% of 1440 cases in three pooled BTSG malignant glioma trials were anaplastic astrocytomas.[63] In addition, patients with anaplastic astrocytomas were simply included along with glioblastoma multiforme patients under the rubric "malignant glioma" in many of the early trials of the RTOG,[24, 64, 65] the BTSG,[31, 46, 66] and the NCOG,[67] often without separate analysis of prognostic factors for the anaplastic astrocytoma group. In some trials, tumors analyzed as "anaplastic astrocytomas" included anaplastic oligodendrogliomas, anaplastic ependymomas, and other tumors.[46] Analyses have pooled patients from these earlier studies[63, 67–71] or from separate cohorts of anaplastic astrocytoma patients[72, 73] in an attempt to define prognostic factors for anaplastic astrocytoma.

Some anaplastic astrocytoma patients have been reported as "long-term survivors," but their tumors were always grouped with those of glioblastoma multiforme patients as "malignant gliomas." As with glioblastoma multiforme, "long-term" has been applied in published series to patients who have survived from 2 years[2] to 10 years,[3] but because the median survival is about 3 years for anaplastic astrocytoma patients,[67, 71] and only 1 year for glioblastoma multiforme patients, these milestones have a different meaning. About one-third of anaplastic astrocytoma patients will live 5 years.[67, 68] Our discussion of prognostic factors in anaplastic astrocytoma will emphasize factors found to be significant in Cox proportional hazards models. Favorable prognostic factors are listed in Table 60–2.

Age

Age is a prognostic factor of undisputed importance in anaplastic astrocytoma, as confirmed by multiple studies.[67–69, 71, 73] The mean age of anaplastic astrocytoma patients in three pooled BTSG trials was 10 years lower than glioblastoma multiforme patients[63]; in the UCSF series, median age was

TABLE 60–2
FAVORABLE PROGNOSTIC FACTORS IN ANAPLASTIC
ASTROCYTOMA

Younger age
Higher Karnofsky Performance Status score
Use of postoperative radiation therapy (probable)
Use of adjuvant chemotherapy (probable)
Location in frontal lobe (probable)

40 years.[67] Although some studies have specified 40 years as the upper age limit for the most favorable prognostic group,[68, 69] in the UCSF series, the risk of mortality at any given time was 2.5 times higher for a 50-year-old (75th age percentile) than for a 33-year-old (25th age percentile). Most multivariate analyses have shown that age remains significant after adjustment for all other known prognostic factors.[67–69, 71]

Duration and Type of Symptoms

Soffietti and co-workers[73] found that absence of a preoperative motor deficit was strongly correlated with longer survival in 102 patients with anaplastic astrocytomas, and that unaltered preoperative level of consciousness was moderately significant. Seizures as a presenting symptom had no prognostic importance. Absence of preoperative motor signs remained significant in the multivariate analysis. In another study, preoperative symptoms for more than 12 months and seizures as sole presenting symptom were favorable indicators, but a multivariate analysis was not performed.[35]

Site and Preoperative Size of Tumor

One study found that tumor location within the frontal lobe and preoperative tumor size less than 5 cm were favorable prognostic indicators for anaplastic astrocytoma patients in a multivariate analysis.[68] A univariate analysis of a cohort of 82 anaplastic astrocytoma patients found the best survival in patients with temporal or frontal lobe tumors.[35]

Karnofsky Performance Status and Related Measures

In the UCSF series,[67] a high postoperative KPS was a highly significant predictor of survival. Other groups have reached similar conclusions.[68, 69, 71, 73] One analysis showed that a second neurologic function classification was even more significant than KPS in predicting survival with anaplastic astrocytoma; both scores were significant in a multivariate analysis.[69]

Extent of Surgery

Several groups have attempted to distinguish the potential benefit of aggressive surgery in anaplastic astrocytoma pa-

tients. The first of three RTOG analyses of anaplastic astrocytoma patients, using data pooled from three prospective trials of malignant glioma, showed that extent of surgery was an important prognostic variable,[71] but a reanalysis of the same data appeared to show that extent of surgery could be replaced by a postoperative neurologic function scale in a multivariate model.[69] The relationship between extensive surgery and postoperative neurologic function was not shown in this study, and the potential importance of tumor location was not addressed. The third RTOG analysis included some of the same patients and concluded that extensive surgery was not a significant predictor of survival.[68] In the UCSF series, extensive surgery was not significantly correlated with longer survival.[67] The relatively small number of patients in these studies and the lack of agreement on the definition of "extensive resection" increase the difficulty of reconciling the disparate conclusions.

Radiation Therapy and Chemotherapy

As discussed earlier, early randomized trials showed longer survival for patients with malignant gliomas treated with radiation therapy.[32, 42] Although no separate analysis of the anaplastic astrocytoma patients participating in these trials has been published, and no prospective randomized trial has ever evaluated the effect of radiation therapy on survival in anaplastic astrocytoma patients, a strong and widely held belief persists that adequate radiation therapy predicts longer survival. Interstitial brachytherapy used after initial radiation therapy did not predict longer survival in the UCSF series.[67]

Randomized trials to evaluate the effect of adjuvant chemotherapy in anaplastic astrocytoma patients are similarly lacking. One study reported a survival advantage in anaplastic astrocytoma patients treated with adjuvant chemotherapy[74] and one did not.[12] A meta-analysis of five trials primarily including patients with anaplastic astrocytoma concluded that a substantial survival benefit was associated with adjuvant chemotherapy.[61] However, no such benefit was found in an analysis of anaplastic astrocytoma patients drawn from three RTOG trials.[69] The use of adjuvant chemotherapy may be a positive prognostic factor in anaplastic astrocytoma, but the published evidence to date remains somewhat inconclusive.

Cure of Anaplastic Astrocytoma

Although more than 20% of anaplastic astrocytoma patients were alive 8 years after diagnosis in the UCSF series,[67] death from tumor and first tumor progression were not uncommon more than 5 years after diagnosis. No large cohort of anaplastic astrocytoma patients followed up for more than 5 years after diagnosis has been reported, and the possibility for cure in anaplastic astrocytoma remains entirely unknown.

ASTROCYTOMA

Only one prospective randomized trial limited to patients with "low-grade" astrocytoma has been published.[75] Nearly

TABLE 60–3
FAVORABLE PROGNOSTIC FACTORS IN ASTROCYTOMA

Younger age
Higher Karnofsky Performance Status score
Lack of contrast enhancement
Lack of gemistocytic histology
Extensive surgical resection (probable)
Use of postoperative radiation therapy after incomplete
resection (probable)

---

all information regarding prognostic factors in this disease is therefore based on retrospective, single-institution series. Because median survival for astrocytoma patients is currently more than 5 years, the concept of ''long-term survival'' is even less clearly defined for astrocytomas than it is for anaplastic astrocytoma. No cohorts of ''long-term'' astrocytoma survivors have been reported.

Gemistocytic astrocytomas and pilocytic astrocytomas are addressed separately; the following discussion applies to ''ordinary'' low-grade astrocytomas. Favorable prognostic factors are summarized in Table 60–3.

Age and Sex

As with glioblastomas multiforme and anaplastic astrocytomas, younger age is generally considered to be an important favorable prognostic factor in astrocytomas. Some authors whose series included both pilocytic and nonpilocytic astrocytomas attributed this favorable effect to the tendency of younger patients to have pilocytic tumors,[76] but a number of large series either excluding pilocytic tumors or containing a very small percentage of them have shown that younger age remains important in predicting longer survival.[75, 77–83] Typical values for 5-year survival with respect to age were given by Medbery and co-workers,[78] who found that 62% of patients younger than 40 years survived for 5 years, compared with only 28% of patients 40 years or older.

The sex of a patient seems unlikely to be important as a prognostic factor. Three studies reported longer survival in women[75, 79, 81] and one reported the opposite.[84] Most authors have found no sex-related difference in survival.[76, 78, 82, 83, 85–87]

Type and Duration of Preoperative Symptoms

Several groups have reported markedly worse survival for patients presenting with decreased level of consciousness or personality change.[76, 79, 87] These patients have constituted only a small minority in most series and may have been principally encountered in the pre-CT era.

The prognostic value of other presenting signs and symptoms is less certain. Patients who present with seizures have had longer survival in a number of series, but no series limited to astrocytoma patients alone has shown this factor to be significant in multivariate analysis.[76, 77, 79, 87] The same can be said of duration of symptoms. One group[87] reported longer survival in patients who presented with focal neuro-

logic deficits; others have found this factor to be a negative indicator[76] or not significant.[77, 80]

Tumor Location, Laterality, and Size

Although one large series reported tumor location in the frontal or temporal lobes as a favorable prognostic indicator in multivariate analysis,[76] it was not statistically significant in several other studies.[79, 80, 86, 87] The side on which the tumor is located has not been reported to have prognostic value.[76, 84, 86, 87] Little attention has been paid to initial tumor size as a prognostic factor. One group[84] found no influence on survival.

Imaging Characteristics: Contrast Enhancement and Cysts

Most astrocytomas do not show enhancement on CT scans or MRI. It has been suggested that astrocytomas that do enhance on preoperative CT scans have a worse prognosis.[77, 80] One study quoted a risk of tumor recurrence 6.8 times higher for patients whose tumors enhanced on CT scans.[77] Other analyses have disputed this conclusion.[81, 86, 88] The presence of a cyst associated with the tumor has sometimes been found to be a favorable indicator in univariate analyses,[76, 80] but not when multivariate analysis is performed. This may be due to confounding with patient age: younger patients are more likely to have cystic tumors.[80]

KPS and Related Measures

A high KPS or other performance measure is a beneficial prognostic factor, whether measured preoperatively[76, 86] or postoperatively.[76, 77, 85, 87] Lack of moderate or severe postoperative neurologic deficit is also favorable.[76]

Treatment-Related Factors: Extent of Surgery, Adjuvant Radiation Therapy, and Chemotherapy

The effects of extensive surgery and adjuvant radiation therapy on prognosis in astrocytoma are very controversial. These much-debated questions are briefly summarized.

It is widely believed that extensive surgical removal results in longer survival for astrocytoma patients. Several large clinical series support this contention,[76, 79, 86, 87] and another found a trend in favor of extensive surgery that was not statistically significant in a multivariate analysis.[82] Other groups have found no significant influence of extensive surgical tumor resection on survival.[75, 78, 80, 81, 83, 84] It is difficult to explain this discordance, unless the sample size necessary to demonstrate the beneficial effect of extensive removal is larger than the typical size of the latter studies. The effectiveness of early surgery, as opposed to a policy of observation, has also been disputed.[89, 90]

Even less agreement exists concerning the benefits of

adjuvant radiation therapy after surgery for astrocytoma. Some retrospective studies specify radiation therapy as a favorable prognostic factor,[81, 84] whereas others do not.[76, 82, 86, 87] It has been suggested that the beneficial effect of radiation therapy on prognosis is limited to older patients.[84, 91]

Adjuvant chemotherapy with lomustine after surgery and radiation therapy failed to improve survival for astrocytoma patients in a randomized trial.[75] No group has reported a favorable influence of adjuvant chemotherapy in this disease.

Cure of Astrocytoma

Laws and colleagues[76] noted in their cohort of 461 astrocytoma patients that by 15 years after diagnosis, the survival curve began to parallel the survival for an age-matched control population. This suggests that at least some patients who survive 15 years after diagnosis of astrocytoma may be cured. It is interesting to note that this phenomenon was not limited to younger patients but extended even to those who were older than 50 years at diagnosis. However, the proportion of patients who reached the 15-year mark varied widely with age at presentation: 15-year survival was about 5% for those older than 50 years, about 10% for those aged 20 to 49 years, and about 70% for those younger than 20 years at time of diagnosis. A substantial fraction of the youngest patients probably had pilocytic tumors, but these figures seem to indicate that in some patients, low-grade astrocytoma is curable with presently available technology. The longest survivor in this series lived 55 years after diagnosis.

GEMISTOCYTIC ASTROCYTOMA

The gemistocytic variant of astrocytoma is uncommon. Westergaard and co-workers[82] found that the incidence of gemistocytic tumors increased linearly with age among a cohort of 218 adults with nonpilocytic astrocytomas. No gemistocytic tumors were seen in patients younger than 20 years, but in the oldest patients (older than 60 years) the proportion rose to 40%. In the UCSF series, patients with the highest proportion of gemistocytes were older than patients with ''mixed'' gemistocytic tumors (49 vs. 38 years).[92] This age distribution may account for the relatively short survival of patients with gemistocytic tumors. In the UCSF series, median survival was less than 3 years.[92] In univariate analyses, younger age, longer duration of preoperative symptoms, seizures as a presenting symptom, and greater extent of resection were favorable prognostic indicators. Other groups have noted a trend toward shorter survival in astrocytoma patients with gemistocytic tumors[84] or found that shorter survival was attributable to older age in these patients.[82]

PILOCYTIC ASTROCYTOMA

Patients with pilocytic astrocytomas have an excellent chance for long-term survival if surgical resection is complete. Favorable prognostic factors are listed in Table 60–4. Because the likelihood of a complete resection varies consid-

TABLE 60–4
FAVORABLE PROGNOSTIC FACTORS IN PILOCYTIC ASTROCYTOMA

Extensive surgical resection
Use of postoperative radiation therapy after incomplete resection (optic chiasm, hypothalamus)

erably based on the location of the tumor, each location is discussed separately.

Cerebellar Tumors

Most astrocytomas of the cerebellum are pilocytic.[93] By 1930, Cushing had already discerned the predilection of these tumors for the cerebellum, the typically young age of the patients, and the favorable prognosis if a complete removal of the tumor could be achieved.[94]

Modern series confirm Cushing's prescient conclusions. In one group of 105 patients with cerebellar pilocytic astrocytomas, some survived 29 years; 83 patients were alive after a median of 16 years of follow-up.[93] Favorable prognostic factors were gross total surgical removal, good neurologic function at diagnosis, and presence of microcysts on microscopic examination. Presence of microcysts and lack of altered consciousness were favorable indicators in another series.[95] Gjerris and Klinken[96] found that 94% of their patients with cerebellar pilocytic astrocytomas survived 25 years. In the UCSF series, no patient thought to have had a complete surgical resection had a tumor recurrence.[97] The remarkable effectiveness of total surgical removal,[98, 99] combined with the high proportion of cases in which this is achieved, has prevented most groups from identifying any other prognostic factor. When the tumor infiltrates the brainstem, complete removal may not be possible,[96, 99] accounting for the less favorable prognosis in these cases.

Pilocytic Astrocytomas of the Optic Nerve, Chiasm, and Hypothalamus

Complete removal is less often achieved for pilocytic astrocytomas in these locations. In an extensive review, Alvord and Lofton[100] noted that patients whose optic nerve tumors were completely excised had an excellent prognosis: 80% were free from tumor recurrence 20 years after diagnosis. Tumors situated less favorably for surgical removal had much higher recurrence rates. Radiation therapy seemed to extend survival, particularly if the dose exceeded 45 Gy.[100] Other groups have reported 10-year survival rates of 90% to 100% in patients treated with adequate doses of radiation.[101–103] Age was a prognostic indicator in the review by Alvord and Lofton; rapid tumor recurrence and death were noted in adult patients.[100] A diagnosis of neurofibromatosis had no clear effect on prognosis.

Pilocytic Astrocytomas of the Cerebral Hemispheres

These uncommon tumors of children and young adults have been the subject of several reports,[104–108] all of which indicate that gross total excisions are correlated with an excellent long-term prognosis. For incompletely excised tumors, radiation therapy has been assumed to improve survival, but proof is lacking.

Late Recurrence and Cure of Pilocytic Astrocytomas

Although many patients with pilocytic astrocytomas survive long term, recurrences have been documented up to 52 years after initial diagnosis.[109–114] These rare events are usually reported to follow subtotal resections with postoperative irradiation of the residual tumor, but exceptions occur. One cerebellar pilocytic astrocytoma recurred 36 years after an apparent gross total resection.[112] Some recurrences are histologically malignant.[109–111, 113] Although it has been suggested that malignant transformation of pilocytic astrocytomas is correlated with postoperative irradiation of residual tumor,[111, 113] this remains unproven. These rare events notwithstanding, the majority of patients who undergo a complete resection of a pilocytic astrocytoma, at least in the cerebellar or cerebral hemispheres, are cured.

SUBEPENDYMAL GIANT CELL ASTROCYTOMA

Little is know concerning long-term survival in patients with this rare tumor. The true subependymal giant cell astrocytoma has been said to occur only in patients with tuberous sclerosis and to have a 15-year survival of about 80%.[115] Those who died were older at diagnosis than those who survived, but not all deaths were due to tumor progression. No other prognostic factors were identified. Histologic features such as necrosis or mitoses are sometimes seen in this tumor, but they seem to lack prognostic significance.[115, 116]

PLEOMORPHIC XANTHOASTROCYTOMA

Pleomorphic xanthoastrocytoma is a very uncommon astroglial tumor first described in 1979.[117] The prognosis is considered to be relatively favorable; the majority of published cases have reported good long-term outcome.[118] A literature review of 71 reported cases found that 76% of patients were alive 10 years after the onset of symptoms.[119] Exceptions were noted, however, particularly when anaplastic histologic features were present.[119] Because of the small number of patients with sufficient follow-up, potential prognostic factors such as extensive surgical resection or use of radiation therapy cannot be identified from the literature.

OLIGODENDROGLIOMA AND OLIGOASTROCYTOMA

Oligodendrogliomas are rare tumors with a relatively slow rate of growth and a good chance for long-term postoperative

TABLE 60–5

FAVORABLE PROGNOSTIC FACTORS IN OLIGODENDROGLIOMA

Younger age
Higher Karnofsky Performance Status score
Non-anaplastic histology
Extensive surgical resection
Use of postoperative radiation therapy after incomplete resection (probable)

survival, as was first recognized by Bailey and Bucy[120] in an analysis of Cushing's surgical series. One of Cushing's patients was alive and well 36 years after operation.[121] Modern series report median survivals of about 7 years.[122–125]

Most retrospective single-institution studies have been too small to identify many prognostic factors. Many studies have included anaplastic oligodendrogliomas and mixed oligoastrocytomas as well as pure oligodendrogliomas. Favorable prognostic factors are listed in Table 60–5.

Histology

Several grading systems for oligodendrogliomas have prognostic value, including the systems of Kernohan,[123] Smith,[31, 126, 127] and the St. Anne-Mayo system.[123, 128] Patients with anaplastic tumors have a significantly shorter survival when graded by any of these systems. Other authors reached the same conclusions using institution-specific criteria of histologic malignancy.[122, 124, 129–131] The prognosis for mixed oligoastrocytomas is roughly similar to that for anaplastic tumors.[124, 125, 132, 133]

Age, Sex, and Race

Young age is a statistically significant favorable prognostic indicator in some series,[122–124, 126] and others show a similar trend.[129, 134] Younger patients were also likely to have lower-grade tumors.[123, 126, 127] Sex of the patient has not been found to be prognostically significant.[122–124, 129, 131, 134] The significance of race is inconclusive. One study showed that black patients had significantly shorter survival than white patients,[29] but this conclusion was based on a small number of nonwhite patients. Another study found no survival difference by race in a univariate analysis.[124]

Presenting Symptoms and Signs

Oligodendroglioma patients typically present with long preoperative histories of seizures. Hemiparesis[129] and cognitive impairment[129, 131] have been reported as unfavorable prognostic signs. Other groups found no influence of presenting symptoms on prognosis.[122, 123]

Location and Size

Two series found frontal or parietal location to be favorable indicators,[123, 126] but this was not confirmed in several other studies.[122, 124, 134] The size of the tumor and the side on which it is located have not been found to be significant.[123]

Imaging Characteristics

Contrast enhancement of the tumor on a preoperative CT scan has been reported to be an unfavorable prognostic indicator.[123] Tumor calcification has been reported as a favorable[123, 124, 134] or neutral[131] factor, and may be more frequent in lower-grade tumors.[124]

Karnofsky Performance Status and Related Measures

Although KPS was not found to be prognostically important in one study,[11] others found that performance measures did predict survival.[130, 134]

Treatment: Surgery, Radiation Therapy, and Chemotherapy

Extensive surgical resection has been reported as a statistically significant beneficial prognostic factor by some groups[32, 123, 130] but not by others.[131] Radiation therapy provided a statistically significant survival benefit in one series[123]; most other studies reported favorable trends that were not statistically significant.[122, 125, 130, 131] Two groups who stratified their analyses of radiation therapy by extent of resection found that the benefit was limited to patients who had not undergone gross total resections.[124, 130] No study has reported any survival advantage for adjuvant chemotherapy, even though some oligodendrogliomas are quite chemosensitive.[135–137]

Mixed Oligoastrocytomas

These uncommon tumors have been studied little. Shaw and co-workers[132, 138] reported that they have a prognosis intermediate between the relatively benign oligodendroglioma and the slightly more aggressive astrocytoma. Favorable indicators in a multivariate analysis were low Kernohan grade, gross total resection, use of postoperative focal irradiation, and radiation dose greater than 50 Gy.[132]

EPENDYMOMA

Intracranial ependymomas are uncommon central nervous system tumors, representing about 3% of primary brain neoplasms.[139] Identification of specific prognostic factors is difficult because of the complex interrelationships among age, location, histology, and the impact of surgery and radiation. Published series often include both adults and children and may lack specific analysis by location. Lack of a uniform histologic grading scale and the use of different postoperative radiation strategies further complicate analysis. Al-

TABLE 60–6
FAVORABLE PROGNOSTIC FACTORS IN EPENDYMOMA

Age >2 yr
Single lesion
Infratentorial location
Extensive surgical resection
Use of postoperative radiation therapy after incomplete resection (probable)

though areas of disagreement persist, recent reports, aided by improved neuroimaging data, have begun to establish some important prognostic factors.[140–143] Our list can be found in Table 60–6.

Age

Studies examining age as a prognostic factor have attempted to demonstrate a difference in survival between adults and children. Some investigators report a poorer prognosis with younger age.[139, 144–146] A recent examination of infratentorial ependymomas demonstrated 5-year survival rates of 76% in adults and 14% in children.[143] Other reviews have found no effect of age on survival,[142, 147, 148] whereas still others have suggested that 5-year survival was actually higher in children than in adults.[149] This disparity may be partly due to failure to specify the age range for "children" or to stratify the analysis by tumor location.

Location

Supratentorial ependymomas have a lower 5-year survival rate than infratentorial tumors.[142, 150, 151] One study found progression-free 10-year survival rates of 48% for patients with infratentorial tumors and 0% for patients with supratentorial lesions,[142] although all of the supratentorial tumors in this series were considered anaplastic. Other series have not found location to be a statistically significant predictor of long-term survival.[139, 149, 152] An analysis of survival for different sites within the posterior fossa found that 5-year survival was significantly poorer for patients with lateral tumors than for those with tumors involving the floor of the fourth ventricle.[153] The presence of multiple lesions within the neuraxis carries a significantly worse prognosis.[152]

Histology

The influence of tumor grade on prognosis varies among studies, partly because multiple grading systems are used; little consensus exists on the histologic factors that define a "high-grade" or "anaplastic" ependymoma.[154, 155] Some studies have documented significantly longer survival for patients with low-grade ependymomas,[139, 142, 147–149, 156] whereas others have found no significant difference between high- and low-grade tumors.[143, 145, 152] A multivariate analysis of several histologic signs commonly attributed to the anaplastic variant did not show a significantly shorter survival for "high-grade" tumors.[155] Another study of "malignant" ependymomas showed no correlation between histologic features and postoperative survival.[154] Investigations of the relationship between survival and mitotic index or in situ bromodeoxyuridine labeling index have shown mixed results.[157, 158] In the UCSF series, ependymomas with a labeling index greater than 1.0% tended to recur more quickly.[159] Survival predictions based on histologic grade remain uncertain; these studies suggest little clinical utility of the current grading schemes.

Extent of Surgical Resection

Although some investigators disagree,[142, 149, 151] most studies suggest a favorable effect of complete surgical resection on postoperative survival. One analysis of 93 primary intracranial ependymoma patients over a 36-year period demonstrated better 5- and 10-year survival rates for those with completely resected low-grade ependymomas.[148] An advantage for extensive resection of high-grade tumors, however, was not detected. Another series of 27 patients showed a 5-year survival rate of 60% for those with complete resections, compared with 31% for incomplete resections.[139] A review of posterior fossa ependymomas[143] showed a trend toward better 5-year survival following gross total resection. In another study, when postoperative imaging (rather than the surgeon's report) was used to determine the extent of resection, the 5-year progression-free survival rate was 75% in patients with complete resections, compared with 0% for patients with radiographically visible residual disease.[145] Although disagreement has occurred among findings of some early studies, most recent series support extensive surgical resection as a favorable prognostic variable.

Radiation Therapy

Treatment with radiation improves postoperative survival for ependymoma.[144, 149, 150] However, the impact on survival of focal, whole-brain, and craniospinal-axis irradiation in relation to location, histology, and risk of leptomeningeal dissemination remains moot.[156] In one multivariate analysis of several clinical characteristics, local field irradiation was found to be the most significant independent prognostic factor in progression-free survival.[142] Another study found no difference in outcome between patients treated with involved-field, whole-brain, or craniospinal radiation after adjustment for postoperative tumor volume as documented by imaging studies.[145]

SUBEPENDYMOMA

Symptomatic subependymomas are very rare tumors that have a favorable postoperative prognosis. Some reports found no tumor progression even after subtotal resections.[160, 161] In the largest series (21 patients over a 40-year period), tumor recurrence was more frequent after subtotal resection.[162] The value of postoperative radiation therapy was unclear, although it has been suggested that tumors with a mixed histology (subependymoma plus ependymoma) may benefit from this treatment.[163] No other prognostic factors have been identified.

REFERENCES

1. Lieberman AN, Foo SH, Ransohoff J, et al: Long term survival among patients with malignant brain tumors. Neurosurgery 1982; 10:450.
2. Phuphanich S, Ferrall S, Greenberg H: Long-term survival in malignant glioma: Prognostic factors. J Fla Med Assoc 1993; 80:181.
3. Salford LG, Brun A, Nirfalk S: Ten-year survival among patients with supratentorial astrocytomas grade III and IV. J Neurosurg 1988; 69:506.
4. Fine HA, Dear KBG, Loeffler JS, et al: Meta-analysis of radiation therapy with and without adjuvant chemotherapy for malignant gliomas in adults. Cancer 1993; 71:2585.
5. Eisenhardt L: Long postoperative survivals in cases of intracranial tumor. Assoc Res Nerv Ment Dis 1935; 16:390.
6. German WJ: The gliomas: A follow-up study. Clin Neurosurg 1959; 7:1.
7. Mahaley SJ Jr, Meftlin C, Natarajan N, et al: National survey of patterns of care for brain-tumor patients. J Neurosurg 1989; 71:826.
8. Chandler KL, Prados MD, Malec M, et al: Long-term survival in patients with glioblastoma multiforme. Neurosurgery 1993; 32:716.
9. McLendon RE, Robinson JS Jr, Chambers DB, et al: The glioblastoma multiforme in Georgia, 1977–1981. Cancer 1985; 56:894.
10. Ullén H, Mattsson B, Collins VP: Long-term survival after malignant glioma: A clinical and histopathological study on the accuracy of the diagnosis in a population-based cancer register. Acta Oncol 1990; 29:875.
11. Byar DP, Green SB, Strike TA: Prognostic factors for malignant glioma. *In* Walker MD (ed): Oncology of the Nervous System. Boston, Martinus Nijhoff, 1983, p 379.
12. Chang CH, Horton J, Schoenfeld D, et al: Comparison of postoperative radiotherapy and combined postoperative radiotherapy and chemotherapy in the multidisciplinary management of malignant gliomas: A joint Radiation Therapy Oncology Group and Eastern Cooperative Oncology Group study. Cancer 1983; 52:997.
13. Devaux BC, O'Fallon JR, Kelly PJ: Resection, biopsy, and survival in malignant glial neoplasms: A retrospective study of clinical parameters, therapy, and outcome. J Neurosurg 1993; 78:767.
14. Duncan GG, Goodman GB, Ludgate CM, et al: The treatment of adult supratentorial high grade astrocytomas. J Neurooncol 1992; 13:63.
15. Franklin CIV: Does the extent of surgery make a difference in high grade malignant astrocytoma? Australas Radiol 1992; 36:44.
16. Kreth FW, Warnke PC, Scheremet R, et al: Surgical resection and radiation therapy versus biopsy and radiation therapy in the treatment of glioblastoma multiforme. J Neurosurg 1993; 78:762.
17. Medical Research Council Brain Tumour Working Party: Prognostic factors for high-grade malignant glioma: Development of a prognostic index. J Neurooncol 1990; 9:47.
18. Simpson JR, Horton J, Scott C, et al: Influence of location and extent of surgical resection on survival of patients with glioblastoma multiforme: results of three consecutive Radiation Therapy Oncology Group (RTOG) clinical trials. Int J Radiat Oncol Biol Phys 1993; 26:239.
19. Winger MJ, Macdonald DR, Cairncross JG: Supratentorial anaplastic gliomas in adults: The prognostic importance of extent of resection and prior low-grade glioma. J Neurosurg 1989; 71:487.
20. Hatanaka H, Sano K, Kitamura K, et al: CT findings in patients with gliomas, surviving more than 10 years. Neurochirurgia (Stuttg) 1984; 27:106.
21. Salcman M, Scholtz H, Kaplan RS, et al: Long-term survival in patients with malignant astrocytoma. Neurosurgery 1994; 34:213.
22. Vertosick FT Jr, Selker RG: Long-term survival after the diagnosis of malignant glioma: A series of 22 patients surviving more than 4 years after diagnosis. Surg Neurol 1992; 38:359.
23. Salcman M: Epidemiology and factors affecting survival. *In* Apuzzo MLJ (ed): Malignant Cerebral Glioma. Park Ridge, Ill, American Association of Neurological Surgeons, 1990, p 95.
24. Nelson DF, Diener-West M, Weinstein AS, et al: A randomized comparison of misonidazole sensitized radiotherapy plus BCNU for

treatment of malignant glioma after surgery: Final report of an RTOG study. Int J Radiat Oncol Biol Phys 1986; 12:1793.

25. Gehan EA, Walker MD: Prognostic factors for patients with brain tumors. Monogr Natl Cancer Inst 1977; 46:189.

26. Cohadon F, Aouad N, Rougier A, et al: Histologic and non-histologic factors correlated with survival time in supratentorial astrocytic tumors. J Neurooncol 1985; 3:105.

27. Vecht CJ, Avezaat CJJ, van Putten WLJ, et al: The influence of the extent of surgery on the neurological function and survival in malignant glioma: A retrospective analysis in 243 patients. J Neurol Neurosurg Psychiatry 1990; 53:466.

28. EORTC Brain Tumor Group: Evaluation of CCNU, VM-26 plus CCNU, and procarbazine in supratentorial brain gliomas: Final evaluation of a randomized study. J Neurosurg 1981; 55:27.

29. Roth JG, Elvidge AR: Glioblastoma multiforme: A clinical survey. J Neurosurg 1960; 17:736.

30. Walker MD, Alexander E Jr, Hunt WE, et al: Evaluation of mithramycin in the treatment of anaplastic gliomas. J Neurosurg 1976; 44:655.

31. Green SB, Byar DP, Walker MD, et al: Comparisons of carmustine, procarbazine, and high-dose methylprednisolone as additions to surgery and radiotherapy for the treatment of malignant glioma. Cancer Treat Rep 1983; 67:121.

32. Walker MD, Green SB, Byar DP, et al: Randomized comparisons of radiotherapy and nitrosoureas for the treatment of malignant glioma after surgery. N Engl J Med 1980; 303:1323.

33. Lowe JS, Palmer J: Statistical prognosis in glioblastoma multiforme: A study of clinical variables and Ki-67 index. Br J Neurosurg 1991; 5:61.

34. Kelly PJ: Stereotactic biopsy and resection of thalamic astrocytomas. Neurosurgery 1989; 25:185.

35. Shingai J, Kanno M: Clinical analysis of glioma: Anaplastic astrocytoma and glioblastoma. In Suzuki J (ed): Treatment of Glioma. Tokyo, Springer-Verlag, 1988, p 153.

36. Reeves GI, Marks JE: Prognostic significance of lesion size for glioblastoma multiforme. Radiology 1979; 132:469.

37. Wood JR, Green SB, Shapiro WR: The prognostic importance of tumor size in malignant gliomas: A computed tomographic scan study by the Brain Tumor Cooperative Group. J Clin Oncol 1988; 6:338.

38. Curran WJ Jr, Scott CB, Weinstein AS, et al: Survival comparison of radiosurgery-eligible and -ineligible malignant glioma patients treated with hyperfractionated radiation therapy and carmustine: A report of Radiation Therapy Oncology Group 83–02. J Clin Oncol 1993; 11:857.

39. Florell RC, Macdonald DR, Irish WD, et al: Selection bias, survival, and brachytherapy for glioma. J Neurosurg 1992; 76:179.

40. Andreou J, George AE, Wise A, et al: CT prognostic criteria of survival after malignant glioma surgery. AJNR 1983; 4:488.

41. Karnofsky DA, Abelmann WH, Craver LF, et al: The use of the nitrogen mustards in the palliative treatment of carcinoma: With particular reference to bronchogenic carcinoma. Cancer 1948; 1:634.

42. Walker MD, Alexander E, Hunt WE, et al: Evaluation of BCNU and/or radiotherapy in the treatment of anaplastic gliomas. J Neurosurg 1978; 49:333.

43. Ducci F, Fabrini MG, Lutzemberg L, et al: Supratentorial malignant gliomas: Results in 280 cases treated by postoperative radiotherapy. Cancer J 1993; 6:163.

44. Halperin EC, Gaspar L, Imperato J, et al: An analysis of radiotherapy data from the CNS Cancer Consortium's randomized prospective trial comparing AZQ to BCNU in the treatment of patients with primary malignant brain tumors. Am J Clin Oncol 1993; 16:277.

45. Schold SC Jr, Herndon JE, Burger PC, et al: Randomized comparison of diaziquinone and carmustine in the treatment of adults with anaplastic glioma. J Clin Oncol 1993; 11:77.

46. Shapiro WR, Green SB, Burger PC, et al: Randomized trial of three chemotherapy regimens and two radiotherapy regimens in postoperative treatment of malignant glioma: Brain Tumor Cooperative Group Trial 8001. J Neurosurg 1989; 71:1.

47. Dinapoli RP, Brown LD, Arusell RM, et al: Phase III comparative evaluation of PCNU and carmustine combined with radiation therapy for high-grade glioma. J Clin Oncol 1993; 11:1316.

48. Bleehen NM, Stenning SP, on behalf of the Medical Research Council Brain Tumour Working Party: A Medical Research Council trial of two radiotherapy doses in the treatment of grades 3 and 4 astrocytoma. Br J Cancer 1991; 64:769.

49. Coffey RJ, Lunsford LD, Taylor FH: Survival after stereotactic biopsy of malignant gliomas. Neurosurgery 1988; 22:465.

50. Nazzaro JM, Neuwelt EA: The role of surgery in the management of supratentorial intermediate and high-grade astrocytomas in adults. J Neurosurg 1990; 73:331.

51. Neuwelt EA, Nazzaro JM, Gumerlock MK: Is there a role for biopsy in the treatment of supratentorial high-grade glioma? Clin Neurosurg 1990; 36:384.

52. Quigley MR, Maroon JC: The relationship between survival and the extent of the resection in patients with supratentorial gliomas. Neurosurgery 1991; 29:385.

53. Ammirati M, Vick N, Liao Y, et al: Effect of the extent of surgical resection on survival and quality of life in patients with supratentorial glioblastomas and anaplastic astrocytomas. Neurosurgery 1987; 21:201.

54. Albert FK, Forsting M, Sartor K, et al: Early postoperative magnetic resonance imaging after resection of malignant glioma: Objective evaluation of residual tumor and its influence on regrowth and prognosis. Neurosurgery 1994; 34:45.

55. Forsting M, Albert FK, Kunze S, et al: Extirpation of glioblastomas: MR and CT follow-up of residual tumor and regrowth patterns. AJNR 1993; 14:77.

56. Fadul C, Wood J, Thaler H, et al: Morbidity and mortality of craniotomy for excision of supratentorial gliomas. Neurology 1988; 38:1374.

57. Prados MD, Gutin PH, Phillips TL, et al: Interstitial brachytherapy for newly diagnosed patients with malignant gliomas: The UCSF experience. Int J Radiat Oncol Biol Phys 1992; 24:593.

58. Wen PY, Alexander E III, Black PM, et al: Long term results of stereotactic brachytherapy used in the initial treatment of patients with glioblastomas. Cancer 1994; 73:3029.

59. Coffey RJ: Boost gamma knife radiosurgery in the treatment of primary glial tumors. Stereotact Funct Neurosurg 1993; 1:59.

60. Loeffler JS, Alexander E III, Shea WM, et al: Radiosurgery as part of the initial management of patients with malignant gliomas. J Clin Oncol 1992; 10:1379.

61. Fine HA: Chemotherapy of astrocytomas in adults. In Black PM, Schoene WC, Lampson LA (eds): Astrocytomas: Diagnosis, Treatment, and Biology. Boston, Blackwell Scientific Publications, 1993, p 86.

62. Bucy PC, Oberhill HR, Siqueira EB, et al: Cerebral glioblastomas can be cured. Neurosurgery 1985; 16:714.

63. Burger PC, Vogel FS, Green SB, et al: Glioblastoma multiforme and anaplastic astrocytoma: Pathologic criteria and prognostic implications. Cancer 1985; 56:1106.

64. Nelson DF, Diener-West M, Horton J, et al: Combined modality approach to treatment of malignant gliomas—re-evaluation of RTOG 7401/ECOG 1374 with long-term follow-up: A joint study of the Radiation Therapy Oncology Group and the Eastern Cooperative Oncology Group. Monogr Natl Cancer Inst 1988; 6:279.

65. Salazar OM, Rubin P, Feldstein ML, et al: High dose radiation therapy in the treatment of malignant gliomas: Final report. Int J Radiat Oncol Biol Phys 1979; 5:1733.

66. Deutsch M, Green SB, Strike TA, et al: Results of a randomized trial comparing BCNU plus radiotherapy, streptozotocin plus radiotherapy, BCNU plus hyperfractionated radiotherapy, and BCNU following misonidazole plus radiotherapy in the postoperative treatment of malignant glioma. Int J Radiat Oncol Biol Phys 1989; 16:1389.

67. Prados MD, Gutin PH, Phillips TL, et al: Highly anaplastic astrocytoma: A review of 357 patients treated between 1977 and 1989. Int J Radiat Oncol Biol Phys 1992; 23:3.

68. Curran WJ Jr, Scott CB, Horton J, et al: Does extent of surgery influence outcome for astrocytoma with atypical or anaplastic foci (AAF)? A report from three Radiation Therapy Oncology Group (RTOG) trials. J Neurooncol 1992; 12:219.

69. Fischbach AJ, Martz KL, Nelson JS, et al: Long-term survival in treated anaplastic astrocytomas. A report of combined RTOG/ECOG studies. Am J Clin Oncol 1991; 14:365.

70. Laramore GE, Martz KL, Nelson JS, et al: Radiation Therapy Oncology Group (RTOG) survival data on anaplastic astrocytomas of the brain: Does a more aggressive form of treatment adversely impact survival? Int J Radiat Oncol Biol Phys 1989; 17:1351.

71. Nelson DF, Nelson JS, Davis DR, et al: Survival and prognosis of patients with astrocytoma with atypical or anaplastic features. J Neurooncol 1985; 3:99.

72. Fulling KH, Garcia DM: Anaplastic astrocytoma of the adult cerebrum: Prognostic value of histologic features. Cancer 1985; 55:928.

73. Soffietti R, Chió A, Giordana MT, et al: Prognostic factors in anaplastic astrocytomas after surgery and conventional radiotherapy. *In* Paoletti P, Takakura K, Walker MD, et al. (eds): Neuro-oncology, Dordrecht, Kluwer Academic Publishers, 1991, p 179.

74. Takakura K, Abe H, Tanaka R, et al: Effects of ACNU and radiotherapy on malignant glioma. J Neurosurg 1986; 64:53.

75. Eyre HJ, Crowley JJ, Townsend JJ, et al: A randomized trial of radiotherapy versus radiotherapy plus CCNU for incompletely resected low-grade gliomas: A Southwest Oncology Group study. J Neurosurg 1993; 78:909.

76. Laws ER Jr, Taylor WF, Clifton MB, et al: Neurosurgical management of low-grade astrocytoma of the cerebral hemispheres. J Neurosurg 1984; 61:665.

77. McCormack BM, Miller DC, Budzilovich GN, et al: Treatment and survival of low-grade astrocytoma in adults—1977–1988. Neurosurgery 1992; 31:636.

78. Medbery CA III, Straus KL, Steinberg SM, et al: Low-grade astrocytomas: Treatment results and prognostic variables. Int J Radiat Oncol Biol Phys 1988; 15:837.

79. North CA, North RB, Epstein JA, et al: Low-grade cerebral astrocytomas: Survival and quality of life after radiation therapy. Cancer 1990; 66:6.

80. Piepmeier JM: Observations on the current treatment of low-grade astrocytic tumors of the cerebral hemispheres. J Neurosurg 1987; 67:177.

81. Shibamoto Y, Kitakabu Y, Takahashi M, et al: Supratentorial low-grade astrocytoma: Correlation of computed tomography findings with effect of radiation therapy and prognostic variables. Cancer 1993; 72:190.

82. Westergaard L, Gjerris F, Klinken L: Prognostic parameters in benign astrocytomas. Acta Neurochir (Wien) 1993; 123:1.

83. Whitton AC, Bloom HJ: Low grade glioma of the cerebral hemispheres in adults: A retrospective analysis of 88 cases. Int J Radiat Oncol Biol Phys 1990; 18:783.

84. Shaw EG, Daumas-Duport C, Scheithauer BW, et al: Radiation therapy in the management of low-grade supratentorial astrocytomas. J Neurosurg 1989; 70:853.

85. Miralbell R, Balart J, Matias-Guiu X, et al: Radiotherapy for supratentorial low-grade gliomas: Results and prognostic factors with special focus on tumour volume parameters. Radiother Oncol 1993; 27:112.

86. Philippon JH, Clemenceau SH, Fauchon FH, et al: Supratentorial low-grade astrocytomas in adults. Neurosurgery 1993; 32:554.

87. Soffietti R, Chió A, Giordana MT, et al: Prognostic factors in well-differentiated cerebral astrocytomas in the adult. Neurosurgery 1989; 24:686.

88. Silverman C, Marks JE: Prognostic significance of contrast enhancement in low-grade astrocytomas of the adult cerebrum. Radiology 1981; 139:211.

89. Cairncross JG, Laperriere NJ: Low-grade glioma. To treat or not to treat? Arch Neurol 1989; 46:1238.

90. Recht LD, Lew R, Smith TW: Suspected low-grade glioma: Is deferring treatment safe? Ann Neurol 1992; 31:431.

91. Vecht CJ: Effect of age on treatment decisions in low-grade glioma. J Neurol Neurosurg Psychiatry 1993; 56:1259.

92. Krouwer HG, Davis RL, Silver P, et al: Gemistocytic astrocytomas: A reappraisal. J Neurosurg 1991; 74:399.

93. Hayostek CJ, Shaw EG, Scheithauer B, et al: Astrocytomas of the cerebellum: A comparative clinicopathologic study of pilocytic and diffuse astrocytomas. Cancer 1993; 72:856.

94. Cushing H: Experiences with the cerebellar astrocytomas: A critical review of seventy-six cases. Surg Gynecol Obstet 1931; 52:129.

95. Leviton A, Fulchiero A, Gilles FH, et al: Survival status of children with cerebellar gliomas. J Neurosurg 1978; 48:29.

96. Gjerris F, Klinken L: Long-term prognosis in children with benign cerebellar astrocytoma. J Neurosurg 1978; 49:179.

97. Wallner KE, Gonzales MF, Edwards MS, et al: Treatment results of juvenile pilocytic astrocytoma. J Neurosurg 1988; 69:171.

98. Kehler U, Arnold H, Muller H: Long-term follow-up of infratentorial pilocytic astrocytomas. Neurosurg Rev 1990; 13:315.

99. Schneider JH Jr, Raffel C, McComb JG: Benign cerebellar astrocytomas of childhood. Neurosurgery 1992; 30:58.

100. Alvord EC Jr, Lofton S: Gliomas of the optic nerve or chiasm: Outcome by patients' age, tumor site, and treatment. J Neurosurg 1988; 68:85.

101. Flickinger JC, Torres C, Deutsch M: Management of low-grade gliomas of the optic nerve and chiasm. Cancer 1988; 61:635.

102. Horwich A, Bloom HJ: Optic gliomas: Radiation therapy and prognosis. Int J Radiat Oncol Biol Phys 1985; 11:1067.

103. Pierce SM, Barnes PD, Loeffler JS, et al: Definitive radiation therapy in the management of symptomatic patients with optic glioma: Survival and long-term effects. Cancer 1990; 65:45.

104. Afra D, Muller W, Slowik F, et al: Supratentorial lobar pilocytic astrocytomas: Report of 45 operated cases, including 9 recurrences. Acta Neurochir (Wien) 1986; 81:90.

105. Clark GB, Henry JM, McKeever PE: Cerebral pilocytic astrocytoma. Cancer 1985; 56:1128.

106. Forsyth PA, Shaw EG, Scheithauer BW, et al: Supratentorial pilocytic astrocytomas: A clinicopathologic, prognostic, and flow cytometric study of 51 patients. Cancer 1993; 72:1335.

107. Garcia DM, Fulling KH: Juvenile pilocytic astrocytoma of the cerebrum in adults: A distinctive neoplasm with favorable prognosis. J Neurosurg 1985; 63:382.

108. Palma L, Guidefti B: Cystic pilocytic astrocytomas of the cerebral hemispheres: Surgical experience with 51 cases and long-term results. J Neurosurg 1985; 62:811.

109. Alpers CE, Davis RL, Wilson CB: Persistence and late malignant transformation of childhood cerebellar astrocytoma: Case report. J Neurosurg 1982; 57:548.

110. Casadei GP, Arrigoni GL, D'Angelo V, et al: Late malignant recurrence of childhood cerebellar astrocytoma. Clin Neuropathol 1990; 9:295.

111. Dirks PB, Jay V, Becker LE, et al: Development of anaplastic changes in low-grade astrocytomas of childhood. Neurosurgery 1994; 34:68.

112. Pagni CA, Giordana MT, Canavero S: Benign recurrence of a pilocytic cerebellar astrocytoma 36 years after radical removal: Case report. Neurosurgery 1991; 28:606.

113. Wisoff HS, Liena JF: Glioblastoma multiforme of the cerebellum five decades after irradiation of a cerebellar tumor. J Neurooncol 1989; 7:339.

114. Yoshizumi MO: Neuro-ophthalmologic signs in a recurrent cerebellar astrocytoma after 48 years. Ann Ophthalmol 1979; 11:1714.

115. Shepherd CW, Scheithauer BW, Gomez MR, et al: Subependymal giant cell astrocytoma: A clinical, pathological, and flow cytometric study. Neurosurgery 1991; 28:864.

116. Chow CW, Klug GL, Lewis EA: Subependymal giant-cell astrocytoma in children: An unusual discrepancy between histological and clinical features. J Neurosurg 1988; 68:880.

117. Kepes JJ, Rubinstein LJ, Eng LF: Pleomorphic xanthoastrocytoma: A distinctive meningocerebral glioma of young subjects with relatively favorable prognosis: A study of 12 cases. Cancer 1979; 44:1839.

118. Thomas C, Golden B: Pleomorphic xanthoastrocytoma: report of two cases and brief review of the literature. Clin Neuropathol 1993; 12:97.

119. Macaulay RJ, Jay V, Hoffman HJ, et al: Increased mitotic activity as a negative prognostic indicator in pleomorphic xanthoastrocytoma: Case report. J Neurosurg 1993; 79:761.

120. Bailey P, Bucy PC: Oligodendrogliomas of the brain. J Pathol Bacteriol 1929; 32:735.

121. Roberts M, German WJ: A long term study of patients with oligodendrogliomas: Follow-up of 50 cases, including Dr. Harvey Cushing's series. J Neurosurg 1966; 24:697.

122. Nijjar TS, Simpson WJ, Gadalla T, et al: Oligodendrogliomas: The Princess Margaret Hospital experience (1958–1984). Cancer 1993; 71:4002.

123. Shaw EG, Scheithauer BW, O'Fallon JR, et al: Oligodendrogliomas: The Mayo Clinic experience. J Neurosurg 1992; 76:428.

124. Shimizu KT, Tran LM, Mark RJ, et al: Management of oligodendrogliomas. Radiology 1993; 186:569.

125. Wallner KE, Gonzales M, Sheline GE: Treatment of oligodendrogliomas with or without postoperative irradiation. J Neurosurg 1988; 68:684.

126. Kros JM, Pieterman H, van Eden CG, et al: Oligodendroglioma: The Rotterdam-Dijkzigt experience. Neurosurgery 1994; 34:959.

127. Ludwig CL, Smith MT, Godfrey AD, et al: A clinicopathological study of 323 patients with oligodendrogliomas. Ann Neurol 1986; 19:15.

128. Daumas-Duport C, Scheithauer B, O'Fallon J, et al: Grading of astrocytomas. A simple and reproducible method. Cancer 1988; 62:2152.

129. Bullard DE, Rawlings CE III, Phillips B, et al: Oligodendroglioma: An analysis of the value of radiation therapy. Cancer 1987; 60:2179.

130. Lindegaard K-F, Mørk SJ, Eide GE, et al: Statistical analysis of clinicopathological features, radiotherapy, and survival in 170 cases of oligodendroglioma. J Neurosurg 1987; 67:224.

131. Sun ZM, Genka S, Shitara N, et al: Factors possibly influencing the prognosis of oligodendroglioma. Neurosurgery 1988; 22:886.

132. Shaw EG, Scheithauer BW, O'Fallon JR, et al: Mixed oligoastrocytomas: A survival and prognostic factor analysis. Neurosurgery 1994; 34:577.

133. Wilkinson IM, Anderson JR, Holmes AE: Oligodendroglioma: An analysis of 42 cases. J Neurol Neurosurg Psychiatry 1987; 50:304.

134. Mørk SJ, Lindegaard KF, Halvorsen TB, et al: Oligodendroglioma: Incidence and biological behavior in a defined population. J Neurosurg 1985; 63:881.

135. Cairncross JG, George ED, MacDonald DR, et al: Aggressive oligodendroglioma: A chemosensitive tumor. Neurosurgery 1992; 31:78.

136. Glass J, Hochberg FH, Gruber ML, et al: The treatment of oligodendrogliomas and mixed oligodendroglioma-astrocytomas with PCV chemotherapy. J Neurosurg 1992; 76:741.

137. Kyritsis AP, Yung WK, Bruner J, et al: The treatment of anaplastic oligodendrogliomas and mixed gliomas. Neurosurgery 1993; 32:365.

138. Shaw EG, Scheithauer BW, O'Fallon JR: Management of supratentorial low-grade gliomas. Oncology 1993; 7:97.

139. Papadopoulos DP, Giri S, Evans RG: Prognostic factors and management of intracranial ependymomas. Anticancer Res 1990; 10:689.

140. Birgisson S, Blöndal H, Björnsson J, et al: Ependymoma: A clinicopathological and immunohistological study. APMIS 1992; 100:294.

141. Ernestus RI, Wilcke O, Schroder R: Intracranial ependymomas: prognostic aspects. Neurosurg Rev 1989; 12:157.

142. Kovalic JJ, Flaris N, Grigsby PW, et al: Intracranial ependymoma long term outcome, patterns of failure. J Neurooncol 1993; 15:125.

143. Lyons MK, Kelly PJ: Posterior fossa ependymomas: report of 30 cases and review of the literature. Neurosurgery 1991; 28:659.

144. Garrett PG, Simpson WJ: Ependymomas: results of radiation treatment. Int J Radiat Oncol Biol Phys 1983; 9:1121.

145. Healey EA, Barnes PD, Kupsky WJ, et al: The prognostic significance of postoperative residual tumor in ependymoma. Neurosurgery 1991; 28:666.

146. Pierre-Kahn A, Hirsch JF, Roux FX, et al: Intracranial ependymomas in childhood—survival and functional results of 47 cases. Childs Brain 1983; 10:145.

147. Afra D, Muller W, Slowik F, et al: Supratentorial lobar ependymomas: Reports on the grading and survival periods in 80 cases, including 46 recurrences. Acta Neurochir (Wien) 1983; 69:243.

148. Vanuytsel LJ, Bessell EM, Ashley SE, et al: Intracranial ependymoma: Long-term results of a policy of surgery and radiotherapy. Int J Radiat Oncol Biol Phys 1992; 23:313.

149. Salazar OM, Castro-Vita H, VanHoutte P, et al: Improved survival in cases of intracranial ependymoma after radiation therapy. Late report and recommendations. J Neurosurg 1983; 59:652.

150. Marks JE, Adler SJ: A comparative study of ependymomas by site of origin. Int J Radiat Oncol Biol Phys 1982; 8:37.

151. Mørk SJ, Loken AC: Ependymoma: a follow-up study of 101 cases. Cancer 1977; 40:907.

152. Rawlings CE III, Giangaspero F, Burger PC, et al: Ependymomas: A clinicopathologic study. Surg Neurol 1988; 29:271.

153. Ikezaki K, Matsushima T, Inoue T, et al: Correlation of microanatomical localization with postoperative survival in posterior fossa ependymomas. Neurosurgery 1993; 32:38.

154. Ross GW, Rubinstein LJ: Lack of histopathological correlation of malignant ependymomas with postoperative survival. J Neurosurg 1989; 70:31.

155. Schiffer D, Chio A, Cravioto H, et al: Ependymoma: Internal correlations among pathological signs: The anaplastic variant. Neurosurgery 1991; 29:206.

156. Bloom HJ: Intracranial tumors: Response and resistance to therapeutic endeavors, 1970–1980. Int J Radiat Oncol Biol Phys 1982; 8:1083.

157. Ilgren EB, Stiller CA, Hughes JT, et al: Ependymomas: A clinical and pathologic study: Part II. Survival features. Clin Neuropathol 1984; 3:122.

158. Nagashima T, Hoshino T, Cho KG, et al: The proliferative potential of human ependymomas measured by in situ bromodeoxyuridine labeling. Cancer 1988; 61:2433.

159. Asai A, Hoshino T, Edwards MS, et al: Predicting the recurrence of ependymomas from the bromodeoxyuridine labeling index. Childs Nerv Syst 1992; 8:273.

160. Artico M, Bardella L, Ciappetta P, et al: Surgical treatment of subependymomas of the central nervous system: Report of 8 cases and review of the literature. Acta Neurochir (Wien) 1989; 98:25.

161. Matsumura A, Ahyai A, Hori A, et al: Intracerebral subependymomas: Clinical and neuropathological analyses with special reference to the possible existence of a less benign variant. Acta Neurochir (Wien) 1989; 96:15.

162. Lombardi D, Scheithauer BW, Meyer FB, et al: Symptomatic subependymoma: A clinicopathological and flow cytometric study. J Neurosurg 1991; 75:583.

163. Vaquero J, Herrero J, Cabezudo JM, et al: Symptomatic subependymomas of the lateral ventricles. Acta Neurochir (Wien) 1980; 53:99.

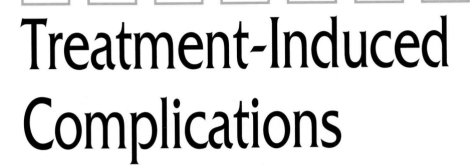

Treatment-Induced Complications

ELLEN E. MACK

CHAPTER 61

Radiation-Induced Tumors

The study of radiation-induced tumors as a distinct entity is greatly hampered by the general difficulty in determining the role of exposure to radiation in the pathogenesis of neoplastic disease. It can never be determined with certainty that the genesis of any particular tumor resulted from the irradiation of normal tissues, because radiographically, pathologically, and clinically, radiation-induced tumors are indistinct from their spontaneously occurring counterparts. The study of radiation-induced neoplasms, therefore, depends heavily on epidemiologic studies. If population-based studies show that a particular neoplasm occurs more frequently than expected in individuals exposed to radiation as compared to nonexposed individuals, then it can be inferred that the tumor is radiation induced. Such epidemiologic findings, in conjunction with the results of research in experimental animals, lend support to the many individual cases of presumed radiation-induced tumors noted throughout the medical literature.

The form of radiation exposure that is most commonly studied is therapeutic irradiation for the treatment of neoplastic disease. However, other forms of radiation exposure must also be considered, including exposures to natural emissions, atomic bomb explosion, nuclear power plant emissions, or medical diagnostic procedures. If a causal relationship exists between radiation exposure and carcinogenesis, then one might expect that exposures to larger amounts of radiation, for example as a result of therapeutic irradiation, are likely to yield more cases of radiation-induced tumors. Indeed, most of the experience reported consists of isolated case reports of patients who have received radiation therapy for a primary neoplasm and later are found to have a second malignancy at a nearby site. Because such double malignancies are a rare event, it is difficult to determine whether they occur by chance. More than likely, the process is multifactorial and includes not only exposure to radiation but also exposure to other recognized and unrecognized carcinogens, as well as a patient's probable inherent susceptibility to the development of neoplastic disease. A genetic predisposition to tumor development is now widely recognized in conditions such as neurofibromatosis and Li-Fraumeni syndrome, and more than likely it exists in many other, as yet unrecognized, forms. It is with these limitations

in mind that the clinical literature on radiation-induced neoplasms must be examined.

To maintain some coherence in the evaluation of individual cases of suspected radiation-induced tumors, certain criteria have been established for acceptance of a tumor as radiation induced: the tumor must occur within the irradiated field or at its margins; it must occur at a reasonable time after the exposure to radiation, and it should be histologically distinct from the original neoplasm. The presence of other evidence of radiation injury, either clinical or pathologic, lends further support to the assumption.[1] Thus, on an individual basis, tumors fulfilling those criteria may be considered radiation induced; but only if their occurrence is found, by statistical or epidemiologic criteria, to be more frequent than expected can one define a radiation-induced neoplasm as a distinct entity. The validity of such a supposition is strengthened if a dose-response relationship can be demonstrated and if studies in experimental animals confirm the ability of radiation exposure to induce the tumor in question.

RADIATION CARCINOGENESIS

Radiation doses are measured in units of gray (Gy), with 1 Gy representing 1 joule per kilogram, which is equivalent to 100 rad. Radiation exposure causes cell killing as a result of ionization of atoms within a cell. The ionization process results in the presence of hydroxy radicals, free electrons, and hydrogen atoms, which interact with nuclear DNA, causing base changes and strand breaks and thereby producing biologic sequelae. The effectiveness of ionization by radiation depends not only on the dose but also on the radiation source within the electromagnetic spectrum. X-rays, γ-rays, electrons, and protons cause low levels of ionization and are therefore referred to as sources of low linear-energy transfer (LET) radiation. Neutrons and heavy charged particles, which are sources of high LET radiation, have a higher rate of ionization and are able to produce more biologic damage. High LET radiation is effective at ionization at all doses, whereas low LET radiation is less effective at low doses of exposure. Often, radiation exposure is expressed in terms of dose equivalence, as both the dose and the degree of LET must be considered in determining the effects on biologic tissues.

The dose of radiation to which an individual is exposed is also quite likely to play a role in the potential for subsequent tumor development; surprisingly, this has never been clearly demonstrated. Many investigators believe that it is the lower doses of radiation exposure that place individuals at risk for tumor development, presumably because higher doses are more likely to result in cell killing rather than more limited cellular damage.[2, 3] This notion is supported by the finding that tumors presumed to be radiation induced are often observed to develop at the margins of the radiation ports[4, 5] and have also been noted to occur after only very small exposures, such as during the treatment of tinea capitis.[6–10]

Host factors are also important in the development of radiation-induced neoplasms. Laboratory studies have shown great variability in radiation-induced carcinogenesis depending on the species and sex of the animal, the tissue irradiated, and the animal's age at the time of exposure. In studies of human survivors of the atomic bomb, it has been noted that specific radiation-induced tumors tend to occur within the population normally at risk for development of that tumor, but they occur more frequently than expected.[2] This observation has also been made of tumors developing after exposure to therapeutic irradiation. For example, radiation-induced meningiomas, like their spontaneous counterparts, occur more frequently in women than men.[11] Although not yet definitively established in human population studies, it appears that age at irradiation may be a factor in the development of secondary malignancies. Such a correlation has been demonstrated for acute lymphoblastic leukemia (ALL), sarcoma, and carcinoma of the breast, lung, and stomach, as persons exposed at a younger age were at a greater risk to develop these radiation-induced malignancies.[2, 12] Less information is available about the role of age at exposure on tumor latency (i.e., the time to tumor development), but in a study on meningiomas induced by exposure to high doses of radiation therapy, a younger age at exposure was associated with a shorter tumor latency.[11] In general, these underlying host factors collectively are thought to play an important role in the carcinogenic potential of radiation.

PATHOGENESIS

The histopathologic changes associated with delayed radiation injury of the brain have been well described.[13] They include: fibrinoid necrosis of the small blood vessels; luminal occlusion of blood vessels secondary to thrombosis, medial fibrosis, and adventitial proliferation; cavitation and coagulative necrosis of the white matter with relative sparing of the gray matter; glial proliferation; and the presence of large, bizarre, multinucleated astrocytes and transformed fibroblasts. Foci of demyelination, which represent an ''early delayed'' effect of irradiation, may no longer be present by the time delayed cerebral necrosis has resulted from radiation exposure.

Kemper and co-workers,[14] in a serial autopsy study of irradiated monkeys, noted changes similar to those described earlier for the human brain. Autopsies performed at the 18-month post-irradiation period showed that necrosis was no longer active, but instead had been replaced by the process of gliosis, a somewhat unexpected finding, as the process of radiation injury was thought to have been completed. However, it is at that time of change from necrosis to gliosis that the first brain tumors were noted to develop in the irradiated monkeys, leading the authors to speculate that radiation exposure may cause a dysregulation of the repair process, which results in excessive gliosis and thereby sets the stage for neoplastic transformation.[14] Pathologic examination of brain tumors thought to be induced by radiation in humans has also shown evidence of radiation injury with delayed radiation necrosis, intense gliosis, and the presence of bizarre, multinucleated, giant glial cells.[1, 10, 15–18] It has been proposed that these giant cells may represent a transformation process from radiation necrosis to neoplasia.[15]

These early theories derived from pathologic observations of radiation-induced tumors in monkeys fit well with the current concept of oncogenesis that both initiators and promoters are required for the process of neoplastic transformation. In general, the initiator is thought to produce a gene mutation and the promotor most likely to cause stimulation of cellular proliferation and/or expression of the mutation. As gene mutation is much more likely to occur in proliferating cells, children would be at much greater risk for neoplastic transformation because glial cell proliferation is considerably more active in young children.[19] Radiation has therefore been proposed as a possible initiator in the process of glioma transformation, especially in susceptible children.[20] Secondary or promotor agents would be necessary to complete the process. These agents remain mostly unknown but could include chemotherapeutic agents, intrathecal methotrexate in particular, which is used to treat most patients who have leukemia. The potentiation of radiation oncogenesis by chemical agents has been well described in reports of laboratory studies.[21]

LABORATORY STUDIES

Perhaps the most compelling evidence of a causal relationship between radiation exposure and neoplastic transformation stems from research in experimental animals performed several decades ago. Most experimental studies have been performed with the *Macaca mulatta* rhesus monkey. This primate serves as an excellent model because the spontaneous occurrence of primary brain tumors is extremely rare in this species; in fact, the first case of a spontaneously occurring glioblastoma multiforme in a monkey has been reported only recently.[22]

In 1958, autopsy studies on rhesus monkeys maintained by the United States Air Force showed that neoplasms were unusual in these animals.[23] Only nine neoplasms were found in a series of 450 autopsies. Of those nine, three were thought to be radiation induced and the remainder were thought to have occurred spontaneously. The radiation-induced neoplasms developed in monkeys who were studied to determine the effects of radiation therapy on cataract formation. Of 112 monkeys receiving whole-brain irradiation, one developed a glioblastoma multiforme, the first time this particular malignancy had been observed in a monkey.[23]

Later studies[24, 25] have also clearly shown the development of glioblastomas in monkeys exposed to whole-body irradiation. The reported incidences range from 7% to 9%, and in one of the studies glioblastoma was noted to be the most common tumor to develop after whole-body irradiation.[25] Extensive evidence of delayed radiation injury of the brain was often noted adjacent to and distant from the tumor.[24]

Monkeys exposed to single-dose radiation have also been noted to develop glioblastoma multiforme. In a study by Kemper and colleagues,[14] rhesus monkeys were irradiated with 1,000, 1,500, or 2,000 rad of whole-brain radiation therapy and some of them were sacrificed every 6 months for 2 years for pathologic study. In the four monkeys receiving 1,500 rad of single-fraction radiation therapy, two developed primary brain tumors that were noted at the time of the 12- and 24-month autopsies. In both cases, the tumors were multifocal.

Similar studies in mice[26] and rats[27] have also shown a considerable increase in the incidence of gliomas in the irradiated animals, although tissues other than the nervous system were more sensitive to the oncogenic effects of radiation in these species. Most of the nervous system tumors were gliomas and included oligoastrocytomas and ependymomas, as well as astrocytomas and glioblastomas.[27] The only report of radiation-induced gliomas, other than astrocytomas or glioblastomas, occurring in monkeys is that by Traynor and Casey,[28] who noted the development of three ependymal tumors (including ependymoblastomas) in *Macaca mulatta* rhesus monkeys receiving 200 to 1,200 rad of whole-body radiation. The studies did not report careful pathologic descriptions, however.

EPIDEMIOLOGIC STUDIES

Little is known about the exposure of individuals to low levels of radiation and the subsequent development of brain tumors, because most epidemiologic studies have focused on higher exposures, such as those obtained from therapeutic irradiation. However, several studies have demonstrated a possible association of low-level radiation exposure, such as that obtained from diagnostic imaging, and brain tumor formation. Such an association has been demonstrated for dental x-ray films,[29, 30] and x-ray films of the shoulder, neck, and head,[31] and as an occupational exposure for dentists and dental nurses working in Sweden.[32] In general, the association is stronger for meningiomas than for gliomas.[29, 33, 34] A small, but significant occupational risk has also been noted for workers at nuclear facilities.[35] Nonionizing radiation, such as the electromagnetic radiation from residential appliances, cathode-ray tubes, and electric power lines, has also been linked to the occurrence of gliomas.[32, 33] In the Adelaide Adult Brain Tumor Study, a fivefold increase in gliomas was seen in women exposed to cathode-ray tubes used in computer video-display terminals.[33]

The best epidemiologic data available are from retrospective analyses of individuals irradiated during childhood for treatment of tinea capitis. Such patients constitute an excellent study population because they do not have a primary malignancy as the reason for radiation exposure, eliminating the bias of an inherent tendency for oncogenesis. The treat-

ment, known as the Adamson-Keinbock (KA) technique, was in wide use until 1959, when griseofulvin became available. It consisted of scalp irradiation resulting in the delivery of approximately 150 cGy to the surface of the brain, 70 cGy to the base of the brain, and 6 cGy to the thyroid gland. Shore and others,[7] in a retrospective analysis of more than 2,000 individuals treated with the KA technique in New York City, found an increased incidence of tumors of the brain, parotid gland, skin, bone, and thyroid gland in irradiated individuals as compared to controls. The onset of the tumors occurred 15 to 20 years after exposure for tumors of the skin and parotid gland, but after only 5 to 10 years for tumors of the brain and thyroid. The incidence of such tumors continued to rise over time and did not show any evidence of leveling off within the 29-year follow-up period. In this cohort, the incidence of brain tumors was 8.3 per 1,000.

In a more extensive study of the effects of radiation exposure on patients with tinea capitis, Ron and co-workers[6] found an eightfold increase in risk for the development of brain tumors in irradiated individuals. The study consisted of a retrospective review of more than 10,000 individuals undergoing the KA treatment in Israel. As compared to controls, irradiated individuals were more likely to develop both benign neural tumors (relative risk [RR] = 9.0) and malignant neural tumors (RR = 4.5). The relative risk of developing a nerve-sheath tumor or meningioma was quite high (RR = 33 and 9.5, respectively), compared to a relative risk of developing a glioma (RR = 2.6). Gliomas, however, tended to develop earlier than meningiomas or nerve-sheath tumors; their mean time to development was 14 years, vs. 21 years for meningiomas and 17 years for nerve-sheath tumors. The risk of developing a radiation-induced tumor was maximal at 15 to 24 years, but was still significantly elevated at 26 years, the point at which follow-up was completed. Additionally, an analysis of individuals repeatedly treated by the KA technique established a dose-response relationship for each type of neural tumor, strengthening the causality link between radiation exposure and tumor development.[6]

The tinea capitis studies lend strong support to the role of radiation therapy in the induction of brain tumors, especially meningiomas and neural sheath tumors. However, most case reports of possible radiation-induced tumors concern patients initially treated for malignant disease. Because secondary tumor development in such patients is likely to depend on more complex risk factors, the role of radiation exposure is more difficult to determine in this cohort. The British Childhood Cancer Research Group found a fivefold overall increase in the risk of a secondary malignancy in a cohort of more than 10,000 survivors of childhood malignancies other than retinoblastoma.[36] More important, if patients were stratified according to the type of therapy received for the first malignancy, excessive risk could be found in patients who had previously received radiation therapy. The relative risk of developing a second malignancy was 3.9 for children not treated with radiation or chemotherapy, but was 5.6 for those who received radiation therapy and 9.3 for those treated with both radiation and chemotherapy. Of interest is that the excessive incidence of secondary tumors in childhood cancer survivors, thought to be attributable to radiation therapy, was most substantial for the survivors of central nervous system (CNS) tumors, which serves to implicate the brain as being particularly prone to radiation carcinogenesis. Overall, the most common types of secondary tumors were those of bone, thyroid, and connective tissue (RR = 18, 16, and 14, respectively), whereas CNS tumors had a lower risk overall (RR = 7). It can be concluded from this study that individuals who develop a malignancy early in life appear to have an inherent risk for further tumor development and, moreover, that exposure to radiation and chemotherapy appears to potentiate the risk of oncogenesis.

Similar results were found in another large British study reviewing 161 children who developed more than one malignancy.[5] In that study, tumors of the CNS were second only to osteosarcomas as the most common type of secondary tumor. Furthermore, the majority of osteosarcomas occurred in association with retinoblastoma and can be explained on that basis. This study also detected a frequent association of acute leukemia and CNS tumors; the CNS tumor occurred as both the primary and secondary tumor in association with leukemia. Sixty-one percent of all secondary tumors and 76% of CNS tumors were associated with radiation therapy and were therefore considered to be radiation induced. Approximately one fourth of the tumors associated with radiation therapy were noted to develop on the edge of the radiation field, lending support to the carcinogenic potential of low doses of radiation therapy.

These findings have been confirmed in American studies as well. Meadows and associates[37] reviewed a large series of children who had more than one malignancy. In approximately half of patients with double malignancy, radiation therapy of the first malignancy was a possible etiology of the second malignancy. In approximately a fourth of patients, a well-recognized genetic predisposition (e.g., neurofibromatosis) was felt to be responsible. However, in the remaining fourth of patients, no discernible etiology for the second malignancy could be found. Within that group, the tumor combination most frequently observed was leukemia or lymphoma with glioma, a finding noted by others as well.[5, 36, 38, 39] That association raises the question of a possible genetic predisposition for the concurrence of these two tumors. In support of this notion is the finding by Farwell and Flannery[40, 41] of a substantially increased incidence of nervous system tumors and hematopoietic malignancies, but not of cancer overall, in relatives of children with CNS tumors. These findings have led to the speculation that the combination of leukemia and CNS tumors may represent a distinct, as yet undescribed, tumor syndrome.[37, 39]

Neglia and co-workers[12] carefully studied the risk of secondary tumor development in patients surviving ALL. In a cohort of 9,720 patients, 43 secondary tumors were detected of which more than half were CNS tumors, including 14 high-grade astrocytomas or glioblastomas multiforme, four primitive neuroectodermal tumors or medulloblastomas, three low-grade astrocytomas or brainstem gliomas, two meningiomas, and one ependymoma. The overall relative risk of developing a secondary neoplasm in children with ALL was 6.9, but that of developing a nervous system tumor was 21.7. A younger age at the time of diagnosis of ALL was associated not only with a higher risk of development of a secondary tumor, but also with a higher risk for the

development of brain tumors in particular. Other studies examining the risk of secondary brain-tumor development in ALL survivors have shown increased risks ranging from 20 to more than 200 (Table 61–1).

These studies lend strong support to the notion that exposure to radiation significantly increases the risk of tumor development, especially tumors of the brain, in individuals with childhood malignancies. Unfortunately, adults are more difficult to study because of the poor survival times associated with the conditions for which they usually receive radiation therapy. However, there are a few situations in which radiation therapy of the brain is used to treat relatively benign tumors, namely pituitary adenomas and meningiomas, for which the life expectancy of patients is normal or near normal. Meningiomas and pituitary adenomas are only rarely associated with other malignancies, minimizing the a possible role of genetic influences on tumor development. These features, plus the use of relatively limited radiation ports in treatment, make patients with these CNS tumors excellent study populations. Two retrospective reviews have demonstrated a risk for the development of radiation-induced gliomas in patients treated for pituitary adenomas.[44, 45] Tsang and colleagues[44] found the relative risk of brain tumor development to be 16 relative to the general population, and all secondary tumors in their series were gliomas. In the series reported by Brada and others,[45] the overall relative risk of developing a brain tumor was 9.4, but the risk for meningeal tumors was higher (RR = 37) than that for gliomas (RR = 8). Gliomas, however, were noted to occur sooner after radiation therapy than meningiomas. In the review of the literature of Brada and co-workers[45] on tumors incurred by pituitary adenoma and craniopharyngioma irradiation, a total of 57 were found, including 12 meningiomas, 24 soft tissue sarcomas, three osteogenic sarcomas, and 18 gliomas. The finding that radiation-induced tumors are more commonly mesenchymal than glial is similar to findings in the tinea capitis studies.[6] Only Jones[46] has failed to confirm an increased risk of secondary gliomas in patients irradiated for pituitary adenomas, leading him to conclude that radiation-induced gliomas were an established entity mostly of individuals irradiated during childhood.

CASE REPORTS OF RADIATION-INDUCED GLIOMAS

By conducting an extensive review of cases of presumed radiation-induced gliomas reported in the English literature

TABLE 61–1

RISK OF SECONDARY BRAIN TUMORS IN PATIENTS WITH ACUTE LYMPHOBLASTIC LEUKEMIA

Series: Author (Year)	No. of Patients	No. of CNS Tumors	Relative Risk
Albo et al[42] (1985)	468	9	226
Fontana et al[18] (1987)	37	3	1
Rimm et al[38] (1987)	592	1	20
Cavin et al[43] (1990)	70	2	125
Neglia et al[12] (1991)	9720	24	22

CNS, central nervous system.

since 1960, we have identified a total of 114 cases (Table 61–2), some of which have been tabulated in previous reviews.[10, 58, 65] Based on the large experience indicating that patients with leukemia may be inherently prone to the development of gliomas, such patients are considered separately in our review. To highlight the small experience of radiation-induced gliomas other than astrocytic tumors, patients with such tumors are also considered separately. The 114 cases have therefore been divided into three groups: 1, astrocytoma or glioblastoma occurring after treatment for conditions other than acute leukemia; 2, any glioma occurring after treatment of acute leukemia; and 3, gliomas other than astrocytoma or glioblastoma occurring after treatment for any condition. Three cases (see Table 61–2) fall into two of the three categories.

In regard to the general features of the 114 reported patients (Table 61–3), the ratio of males to females is 1.41:1 overall, 1.06:1 for the patients with leukemia, and 1.82:1 for other patients developing astrocytic tumors. Tumors occurred from 1 to 61 years after radiation therapy with a median latency of 7 years (mean, 10.1 years). Patients with leukemia tended to develop a secondary glioma earlier than other patients, with a median latency of 6 to 7 years vs. 9 years for the other patients (mean, 6.8 vs. 12.7 years). Moreover, leukemia survivors all developed gliomas within a rather narrow time range, from 4 to 11 years after therapy, whereas the other patients were still noted to develop gliomas 20 to 60 years after exposure. Whether this lack of late development of gliomas in leukemia survivors is merely a function of follow-up and reporting techniques or is a result of other risk factors remains unknown. The tumor latencies for the patients without leukemia shows a bimodal distribution, with peaks at 5 to 8 years and 21 to 28 years. Kitanaka and associates[66] first made this observation and suggested that two distinct mechanisms may be involved in the induction of radiation gliomas by radiation therapy. Nonetheless, the continued very late observation of secondary glioma development is important because it indicates that exposure to radiation may have lifelong or permanent sequelae.

The observation that patients with leukemia tended to develop gliomas earlier than other patients may be due to many factors, including the younger age at exposure, the concurrent use of chemotherapy, and possible genetic predisposition in leukemia patients. To assess the role of concurrent chemotherapy, the latency of tumor formation in patients without leukemia was compared for those treated with or without chemotherapy. In the nine patients receiving adjuvant chemotherapy, the median latency was 6 years (mean, 7.6 years) compared to a median latency of 8 years (mean, 13.6 years) in the 53 patients not receiving chemotherapy. This finding lends support to the notion that chemotherapy acts synergistically with radiation therapy in the pathogenesis of gliomas.

Although there is strong suspicion that the individual's age at the time of exposure to radiation plays a role in oncogenesis, analysis of these data did not show a correlation between age at irradiation and tumor latency. Whether younger age is associated with a greater chance of development of a radiation-induced tumor cannot be determined from these data, as they are merely a collection of isolated case reports. The large number of case reports of secondary gliomas in childhood cancer survivors, however, has led others to speculate that young children are more prone than adults to the development of radiation-induced tumors.[20]

The 114 tumors reported consist of 43 glioblastomas multiforme, 27 anaplastic astrocytomas, 19 astrocytomas, 4 oligoastrocytomas, 4 gliosarcomas, 3 ependymomas, and 14 gliomas or astrocytomas not otherwise specified (NOS). Of the tumors specified as to grade, 77% are high-grade tumors, including glioblastoma, anaplastic astrocytoma, mixed anaplastic tumors, and gliosarcoma. This spectrum of brain tumors is not significantly different from that seen in the general population as determined by autopsy series.[87] The rather young age at which glioblastoma multiforme occurs in these irradiated patients does differ from the pattern seen in populations with spontaneously occurring tumors. The median age of diagnosis of glioblastoma was 30 years in the group that did not have leukemia and 10 years in the leukemia group. Gliomas occurred within the spine in four patients treated for Hodgkin's disease, thyroid carcinoma, and tuberculosis, corresponding to the ports of irradiation.

Radiation-induced gliomas, as compared to their spontaneously occurring counterparts, are more commonly multifocal, as seen in 10% of the patients in this series.[87] The majority of multifocal cases developed in the cohort treated for acute leukemia, where multifocal gliomas were noted in 20% of patients. This strikingly high incidence of multifocal tumors in patients with leukemia is most likely a consequence of many factors, including a genetic predisposition to develop gliomas,[37] large fields of exposure secondary to the use of cranial or craniospinal irradiation, and the use of systemic and intrathecal chemotherapy in conjunction with radiation therapy. Of interest is that multifocal gliomas have also been noted in patients with multiple sclerosis and progressive multifocal leukoencephalopathy, both conditions characterized by patchy areas of demyelination and gliosis, which are reminiscent of the pathologic changes seen in the leukoencephalopathy associated with the use of radiation therapy and intrathecal chemotherapy in patients with leukemia.[39] Multifocal tumors were seen in only 3% of patients without leukemia who were receiving radiation therapy, a value similar to that for patients with spontaneously occurring gliomas.[87]

A correlation of radiation dose with the period of tumor latency was not performed because typically insufficient information was available to reliably make such calculations. Although the dose of radiation therapy administered was provided in most case reports, no information was available regarding the dose per fraction of radiation, the number of fractions, or the time over which ionizing radiation was administered. These factors all play a role in the biologic effect of ionizing radiation. Moreover, because the exact location of the secondary tumor in relationship to the isodose curves generated from radiation therapy of the primary malignancy was almost never provided, it was not possible to determine the actual amount of radiation exposure at the site of tumor development. As many tumors are noted to appear at the periphery of the radiation ports, this value is only a small percentage of the total dose of radiation therapy reported. Indeed, analysis performed in the past has failed to show a relationship between radiation dose and tumor latency.[10, 58]

Text continued on page 733

TABLE 61-2
CASE REPORTS OF RADIATION-INDUCED GLIOMAS

Case No.	Age at RT (yr)	Sex	Radiation Dose (rad)	Primary Diagnosis	Latency (yr)	Secondary Diagnosis	Chemotherapy	Author (Year)
1	11	M	400	Cervical adenitis	11	Glioblastoma	No	Saenger et al[47] (1960)
				Astrocytic Tumors Induced by Radiation Therapy (Patients Without Leukemia)				
2	4	M	140	Tinea capitis	4	Astrocytoma	No	Albert et al[9] (1966)
3	10	M	140	Tinea capitis	1	Astrocytoma	No	Albert et al[9] (1966)
4	10	M	250	Tinea capitis	6	Astrocytoma	No	Shore et al[7] (1976)
5	8	M	140	Tinea capitis	26	Astrocytoma	No	Shore et al[7] (1976)
6	7	M	140	Tinea capitis	5	Glioma, NOS	No	Shore et al[7] (1976)
7	22	M	5,400	Craniopharyngioma	6	Glioblastoma	No	Komaki et al[48] (1977)
8	9	F	6,007	Craniopharyngioma	6	Anaplastic astrocytoma	No	Sogg et al[49] (1978)
9	10/12	M	5,000	Medulloblastoma	11	Anaplastic astrocytoma	No	Kleriga et al[17] (1978)
10	10	M	4,000	Pineal teratoma	25	Glioblastoma	No	Robinson[50] (1978)
11	36	M	2,750	Meningioma	21	Anaplastic astrocytoma	No	Robinson[50] (1978)
12	1	F	3,960	Ependymoma	5	Glioblastoma	No	Bachman & Ostrow[51] (1978)
13	44	M	4,480	Glomus jugulare tumor	8	Anaplastic astrocytoma	No	Preissig et al[16] (1979)
14	20	F	Chest fluoroscopy	Tuberculosis	25	Astrocytoma, spinal	No	Steinbok[52] (1980)
15	21	M	4,969	Hodgkin's disease	5	Glioblastoma, spinal	No	Clifton et al[53] (1980)
16	5	M	3,000	Medulloblastoma	13	Glioblastoma	No	Pearl et al[54] (1980)
17	4	F	3,500	Medulloblastoma	15	Astrocytoma	No	Cohen et al[15] (1981)
18	17	F	4,000	Metastatic choriocarcinoma	6	Glioblastoma, multifocal	Yes	Barnes et al[55] (1982)
19	5/12	F	1,400	Retinoblastoma	8	Glioblastoma	No	Snead et al[56] (1982)
20	38	M	4,900	Pituitary adenoma	14	Glioblastoma	No	Piatt et al[57] (1983)
21	25	M	4,500	Pituitary adenoma	10	Glioblastoma	No	Piatt et al[57] (1983)
22	?	M	?	Meningioma	5	Glioma, NOS	No	Farwell & Flannery[41] (1984)
23	?	M	?	Lymphoma	1	Glioblastoma	No	Farwell & Flannery[41] (1984)
24	10/52	F	1,610	Scalp hemangioma	24	Astrocytoma	No	Zochodne et al[1] (1984)
25	11	M	5,900	Craniopharyngioma	25	Glioblastoma	No	Liwnicz et al[58] (1985)
26	2	M	3,500	Ependymoma	14	Glioblastoma	No	Liwnicz et al[58] (1985)
27	2/52	M	5,500	Retinoblastoma	12	Glioblastoma	No	Liwnicz et al[58] (1985)
28	5	M	1,800	Lymphoma	5	Anaplastic astrocytoma	Yes	Liwnicz et al[58] (1985)
29	39	F	5,000	Pituitary adenoma	5	Glioblastoma	No	Okamoto et al[59] (1985)
30	5	M	6,000	Craniopharyngioma	14	Glioblastoma	No	Maat-Schieman et al[60] (1985)
31	10	M	3,200	Lymphoma	7	Glioblastoma	Yes	Marus et al[4] (1986)
32	52	F	4,500	Pituitary adenoma	6	Anaplastic astrocytoma	No	Marus et al[4] (1986)
33	19	F	4,200	Thyroid carcinoma	23	Anaplastic astrocytoma, spinal	No	Marus et al[4] (1986)
34	2	F	1,800	Retinoblastoma	4	Glioblastoma	Yes	Marus et al[4] (1986)
35	13	M	6,000	Medulloblastoma	6	Glioblastoma	Yes	Schmidbauer et al[61] (1987)
36	2	F	5,460	Craniopharyngioma	5	Glioblastoma	No	Ushio et al[62] (1987)
37	33	M	5,500	Pituitary adenoma	8	Anaplastic astrocytoma	No	Hufnagel et al[63] (1988)

Table continued on following page

TABLE 61–2
CASE REPORTS OF RADIATION-INDUCED GLIOMAS (Continued)

Case No.	Age at RT (yr)	Sex	Radiation Dose (rad)	Primary Diagnosis	Latency (yr)	Secondary Diagnosis	Chemotherapy	Author (Year)
38	16	F	5,000	Fibrosarcoma	11	Anaplastic astrocytoma	Yes	Dierssen et al[64] (1988)
39	15	M	1,800	Chronic otitis media	11	Astrocytoma	No	Dierssen et al[64] (1988)
40	28	M	6,000	Pituitary adenoma	6	Anaplastic astrocytoma	No	Dierssen et al[64] (1988)
41	27	M	9,500	Pituitary adenoma	22	Glioblastoma	No	Shapiro et al[65] (1989)
42	13	M	3,400	Germinoma	7	Anaplastic astrocytoma	No	Kitanaka et al[66] (1989)
43	7	F	6,000	Craniopharyngioma	16	Anaplastic astrocytoma	Yes	Kitanaka et al[66] (1989)
44	11	M	4,000	Sarcoma	7	Anaplastic astrocytoma	No	Zampieri et al[67] (1989)
45	45	F	5,000	Pituitary adenoma	9	Anaplastic astrocytoma	No	Zampieri et al[67] (1989)
46	55	M	4,750	Pituitary adenoma	7	Glioblastoma	No	Flickinger et al[68] (1989)
47	31	M	4,250	Germinoma	8	Anaplastic astrocytoma	No	Tamura et al[69] (1989)
48	2	F	140	Tinea capitis	61	Glioblastoma	No	Soffer et al[8] (1990)
49	?	F	140	Tinea capitis	40	Astrocytoma	No	Soffer et al[8] (1990)
50	4	F	140	Tinea capitis	36	Astrocytoma	No	Soffer et al[8] (1990)
51	19	M	4,000	Hodgkin's disease	7	Anaplastic astrocytoma, spinal	No	Bazan et al[70] (1990)
52	24	F	4,500	Pituitary adenoma	9	Glioblastoma	No	Cavin et al[43] (1990)
53	8	M	140	Tinea capitis	26	Glioblastoma	No	Salvati et al[10] (1991)
54	14	M	5,000	Ganglioglioma	13	Glioblastoma	No	Case Records Mass. General[71] (1991)
55	34	M	4,000	Pituitary adenoma	28	Anaplastic astrocytoma, multifocal	No	Jones[46] (1991)
56	47	F	4,500	Pituitary adenoma	12	Glioblastoma	No	Jones[46] (1991)
57	54	M	>4,000	Pituitary adenoma	6	Glioblastoma	No	Brada et al[45] (1992)
58	40	F	>4,000	Pituitary adenoma	7	Glioblastoma	No	Brada et al[45] (1992)
59	26	M	4,250	Pituitary adenoma	10	Brainstem glioma	No	Tsang et al[44] (1993)
60	34	F	5,000	Pituitary adenoma	10	Glioblastoma	No	Tsang et al[44] (1993)
61	42	M	5,000	Pituitary adenoma	15	Glioblastoma	No	Tsang et al[44] (1993)
62	38	M	5,000	Pituitary adenoma	8	Anaplastic astrocytoma	No	Tsang et al[44] (1993)
Gliomas Induced by Radiation Therapy (Patients With Leukemia)								
63	3	?	2,623	ALL	6	Astrocytoma	Yes	Walters[72] (1979)
64	2	M	2,400	ALL	5	Glioblastoma	Yes	Chung et al[73] (1981)
65	4	F	3,400	ALL	5	Glioblastoma, multifocal	Yes	Sanders et al[74] (1982)
66	3	F	2,400	ALL	6	Anaplastic astrocytoma, multifocal	Yes	Anderson & Treip[75] (1984)
67	3	F	2,400	ALL	9	Astrocytoma, multifocal	Yes	Judge et al[76] (1984)
68	6	F	2,400	ALL	7	Anaplastic astrocytoma	Yes	Raffel et al[77] (1985)
69–77	≤5	5 M, 4 F	2,400	ALL	≤7	4 Astrocytoma, 4 glioma (NOS), 1 ependymoma	Yes	Albo et al[42] (1985)

Case	Age (yr)	Sex	Dose (rad)	Primary diagnosis	Induced tumor	Latency (yr)		Reference
78	8	F	2,000	ALL	Astrocytoma, spinal	4	Yes	Malone et al[78] (1986)
79	19	M	2,516	ALL	Astrocytoma	5	Yes	Malone et al[78] (1986)
80	6	F	2,400	ALL	Anaplastic astrocytoma	5	Yes	Malone et al[78] (1986)
81	3	M	4,800	ALL	Anaplastic astrocytoma	8	Yes	McWhirter et al[79] (1986)
82	2	F	2,400	ALL	Astrocytoma, multifocal	9	Yes	Edwards et al[80] (1986)
83	5	F	2,400	ALL	Astrocytoma	5	Yes	Edwards et al[80] (1986)
84	3	M	4,800	ALL	Glioblastoma	7	Yes	Edwards et al[80] (1986)
85	4	M	2,400	ALL	Anaplastic astrocytoma	4	Yes	Edwards et al[80] (1986)
86	6	M	2,400	ALL	Glioblastoma/oligodendroglioma, multifocal	11	Yes	Fontana et al[18] (1987)
87	6	F	2,400	ALL	Anaplastic astrocytoma, multifocal	10	Yes	Fontana et al[18] (1987)
88	3	M	2,400	ALL	Glioblastoma, multifocal	6	Yes	Fontana et al[18] (1987)
89	?	?	2,400	ALL	Astrocytoma, NOS	5	Yes	Kingston et al[5] (1987)
90	?	?	2,400	ALL	Astrocytoma, NOS	4	Yes	Kingston et al[5] (1987)
91	?	?	2,400	ALL	Astrocytoma, NOS	5	Yes	Kingston et al[5] (1987)
92	?	?	2,400	ALL	Astrocytoma, NOS	6	Yes	Kingston et al[5] (1987)
93	?	?	2,400	ALL	Astrocytoma, NOS	9	Yes	Kingston et al[5] (1987)
94	?	?	2,400	ALL	Astrocytoma, NOS	7	Yes	Kingston et al[5] (1987)
95	5	M	2,400	ALL	Anaplastic astrocytoma, multifocal	10	Yes	Rimm et al[38] (1987)
96	3	M	2,400	ALL	Oligoastrocytoma	11	Yes	Palma et al[20] (1988)
97	3	M	4,800	ALL	Glioma, NOS	7	Yes	Shapiro et al[65] (1989)
98	2	F	2,400	ALL	Glioma, multifocal	9	Yes	Shapiro et al[65] (1989)
99	5	F	2,400	ALL	Anaplastic astrocytoma	6	Yes	Shapiro et al[65] (1989)
100	4	M	2,400	ALL	Anaplastic astrocytoma	4	Yes	Shapiro et al[65] (1989)
101	6	F	2,400	ALL	Glioblastoma	4	Yes	Shapiro et al[65] (1989)
102	1	M	2,400	ALL	Glioblastoma	9	Yes	Cavin et al[43] (1990)
103	3	F	2,400	ALL	Glioblastoma	7	Yes	Cavin et al[43] (1990)
104	12	M	2,400	ALL	Glioblastoma	6	Yes	Salvati et al[10] (1991)
105	10	F	2,400	ALL	Glioblastoma	11	Yes	Salvati et al[10] (1991)
106	3	M	1,800	AML	Glioblastoma	10	Yes	Zagzag et al[81] (1992)

Radiation-Induced Gliomas Other than Astrocytomas

Case	Age (yr)	Sex	Dose (rad)	Primary diagnosis	Induced tumor	Latency (yr)		Reference
107	<1	?	550	Histiocytosis	Ependymoma	15	Yes	Haselow et al[3] (1978)
108	36	M	5,814	Meningioma	Gliosarcoma	1	No	Averback[82] (1978)
109	52	F	5,400	Pituitary adenoma	Gliosarcoma	1	No	Averback[82] (1978)
110	25	F	4,200	Pituitary adenoma	Ependymoma	6	No	Anderson & Triep[75] (1984)
77*	≤5	?	2,400	ALL	Ependymoma	≤7	Yes	Albo et al[42] (1985)

Table continued on following page

TABLE 61–2
CASE REPORTS OF RADIATION-INDUCED GLIOMAS *(Continued)*

Case No.	Age at RT (yr)	Sex	Radiation Dose (rad)	Primary Diagnosis	Latency (yr)	Secondary Diagnosis	Chemotherapy	Author (Year)
111	32	M	5,600	Meningioma	10	Oligodendroglioma/ Glioblastoma	No	Zuccarello et al[83] (1986)
86*	6	M	2,400	ALL	11	Oligodendroglioma/ Glioblastoma, multifocal	Yes	Fontana et al[18] (1987)
112	26	M	6,600	Pituitary adenoma	12	Anaplastic oligodendroglioma	No	Huang et al[84] (1987)
96*	3	M	2,400	ALL	11	Oligoastrocytoma	Yes	Palma et al[20] (1988)
113	27	F	1 cm³ Thorotrast	Cerebral abscess	21	Gliosarcoma	No	Reid et al[85] (1988)
114	26	F	5,000	Mucoepidermoid carcinoma	8	Gliosarcoma	No	Beute et al[86] (1991)

*Case listed more than once.
NOS, not otherwise specified; ALL, acute lymphoblastic leukemia; AML, acute myelogenous leukemia.

TABLE 61–3
SUMMARY OF 114 CASES OF RADIATION-INDUCED GLIOMAS

Characteristic	All Patients	Patients Without Leukemia			Patients With Leukemia
		Total	CXT+	CXT−	
Sex					
M	62	40			19
F	44	22			18
Tumor latency					
No. of patients	106	62	9	53	44
Median (years)	7	9	6	8	6–7
Range (years)	1–61	1–61	1–16	1–61	4–11
Tumor histology					
Glioblastoma multiforme	43				
Anaplastic astrocytoma	27				
Astrocytoma	19				
Oligoastrocytoma	4				
Ependymoma	3				
Glioma, NOS	14				
Gliosarcoma	4				
Total lesions	114				
Multifocal lesions, No. (%)	11 (10)	2 (3)			9 (20)

NOS, Not otherwise specified; CXT+, patients who underwent chemotherapy; CXT−, patients who did not have chemotherapy.

Little is known about the clinical outcome of patients with radiation-induced gliomas because most reports do not provide this information. Shapiro and co-workers,[65] in their analysis of cases of radiation-induced gliomas, did address this issue, however, and found that such patients had shorter survival times than patients with spontaneously occurring gliomas. However, patients treated comparably to those with spontaneously occurring tumors had expected survival times. Typically, patients with radiation-induced gliomas receive less aggressive therapy because of their physicians' concerns about cerebral radiation necrosis and because of concerns of their family regarding further psychosocial hardships for the patient.

Although the cases summarized in Table 61–2 represent an extensive review of the literature, some cases of possible radiation-induced gliomas were not included because established criteria were not met. In particular, cases of anaplastic astrocytoma or glioblastoma thought to occur from radiation therapy for primary astrocytomas were not included because the histologic characteristics of the two tumors do not differ significantly and anaplastic progression could not be ruled out. However, the evidence in at least some of these cases is sufficient to invoke radiation therapy as a likely pathogenetic factor. Dirks and colleagues[88] reviewed a series of high-grade gliomas developing in patients with primary low-grade astrocytic tumors, mostly pilocytic astrocytomas, optic gliomas, and cerebellar gliomas—tumors thought not to progress to a malignant state. They make a compelling argument that those patients should be included among patients with radiation-induced gliomas. In their review of 55 children with optic/hypothalamic glioma, only children treated with radiation therapy (i.e., 5 of 30 patients) had later development of higher-grade tumors, whereas none of the patients who were not treated with radiation therapy had malignant degeneration. In this extensive review of the literature, these authors did not find a single case of malignant transformation of either a low-grade cerebellar astrocy-

toma or a pilocytic optic chiasmatic tumor in the absence of radiation therapy.[88] This lends support to the role of radiation therapy in the malignant degeneration of low-grade astrocytomas and warrants their inclusion in the growing list of radiation-induced gliomas.

CONCLUSION

Although radiation-induced meningiomas and cranial sarcomas have long been accepted as distinct entities, the acceptance of radiation-induced gliomas as valid clinical diagnostic category has been slow to develop. As this review indicates, however, all criteria for the inclusion of gliomas as radiation-induced tumors have been met. In addition to a growing literature of individual case reports, large epidemiologic studies have confirmed an increased risk of glial tumor development after radiation exposure, and some studies have even demonstrated a dose-response relationship. Laboratory studies in animals, especially in primates, also show a high incidence of malignant gliomas in irradiated animals.

Several features of radiation-induced gliomas are distinctive. The risk of developing a radiation-induced glioma is lower than the risk of developing a radiation-induced meningioma, as has been demonstrated in the case of low-exposure studies (dental x-rays), moderate-dose studies (tinea capitis treatment), and high-dose exposures (treatment of pituitary adenomas). Studies have also shown that gliomas occur earlier after radiation therapy than do meningiomas, but that the increased risk of tumor development is long-term, perhaps even lifelong. Certain patients are at particular risk to develop radiation-induced gliomas, such as patients with ALL, in whom a genetic predisposition for glioma development may be compounded by exposure to radiation and chemotherapy. Indeed, in those patients, the more common radiation-induced mesenchymal tumors have only rarely been reported.[18]

Radiation-induced gliomas, therefore, are a distinct entity on the grounds of clinical, epidemiologic, and basic experimental research. Their recognition is important so that further studies can elucidate the pathogenesis of the radiation-induced and spontaneously occurring forms of gliomas. More than likely, their incidence will continue to increase as long as radiation therapy is used to control oncologic disease more effectively.

REFERENCES

1. Zochodne DW, Cairncross G, Arce FP, et al: Astrocytoma following scalp radiotherapy in infancy. Can J Neurol Sci 1984; 11:475.
2. Kohn HI, Fry RJ: Radiation carcinogenesis. N Engl J Med 1984; 310:504.
3. Haselow RE, Nesbit M, Dehner LP, et al: Second neoplasms following megavoltage radiation in a pediatric population. Cancer 1978; 42:1185.
4. Marus G, Levin CV, Rutherfoord GS: Malignant glioma following radiotherapy for unrelated primary tumors. Cancer 1986; 58:886.
5. Kingston JE, Hawkins MM, Draper GJ, et al: Patterns of multiple primary tumours in patients treated for cancer during childhood. Br J Cancer 1987; 56:331.
6. Ron E, Modan B, Boige JD, et al: Tumors of the brain and nervous system after radiotherapy in childhood. N Engl J Med 1988; 319:1033.
7. Shore RE, Albert RE, Pasternack BS: Follow-up study of patients treated by x-ray epilation for tinea capitis: Resurvey of post-treatment illness and mortality experience. Arch Environ Health 1976; 31:17.
8. Soffer D, Gomori M, Pomeranz S, et al: Gliomas following low-dose irradiation to the head: Report of three cases. J Neurooncol 1990; 8:67.
9. Albert RE, Omran AR, Brauer EW, et al: Follow-up study of patients treated by x-ray for tinea capitis. Am J Public Health 1966; 56:2114.
10. Salvati M, Artico M, Caruso R, et al: A report on radiation-induced gliomas. Cancer 1991; 67:3927.
11. Mack EE, Wilson CB: Meningiomas induced by high-dose cranial irradiation. J Neurosurg 1993; 79:28.
12. Neglia JP, Meadows AT, Robison LL, et al: Second neoplasms after acute lymphoblastic leukemia in childhood. N Engl J Med 1991; 325:1330.
13. Rottenberg DA, Chernik NL, Deck MDF, et al: Cerebral necrosis following radiotherapy of extracranial neoplasms. Ann Neurol 1977; 1:339.
14. Kemper TL, O'Neill R, Caveness WF: Effects of single dose supervoltage whole brain radiation in Macaca mulatta. J Neuropathol Exp Neurol 1977; 36:916.
15. Cohen MS, Kushner MJ, Dell S: Frontal lobe astrocytoma following radiotherapy for medulloblastoma. Neurology 1981; 31:616.
16. Preissig SH, Bohmfalk GL, Reichel GW, et al: Anaplastic astrocytoma following radiation for a glomus jugulare tumor. Cancer 1979; 43:2243.
17. Kleriga E, Sher JH, Nallainathan S, et al: Development of cerebellar malignant astrocytoma at site of a medulloblastoma treated 11 years earlier. J Neurosurg 1978; 49:445.
18. Fontana M, Stanton C, Pompili A, et al: Late multifocal gliomas in adolescents previously treated for acute lymphoblastic leukemia. Cancer 1987; 60:1510.
19. Schmidbauer M, Budka H, Bruckner R, et al: Glioblastoma developing at the site of a cerebellar medulloblastoma treated 6 years earlier. J Neurosurg 1987; 67:915.
20. Palma L, Vagnozzi R, Armino L, et al: Post-radiation glioma in a child: Case report and review of the literature. Childs Nerv Syst 1988; 4:296.
21. Vogel HH, Zaldivar R: Cocarcinogenesis: The interaction of chemical and physical agents. Radiat Res 1971; 47:644.
22. Solleveld HA: Brain tumors in man and animals: Report of a workshop. Environ Health Perspect 1986; 68:155.
23. Kent SP, Pickering JE: Neoplasms in monkeys (Macaca mulatta): Spontaneous and irradiation-induced. Cancer 1958; 11:138.
24. Haymaker W, Rubinstein LJ, Miquel J: Brain tumors in irradiated monkeys. Acta Neuropathol (Berl) 1972; 20:267.
25. Krupp JH: Nine-year mortality experience in proton-exposed Macaca mulatta. Radiat Res 1976; 67:244.
26. Castanera TJ, Jones DC, Kimeldord DJ, et al: The influence of whole-body exposure to x-rays or neutrons on the life span distribution of tumors among male rats. Cancer Res 1968; 28:170.
27. Knowles JF: Radiation-induced nervous system tumours in the rat. Int J Radiat Biol 1982; 41:79.
28. Traynor JE, Casey HW: Five year follow-up of primates exposed to 55 MeV protons. Radiat Res 1971; 47:143.
29. Preston-Martin S, Mack W, Henderson BE: Risk factors for gliomas and meningiomas in males in Los Angeles County. Cancer Res 1989; 49:6137.
30. Neuberger JS, Brownson RC, Morantz RA, et al: Association of brain cancer with dental x-rays and occupation in Missouri. Cancer Detect Prev 1991; 15:31.
31. Burch JD, Craib KJP, Choi BCK, et al: An exploratory case-control study of brain tumors in adults. J Natl Cancer Inst 1987; 78:601.
32. Wrensch M, Bondy ML, Wiencke J, et al: Environmental risk factors for primary malignant brain tumors: A review. J Neurooncol 1993; 17:47.
33. Ryan P, Lee MW, North B, et al: Risk factors for tumors of the brain and meninges: Results from the Adelaide Adult Brain Tumor Study. Int J Cancer 1992; 51:20.
34. Ryan P, Lee MW, North B, et al: Amalgam fillings, diagnostic dental x-rays and tumours of the brain and meninges. Eur J Cancer B Oral Oncol 1992; 28B:91.
35. Alexander V: Brain tumor risk among United States nuclear workers. Occup Med (Oxf) 1991; 6:695.
36. Hawkins MM, Draper GJ, Kingston JE: Incidence of second primary tumours among childhood cancer survivors. Br J Cancer 1987; 56:339.
37. Meadows AT, D'Angio GJ, Miké V, et al: Patterns of second malignant neoplasms in children. Cancer 1977; 40:1903.
38. Rimm IJ, Ki FC, Tarbell NJ, et al: Brain tumors after cranial irradiation for childhood acute lymphoblastic leukemia: A 13 year experience from the Dana-Farber Cancer Institute and The Children's Hospital. Cancer 1987; 59:1506.
39. Shapiro S, Mealey J: Late anaplastic gliomas in children previously treated for acute lymphoblastic leukemia. Pediatr Neurosci 1989; 15:176.
40. Farwell J, Flannery JT: Cancer in relatives of children with central nervous system neoplasms. N Engl J Med 1984; 311:749.
41. Farwell J, Flannery JT: Second primaries in children with central nervous system tumors. J Neurooncol 1984; 2:371.
42. Albo V, Miller D, Leiken S, et al: Nine brain tumors as a late effect in children "cured" of acute lymphoblastic leukemia from a single protocol study (141). Proc Am Soc Clin Oncol 1985; 4:172.
43. Cavin LW, Dalrymple GV, McGuire EL, et al: CNS tumor induction by radiotherapy: A report of four new cases and estimate of dose required. Int J Radiat Oncol Biol Phys 1990; 18:399.
44. Tsang RW, Laperriere NJ, Simpson WJ, et al: Glioma arising after radiation therapy for pituitary adenoma. Cancer 1993; 72:2227.
45. Brada M, Ford D, Ashley S, et al: Risk of second brain tumour after conservative surgery and radiotherapy for pituitary adenoma. Br Med J 1992; 304:1343.
46. Jones A: Radiation oncogenesis in relation to the treatment of pituitary tumours. Clin Endocrinol (Oxf) 1991; 35:379.
47. Saenger EL, Silverman FN, Sterling TD, et al: Neoplasia following therapeutic irradiation for benign conditions in childhood. Radiology 1960; 74:889.
48. Komaki S, Komaki R, Choi H, et al: Radiation- and drug-induced intracranial neoplasm with angiographic demonstration. Neurol Med Chir 1977; 17:55.
49. Sogg RL, Donaldson SS, Yorke CH: Malignant astrocytoma following radiotherapy of a craniopharyngioma. J Neurosurg 1978; 48:622.
50. Robinson RG: A second brain tumour and irradiation. J Neurol Neurosurg Psychiatry 1978; 41:1005.
51. Bachman DS, Ostrow PT: Fatal long-term sequela following radiation "cure" for ependymoma. Ann Neurol 1978; 4:319.
52. Steinbok P: Spinal cord glioma after multiple fluoroscopies during artificial pneumothorax treatment of pulmonary tuberculosis. J Neurosurg 1980; 52:838.
53. Clifton MD, Amromin GD, Perry MC, et al: Spinal cord glioma following irradiation for Hodgkin's disease. Cancer 1980; 45:2051.
54. Pearl GS, Mirra SS, Miles ML: Glioblastoma multiforme occurring 13 years after treatment of a medulloblastoma. Neurosurgery 1980; 6:546.
55. Barnes AE, Liwnicz BH, Schellhas HF, et al: Successful treatment of placental choriocarcinoma metastatic to brain followed by primary brain glioblastoma. Gynecol Oncol 1982; 13:108.

56. Snead OC, Acker JD, Morawetz RW, et al: High resolution computerized tomography with coronal and sagittal reconstruction in the diagnosis of brain tumors in children. Childs Brain 1982; 9:1.

57. Piatt JH, Blue JM, Schold SC, et al: Glioblastoma multiforme after radiotherapy for acromegaly. Neurosurgery 1983; 13:85.

58. Liwnicz BH, Berger TS, Liwnicz R, et al: Radiation-associated gliomas: A report of four cases and analysis of postradiation tumors of the central nervous system. Neurosurgery 1985; 17:436.

59. Okamoto S, Handa H, Yamashita J, et al: Postirradiation brain tumors. Neurol Med Chir 1985; 5:528.

60. Maat-Schieman MLC, Bots GTAM, Thomeer RTWM, et al: Malignant astrocytoma following radiotherapy for craniopharyngioma. Br J Radiol 1985; 58:480.

61. Schmidbauer M, Budka H, Bruckner R, et al: Glioblastoma developing at the site of a cerebellar medulloblastoma treated six years earlier. J Neurosurg 1987; 67:915.

62. Ushio Y, Arita N, Yoshimine T, et al: Glioblastoma after radiotherapy for craniopharyngioma: Case report. Neurosurgery 1987; 21:33.

63. Hufnagel TJ, Kim JH, Lesser R, et al: Malignant glioma of the optic chiasm eight years after radiotherapy for prolactinoma. Arch Ophthalmol 1988; 106:1701.

64. Dierssen G, Alvarez G, Figols J: Anaplastic astrocytomas associated with previous radiotherapy: Report of three cases. Neurosurgery 1988; 22:1095.

65. Shapiro S, Mealey J, Sartorius C: Radiation-induced intracranial malignant gliomas. J Neurosurg 1989; 71:77.

66. Kitanaka C, Shitara N, Nakagomi T, et al: Postradiation astrocytoma: Report of two cases. J Neurosurg 1989; 70:469.

67. Zampieri P, Zorat PL, Mingrino S, et al: Radiation associated cerebral gliomas: A report of two cases and review of the literature. J Neurosurg Sci 1989; 33:271.

68. Flickinger JC, Nelson PB, Martinez AJ, et al: Radiotherapy of nonfunctional adenomas of the pituitary gland: Results with long-term follow-up. Cancer 1989; 63:2409.

69. Tamura T, Nakamura S, Shirata K, et al: Cerebellar malignant glioma after radiation therapy for suprasellar germinoma. Neurol Med Chir 1989; 29:2239.

70. Bazan C, New PZ, Kagan-Hallet KS: MRI of radiation-induced spinal cord glioma. Neuroradiology 1990; 32:331.

71. Case records of the Massachusetts General Hospital (case 23–1991). N Engl J Med 1991; 324:1651.

72. Walters TR: Childhood acute lymphocytic leukemia with a second primary neoplasm. Am J Pediatr Hematol Oncol 1979; 1:285.

73. Chung CK, Stryker JA, Cruse R, et al: Glioblastoma multiforme following prophylactic cranial irradiation and intrathecal methotrexate in a child with acute lymphocytic leukemia. Cancer 1981; 47:2563.

74. Sanders J, Sale GE, Ramberg R, et al: Glioblastoma multiforme in a patient with acute lymphoblastic leukemia who received a marrow transplant. Transplant Proc 1982; 14:770.

75. Anderson JR, Treip CS: Radiation-induced intracranial neoplasms: A report of three cases. Cancer 1984; 53:426.

76. Judge MR, Eden OB, O'Neill P: Cerebral glioma after cranial prophylaxis for acute lymphoblastic leukemia. Br Med J 1984; 289:1038.

77. Raffel C, Edwards MSB, Davis RL, et al: Postirradiation cerebellar glioma. J Neurosurg 1985; 62:300.

78. Malone M, Lumley H, Erdohazi M: Astrocytoma as a second malignancy in patients with acute lymphoblastic leukemia. Cancer 1986; 57:1979.

79. McWhirter WR, Pearn JH, Smith G, et al: Cerebral astrocytoma as a complication of acute lymphoblastic leukaemia. Med J Aust 1986; 145:96.

80. Edwards MK, Terry JG, Montebello JF, et al: Gliomas in children following radiation therapy for lymphoblastic leukemia. Acta Radiol Suppl 1986; 369:6513.

81. Zagzag D, Miller DC, Cangiarella J, et al: Brainstem glioma after radiation therapy for acute myeloblastic leukemia in a child with Down syndrome: Possible pathogenetic mechanisms. Cancer 1992; 70:1188.

82. Averback P: Mixed intracranial sarcomas: Rare forms and a new association with previous radiation therapy. Ann Neurol 1978; 4:229.

83. Zuccarello M, Sawaya R, deCourten-Myers G: Glioblastoma occurring after radiation therapy for meningioma: Case report and review of literature. Neurosurgery 1986; 19:114.

84. Huang CI, Chiou WH, Ho DM: Oligodendroglioma occurring after radiation therapy for pituitary adenoma. J Neurol Neurosurg Psychiatry 1987; 50:1619.

85. Reid PM, Barber PC, Phil D: Gliosarcoma developing in close relationship to an abscess cavity injected with Thorotrast. Surg Neurol 1988; 29:67.

86. Beute BJ, Fobben ES, Hubschmann O, et al: Cerebellar gliosarcoma: Report of a probable radiation-induced neoplasm. AJNR Am J Neuroradiol 1991; 12:554.

87. Russell DS, Rubinstein LJ: Pathology of Tumors of the Nervous System, ed 5. Baltimore, Williams & Wilkins, 1989.

88. Dirks PB, Jay V, Becker LE, et al: Development of anaplastic changes in low-grade astrocytomas of childhood. Neurosurgery 1994; 34:68.

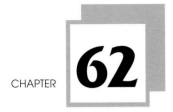

DENNIS C. SHRIEVE

PHILIP H. GUTIN

DAVID A. LARSON

CHAPTER **62**

Central Nervous System Toxic Effects of Radiotherapy

Spinal cord and brain are often irradiated during the course of radiation therapy for a primary or metastatic neoplasm involving the central nervous system (CNS) or during the treatment of non-CNS malignancies, such as head and neck cancers, lung cancers, or lymphomas. The mechanisms of CNS damage resulting from radiation are poorly understood. Unfortunately, much of the literature on the tolerance of CNS to therapeutic irradiation is anecdotal, and it is difficult to assign a precise risk to any clinical situation. Although some sequelae of CNS irradiation may be unavoidable, adherence to standard guidelines will prevent complications in the vast majority of patients treated.

RADIATION-ASSOCIATED TOXIC EFFECTS

Brain

In general, toxic effects associated with irradiation of the human brain are categorized according to the time at which they become apparent:

1. *Acute reactions* occur during radiation therapy.

2. *Early-delayed reactions* occur within weeks of radiation.

3. *Late reactions* occur months to years following treatment.

ACUTE REACTIONS

Acute reactions associated with irradiation of brain tumors are usually not severe. The most common acute side effect of cranial irradiation is hair loss, which is associated with the local dose to the scalp. Other acute effects of cranial irradiation are associated with increased edema or intracranial pressure caused by an acute reaction of the tumor to treatment. Pre-existing neurologic deficits may worsen or a clinical syndrome may appear that is consistent with an increase in intracranial pressure. The appearance of such early effects is usually associated with significant postopera-

tive residual tumor and critical location. These effects are usually minimized by administration of corticosteroids.[1]

Acute reactions occur infrequently with the use of conventional daily dose fractionation (1.8 to 2.0 Gy/day). Higher daily doses up to 6 Gy are also well tolerated with appropriate reduction in total dose.[2] However, larger single daily fractions to large volumes are poorly tolerated. Acute complications (nausea, headache, fever) may occur in up to 50% of patients who receive treatment to the whole brain with 10 Gy as a single fraction or with 15 Gy in two fractions over 3 days.[3, 4] Life-threatening herniation may occur in 10% of patients so treated.

EARLY-DELAYED REACTIONS

Subacute effects of cranial irradiation are related to transient demyelination mediated by radiation injury to oligodendrocytes or through alterations in capillary permeability. The most common clinical manifestations are a transient syndrome of somnolence, anorexia, and irritability following cranial irradiation (somnolence syndrome). Occasionally new neurologic symptoms may develop in patients during the subacute period.

The *somnolence syndrome* is well described in pediatric patients with acute lymphoblastic leukemia (ALL) following whole-brain irradiation and usually occurs within 10 weeks of the end of treatment.[5, 6] The syndrome is more commonly recognized in children younger than 3 years. An associated protein elevation and pleocytosis of the cerebrospinal fluid may be present. However, lack of focal neurologic manifestations is typical. Up to 75% of children receiving prophylactic cranial irradiation for ALL may develop the syndrome. The impact of fraction size on this incidence is not clear.[5, 7] Somnolence syndrome is a self-limiting process, but patients may benefit from administration of steroids. The occurrence of somnolence syndrome in patients with ALL does not appear to have an impact on the rate of relapse, survival, or development of late sequelae.[7, 8] This syndrome occurs only rarely in patients treated with limited fields for primary brain tumors.

The development of new neurologic deficits in the subacute period following cranial irradiation is uncommon. Several reports of small numbers of patients in whom *transient* symptoms of nausea, vomiting, ataxia, dysphagia, or dysarthria develop approximately 10 weeks following cranial radiotherapy suggest that management decisions based on such symptoms should be made cautiously during this time.[9, 10] Such symptoms do not necessarily indicate treatment failure. Administration of corticosteroids may be effective in relieving symptoms.

LATE EFFECTS

Late effects following cranial irradiation occur within several months or up to many years following treatment. Clinical and radiographic changes vary from asymptomatic changes of the white matter and vasculature[11] to changes in cognitive abilities,[12] hypothalamic pituitary dysfunction,[13] cranial neuropathy, frank tissue necrosis, and second malignancies. Development of hypothalamic-pituitary dysfunction, cognitive deficits, and second tumors following CNS irradiation are discussed in detail in other chapters.

The pathogenesis of the various late effects of radiotherapy has not been well elucidated. It is likely that several mechanisms are involved, including demyelination secondary to injury to the oligodendrocytes,[14, 15] damage to small and medium-sized blood vessels,[16–18] release of factors (e.g., cytokines) from injured cells, and an immunologic response.[19]

RADIATION NECROSIS

Sheline and co-workers[20] examined 80 cases of cerebral necrosis following cranial irradiation. The interval from completion of radiotherapy to development of necrosis ranged from 4 months to 7.5 years. The total radiation dose, daily dose, and overall treatment time were documented for all patients. Plotting the total dose vs. the number of fractions for each case of necrosis described a line representing the threshold for radionecrosis. The authors defined the term *neuret* as follows:

$$\text{Neuret} = D \times N^{-0.41} \times T^{-0.03}$$

where *D, N,* and *T* represent the total dose, number of fractions, and overall time, respectively. From this analysis one finds that the threshold dose for necrosis is 35 Gy in 10 fractions, 60 Gy in 35 fractions, and 76 Gy in 60 fractions when treatments are given 5 days/week. This threshold corresponds to approximately 1250 neuret. This work indicated the relative importance of number of fractions (and, therefore, dose per fraction) in determining risk of late effects following radiotherapy. Daily dose and total dose have been reconfirmed to be the most important factors determining risk of radionecrosis by Marks and others.[21] They suggested that a dose biologically equivalent to 54 Gy in 30 fractions represented the threshold for radionecrosis. A reanalysis of these data indicated no cases of necrosis in 51 patients receiving 57.6 Gy or less; necrosis was present in two of 60 patients (3.3%) treated with doses of 57.6 to 64.8 Gy and in five of 28 patients (18%) following doses of 64.8 to 75.6 Gy.[22]

These clinical studies form the basis of what is considered to be standard radiotherapy for intracranial tumors. Benign or low-grade tumors receive 54 Gy in 30 fractions, which carries virtually no risk of radionecrosis but is efficacious in a wide range of diseases, including meningiomas and low-grade gliomas. This dose corresponds to the more conservative recommendation of Marks and associates.[21] Malignant gliomas (anaplastic astrocytomas and glioblastoma multiforme) are less well-controlled by 54 Gy, and the aggressiveness of the disease warrants a higher dose and a small risk of necrosis. A standard dose would be 60 Gy in 30 to 33 fractions, corresponding to a dose just above the threshold established by Sheline and co-workers.[20]

CRANIAL NEUROPATHY

Fraction size has been found to be of primary importance when considering radiation tolerance of optic nerve and other cranial nerves. Harris and Levene[23] showed clearly that daily doses in excess of 250 cGy were associated with an increased risk of visual loss in patients irradiated for pituitary adenoma or craniopharyngioma. Goldsmith and colleagues[24] applied the neuret formula to the analysis of radiation-induced optic neuropathy and found that fraction size was much more important than overall time. They proposed a model defining the *optic ret* as follows:

$$\text{Optic ret} = D \times N^{-0.53}$$

where the term for overall time has been omitted, emphasizing the relative importance of fraction size. Goldsmith and others[24] have recommended a threshold dose for optic neuropathy of 890 optic ret, which corresponds to 54 Gy in 30 fractions. Parsons and co-workers[25] recently reported no incident of optic neuropathy in 106 patients receiving doses less than 59 Gy.[25] In patients receiving higher doses, an 11% risk of optic neuropathy was found when dose per fraction was less than 1.9 Gy and 47% for higher doses per fraction. These findings emphasize the importance of dose per fraction and are consistent with the recommendations of Goldsmith and co-workers.[24]

The previous formulas for *neuret* and *optic ret* appear to be useful guidelines for establishment of dose regimens that avoid cerebral necrosis or optic neuropathy in a vast majority of cases. However, caution should be used when extrapolating to either very small numbers of fractions (e.g., radiosurgery) or large numbers of fractions (e.g., hyperfractionated radiotherapy). The effect of treatment volume is also an important consideration not accounted for in these models.

NECROTIZING LEUKOENCEPHALOPATHY AND MINERALIZING MICROANGIOPATHY

Necrotizing leukoencephalopathy (disseminated necrotizing leukoencephalopathy or subacute leukoencephalopathy) presents as progressive development of disorientation, memory loss, changes in personality, or frank dementia. First described in children treated for ALL, it is seen in up to 15% of such children receiving cranial irradiation and methotrexate.[26] Development of nonenhancing, periventricular hypodensities on CT progressing to ventricular dilatation and broadening of the sulci are the radiographic hallmarks. Histopathologically, lesions are characterized by demyelination, multifocal coagulation necrosis, and gliosis. Most children who survive the syndrome suffer some permanent neurologic deficit. Although classically described in children, leukoencephalopathy may also be seen in adults treated with cranial radiotherapy, with or without chemotherapy.[27, 28]

Mineralizing microangiopathy presents as headache, focal seizure, ataxia, behavioral changes, or motor disability. A computed tomographic (CT) scan may show calcification of the basal ganglia. Histopathologic analysis may show occlusion of small blood vessels by calcium deposits, with surrounding brain tissue being mineralized and necrotic.[29]

COGNITIVE EFFECTS

The risk of treatment-induced cognitive disability following radiotherapy for brain tumors has not been well quantified. Cranial irradiation has been associated with learning disabilities in the setting of low-dose whole-brain radiotherapy in very young children with leukemia.[12] Clearly, high-dose whole-brain radiotherapy may result in dementia in some patients treated for brain metastases, but the incidence is not precisely known.[30] Effects of partial brain radiotherapy on memory, intellect, or other testable measures of cognitive function are not predictable in either pediatric or adult populations.[31] Factors such as patient age, tumor site and volume, radiation dose, and previous treatment with surgery and/or chemotherapy are co-variables that make evaluation of the effects of radiotherapy difficult.[12] Careful neuropsychological testing of patients with long potential follow-up is required to more precisely define the risk to patients undergoing partial brain radiotherapy.

RADIOGRAPHIC CHANGES FOLLOWING CRANIAL RADIOTHERAPY

Late radiation injury may present radiographically as focal necrosis or diffuse white matter changes. Focal necrosis appears on imaging as a low-density region with mass effect and irregular contrast enhancing margins surrounded by edema. This pattern is often difficult to distinguish from focally recurrent tumor. Positron emission tomography (PET) or single-photon emission computed tomography (SPECT) may be useful in making this distinction.[32, 33]

Diffuse white matter changes present radiographically as bilateral low-density regions involving much of the hemispheric white matter. Such changes seen in patients following irradiation are usually indistinguishable from white matter changes seen in aging, non-irradiated patients or in those with cerebral vascular disease. Determining the precise incidence of such changes following radiotherapy depends on the criteria used in defining injury.[34, 35] The incidence certainly increases with increasing dose, volume irradiated, interval since radiotherapy, and patient age. Clinically significant deficits may be associated with these radiographic changes, or patients may be asymptomatic.[36] Diffuse white matter changes may occur at lower doses and with a longer latent period than for focal necrosis. Associated cerebral atrophy may occur.[28]

Spinal Cord

Radiation myelopathies may be subcategorized as follows:

1. *Transient radiation myelopathies* appear within 12 months of radiotherapy.

2. *Delayed radiation myelopathies* occur later that 12 months following radiotherapy.

Radiation tolerance of the spinal cord is a dose-limiting factor in the treatment of many malignancies: intrinsic spinal cord tumors, spinous metastases, Hodgkin's lymphoma, and carcinoma of the head and neck, esophagus, and lung. As with radiation-induced damage to brain parenchyma, the risk of spinal cord injury increases with increasing dose per fraction and total radiation dose. Radiation-associated myelopathy may occur within months of radiotherapy and be transient in nature, or it may have a delayed time of onset and be permanent in nature.

TRANSIENT RADIATION MYELOPATHY

Transient radiation-induced myelopathy is described by patients as "electric shocks" radiating from the spine down the upper extremities on flexion of the neck (Lhermitte's sign). It has been reported to occur in up to 15% of patients following mantle irradiation for Hodgkin's disease.[37] The proposed mechanism involves transient demyelination of the posterior columns or spinothalamic tracts within the irradiated volume. This suggests a direct effect of radiotherapy on the slowly proliferating oligodendrocytes and a transient reduction in myelin production. This classic clinical picture is usually self-limiting when standard doses of radiation have been used.

DELAYED RADIATION MYELOPATHY

Patients with delayed radiation myelitis typically present with a several months' history of progressive neurologic signs and symptoms, such as paresthesias and decreased pain and temperature sensation. In terms of latent period following radiotherapy, a bimodal distribution may be noted, with peaks at 13 and 26 months.[38] Symptoms are usually progressive over a 6-month period and eventually involve all systems below the affected level.

The mechanism involves white matter damage. A dual mechanism of spinal cord injury following radiation has been suggested. Extensive demyelination is associated with damage to oligodendrocytes. This process corresponds to a shorter latent period and effects may be transient or progressive, leading to white matter necrosis. A separate mechanism involves damage to the vascular endothelium. Resultant changes in permeability may induce white matter injury and lead to necrosis.[39] Wara and co-workers[40] described the time-dose relationship for radiation-induced spinal cord injury. They used an effective single dose (ED) as follows:

$$ED = D(cGy) \times N^{-0.377} \times T^{-0.058}$$

Based on this formula, the authors suggested that doses of 20 Gy in 5 fractions, 30 Gy in 10 fractions, and 50 Gy in 20 fractions were safe. This corresponds to a single effective dose of about 1,000 Gy, and was thought to be associated with a 1% incidence of myelopathy. In practice, the risk is probably much lower. In a review of patients receiving radiotherapy to the cervical spine, Marcus and Million[41] found that myelopathy developed in 2 of 1,112 (0.18%) who received a dose of 30 to 60 Gy. It has been estimated that the dose of standard fractionated radiotherapy that would be associated with a 5% incidence of spinal cord injury is 57 to 61 Gy.[42]

No effective treatment exists for delayed radiation myelopathy. Long-term survival is possible; however, the risk of death from complications associated with thoracic and cervical cord injuries is 30% and 70% respectively.[43]

REFERENCES

1. Plowman PN, Fuentos J, Harnett AN: Early radiation swelling remains a problem in the management of paediatric brain tumours. Br J Radiol 1987; 60:931.
2. Borgelt B, Gelber R, Kramer S, et al: The palliation of brain metastases: Final results of the first two studies by the Radiation Therapy Oncology Group. Int J Radiat Oncol Biol Phys 1980; 6:1.
3. Hindo WA, DeTrana FA III, Lee M-S, et al: Large dose increment irradiation in treatment of cerebral metastases. Cancer 1970; 26:138.
4. Young DF, Posner JB, Chu F, et al: Rapid-course radiation therapy of cerebral metastases: Results and complications. Cancer 1974; 34:1069.
5. Littman P, Rosenstock J, Gale G, et al: The somnolence syndrome in leukemic children following reduced daily dose fractions of cranial irradiation. Int J Radiat Oncol Biol Phys 1984; 10:1851.
6. Freeman JE, Johnston PGB, Voke JM: Somnolence after prophylactic cranial irradiation in children with acute lymphoblastic leukemia. Br Med J 1973; 4:523.
7. Parker D, Malpas JS, Sandland R, et al: Outlook following "somnolence syndrome" after prophylactic cranial irradiation. Br Med J 1978; 1:554.
8. Trautman PD, Erickson C, Shaffer D, et al: Prediction of intellectual deficits in children with acute lymphoblastic leukemia. J Dev Behav Pediatr 1988; 9:122.
9. Boldrey E, Sheline GE: Delayed transitory clinical manifestations after radiation treatment of intracranial tumors. Acta Radiol 1966; 5:5.
10. Hoffman WF, Levin VA, Wilson CB: Evaluation of malignant glioma patients during the postirradiation period. J Neurosurg 1979; 50:624.
11. Leibel SA, Sheline GE: Tolerance of the brain and spinal cord to conventional irradiation. In Gutin PH, Leibel SA, Sheline GE (eds): Radiation Injury to the Nervous System. New York, Raven, 1991, p 239.
12. Mulhern RK, Ochs J, Kun LE: Changes in intellect associated with cranial radiation therapy. In Gutin PH, Leibel SA, Sheline GE (eds): Radiation Injury to the Nervous System. New York, Raven, 1991, 325.
13. Constine LC, Woolf PD, Cann D, et al: Hypothalamic-pituitary dysfunction after radiation for brain tumors. N Engl J Med 1993; 328:87.
14. Zeman W, Samorajski T: Effects of irradiation on the nervous system. In Berdjis CC (ed): Pathology of Irradiation. Baltimore, Williams & Wilkins, 1971, p 213.
15. Zeman W: Disturbance of nucleic acid metabolism preceding delayed radionecrosis of nervous tissue. Proc Natl Acad Sci USA 1963; 50:626.
16. Hopewell JW, Wright EA: The nature of latent cerebral irradiation damage and its modification by hypertension. Br J Radiol 1970; 43:161.
17. Hopewell JW: The late vascular effects of radiation. Br J Radiol 1974; 47:157.
18. Martins AN, Johnston JS, Henry JM, et al: Delayed radiation necrosis of the brain. J Neurosurg 1977; 47:336.
19. Lampert PW, Tom MI, Rider WD: Disseminated demyelination of the brain following Co60 (gamma) radiation. Arch Pathol 1959; 68:322.
20. Sheline GE, Wara WM, Smith V: Therapeutic irradiation and brain injury. Int J Radiat Oncol Biol Phys 1980; 6:1215.
21. Marks JE, Baglan RJ, Prassad SC, et al: Cerebral radionecrosis: Incidence and risk in relation to dose, time, fractionation and volume. Int J Radiat Oncol Biol Phys 1981; 7:243.
22. Levin VA, Sheline GE, Gutin PH: Neoplasms of the central nervous system. In DeVita VT, Hellman S, Rosenberg SA (eds): Cancer: Principles and Practice of Oncology. Philadelphia, JB Lippincott, 1989, p 1557.
23. Harris JR, Levene MB: Visual complications following irradiation for pituitary adenomas and craniopharyngiomas. Radiology 1976; 120:167.
24. Goldsmith BJ, Rosenthal SA, Wara WM, et al: Optic neuropathy after irradiation of meningioma. Radiology 1992; 185:71.
25. Parsons JT, Bova FJ, Fitzgerald CR, et al: Radiation neuropathy after megavoltage external-beam irradiation: Analysis of time-dose factors. Int J Radiat Oncol Biol Phys 1994; 30:755.
26. Bleyer WA, Griffin TW: White matter necrosis, microangiopathy and intellectual abilities in survivors of childhood leukemia: Association with central nervous system irradiation and methotrexate therapy. In Gilbert HA, Kagan AR (eds): Radiation Damage to the Nervous System. New York, Raven, 1980, p 155.
27. Lee Y, Nauert C, Glass JP: Treatment-related white matter changes in cancer patients. Cancer 1986; 57:1473.
28. Styopoulos LA, George AE, de Leon MJ, et al: Longitudinal CT study of parenchymal brain changes in glioma survivors. Am J Neuroradiol 1988; 9:517.
29. Price RA, Birdwell DA: The central nervous system in childhood leukemia: III. Mineralizing microangiopathy and dystrophic calcifications. Cancer 1978; 42:717.
30. DeAngelis LM, Delattre J-Y, Posner JB: Radiation-induced dementia in patients cured of brain metastases. Neurology 1989; 39:789.
31. Maire J-P, Coudin B, Guerin J, et al: Neuropsychologic impairment in adults with brain tumors. Am J Clin Oncol 1987; 10:156.
32. Carvalho PA, Schwartz RB, Alexander E III, et al: Detection of recurrent gliomas with quantitative thallium-201/technetium-99m HMPAO single-photon emission computed tomography. J Neurosurg 1992; 77:565.
33. Valk PE, Budinger TF, Levin VA, et al: PET of malignant cerebral tumors after interstitial brachytherapy. J Neurosurg 1988; 69:830.
34. Tsuruda JS, Kortman KE, Bradley WG, et al: Radiation effects on cerebral white matter: MRI evaluation. AJR 1987; 8:431.
35. Constine LS, Konski A, Ekholm S, et al: Adverse effects of brain irradiation correlated with MR or CT imaging. Int J Radiat Oncol Biol Phys 1988; 15:319.
36. Curran WJ, Hecht-Leavitt C, Schut L, et al: Magnetic resonance imaging of cranial radiation lesions. Int J Radiat Oncol Biol Phys 1987; 13:1093.
37. Carmel RJ, Kaplan HS: Mantle irradiation in Hodgkin's disease: An analysis of technique, tumor eradication and complications. Cancer 1976; 37:2813.
38. Schultheiss TE, Higgins EM, El-Mahdi AM: The latent period in clinical radiation myelopathy. Int J Radiat Oncol Biol Phys 1984; 10:1109.
39. Delattre JY, Rosenblum MK, Thaler HT, et al: A model of radiation myelopathy in the rat: Pathology, regional capillary permeability changes and treatment with dexamethasone. Brain 1988; 111:1319.
40. Wara WM, Phillips TL, Sheline GE, et al: Radiation tolerance of the spinal cord. Cancer 1975; 35:1558.
41. Marcus RB, Million RR: The incidence of myelitis after irradiation of the cervical spinal cord. Int J Radiat Oncol Biol Phys 1990; 19:3.
42. Schultheiss TE: Spinal cord radiation "tolerance": Doctrine versus data. Int J Radiat Oncol Biol Phys 1990; 19:219.
43. Schultheiss TE, Stephens LC, Peter LJ: Survival in radiation myelopathy. Int J Radiat Oncol Biol Phys 1986; 12:1765.

RAYMOND K. MULHERN

LARRY E. KUN

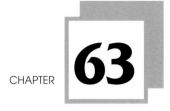

CHAPTER **63**

Cognitive Deficits*

This chapter discusses cognitive "late effects" that are associated with intracranial glioma and its treatment. The study of late effects presupposes that patients are long-term survivors of the disease, if not permanently cured. Late effects are temporally defined as occurring after the successful completion of medical therapy, usually 2 or more years from the time of diagnosis. It is generally assumed that late effects are chronic, if not progressive, in their course. This definition serves to separate late effects from those effects of disease and treatment that are acute or subacute and time-limited, such as chemotherapy-induced nausea and vomiting or temporary cognitive changes induced by cranial irradiation.[1]

Research interest in cognitive late effects, as well as in neurologic and other functional late effects, has shown an increase commensurate with improvements in effective therapy. For example, in the mid-1960s, when few children were cured of acute lymphoblastic leukemia (ALL), questions relating to the ultimate academic or vocational performance of long-term survivors were trivial compared to the need for improved therapy. In contrast, more than 60% of children diagnosed with ALL today can be cured,[2] and issues relating to quality of life of long-term survivors have now received increased emphasis.[3] At least comparable attention has been paid to neuropsychological status in primary CNS tumors. Functional changes attributed to radiation therapy in pediatric low-grade gliomas have stimulated much of the interest in surgical or initial chemotherapeutic approaches. In adults with malignant gliomas, investigations of more aggressive radiation techniques have been accompanied by studies of neurocognitive outcome, despite the limited likelihood of disease control.[4, 5]

Neurocognitive or neuropsychological late effects, as a subset of psychological late effects, are defined by a special emphasis on pathological changes in the CNS secondary to tumor or to its treatment, that result in changes in thinking and behavior. The most often studied behavioral correlates include intellect, memory, and academic performance. At best, research designs are quasi-experimental because of

limitations in controlling essential features of the patient's disease and medical therapy. For example, in contrast to traditional manipulations of independent variables in psychological research, one cannot control who will be diagnosed with cancer, when the diagnosis will be made, what type of cancer will develop, what type of CNS therapy will be given, or how the patient will respond to therapy. Although some of these factors may be controlled with appropriate comparison groups or statistical analyses, one generally cannot expect the same level of rigor as is possible in samples of patients without life-threatening disease. Without question, the most troublesome issue resulting from this lack of experimental control is determining the degree to which patient samples are representative and can therefore be considered valid for generalization of results.[6] Other problems that hamper research progress include the delayed onset of treatment-induced encephalopathies and the insensitivity of methods of assessment.[7]

This chapter discusses the evidence for neuropsychological deficits associated with primary intracranial gliomas. Literature on CNS therapies in ALL and treatment of brain metastases from extraneural cancers is reviewed elsewhere.[8, 9] It is worth noting that the treatment received by patients now participating in late effects studies may have further evolved for today's newly diagnosed patient. One must therefore select information from late effects studies that is pertinent to clinical questions currently being asked about tumor- or treatment-related toxic effects. We focus first on issues of general importance in determining cognitive deficits among survivors of brain tumors, because many of these issues are independent of tumor histology.[10–13] Next, the discussion focuses on studies of patients surviving gliomas.[14–25] The studies reviewed are outlined in Table 63–1.

FACTORS GENERALLY ASSOCIATED WITH LATE COGNITIVE CHANGES

A recent review of intellectual outcomes among children treated for brain tumors was reported by Mulhern and co-workers.[6] The review included 22 studies of the neuropsychological status in 544 children surviving treatment of brain

*Preparation of this chapter was supported in part by the American Lebanese Syrian Associated Charities and grants CA 21765 and CA 20180 from the National Cancer Institute.

TABLE 63–1
SUMMARY OF STUDIES REVIEWED FOR COGNITIVE DEFICITS AMONG SURVIVORS

Study	Sample*	Tumor Histology	Tumor Location	Treatment Following Surgery	Follow-up Interval	Neurocognitive Toxicity	Risk Factors†
Mixed Series							
Ellenberg et al[10]	43 Children	Varied	Varied	23 CFRT + LRT 14 LRT	≤4 yr	Lowered IQ distribution	Early childhood treatment (+) RT volume (+) Cerebral tumor location (+) Hydrocephalus at diagnosis (±) Degree of resection (−) Time elapsed from treatment (+)
Jennoun & Bloom[11]	62 Children	Varied	Varied	8 Chemotherapy + RT 13 CRT + LRT 49 LRT	3–20 yr	Lowered IQ distribution	Early childhood treatment (+) RT volume (NS) Cerebral tumor location (NS) Hydrocephalus at diagnosis (±) Gender (−)
Mostow et al[12]	342 Children	Varied	Varied	185 ?RT	>5 yr	Lowered QL	Early childhood treatment (+) RT (+) Cerebral tumor location (+) Male gender (+)
Marie[13]	49 Adults	Varied	Varied	42 LRT or SRT 7 CRT + LRT 39 Chemotherapy	0.8–11 yr	Minimal IQ changes	Late adulthood treatment (+) Time elapsed from treatment (−)
Glioma Series							
Cavazzuti et al[14]	20 Children	Various glioma	10 L Temporal 10 R Temporal lobe	11 RT	10–12 mo	Changes in memory and IQ	L/R hemisphere tumor location (+) RT (+)
Mulhern et al[15]	7 Children	II–III Astrocytoma	Temporal lobe	9 Surgery only 1 CRT + LRT 6 LRT	2–7 yr	Lowered IQ distribution Academic problems	Early childhood treatment (+) RT volume (+) Perioperative complications (+) Seizures (+)
Hirsch et al[16]	42 Children	22 Astrocytoma 20 Oligodendroglioma	Cerebral hemisphere	None	0.5–17 yr	29% with IQ <80	RT (+)
Riva et al[17]	15 Children	8 Medulloblastoma 7 Astrocytoma	Posterior fossa	8 CRT + LRT 7 None	>2 yr >3 yr	Medulloblastoma: mean IQ = 74.6 Astrocytoma: mean IQ = 105.8	RT (+)
Carpentieri & Mulhern[18]	14 Children	Various glioma	7 L Temporal 7 R Temporal	6 LRT	1.5–5.5 yr	Decreased intellect Dyslexia in 3 Verbal memory problems in 7	Early childhood treatment (+) RT (+) L/R hemisphere tumor location (+)
Mulhern et al[19]	16 Children	Various glioma	Brainstem	4 LRT 5 HFLRT (70.2 Gy)	1–5 yr	Cognitive deficits in 3	Early childhood treatment (NS) RT (±) Perioperative complications (+)
North et al[20]	12 Adults 18 Children	I–II Astrocytoma	Supratentorial	? None ? LRT	2–12 yr	Minimal in adults IQ < 70 in 9 children Poor functional status in 7	Early childhood treatment (+) RT (+)
Seiler[21]	14 Adults	III–IV Astrocytoma	Supratentorial	CRT + LRT + Chemotherapy	>2.5 yr		Time elapsed from treatment (+) Hydrocephalus (+) Neuroimaging changes (+)
Trojanowski et al[22]	198 Adults	149 Anaplastic glioma 49 Differentiated glioma	Supratentorial	104 LRT 94 LRT + Lomustine	2 yr	No QL differences between groups	Age at treatment (+) RT (NS) Cerebral tumor location (+) Gender (NS)
Imperato et al[23]	9 Adults	7 Glioblastoma 2 Anaplastic astrocytoma	Unspecified	8 CRT + LRT 1 LRT 7 Chemotherapy	>2 yr	Profound dementia in 2 Moderate cognitive dysfunction in 3 Specific memory dysfunction in 3 1 Normal	
Kleinberg et al[24]	30 Adults	Various glioma	Varied	12 CRT + LRT 2 CRT 16 LRT	1–10 yr	Decreased QL scores in 3 Decreased memory function in 3	RT volume (NS)
Lieberman et al[25]	8 Adults	Malignant astrocytoma	Cerebrum	8 CRT + LRT + Chemotherapy	>2 yr	3 Unable to work Decreased memory function in 2	Time elapsed from treatment (+) Neuroimaging changes (+)

*Age range at time of treatment.
†Presence of direct effect (+), inverse effect (−), ambiguous findings (±), or absence of effect (NS) on neurocognitive outcomes from risk factor investigated.
LRT, local radiation therapy; CRT, cranial radiation therapy; HFLRT, hyperfractionated LRT; IQ, intelligence quotient; and QL, quality of life.

tumors. A quantitative reanalysis of IQ data from 403 children investigated the impact of age, tumor location, and cranial (whole-brain) radiation therapy (CRT). Although the mean IQ was 91.0, particular subgroups were clearly at greater risk. In particular, children who received CRT when they were younger than 4 years were very vulnerable to intellectual loss compared to older children (means, 73.4 vs. 87.0). The impact of tumor location was equivocal. Qualitative review of studies not appropriate for reanalysis suggested that perioperative insults, hydrocephalus, chemotherapy, time elapsed from treatment, and chronic neurologic deficits were frequently associated with IQ loss.

A comprehensive assessment of risk factors in children was conducted in a longitudinal design by Ellenberg and associates[10] A total of 43 children with various brain tumors were followed up with serial IQ testing. Univariate analyses found significantly lower IQs among children who were younger at treatment, received a greater RT volume, and had cerebral (vs. posterior fossa) tumors. IQ deficits were greater when more time had elapsed after treatment. Multivariate analysis revealed that IQ at 1 month following diagnosis, age at treatment, and RT volume accounted for 80% of the variance in IQ scores 1 to 4 years later.

Jannoun and Bloom[11] provided neuropsychological follow-up 3 to 20 years after irradiation in 62 children with a variety of brain tumors. Tumor location, RT volume (limited vs. full CRT), and patient gender had no discernible effect on IQ outcomes. The age of the patient at the time of treatment was the most powerful determinant of ultimate IQ, with those younger than 5 years being at greatest risk (mean IQ, 72), those 6 to 11 years old being at intermediate risk (mean IQ, 93), and those older than 11 years functioning solidly in the normal range (mean IQ, 107). Although not statistically significant, children presenting with hydrocephalus had a 10-point decrement in IQ compared with those with normal intracranial pressure.

The quality of life in survivors of pediatric brain tumors was reported by Mostow and colleagues[12] who studied 342 adults who had been treated for brain tumors before age 20 years and who had survived 5 years or more. When compared to their siblings, survivors were at significantly greater risk for unemployment, chronic health problems, and inability to operate a motor vehicle. Specific risk factors included male gender, supratentorial tumors, and treatment that included RT. Treatment at a younger age was associated with a greater risk of poor school achievement, never being employed, and never being married.

With regard to adult patients, Crossen and co-workers[7] reviewed 29 studies reporting neurobehavioral outcomes among 748 adults following therapeutic CRT for primary and metastatic brain neoplasms. They reported that 92 survivors (12%) manifested neurobehavioral syndromes severe enough to be classified as dementia, and that an additional 44 patients (6%) had significantly reduced quality of life attributed to neurobehavioral symptoms associated with CRT. The review suggested that the elderly as well as the very young are more susceptible to radiation-induced brain injury and dementia. The authors speculate that in older patients, coexisting high blood pressure and high cholesterol may predispose to greater vascular damage following CRT.

A series by French researchers of 49 adult patients related serial IQ assessments 1 to 11 years following postoperative RT, with or without chemotherapy, for malignant brain tumors defined a fluctuating course with minimal long-term deficits among most surviving patients.[13] Late improvement in intellectual function was noted, especially in patients younger than 30 years; most patients returned to previous occupations.

Based on our clinical experience and on the recent reviews and studies of children and adults with brain tumors, we will discuss the following variables as they relate to cognitive outcome among patients surviving glioma: age at the time of treatment, time elapsed since completion of treatment, hydrocephalus, tumor location, RT, chemotherapy, and miscellaneous factors mentioned less frequently in the literature, such as seizures and operative complications.

MECHANISMS AND EVIDENCE FOR LATE COGNITIVE CHANGES

Post-treatment Interval and Neurocognitive Changes

Time elapsed since exposure appears to be an important parameter in evaluating outcome. Changes in intellect and functional status may not be manifest until a year or more following completion of therapy, and ultimate deficits in functional levels may not be apparent until years later.[6, 10] In mixed series of children[10] and adults,[13] as well as in studies of adults surviving malignant glioma,[11, 23] delayed and progressive deterioration in cognitive status has been noted following completion of treatment. Psychometric examinations with or without concurrent neuroimaging changes of white matter degeneration and cortical atrophy have antedated overt changes in quality of life or functional status.[5, 21, 23] In children with medulloblastoma, reports have conflicted and have indicated either stability[26] or further decline[27] in intellectual parameters beyond 2 to 4 years post-treatment. Progressive decline in academic performance among young children may relate to relative lack of newly acquired skills and knowledge in comparison to that of peers at a time of normally rapid learning. In adults, cognitive changes were seen 1 to 2 years following treatment for malignant glioma with CRT and aggressive chemotherapy following surgical resection.[4]

Age

MECHANISM

The patient's age at the time of exposure is undoubtedly an important variable in considering the potential sources of brain damage. Very young children treated for cancer, especially those younger than 4 years, are exposed to potentially neurotoxic agents during a time of accelerated neuroanatomic and psychological development. Some of these neurotoxic events may be focal in nature, such as tumor and associated mass effect as well as volume-specific RT; others may have a diffuse impact, such as full CRT or chemotherapy. The prevailing opinion is that very young children are at greater risk, as the CNS is still developing anatomically and functionally. Particularly in the young, diffuse insults may result in greater relative functional deficits; the brain's greater adaptive capacity to shift developing functions to unimpaired areas may mitigate exposure to focal insults. At the opposite end of the age spectrum, older adults may be at increased risk for cognitive dysfunction due to more limited "brain reserve" with earlier CNS insults or cumulative subclinical damage.[15]

EVIDENCE FOR COGNITIVE CHANGES

Among the reviews and studies cited earlier, all found that the patient's age at the time of treatment correlated significantly with the degree of cognitive deficit. Children at or below the preschool years were at especially high risk for cognitive sequelae, and these deficits were usually manifest within 4 years of completion of treatment.[10–12] In one series of adults, patients treated after age 50 years showed less recovery of function following treatment than did patients younger than 30 years.[13] Three of five studies that analyzed cognitive outcome in patients with gliomas as a function of age at treatment found age to be important.[15, 18–20] All patients were children who had received surgical excision with or without local supratentorial RT to the region of the tumor. For children with tumors outside the cerebral hemisphere (e.g., medulloblastoma), full CRT has been associated with an age-related decline in cognitive function in numerous series. The increased relationship between age at treatment and degree of intellectual deficit had been noted in some of the earlier data that related to outcome.[28, 29] Other prospective series indicate significant cognitive deficits largely in children younger than 5 to 7 years.[11, 16, 27, 30]

In addition to declines in IQ, specific problems with school achievement,[15] dyslexia,[18] and memory functions[18] were reported among children surviving temporal lobe gliomas. Both in children and adults, alterations in memory and attention are often apparent, and they appear to be most pronounced among young children.[4, 15]

Hydrocephalus

MECHANISMS

Hydrocephalus, defined here as ventricular dilatation with increased intracranial pressure, is common as a presenting feature in newly diagnosed patients, especially those with obstruction of CSF flow through the fourth ventricle. This phenomenon is more common among children than among adults with intracranial tumors, largely because of the greater prevalence of posterior fossa tumors in the younger age group.[31] Suprasellar tumors in both children and adults are often associated with hydrocephalus. If untreated, brain edema and periventricular white matter and vascular damage result. The association of chronic hydrocephalus with learning disability and mental retardation among children without brain tumors is well documented.[32] However, the effects of episodic and temporary increases in intracranial pressure are not well understood.

EVIDENCE FOR COGNITIVE CHANGES

Hydrocephalus has been variably reported as a risk factor for cognitive deficits in the setting of brain tumors. In mixed series of patients studied by Ellenberg and associates,[10] 28 of 43 children presented with hydrocephalus at diagnosis. IQ deficits were documented at 1 and 4 months following tumor excision whether or not a shunt was required. All children showed gains, but those who received a shunt showed the greatest gains, which suggests that their initial IQ scores in part reflected the effects of excess intracranial pressure. Hydrocephalus at diagnosis had no significant effect on IQ measured 1 to 4 years later. In a later series of a heterogeneous group of children, 40 who presented with hydrocephalus at diagnosis were compared with 22 who had normal ventricles, and no differences were found between the two groups with regard to mean IQ at follow-up; however, children who presented with hydrocephalus were twice as likely to be functioning in the intellectually deficient range (IQ < 70).[11] In children with medulloblastoma, insertion of a ventriculoperitoneal shunt was associated with less pronounced intellectual and academic deficits at follow-up.[26] Only one study of patients with gliomas analyzed outcomes based on hydrocephalus. Seiler[21] noted an association between late ventriculomegaly among long-term survivors of supratentorial malignant glioma and poor functional status. Ventriculomegaly in this setting related to cortical atrophy, which was attributed to a combined result of RT and chemotherapy.

Tumor Location

MECHANISMS

Infiltrative tumors invade and destroy normal brain structures, whereas noninvasive or encapsulated tumors displace and compress normal brain structures. Subsequent alterations of brain function related to the area of insult may be transient, durable, or progressive. The manner in which tumor effects are manifested neuropsychologically may depend on the developmental stage of a child. Cognitive theories of the functional organization of the brain have focused on adult-onset disorders involving the cerebral hemispheres, which consistently demonstrate gross differences between insults to language-dominant vs. non–language-dominant hemispheres and even between geographically proximal areas (e.g., anterior vs. posterior temporal lobe).[33]

EVIDENCE FOR COGNITIVE CHANGES

Two of the three studies cited in Table 63–1 that investigated tumor location as a risk factor had positive findings.[10, 12] In each instance, patients who survived tumors of the cerebral hemispheres had lower IQ and/or quality of life than those with noncerebral tumors. A study of adult glioma patients treated with local RT found that those with tumors of the cerebral hemispheres had poorer quality of life than those with noncerebral tumors. In two different studies of children treated for temporal lobe tumors with surgery, with or without RT, memory deficits and other cognitive changes have been associated with tumor location (i.e., language-dominant or non–language-dominant cerebral hemisphere).[14, 18]

Recently, investigators from France have reported a cohort of 42 consecutively diagnosed children with low-grade cerebral hemispheric gliomas.[16] Children were treated with surgery alone, which constituted an important "standard" for evaluating the late effects of other forms of treatment. Long-term follow-up revealed that 29% of children had IQ levels below 80, often accompanied by major problems in school. Although the authors did not associate a 20% incidence of poorly controlled postoperative seizures with low IQ or school problems, this additional influence cannot be ruled out. In contrast, Riva and associates[17] reported normal IQ among children with posterior fossa (largely cerebellar) astrocytoma similarly managed with surgery alone, which implies that tumor location is important in non-irradiated children. In contrast, cognitive decline has been documented in children with low-grade tumors of the brainstem following often limited surgery, with or without local RT.[19]

Cranial Radiation Therapy

MECHANISMS

The goal of RT is the selective destruction of neoplastic cells. The effects of radiation on neoplastic and normal tissues vary with treatment factors and the kinetics of the target tissue. Cells of more rapidly growing normal organ systems are more vulnerable to the adverse effects of radiation.[34] Radiation effects on the nervous system are, accordingly, most pronounced on the supporting glial and endothelial cells.[35] Although previously considered to be "resistant" to deleterious radiation-related changes, the slowly replicating cell systems of the CNS are now recognized as being relatively sensitive to irradiation. Significant effects are apparent only some time after exposure. Alterations that occur 6 months to several years after treatment include morphologic (atrophy, calcification, white matter degeneration, necrosis) and functional (encephalopathy, neuropsychological deterioration, focal neurologic deficits) changes. Factors related to late complications include host factors (tumor, age, diabetes mellitus, hypertension), radiation parameters (particularly individual fraction size, potential dose inhomogeneity, and treatment volume), and associated treatments, such as chemotherapy and surgery. Perhaps the most serious, if least common, late CNS alteration is post-irradiation cerebral necrosis. Most often reported 6 months to 2 years posttreatment,[35] changes related to focal radiation necrosis on computed tomography (CT) or magnetic resonance imaging (MRI) are reported to correlate with the dose and dosimetric distribution. Both the total dose and fraction size affect the frequency of this occurrence. Necrosis in this setting is virtually unreported after doses up to 50 to 55 Gy given with standard fractionation (180 to 200 cGy once daily).[36, 37] CNS effects, as reported for the brain, spinal cord, and optic nerves, are relatively more dependent on fraction size than are those of other normal tissues.[38, 39] Daily increments in excess of 220 to 250 cGy are associated with an increased risk of late necrosis, as are limited-volume dose-intensive radiation techniques (i.e., interstitial brain implants and stereotactic radiosurgery).[38, 40]

Following irradiation, CT and MRI demonstrate white matter changes that vary directly with the radiation dose.[5, 41] Changes are often limited to the high-dose radiation volume, but they may progress from focal to diffuse "encephalopathy"

and include significant volumes of one or both cerebral hemispheres.

EVIDENCE FOR COGNITIVE CHANGES

The late deleterious effects of RT for brain tumors in children and adults have been demonstrated using a variety of designs, but the primary design has compared the effect of the presence vs. the absence of RT as a treatment component or has compared local RT to full CRT. Given the previous discussion of mechanisms of action, studies relating total dose and fraction size to cognitive function would be important.

Some adult data indicate a correlation to dose despite differences in fraction size (i.e., 120 to 150 cGy/fraction) in a malignant glioma trial using twice-daily irradiation.[26] The effect of both dose and volume had been related to imaging changes in children and adults.[41] The relationship between neuroimaging abnormalities and functional or neurocognitive status is less direct.[5, 26, 41] One can anticipate that the effects of frank necrosis are size and site dependent. The impact of white matter abnormalities or "encephalopathy" are often pronounced, are related to general cognitive or functional levels, and are often difficult to quantify.[5, 26, 41]

Although one mixed series of children failed to detect an effect of RT volume,[11] Ellenberg and co-workers[10] found that the IQ values of children given CRT were significantly lower than those given local RT or no RT; the latter groups did not differ from each other. Other studies suggest a site- or volume-dependent relationship regarding IQ deficits in children.[42, 43] The very long-term follow-up by Mostow and others[12] of adults who had been treated during childhood found that the use of RT as part of the treatment regimen was associated with an almost threefold increase in the risk of chronic unemployment. Five of the eight studies of patients who survived glioma found evidence of deleterious effects of RT on ultimate cognitive function,[14, 15, 17, 18, 20] and in one study the effects were equivocal.[19] In general, the findings indicate that patients who require CRT attain a lower level of cognitive function and quality of life than those treated with local RT or no RT. However, at least two qualifications to this statement must be made. First, this relationship appears to be mediated by age (younger children have a greater risk for deterioration, as noted previously). Second, the combination of CRT with particular types of systemic chemotherapy may be devastating, even to adults with no other apparent risks for cognitive dysfunction.[21, 25] Two studies from our group illustrate the potential for unexpected cognitive changes on children treated with local RT for brainstem gliomas[19] and gliomas of the temporal lobes,[18] apparently related to the impact on normal temporal lobe areas.

Chemotherapy

MECHANISMS

Neurotoxicity has been related to several chemotherapeutic agents. Effects are generally acute and often self-limited for the CNS, as typified by encephalopathies attributed to electrolyte disturbance (e.g., with cisplatin) or direct drug effects (e.g., methotrexate or ifosfamide).[44]

Reduction of RT-induced brain damage has been used to justify the use of primary chemotherapy with malignant or low-grade brain tumors, especially for very young children.[45, 46] Neurotoxic effects of chemotherapy in this clinical setting may relate to later functional change, as in dose-related sensorineural hearing loss associated with cisplatin. Hearing loss extending into the speech frequencies can limit normal cognitive development and academic progress in children. In one study of infants and very young children treated for brain tumors with pre-irradiation chemotherapy, physical and psychological growth was abnormal in the majority of children and showed no "catch-up" effect during the time that CRT was delayed.[47]

EVIDENCE FOR COGNITIVE CHANGES

In the series of Jannoun and Bloom[11] of mixed intracranial tumors of children receiving neuraxis RT, eight of the 13 patients also received chemotherapy. The chemotherapy was not specified, and patient function was not analyzed using chemotherapy exposure as a potential risk factor. Interpretation of the effects of whole brain irradiation in this series is complicated by the high proportion of patients who also received chemotherapy.

In their study of 49 adult patients with tumors of various histologic types, Marie and colleagues[13] reported that 39 had received chemotherapy (primarily vincristine, teniposide, and carmustine or lomustine) following RT, but late toxic response data were not reported.[13] Adult survivors of malignant gliomas received chemotherapy in four studies of late cognitive effects. All 14 survivors in the Seiler[21] study had been treated with teniposide and carmustine, with or without procarbazine and bleomycin, following CRT; six of the 14 showed slowly evolving deterioration of cognitive function without focal neurologic signs, increased intracranial pressure, or recurrent tumor 1 to 2 years following surgery. All of these patients had radiographic changes correlated with dementia, including cortical atrophy, leukoencephalopathy, and periventricular changes attributed to the synergistic effects of combined CRT and chemotherapy.

In a randomized study of 198 patients that compared local RT to local RT plus lomustine following surgery for malignant supratentorial glioma, Trojanowski and co-workers[22] reported on the status of survivors at 6, 12, and 24 months. No significant differences between groups with regard to duration of survival, Karnofsky performance status scores, or specially constructed neuropsychological quality-of-life scores were found. Of the nine survivors reported by Imperato and associates,[23] seven had received carmustine or lomustine with or without diaziquone and procarbazine after RT. Only one patient, who had received carmustine alone, retained normal cognitive function.

Lieberman and colleagues[25] reported on eight of 57 patients surviving 2 years or more after treatment for malignant astrocytomas of the cerebral hemispheres. All patients had received CRT followed by carmustine, with or without methylprednisolone, methylprednisolone, or procarbazine. Quality of life as assessed by the Karnofsky performance scale and psychometric testing was characterized as good until signs of disease progression occurred; seven of the eight eventually died of recurrent tumor (four), second primary tumor (one), or cardiac complications (two). It is interesting to note that in the four cases of tumor recurrence, psychometric testing changes antedated neurologic signs and symptoms as well as neuroimaging changes. The impact of chemotherapy or its potential augmentation of radiation-related injury is impossible to sort out in the available data.

Other Sources of CNS Insult

Other factors that may affect cognitive performance following treatment for brain tumors are mentioned only sporadically in the literature. These include family socioeconomic resources, premorbid levels of functioning, chronic sensory and motor deficits, and seizures. For example, in children without brain tumors, poorly controlled seizures are associated with abnormal intellectual and academic development.[48] Poorly controlled seizures among children surviving temporal lobe astrocytomas are associated with psychopathology and poor academic achievement.[15]

Surveys have found that 25% to 30% of surviving patients have clinically significant visual (optic atrophy, hemianopsia), auditory, and motor disabilities (hemiparesis, ataxia) or seizures that grossly affect performance of age-appropriate activities of daily living, such as self-care and socialization.[49] The precise origin of these complications is often unknown, but chronic increased intracranial pressure, operative complications, and cisplatin-induced hearing loss are not uncommon. These deficits indirectly affect patient functional status because of the limitations placed on input and performance of tasks rather than on cognitive processing itself.

SUMMARY

In summary, cognitive outcomes following treatment for gliomas and other brain tumors are a result of multiple factors; in addition complex potential interactions exist among risk factors.[10] Unfortunately, the probability of long-term survival and the probability of chronic cognitive deficits appear to be inversely related. For children and adults treated for low-grade gliomas, survival is often excellent with surgical resection alone. In the absence of complications such as poorly controlled seizures or sensory deficits, the quality of life of these patients may be virtually normal. In extreme contrast are those patients with malignant gliomas with dismal prognosis despite more aggressive therapy, including surgery, RT, and chemotherapy. Although variable in reported prevalence, the risk for dementia and less severe cognitive changes is significant, especially in very young and elderly patients. Similar forms of cognitive toxic effects may arise from either RT or chemotherapy; their combined effects can take a devastating toll on cognitive function, especially when cortical atrophy is present. Among these patients, it is difficult to define the costs in terms of quality of life for achieving increased duration of survival.

Brain Reserve Capacity as a Conceptual Model

The concept of "brain reserve capacity" has recently been proposed by Satz[50] to explain individual variation in the behavioral manifestation of signs and symptoms of brain damage. Using a model derived from adult studies of progressive neurologic diseases that result in dementia (Alzheimer's disease, Parkinson's disease, AIDS), the author proposes that each individual has a unique threshold for tolerance of brain damage before signs and symptoms are noted. Cumulative effects of brain insults that remain below the individual threshold allow a person to remain asymptomatic, and clinical symptoms become apparent once the threshold is reached. Patients with greater brain reserve capacity will be more resilient (i.e., have a higher threshold) to the effects of any specific brain insult than will those with lesser reserve capacity. Brain reserve capacity can be estimated neuroanatomically (CT, MRI) by normal brain volume and functionally by intellectual and educational attainment.

The concept of brain reserve capacity discussed by Satz[50] did not make reference to brain damage or brain tumors on childhood. However, it is relevant to the present research discussion in that it provides a useful framework to explain variability in cognitive function among patients who have received virtually identical medical treatment. Several hypotheses follow from the reserve capacity model that have received some support. One hypothesis is that patients who are more cognitively and neurologically intact prior to a particular form of therapy, such as CRT, will have a better functional outcome. The regression analysis of IQ function by Ellenberg and colleagues[10] 4 years following treatment for childhood brain tumor revealed that postoperative IQ was the best predictor, alone accounting for 62% of the variance. Our group has recently analyzed pre- and post-CRT IQ data for children with ALL; initial IQ accounted for greater than 80% of IQ variance among long-term survivors.[51]

Quality-Adjusted Survival

The current research literature on late effects of treatment of gliomas, and of cancer in general, is limited by the absence of an accepted method of quantifying quality of life and by the absence of a method for combining quality and duration of survival in a meaningful manner. Some progress has been made in this regard with adult women with breast cancer, but this method has yet to be applied to the treatment of brain tumors.

For example, following mastectomy, 463 women were randomized to receive either chemoendocrine therapy for 1 year, endocrine therapy alone for 1 year, or no adjuvant therapy.[52] Overall survival (OS) was significantly better in the chemoendocrine therapy group than in the other two groups. OS was then divided into time with toxic effects (TOX), time without symptoms and toxic efects (TWiST), and time after systemic relapse (REL). Quality-adjusted survival (Q-TWiST) was defined as the sum of TOX and REL, weighted by coefficients (0.0 to 1.0) derived from patients' subjective comparisons to TWiST. An analysis comparing the treatments in terms of the quality-of-life benefits relative to a delay in disease progression and the costs due to adverse events was performed for all values of utility weights. This "threshold" function displays points at which treatment

alternatives are equivalent for combinations of the weighted values of TOX and REL. For most coefficients, the Q-TWiST analysis also favored the chemoendocrine treatment group. This system can also be used to generate statements with acceptable statistical confidence intervals such as: for patient A, who would give up 1 month of life from a year after disease progression to gain time without symptoms of disease or toxic effects, treatment X will provide a gain of 4 days in quality-adjusted survival over treatment Y. We think that similar analyses of alternative treatments for malignant glioma and other types of brain tumors would also be useful.

CONCLUSIONS

Significant progress has been made in the past decade in recognizing the importance of cognitive status and other psychological factors to the quality of life of children and adults receiving treatment for brain tumors. Patient-, disease-, and treatment-related risk factors for alterations in cognitive function have been identified. Furthermore, known sources of risk (e.g., CRT in early childhood) have stimulated modifications in treatment approaches and indicate the importance of clinical surveillance of neuropsychological and overall functional capabilities. However, further research in this area is limited by the absence of an integrative model of patient vulnerability and the absence of a systematic method to balance quality and duration of survival. These issues are discussed in more detail in the following paragraphs.

Recommendations for Patient Care

Treating physicians at major medical centers, most often pediatric or medical oncologists and radiation oncologists, are generally aware of the risks for neuropsychological problems among children and adults with brain tumors. However, considerable variability exists among institutions as to how these potential risks affect patient care. The following recommendations are based on the clinical experience of the authors and the present literature.

1. Available knowledge about the potential for adverse neuropsychological late effects of tumors and various treatment options must be made explicit to adult patients, to parents of child patients, and to the child, if he or she is old enough to assist in decision making. This is especially important in situations in which the patient is receiving "standard" treatment that is not part of a research study that has been approved by a human subjects review board. Monitoring how risks and benefits are described to patients whose informed consent is required for prospective protocols is a major responsibility of internal review boards. Particularly in an era of evolving treatment options, similar attention to potential functional alteration is critical in "standard care" situations.

2. A formal plan of prospective surveillance of neuropsychological status should be set forth for each patient based on known or suspected risk for problems. This assumes that

a qualified psychologist has been identified as a consultant to the institution. For example, a middle-aged adult with a supratentorial low-grade glioma that is treated with surgery alone may require formal assessment only once or twice during the 2-year period following diagnosis, with the focus being evidence of loss of abilities. In contrast, a young child with the same tumor and treatment should have a neuropsychological evaluation scheduled at the completion of therapy and 3 to 5 years later, whereas an infant with a brain tumor should probably be evaluated every 6 months until the age of 3 or 4 years, and then yearly until 5 years after therapy. Such plans should not depend on the presentation of symptoms, because presymptomatic assessments often allow for early educational interventions that may minimize deficits.[8]

3. Formal consultative arrangements should be made between the treating physician and the psychologist to clarify methods of information exchange. As obvious as this may seem, problems with the timely communication of patient information can limit the quality of patient care. A social worker from the cancer center or a psychologist should be designated as a liaison with the child's school and other community service agencies. For children with complex medical conditions and concurrent neuropsychological problems, timely communication of accurate information can avoid misunderstandings that have important implications for the child's quality of life.

REFERENCES

1. Armstrong C, Mollman J, Corn BW, et al: Effects of radiation therapy on adult brain behavior. Neurology 1993; 43:1961.
2. Neglia JP, Robison LL: Epidemiology of the childhood acute leukemias. Pediatr Clin North Am 1988; 35:675.
3. Green DM, D'Angio GJ: Late Effects of Treatment for Childhood Cancer. New York, Wiley-Liss, 1992.
4. Archibald YM, Lunn D, Ruttan LA, et al: Cognitive functioning in long-term survivors of high grade glioma. J Neurosurg 1994; 80:247–253.
5. Corn BW, Yousem DM, Scott CB, et al: White matter changes are correlated significantly with radiation dose. Cancer 1994; 74:2828–2835.
6. Mulhern RK, Hancock J, Fairclough D, et al: Neuropsychological status of children treated for brain tumors: A critical review and integrative analysis. Med Pediatr Oncol 1992; 20:181.
7. Crossen JR, Garwood D, Glastein E, et al: Neurobehavioral sequelae of cranial irradiation in adults: A review of radiation-induced encephalopathy. J Clin Oncol 1994; 12:627.
8. Mulhern RK: Neuropsychological late effects. In Bearison DJ, Mulhern RK (eds): Pediatric Psychooncology. New York, Oxford University Press, 1994, pp 215–222.
9. DeAngelis LM, Delattre JY, Posner JB: Radiation-induced dementia in patients cured of brain metastases. Neurology 1989; 39:789–796.
10. Ellenberg L, McComb JG, Siegel SE, et al: Factors affecting intellectual outcome in pediatric brain tumor patients. Neurosurgery 1987; 21:638.
11. Jannoun L, Bloom HJG: Long-term psychological effects in children treated for intracranial tumors. Int J Radiat Oncol Biol Phys 1990; 18:747.
12. Mostow EN, Byrne J, Connelly RR, et al: Quality of life in long-term survivors of CNS tumors of childhood and adolescence. J Clin Oncol 1991; 9:592.
13. Marie JP, Coudin B, Guerin J, et al: Neuropsychologic impairment in adults with brain tumors. Am J Clin Oncol 1987; 10:156.
14. Cavazzuti V, Winston K, Baket R, et al: Psychological changes following surgery for tumors in the temporal lobe. J Neurosurg 1980; 53:618–626.
15. Mulhern RK, Kovnar EK, Kun LE, et al: Psychologic and neurologic function following treatment for childhood temporal lobe astrocytoma. J Child Neurol 1988; 3:47.
16. Hirsch JF, Rose CS, Pierre-Kahn A, et al: Benign astrocytic and oligodendrocytic tumors of the cerebral hemispheres in children. J Neurosurg 1989; 70:568.
17. Riva D, Pantaleone C, Milani N, et al: Impairment of neuropsychological functions in children with medulloblastomas and astrocytomas in the posterior fossa. Childs Nerv Syst 1989; 5:107.
18. Carpentieri S, Mulhern RK: Patterns of memory dysfunction among children surviving temporal lobe tumors. Arch Clin Neuropsychol 1993; 8:345–357.
19. Mulhern RK, Heideman RL, Khatib ZA, et al: Quality of survival among children treated for brain stem glioma. Pediatr Neurosurg 1994; 20:226–232.
20. North CA, North RB, Epstein JA, et al: Low-grade cerebral astrocytomas: Survival and quality of life after radiation therapy. Cancer 1990; 66:6.
21. Seiler RW: Late results of multimodality therapy of high-grade supratentorial astrocytomas. Surg Neurol 1981; 15:88.
22. Trojanowski T, Peszynsik J, Krzysztof M, et al: Quality of survival of patients with brain gliomas treated with postoperative CCNU and radiation therapy. J Neurosurg 1989; 70:18.
23. Imperato JP, Paleologos NA, Vick NA: Effects of treatment on long-term survivors with malignant astrocytomas. Ann Neurol 1990; 28:818.
24. Kleinberg L, Wallner K, Malkin MG: Good performance status of long-term disease-free survivors of intracranial glioma. Int J Radiat Oncol Biol Phys 1993; 26:129.
25. Lieberman AN, Foo SH, Ransohoff J, et al: Long term survival among patients with malignant brain tumors. Neurosurgery 1982; 10:450.
26. Johnson DL, McCabe MA, Nicholson HS, et al: Quality of long-term survival in young children with medulloblastoma. J Neurosurg 1994; 80:1004–1010.
27. Hoppe-Hirsch E, Renier D, Lellouch-Tubiana A, et al: Medulloblastoma in childhood: Progressive intellectual deterioration. Childs Nerv Syst 1990; 6:60–65.
28. Bloom HCG, Wallace ENK, Henk J: The treatment and prognosis of medulloblastoma in children. AJR 1969; 105:43–62.
29. Hirsch JF, Renier C, Czernichow P: Medulloblastoma in childhood: Survival and functional results. Acta Neurochir 1979; 48:1–15.
30. Radcliffe J, Packer R, Atkins T, et al: Three- and four-year cognitive outcome in children with noncortical brain tumors treated with whole-brain radiotherapy. Ann Neurol 1992; 32:551–554.
31. Klein DM. Principles of neurosurgery. In Cohen M, Duffner P (eds): Brain Tumors in Children. New York, Raven Press, 1984, p 92.
32. Wills KE: Neuropsychological functioning in children with spina bifida and/or hydrocephalus. J Clin Child Psychol 1994; 22:247.
33. Filskov SB, Grimm BH, Lewis JA: Brain-behavior relationships. In Boll T, Filskov SB (eds): Handbook of Clinical Neuropsychology. New York, John Wiley, 1981, p 39.
34. Kun LE: Principles of radiation therapy. In Cohen M, Duffner P (eds): Brain Tumors in Children, ed 2. New York, Raven Press, 1993.
35. van der Kogel AJ: Central nervous system radiation injury in small animal models. In Gutin PH, Leibel SA, Sheline GE (eds): Radiation Injury to the Nervous System. New York, Raven Press, 1991, p 91.
36. Leibel SA, Sheline GE: Tolerance of the brain and spinal cord to conventional irradiation. In Gutin P, Leibel S, Sheline G (eds): Radiation Injury to the Nervous System. New York, Raven Press, 1991, p 239.
37. Mikhael MA: Radiation necrosis of the brain: Correlation between computed tomography, pathology, and dose distribution. J Comput Assist Tomogr 1978; 2:71.
38. Sheline GE, Wara WM, Smith V: Therapeutic irradiation and brain injury. Int J Radiat Oncol Biol Phys 1980; 6:1215.
39. Wigg DR, Koschel K, Hodgson GS: Tolerance of the mature human central nervous system to photon irradiation. Br J Radiol 1981; 54:787.
40. Marks JE, Baglan RJ, Prassad SC, et al: Cerebral radionecrosis: Incidence and risk in relation to dose, time, fractionation and volume. Int J Radiat Oncol Biol Phys 1981; 7:243.
41. Constine LS, Konski A, Ekholm S, et al: Adverse effects of brain irradiation correlated with MR and CT imaging. Int J Radiat Oncol Biol Phys 1988; 15:319–330.
42. Kun LE, Mulhern RK, Crisco JJ: Quality of life in children treated for brain tumors: Intellectual, emotional, and academic function. J Neurosurg 1983; 58:1–6.

43. Carpentieri S, Mulhern RK, Douglas SM, et al: Behavioral resiliency among children surviving brain tumors: A longitudinal study. J Clin Child Psychol 1994; 22:236–246.

44. Poplack DG, Brouwers P: Adverse sequalae of central nervous system therapy. Clin Oncol 1985; 4:263.

45. Duffner P, Horowitz M, Krischer J, et al: Postoperative chemotherapy and delayed radiation in children less than 3 years of age with malignant brain tumors: A Pediatric Oncology Group Study. N Engl J Med 1993; 328:1725–1731.

46. Packer RJ, Sutton LN, Bilaniuk LT, et al: Treatment of chiasmatic/hypothalamic gliomas of childhood with chemotherapy: An update. Ann Neurol 1988; 32:551–554.

47. Mulhern RK, Horowitz ME, Kovnar EH, et al: Neurodevelopmental status of infants and young children treated for brain tumors with pre-irradiation chemotherapy. J Clin Oncol 1989; 7:1660.

48. Bourgeois BTD, Prensky AL, Palkes HS, et al: Intelligence in epilepsy: A prospective study in children. Ann Neurol 1983; 14:438.

49. Mulhern RK, Crisco JJ, Kun LE: Neuropsychological sequelae of childhood brain tumors: A review. J Clin Child Psychol 1983; 12:66.

50. Satz P: Brain reserve capacity on symptom onset after brain injury: A formulation and review of evidence for threshold theory. Neuropsychology 1993; 7:273.

51. Kumar P, Mulhern RK, Regine WF, et al: Prospective neurocognitive evaluation of children treated with additional chemotherapy and craniospinal irradiation following isolated central nervous system relapse in acute lymphoblastic leukemia. Int J Radiat Oncol Biol Phys 1995; 31:561–566.

52. Goldhirsch, A, Gelber R, Simes, et al: Costs and benefits of adjuvant therapy in breast cancer: A quality-adjusted survival analysis. J Clin Oncol 1989; 7:36.

PAUL M. KANEV

PAULA M. HALE

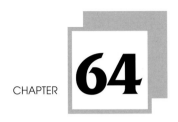

CHAPTER **64**

Endocrinologic Dysfunction Following Adjunct Tumor Therapy

Endocrine complications of adjuvant tumor therapy have been recognized since the 1960s. Comprehensive hormonal studies have demonstrated dose-dependent irradiation changes in pituitary and hypothalamic function. Primary or secondary hypothyroidism is recognized in nearly three-quarters of patients treated for medulloblastoma,[47] and independent of tumor histology, growth hormone (GH) deficiency develops in most patients following whole-brain and posterior fossa radiation therapy.[24, 31] Supplementation with pituitary-derived growth hormone has been linked with Creutzfeldt-Jakob disease, leading to withdrawal of this hormone in most countries in the mid-1980s.[11, 26, 32, 70] Recombinant biosynthetic GH replacement therapy became available in 1985, and some treated patients have achieved normal growth velocities.[15, 31] GH supplementation has not been associated with tumor recurrence or progression of residual disease.[14, 39, 48]

The overall mortality of primary brain tumors has steadily decreased, and the prognosis for medulloblastoma 5 and 10 years after resection, irradiation, and chemotherapy is approaching 60% to 85%.[30, 49] As the prognosis for brain tumors improves and more aggressive adjuvant therapy is utilized, greater attention must be focused on the long-term sequelae of treatment. This chapter reviews the clinical presentation and the treatment of hormone deficiencies.

GROWTH HORMONE DEFICIENCY

Frequency of Hormone Deficiency

Of the hypothalamic-pituitary system, the growth hormone axis is the most sensitive to the effects of irradiation. Growth hormone deficiency following radiation therapy for brain tumors has been documented since the 1960s. In 1969, Bloom and co-workers[5] reported GH deficiency among 65% of 82 medulloblastoma patients with long-term survival. Shalet and others[60] demonstrated GH deficiency among 50% of 14 patients who underwent endocrine studies. Growth velocity decelerated during the second year following tumor resection and was most common following treatment for medulloblastoma and ependymoma. Brown and colleagues[10] investigated 13 patients with medulloblastoma after surgery and craniospinal radiation. Four of these patients received chemotherapy and poor growth was confirmed in all children, and partial or complete GH deficiency was documented in four males and five females. In a later study reported by Park and associates,[50] 47% of the 35 long-term survivors of medulloblastomas treated at the Hospital for Sick Children, Toronto, were in less than the third percentile in height. Comprehensive endocrine study of these patients confirmed panhypopituitarism in 11 children and hypothyroidism and GH deficiency in four patients. Among a group of patients studied by Lannering and co-workers,[34] decreased pulsatile GH secretion was demonstrated in 16 children following tumor therapy. In this series, ten children received GH replacement and had mean growth velocity of 8.3 cm/year without acceleration of bone age. Only two patients experienced catch-up growth.

Further studies in patients treated for brain tumors in childhood with radiation therapy revealed that a high proportion of survivors had short stature and GH deficiency. Haider and associates[28] reported results of comprehensive endocrinologic studies in 18 children with brain tumors including six patients with optic nerve gliomas. Depressed GH levels were recorded in each patient with optic glioma following radiation therapy. Normal growth continued in three children who had neurofibromatosis and precocious puberty. In another study of children with optic nerve glioma, each suffered GH deficiency in the years subsequent to radiation exposure exceeding 4,500 cGy.[8] Five patients with hypothalamic gliomas, reported by Taylor and colleagues,[68] developed GH deficiency and panhypopituitarism within 1 year following irradiation.

A review of 123 children with brain tumors[31] demonstrated GH deficiency in 40% of the survivors who received radiation therapy. The children at greatest risk were those who had had treatment for medulloblastoma, ependymoma, and craniopharyngioma. The onset of short stature began in the first year after completing radiation therapy, and the mean interval from tumor diagnosis until confirmation of GH deficiency was 26 months in boys and 17 months in girls. GH failure was twice as common after focal infratentorial and craniospinal radiation therapy when adjuvant chemotherapy was involved. The sensitivity of screening with insulin-like growth factor 1 (IGF1) for GH deficiency was 92%.

Diagnosis of Growth Hormone Deficiency

The classical criteria for growth hormone deficiency include short stature, inadequate growth velocity, and subnormal response to pharmacologic stimulation (peak GH levels less than 10 ng/mL).[52] Insulin-induced hypoglycemia is the most potent stimulus for GH secretion. The test is usually performed during an inpatient hospitalization and carries a 10% incidence of seizures. The test may be particularly hazardous in children who are GH deficient and may already be prone to development of hypoglycemia and who, following surgery, have an increased risk for seizures. Stimulation of GH also follows exercise, arginine infusion, and administration of levodopa, propranolol, glucagon, and clonidine. Donaldson and others[21] have concluded that measurement of pulsatile GH on a single night was the most sensitive assay of endogenous GH secretion. In another study by Mauras and co-workers,[44] provocative testing, however, was more sensitive than pulsatile GH assay. Urinary measurement of GH has not proved sensitive enough to determine hormone deficiency.[71]

Monitoring of serum IGF1 levels may accurately screen for GH deficiency, and it correctly predicts subnormal response to provocative stimulation studies.[18, 54, 69] The screening effectiveness of IGF1, however, may be compromised by steroids, diabetes, low body weight, and decreased protein or caloric intake. Normal thyroid function must be confirmed for accurate interpretation. To confirm GH deficiency, we advocate careful measurement of patient height and weight during neuro-oncology clinic follow-up visits and sampling of thyroxine (T_4), thyroid-stimulating hormone (TSH), and IGF1 every 6 months. If a deceleration in growth velocity is observed, we recommend overnight sampling of pulsatile GH secretion followed by pharmacologic testing with two provocative agents. In our institution we sample GH following stimulation with levodopa (10 mg/kg, at 30, 60, and 90 minutes) and clonidine (0.15 mg/m^2, up to a maximum dose of 0.1 mg, at 60, 90 and 120 minutes).

Etiology of Growth Hormone Deficiency

The mechanism of radiation-induced hormone deficiency may include direct cell injury to the hypothalamus or pituitary gland, vascular injury within the hypophyseal-pituitary portal system, or injury to the catecholaminergic or serotonergic pathways to the hypothalamus. Receptor-binding studies have demonstrated the presence of hypothalamic and suprahypothalamic GH receptors in the CNS of fish species,

birds, and mammals.[56] The hypothalamus may have a greater radiation vulnerability than the pituitary gland.[42, 62] Prolactin levels are commonly increased following irradiation, and in many cases, normal pituitary secretion may follow stimulation with trophic hormones, such as growth hormone–releasing hormone (GH-RH) and thyrotropin-releasing hormone (TRH).[54]

It has not been possible to identify the radiation dose sensitivity of the hypothalamic-pituitary region. Laboratory studies in monkeys demonstrated impaired GH response to insulin hypoglycemia following 2,400 cGy of cranial irradiation delivered over 2 weeks in 10 fractions.[13] A similar threshold exposure of 2,500 to 3,000 cGy delivered in 16 fractions over 3 weeks in a group of children with primary brain tumors was observed by Shalet and co-workers[61] to be the threshold for the onset of endocrine dysfunction. Sanders and others[58] have reported a 43% incidence of GH deficiency among 25 patients who received 1,000 to 1,700 cGy of total-body irradiation prior to bone marrow transplantation, which suggests that the endocrine axis sensitivity is much lower than previously thought. Clayton and Shalet[15] reported a 74% incidence of GH deficiency among 82 children with brain tumors who completed radiation therapy. Independent risk variables influencing peak GH concentration were radiation dose and the time from irradiation.

GH deficiency following single-fraction gamma-knife radiation therapy in 324 patients younger than 17 years has not been present according to observations of Steiner,[66] which suggests that GH deficiency is a result of the complex relationships among the radiation dosage, the volume of treated tissue, and the number of treatment fractions. Data regarding whether the hypothalamic-pituitary axis is more vulnerable in younger patients are conflicting,[15, 16, 27, 31, 53] although two prospective studies suggest that acquired GH deficiency following radiation exposure exceeding 3,000 cGy begins more rapidly in children than in adults.[33]

Decreased growth velocity is common during chemotherapy[45] and is most likely related to decreased protein-calorie intake. Hypothalamic and pituitary function, however, appear refractory to chemotherapy.[68] Among patients treated in Seattle, adjuvant chemotherapy enhanced GH failure in patients who completed craniospinal and posterior fossa radiation therapy, although the effectiveness of GH supplementation was not impaired.[31]

The time of onset of GH deficiency following radiation therapy remains uncertain. Shalet[59] conducted a prospective study of 14 patients and demonstrated GH failure in six patients at 1 year following radiation therapy, with an additional patient manifesting GH insufficiency during the second year. In another prospective study by Duffner and associates,[24] GH deficiency was demonstrated as early as 3 months following radiation therapy. The deficits were progressive over time and occurred in nearly all children within 1 year of tumor radiation therapy. Three of seven patients studied by Brauner and co-workers[9] had GH deficiency 2 years after radiation therapy. A later prospective study of 27 children conducted by Sulmont and others[67] demonstrated abnormal GH responses to provocative testing in 58% of patients 2 years after treatment. In that series, craniospinal irradiation led to greater height losses than did cranial irradiation alone. Oberfield and colleagues[47] prospectively studied

19 patients with medulloblastomas and recorded decreased growth velocities in 14 children. The falloff in growth velocity was observed as early as 6 months following treatment. Provocative studies confirmed abnormal thyroid function in each child with growth rate disturbance, whereas normal GH secretion was demonstrated in ten patients.

We prospectively studied endocrinologic function in 31 children with newly diagnosed brain tumors at St. Christopher's Hospital for Children, Philadelphia. Histopathologic findings were confirmed at craniotomy in 27 patients, and diagnosis of brainstem or optic pathway tumors was made by MRI in four children. Sixteen children completed radiation therapy, and the exposure to the posterior hypothalamus in each patient exceeded 2,400 cGy. Adjuvant protocol chemotherapy supplemented irradiation in ten children, and complete tumor resection was accomplished in nine patients.

All patients maintained normal growth during the first 6 months following tumor diagnosis and treatment. Five of 16 patients had a decline in growth velocity when compared with the pretreatment growth rate 6 to 9 months following the completion of irradiation. An additional six patients had a decline in growth velocity 9 to 12 months after finishing radiation exposure. In all cases, the decline in growth was less than 1 SD below the initial height. Normal growth continued in each patient following complete tumor resection or in each patient who received primary chemotherapy.

GH deficiency developed in all prepubertal patients during the first year following completion of irradiation. Following the completion of radiation therapy, a progressive decline in IGF1 and a failure to respond to provocative GH stimulation over time were noted. Confirming the previous findings of Duffner and colleagues,[24] three of 16 patients had GH deficiency as early as 3 months following irradiation, and it was present in 13 of 16 patients after 1 year. In each case, subnormal IGF1 levels for age correctly predicted GH deficiency and failure to respond to provocative stimulation. Hypothyroidism was present in 50% of patients following radiation therapy, which is similar to the results of Oberfield and co-workers.[47] In contrast to the results of Brauner and others,[9] our data suggested that GH failure may precede declining growth by a significant interval. This latency period could be an ideal time to initiate an endocrinologic evaluation. Early hormone replacement may prevent the falloff in growth velocity and failure to achieve catch-up growth that are common when replacement hormone therapy is delayed.

Replacement Therapy

GH therapy in children with idiopathic GH deficiency has achieved standard deviation catch-up growth with velocities reaching 12.8 cm/year.[29] This treatment success has not been duplicated in patients receiving GH replacement for radiation-induced hormone deficiency. Sulmont and associates[67] concluded that GH therapy did not improve the standard deviation score in patients who received cranial irradiation. Lannering and co-workers,[34] however, reported catch-up growth in two of ten children treated with GH following radiation therapy, and improvement in height percentile was seen in eight of 25 patients treated in Seattle.[31]

The success of hormone replacement therapy among patients treated in Seattle was influenced by simultaneous thyroid hormone replacement and early GH replacement, in agreement with the conclusions of Sulmont and colleagues[67] and Clayton and Shalet.[15] Two children began supplementation within 1 year of completing radiation therapy and experienced catch-up growth to their original height percentile within 18 months. Three of eight patients who received levothyroxine experienced an acceleration in growth velocity after beginning thyroid replacement therapy. Careful monitoring and serial maintenance of normal thyroid function is required to achieve the maximum effectiveness of GH replacement.

The success of treatment with recombinant GH appears to be independent of sex, radiation therapy portals, and chemotherapy. Recently, Shalet and others[63] evaluated the effectiveness of GH therapy in a group of patients with tumors following radiation therapy. Final height above the third percentile was reached in half of the patients, and the growth velocity was 5.6 to 7.4 cm/year during hormone treatment.

GH supplementation is recommended with Protropin (Genentech, San Francisco) or Humatrope (Eli Lilly, Indianapolis). Each preparation is administered as a subcutaneous injection on 6 of 7 days. The recommended doses of the two products differ slightly; in our institution, the Protropin dose is 0.05 mg/kg/day, whereas the Humatrope is administered in a dose of 0.03 mg/kg/day. To achieve the maximum benefit of replacement therapy, dosage is adjusted to current body weight on each quarterly neuro-oncology follow-up visit.

Treatment Recommendations

An analysis by Clayton and associates[14] concluded that recombinant GH replacement therapy did not contribute to late tumor relapse of leukemias, medulloblastomas, or gliomas. A recent long-term study reported by Ogilvy-Stuart and colleagues,[48] which included many of these patients, demonstrated decreased tumor recurrence rates in children with medulloblastoma, other brain tumors, and acute lymphocytic leukemia (ALL) who received GH. The authors suggested that GH offered a protective effect against the risk of relapse. They concluded that hormone supplementation appeared safe at any age but recommended critical surveillance and monitoring of tumor recurrence. Hormone supplementation had no influence on neuroradiologic imaging studies.

No cases have been reported of radiation-induced GH deficiency resolving over time. Given the apparent safety of GH use, we advocate early replacement therapy to achieve the maximum benefits of GH therapy. We recommend initiation of hormone supplementation on confirmation of hormone deficiency in all patients with decelerating growth velocity who are without evidence of residual disease 18 months following the completion of surgery and appropriate adjuvant therapy. Early use of GH is also advocated in children with low-grade tumors and residual disease, such as optic pathway or cerebellar astrocytomas, for which prognosis is very favorable.

THYROID HORMONE DEFICIENCY

Frequency of Thyroid Hormone Deficiency

Although less common than GH deficiency, thyroid dysfunction has also been reported in children and adults who have received craniospinal irradiation. Children who received radiation to the spinal axis are at risk for the development of primary hypothyroidism secondary to thyroid gland injury. Radiation of the thyroid gland has been associated with the development of compensated hypothyroidism, clinical hypothyroidism, chronic lymphocytic thyroiditis, and thyroid neoplasms.[25, 27]

Craniospinal irradiation can result in damage to the pituitary gland or hypothalamus, causing secondary or tertiary hypothyroidism. A number of studies have suggested that the hypothalamus is more sensitive to damage from irradiation than is the pituitary gland.[62] The total dose of radiation delivered to the hypothalamic-pituitary region is a major determinant of the speed of onset and incidence of anterior pituitary deficiency. The fraction size, as well as the total radiation dose, is important in determining the extent of damage to the hypothalamic-pituitary axis.[39] Oberfield and co-workers[47] reported a high incidence of thyroid dysfunction in children who received craniospinal irradiation for medulloblastoma. More than two-thirds of the 22 patients studied were shown to have thyroid dysfunction, and abnormal thyroid hormone levels were documented from less than 6 months to 6½ years after therapy. In most cases thyroid dysfunction was primary, involving the thyroid gland, and compensated.

In another study, thyroid function was evaluated in 119 children with tumors distant from the hypothalamic pituitary region.[41] The prevalence of primary thyroid dysfunction was 28%, compared with only 3% for secondary dysfunction. Although little is known about the effects of high doses of chemotherapy on thyroid function, a significantly higher prevalence of primary thyroid dysfunction was seen in patients who received combination chemotherapy and spinal irradiation than after spinal irradiation alone.

In another study of 13 patients with medulloblastoma following surgery and craniospinal irradiation,[10] seven patients were shown to have elevated TSH levels with normal T₄ levels and were clinically euthyroid. All seven patients demonstrated excessive TSH response to TRH, a sign of primary thyroid dysfunction and an increased pituitary TSH reserve. Pasqualini and others[51] have suggested that thyroid dysfunction occurs frequently in all children following comprehensive treatment for medulloblastoma. Nine of 13 patients they studied had an elevated TSH response after TRH, which indicated the presence of either primary or hypothalamic (tertiary) disease.

Secondary or pituitary hypothyroidism is less common than primary dysfunction but occurs more frequently as the total radiation exposure of the hypothalamic-pituitary axis is increased. The rapidity of onset of TSH deficiency is dose dependent,[39] but the actual dose of radiation required to produce endocrine dysfunction has not been conclusively demonstrated. Duffner and co-workers[23] reported that children who received at least 3,000 cGy to the spine developed primary hypothyroidism, whereas a dose of at least 5,500 cGy to the whole brain resulted in TSH deficiency as well as GH and adrenocorticotropin (ACTH) deficiency.[23]

A high incidence of lymphocytic thyroiditis is observed after thyroid irradiation. In a series of 416 patients with a history of thyroid irradiation and suspected thyroid dysfunction, 20% had antimicrosomal antibodies and 9% had antithyroglobulin antibodies.[20] Thyroid antibodies in five of 11 patients with medulloblastoma were reported in another study by Pasqualini and colleagues.[51] Chronic lymphocytic thyroiditis may progress with time into hypothyroidism.

Diagnosis of Thyroid Hormone Deficiency

Evaluation of thyroid function should include the measurement of serum T₄, TSH, and triiodothyronine (T₃). If an isolated elevation of TSH occurs, measurement of antimicrosomal and antithyroglobulin antibodies is important in diagnosing chronic lymphocytic thyroiditis. A TRH stimulation test is not necessary for confirmation of hypothyroidism following craniospinal irradiation. In primary hypothyroidism, an elevated TSH level with a normal (compensated) or low serum T₄ level is seen. In secondary-pituitary, or tertiary-hypothalamic hypothyroidism, a low serum T₄ level with normal or low TSH levels are present.

Etiology of Thyroid Hormone Deficiency

Patients who receive craniospinal irradiation for brain tumors are at risk for development of primary hypothyroidism from radiation injury to the thyroid gland. Hormone deficiency may occur following radiation damage to the thyroid follicular cells, the supporting stroma, or the microvasculature. As with GH administration, cranial irradiation can result in pituitary or hypothalamic hypothyroidism. The mechanisms of injury may include damage to the pituitary cells, which secrete TSH; impaired hypothalamic secretion of TRH; pituitary stroma injury; or vascular changes, which impair delivery of hypothalamic releasing factors.[19]

Treatment Recommendations

The majority of patients who manifest hypothyroidism secondary to craniospinal irradiation have subclinical hypothyroidism. Animal studies by Lindsay and associates[38] demonstrated that elevation of TSH may increase the formation of thyroid gland tumors, and the risks of developing thyroid tumors following radiation exposure of the gland may be increased by longstanding elevation of TSH. We recommend, therefore, that even modest elevations of TSH be suppressed with levothyroxine supplementation. An initial levothyroxine dose of 0.05 to 0.10 mg/day is adjusted according to patient age and weight. Although levothyroxine reduces TSH levels to normal, no long-term evidence exists to support a protective effect on the risk of thyroid carcinoma.

Patients who have received a radiation dose exceeding

1,000 cGy to the neck should undergo thyroid screening examination every 6 months for at least 3 years. Evaluation should include careful physical examination of the thyroid gland and serial assay of serum T_4 and TSH levels. On confirmation of thyroid hormone deficiency, supplementation is initiated with oral levothyroxine, 0.05 to 0.10 mg/day, and follow-up endocrinologic evaluation is scheduled every 6 months.

GONDADOTROPIN DEFICIENCY AND GONADAL DYSFUNCTION

Frequency of Gonadotropin and Gonadal Dysfunction

Cranial irradiation may alter gonadotropin secretion in diverse ways. Irradiation of the hypothalamic-pituitary axis can result in gonadotropin deficiency or hyperprolactinemia.[55] Elevated prolactin levels, which can alter normal reproductive physiology, have been reported in adults who have completed high doses of cranial irradiation,[55] whereas similar changes have been infrequent in children and adolescents. Precocious puberty has been reported following high-dose cranial irradiation administered for brain tumors distant from the hypothalamic-pituitary axis and following low doses given to children with ALL.[7, 35] Radiation targeted to the abdomen, spine, or gonads may produce primary gonadal dysfunction. Primary gonadal dysfunction may also result from diverse chemotherapeutic agents, with or without irradiation.

Gonadotropin deficiency may result in either a lack of or an interruption in pubertal development. As with other hormone deficiencies, the risk of gonadotropin deficiency is linked to the radiation dosage. The hypothalamic neurons that secrete gonadotropin-releasing hormone (GnRH) and the pituitary gonadotropes are relatively resistant to the biologic effects of radiation exposure of less than 2,400 cGy, especially in prepubertal patients.[44, 65] In a study of 45 children who received cranial irradiation for treatment of head and neck tumors and medulloblastoma, five children developed GnRH deficiency.[55] Following comprehensive treatment for brain tumors distant from the hypothalamic-pituitary region, Livesy and co-workers[40] studied gonadotropin secretion in 93 patients: 51 males and 42 females. Hypogonadotropic hypogonadism occurred in 5.8% of postpubertal patients. Two of these seven male patients had pineal region tumors, which are known to interfere with gonadotropin secretion; this suggests that the prevalence of treatment-associated gonadotropin deficiency in the study may be overestimated.

Ahmed and colleagues[1] studied ten males and seven females with medulloblastoma following craniospinal irradiation alone or in combination with adjuvant chemotherapy. Primary gonadal dysfunction was observed in the nine children who received a combination of craniospinal irradiation and nitrosourea chemotherapy. Gonadal dysfunction was not observed following irradiation alone, which suggests that nitrosoureas may cause severe gonadal injury.

In the testes, spermatogonia are more susceptible than Leydig cells to damage from irradiation. Exposure as low as 20 cGy may cause temporary sterility in adults. Increased irradiation to the testes results in a decrease in recovery capacity and an increase in the delay of recovery, whereas chance of recovery is little when exposure exceeds 600 cGy.[6] Leydig cell insufficiency occurs in the majority of children treated with direct bilateral testicular irradiation for ALL. The severity of the damage is correlated with the age at exposure, and younger patients appear more vulnerable.

Irradiation of the prepubertal testis may lead to changes in gonadotropin levels during the prepubertal years. After an exposure of 2,400 cGy of testicular irradiation, basal plasma follicle-stimulating hormone (FSH) levels were elevated in some prepubertal and in all pubertal patients studied by Brauner and co-workers.[6] In some patients, gonadotropin levels were elevated only after puberty began. Spontaneous pubertal virilization does occur in some children who have sustained gonadal damage, and it is accompanied by compensated Leydig cell dysfunction.

Radiation damage to the ovaries occurs more frequently in older than in younger women. The population of oocytes is finalized at birth and decreases with age, resulting in an increased susceptibility to radiation damage in older women. The dose of radiation that causes permanent sterility is related to patient age and the number of remaining oocytes at the time of irradiation. It is possible, however, to induce permanent sterility in women of any age with a single exposure exceeding 600 cGy.

Cyclophosphamide and alkylating agents have been associated with gonadal damage. The degree and the permanence of the injury depends on patient age, total dose of drug received, and duration of treatment.[6, 12, 43] Irrespective of pubertal status, the ovaries are sensitive to effects of chemotherapy. Nicosia and others[46] studied the gonadal histologic characteristics of 21 prepubertal and pubertal females who received radiation therapy to the entire abdomen, pelvis, or inguinal region, with or without chemotherapy, for non-leukemia cancers. More than 50% of the patients, regardless of age, had a reduced number of ovarian follicles compared with age-matched controls. This decrease followed chemotherapy and was enhanced when treatment also included irradiation.

Cranial irradiation can lead to gonadotropin dysfunction, resulting in precocious puberty.[7] Precocious puberty has been reported in patients receiving cranial irradiation with exposure as low as 1,800 cGy.[35] Early puberty development with low-dose cranial irradiation is most common in young girls; the younger the child is when irradiation is completed, the more likely it is that a disturbance in the timing of puberty will occur.[62]

Etiology of Gonadal Dysfunction

Comprehensive treatment of brain tumors with irradiation and/or chemotherapy may result in gonadal dysfunction caused by primary gonadal injury or hypothalamic-pituitary dysfunction. As with other hormones, the hypothalamus appears to be more vulnerable than the pituitary to irradiation. Radiation exposure of 5,000 to 6,500 cGy to the pituitary and hypothalamus may result in severe gonadotropin deficiency.[55] Isolated gonadotropin deficiency is quite rare and is closely linked with GH deficiency.

Spinal axis radiation therapy may cause injury to the ovaries or the testes. The testes are more vulnerable to damage by cytotoxic agents than are the ovaries. Despite a profound impact of cyclophosphamide or nitrosoureas on the germinal epithelium of the testes, pubertal development may progress normally, because the severity of testosterone insufficiency and damage to the Leydig cell is quite variable.[17] Few patients require androgen therapy. Following administration of cyclophosphamide, a dose-dependent oligospermia or azoospermia occurs, and sperm density is inversely linked with the cumulative dose.[17] Subtle injury to the Leydig cell has been observed; the ovary, however, suffers injury that includes reduction in the number of follicles, stromal fibrosis, vascular proliferation, and thickening.[46]

Diagnosis of Gonadotropin and Gonadal Dysfunction

Patients who have completed comprehensive tumor therapy should be evaluated for gonadotropin deficiency or gonadal failure if they fail to progress through puberty at the appropriate age. Boys younger than 9 years and girls younger than 8 years who exhibit early signs of sexual development should be evaluated for precocious puberty.

In contrast to GH deficiency, which is often apparent in the first year following comprehensive tumor therapy, gonadal abnormalities may not be diagnosed until a child reaches either puberty or adulthood. An increase in plasma FSH reflects damage to the germinal cells of the testis or ovary, and damage to the Leydig cells of the testis or the theca cells of the ovary may result in an increased luteinizing hormone concentration. Elevated serum FSH is the most sensitive indicator of gonadal damage; the level varies widely with patient age and the extent of injury.[71]

If precocious puberty is suspected on the basis of clinical findings, the diagnosis is confirmed by demonstrating a pubertal gonadotropin response to GnRH dynamic testing.

Treatment and Recommendations

Children who have gonadal failure or hypothalamic or pituitary gonadal dysfunction should be treated with the appropriate sex steroid at the time at which normal pubertal development would occur. Monthly intramuscular testosterone enanthate injections in slowly increasing doses results in appropriate pubertal virilization in males. Young females should receive an estrogen preparation, initially at a low dose that is ultimately increased, and progesterone should be added in a cyclical manner.

Children who manifest early puberty should be treated with a GnRH analog, such as Lupron (TAP Pharmaceuticals, Deerfield, Ill.). The effects of Lupron include suppression of further pubertal development, some regression of sexual development, and possibly a reduced rate of epiphyseal maturation.

ADRENOCORTICOTROPIN DYSFUNCTION

Frequency of Adrenocorticotropin Dysfunction

Symptomatic ACTH deficiency is a rare complication of cranial irradiation.[54] Subnormal stimulated cortisol levels have been observed following cranial irradiation, whereas the long-term effects of adrenal exposure following craniospinal axis irradiation are unknown. In a study of 78 children treated with multi-agent chemotherapy, with or without irradiation, prior to bone marrow transplantation for hematologic malignancies, adrenal function was noted to be subnormal in 24% of the patients. Although these patients were asymptomatic, a subnormal plasma 11-deoxycortisol level was demonstrated after metyrapone stimulation.[57] As with other hormone deficiencies, ACTH deficiency is related to the dose of cranial radiation. Following pituitary irradiation in 141 adult patients, the incidence of ACTH deficiency was greater among patients who received 3,500 to 4,500 cGy than in those who received 2,000 cGy.[39]

Diagnosis and Treatment

The evaluation of the hypothalamic-pituitary-adrenal axis requires demonstration of diurnal cortisol rhythms, increased cortisol levels following insulin-induced hypoglycemia, and metyrapone testing. Following confirmation of adrenal insufficiency, daily hydrocortisone replacement therapy is initiated with 10 to 12.5 mg/m² in two divided doses. In the event of minor illness in the patient, the dose should be doubled and should be administered three or four times daily. In situations of greater physiologic stress, especially during surgery or episodes of sepsis, the dose of hydrocortisone should be fivefold to tenfold greater than the maintenance dose, and it should be administered parenterally in three or four divided doses.

CONCLUSIONS

Following comprehensive brain tumor therapy, patients are at risk for development of hypothalamic-pituitary dysfunction.[23] The total radiation dose, fractionation schedule, and duration of therapy are important variables that influence the risk of endocrinologic dysfunction after irradiation. Protocol administration of chemotherapeutic agents can lead to direct gonadal damage and may sensitize the hypothalamus or pituitary to the ionizing effects of radiation.

Endocrinologic evaluation should be performed before and after surgery and comprehensive brain tumor therapy. Endocrine failure may occur anytime from shortly after treatment to many years later, and long-term surveillance of hormone function is required. Baseline studies should include thyroid function tests, serum IGF1 levels, and x-rays of the hand and wrist for bone age determination. It is very helpful when prior growth curves are available for comparison. During neuro-oncology follow-up, linear growth should be recorded each 3 to 6 months and serial IGF1 and thyroid function screening levels sampled. When a patient's growth velocity begins to decelerate, or if IGF1 levels decrease, further evaluation for GH deficiency is indicated. Additional static and provocative assays test the function of the thyroid and the hypothalamic-pituitary-adrenal and hypothalamic-pituitary-gonadal axes.

Early diagnosis and supplementation of GH or other hormone deficiencies can successfully facilitate growth to nearly normal height. With preservation of stature and normal puberty development, patients may view themselves more positively and be better able to integrate within their families and in school, employment, and social communities.

REFERENCES

1. Ahmed SR, Shalet SM, Campbell RH, et al: Primary gonadal damage following treatment of brain tumors in childhood. J Pediatr 1983; 103:562–565.
2. Albini CH, Sotos J, Sherman B, et al: Diagnostic significance of urinary growth hormone measurements in children with growth hormone failure: Correlation between serum and urine growth hormone. Pediatr Res 1991; 29:619–622.
3. Arslanian SA, Becker DJ, Lee PA, et al: Growth hormone therapy and tumour recurrence. AJDC 1985; 139:347–350.
4. Barnes ND: Effects of external irradiation on the thyroid gland in childhood. Horm Res 1988; 30:84–89.
5. Bloom HJ, Wallace EN, Henk JM, et al: The treatment and prognosis of medulloblastoma in children: A study of 82 certified cases. AJR 1969; 105:43–62.
6. Brauner R, Caltabiano P, Rappaport R, et al: Leydig cell insufficiency after testicular irradiation for acute lymphoblastic leukemia. Horm Res 1988; 30:111–114.
7. Brauner R, Czernichow P, Rappaport R: Precocious puberty after hypothalamic and pituitary irradiation in young children. N Engl J Med 1984; 311:920.
8. Brauner R, Malandry F, Rappaport R, et al: Sequential occurrence of endocrine disturbances in children treated for optic gliomas. Pediatr Res 1988; 23:111.
9. Brauner R, Rappaport R, Prevot C, et al: A prospective study of the development of growth hormone deficiency in children given cranial irradiation, and its relation to statuary growth. J Clin Endocrinol Metabol 1989; 68:346–351.
10. Brown H, Lee TJ, Eden OB, et al: Growth and endocrine function after treatment for medulloblastoma. Arch Dis Child 1983; 58:722–727.
11. Brown P, Gajdusek DC, Gibbs CJ Jr, et al: Epidemic of Creutzfeldt-Jakob disease from human growth hormone therapy. N Engl J Med 1985; 313:728–731.
12. Chapman RM: Effects of cytotoxic therapy on sexuality and gonadal function. Semin Oncol 1982; 9:84–92.
13. Chrousos GO, Poplack D, Brown T, et al: Effects of cranial radiation on hypothalamic-adenohypophyseal function: Abnormal growth hormone secretory dynamics. J Clin Endocrinol Metabol 1982; 54:1135–1139.
14. Clayton PE, Shalet SM, Gattamaneni HR, et al: Does growth hormone cause relapse of brain tumors? Lancet 1987; 1:711–713.
15. Clayton PE, Shalet SM: Dose dependency of time of onset of radiation-induced growth hormone deficiency. J Pediatr 1991; 118:226–228.
16. Clayton PE, Shalet SM, Price DA: Growth response to growth hormone therapy following cranial irradiation. Eur J Pediatr 1988; 147:593–596.
17. Clayton PE, Shalet SM, Price DA, et al: Gonadal function after chemotherapy and irradiation for childhood malignancies. Horm Res 1988; 30:104–110.
18. Costin G: Effects of low-dose cranial radiation on growth hormone secretory dynamics and hypothalamic function. AJDC 1988; 142:847–852.
19. Constine LS, Woolf PD, Cann D, et al: Hypothalamic-pituitary dysfunction after radiation for brain tumors. N Engl J Med 1993; 328:87–94.
20. DeGroot LJ, Reilly M, Pinnameneni K, et al: Retrospective and prospective study of radiation induced thyroid disease. Am J Med 1983; 74:852–862.
21. Donaldson DL, Pan F, Hollowell JG: Reliability of stimulated and spontaneous growth hormone (GH) levels for identifying the child with low GH secretion. J Clin Endocrinol Metabol 1991; 72:647–652.
22. Duffner PK, Cohen ME: Long-term consequences of CNS treatment for childhood cancer: II. Clinical consequences. Pediatr Neurol 1991; 7:237–242.
23. Duffner PK, Cohen ME, Anderson SW, et al: Long-term effects of treatment on endocrine function in children with brain tumors. Ann Neurol 1983; 14:528–532.
24. Duffner PK, Cohen ME, Voorhees ML: Long-term effects of cranial irradiation on endocrine function in children with brain tumors: A prospective study. Cancer 1985; 56:2189–2193.
25. Fleming D, Black TL, Thompson EI, et al: Thyroid dysfunction and neoplasia in children receiving neck irradiation for cancer. Cancer 1985; 55:1190.
26. Gibbs CJ, Joy A, Heffner R, et al: Clinical and pathological features and laboratory confirmation of Creutzfeldt-Jakob disease in a recipient of pituitary-derived human growth hormone. N Engl J Med 1985; 313:734–738.
27. Green DM, Brecher ML, Yakar D, et al: Thyroid function in pediatric patients after neck irradiation for Hodgkin's disease. Med Pediatr Oncol 1980; 8:127.
28. Haider A, Cullen JW, Ellerbeck JA, et al: Pituitary function in children and adolescents following treatment for glial tumors. J Pediatr Endocrinol 1989; 3:205–211.
29. Heinrich JJ, Martinez AS, Domene H, et al: Treatment of hypopituitary children with synthetic met-growth hormone (Somatrem): Two years experience. J Pediatr Endocrinol 1991; 4:7–18.
30. Inoya H, Takakura K, Epstein F, et al: Treatment of medulloblastoma. *In* Kageyama N, et al (eds): Intracranial Tumors in Infancy and Childhood. Basel, Switzerland, Karger, 1987, pp 91–99.
31. Kanev PM, Lefebvre JF, Mauseth RS, et al: Growth hormone deficiency following radiation therapy of primary brain tumors in children. J Neurosurg 1991; 74:743–748.
32. Koch TK, Berg BO, DeArmand SJ, et al: Creutzfeldt-Jakob disease in a young adult with idiopathic hypopituitarism: Possible relation to the administration of cadaveric human growth hormone. N Engl J Med 1985; 313:731–733.
33. Lam KSL, Tse VKC, Wang C, et al: Early effects of cranial irradiation on hypothalamic pituitary function. J Clin Endocrinol Metabol 1987; 64:418–424.
34. Lannering B, Marky I, Mellander L: Growth hormone secretion and response to growth hormone therapy after treatment for brain tumor. Acta Paediatr Scand 1988; 343(suppl):146–151.
35. Leiper AD, Stanhope R, Kitching P, et al: Precocious puberty associated with treatment of acute lymphoblastic leukemia. Arch Dis Child 1987; 62:1107–1112.
36. Leiper AD, Stanhope R, Preece MA, et al: Precocious or early puberty and growth failure in girls treated for acute lymphoblastic leukemia. Horm Res 1988; 30:72–76.
37. Lentz RD, Bergstein J, Steffes MW, et al: Postpubertal evaluation of gonadal function following cyclophosphamide therapy before and during puberty. J Pediatr 1977; 91:385–394.
38. Lindsay S, Sheline GE, Potter GD, et al: Induction of neoplasia in the thyroid gland of the rat by x-irradiation of the gland. Cancer Res 1961; 21:9–16.
39. Littley MD, Shalet SM, Beardwell CG, et al: Radiation induced hypopituitarism is dose dependent. Clin Endocrinol 1989; 31:363–373.
40. Livesey EA, Brook CG: Gonadal dysfunction after treatment of intracranial tumors. Arch Dis Child 1988; 63:495–500.
41. Livesey EA, Brook CG: Thyroid dysfunction after radiotherapy and chemotherapy of brain tumors. Arch Dis Child 1989; 64:593–595.
42. Lustig RH, Schriock EA, Kaplan SL, et al: Effect of growth hormone-releasing factor on growth hormone release in children with radiation induced growth hormone deficiency. Pediatrics 1985; 76:274–279.
43. Maquire L: Fertility and cancer therapy. Postgrad Med 1979; 65(5 suppl):293–299.
44. Mauras N, Sabio H, Rogol AD: Neuroendocrine function in survivors of childhood leukemia and non-Hodgkin's lymphoma: A study of pulsatile growth hormone and gonadotropin secretions. Am J Pediatr Hematol Oncol 1988; 10:9–17.
45. Mulhern RK, Horowitz ME, Kovnar EH, et al: Neurodevelopmental

status of infants and young children treated for brain tumors with preirradiation chemotherapy. J Clinical Oncol 1989; 7:1660–1666.

46. Nicosia SV, Matus-Ridley M, Meadows AT: Gonadal effects of cancer therapy in girls. Cancer 1985; 55:2364–2372.

47. Oberfield SE, Allen JC, Pollack J, et al: Long-term endocrine sequelae after treatment of medulloblastoma: Prospective study of growth and thyroid function. J Pediatr 1986; 108:219–223.

48. Ogilvy-Stuart AL, Ryder WDJ, Gattamaneni HR, et al: Growth hormone and tumour recurrence. Br Med J 1992; 304:1601–1604.

49. Packer RJ, Sutton LN, Goldwein JW, et al: Improved survival with the use of adjuvant chemotherapy in the treatment of medulloblastoma. J Neurosurg 1991; 74:433–440.

50. Park TS, Hoffman HJ, Hendrick EB, et al: Medulloblastoma: Clinical presentation and management. J Neurosurg 1983; 58:543–552.

51. Pasqualini T, Diez B, Domene H, et al: Long-term endocrine sequelae after surgery, radiotherapy, and chemotherapy in children with medulloblastoma. Cancer 1987; 59:801–806.

52. Pavord SR, Girach A, Price DE, et al: A retrospective audit of the combined pituitary function test, using the insulin stress test, TRH and GnRH in a district laboratory. Clin Endocrinol 1992; 36:135–139.

53. Pomerede R, Czernichow P, Zucker JM, et al: Incidence of anterior pituitary deficiency after radiotherapy at an early age: Study in retinoblastoma. Acta Paediatr Scand 1984; 73:115–119.

54. Rappaport R, Brauner R: Growth and endocrine disorders secondary to cranial irradiation. Pediatr Res 1989; 25:561–567.

55. Rappaport R, Brauner R, Czernichow P, et al: Effect of hypothalamic and pituitary irradiation on pubertal development of children with brain tumors. J Clin Endocrinol Metabol 1982; 54:1164–1168.

56. Sanchez JP, Smal J, Le Bail PY: Localization and characterization of growth hormone binding sites in the central nervous system of a teleost fish (*Oncorhynchus mykiss*). Growth Regul 1991; 1:145–152.

57. Sanders JE, Pritchard S, Mahoney P, et al: Growth and development following marrow transplantation for leukemia. Blood 1986; 68:1129–1135.

58. Sanders JE, Buckner CD, Sullivan K, et al: Growth and development after bone marrow transplantation. *In* Buckner CD, Gale RP, Lucarelli G, et al (eds): Advances and Controversies in Thalasemia Therapy: Bone Marrow Transplantation and Other Approaches. New York, Alan R. Liss, 1989; pp 375–382.

59. Shalet SM: Irradiation-induced growth failure. Clin Endocrinol Metabol 1986; 15:591–605.

60. Shalet SM, Beardwell CA, Aarons BM, et al: Growth impairment in children treated for brain tumors. Arch Dis Child 1978; 53:491–494.

61. Shalet SM, Beardwell CG, Pearson D, et al: The effect of varying doses of cerebral irradiation in growth hormone production in childhood. Clinical Endocrinol 1976; 5:287–290.

62. Shalet SM, Clayton PE, Price DA: Growth and pituitary function in children treated for brain tumors and acute lymphocytic leukemia. Horm Res 1988; 30:53–61.

63. Shalet SM, Clayton PE, Price DA: Growth impairment following treatment for childhood brain tumors. Acta Paediatric Scand 1988; 343(suppl):137–145.

64. Silink M: Alternative methods of diagnosis of growth hormone deficiency. J Pediatr Endocrinol 1992; 5:43–52.

65. Siris ES, Leventhal BG, Vaitukaitis JL, et al: Effects of childhood leukemia and chemotherapy on puberty and reproductive function in girls. N Engl J Med 1976; 294:1143–1146.

66. Steiner L: Personal communication, 1994.

67. Sulmont V, Brauner R, Fontoura M, et al: Response to growth hormone treatment and final height after cranial or craniospinal irradiation. Acta Paediatr Scand 1990; 79:542–549.

68. Taylor SL, Kaplan SL, Conte FA, et al: The endocrine morbidity of hypothalamic gliomas. Abstract presented at the 20th winter meeting, Pediatric Section—American Association of Neurological Surgeons. Boston, December 1991.

69. Van Vliet G, Styne DM, Kaplan SL, et al: Growth hormone treatment for short stature. N Engl J Med 1983; 309:1017–1022.

70. Will RG: An overview of Creutzfeldt-Jakob disease associated with the use of human pituitary growth hormone. Dev Biol Stand 1991; 75:85–86.

71. Winter JS, Faiman C: Serum gonadotropin concentrations in agonadal children and adults. J Clin Endocrinol Metabol 1972; 35:561–564.

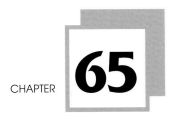

CHAPTER **65**

Systemic Sequelae of Chemotherapy for Gliomas

Because current chemotherapeutic agents are only modestly effective in controlling most gliomas, it is imperative that the physician treating the patient be familiar with the potential toxic effects of therapy. One must evaluate the potential benefits and harms of the proposed intervention to make appropriate treatment recommendations. Furthermore, safe and effective use of combinations of drugs depends in part on choosing agents that have different toxic effects. This chapter reviews the toxic effects of the most commonly used chemotherapeutic agents. It does not discuss the many drugs that are not used with regularity nor does it review drugs that are available only through experimental protocols. Specifically, the nitrosoureas (BCNU [carmustine] and CCNU [lomustine]), procarbazine, vincristine, and the platinum analogues (cisplatin and carboplatin), are reviewed.

NITROSOUREAS

Carmustine is probably the most commonly prescribed chemotherapeutic agent used in the treatment of gliomas. Both conventional doses and high-dose regimens with autologous bone marrow rescue have been employed. It can be given either by intravenous or intra-arterial routes. Toxic effects vary, depending on the dose and the route of administration. The toxic effects of conventional intravenous administration, high-dose regimens with bone marrow transplantation, and intra-arterial administration, respectively, are reviewed here.

Conventional Intravenous Administration

For gliomas, carmustine is commonly administered intravenously at a dose of 200 mg/m^2 on 1 day or 80 mg/m^2 for 3 consecutive days every 6 to 8 weeks. At these doses, the most common acute toxic effects are local venous irritation at the site of the infusion, nausea, and vomiting.[1] The venous irritation may be lessened by slowing the infusion rate or by wrapping the arm with a heating pad. With the administration of antiemetic agents with antiserotonergic properties, such as ondansetron and granisetron, nausea and vomiting with single-agent carmustine therapy is uncommon. When it occurs, patients usually experience symptoms within 2 to 6 hours, with resolution of symptoms within 24 hours. Emesis is seldom a substantial problem when antiemetics are used appropriately.

Myelosuppression is usually the dose-limiting toxic effect of conventional intravenous carmustine therapy.[1, 2] Myelosuppression is characteristically delayed 3 to 6 weeks following drug administration, with thrombocytopenia occurring first, followed by leukopenia. Spontaneous resolution of cytopenia usually occurs in 6 to 8 weeks, allowing for repetitive dosing. However, cumulative myelosuppression often occurs, requiring dose reduction and increased intervals between treatments. It is necessary to monitor leukocyte and platelet counts following each cycle of treatment, because myelosuppression often becomes progressively more severe with each dose. Myelosuppression may be complicated by life-threatening or fatal infection or hemorrhage. Leukopenia with infection is the most common fatal complication of carmustine therapy.

Hemorrhage is significantly less common, although platelet transfusions prophylactically for platelets less than 20,000/µL) may be required. Occasionally, leukocyte and platelet counts never return to sufficiently high levels to permit additional chemotherapy. The utility and timing of administration of colony stimulating factors, such as granulocyte–colony-stimulating factor (G-CSF) and granulocyte-macrophage colony-stimulating factor (GM-CSF) have not been adequately evaluated with regard to the nitrosoureas. This issue is under investigation.[3]

Increased myelosuppression has also been reported with carmustine and other drugs, particularly cimetidine.[4] Because administration of anticonvulsants, especially carbamazepine and phenytoin, may also result in myelosuppression, unusually severe, prolonged, or progressive cytopenia should alert the clinician to consider switching or discontinuing the other drugs if the risk to the patient becomes significant.

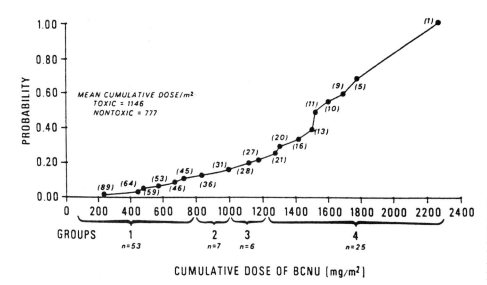

Figure 65–1 Correlation of carmustine (BCNU) pulmonary toxic response and total cumulative dose. (From Aronin PA, Mahaley MS Jr, Rudnick SA, et al: Prediction of BCNU pulmonary toxicity in patients with malignant gliomas. N Engl J Med 1980;303:183–188.)

Another relatively common subacute toxic effect of carmustine is elevation of the hepatic enzymes, usually the transaminases, such as aspartate aminotransferase (AST). Transaminase elevation is most commonly asymptomatic and mild. It is typically reversible with discontinuation of treatment.[1] Patients may tolerate additional carmustine if the dose is reduced in relation to the transaminase elevation. Patients occasionally experience symptoms of clinical hepatitis, such as nausea, vomiting, fatigue, anorexia, and weight loss. Continued administration of carmustine under those circumstances may result in substantial hepatic toxic effects. Occasionally, hepatic toxic effects will preclude continued use of the drug.

Carmustine and other nitrosoureas may cause renal insufficiency,[1] usually manifested by an asymptomatic rise in blood urea nitrogen (BUN) or creatinine levels. These changes seem to be more prominent with increased cumulative doses and may appear following cessation of therapy.[5–7] When the total cumulative dose is limited, clinically significant renal toxic effects appear to be minimal.

Pulmonary toxic effects, first reported in 1976,[8] can be a fatal complication of carmustine chemotherapy. The incidence of this complication has been estimated to be 10% to 30% in patients given sufficiently high doses.[9–12] The risk of pulmonary toxic effects increases with total cumulative dose, with excessive risk occurring at total doses above 1,200 to 1,500 mg/m^2 (Fig. 65–1). Patients with underlying pulmonary disease are at increased risk of toxic response.

The pathologic process probably begins as an interstitial inflammatory process, resulting in diminished oxygen transfer from the alveoli to the interstitial capillaries (Fig. 65–2). Patients may be asymptomatic at this stage, with detection possible only through screening pulmonary function studies. Patients may also develop a nonproductive cough, dyspnea, and tachypnea. Progressive pulmonary injury may occur with or without additional doses of carmustine, resulting in pulmonary fibrosis with severe dyspnea, tachycardia, respiratory insufficiency, and death. In advanced cases, pathologic examination reveals abundant fibrous connective tissue within the alveolar septa, absence of inflammation, hyperplasia of the type II alveolar lining cells, and proliferation of visceral pleura connective tissue.

Physical examination of the chest may be normal or basilar or diffuse rales and rhonchi may be present. Pulmonary function studies generally reveal lowered carbon monoxide diffusion capacity (DL$_{CO}$), a measure of transcapillary gas exchange. If the process is more advanced or fulminant, pulmonary function studies may demonstrate a pattern of restrictive lung disease, including reduced lung volumes and vital capacity. Arterial blood gases may show an increased alveolar/arterial oxygen gradient, with or without low oxygen levels. Chest x-ray may be normal initially or may show unilateral or bilateral interstitial infiltrates in a reticulonodular pattern, with or without pleural effusions (Fig. 65–3). In the setting of leukopenia and corticosteroid administration, one must also consider an opportunistic infection in the differential diagnosis. Bronchoalveolar lavage and lung biopsy may be necessary to establish the diagnosis under these circumstances.

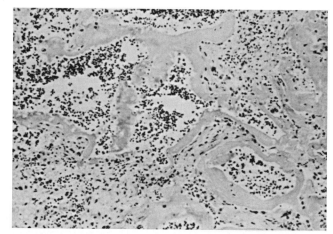

Figure 65–2 Photomicrograph of lung tissue from patient showing inflammatory changes, dense hyaline membranes, and interstitial edema associated with carmustine (BCNU) pulmonary toxic effects. (From Litam JP, Dail DH, Spitzer G, et al: Early pulmonary toxicity after administration of high-dose BCNU. Cancer Treat Rep 1981;65:39–44.)

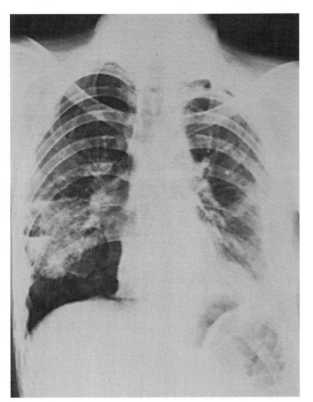

Figure 65–3 Chest x-ray showing bilateral pulmonary fibrosis and a small right pneumothorax in a patient who had received carmustine (BCNU). (From Holoye PY, Jenkins DE, Greenber SD: Pulmonary toxicity in long-term administration of BCNU. Cancer Treat Rep 1976;60:1691–1694.)

If the diagnosis of carmustine-induced pulmonary toxic response is suspected, no further treatment should be administered until the diagnosis is clarified. If the diagnosis is confirmed, patients should be given corticosteroids if they are not already receiving them. The condition may or may not reverse with corticosteroids. In general, pulmonary toxic effects are more amenable to treatment if diagnosed early in their evolution. If frank pulmonary fibrosis has occurred, the condition is irreversible.

Because of the potential severity of the complication and because of the availability of successful treatment if it is diagnosed early, some clinicians advocate the routine use of sequential screening DL_{CO} determinations in asymptomatic patients, and most recommend obtaining pulmonary function studies in patients with a history of pulmonary disease. For patients receiving therapy, a DL_{CO} less than 50% of predicted is considered a contraindication to further treatment, even in the absence of symptoms. Patients should continue to be evaluated following the completion of therapy, because pulmonary symptoms may appear up to several years later.[13, 14]

Another potential long-term effect of carmustine therapy is gonadal dysfunction. In females, chemotherapy-induced gonadal injury depends on the patient's age[15–17] and the cumulative dose of drug.[18] Although prepubertal girls may exhibit biochemical evidence of primary ovarian dysfunction, most progress normally through puberty and ovarian function appears to return to normal.[19] However, adult women commonly exhibit evidence of primary ovarian dys-

function, manifested symptomatically as amenorrhea, vaginal dryness with dyspareunia, diminshed libido, and hot flashes. Laboratory studies may reveal low circulating estrogen levels with elevated gonadotropins, luteinizing hormone (LH) and follicle-stimulating hormone (FSH). Older premenopausal women treated with higher doses of alkylating agents appear most likely to develop primary ovarian failure.

In addition to interference with ovarian endocrine function, damage to ovarian follicles may occur. Biopsy findings include absence of ova and follicles with thickening of the tunica albuginea and stromal hyalinization.[20] Infertility may or may not be permanent. Women should be informed of the risk of permanent premature ovarian failure and its consequences. The utility of reproductive technologies to induce multiple follicles and harvest oocytes for cryopreservation has not been explored.

The diagnosis of ovarian dysfunction from carmustine therapy may be complicated by other causes of ovarian dysfunction, such as hypothalamic or pituitary dysfunction caused by the brain tumor itself, endocrinopathy related to corticosteroids, or alterations related to cranial irradiation. Pregnancy is unlikely in the event of carmustine-induced ovarian failure, but it may be possible in the case of hypothalamic or pituitary dysfunction. Oral contraceptive or other estrogen and progesterone replacement may alleviate symptoms of menstrual irregularities, vaginal dryness, change in libido, and hot flashes. However, the increased risk of thromboembolic events associated both with hormone replacement and brain tumors must be considered.

Gonadal dysfunction in males is usually manifested by oligospermia. The incidence of sterility following carmustine therapy is unclear. Many patients succumb to the tumor, and posttreatment studies in survivors have not been performed. However, if one extrapolates information obtained from the laboratory and from experience in the treatment of boys and men with Hodgkin's disease and testicular carcinoma, certain generalizations can be inferred. First, alkylators appear particularly potent in damaging seminiferous tubules. The incidence of oligospermia is very high following 1 to 2 cycles of chemotherapy and remains high throughout treatment.[21, 22] Recovery following completion of chemotherapy is variable. Prepubertal males are less likely to become infertile than are postpubertal males. Higher doses of alkylators are associated with higher risk of oligospermia. Men should be informed of the potential for permanent sterility and referred for consideration of semen cryopreservation if desired. Given current reproductive endocrinology capabilities, semen cryopreservation is unlikely to delay initiation of chemotherapy. The pregnancy rate following semen cryopreservation and subsequent insemination is unknown.

Leydig cell damage with lowered testosterone levels is uncommon, and most males progress through puberty normally and maintain normal LH and testosterone levels during and following chemotherapy. In brain tumor patients, however, the use of cranial radiation complicates the evaluation of delayed puberty, impotence, and oligospermia, because both the hypothalamus and pituitary may be damaged from radiation, whereas only the testes are affected by chemotherapy. Laboratory evaluation should include both testosterone and gonadotropin levels, because simple replacement of testosterone may restore sexual function to pretreatment status.

Alkylators such as carmustine are known to be leukemogenic.[23] Myelofibrosis,[24] secondary myelodysplasia (MDS), and acute leukemia (AL) following treatment of glioma patients with nitrosourea chemotherapy have all been reported.[25–28] The median time to the development of MDS/AL is approximately 4 to 5 years, ranging from less than 1 to more than 25 years. A large percentage of patients who develop secondary MDS (55% to 84%) subsequently experience transformation to acute leukemia. Median survival following diagnosis of secondary MDS or AL is approximately 10 months. Either disorder is notoriously refractory to treatment. Presenting symptoms include fatigue, fever, bruising, or hemorrhage. Physical signs include pallor and bruises. Less commonly, patients may exhibit hepatomegaly, splenomegaly, lymphadenopathy, gingival hypertrophy, skin infiltration, or neurologic abnormalities related to CNS infiltration by leukemic cells. Peripheral blood findings are characterized predominantly by anemia and thrombocytopenia and, less commonly, leukopenia. Bone marrow examination most commonly reveals hypercellularity, although hypocellularity or normocellularity may be present. In secondary MDS, the marrow most closely resembles refractory anemia with excess blasts as described in the French-American-British classification for primary MDS/AL. However, morphologic differences exist in the appearance of the cells compared with those of de novo MDS, and precise classification is difficult. Similarly, the marrow in secondary AL is most commonly of the M1–M2 or M4 type, but morphologic differences between secondary and primary AL exist. Partial or complete losses of chromosome 5, and especially of chromosome 7, are characteristic of secondary MDS/AL; these losses occur in 50% to 97% of patients. The molecular mechanisms of secondary leukemogenesis are under investigation.

The incidence of secondary MDS/AL in brain tumor patients treated with nitrosourea chemotherapy is uncertain. Greene and co-workers[25] reported two cases of AL in 1,628 patients treated with carmustine. However, only 290 patients were observed for 2 years or longer. It is likely that the incidence is higher in patients who survive longer. For example, in patients with lung cancer treated with combination chemotherapy containing a nitrosourea, rates of secondary MDS/AL as high as 14% at 4 years and 25% at 3 years have been reported.[23] Possible factors that increase the incidence of secondary MDS/AL include older age (over 60 years), the use of multiple alkylators (such as nitrosourea plus procarbazine), and higher total cumulative dose and/or prolonged duration of therapy. These factors are particularly important when considering adjuvant chemotherapy with regimens such as procarbazine, CCNU, and vincristine for patients with more indolent tumors, such as low-grade or anaplastic astrocytoma and oligodendroglioma. Such patients must be informed of the potential risk of developing MDS/AL as well as of the uncertainties of the magnitude of risk.

Alkylators have long been known to be teratogenic.[29, 30] The risk of fetal loss or malformation is greatest if drugs are administered during the first trimester of pregnancy. Increased risk of congenital abnormalities related to chemotherapy administration during the second and third trimesters has been difficult to demonstrate. The risk of other abnormalities later in life, such as sterility or increased risk of malignancy, cannot be excluded, and women with childbearing potential should be advised of the risks and uncertainties of receiving chemotherapy at any time during pregnancy. In contrast, there is no indication that children born to women who have received chemotherapy prior to pregnancy have any increased risk of congenital abnormalities or malignancy.[31] Additional data are necessary to confirm these preliminary observations.

Lomustine is available only in oral formulation. Its toxic effects are essentially identical to those of carmustine, namely, nausea and vomiting; delayed and cumulative myelosuppression; pulmonary, hepatic, and renal toxic effects; leukemogenesis; teratogenicity; and gonadal dysfunction. The evidence that lomustine produces pulmonary toxic effects is limited to case reports, as no large series employing lomustine have reported pulmonary toxic effects.[12]

High-Dose Nitrosourea With Bone Marrow Transplantation

Because myelosuppression is often the dose-limiting toxic effect of carmustine, several investigators have examined the utility of high-dose carmustine followed by autologous bone marrow rescue. In these studies, doses of carmustine could be administered that ranged from 600 to 1,400 mg/m². As expected, myelosuppression could be ameliorated but not eliminated.[32–36] Typically, myelosuppression occurred earlier than with standard doses (1 week vs. 3 to 4 weeks), and deaths from sepsis during the period of myelosuppression occurred in most series despite the use of autologous marrow support. Interestingly, one report described late marrow failure following marrow engraftment,[36] which was attributed to premature marrow reinfusion before carmustine had cleared from the serum.

In addition to myelosuppression, pulmonary toxic effects were prevalent and became the dose-limiting toxic effect, occurring in up to 22% of patients. Other toxic effects included transaminasemia with occasional clinically symptomatic chemical hepatitis and hepatic failure. Acute facial flushing with tachycardia and hypotension during the infusion also occurred, as did acute and chronic encephalopathy. Hochberg and co-workers[32] concluded that doses of 1,400 mg/m² were associated with unacceptable CNS toxic effects.

In summary, high-dose carmustine with autologous bone marrow transplantation is feasible, permitting dose escalation for one or two courses at levels threefold to sixfold higher than conventional intravenous dosing. Dose-limiting toxic effects appear to be interstitial pneumonitis rather than myelosuppression. Fatal toxic effects include sepsis, pulmonary failure, and hepatic failure. The high rate of severe and fatal toxic effects makes this approach extremely hazardous.

Intracarotid Carmustine

The intracarotid administration of carmustine has resulted in toxic effects specific for that method of administration. In addition to myelosuppression, intracarotid carmustine causes ocular and central nervous system toxic responses. Early studies documented moderate to severe ipsilateral eye pain during the infusion in nearly all patients treated.[37] In addition, phase II studies demonstrated ipsilateral visual loss as a delayed complication of treatment occurring in 25% to 65% of patients treated.[37–40] Amaurosis can occur at the time of treatment with return of vision following therapy, or visual loss may begin several weeks from the start of therapy and continue to progress to irreversible blindness. Funduscopic findings include nerve fiber layer hemorrhages and infarctions ipsilateral to the side of infusion, along with cilioretinal artery occlusion, choroidal thrombi, and papillitis. Secondary glaucoma and a dilated, fixed pupil without other evidence of third nerve damage have also been reported. The mechanism of damage appears to be retinal vasculitis, as fluoroscein angiograms have shown both periarterial and perivenous leakage (Fig. 65–4).[40] In an attempt to prevent ocular toxic effects, investigators have utilized supraophthalmic intracarotid infusion of carmustine.[41, 42] Although ocular toxic response was minimized in these trials, central nervous system toxic response continued to occur.

Central nervous system toxic response has been reported using high-dose carmustine with autologous bone marrow transplant. Early studies demonstrated evidence of central nervous system toxic effects using intracarotid carmustine as well. In an early phase II trial, 7 of 36 patients demonstrated low-attenuation white matter changes on follow-up computed tomographic (CT) scans. Two of these seven patients experienced increased frequency of seizures and severe hemiparesis in the absence of tumor progression.[43] Subsequent publications described clinical and pathologic sequelae consistent with drug-induced leukoencephalopathy.[44–47] The appearance of neurotoxic response commonly occurs several weeks following treatment and consists of focal neurologic deficits corresponding to the vascular distribution infused with carmustine with associated generalized cognitive decline. Characteristic CT scan changes include low attenuation within the vascular distribution of the infusion. These changes may be associated with ventricular compression and midline shift; gyral and ventricular enhancement; and eventual calcification, permanent white matter hypodensity, and ventricular dilatation.

Neuropathologic features include severe hemispheric edema, swollen axons, coagulative and hemorrhagic white matter necrosis, fibrinoid vascular necrosis, and bizarre cellular morphology within the carmustine perfusion territory. Encephalopathy occurred in 9.5% of 153 patients treated in a large phase III trial that compared the efficacy of intravenous and intra-arterial carmustine therapy.[47] In this trial, it is also interesting to note that the frequency of systemic sequelae (myelosuppression with infection, altered hepatic and renal function, and pulmonary toxic effects) were similar in the intravenous and intra-arterial treatment groups.

PROCARBAZINE

Procarbazine is an oral agent classified as a nonclassic alkylating agent. It is usually administered daily for 14 to 21 days, followed by 1 week or more without therapy. Its toxic effects are similar to those of other alkylators, such as the nitrosoureas. As with carmustine and lomustine, myelosuppression is the dose-limiting toxic effect. However, the pattern of myelosuppression is different from that of the nitrosoureas in that the nadir leukocyte and platelet counts occur 7 to 14 days following completion of the course of therapy, and the marked cumulative toxic effects seen with the nitrosoureas is not evident. Procarbazine may also cause hemolytic anemia in patients with glucose-6-phosphate dehydrogenase deficiency.[48] Nausea and vomiting occur regularly with procarbazine unless antiemetics are administered prophylactically. Vomiting is more common in the first few days of a multiple-day course, tending to lessen as the course progresses. The use of antiemetics routinely for the first 3

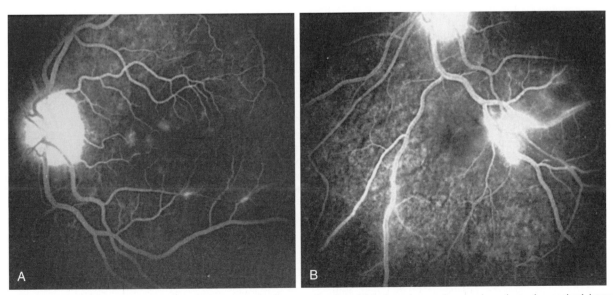

Figure 65–4 *A,* Intravenous fluorescein angiogram showing focal areas of periarterial leakage in macular area in patient who received intracarotid chemotherapy. *B,* Intravenous fluorescein angiogram showing areas of perivenous leakage in patient who received intracarotid chemotherapy. (From Miller DF, Bay JW, Lederman RJ, et al: Ocular and orbital toxicity following intracarotid injection of BCNU (carmustine) and cisplatinum for malignant gliomas. Ophthalmology 1985;92:402–406.)

days or more, or starting with a lower dose of procarbazine and progressing to higher doses during each cycle, may help lessen the degree of nausea and emesis. Like the nitrosoureas, procarbazine alone sometimes causes alopecia.

Allergic skin reactions and allergic interstitial pneumonitis have been reported with procarbazine.[49–53] These reactions appear to be treatable with corticosteroid administration. Patients may continue treatment with procarbazine following mild skin reactions, but severe skin reactions or interstitial pneumonitis pose sufficient risk to the patient that further administration under these circumstances would rarely be appropriate.

Procarbazine is a monoamine oxidase inhibitor with metabolism by the hepatic mitochondrial oxidase enzymes. These properties may result in direct central nervous system depression,[54] as noted when patients receive the intravenous formulation, and may potentiate the sedative effects of other agents metabolized by the same enzymes, notably phenobarbital and phenytoin.[55, 56] Such interactions may impair catabolism of these anticonvulsants and other CNS depressants, such as narcotics, phenothiazines, and sedative-type medications, thereby increasing their CNS depressant activity. Conversely, pretreatment with drugs metabolized by the hepatic microsomal enzyme system may increase the cytotoxic effects of procarbazine.[57] Theoretically, patients may be predisposed to hypertensive reactions if they are also receiving tricyclic antidepressants of or sympathomimetic agents or if they consume foods rich in tyramine such as red wine, bananas, ripe cheeses, and yogurt. Also, patients may experience a disulfuram-like reaction consisting of facial flushing, sweating, and headaches if they consume alcohol while taking procarbazine. Patients should be informed of the potential drug interactions, counseled regarding dietary and alcohol consumption, and monitored regularly with regard to serum anticonvulsant levels when treated with procarbazine.

Gonadal dysfunction in females and males has been noted clinically in patients treated with procarbazine for Hodgkin's disease, as noted previously. Because procarbazine is commonly given with another alkylator for Hodgkin's disease (nitrogen mustard) and gliomas (CCNU), it is difficult to separate the differential effects of procarbazine from the other alkylator. However, preclinical studies show procarbazine to be a potent suppressor of spermatogenesis.[58, 59] It is reasonable to conclude that procarbazine itself has potent gonadal effects that may or may not be reversible. It is particularly important to discuss the potential for infertility with younger patients with more indolent glioma so that they may assess their willingness to proceed with therapy and plan for assisted reproductive technologies should infertility result from treatment.

Teratogenic, leukemogenic, and carcinogenic effects of procarbazine are similar to those of the nitrosoureas, as discussed previously. Similar to the situation with gonadal toxic effects, the contribution of procarbazine to secondary malignancies and fetal malformation when administered with other alkylators cannot be distinguished clearly. Again, preclinical studies document the mutagenicity[60] and teratogenicity[61] of procarbazine, suggesting that procarbazine plays a substantial role in the clinical manifestations of these late toxic responses.

VINCRISTINE

Unlike the alkylators, vincristine has negligible myelosuppressive effects, making it an ideal agent to combine with other agents. Instead, its principal toxic effect is neurologic. The dose-limiting toxic effect of vincristine is peripheral neuropathy, which becomes progressively worse with cumulative administration of the drug.[62] Characteristically, the peripheral neuropathy presents first as asymptomatic loss of deep tendon reflexes—especially ankle jerks—and lowered vibratory perception threshold; this is followed by symmetrical paresthesias and numbness of the toes and fingertips, with progressively proximal extension over time. Weakness may occur as the neuropathy worsens. If a patient experiences severe sensory changes or if motor dysfunction occurs, it is usually necessary to permanently discontinue vincristine administration. The neuropathy may worsen, remain stable, or improve following discontinuation of therapy.

With higher dose administration, patients may also experience abdominal cramping, constipation, and ileus. On occasion, these side effects may necessitate hospitalization for symptomatic relief. Jaw pain may also occur shortly after administration of vincristine. Rarely, cranial nerve dysfunction with diplopia, hoarseness, dysphagia, or facial palsy may occur, usually, again, with higher doses (exceeding 2 mg/m^2 per dose). Central nervous system symptoms of depression, confusion, and insomnia have been reported, as have autonomic neuropathy associated with orthostatic hypotension.[63]

The only non-neurologic side effect noted with any significant degree of frequency is the syndrome of inappropriate secretion of antidiuretic hormone (SIADH).[64] This syndrome usually remits spontaneously in 2 to 3 days and usually requires no particular intervention.

PLATINUM ANALOGUES

Cisplatin and carboplatin, though chemically similar, have markedly different spectra of toxic responses. The most common toxic effects of cisplatin include nausea, vomiting, renal dysfunction, peripheral neuropathy, and ototoxic effects with relatively less myelosuppression. Cisplatin, like carmustine, has been administered via the intracarotid route with resulting ototoxic and central neurotoxic effects. By contrast, carboplatin rarely causes nausea, vomiting, nephrotoxic, neurotoxic, or ototoxic effects, but it is limited by myelosuppression. We review the toxic effects of conventional intravenous administration of cisplatin, intracarotid cisplatin, and carboplatin.

Intravenous Cisplatin

The most immediate side effect following administration of intravenous cisplatin is nausea and vomiting. It is one of the most emetic chemotherapeutic agents in use. Many studies of antiemetic agents use cisplatin-induced emesis to assess the effectiveness of the agents under study. With the availability of antiserotonergic agents, such as ondansetron and granisetron, emesis can be lessened in some, but not all, patients. It is usually possible to prevent the acute nausea and vomiting that occurs within 24 hours of administration, but delayed nausea and vomiting 48 to 120 hours after completion of therapy remains problematic for some patients. Furthermore, emesis seems more common with the last days of a multiple-day dosing schedule of cisplatin, compared with the first 1 or 2 days. Tachyphylaxis to antiserotoninergic agents is common, rendering emesis more difficult to control.

Nausea and vomiting are now less commonly the dose-limiting toxic effects of cisplatin, whereas nephrotoxic response remains a persistent, though manageable, problem. Commonly, patients experience transient elevation of the serum creatinine 1 to 2 weeks following administration of cisplatin, followed by return to normal or near-normal values.[65] Vigorous hydration, mannitol administration, and use of furosemide before and after chemotherapy lessen the probability and severity of renal dysfunction.[66, 67] Concomitant administration of other nephrotoxic agents, such as aminoglycosides or amphotericin B, may increase the risk of renal toxic effects.

Renal toxic response may appear either as reduced glomerular filtration rates (GFR) with decreased creatinine clearance and increased serum creatinine levels or as a tubular defect with hypomagnesemia and other electrolyte abnormalities.[68, 69] In the case of mildly reduced GFR, patients may continue treatment at full or reduced dosage, depending on the severity of renal damage. Similarly, mild renal tubular deficits can often be managed by electrolyte replacement in the form of oral magnesium, potassium, and/or bicarbonate. Uncommonly, the patient may develop chronic renal failure sufficiently severe to require dialysis. The mechanism of renal insufficiency appears to be direct toxic effects to specific renal brush border enzymes and renal tubular epithelium (Fig. 65–5).[67, 70]

Similar to vincristine, cisplatin may cause a symmetrical peripheral neuropathy involving the distal extremities, which is manifested by decreased ankle jerks, loss of vibratory

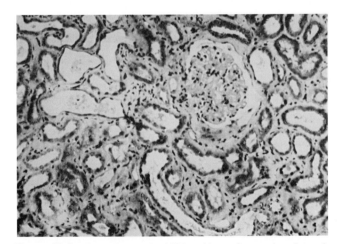

Figure 65–5 Photomicrograph of kidney biopsy from patient 5 months after cisplatin therapy showing dilation of the proximal and distal tubules with flattening of the lining cells and interstitial fibrosis. (From Dentino M, Luft FC, Yum MN, et al: Long-term effect of cis-diamminedichloride platinum (CDDP) on renal function and structure in man. Cancer 1978;41:1274–1281.)

sensation, paresthesias, and numbness of the fingertips and toes, followed by progressively proximal involvement of the limbs.[71, 72] Motor involvement follows unless the drug is discontinued. Following discontinuation, the neuropathy may improve, stabilize, or continue to worsen.[73, 74] In general, however, if cisplatin is discontinued prior to the onset of severe sensory changes or any motor changes, the residual toxic effects are not disabling.

In addition to the peripheral neurotoxic effects, cisplatin may result in sensorineural hearing loss.[75, 76] As with the neuropathy, the onset is subacute, initially presenting as tinnitus; it progresses to increasingly severe high-frequency hearing loss and then to deafness if drug therapy is continued. Like the peripheral neuropathy, ototoxic effects may improve, stabilize, or worsen following discontinuation of drug therapy. No preventive measures are available to prevent hearing loss, so the clinician must remember to question the patient prior to each dose of cisplatin regarding symptoms of hearing loss. Alternatively, serial audiograms may detect presymptomatic changes in high-frequency hearing.

In comparison with the classic alkylating agents, cisplatin has relatively less myelosuppression, making it an attractive agent to combine with more myelosuppressive agents. At higher doses, cisplatin causes thrombocytopenia to a greater extent than leukopenia.[77] The nadir leukocyte and platelet counts typically occur 7 to 14 days following drug administration, with recovery within 3 weeks. In addition, cisplatin may cause significant anemia,[78] probably by direct suppression of marrow erythroid precursors. The anemia may require several months to correct itself following discontinuation of cisplatin, and it is occasionally severe enough to warrant red blood cell transfusion.

Although secondary leukemias have been reported,[79, 80] they seem to occur less frequently with cisplatin than with the classic alkylators and procarbazine. Similarly, gonadal toxic effects with infertility appear to be less of a problem with cisplatin than with other alkylator-containing regimens.[81, 82]

Intracarotid Cisplatin

Systemic toxic effects with intracarotid cisplatin that are similar to those with intravenous cisplatin have been reported, including mild myelosuppression, nausea and vomiting, auditory toxic effects, nephrotoxic effects, and hypomagnesemia.[83–85] In addition, toxic effects similar to those with intracarotid carmustine have been observed with intracarotid cisplatin. Severe ocular and central nervous system toxic effects have been reported. Ocular toxic effects consisted of orbital pain and transient or permanent ipsilateral or bilateral decreased visual acuity, including permanent blindness. Neuro-ophthalmologic examinations and fluoroscein angiography have demonstrated retinal vasculitis and ischemic optic neuropathy. Central nervous system toxic effects include seizures immediately following treatment, including status epilepticus leading to permanent encephalopathy and coma. Transient or permanent focal neurologic damage may occur, including hemiparesis or aphasia. The focal deficits may result either from emboli or direct central nervous system toxic response. Delayed encephalopathic changes may also occur, with CT scan showing diffuse ipsilateral hemispheric low-attenuation changes. The frequency of central nervous system toxic effects is unclear, but it may be lower than that seen with intracarotid carmustine.[86] Even if the frequency of these complications is relatively low, their severity would require that the treatment result in substantially meaningful clinical benefits to justify the risk to the patient.

Carboplatin

Unlike cisplatin, carboplatin seldom results in significant emesis or neurotoxic, nephrotoxic, or ototoxic effects. However, myelosuppression limits the dose of carboplatin and makes combination therapy with other myelosuppressive agents more difficult. Toxic response consists primarily of leukopenia, but thrombocytopenia can also be dose-limiting. Similar to the nitrosoureas, myelosuppression with carboplatin can be cumulative and delayed. Attempts to escalate the dose of carboplatin using colony-stimulating factors and bone marrow transplantation are ongoing.[87]

CONCLUSION

Despite extensive efforts to find effective agents for the treatment of gliomas, the number of currently available agents and their clinical benefit remains extremely limited. Because the adverse effects of these agents can be substantial, it is necessary that clinicians treating glioma patients understand these limitations and weigh carefully the toxic effects against the potential benefits. It is also important that clinicians evaluating new agents be aware of potential consequences and report toxic effects clearly to develop effective and safe therapies in the future.

REFERENCES

1. De Vita VT, Carbone PP, Owens AH Jr, et al: Clinical trials with 1,3–bis(2-chloroethyl)-1-nitrosourea, NSC–409962. Cancer Res 1965; 25:1876–1881.
2. Buckner JC, Cascino TL, Schomberg PS, et al: Toxicity of interferon-alpha (IFN-α), BCNU, and radiation (RT) in high-grade glioma patients. J Neurooncol 1993;15:S6.
3. Rampling R, Steward W, Paul J, et al: rhGM-CSF ameliorates neutropenia in patients with malignant glioma treated with BCNU. Br J Cancer 1994;69:541–545.
4. Volkin RL, Shadduck RK, Winkelstein A, et al: Potentiation of carmustine-cranial irradiation-induced myelosuppression by cimetidine. Arch Intern Med 1982;142:243–245.
5. Harmon WE, Cohen HJ, Schneeberger EE, et al: Chronic renal failure in children treated with methyl CCNU. N Engl J Med 1979;300:1200–1203.
6. Schact RG, Baldwin DS: Chronic interstitial nephritis and renal failure due to nitrosourea therapy. Kidney Int 1978;14:661.
7. Silver RKB, Morton DL: CCNU nephrotoxicity following sustained remission in oat cell carcinoma (letter). Cancer Treat Rep 1978;63:226–227.
8. Holoye PY, Jenkins DE, Greenber SD: Pulmonary toxicity in long-term administration of BCNU. Cancer Treat Rep 1976;60:1691–1694.
9. Weinstein AS, Diener-West M, Nelson DF, et al: Pulmonary toxicity of carmustine in patients treated for malignant glioma. Cancer Treat Rep 1986;70:943–946.
10. Aronin PA, Mahaley MS Jr, Rudnick SA, et al: Prediction of BCNU

11. Selker RG, Jacobs SA, Moore PB, et al: 1,3-Bis(2-chloroethyl)-1-nitrosourea (BCNU)-induced pulmonary fibrosis. Neurosurgery 1980; 7:560–565.
12. Smith AC: The pulmonary toxicity of nitrosoureas. Pharmacol Ther 1989;41:443–460.
13. O'Driscoll BR, Hasleton PS, Taylor PM, et al: Active lung fibrosis up to 17 years after chemotherapy with carmustine (BCNU) in childhood. N Engl J Med 1990;323:378–382.
14. Limper AH, McDonald JA: Delayed pulmonary fibrosis after nitrosourea therapy (editorial). N Engl J Med 1990;323:407–409.
15. Schilsky RL, Sherins RJ, Hubbard SM, et al: Long-term follow-up of ovarian function in women treated with MOPP chemotherapy for Hodgkin's disease. Am J Med 1981;71:552–556.
16. Andrieu JM, Ochoa-Molina ME: Menstrual cycle, pregnancies and offspring before and after MOPP therapy for Hodgkin's disease. Cancer 1983;52:435–438.
17. Lacher MJ, Toner K: Pregnancies and menstrual function before and after combined radiation (RT) and chemotherapy (TVPP) for Hodgkin's disease. Cancer Invest 1986;4:93–100.
18. Rivkees SA, Crawford JD: The relationship of gonadal activity and chemotherapy-induced gonadal damage. JAMA 1988;259:2123–2125.
19. Clayton PE, Shalet SM, Price DA, et al: Ovarian function following chemotherapy for childhood brain tumors. Med Pediatr Oncol 1989;17:92–96.
20. Miller JJ, Williams GF, Leissring JC: Multiple late complications of therapy with cyclophosphamide including ovarian destruction. Am J Med 1971;50:530.
21. Waxman JHX, Terry YA, Wrigley PFM, et al: Gonadal function in Hodgkin's disease: Long-term follow-up of chemotherapy. Br Med J 1982;285:1612–1613.
22. Schilsky RL, Lewis BH, Sherins RJ, et al: Gonadal dysfunction in patients receiving chemotherapy for cancer. Ann Intern Med 1980;93:109–114.
23. Levine EG, Bloomfield CD: Leukemias and myelodysplastic syndromes secondary to drug, radiation, and environmental exposure. Semin Oncol 1992;19:47–84.
24. McKenney SA, Fehir KM: Myelofibrosis following treatment with a nitrosourea for malignant glioma. Cancer 1986;58:1426–1427.
25. Greene MH, Noice JD, Strike TA: Carmustine as a cause of acute nonlymphocytic leukemia. N Engl J Med 1985;313:579.
26. Cohen RJ, Wiernik PH, Walker MD: Acute nonlymphocytic leukemia associated with nitrosourea chemotherapy: Report of two cases. Cancer Treat Rep 1976;60:1257–1261.
27. Vogel SE: Acute leukemia complicating treatment of glioblastoma multiforme. Cancer 1978;4:333–336.
28. Genot JY, Krulik M, Poisson M: Two cases of acute leukemia following treatment of malignant glioma. Cancer 1983;52:222–226.
29. Garrett MJ: Teratogenic effects of combination chemotherapy. Ann Intern Med 1974;80:667.
30. Nicholson HO: Cytotoxic drugs in pregnancy. Obstet Gynaecol Br J 1968;75:307–312.
31. Holmes GE, Holmes FF: Pregnancy outcome of patients treated for Hodgkin's disease. Cancer 1978;41:1317–1322.
32. Hochberg FH, Parker LM, Takvorian T, et al: High-dose BCNU with autologous bone marrow rescue for recurrent glioblastoma multiforme. J Neurosurg 1981;54:455–460.
33. Phillips GL, Wolff SN, Fay JW, et al: Intensive 1,3-bis(2-chloroethyl)-1-nitrosourea (BCNU) monochemotherapy and autologous marrow transplantation for malignant glioma. J Clin Oncol 1986;4:639–645.
34. Wolff SN, Phillips GL, Herzig GP: High-dose carmustine with autologous bone marrow transplantation for the adjuvant treatment of high-grade gliomas of the central nervous system. Cancer Treat Rep 1987;71:183–185.
35. Johnson DB, Thompson JM, Corwin JA, et al: Prolongation of survival for high-grade malignant gliomas with adjuvant high-dose BCNU and autologous bone marrow transplantation. J Clin Oncol 1987;5:783–789.
36. Mbidde EK, Selby PJ, Perren TJ, et al: High dose BCNU chemotherapy with autologous bone marrow transplantation and full dose radiotherapy for grade IV astrocytoma. Br J Cancer 1988; 58:779–782.
37. Greenberg HS, Ensminger WD, Seeger JF, et al: Intra-arterial BCNU chemotherapy for the treatment of malignant gliomas of the central nervous system: A preliminary report. Cancer Treat Rep 1981;65:803–810.

38. Grimson BS, Mahaley MS Jr, Dubey HD, et al: Ophthalmic and central nervous system complications following intracarotid BCNU (carmustine). J Clin Neuroophthalmol 1981;1:261–264.

39. Shingleton BJ, Bienfang DC, Albert DM, et al: Ocular toxicity associated with high-dose carmustine. Arch Ophthalmol 1982;100:1766–1772.

40. Miller DF, Bay JW, Lederman RJ, et al: Ocular and orbital toxicity following intracarotid injection of BCNU (carmustine) and cisplatinum for malignant gliomas. Ophthalmology 1985;92:402–406.

41. Hochberg FH, Pruitt AA, Beck DO, et al: The rationale and methodology for intra-arterial chemotherapy with BCNU as treatment for glioblastoma. J Neurosurg 1985;63:876–880.

42. Foo S, Choi I, Berenstein A, et al: Supraophthalmic intracarotid infusion of BCNU for malignant glioma. Neurology 1986;36:1437–1444.

43. Greenberg HS, Ensminger WD, Chandler WF, et al: Intra-arterial BCNU chemotherapy for treatment of malignant gliomas of the central nervous system. J Neurosurg 1984;61:423–429.

44. Mahaley MS Jr, Whaley RA, Blue M, et al: Central neurotoxicity following intracarotid BCNU chemotherapy for malignant gliomas. J Neurooncol 1986;3:297–314.

45. Kleinschmidt-DeMasters BK: Intracarotid BCNU leukoencephalopathy. Cancer 1986;57:1276–1280.

46. Rosenblum MK, Delattre JY, Walker RW, et al: Fatal necrotizing encephalopathy complicating treatment of malignant gliomas with intra-arterial BCNU and irradiation: A pathological study. J Neurooncol 1989;7:269–281.

47. Shapiro WR, Green SB, Burger PC, et al: A randomized comparison of intra-arterial versus intravenous BCNU, with or without intravenous 5-fluorouracil, for newly diagnosed patients with malignant glioma. J Neurosurg 1992;76:772–781.

48. Sponzo RW, Arseneau J, Canellos GP: Procarbazine-induced oxidative haemolysis: Relationship to in vivo red cell survival. Br J Haematol 1974;27:587–595.

49. Jones SE, Moore M, Blank N, et al: Hypersensitivity of procarbazine (Matulane) manifested by fever and pleuro-pulmonary reaction. Cancer 1972;29:498–500.

50. Lokich JJ, Moloney WC: Allergic reaction to procarbazine. Clin Pharmacol Ther 1972;13:573–574.

51. Dohner VA, Ward HP, Standord RE: Alveolitis during procarbazine, vincristine, and cyclophosphamide therapy. Chest 1972;62:636–639.

52. Farney RJ, Morris AH, Armstrong JD Jr, et al: Diffuse pulmonary disease after therapy with nitrogen mustard, vincristine, procarbazine, and prednisone. Am Rev Respir Dis 1977;115:135–145.

53. Garbes ID, Henderson ES, Gomez GA, et al: Procarbazine-induced interstitial pneumonitis with a normal chest x-ray: A case report. Med Pediatr Oncol 1986;14:238–241.

54. Chabner BA, Sponzo R, Hubbard S, et al: High dose intermittent intravenous infusion of procarbazine (NSC–77213). Cancer Chemother Rep 1973;57:361–363.

55. Lee IP, Lucier GW: The potentiation of barbiturate-induced narcosis by procarbazine. J Pharmacol Exp Ther 1976;196:586–593.

56. Eade NR, MacLeod SM, Renton KW: Inhibition of hepatic microsomal drug metabolism by the hydrazine Ro 4–4602, MK 486, and procarbazine hydrochloride. Can J Physiol Pharmacol 1972;50:721–724.

57. Shiba DA, Weinkam RJ: The in vivo cytotoxic activity of procarbazine and procarbazine metabolites against L1210 ascites leukemia cells and CDF₁ mice and the effects of pretreatment with procarbazine, phenobarbital, diphenylhydantoin, and methylprednisolone upon in vivo procarbazine activity. Cancer Chemother Pharmacol 1983;11:124–129.

58. Parvinen L: Early effects of procarbazine (N-isopropyl-L-(2-methylhydrazino)-p-toluamide hydrochloride) on rat spermatogenesis. Exp Mol Pathol 1979;30:1–11.

59. Yost GS, Horstman MG, El Walily AF, et al: Procarbazine spermatogenesis toxicity: Deuterium isotope effects point to regioselective metabolism in mice. Toxicol Appl Pharmacol 1985;80:316–322.

60. Gatehouse DG, Paes DJ: A demonstration of the in vitro bacterial mutagenicity of procarbazine, using the microtitre fluctuation test and large concentrations of S9 fraction. Carcinogenesis 1983;4:347–352.

61. Chaube S, Murphy ML: Fetal malformations produced in rats by N-isopropyl-α-(2-methylhydrazino)-p-toluamide hydrochloride (procarbazine). Teratology 1969;2:23–32.

62. Weiss HD, Walker MD, Wiernik PH: Neurotoxicity of commonly used antineoplastic agents. N Engl J Med 1974;291:127–133.

63. Roca E, Bruera E, Politi PM, et al: Vinca alkaloid-induced cardiovascular autonomic neuropathy. Cancer Treat Rep 1985;69:149–151.

64. Robertson GL, Bhoopalam N, Zelkowitz LJ: Vincristine neurotoxicity and abnormal secretion of antidiuretic hormone. Arch Intern Med 1973;132:717–720.

65. Dentino, M, Luft FC, Yum MN, et al: Long term effect of cis-diamminedichloride platinum (CDDP) on renal function and structure in man. Cancer 1978;41:1274–1281.

66. Hayes DM, Cvitkovic E, Golbey RB, et al: High dose cis-platinum diammine dichloride: Amelioration of renal toxicity by mannitol diuresis. Cancer 1977;39:1372–1381.

67. Pera MR Jr, Zook BC, Harder HC: Effects of mannitol or furosemide diuresis on the nephrotoxicity and physiological disposition of cis-dichlorodiammineplatinum-(II) in rats. Cancer Res 1979;39:1269–1278.

68. Goren MP, Wright RK, Horowitz ME: Cumulative renal tubular damage associated with cisplatin nephrotoxicity. Cancer Chemother Pharmacol 1986;18:69–73.

69. Safirstein R, Winston J, Goldstein M, et al: Cisplatin nephrotoxicity. Am J Kidney Dis 1986;8:356–367.

70. Dobyan DC, Levi J, Jacobs C, et al: Mechanism of cis-platinum nephrotoxicity: II. Morphologic observations. J Pharmacol Exp Ther 1980;213:551–556.

71. von Hoff DD, Schilsky R, Reichert CM, et al: Toxic effects of cis-diamminedichloroplatinum (II) in man. Cancer Treat Rep 1979; 63: 1527–1531.

72. Elderson A, Gerritsen van der Hoop R, Haanstra W, et al: Vibration perception and thermoperception as quantitative measurements in the monitoring of cisplatin induced neurotoxicity. J Neurol Sci 1989;93:167–174.

73. Hansen SW, Hewlet-Larsen S, Trojaborg W: Long-term neurotoxicity in patients treated with cisplatin, vinblastine, and bleomycin for metastatic germ cell cancer. J Clin Oncol 1989;7:1457–1461.

74. Grunberg SM, Sonka S, Stevenson LL, et al: Progressive paresthesias after cessation of therapy with very high-dose cisplatin. Cancer Chemother Pharmacol 1989;23:62–64.

75. Boheim K, Bichler E: Cisplatin-induced ototoxicity: Audiometric findings and experimental cochlear pathology. Archive of Otorhinolaryngol 1985;242:1–6.

76. Schaefer SD, Post JD, Close LG, et al: Ototoxicity of low- and moderate-dose cisplatin. Cancer 1985;56:1934–1939.

77. Rothmann SA, Paul P, Weick JK, et al: Effect of cis-diamminedichloroplatinum on erythropoietin production and hematopoietic progenitor cells. Int J Cell Cloning 1985;3:415–423.

78. Kumar L, Dua H: Cisplatin induced anaemia (letter). NZ Med J 1987;100:81.

79. Pogliani EM, Pioltelli P, Rossini F, et al: Acute leukaemia following cisplatin for ovarian cancer (letter). Haematologica 1987;72:184–185.

80. Bassett WB, Weill RB: Acute leukemia following cisplatin for bladder cancer (letter). J Clin Oncol 1986;4:614.

81. Roth BJ, Einhorn LH, Greist A: Long-term complication of cisplatin-based chemotherapy for testis cancer. Semin Oncol 1988;15:345–350.

82. Hansen PV, Glavind K, Panduro J, et al: Paternity in patients with testicular germ cell cancer: Pretreatment and post-treatment findings. Eur J Cancer 1991;27:1385–1389.

83. Stewart DJ, Wallace S, Feun L, et al: A phase I study of intracarotid artery infusion of cis-diamminedichloroplatinum (II) in patients with recurrent malignant intracerebral tumors. Cancer Res 1982;42:2059–2062.

84. Feun LG, Wallace S, Stewart DJ, et al: Intracarotid infusion of cis-diamminedichloroplatinum in the treatment of recurrent malignant brain tumors. Cancer 1984;54:794–799.

85. Newton HB, Page MA, Junck L, et al: Intra-arterial cisplatin for the treatment of malignant gliomas. J Neurooncol 1989;7:39–45.

86. Shapiro WR: Chemotherapy of malignant gliomas: Studies of the BTCG. Rev Neurol 1992;148:428–434.

87. Calvert AH, Newell DR, Gore ME: Future directions with carboplatin: Can therapeutic monitoring, high-dose administration, and hematologic support with growth factors expand the spectrum compared with cisplatin? Semin Oncol 1992;19(1), suppl 2:155–163.

LLOYD I. MALINER

STEPHEN K. POWERS

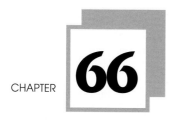

CHAPTER **66**

Deep Venous Thrombosis and Pulmonary Embolism

Thromboembolic disease (TE) is a well-known cause of morbidity and mortality, especially in the postoperative patient population. TE is also a common complication in patients with neoplastic disease, possibly being the second major cause of mortality in patients with solid tumors.[49] The combination of a postoperative patient with a tumor, especially a brain tumor, is of special consideration. Concern has been expressed that as a group, brain tumor patients are more susceptible to development of TE complications due to a variety of factors that include brain tissue components, malignant tissue products, neurologic system interface, and adjuvant treatment modalities. In addition, the treatment of TE can lead to hemorrhagic complications, especially intracranial hemorrhage, which can be particularly devastating in the postoperative brain tumor patient.

Thromboembolic complications have long been, and still are, an active topic of study. However, as is often the case in medicine, clinical studies in this area have varied greatly in method as well as results. The amount of data is enormous, covering all situations from spontaneous TE to TEs that have occurred specifically within 3 postoperative weeks in malignant glioma patients. As expected, the latter studies, which are focused on a particular patient subgroup, are fewer in number and involve smaller populations. This is especially significant because the rate of fatal pulmonary embolism (PE), the endpoint of concern with TE, is less than 1%, therefore necessitating huge numbers of patients to produce meaningful results. The studies also vary in character, with many meta-analyses and retrospective studies vs. few prospective and randomized control trials with systematic TE screening. Therefore, conclusions drawn from these studies are usually implied and are rarely absolute.

INCIDENCE

Without prophylaxis, the incidence of postoperative deep venous thrombosis (DVT) is 25% in general surgical patients, 50% in orthopedic patients, and 45% to 60% in patients with abdominal malignancies.[42] The majority of DVTs are asymptomatic. The incidence of PE in postoperative patients is 1.6%, and the rate of fatal PE is 0.86%,[13] with estimates that 14% to 45% of PEs are clinically undetected.[37, 42]

In the neurosurgical patient population, the incidence of DVT is 29% to 43%, with only 3% to 6% being symptomatic,[14] and the incidence of PE is 0% to 5%, with 9% to 50% of these being fatal.[23] An autopsy study found a 27.5% DVT rate in brain tumor patients vs. a 17% rate in a control group (no malignancy), and 93% of the patients with DVT had PE.[29] Specifically, patients with malignant glioma have a symptomatic TE incidence rate of 10% to 36%,[6, 11, 12, 14, 15] which reached 60% with routine screening in one study.[47] Similar rates of occurrence of TE as a postoperative complication (19% to 27%) and related solely to the presence of the glioma (4% to 28%) suggest that nonsurgical factors play a major role in the development of TE for brain tumor patients.[6, 11, 12, 29] Overall, the relative incidence of TE in glioma patients is felt to be greater than that of either general neurosurgical patients or other brain tumor patients, but not of meningioma patients (Table 66–1). Appropriate prophylaxis, however, decreases the TE rate by 50% to 75% for an incidence of less than 10%.[23, 42]

PREDISPOSING FACTORS

A number of factors have been suggested to increase the risk of TE, but only the following have been documented: advanced age; previous TE; leg weakness or immobility; varicose veins; cardiac disease (especially congestive heart failure); malignancy; use of oral contraceptives; pregnancy; myeloproliferative disorders;[42] and deficiency of protein C, protein S, or antithrombin III.[23] In general, any condition resulting in venous stasis of the lower extremities or a hypercoagulable state should lead the physician to suspect a greater risk of thromboembolic complications in the postoperative period. Age seems to be the most important risk

TABLE 66–1
INCIDENCE OF THROMBOEMBOLIC EVENTS (TE) IN MALIGNANT GLIOMA PATIENTS

Study (Year)	No. of Patients	Prophylaxis	TE Screening	Time from Surgery (wk)	Incidence of TE (%)			
					Malignant Glioma	Metastases	Meningioma	Total
Buckner & Quevedo (1992)[6]	64	Aspirin	No	<12	18	—	—	18
Cheruku et al (1991)[11]	77	—	No	>3	19	—	—	19
Choucair et al (1987)[12]	915	None	No	>6	4	—	—	4
Constantini et al (1991)[14]	492	None	No	<3	10	10	5	6
Dhami et al (1993)[15]	68	None	No	>52	19	—	—	19
Kayser-Gatchalian & Kayser (1975)[29]	334	—	Yes	—	32	—	30	27.5
Levi et al (1991)[32]	1,703	Mixed	No	<4	1.0	1.0	3.1	1.6
Muchmore et al (1989)[38]	23	—	No	>4	22	—	—	22
Ruff & Posner (1983)[45]	268	None	No	<3	36	—	—	36
	117	SPCS	No	<6	10	—	—	10
Sawaya et al (1992)[47]	46	None	Yes	<2	20	72	60	44

SPCS, sequential pneumatic compression stockings; TE, thromboembolism.

factor in the development of DVT in both the general surgical and neurosurgical populations. An increased incidence of TE is also seen in patients older than 40 years with prolonged immobilization. Neurosurgical patients have the additional risk factors of prolonged operations, steroid use, prolonged bedrest, malignancy, dehydration, and the release of cerebral thromboplastic substances.[42] The increase in the risk of DVT in neurosurgical patients with operations lasting longer than 4 hours is twofold.[41] Also, the risk of postoperative TE is greater after the removal of supratentorial compared to infratentorial tumors, especially malignant gliomas,[14] possibly due to direct hypothalamic-mediated neural control of the coagulation system.[14, 49] However, the risk of developing DVT after either spinal or intracranial operations is the same.[42]

Although much of the reported data seem contradictory, the incidence of TE in patients with brain tumors is generally thought to be increased over that in the general neurosurgical population. Several studies suggest that the degree of malignancy, length of surgery, presence of paresis, and use of chemotherapy increase the risk of TE,[1, 11, 14, 15, 23, 33, 45, 47] but the same parameters were not found to be significant in other studies.[15, 29, 47] The general consensus is that TE risks in brain tumor patients are increased age, tumor presence (meningiomas are the worst), and history of paresis, surgery, and chemotherapy. It is interesting to note that although the risk is not directly related to paresis, and patients are usually ambulatory at the time of occurrence, DVT has a propensity to occur in the limb that was originally paretic.[11, 14, 15] The interval between surgery and the development of TE averages between 1 and 6 weeks,[11, 15, 32] though in some studies the risk of TE development continues beyond 2 months after surgery.[12] Furthermore, in an autopsy study, the development of TE did not even correlate to whether the patient had had surgery.[29] Another TE risk factor is chemotherapy, which is felt to act mainly by causing direct endothelial damage.[15]

Several inherent factors of normal and neoplastic brain tissue are possibly contributory to the TE risk. Brain tissue contains high levels of thromboplastin, which is potentially released with tumor invasion and necrosis; this has not been proven, however, because thromboplastin levels are not clinically measurable.[49, 50] Several Eastern European studies have reported a variety of abnormal hemostatic parameters in brain tumor patients that include increased platelet adhesiveness; hyperfibrinogenemia; shortened thromboelastogram; decreased levels of clotting factors II, V, and VII; and increased fibrinolysis as measured by the euglobulin fraction of plasma.[48, 49] However, only an elevated prothrombin time has been confirmed as a significant finding in the hemostatic profile of preoperative and postoperative brain tumor patients with TE.[48] Glioma tissue itself is purported to have active hemostatic properties. A consumption coagulopathy with glioblastoma multiforme has been demonstrated using a guinea pig model.[48, 49] Also, a direct association exists between glial tumor invasiveness and high levels of plaminogen activators and fibrinolysis inhibitors,[22, 50] as well as plasmin inhibitors (CSF alpha-one-antitrypsin) in tissue cultures.[49]

MECHANISM OF CLOT FORMATION

Figure 66–1 illustrates the mechanisms of the coagulation system. Platelets, the first line of defense in the normal hemostatic mechanism, are activated only after the vascular endothelial lining has been damaged. The adhesiveness (ability to stick to nonplatelet surfaces) and aggregation (ability to stick to one another) of platelets assist in this hemostatic function. The second line of normal hemostatic defense is the fibrin plug. This system is activated by either the intrinsic pathway, which requires only blood components, or the extrinsic pathway, which requires thromboplastins released from tissue for activation.

Clot formation in the intrinsic pathway begins with the sequential activation of four "hemophilioid factors" (so-called because of the hemophilic states that exist with decreased activity of factors VIII, IX, and XI) caused by phospholipids that probably come from platelets. Each step in the clotting cascade begins when an inactive plasma protein factor is changed into an enzymatically active form, which activates the next factor in the sequence. Calcium is involved in these reactions. Activated factor VIII activates

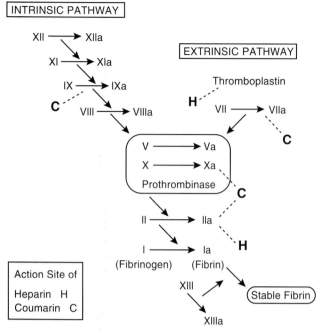

Figure 66–1 Coagulation system, with sites of heparin and coumarin action indicated. From Powers SK, Maliner LI: Prevention and treatment of thromboembolic complications in a neurosurgical patient. *In* Wilkins RH, Rengachary SS eds: Neurosurgery, ed 2. New York, McGraw-Hill, 1994.

factors V and X; with platelet phospholipids and calcium, factors V and X form a four-way complex that has prothrombinase activity, and converts prothrombin (II) to thrombin (IIa), the latter of which then converts fibrinogen (I) to fibrin. However, at this point the fibrin clot is soft and fragile, and without the presence of activated factor XIII it would disintegrate rapidly in plasma. The extrinsic clotting pathway is initiated by the activation of factor VII by either tissue phospholipids or thromboplastin. Factor VII in turn activates the formation of the prothrombinase complex (factor Va–factor Xa–phospholipid–calcium) that converts prothrombin to thrombin and then forms fibrin, which is finally stabilized by factor XIIIa. The intrinsic and extrinsic pathways converge at clotting factor X, which is the point in the mechanism at which low-dose heparin prevents the formation of thrombi.[42]

Blood clots that form in the veins of the pelvis and lower extremities (DVT) consist primarily of fibrin, erythrocytes, a few white blood cells, and some platelets that are randomly distributed throughout the venous plug. In contrast to the products of arterial thrombosis, platelets and platelet debris are rarely found in venous thrombi; activation of platelets by vascular endothelial injury that takes place in arterial thrombosis is not important in this sequence.

CLINICAL FEATURES

DVT often develops without obvious symptoms or signs; in fact, only 10% to 17% of DVTs are clinically apparent. Not uncommonly, the first indicators of DVT are those observed with PE. A variety of clinical signs may be present, including edema, increased calf girth, local deep tenderness (Pratt's sign), and pain with dorsiflexion or plantar flexion (Homan's sign); but these clinical signs are both insensitive and nonspecific, and their absence does not indicate the absence of venous thrombosis. One study found the TE incidence to be 2% to 36% with clinical detection, and 23% to 45% with screening of neurosurgery patients.[32] Likewise, the majority of patients with PE are known to have symptoms and signs that are relatively nonspecific and may mimic any number of cardiopulmonary abnormalities, or there may be no warning whatsoever. A somewhat unexpected finding is that at least 40% of patients with DVT have asymptomatic PE.[37] PE is one of the few causes of "sudden death" and is the third most common cause of death in the United States.[30] In one study of postoperative neurosurgery patients, 37% of patients diagnosed with PE died; 6 out of 7 patients died within minutes to hours of the onset of symptoms.[14]

The sudden onset of dyspnea in a postoperative patient should suggest the diagnosis of PE. Dyspnea is seen in 81% of the patients with PE, and the intensity of this complaint by patients tends to be out of proportion to the degree of the objective abnormal findings. Pleuritic chest pain occurs in approximately three-fourths of patients; but it is not often associated with hemoptysis, which occurs in approximately one-third of all patients with PE and indicates pulmonary infarction. Other symptoms commonly seen with PE are apprehension, a dry and hacking cough, diaphoresis, and, occasionally, syncope (with a massive PE). However, the overall value of clinical symptoms tends to be more for ruling out a PE as opposed to making the definitive diagnosis.

The most frequent physical finding in PE is tachypnea, with a respiratory rate of greater than 16 per minute. Tachycardia is also seen, with a heart rate greater than 100 beats per minute. A direct relationship tends to be seen between the size of the embolic process and the increase in the heart rate. Almost half of the patients are febrile, but temperature is usually only modestly elevated (100 to 102°F) and does not have the "spiking" nature of a fever seen with a systemic infectious process. A temperature greater than 103°F should suggest an origin other than thromboembolism. Gallop heart sounds (S_3 and S_4) occur in one-third of patients with extensive embolic obstruction and reflect abnormal right ventricular hemodynamics. Cyanosis is uncommon and occurs only in patients with severe hypoxemia from extensive embolic obstruction.[42]

DIAGNOSTIC TESTS

The objective of diagnostic evaluation for PE is to either confirm the physician's clinical suspicion or exclude the presence of disease as expeditiously as possible, as the mortality of untreated PE (to 50%) is three to four times higher than in patients treated with conventional anticoagulation (8%) or thrombolytic therapy. Routine laboratory studies offer little in the diagnosis of PE. A nonspecific elevation of lactate dehydrogenase and serum bilirubin in the presence of normal serum glutamic oxalacetic transaminase are often noted.[42] The platelet count may be helpful, but only in that a PE is less likely with an above-baseline platelet count.[36] The electrocardiogram will be abnormal in 30% of PE patients,[39] but the findings are nonspecific. Chest x-rays are notoriously unhelpful during the acute phase. They may demonstrate pulmonary infiltration and evidence of pleural effusion if infarction has occurred, but not until 12 to 36 hours after the event. Massive emboli are often associated with arterial hypoxemia, hypocapnia, and respiratory alkalosis.[42]

The most common and valuable diagnostic method is the combination of ventilation and perfusion (V/Q) lung scans, which demonstrate a mismatch of pulmonary blood flow with ventilated lung. Based on retrospective and prospective analyses, when there is clinical suspicion of TE, high probability and low probability V/Q scans are 85% accurate in the diagnosis of the existence or exclusion of PE. When a low probability V/Q scan is paired with no clinical suspicion, the probability of PE is less than 5%.[30]

In patients with underlying heart or lung disease whose clinical presentation may be nonspecific and compatible with exacerbation of an underlying disease, or whose V/Q scans may be less specific, angiography is most helpful. Selective pulmonary angiography is the only means by which anatomic information about the pulmonary vasculature can be obtained, and it remains the gold standard for the diagnosis of PE. However, pulmonary angiography is an invasive procedure and carries an overall mortality of 1% when performed by experienced personnel.[42] A safer alternative may be pulmonary magnetic resonance imaging (MRI), magnetic resonance pulmonary angiography, or spiral computed tomography (CT) pulmonary angiography, techniques that show promise in recent studies but are still under evaluation.[16, 21, 26, 54]

Most patients who die from PE will have evidence of DVT of the legs at autopsy. Because of this observation, the assessment of the deep venous system with various noninvasive techniques may aid in the indirect diagnosis of PE, and it has even been shown to improve the specificity of the diagnosis. The ^{125}I-fibrinogen uptake test is the most sensitive technique for detecting active thrombosis in calf veins. It is the most useful clinical test for establishing the activity of thrombosis in patients in whom recurrence of active venous thrombosis is suspected. However, the technique is insensitive to thrombi that are not actively forming and can be confused by leg wounds, hematomas, or inflammatory conditions. The technique is also insensitive to proximal thigh vein thrombosis and particularly to thrombi in the iliac veins. Furthermore, a complete study takes hours to perform.[42]

Doppler ultrasound, which involves a sound pattern recognition, has become the examination of choice in many institutions, as its use has become more widespread and the technicians performing the studies more experienced. This method has a 95% accuracy for either the identification or exclusion of DVT as compared with contrast phlebography. The technique detects alterations in the normal phasic flow characteristics of the extremities and is, hence, quite nonspecific. Any condition that affects venous outflow will result in doppler venous abnormalities. This technique is being further expanded with triplex imaging and color Doppler studies.[39] Another noninvasive technique is plethysmography, which is very sensitive but not so specific, so that it is most helpful if findings are negative.[20] Liquid crystal

thermography, with a 96% negative predictive value, is relatively new and unavailable.[9] Radionuclide phlebography may be as reliable as contrast phlebography;[35] however venography, which is an invasive procedure, remains the gold standard diagnostic study for DVT.

TREATMENT

The treatment for non-massive PE and proximal (above-the-knee) DVT consists of acute intravenous (IV) heparin anticoagulation followed by 3 to 6 months of oral warfarin to maintain anticoagulation. Distal (below-the-knee) DVT can be monitored without anticoagulation, because it is not directly associated with PE, though it can propagate proximally. Anticoagulation is usually initiated with an IV heparin bolus of 5,000 to 10,000 units (75 to 100 units/kg) followed by a continuous IV drip of 1,000 to 2,000 units/hour to maintain an activated partial thromboplastin time 100% to 150% above normal. Warfarin therapy is usually initiated with a single dose of 10 mg followed by doses varying from 5 to 10 mg nightly, with an anticipated maintenance of 2.5 to 5 mg nightly by the fourth or fifth day. Warfarin therapy has traditionally been monitored by the prothrombin time (PT), but this has been found to be accurate in only 8% to 20% of laboratories due to variations in the laboratory thromboplastin assay. This variation is corrected by using the international normalized ratio (INR) (which is the patient's PT divided by the control PT, and all raised to the power of the international sensitivity index of the thromboplastin), with a goal of 2 to 3 being appropriate.[7] More recent studies have shown effective anticoagulation being achieved within a shorter timespan when warfarin was started simultaneous to or 1 day after initiation of heparin therapy.[19, 28, 29, 44] There is a theoretical risk of inducing a hypercoaguable state with the initiation of warfarin due to the inhibition of protein C, a vitamin K-dependent factor that is itself an inhibitor of the coagulation cascade;[44, 46] but the heparin seems to provide protection.

Anticoagulant therapy is the mainstay of management for TE. Unfortunately, patients who have undergone either intracranial or of intraspinal operations are at high risk for clinical catastrophe from a major hemorrhage into the operative site in conjunction with anticoagulant therapy. This risk is an important issue in the treatment of TE in any patient with a glioma. Even those patients who have not had recent procedures or therapy are at risk for hemorrhaging into the tumor.[29, 42] However, an untreated PE is potentially more devastating to the patient. It has been reported that the mortality of PE in postoperative glioma patients is 1% in those who received anticoagulant therapy vs. 50% in those who were not treated.[45]

It can be concluded from available data[1, 11, 12, 14, 15, 45] that full anticoagulation is safe in both the nonoperative and postoperative glioma patients, including those receiving adjuvant radiation or chemotherapy (Table 66–2). In fact, the incidence of intracranial hemorrhage in anticoagulated neurosurgical patients does not exceed the incidence of spontaneous intracranial hemorrhages in brain tumor patients (1% to 4%), though the severity of the hemorrhage has not been addressed.[12, 45] Furthermore, gastrointestinal hemorrhages

TABLE 66-2
ANTICOAGULATION IN MALIGNANT GLIOMA PATIENTS

Study (Year)	No. of Patients	Time From Surgery (wk)	Complications (%)	Recurrent TE (%)	Intracranial Hemorrhage (%)	Mortality (%)
Altschuler et al (1990)[1]	23	>1	4	17*	0	—
Cheruku et al (1991)[11]	8	>3	25	0	12†	—
Choucair et al (1987)[12]	22	>6	0	0	0	—
Constantini et al (1991)[14]	12	<2	17	17	8‡	8
Dhami et al (1993)[15]	8	—	38	12*	0	—
Ruff & Posner (1983)[45]	103	—	1	1	2§	1

TE, thromboembolism.
*Patient was receiving anticoagulant therapy at time.
†Occurred 8 weeks into anticoagulation therapy.
‡Occurred 5 days postoperatively and required surgical treatment.
§Due to intracranial hemorrhage, but control population had 2% mortality from same.

made up the majority of hemorrhagic complications in clinical postoperative neurosurgical studies. Unfortunately, the question that none of these studies systematically addressed was how soon after surgery anticoagulation can safely be initiated. Anecdotal reports have been published of full anticoagulation without complications within 7 days,[1, 51] and even within 24 hours,[47] of intracranial procedures. This is countered by a rat study that found an increased rate of intracranial hemorrhage when anticoagulation occurred within the first week after craniotomy.[47] More intuitively accepted waiting periods of 1 to 3 weeks have been presented,[23, 51] but no conclusive evidence supports this position. Because heparin anticoagulation does not cause lysis of established clots (it only prevents their extension), early institution of heparin anticoagulation for the treatment of TE seems reasonable.

An acceptable alternative TE treatment option is placement of a vena caval filter to prevent PE or further PE in the face of lower extremity DVT. Vena caval ligation is no longer a standard therapeutic option. Vena caval filter placement is well supported in the neurosurgical literature,[23, 38, 42, 51] with one study showing no difference in complication or subsequent PE rate in a comparison of a limited number of glioma patients treated with filters vs. anticoagulation therapy.[38] However, filters do have their own associated morbidity including the need for an invasive procedure (now a percutaneous process), leg edema, vena caval obstruction, and continued embolic events; and anticoagulation is still recommended as the long-term treatment.[23, 38] Also, filters provide no protection from upper extremity DVTs, which occur in 2% of patients,[45] nor do they prevent propagation of existing PE.

The most effective treatment of TE is thrombolysis with streptokinase and urokinase, which are plasminogen activators. Their benefit is reflected in better improvement in the abnormal hemodynamics of the right ventricle and pulmonary circulation than is seen with heparin. However, there is no difference in the mortality rate from PE between patients treated with fibrinolytic agents and those treated with heparin. Also, significant hemorrhagic complications occur in 5% to 9% of unoperated patients who receive either urokinase or streptokinase, which is much higher than that for high-dose heparin. The hemorrhagic risk associated with thrombolysis has been evaluated by the National Institutes of Health (NIH). The NIH defined the absolute contraindications for thrombolysis to include an active internal bleeding state or a recent (within 2 months) cerebrovascular process or procedure.[8] A more remote (greater than 2 months) cerebrovascular process should be considered a very strong but relative contraindication, with the decision to use thrombolytic agents based on the risk-benefit status. Another relative contraindication includes any recent invasive procedure involving a body cavity (for example, the spinal canal) or vessel that cannot be compressed for a long period, unless the risk of the thromboembolic process overrides the risk of bleeding.[42]

PROPHYLAXIS

The prophylaxis of thromboembolic complications has long been an active topic of study. As previously mentioned, the studies vary greatly in method as well as in results, and conclusions are more implied than absolutely proven, especially on the topic of TE prophylaxis. What is clear is that prophylaxis works; it decreases the incidence of DVT by 50% to 75%.[23, 42]

Prophylactic methods are easily divided into two major groups: mechanical and pharmacologic. Mechanical methods are popular because they have no risk of hemorrhagic complications. Earlier methods of mechanical prophylaxis, which include early ambulation, leg elevation, physiotherapy, and elastic stockings, have been shown not to prevent DVT.[41] Current popular mechanical modes of prophylaxis include graduated elastic stockings (GES) and sequential pneumatic compression stockings (SPCS), both of which have been proven effective. Their effectiveness, and that of all prophylactic methods, is dependent on their use throughout the TE risk period, that is, they must be applied in the operating room and worn until the patient is fully ambulatory.[9] These systems have both been shown to function, with no significant difference in efficacy,[13, 24] by increasing blood flow in the proximal femoral veins and eliminating venous stasis.[31, 39] The effect of either method on PE risk specifically is not known. The SPCS is also felt to have the added benefit of stimulating the fibrinolytic system, supposedly in proportion to the amount of tissue involved.[9] This led to the idea that thigh-high devices would be more effective than knee-high, but this has been disproven for both GES and SPCS.[31, 40] Another common assumption that has been disproven regards the systems having an additive effect,[39, 52] although we combine their use in our clinical practice, because one system invariably seems to be off the patient at any given time. A different mechanical method is the vena cava filter (umbrella), which requires an operative (percutaneous) procedure. Traditionally this technique has been reserved for patients with documented DVT who are unable to tolerate, or are recalcitrant to, pharmacologic PE protection. However, some work suggests a role for filter placement prophylactically in patients at high risk for TE.[42]

Pharmacologic prophylaxis includes a variety of agents that interfere with clot formation. Antiplatelet agents such as aspirin and dipyridamole have previously been evaluated, and at least aspirin has conclusively been shown to be ineffective. Warfarin is effective, and convenient, but has the drawbacks of hemorrhagic complications and a long half-life. The standard method of TE prophylaxis, against which all other methods are measured, is subcutaneously administered low-dose heparin (LDH), whose efficacy in prevention of both DVT and PE is indisputable. The customary prophylactic dose is 5,000 units, given two or three times daily, beginning preoperatively and continuing until the patient is ambulatory. Use of LDH has not become routine in all neurosurgical patients because of the concern over postoperative hemorrhage. However, LDH has been thoroughly evaluated in several cohorts of neurosurgical patients, ranging from nonoperative hematomas to postoperative brain tumor patients, and its safety has been established.[2, 4, 13, 17, 18]

The concern for hemorrhagic complications has led to the study of variations of LDH therapy, including ultra-low-dose heparin (ULDH) and low-molecular-weight heparin (LMWH). The ULDH method achieves comparable prevention by utilizing a continuous intravenous (IV) drip of a doseapproximately equivalent to a routine IV flush (1 unit/kg/hour), but this method is inconvenient and not well favored.[41, 42] However, LMWH, a group of low-molecular-weight fragments of depolymerized heparin, is the focus of current study. These fragments are designed to have a longer half-life, produce fewer hemorrhagic complications, have better bioavailability, produce less platelet interaction, and initiate less lipolysis.[5, 33, 43] The major interest, however, is the greater ratio of antithrombotic to anticoagulant activity, and the theoretically lower risk of hemorrhagic complications.[13] The conclusions obtained by grouping results from the limited studies of each particular LMWH (which may not be appropriate due to their similar but not identical activities) have been favorable. They are at least as effective as LDH with no more, and possibly fewer, hemorrhagic complications.[3, 9, 25, 27] Unfortunately only one LMWH is currently approved for use in the United States, though several are available in Europe.

Two other prophylactic medications are dihydroergotamine (DHET), used with LDH, and dextran. The LDH-DHET combination has been shown to be more effective than LDH alone, but it has significant side effects, including cardiac and peripheral vasospasm.[13, 34] Dextran, however, has been found to provide no better, and possibly worse, TE protection than LDH, with more complications.[13] When compared to LDH, dextran not only increases the risk for hemor-

rhage, it also has a higher incidence of anaphylaxis, potentially leads to vascular overload, and is known to increase cerebral edema in regions of incompetent blood-brain barrier. Dextran is, therefore, not a favorable choice for TE prophylaxis in neurosurgical patients.

The two most popular methods of TE prophylaxis are LDH and SPCS, and these have been compared. A recent study of neurosurgery patients favored LDH, but the study itself was retrospective and based on clinically detected DVT (as opposed to screening).[18] The majority of studies have found no difference between LDH and SPCS. Again, no good data are available on the ability of SPCS to prevent PE.[13, 18, 39] The general conclusion is that LDH is currently the most effective method of TE prophylaxis and is safe in postcraniotomy patients, with SPCS being nearly as effective and very safe. LMWH is exciting and will possibly replace LDH; the main obstacle at this point is their availability and the lack of neurosurgical trials.

CONCLUSIONS

Thromboembolic complications are of significant concern in the neurosurgical patient, especially in those with intracranial malignant gliomas. Prevention is the key to successful management of the TE risk. The mainstay of TE prophylaxis is GES, which should be applied as part of the routine surgical preparation. The next level of protection, appropriate for any craniotomy or procedure that lasts a few hours, is SPCS; these should also be placed intraoperatively and worn throughout the nonambulatory periods. For patients with greater risks, such as morbid obesity or full paralysis, administration of LDH (and possibly LMWH) should be implemented preoperatively or early in the postoperative period. Any suspicion of TE warrants investigation, or in the case of suspected PE, immediate treatment before conclusive diagnosis (especially if the risk for hemorrhage is remote—more than 3 weeks from surgery). In the event of proven DVT or PE, appropriate treatment should be implemented without hesitation. Full anticoagulation for patients more than 1 week from surgery is safe and appropriate, and in earlier TE events, either anticoagulation or vena cava filter placement can be considered.

REFERENCES

1. Altschuler E, Moosa H, Selker RG, et al: The risk and efficacy of anticoagulant therapy in the treatment of thromboembolic complications in patients with primary malignant brain tumors. Neurosurgery 1990; 27:74–77.
2. Barnett HG, Clifford JE, Llowllyn RC: Safety of mini-dose heparin administration for neurosurgical patients. J Neurosurg 1977; 47:27–30.
3. Bergqvist D: Review of clinical trials of low molecular weight heparins. Eur J Surg 1992; 158:67–78.
4. Boeer A, Voth E, Henze TH, et al: Early heparin therapy in patients with spontaneous intracerebral hemorrhage. J Neurol Neurosurg Psychiatry 1991; 54:466–467.
5. Bucci MN, Papadopoulos SM, Chen JC, et al: Mechanical prophylaxis of venous thrombis in patients undergoing craniotomy: A randomized trial. Surg Neurol 1989; 32:285–288.
6. Buckner JC, Quevedo F: Thromboembolism in high-grade glioma patients (abstract). Neurology 1992; 42(suppl 3):459.
7. Bussey HI, Force RW, Bianco TM, et al: Reliance on prothrombin

time ratios causes significant errors in anticoagulation therapy. Arch Intern Med 1992; 152:278–282.

8. Cachecho R, Grindlinger G, Dennis R, et al: Deep venous thrombosis and pulmonary embolism in patients with severe head injury (abstract). Chest 1992; 102:119S.

9. Caprini JA, Arcelus JI, Traverso CI, et al: Low molecular weight heparins and external pneumatic compression as options for venous thromboembolism prophylaxis: A surgeon's perspective. Semin Thromb Hemost 1991; 17:356–366.

10. Cerrato D, Ariano C, Fiacchino F: Deep vein thrombosis and low-dose heparin prophylaxis in neurosurgical patients. J Neurosurg 1978; 49:378–381.

11. Cheruku R, Tapazoglou E, Ensley J, et al: The incidence and significance of thromboembolic complications in patients with high-grade gliomas. Cancer 1991; 68:2621–2624.

12. Choucair AK, Silver P, Levin VA: Risk of intracranial hemorrhage in glioma patients receiving anticoagulant therapy for venous thrombolism. J Neurosurg 1987; 66:357–358.

13. Clagett GP, Reisch JS: Prevention of venous thromboembolism in general surgical patients. Ann Surg 1988; 208:227–240.

14. Constantini S, Kornowski R, Pomeranz S, et al: Thromboembolic phenomena in neurosurgical patients operated upon for primary and metastatic brain tumours. Acta Neurochir 1991; 109:93–97.

15. Dhami MS, Bona RD, Calogero JA, et al: Venous thromboembolism and high grade gliomas. Thromb Haemost 1993; 70:393–396.

16. Erdman WA, Peshock RM, Redman HC, et al: Pulmonary embolism: Comparison of MR images with radionuclide and angiographic studies. Radiology 1994; 190:499–508.

17. Eriksson BI, Kalebo R, Anthmyr BA, et al: Prevention of deep-vein thrombosis and pulmonary embolism after total hip replacement. J Bone Joint Surg Am 1991; 73:484–493.

18. Frim D, Barker II FG, Poletti CE, et al: Postoperative low-dose heparin decreases thromboembolic complications in neurosurgical patients. Neurosurgery 1992; 30:847–854.

19. Gallus A, Jackaman J, Tillett J, et al: Safety and efficacy of warfarin started early after submassive venous thrombosis or pulmonary embolism. Lancet 1986; 2(8519):1293–1296.

20. Glew D, Cooper T, Mitchelmore AE, et al: Impedance plethysmography and thrombo-embolic disease. Br J Radiol 1992; 65:305–308.

21. Grist TM, Sostman HD, MacFall JR, et al: Pulmonary angiography with MR imaging: Preliminary clinical experience. Radiology 1993; 189:523–530.

22. Gross JL, Behrens DL, Mullins DE, et al: Plasminogen activator and inhibitor activity in human glioma cells and modulation by sodium butyrate. Cancer Res 1988; 48:291–296.

23. Hamilton MG, Hull RD, Pineo GF: Venous thromboembolism in neurosurgery and neurology patients: A review. Neurosurgery 1994; 34:280–296.

24. Hansberry KL, Thompson IM, Bauman J, et al: A prospective comparison of thromboembolic stockings, external sequential pneumatic compression stockings and heparin sodium/dihydroergotamine mesylate for the prevention of thromboembolic complications in urological surgery. J Urol 1991; 145:1205–1208.

25. Hass S, Flosbach CW: Prevention of post-operative thromboembolism in general surgery with enoxaparin: Preliminary findings. Acta Chir Scand Suppl 1990; 556:96–102.

26. Hatabu H, Gefter WB, Listerud J, et al: Pulmonary MR angiography utilizing phased-array surface coils. J Comput Assist Tomogr 1992; 16:410–417.

27. Hirsh J, Levine MN: Low molecular weight heparin. Blood 1992; 79:1–17.

28. Hull RD, Raskob GE, Rosenbloom D, et al: Heparin for 5 days compared with 10 days in the initial treatment of proximal venous thrombosis. N Engl J Med 1990; 322:1260–1264.

29. Kayser-Gatchalian MC, Kayser K: Thrombosis and intracranial tumors. J Neurol 1975; 209:217–224.

30. Kelly MA, Carson JL, Palevsky HI, et al: Diagnosing pulmonary embolism: New facts and strategies. Ann Intern Med 1991; 114:300–306.

31. Lawrence D, Kakkar VV: Graduated, static, external compression of the lower limb: A physiological assessment. Br J Surg 1980; 67:119–121.

32. Levi ADO, Wallace MC, Bernstein M, et al: Venous thromboembolism after brain tumor surgery: A retrospective review. Neurosurgery 1991; 28:859–863.

33. Levine MN, Hirsh J, Gent M, et al: Prevention of deep vein thrombosis after elective hip surgery. Ann Intern Med 1991; 114:545–551.

34. Lindblad B: Prophylaxis of postoperative thromboembolism with low dose heparin alone or in combination with dihydroergotamine. Acta Chir Scand Suppl 1988; 543:31–42.

35. Miller TA: Physiologic Basis of Modern Surgical Care. Mosby–Year Book, 1988, pp 141–142, 866–871.

36. Monreal M, Lafoz E, Casals A, et al: Platelet count and venous thromboembolism. Chest 1991; 100:1493–1496.

37. Moser KM, Fedullo PF, Litte-John JK, et al: Frequent asymptomatic pulmonary embolism in patients with deep venous thrombosis. JAMA 1994; 271:223–225.

38. Muchmore JH, Dunlap JN, Culicchia F, et al: Deep vein thrombophlebitis and pulmonary embolism in patients with malignant gliomas. South Med J 1989; 82:1352–1356.

39. Persson AV, Davis RJ, Villavicencio JL: Deep venous thrombosis and pulmonary embolism. Surg Clinic North Am 1991; 71:1195–1209.

40. Porteous MJ, Nicholson EA, Morris LT, et al: Thigh length versus knee length stockings in the prevention of deep vein thrombosis. Br J Surg 1989; 76:296–297.

41. Powers SK, Edwards SB: Prophylaxis of thromboembolism in the neurosurgical patient: A review. Neurosurgery 1982; 10:509–513.

42. Powers SK, Maliner LI: Prevention and treatment of thromboembolic complications in a neurosurgical patient, in Wilkins RH, Rengachary SS (eds): Neurosurgery, ed 2. New York, McGraw-Hill, 1994.

43. Prandoni P, Lensing AWA, Buller HR, et al: Comparison of subcutaneous low-molecular-weight heparin with intravenous standard heparin in proximal deep-vein thrombosis. Lancet 1992; 339:441–445.

44. Rosielly RA, Chan CK, Tencza F, et al: Timing of oral anticoagulation therapy in the treatment of angiographically proven acute pulmonary embolism. Arch Intern Med 1987; 147:1469–1473.

45. Ruff RL, Posner JB: Incidence and treatment of peripheral venous thrombosis in patients with glioma. Ann Neurol 1983; 13:334–346.

46. Sabiston DC: Sabiston's Essentials of Surgery. Philadelphia, WB Saunders, 1987, pp 83–85, 941–942.

47. Sawaya R, Zuccarello M, Elkalliny M, et al: Postoperative venous thromboembolism and brain tumors: I. Clinical profile. J Neurooncol 1992; 14:119–125.

48. Sawaya R, Glas-Greenwalt P: Postoperative venous thromboembolism and brain tumors: II. Hemostatic profile. J Neurooncol 1992;14:127–134.

49. Sawaya R, Decourteen-Meyers G, Copeland B: Massive preoperative pulmonary embolism and suprasellar brain tumor: Case report and review of the literature. Neurosurgery 1984; 15:566–570.

50. Sawaya R, Cummins CJ, Kornblith PL: Brain tumors and plasmin inhibitors. Neurosurgery 1984; 15:795–800.

51. Swann KW, Black PM, Baker MF: Management of symptomatic deep venous thrombosis and pulmonary embolism on a neurosurgical service. J Neurosurg 1986; 64:563–567.

52. Turpie AGG, Hirsh J, Gent M, et al: Prevention of deep vein thrombosis in potential neurosurgical patients. Arch Intern Med 1989;149:679–681.

53. Willis BK: Timing of anticoagulant therapy for thromboembolic complications after craniotomy for brain tumors (letter). Neurosurgery 1991; 28:929.

54. Gefter WB, Hatabu H, Holland GA, et al: Pulmonary thromboembolism: Recent developments in diagnosis with CT and MR imaging. Radiology 1995; 197:561–574.

Index

Note: Page numbers in *italics* refer to figures; page numbers followed by t refer to tables.

ISBN 0-7216-4825-8

9 780721 648255

90038